American Academy of Child and Adolescent Psychiatry

American Psychiatric Press

TEXTBOOK OF CHILD & ADOLESCENT PSYCHIATRY

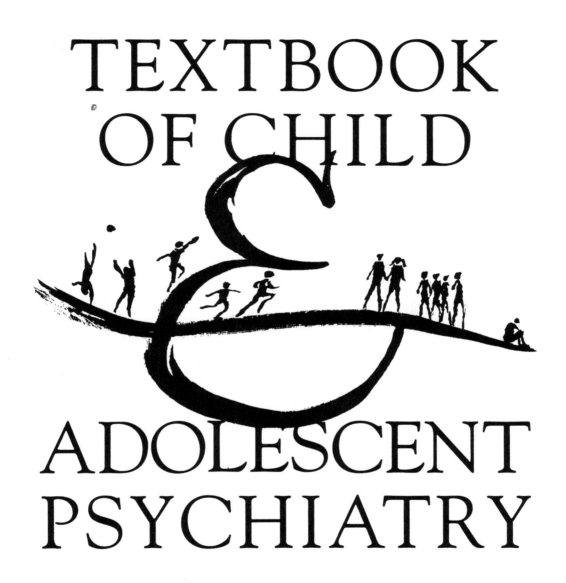

Edited by

Jerry M. Wiener, M.D.
Leon Yochelson Professor and Chairman
Department of Psychiatry and Behavioral Sciences
Professor of Pediatrics
The George Washington University School of Medicine
Washington, DC

Note: The authors have worked to ensure that all information in this book concerning drug dosages, schedules, and routes of administration is accurate as of the time of publication and consistent with standards set by the U.S. Food and Drug Administration and the general medical community. As medical research and practice advance, however, therapeutic standards may change. For this reason and because human and medical errors sometimes occur, we recommend that readers follow the advice of a physician who is directly involved in their care or the care of a member of their family.

Books published by the American Psychiatric Press, Inc., represent the views and opinions of the individual authors and do not necessarily represent the policies and opinions of the Press or the American Psychiatric Association.

American Psychiatric Press, Inc.
1400 K Street, N.W., Washington, DC 20005

Library of Congress Cataloging-in-Publication Data
Textbook of child and adolescent psychiatry / edited by Jerry M. Wiener.—1st ed.
    p.   cm.
Includes bibliographical references.
Includes index.
ISBN 0-88048-296-6 (alk. paper)
    1. Child psychiatry.   2. Adolescent psychiatry.   I. Wiener, Jerry M., 1933–   .
    [DNLM: 1. Mental Disorders—in adolescence.   2. Mental Disorders—in infancy & childhood.
WS 350 T355]
RJ45.T433   1991
618.92′89—dc 20
DNLM/DLC
for Library of Congress   91-4548
                                                                                                                          CIP

British Library Cataloguing in Publication Data
A CIP record is available from the British Library.

Contents

Section VI: Anxiety Disorders

Section VII: Eating and Nutritional Disorders

Section VIII: Tic and Movement Disorders

Section IX: Disorders in Somatic Function

Contributors

Ann Aldershof, Sc.B., Ph.D.
Research Associate, Project Director
Adolescent Language Research Project
Bradley Hospital
Providence, Rhode Island

Thomas F. Anders, M.D.
Professor of Psychiatry and Human Behavior
Brown University;
Psychiatrist-in-Chief
Bradley Hospital
Providence, Rhode Island

Paul Andreason, M.D., M.S.
Senior Staff Fellow
National Institute of Mental Health
Bethesda, Maryland

George W. Bailey, M.D.
Associate Clinical Professor of Psychiatry and
    Pediatrics
The George Washington University School of
    Medicine
Washington, DC

Joan K. Barber, M.D.
Associate Professor of Psychiatry and Behavioral
    Sciences
The George Washington University School of
    Medicine
Washington, DC

Ida Sue Baron, Ph.D.
Clinical Neuropsychologist
Potomac, Maryland

Myron L. Belfer, M.D.
Professor and Chairman
Department of Psychiatry
The Cambridge Hospital
Harvard Medical School
Cambridge, Massachusetts

Jules Bemporad, M.D.
Director of Education
The New York Hospital–Cornell Medical Center
    Westchester Division;
Professor of Clinical Psychiatry
Cornell University Medical College
White Plains, New York

Eugene V. Beresin, M.D.
Director, Child Psychiatry Residency Training
    Program
Massachusetts General Hospital;
Assistant Professor of Psychiatry
Harvard Medical School
Boston, Massachusetts

Irving N. Berlin, M.D.
Professor of Psychiatry and Pediatrics
University of New Mexico School of Medicine
Albuquerque, New Mexico

Barbara Bettes, Ph.D
Research Fellow in Child Psychology
Columbia University College of Physicians and
    Surgeons
New York, New York

Joseph Biederman, M.D.
Director, Pediatric Psychopharmacology
Massachusetts General Hospital;
Associate Professor of Psychiatry
Harvard Medical School
Boston, Massachusetts

Hector R. Bird, M.D.
Deputy Director of Child Psychiatry
New York State Psychiatric Institute;
Clinical Professor of Psychiatry
Columbia University College of Physicians and
    Surgeons
New York, New York

Larry K. Brown, M.D.
Assistant Professor of Psychiatry and Human
  Behavior
Brown University;
Director, Child Psychiatry Consult Service
Rhode Island Hospital
Providence, Rhode Island

Magda Campbell, M.D.
Professor of Psychiatry
Director, Division of Child and Adolescent
  Psychiatry
New York University Medical Center
New York, New York

Irene Chatoor, M.D.
Director, Eating Disorders Program
Children's National Medical Center;
Associate Professor of Psychiatry and Behavioral
  Sciences and of Pediatrics
The George Washington University School of
  Medicine
Washington, DC

Donald J. Cohen, M.D.
Director, Yale Child Study Center
Irving B. Harris Professor of Child Psychiatry,
  Pediatrics, and Psychology
New Haven, Connecticut

Richard L. Cohen, M.D.
Professor Emeritus of Child Psychiatry
University of Pittsburgh School of Medicine
Pittsburgh, Pennsylvania

Leslie M. Conroy, M.D.
Assistant Professor of Clinical Psychiatry
The University of Chicago
Chicago, Illinois

Anthony J. Costello, M.D.
Professor of Psychiatry
University of Massachusetts
Worcester, Massachusetts

Susan Delavan Cunningham, M.D.
Assistant Professor of Psychiatry
Michigan State University
East Lansing, Michigan

James Egan, M.D.
Clinical Professor of Psychiatry and Behavioral
  Sciences and of Pediatrics
The George Washington University School of
  Medicine
Washington, DC

Norbert B. Enzer, M.D.
Professor and Chairman
Department of Psychiatry
Michigan State University
East Lansing, Michigan

Thomas D. Eppright, M.D.
Fellow in Child Psychiatry
The University of Missouri School of Medicine
Columbia, Missouri

L. Erlenmeyer-Kimling, Ph.D.
Professor, Departments of Psychiatry and of
  Human Genetics and Development
Columbia University College of Physicians and
  Surgeons
New York, New York

Carl Feinstein, M.D.
Clinical Director, Bradley Hospital;
Associate Professor of Psychiatry and Human
  Behavior
Brown University Program in Medicine
Providence, Rhode Island

Gregory K. Fritz, M.D.
Director of Child and Family Psychiatry
Rhode Island Hospital, Providence;
Professor of Psychiatry and Human Behavior
Brown University Program in Medicine
Providence, Rhode Island

Mohammad Ghaziuddin, M.D.
Lecturer in Child Psychiatry
Child and Adolescent Psychiatry Service
The University of Michigan Medical Center
Ann Arbor, Michigan

Arthur H. Green, M.D.
Clinical Associate Professor of Psychiatry
Columbia University College of Physicians and
  Surgeons
New York, New York

Richard Green, M.D., J.D.
Professor of Psychiatry in Residence
Professor of Law in Residence
University of California, Los Angeles
Los Angeles, California

Laurence L. Greenhill, M.D.
Associate Professor of Clinical Psychiatry
Division of Child and Adolescent Psychiatry
Columbia University College of Physicians and
  Surgeons
New York, New York

Stanley I. Greenspan, M.D.
Clinical Professor of Psychiatry and Pediatrics
The George Washington University School of
  Medicine
Washington, DC

James C. Harris, M.D.
Director, Developmental Neuropsychiatry
Associate Professor of Psychiatry, Pediatrics, and
  Mental Hygiene
Division of Child and Adolescent Psychiatry
Johns Hopkins School of Medicine
Baltimore, Maryland

Robert L. Hendren, D.O.
Director, Division of Child and Adolescent
  Psychiatry
Associate Professor of Psychiatry and Pediatrics
University of New Mexico School of Medicine
Albuquerque, New Mexico

David B. Herzog, M.D.
Director, Eating Disorders Unit
Massachusetts General Hospital;
Associate Professor of Psychiatry
Harvard Medical School
Boston, Massachusetts

Steven L. Jaffe, M.D.
Associate Professor of Psychiatry
Emory University;
Director, Adolescent Psychiatric and Chemical
  Dependency Programs
C.P.C.-Parkwood Hospital
Atlanta, Georgia

Michael Jellinek, M.D.
Chief, Child Psychiatry Service
Director, Outpatient Psychiatry
Massachusetts General Hospital;
Associate Professor of Psychiatry (Pediatrics)
Harvard Medical School
Boston, Massachusetts

Bernard Kahan, M.D.
Medical Director, Medical/Psychiatric Unit
Egleston Hospital;
Assistant Professor of Psychiatry
Emory University
Atlanta, Georgia

Lawrence C. Kaplan, M.D.
Director, Birth Defects Center
Children's Hospital;
Assistant Professor of Pediatrics
Harvard Medical School
Boston, Massachusetts

Javad H. Kashani, M.D.
Director of Child and Adolescent Services
Mid-Missouri Mental Health Center;
Professor of Psychiatry, Psychology, Pediatrics,
  and Medicine
The University of Missouri School of Medicine
Columbia, Missouri

Alan E. Kazdin, Ph.D.
Professor of Psychology
Yale University
New Haven, Connecticut

Paulina F. Kernberg, M.D.
Director, Child and Adolescent Psychiatry
The New York Hospital–Cornell Medical Center
  Westchester Division;
Associate Professor of Psychiatry
Cornell University Medical College
White Plains, New York

Clarice J. Kestenbaum, M.D.
Training Director, Division of Child and
  Adolescent Psychiatry
Clinical Professor of Psychiatry
Columbia University College of Physicians and
  Surgeons
New York, New York

Robert A. King, M.D.
Assistant Professor of Child Psychiatry
Yale Child Study Center
New Haven, Connecticut

Sharon C. Kowalik, M.D., Ph.D.
Resident in Psychiatry
New York University Medical Center
New York, New York

Markus J. P. Kruesi, M.D.
National Institute of Mental Health
Bethesda, Maryland

James F. Leckman, M.D.
Nelson Harris Professor of Child Psychiatry and
  Pediatrics
Yale Child Study Center
New Haven, Connecticut

Henrietta L. Leonard, M.D.
Senior Staff Fellow
Child Psychiatry Branch
National Institute of Mental Health
Bethesda, Maryland

Bennett L. Leventhal, M.D.
Professor of Psychiatry and Pediatrics
The University of Chicago Medical School
Chicago, Illinois

Dorothy Otnow Lewis, M.D.
Clinical Professor of Psychiatry
Yale Child Study Center
New Haven, Connecticut;
Professor of Psychiatry
New York University School of Medicine
New York, New York

Melvin Lewis, M.B.,B.S., F.R.C.Psych., D.C.H.
Director of Medical Studies
Professor of Pediatrics and Psychiatry
Yale Child Study Center
New Haven, Connecticut

Carl P. Malmquist, M.D.
Professor of Social Psychiatry
University of Minnesota School of Medicine
Minneapolis, Minnesota

Charles A. Malone, M.D.
Director of Graduate and Undergraduate
  Education
Bradley Hospital;
Professor of Psychiatry and Human Behavior
Brown University Program in Medicine
Providence, Rhode Island

John S. March, M.D., M.P.H.
Assistant Professor of Psychiatry
Director, Program in Childhood and Adolescent
  Anxiety Disorders
Duke University Hospital
Durham, North Carolina

Edgardo Menvielle, M.D.
Assistant Professor of Psychiatry and Behavioral
  Sciences and of Pediatrics
The George Washington University School of
  Medicine
Washington, DC

Kerim Munir, M.B.,B.S., M.P.H.
Lecturer on Psychiatry
Department of Psychiatry
The Cambridge Hospital
Harvard Medical School
Cambridge, Massachusetts

Kathi Nader, D.S.W.
Director of Evaluation
Program in Trauma, Violence and Sudden
  Bereavement
Neuropsychiatric Institute and Hospital
University of California, Los Angeles
Los Angeles, California

Cynthia R. Pfeffer, M.D.
Chief, Child Psychiatry Inpatient Unit
New York Hospital–Cornell Medical Center
  Westchester Division;
Professor of Psychiatry
Cornell University Medical College
White Plains, New York

Robert S. Pynoos, M.D., M.P.H.
Associate Professor and Director
Program in Trauma, Violence and Sudden
  Bereavement
Department of Psychiatry
University of California, Los Angeles
Los Angeles, California

Judith L. Rapoport, M.D.
Chief, Child Psychiatry Branch
National Institute of Mental Health
Bethesda, Maryland;
Clinical Professor of Psychiatry and Pediatrics
The George Washington University School of
  Medicine
Washington, DC

Rebecca E. Rieger, Ph.D.
Clinical Psychologist
Bethesda, Maryland;
Clinical Professor of Psychiatry (Psychology)
The George Washington University School of
  Medicine
Washington, DC

John E. Schowalter, M.D.
Albert J. Solnit Professor of Child Psychiatry and
  Pediatrics
Chief of Child Psychiatry
Yale Child Study Center
New Haven, Connecticut

David Shaffer, M.B.,B.S., F.R.C.P.,
  F.R.C.Psych.
Irving Philips Professor of Child and Adolescent
  Psychiatry
Columbia University College of Physicians and
  Surgeons
New York State Psychiatric Institute
New York, New York

Theodore Shapiro, M.D.
Director of Child and Adolescent Psychiatry
Professor of Psychiatry in Pediatrics
Cornell University Medical College
New York, New York

G. Pirooz Sholevar, M.D.
Professor and Director
Division of Child, Adolescent and Family
  Psychiatry
Department of Psychiatry and Human Behavior
Jefferson Medical College
Philadelphia, Pennsylvania

John B. Sikorski, M.D.
Associate Clinical Professor
Child and Adolescent Service
Department of Psychiatry
University of California, San Francisco
San Francisco, California

Elizabeth Kay Spencer, M.D.
Research Assistant Professor in Psychiatry
New York University Medical Center
New York, New York

Ludwik S. Szymanski, M.D.
Director of Psychiatry
Developmental Evaluation Center
Children's Hospital;
Assistant Professor of Psychiatry
Harvard Medical School
Boston, Massachusetts

Luke Y. Tsai, M.D.
Chief of Child and Adolescent Psychiatry Service
Associate Professor of Psychiatry and Pediatrics
The University of Michigan Medical Center
Ann Arbor, Michigan

Thomas Walsh, M.D.
Associate Clinical Professor of Psychiatry and
  Behavioral Sciences and of Pediatrics
The George Washington University School of
  Medicine
Washington, DC

Elizabeth Weller, M.D.
Director of Child and Adolescent Psychiatry
Professor of Psychiatry and Pediatrics
Ohio State University School of Medicine
Columbus, Ohio

Ronald A. Weller, M.D.
Director of Training and Education
Professor of Psychiatry
Ohio State University School of Medicine
Columbus, Ohio

Jerry M. Wiener, M.D.
Leon Yochelson Professor and Chairman
Department of Psychiatry and Behavioral
  Sciences
Professor of Pediatrics
The George Washington University School of
  Medicine
Washington, DC

Daniel T. Williams, M.D.
Director, Pediatric Neuropsychiatry Service
Columbia-Presbyterian Medical Center;
Associate Clinical Professor of Psychiatry
Columbia University College of Physicians and
  Surgeons
New York, New York

Joseph L. Woolston, M.D.
Associate Clinical Professor of Child Psychiatry
Yale Child Study Center
New Haven, Connecticut

Alayne Yates, M.D.
Chief of Child Psychiatry
Professor of Psychiatry and Pediatrics
College of Medicine,
University of Arizona
Tucson, Arizona

Alan J. Zametkin, M.D.
Senior Staff Psychiatrist
Section on Clinical Brain Imaging
Laboratory of Cerebral Metabolism
National Institute of Mental Health
Bethesda, Maryland

Kenneth J. Zucker, Ph.D.
Head, Child and Adolescent Gender Identity
  Clinic
Child and Family Studies Centre
Clarke Institute of Psychiatry
Toronto, Ontario, Canada

Introduction

At the beginning of the decade of the 1990s, on the threshold of a new century, the field of child and adolescent psychiatry is itself almost 100 years old. It had its beginnings in the early 1900s when pioneers in pediatrics, psychiatry, and psychology became interested in the children and adolescents who were being processed by the juvenile courts and by social agencies in charge of neglected, delinquent, orphaned, and destitute children. At the time, these young people were not thought of as mentally ill, but as victims of circumstance.

As psychoanalytic theory began to become more widely known, delinquency and other behaviors increasingly came to be viewed from its perspective. As psychoanalytic theory shifted and became more developmentally oriented, the psychodynamic understanding and treatment of child and adolescent disorders flourished and predominated. There were, after all, no significant competing or complementary theories, and therefore little emphasis on diagnostic classification or differential therapeutics until well into the 1960s, when neurobiological theories were beginning to take hold.

The literature of child and adolescent psychiatry for its first 60 years largely consisted of anecdotal case reports, small series of cases illustrating common underlying psychodynamic themes, and methodologically unsophisticated treatment studies. Although it is true that psychoactive medication was first used to treat children with behavior disorders in 1937, and refinements in this treatment occurred well into the 1970s, there was no significant additional medication usage until the 1960 treatment of enuresis with the antidepressant imipramine. Before that, in the mid-1950s, the so-called biological revolution had begun in general psychiatry and gradually increased in importance until biological theories and treatments established themselves as the dominant force in the explanation and treatment of almost all, if not all, the major psychiatric disorders. One most significant hallmark of this revolutionary change came with the development of Feighner's (1972) diagnostic criteria in the early 1970s and the subsequent development of a descriptively based, atheoretical, multiaxial system introduced in the Diagnostic and Statistical Manual of Mental Disorders, 3rd Edition (American Psychiatric Association 1980). This sea change in the importance of reliable diagnostic criteria focusing on observable and reportable description was accompanied by the publication of the first textbook on child and adolescent psychopharmacology (Wiener 1977) and by several textbooks or manuals that have reflected DSM-III and DSM-III-R (American Psychiatric Association 1987) classification and broader approaches to treatment.

This volume, then, arose out of a sense that the field had developed to the point of a need for a clinically focused textbook that would encompass the state of the art and the science, and be useful to the student, general resident, career resident in child and adolescent psychiatry, clinician, and also pediatrician.

Section I describes the field of child and adolescent psychiatry: its development as a subspecialty, the emergence and evolution of its classification schemes, and informed speculations about its future development. This section is important for the understanding of the roots and soil from which has grown the current practice of child and adolescent psychiatry and the role of the American Academy of Child and Adolescent Psychiatry in that development. As such, it is of particular interest and useful to those who have chosen child and adolescent psychiatry as a career and to those considering such a career choice.

Section II includes 12 chapters on the assessment and diagnostic process in child and adolescent psychiatry. It begins with a thorough and balanced overview of normal growth and development, which sets the stage for chapters covering the concepts of diagnostic classification and detailed discussions of clinical interviewing at each developmental stage—infancy, childhood, and adolescence—each chapter developed by senior, experienced clinicians and teachers. There are special chapters on parent and family interviews; on the use of standardized assessment instruments as an increasingly important clinical (and not just research) tool; on the use of psychological testing, with a special focus on neuropsychological assessment; and on laboratory and diagnostic testing, the latter including a discussion of the current state and use of diagnostic imaging. This section closes with special chapters on the diagnostic formulation and the presentation of findings to the parents and patient, an important skill often overlooked. This entire section is a reemphasis and affirmation of the biopsychosocial model in the conducting of a careful and systematic diagnostic assessment, integrating knowledge and information from all levels: biological, developmental, psychodynamic, cognitive, family, and social.

Sections III through IX cover clinical disorders. They closely follow DSM-III-R classification but add considerable differentiation, detail, and variety to the DSM-III-R categories to encompass the entire range of the clinical disorders seen in child, adolescent, and family disorders. To the maximum extent possible, each clinical chapter is organized by the inclusion of DSM-III-R diagnostic criteria, clinical findings, differential diagnosis, epidemiology, etiology, clinical courses, and prognosis. Each clinical chapter is authored by an outstanding authority(s), usually a clinician-researcher with extensive direct, hands-on clinical experience with that disorder.

Section X covers special issues in childhood and adolescence, including substance abuse, gender identity and psychosexual disorders, adjustment and reactive disorders, physical and sexual abuse, acquired immunodeficiency syndrome, suicide, the concept of personality disorders in childhood, and forensic psychiatry. These special issues identify many of the patients seen in clinical practice who cut across or fall outside the more traditional diagnostic categories.

Naturally, Section XI deals with treatment. Treatment approaches now might be divided into 1) those more typically done *with* the patient (psychodynamic, psychoanalytic, family, group); 2) those requiring something done *to* the patient (psychopharmacology, some forms of behavior modification) and requiring less of the patient's active motivation and cooperation; and 3) those more in-between or midpoint on the spectrum (hypnosis and a number of behavior modification approaches). Although the divisions are not clear-cut, and there are many areas of overlap, one can still think of the various treatment approaches along these lines. Each chapter, as with the clinical disorders, reflects the in-depth experience each author brings to the particular treatment. At the same time, the clinician will recognize and the trainee must be reminded that, in most circumstances, no single treatment is sufficient and that a proper sequence or combination of treatments must be integrated into a systematic plan. It is this integrative capacity that most separates the physician from the nonphysician and the specialist from the generalist.

This is a rapidly changing field; we are in a period of major advances through expanded research into an understanding of epidemiology, diagnosis, and treatment. In that sense, any textbook must be read as a foundation and structure onto which new information can be attached as acquired from the current literature. This text, used in that way, will amply reward the reader with the solid core of child and adolescent psychiatry.

As to the preparation and editing of this volume, William James observed that "Whenever two people meet there are really six people present. There is each man as he sees himself, each man as the other person sees him, and each man as he really is." Imagine, then, what happens when one meets (figuratively and literally) with the 78 authors of 56 chapters—an experience with a unique collection of experts and authorities as seen by themselves, by their editor, and as they really are, although the latter is in fact never actually knowable. However challenging, sometimes frustrating, and occasionally maddening, the experience overall has been one of great satisfaction with both collegial and intellectual rewards. No small part of these rewards came from my association with the members of the Editorial Board, without whose able assistance whatever merit is to be found in this volume would not have been possible.

Jerry M. Wiener, M.D.

References

American Psychiatric Association: Diagnostic and Statistical Manual of Mental Disorders, 3rd Edition. Washington, DC, American Psychiatric Association, 1980

American Psychiatric Association: Diagnostic and Statistical Manual of Mental Disorders, 3rd Edition, Revised. Washington, DC, American Psychiatric Association, 1987

Feighner JP, Robins E, Guze SB, et al: Diagnostic criteria for use in psychiatric research. Arch Gen Psychiatry 26:57–63, 1972

Wiener JM (ed): Psychopharmacology of Childhood and Adolescent Disorders. New York, Basic Books, 1977

Section I

The Field of Child and Adolescent Psychiatry

Chapter 1

Classification of Child and Adolescent Psychiatric Disorders: A Historical Review

Jerry M. Wiener, M.D.

Two particular developments, more than any others, have affected the shape and identity of modern psychiatry: the biological revolution, ushered in by the discovery in 1952 of the antipsychotic properties of chlorpromazine, and (distinctly related to the first) the diagnostic revolution, ushered in by the introduction of Feighner's (1972) diagnostic criteria in the early 1970s, and crystallized by the publication in 1980 of the *Diagnostic and Statistical Manual of Mental Disorders*, 3rd Edition (DSM-III) (American Psychiatric Association 1980).

Clearly, of course, diagnostic classification did not begin with DSM-III; in regard to childhood and adolescent disorders, it could be said to have had its formal beginning with the publication by Leo Kanner (1935) of the first English language textbook of child psychiatry. Kanner listed several diagnostic principles, promulgated by Adolf Meyer, that seem remarkably contemporary, including: 1) working with concrete, objectively demonstrable facts; 2) recognizing a multiplicity of factors at play; 3) using a practical application, in the sense of sober scientific work that can be taught and learned; and 4) "using a terminology which can be made accessible to, and understood by, everyone whose capacity for clear, logical thinking and common sense has not been blunted by one-sided preoccupations" (p. 12).

Kanner (1935) referred to all disorders in terms of various categories of "personality difficulties."

The first group included those difficulties caused by or sequels to structural brain disorders or damage, such as tumors, trauma, or infection. The next group was those organic disorders that were reversible or potentially so, including delirium, hallucinosis, stupor, and coma. Next came categories of endocrinopathies, and then what came to be known as psychosomatic disorders, followed by somatoform and conversion disorders affecting each of the various organ and sensory systems. These all were referred to as "involuntary part-dysfunctions" and included such diverse phenomena as migraine headaches, psychogenic vomiting, tics, and hallucinations.

The final and largest section referred to "difficulties" expressed as "whole-dysfunctions" and included, among other categories, mental retardation, disorders of speech (a major category), habits, sleeping disturbances, "antisocial trends" (e.g., disrespect, lying, destructiveness, cruelty), sexual difficulties, "attack disorders" (e.g., epilepsy, breath-holding, fainting spells), the "minor psychoses" (e.g., obsessive states, hysteria), and the "major psychoses" (covered in 18 pages). Of interest is a final section on children's suicides.

The third (and final) edition of Kanner's (1957) textbook addressed the limitations of available diagnostic classification, particularly the insufficiency of descriptive categories. Kanner observed that, in psychoanalysis, "diagnosis is the result of, rather than preliminary to therapy" (p. 205). In this edition, in the section of the book on phenomenology, "personality problems" arise from "physical illness," "psychosomatic problems," and "problems of behavior."

The problems arising from physical illness were categorized under: 1) structural and metabolic disorders, 2) the epilepsies, 3) transient affections (e.g., delirium, hallucinosis, stupor), 4) chorea, and 5) the endocrinopathies (including the "sex glands").

Psychosomatic problems included diverse affections under each of the major organ systems, ranging from migraine headaches to hypertension, fainting, asthma, ulcerative colitis, tics, and hallucinations. Since there was no theoretical underpinning to this section, it was organized by organ system.

Problems of behavior constituted the final and largest grouping. It dealt with such categories as eating behavior (e.g., anorexia nervosa, rumination), sleeping behavior (e.g., nightmares, sleepwalking, narcolepsy), speech and language, habits, scholastic performance, sexual behavior, anger, jealousy, fear, anxiety attacks, hypochondriasis, obsession and compulsions, hysteria, delinquency (a large chapter), hospitalism, schizophrenia (including a chapter on Kanner's concept of early infantile autism), and, once again at the end, suicide. By this edition, the concept of disorders was far broader and sophisticated—indeed, if anything, overinclusive, reflecting perhaps the lack of any clear etiologies for a majority of the described conditions. The influence of psychoanalytic theory is considerably in evidence. In addition, there is a wealth of astute observation, clinical wisdom, and sound advice. The classification system remained, however, largely phenomenological because little of an overall conceptual framework was available.

Moving backward just a bit, the first *Diagnostic and Statistical Manual of Mental Disorders* (DSM-I) was published in 1952 by the American Psychiatric Association (APA). Prior to this, the APA had promulgated a classification of mental disease that was primarily a statistical instrument for use in state hospitals. Of related interest is that the "Standard Classified Nomenclature of Disease" for all of medicine first appeared only in 1933, and DSM-I constituted the section on "Diseases of the Psychobiologic Unit" from the Fourth Edition (National Conference on Medical Nomenclature 1952) of the *Standard Nomenclature of Diseases and Operations*. This first diagnostic manual incorporated the experiences of psychiatry in World War II (e.g., under "gross stress reaction") and came after the

founding of the National Institute of Mental Health. However, of the 28 members of the APA Committee on Nomenclature and Statistics, which was responsible for developing DSM-I between 1946 and 1951, none were identified primarily with child and adolescent psychiatry. It is then perhaps not surprising that DSM-I included very little mention of disorders in childhood or adolescence, containing so little in the way of descriptive material or diagnostic criteria as to indicate the relatively low priority accorded to diagnostic classification by American psychiatry at that time. Obviously, many childhood disorders could be classified under many general headings—such as acute and chronic brain disorders (both due to various conditions); mental deficiency; psychotic reactions; and psychophysiologic, psychoneurotic, personality, and transient situational personality reactions. There were only four categories in which childhood or adolescence was a specific condition in the nomenclature: 1) chronic brain syndrome associated with birth trauma; 2) schizophrenic reaction, childhood type; 3) special symptom reactions such as learning disturbance, enuresis, and somnambulism; and 4) the "adjustment reactions" of infancy, childhood (habit disturbance, conduct disturbance, neurotic traits), and adolescence.

DSM-I itself was influenced significantly by psychoanalytic theory. As observed by Kanner (1957), diagnosis followed therapy rather than initiated it in psychoanalysis. It is not surprising that DSM-I had little if any impact on the practice of psychiatry in general, or on child and adolescent psychiatry in particular, since it was neither strongly phenomenological nor conceptual in organization.

Recognizing a major need for an adequate classification of disorders in children and adolescents, the Group for the Advancement of Psychiatry (GAP) Committee on Child Psychiatry published its classification in 1966. In considering the GAP classification as a major advance, it is relevant to note that a large number of classification schemes had been advanced and were in isolated usage in the field of child and adolescent mental and emotional disorders. In fact, the appendix of the GAP classification identified 24 previous systems containing varying degrees of detail and differences in approach, including proposals by Kanner, Nathan Ackerman, Chess, Pacella, Pearson, and Rose. These various approaches made differing contributions to the GAP system.

The GAP classification provides a broad, inclusive, biopsychosocial and developmental framework within which to include interactive, etiologic, and phenomenological considerations. There are nine major categories (number 10 is the ubiquitous "other") arranged roughly in a hierarchy of least to most serious, and from the most environmental-experiential through internalized-psychological to those disorders with the most somatic factors:

1. Healthy responses
2. Reactive disorders
3. Developmental deviations
4. Psychoneurotic disorders (with a clear psychoanalytic etiologic presumption)
5. Personality disorders
6. Psychotic disorders
7. Psychophysiologic disorders
8. Brain syndromes
9. Mental retardation

All these categories except numbers 6, 8, and 9 are discussed in terms of the interaction between developmental level and psychodynamic issues. The proposed classification is supplemented by a very long, detailed symptom list of problem behaviors, which is used to fill in the classification. Finally, the GAP classification was and remains the only major system to categorize from least serious (healthy responses) to most serious (mental retardation), rather than the other way around.

DSM-II (American Psychiatric Association 1968) appeared 2 years after the GAP classification and was intended to coincide with ICD-8 (World Health Organization 1969). It represented some major changes and degrees of improvement over DSM-I, but from the point of view of child and adolescent disorders, continued to suffer from the lack of input by child psychiatrists; only 2 of the 39 members of the committee between 1946 and 1967 were child psychiatrists. The major overall changes in DSM-II included dropping the term *reaction* from many of the categories (e.g., "schizophrenia" rather than "schizophrenic reaction"), and specifically trying "to avoid terms which carry with them *implications* regarding either the nature of a disorder or its causes" and to be "explicit about causal assumptions when they are integral to a diagnostic concept" (p. viii). DSM-II was organized into 10 categories instead of the 3 large groupings in DSM-I, and the personality disorders category was expanded and emphasized more. Multiple diagnoses, especially associated medical conditions, were encouraged, and the qualifying phrases of "acute" and "chronic," "not psychotic," and "degree of severity" (mild, mod-

erate, severe) were added. Although not specifically addressed as an issue in the supporting text, DSM-II in fact did reflect the growing importance of biological theories and research findings in understanding mental disorders and the growing challenge to psychoanalytic theory as sufficiently or even predominantly explanatory. Thus while the neuroses were still presented as etiologically known, the affective and psychotic disorders, as well as some other disorders, were definitely unbundled from etiologic assumptions. Descriptive phenomenology assumed a larger role than it had previously. In addition, the substitution of "sexual orientation disturbance" for homosexuality was one controversial element in the revision.

In regard to child and adolescent disorders, DSM-II did represent progress. Mental retardation was moved to be the very first category. Schizophrenia, childhood type, remained, as did an expanded section of "special symptoms" and transient situational disturbances. The major change was the addition of "behavior disorders of childhood and adolescence," subclassified into the following:

1. Hyperkinetic reaction of childhood (or adolescence)
2. Withdrawing reaction of childhood (or adolescence)
3. Overanxious reaction of childhood (or adolescence)
4. Runaway reaction of childhood (or adolescence)
5. Unsocialized aggressive reaction of childhood (or adolescence)
6. Group delinquent reaction of childhood (or adolescence)
7. Other reaction of childhood (or adolescence)

This entire category was intended to classify disorders or patterns intermediate between transient situational disturbances and the presumably more stable and structured pathology of the psychoses, neuroses, and personality disorder categories. Although the absence of adequate descriptive, epidemiologic, and prognostic data later made this rationale erroneous, the addition of this category was an important recognition of a broader and more specific range of psychopathologies in children and adolescents.

In its etiologic leaning, in its greater reliance on description rather than dynamics, and in its inclusion of Robert Spitzer, M.D., as a consultant, DSM-II laid the groundwork and set the stage for the development of the revolutionary DSM-III (American Psychiatric Association 1980). DSM-III represented and became the hallmark of the dramatic changes that had occurred in psychiatry during the previous 20 years, referred to as the "biological revolution." DSM-III departed from DSM-II in the following ways.

First, except where etiology was clearly known, as in organic mental disorders or in adjustment disorder (reaction to a psychosocial stress), no assumptions as to etiology were included. The approach is instead atheoretical as to etiology and pathophysiology.

Second, DSM-III was comprehensively descriptive and categorical and provided specific diagnostic criteria for each disorder (albeit acknowledging that the criteria had not been validated for many of the disorders).

Third, DSM-III introduced a five-part multiaxial system that allowed for the coding of physical disorders, psychosocial stressors, and highest level of adaptive functioning in the past year, in addition, of course, to the coding of disorders on Axis I and Axis II. The basic message of DSM-III was that diagnosis now made a difference for both clinical care and research, that a common language needed to be used, and that a diagnosis could and should increasingly inform treatment planning and prognosis, rather than be considered unimportant.

For the field of child and adolescent psychiatry, DSM-III introduced as its first Axis I category "disorders usually first evident in infancy, childhood, or adolescence," which included the following:

- Mental retardation
- Attention-deficit disorder (with and without hyperactivity)
- Conduct disorder (with five subtypes)
- Anxiety disorders (i.e., separation anxiety, avoidant, and overanxious)
- "Other" disorders of infancy, childhood, or adolescence (i.e., reactive attachment, schizoid, elective mutism, oppositional, and identity disorders)
- Eating disorders
- Stereotyped movement disorders (including tic disorders and Tourette's syndrome)
- Other disorders with physical manifestations (i.e., stuttering, enuresis, encopresis, sleepwalking, and sleep terror)
- Pervasive developmental disorders (e.g., infantile autism).

"Specific developmental disorders" (e.g., reading, arithmetic) were to be coded on Axis II. The adult personality disorder diagnoses could not be made until late adolescence (although by definition they were acknowledged to begin in childhood and early adolescence). Diagnoses such as schizophrenia, affective disorders, organic disorders, and anxiety disorders were to be made in children and adolescents by applying the same criteria required for the diagnosis in adults.

To the extent that any relevant information was known, each clinical disorder or entity included the characteristics of essential features, associated features, age at onset, course, impairment, complications, predisposing factors, prevalence, sex ratio, familial pattern, and differential diagnosis. The frequent absence or paucity of information in many or most of these categories in many or most disorders arising in childhood or adolescence served to point the way to badly needed research. Indeed DSM-III was the product of a quantum leap in scientific research in psychiatry, and then served to identify major deficits in our knowledge.

It took 16 years to move from DSM-I to DSM-II, another 12 years from DSM-II to DSM-III, but only 7 years from DSM-III to DSM-III-R (American Psychiatric Association 1987); DSM-IV is actively in preparation for a 1993 publication. DSM-III-R was stimulated by both the clinical and the research use of DSM-III, leading to new data about some disorders and revealing problems or inconsistencies in the use of other categories.

The major principles guiding DSM-III-R were the same as for DSM-III. Some important changes occurred in the sections covering disorders usually first evident in infancy, childhood, or adolescence. First, because they were considered chronic, the developmental disorders were shifted from Axis I to Axis II. These disorders include: 1) mental retardation, 2) pervasive developmental disorders (autistic disorder), and 3) specific developmental disorders (including academic, language, and motor skills disorders).

In the Axis I disorders, there are now eight rather than nine headings, with some significant reorganizations (see Table 1-1).

It has been a matter of considerable controversy whether DSM-III-R represents an improvement or a worsening of the problems found in DSM-III. The rationale of the groupings has come into question. The absence of an axis or mechanism by which to include either psychodynamic or family consider-

Table 1-1. DSM-III-R Axis I disorders

1. Disruptive behavior disorders—a new terminology, not found in DSM-III
   a. Attention-deficit hyperactivity disorder—a name change from DSM-III
   b. Conduct disorder (group, solitary aggressive, and undifferentiated types)
   c. Oppositional defiant disorder
2. Anxiety disorders of childhood or adolescence—no change
3. Eating disorders—no significant change
4. Gender identity disorders—a new category
   a. Gender identity disorder of childhood
   b. Transsexualism
   c. Gender identity disorder of adolescence or adulthood, nontranssexual type
   d. Gender identity disorder not otherwise specified (NOS)
5. Tic disorders—instead of stereotyped movement disorders, otherwise minor and nonsignificant changes
6. Elimination disorders (includes encopresis and enuresis)—a new category
7. Speech disorders not elsewhere classified (includes cluttering and stuttering)—also a new category
8. Other disorders of infancy, childhood, or adolescence, including:
   a. Elective mutism
   b. Identity disorder
   c. Reactive attachment disorder of infancy or early childhood
   d. Stereotypy/habit disorder
   e. Undifferentiated attention-deficit disorder

ations has been particularly troubling for application to child and adolescent disorders.

However, the extensive involvement of child and adolescent psychiatry from the very beginning of the development of DSM-IV (on the oversight committee, the task force itself, and on many if not all of the working groups) promises that improvements will be made in the relevance, rationale, and usefulness of DSM-IV for infant, child, adolescent, and family-related disorders.

References

American Psychiatric Association: Diagnostic and Statistical Manual of Mental Disorders, 1st Edition. Washington, DC, American Psychiatric Association, 1952

American Psychiatric Association: Diagnostic and Statistical Manual of Mental Disorders, 2nd Edition. Washington, DC, American Psychiatric Association, 1968

American Psychiatric Association: Diagnostic and Statistical Manual of Mental Disorders, 3rd Edition. Washington, DC, American Psychiatric Association, 1980

American Psychiatric Association: Diagnostic and Statistical Manual of Mental Disorders, 3rd Edition, Revised. Washington, DC, American Psychiatric Association, 1987

Feighner JP, Robins E, Guze SB, et al: Diagnostic criteria for use in psychiatric research. Arch Gen Psychiatry 26:57–63, 1972

Group for the Advancement of Psychiatry: Psychopathological Disorders in Childhood: Theoretical Considerations and a Proposed Classification. New York, Group for the Advancement of Psychiatry, Vol 6, 1966, p 62

Kanner L: Child Psychiatry, 1st Edition. Baltimore, MD, Charles C Thomas, 1935

Kanner L: Child Psychiatry, 3rd Edition. Baltimore, MD, Charles C Thomas, 1957

National Conference on Medical Nomenclature: Standard Classified Nomenclature of Diseases, 4th Edition. New York, Blakiston, 1952

World Health Organization: International Classification of Diseases, 8th Revision. Geneva, World Health Organization, 1969

Chapter 2

Development of the Subspecialty of Child and Adolescent Psychiatry

Irving N. Berlin, M.D.

This chapter is an effort to tie together some of the historical influences that ultimately led to the subspecialty of child and adolescent psychiatry and the proximate events and people responsible for the establishment of subspecialty boards in child psychiatry. Because many of the pioneers in child and adolescent psychiatry were known to me, I have mentioned their names and contributions. I will try to bring into historical perspective the development of psychotherapy and some of the other therapeutic methods utilized in our field as well as aspects of early research significant to the growth of this subspecialty.

Child psychiatry as a clinical entity can be said to have begun with the work of William Healy in Chicago with juvenile delinquency and with the founding of the Juvenile Psychopathic Institute in Chicago in 1909. This will be discussed in greater detail later in this chapter.

Child psychiatry as a clinical subspecialty of psychiatry can be said to have begun with the formation of the American Academy of Child Psychiatry in 1952.

The Role of the Academy of Child Psychiatry

Child psychiatry as a subspecialty began with the formation of the Academy of Child Psychiatry in 1952. Its founders were all members of the American Orthopsychiatric Association (Ortho), which was founded by psychiatrists in 1924 as a place to discuss clinical issues, especially those having to do with children and adolescents. Karl Menninger, David Levy, and Sheldon Glueck were among the founders. A decade later, Ortho became an interdisciplinary organization (Crutcher 1943; Lowrey 1955; Witmer 1940). In 1951, George Gardner was president of Ortho, and James Cunningham was President of the American Association of Psychiatric Clinics for Children (Lowrey 1955). This latter organization had become the standard-setting body for child psychiatry practice and training in clinics in the United States. On May 7, 1951, when Ortho was meeting in Cincinnati, George Gardner and Mabel Ross convened a meeting of the leading child psychiatrists present. These distinguished child psychiatrists were directors of child guidance clinics or faculty of the several medical schools with affiliated child psychiatry clinics. Gardner, for example, was director of the Judge Baker Child Guidance Center in Boston and a member of the Harvard Medical School faculty in the Department of Psychiatry (American Academy of Child Psychiatry 1962; Lowrey 1944).

The child psychiatrists who met were Drs. George Gardner, Mabel Ross, James Cunningham, Frank Curran, Spafford Ackerly, Lauretta Bender, Leo Kanner, Edward Liss, John Rose, Frederick Allen, William Langford, Jules Coleman, Margaret Gerard, Stanislaus Szurek, Othilda Krug, Hyman Lippman, and Reynold Jenson. This group issued a call to all child psychiatrists in the United States to plan the formation of the Academy of Child Psychiatry. On February 24, 1952, 96 child/adolescent psychiatrists, some of them psychoanalysts, met to discuss the purpose and function of an Academy of Child Psychiatry.

On May 12, 1952, at Atlantic City, another meeting was held; six members of the organizing committee became the first council. Dr. George Gardner was the first president. The president-elect was Frederick Allen; the secretary was Frank Curran; and the treasurer was Mabel Ross. The first meeting of the Academy of Child Psychiatry occurred in February 1953 in Cleveland, Ohio (American Academy of Child Psychiatry 1962).

This organization was clearly a medical organization whose purpose was to delineate the scope of child psychiatry and its practice. It also emphasized the need to have such specialty practice recognized by medicine and psychiatry. The Academy of Child Psychiatry set standards of training and practice and also endorsed the promotion and advancement of prevention, treatment, research, and teaching in child psychiatry.

The constitution and bylaws established two classes of membership: fellows and associate members. Membership was by invitation only. Those individuals who began their training in child psychiatry after 1946 had to be diplomates of the board and had to have 2 years of training in child psychiatry in addition to their general psychiatry training. The setting for training in child psychiatry had to be deemed adequate by the organization. Invitations to membership required 5 years of practice in the field; one had to have made a significant contribution to child psychiatry and also demonstrated competence in the field as a practitioner, teacher, trainer, researcher in child psychiatry, or administrator of a clinic or of a governmental child psychiatry office.

The associate members were those distinguished physicians who had made significant contributions to the field but could not meet the specifications of training and certification (American Academy of Child Psychiatry 1962).

In 1969, under the leadership of Sidney Berman, the Academy of Scholars' concept, which had excluded most child psychiatrists from the Academy, was considerably broadened by new membership criteria voted on by the members. Eligibility now required completion of child psychiatry training in an accredited program and an affirmation of a current professional interest and work in child psychiatry. This change made the Academy representative of child psychiatry in the nation and made it a more influential organization on behalf of children (Berman 1970; Slaff 1989).

The American Psychiatric Association's Role

There was simultaneous activity in the American Psychiatric Association, which also contributed to the establishment of a subspecialty in child psychiatry. In 1943, the American Psychiatric Association appointed a Committee on Psychopathology of Childhood, which in 1949 became the Committee on Child Psychiatry. In 1952, this committee, chaired by Dr. George Gardner, petitioned the Council of the American Psychiatric Association for endorsement of subspecialty certification in child psychiatry. That petition was turned down. In 1957, the Committee on Child Psychiatry, together with a committee from the American Academy of Child Psychiatry, gained the endorsement of the American Psychiatric Association to request the American Board of Psychiatry and Neurology to form a subspecialty Board in Child Psychiatry (American Psychiatric Association 1964).

Creation of the Committee on Certification in Child Psychiatry

In 1958, the American Board of Psychiatry and Neurology requested that the six members of the Council of the Academy of Child Psychiatry meet with them to work out the mechanism for a subspecialty committee on certification in child psychiatry. The Committee on Certification in Child Psychiatry was created in 1959. The chairman was Frederick Allen; William Langford was vice-chairman and Franklin Robinson was secretary. Othilda Krug, Frank Curran, and Hyman Lippman were the other board members, with James C. Hugh as the representative from the American Board of Pediatrics (American Psychiatric Association 1964).

In 1960, the Subcommittee on Child Psychiatry of the Residency Review Committee in Psychiatry was established. It developed training criteria and began to examine child psychiatry training programs (Wiener 1988).

Other Factors in the Development of Child Psychiatry as a Subspecialty

In 1940, Witmer described the concern of the National Committee on Mental Hygiene when so many thousands of soldiers in World War I suffered from "shell shock." Dr. George Stevenson and others began to point to the need for preventive treatment of children and adolescents and influenced the Commonwealth Fund and the Rockefeller Foundation to sponsor the development of child guidance clinics, which began in the late 1920s and early 1930s. In the mid-1930s, the rise of Hitler in Germany and his invasion of Austria resulted in an exodus of psychoanalysts from Germany and Austria to the United States. This also was the time of the Great Depression. The only positions open to many of these psychoanalysts were in the child guidance clinics and the universities. Thus began a melding of psychoanalytic ideas about psychotherapy of children along with ideas already developed in the many child guidance clinics established, especially because of the earlier work of Healy (Healy and Bronner 1952; Levy 1968). The pattern of service delivery in Frederick Allen's Philadelphia Child Guidance Clinic was typical. A psychiatrist treated the child; a social worker consulted with the mother or parents; and a psychologist did the testing. Family involvement in the child guidance clinics evolved, in part, from Adolph Meyer's convictions that one could study and understand the whole child only by also working with the family, and from Healy and Bronner's work with delinquents (Berlin 1964; Crutcher 1943; Healy and Bronner 1952; Noshpitz 1979). In 1930, Meyer asked Leo Kanner to form the first "pediatric psychiatry clinic." The Child Psychiatry section of the Harriet Lane Pediatric Clinic at Johns Hopkins was the precursor of the university divisions of child psychiatry (Kanner 1960b).

In 1935, Leo Kanner published the first textbook of child psychiatry. In it was the first official use of the term child psychiatry. In 1942, Frederick Allen's book, *Psychotherapy with Children*, was published. In the late 1930s and early 1940s, Adelaide Johnson and Stanislaus Szurek at the Institute for Juvenile Research in Chicago began to test the effectiveness of collaborative therapy for both the neurotic child and his or her parents (Szurek et al. 1942). In 1948, under Allen's leadership, 54 child guidance clinics banded together to form the American Association of Psychiatric Clinics for Children to develop standards for clinic operations, services,

and training. Once the Committee on Certification was formed, this organization no longer had influence on child psychiatrists' training and eventually gave up its standard setting and clinic evaluation function.

An important stimulus to child psychiatry as a subspecialty occurred in 1949 with the creation of the National Institute of Mental Health, directed by Dr. Robert Felix, a prominent psychiatrist. From the National Institute of Mental Health, training branch came stipends for training in psychiatry, child psychiatry, psychology, and social work (American Psychiatric Association 1964).

In 1963, a conference on training in child psychiatry was called, sponsored by the American Psychiatric Association and the Association of American Medical Colleges. That conference sought to lay out the essentials of a curriculum and to specify areas that were necessary to child psychiatry training as well as areas that might be elective. At that time there were about 200 board-certified child psychiatrists, most of them members of the Academy and about another 200 individuals in training.

As a participant in that conference, I can recall the comments and presentations from pioneers in the field like Leo Kanner, George Gardner, Frank Curran, Othilda Krug, Eveoleen Rexford, Adelaide Johnson, and Irene Josselyn. I was struck with the dedication of this group of eminent child psychiatrists but also with the sense of intimacy, good humor, and respect that permeated their relationships. It should be noted that, of this group, more than half were in charge of university child psychiatric inpatient and outpatient settings (American Psychiatric Association 1964).

The Evolution of Various Therapies and Research: Its Influence on the Development of Child Psychiatry as a Subspecialty

Psychotherapy

For many years, psychoanalysis formed the theoretical base of child psychiatry. Influenced by Anna Freud (1928, 1946) and by Melanie Klein (1932), play therapy began as an effort to discover the unconscious conflicts revealed in the child's play. By contrast, Allen (1942) and others emphasized the therapeutic effect of the formation of a new and healthier relationship between an adult and the child. In 1947, Virginia Axline, a student of Carl Rogers, wrote her book *Play Therapy*. She emphasized the priority of helping children work through conflicts without much interpretation but instead with an empathic understanding of the children's problems while at the same time communicating that awareness. In 1950, Erik Erikson wrote *Childhood and Society*, which brought ego psychology, introduced by Anna Freud in 1936, into the forefront as an important factor in understanding development and psychopathology in children and adolescents. Solomon (1948) introduced structured play techniques. Levy (1939, 1959) described release therapy and his experiences at a demonstration clinic designed to treat disturbed mothers and young children. Lippman (1961), in his book *Treatment of the Child in Emotional Conflict*, synthesized many of these ideas.

Family and Group Therapy

Beginning with Ackerman's papers in 1938, family therapy began to have its impact on psychiatry and child psychiatry (Ackerman 1958). In the late 1950s and early 1960s, Don Jackson, Gregory Bateson, Bowen, Laing, Lidz, Wynne, and others began to develop family therapy theory, and the books of Ackerman (1958) and Satir (1963) on clinical applications of family therapy were major influences on its growth (Whiteside 1979).

Group therapy had its start with Slavson's (1943) work. He described group activity therapy with latency-aged children. In 1936, Bender and Waltman described their work with psychotic children in group therapy. In 1954, Gisela Konopka, a professor of social work, published her book on group therapy with adolescent girls. Throughout the 1950s, 1960s, and 1970s, a good many child psychiatrists helped develop the theory and practice of group therapy with children and adolescents (Kraft 1979).

Behavior Therapy

Behavior therapy has been described as starting with the work of Pavlov on conditioned reflexes in animals. The noted psychologist Watson applied learning principles to alter children's behavior patterns. Thorndike's learning theory described the "law of effect," which emphasized the influence of reinforcing consequences on behavior. B. F. Skinner then used these ideas to develop the behavioral

psychology of operant conditioning. Joseph Wolpe (1952) in turn helped develop the methodology. The development of social learning theory by Ferster along with Zigler and others provided new explanations of development and psychopathology. The behavioral therapy methods as described by Luria and Lazarus include cognitive learning theory and practice (McGee and Saidel 1979). Imitative learning through modeling, as described by Bandera and Walters (1963) and others, provides a cognitive awareness of how behavior can be altered through emulation. These various behavioral interventions based on learning theory arose in part as a reaction to the less empirical and more subjectively based theory and practice of psychoanalysis, and originated primarily with academic psychologists (Krasner 1971; McGee and Saidel 1979).

Mental Health Consultation and Crisis Intervention

Child psychiatrists and child and adult analysts have developed both the theory and applications of the models for mental health consultation and crisis intervention. Lindeman (1944), one of the pioneers, worked primarily in the area of crisis intervention with families and individuals who experienced overwhelming stress. More recently, the treatment of children and families who have experienced catastrophic events has been dealt with as a field of its own, with different therapeutic strategies utilizing psychodynamic, behavioral, and pharmacologic approaches (Lindeman 1944; Noshpitz 1979).

Many of the pioneers who developed mental health consultation methodology were child psychiatrists: Jules Coleman at Yale in 1947 (see Coleman 1953), Gerald Caplan at the Harvard School of Public Health in 1956 (see Caplan 1970), Viola Bernard at Columbia in 1954 (see also Bernard 1964), and I. N. Berlin at the University of California in 1956.

These efforts led to the teaching and training of child psychiatry residents in school and agency mental health consultation.

Delinquency Research and Treatment Strategies

Since the 1800s, delinquency has been and still is one of the most serious and poorly understood and poorly treated problems of childhood and, especially, adolescence.

William Healy, a neurologist, was encouraged by philanthropists who were influenced by Adolph Meyer and William James, and by those working with the courts in Chicago, to study and try to treat delinquency. In 1909 Healy founded the Juvenile Psychopathic Institute in Chicago, later to be named the Institute for Juvenile Research. This was the first child guidance clinic in America. In 1915, Healy published his first findings in *The Individual Delinquent*. In 1917, Healy and his collaborator, Augusta Bronner, dissatisfied with the role of the juvenile court in Chicago, were encouraged to move to Boston. There they founded the Judge Baker Foundation, later named the Judge Baker Guidance Center. In his first book, Healy described the role of social and developmental factors in the etiology of delinquency. He emphasized the team concept of psychiatrist, psychologist, and social worker collaborating both in gathering data and in working with the delinquent and his or her family. *New Light on Delinquency and Its Treatment*, coauthored by Healy and Bronner, was published in 1936. In this volume, the authors documented the role of dysfunctional families and adverse social conditions, such as poverty and ghetto living, as being significant to the origins of delinquency (Gardner 1972; Noshpitz 1962).

The understanding and the treatment of delinquents were also of major concern to child psychiatrists and analysts. Szurek (1942) and Johnson (1949) described superego lacunae in adolescents resulting from unconscious parental permission for delinquent acts. In 1952, this thesis was amplified in the Johnson and Szurek work on the genesis of antisocial behavior. In 1955, Bettelheim wrote *Truants From Life*. In 1957, 1958, and 1963, Rexford, Van Amerongen, and Josselyn reported their clinical work with impulsive acting out in children. The talented educator and psychoanalyst Fritz Redl together with Wineman studied delinquent adolescent boys and wrote *The Aggressive Child* in 1937, *Children Who Hate* in 1951, and *Controls From Within* in 1952. Redl pioneered the use of group therapy with delinquents, first at his famous Michigan summer camp and later at Pioneer House in Detroit. He also described many of the principles of residential treatment (Noshpitz 1979; Redl 1959). In the early 1950s, the Gluecks' studies of juvenile delinquency published in 1959 and 1970 implicated poverty as one of its causes. In 1962, Noshpitz, who had worked with Redl, described his group's stud-

ies of hyperaggressive children. Always a great concern of American society, delinquent antisocial behavior has been studied since the early 1800s and is still an important area of research. The pioneering work of Kempe et al. (1962) has clarified the role of physical abuse as an etiologic factor in some delinquent behavior.

The Psychotic Child

In 1942, Lauretta Bender described her experiences beginning in 1935 at Bellevue Hospital in New York City. As the director of one of the first child psychiatric wards for the treatment of childhood schizophrenia, Bender, through her extremely astute observations, pointed to a combination of genetic and environmental etiologic factors.

In 1943 and 1944, Leo Kanner described early infantile autism and also described the presumed etiologic "refrigerator-like" characteristics of these children's parents, which later he noted to be an inaccurate conclusion. In 1952, Margaret Mahler described autistic and symbiotic infantile psychoses. Previously, Potter (1933) and Bradley (1941) had described the characteristics of schizophrenia in children whom they had treated in hospital settings (Bender 1942; Kanner 1943, 1960a; Mahler 1952). Fish et al. (1968) then described the various characteristics and classification of this disorder.

In 1953, Jones described the therapeutic community. In the 1950s and early 1960s, Bruno Bettelheim and Emmy Sylvester of the orthogenic school in Chicago coined the term *milieu* to describe their setting; Bettelheim was one of the major proponents of a psychotherapeutic approach to childhood psychoses (Bettelheim 1950; Bettelheim and Sylvester 1949). In California, Szurek and Ekstein described their inpatient psychotherapeutic treatment efforts with psychotic children that involved intensive psychotherapy with each child (Ekstein and Wallerstein 1956; Szurek 1956). For Szurek and others, treatment involved both the child and the parents.

The biological genetic determinants of childhood psychoses have become manifest in the last two decades. Bender (1938, 1942), Goldfarb (1956), and Fish and Alper (1962) are some of the researchers who have described some of these early biological manifestations. In 1957, Chapman described early infantile autism in twins.

Research Important to Child Psychiatry as a Subspecialty

Piaget's (1926) important research in cognitive development laid a foundation for later research. In 1941 at the Yale Child Study Center, Arnold Gessell, along with C. S. Amatruda, developed the first scales for measuring developmental stages of physical, cognitive, and psychological development (Kanner 1960b). Infant psychiatry, as it is known today, began with the very illuminating research of René Spitz. In 1945, Spitz described the results of early deprivation of mothering in infancy. In his article on "Anaclitic depression," Spitz (1946) clearly delineated the devastating effects of prolonged separation from the mother in the second half of the first year. Bergman and Escalona (1949) also described the effects of separation and stress in young children. Levy (1937) described primary affect hunger in young children. John Bowlby's seminal work for the World Health Organization in 1951 and his later volumes on attachment (1969, 1973) further emphasized the critical nature of the mother-child relationship in infancy. The words *attachment* and *bonding* became important descriptions of a close relationship between an infant (or child or adolescent) and an adult that supported normal development. Brazelton and others were able to observe and capture on film the early competence of the infant and how the infant's interaction with the mother influenced maternal behavior (Brazelton et al. 1966). In 1946, Benjamin Spock's *Baby and Child Care* introduced psychodynamic principles of development to the general public and became a best-seller.

A number of longitudinal studies produced important data, including prospective studies by Chess, Thomas, and Birch on temperamental differences in children (Chess et al. 1963; Thomas et al. 1968). Emmy Werner, a psychologist, and her colleagues did a prospective study on a cohort of infants born on the Island of Kauai (Werner et al. 1971). Having followed them for 30 years, she was able to document the effects of neurologic dysfunction in infancy on the subsequent development of these children.

Psychopharmacologic research, beginning with the discovery of chlorpromazine by Delay in France in 1937 and of lithium by Cade in Australia in 1949, was important to the development of the field. The subsequent research on the use of various pharmacotherapeutic agents—in minimal brain dysfunction (now attention-deficit disorder or attention-deficit hyperactivity disorder), childhood psychoses, childhood and adolescent depressions, Tourette's syndrome, anorexia and bulimia, and obsessive-compulsive disorder—has made pharmacotherapy very important in child psychiatry. However, its major impact on the practice of the subspecialty is relatively recent (Cade 1949; Campbell 1979) but growing.

Conclusion

The subspecialty of child psychiatry has a long history, beginning with the child guidance movement in the late 1920s and 1930s. The large number of draftees rejected for psychiatric reasons during World War II and the great frequency of mental illness in the armed services led to a resurgence of interest in the mental health of children and adolescents. To a large extent, child psychiatry in the 1950s and 1960s moved from the child guidance clinics to the university medical schools. The purely psychotherapeutic treatment model was altered as basic research in the epidemiology of mental illnesses and in the biological and biochemical aspects, especially genetic research, began to shed light on important variables in the etiology of mental illness. Psychopharmacology became a common treatment for certain mental illnesses of childhood and adolescence. Child psychiatry is now a well-established and vigorous subspecialty.

References

Ackerman NW: The Psychodynamics of Family Life. New York, Basic Books, 1958

Allen F: Psychotherapy With Children. New York, WW Norton, 1942

American Academy of Child Psychiatry: The history of the American Academy of Child Psychiatry. Journal of the American Academy of Child Psychiatry 1:196–202, 1962

American Psychiatric Association: Career Training in Child Psychiatry. Washington, DC, American Psychiatric Association, 1964

Axline VM: Play Therapy. New York, Ballantine, 1947

Bandera A, Walters R: Social Learning and Personality Development. New York, Holt, Rinehart, 1963

Bender L: A Visual-Motor Gestalt Test With Children and Its Clinical Use (Monogr No 2). New York, American Orthopsychiatric Association, 1938

Bender L: Childhood Schizophrenia. Nervous Child 1:138–140, 1942

Bender L, Waltman AS: The use of puppet shows as a psychotherapeutic method for behavior problems in children. Journal of the American Orthopsychiatric Association 6:341–348, 1936

Bergman P, Escalona S: Unusual sensitivities in very young children. Psychiatric Study of the Child 2:333–353, 1949

Berlin IN: Some learning experiences as a psychiatric consultant in the schools. Mental Hygiene 40:215–236, 1956

Berlin IN: A history of challenges in child psychiatry training. Mental Hygiene 48:558–565, 1964

Berman S: Epilogue and a new beginning. Journal of the American Academy of Child Psychiatry 9:193–201, 1970

Bernard V: Psychiatric consultation in the social agency. Child Welfare 33:3–8, 1954

Bernard VW: Roles and functions of child psychiatrists in social and community psychiatry. Journal of the American Academy of Child Psychiatry 3:165–176, 1964

Bettelheim B: Love Is Not Enough: The Treatment Of Emotionally Disturbed Children. Glencoe, IL, Free Press, 1950

Bettelheim B: Truants From Life. Glencoe, IL, Free Press, 1955

Bettelheim B, Sylvester E: Milieu therapy: indications and illustrations. Psychoanal Rev 36:54–67, 1949

Bowlby J: Maternal Care and Mental Health (Monogr Ser No 2). Geneva, World Health Organization, 1951

Bowlby J: Attachment and Loss, Vol 1: Attachment. New York, Basic Books, 1969

Bowlby J: Attachment and Loss, Vol 2: Separation: Anxiety and Anger. London, Hogarth Press, 1973

Bradley C: Schizophrenia in Childhood. New York, Macmillan, 1941

Brazelton TB, Scholl ML, Robey JS: Visual responses in the newborn. Pediatrics 37:284–290, 1966

Cade JFJ: Lithium salts in the treatment of psychotic excitement. Med J Aust 2:349–352, 1949

Campbell M: Psychopharmacology, in Basic Handbook of Child Psychiatry, Vol 3. Edited by Noshpitz JD. New York, Basic Books, 1979, pp 376–409

Caplan G: Mental health consultation in the schools, in Elements of a Community Mental Health Program. Edited by Caplan G. New York, Milbank Memorial Fund, 1956, pp 77–85

Caplan G: The Theory and Practice of Mental Health Consultation. New York, Basic Books, 1970

Chapman AH: Early infantile autism in identical twins: report of a case. Archives of Neurology and Psychiatry 78:621–623, 1957

Chess S, Thomas A, Rutter M, et al: Interaction of temperament and environment in the production of behavioral disturbances. Am J Psychiatry 120:142–147, 1963

Coleman JV: The contribution of the psychiatrist to the social worker and to the client. Mental Hygiene 37:249–258, 1953

Crutcher R: Child psychiatry: a history of its development. Psychiatry 6:191–201, 1943

Ekstein R, Wallerstein J: Observations on the psychology of borderline and psychotic children. Psychoanal Study Child 11:166–235, 1956

Erikson EH: Childhood and Society. New York, WW Norton, 1950

Fish B, Alper M: Abnormal states of consciousness and muscle tone in infants born to schizophrenic mothers. Am J Psychiatry 119:439–445, 1962

Fish B, Shapiro T, Campbell M, et al: A classification of schizophrenic children under five years. Am J Psychiatry 124:1415–1423, 1968

Freud A: Introduction to the Technique of Child Analysis. New York, Nervous and Mental Disease Publishing, 1928

Freud A: The Ego and the Mechanisms of Defense. New York, International Universities Press, 1946

Gardner GE: William Healy, 1869–1963. Journal of the American Academy of Child Psychiatry 11:1–29, 1972

Glueck S: The Problem of Delinquency. Boston, MA, Houghton Mifflin, 1959

Glueck S, Glueck E: Toward a Typology of Juvenile Offenders. New York, Grune & Stratton, 1970

Goldfarb W: Receptor preference in schizophrenic children. Archives of Neurology and Psychiatry 76:643–652, 1956

Healy W: The Individual Delinquent. Boston, MA, Little, Brown, 1915

Healy W, Bronner AF: New Light on Delinquency and Its Treatment. New Haven, CT, Yale University Press, 1952

Johnson A: Sanctions for superego lacunae of adolescents, in Search Lights on Delinquency. Edited by Eissler K. New York, International Universities Press, 1949, pp 225–245

Johnson AM, Szurek SA: The genesis of antisocial acting out in children and adults. Psychoanal Q 21:323–343, 1952

Jones M: The Therapeutic Community: A New Treatment Method in Psychiatry. New York, Basic Books, 1953

Josselyn IM: A type of predelinquent behavior. Am J Orthopsychiatry 28:606–612, 1958

Kanner L: Child Psychiatry. Springfield, IL, Charles C Thomas, 1935

Kanner L: Autistic disturbances of affective contact. Nervous Child 2:217–250, 1943

Kanner L: Early infantile autism. J Pediatr 25:211–217, 1944

Kanner L: Arnold Gesell's place in the history of developmental psychology and psychiatry, in Child Development and Child Psychiatry (Psychiatric Research Reports No 13). Edited by Shagass C, Pasamanick B. Washington, DC, American Psychiatric Association, 1960a, pp 1–9

Kanner L: Child psychiatry: retrospect and prospect. Am J Psychiatry 117:15–22, 1960b

Kempe CH, Silverman FN, Steele BF, et al: The battered child syndrome. JAMA 181:17–24, 1962

Klein M: The Psychoanalysis of Children. New York, WW Norton, 1932

Konopka G: Group Work in the Institution: A Modern Challenge. New York, Whiteside & Wimorrow, 1954

Kraft IA: Group therapy, in Basic Handbook of Child Psychiatry, Vol 3. Edited by Noshpitz JD. New York, Basic Books, 1979, pp 159–180

Krasner IA: Behavior therapy. Annu Rev Psychol 22:483–531, 1971

Levy DM: Primary affect hunger. Am J Psychiatry 94:643, 1937

Levy DM: Release therapy. Am J Orthopsychiatry 9:713–736, 1939

Levy DM: The Demonstration Clinic for the Psychological Study and Treatment of Mother and Child in Medical Practice. Springfield, IL, Charles C Thomas, 1959

Levy DM: Beginnings of the child guidance movement. Am J Orthopsychiatry 38:799–804, 1968

Lindeman E: Symptomatology and management of acute grief. Am J Psychiatry 101:141–148, 1944

Lippman HS: Treatment of the Child in Emotional Conflict. New York, Blakiston, 1961

Lowrey LG: Psychiatry for children: a brief history of developments. Am J Psychiatry 101:375–388, 1944

Lowrey LG: The contribution of orthopsychiatry to psychiatry: brief historical note. Am J Orthopsychiatry 25:475–478, 1955

Mahler M: On child psychosis and schizophrenia: autistic and symbiotic infantile psychosis. Psychoanal Study Child 7:286–305, 1952

McGee JP, Saidel DH: Individual behavior therapy, in Basic Handbook of Child Psychiatry, Vol 3. Edited by Noshpitz JD. New York, Basic Books, 1979, pp 72–107

National Conference on Medical Nomenclature: Standard Classified Nomenclature of Diseases, 4th Edition. New York, Blakiston, 1952

Noshpitz JD: Notes on the theory of residential treatment. Journal of the American Academy of Child Psychiatry 1:284–296, 1962

Noshpitz JD: History of childhood and child psychiatry in the twentieth century (typescript). Washington, DC, Washington University School of Medicine, 1979

Piaget J: The Language and Thought of the Child. New York, Harcourt Brace, 1926

Potter H: Schizophrenia in children. Am J Psychiatry 8:1253–1270, 1933

Redl F: A strategy and technique of the life space interview. Am J Orthopsychiatry 29:1–18, 1959

Redl F, Wineman D: The Aggressive Child. Springfield, IL, Illinois Free Press, 1937

Redl F, Wineman D: Children Who Hate. Glencoe, IL, Free Press, 1951

Redl F, Wineman D: Controls From Within. Glencoe, IL, Free Press, 1952

Rexford EN: A developmental concept of the problems of acting out. Journal of the American Academy of Child Psychiatry 2:6–21, 1963

Rexford EN, Van Amerongen ST: The influence of unresolved maternal oral conflicts upon impulsive acting out. Am J Orthopsychiatry 28:606–612, 1958

Satir V: Conjoint Family Therapy: A Guide. Palo Alto, CA, Science and Behavior Books, 1963

Slaff B: History of child and adolescent psychiatry ideas and organizations in the United States: a twentieth century review. Adolesc Psychiatry 16:31–52, 1989

Slavson SR: An Introduction to Group Therapy. New York, Commonwealth Fund, 1943

Solomon JC: Play techniques. Am J Orthopsychiatry 18:402–413, 1948

Spitz RA: Hospitalism: an inquiry into the genesis of psychiatric conditions in early childhood. Psychoanal Study Child 1:53–74, 1945

Spitz RA: Anaclitic depression. Psychoanal Study Child 2:313–342, 1946

Spock B: Baby and Child Care. New York, Pocket Books, 1946

Szurek SA: Notes on the genesis of psychopathic personality trends. Psychiatry 5:1–6, 1942

Szurek SA: Childhood schizophrenia: psychotic episodes and psychotic maldevelopment. Am J Orthopsychiatry 26:519–543, 1956

Szurek SA, Johnson A, Falstein E: Collaborative psychiatric therapy of parent-child problems. Am J Orthopsychiatry 12:511–516, 1942

Thomas A, Chess S, Birch HG: Temperament and Behavior Disorders in Children. New York, New York University Press, 1968

Werner EE, Bierman JM, French FE: The Children of Kauai. Honolulu, HI, University of Hawaii Press, 1971

Whiteside MF: Family therapy, in Basic Handbook of Child Psychiatry, Vol 3. Edited by Noshpitz JD. New York, Basic Books, 1979, pp 117–158

Wiener JM: The future of child and adolescent psychiatry: if not now, when? J Am Acad Child Adolesc Psychiatry 27:8–10, 1988

Witmer HL: Psychiatric Clinics for Children. New York, Commonwealth Fund, 1940

Wolpe J: Experimental neurosis as learned behavior. Br J Psychol 43:243–268, 1952

Chapter 3

Future Trends in Child and Adolescent Psychiatry

Richard L. Cohen, M.D.

The task of this chapter is to make some considered projections about the field of child and adolescent psychiatry. Is such an essay justifiable within the body of a major text? The answer to this question can be affirmative only if we reach an acceptable level of reliability with our predictions. This is best achieved by keeping one eye intently trained on the past. We need constant reminders that we have all, at one time or another, jumped on bandwagons only to learn of our folly later. As Chess (1988) has stated, "The search for simple formulas that can be applied like cookbook recipes to all children and adolescents is, indeed, a search for 'fool's gold' " (p. 6).

There are distinct and definable patterns in the life histories of all medical specialties. Although these may differ in some ways that are specialty-specific, the developmental progression from polymorphic infancy to well-integrated maturity is universal. There is no reason to expect that child and adolescent psychiatry will be an exception, particularly since its historical development to date is consistent with that of other relatively new medical disciplines.

There is, of course, the risk embodied in presenting any data-free work that the wish will be father to the thought, that fantasy will triumph over wisdom, and that science will take a backseat to dogma. With the fervent prayer that I have resisted these demons, the following observations are offered.

To begin, three tenets should guide our projections about the future because they have always influenced the form and substance of medical practice. First, physicians have roles assigned to them by society (both through traditional community standards and by governmental law and regulations). Second, in most industrialized nations, the practice of medicine is a professional service that responds to competitive forces in the marketplace and to developments in the international medical-industrial complex. Third, the torrent of new information and technologies emerging from our biomedical and behavioral research enterprise makes patient care increasingly complex and constantly modifies what is "standard of practice."

In the "real world," these three factors usually interact with each other to produce any given outcome. This makes reliable prediction even riskier. For instance, the injunctions of strict confidentiality must be reconsidered in light of the Tarasoff decision. Reimbursement for inpatient care based on a prospective payment formula may result in recourse to clinically less effective community resources. Managed care practices may result in de facto rationing of medical services, clinical indications notwithstanding. For purposes of this chapter, however, we will consider each of these three areas individually.

Changing Societal Attitudes

The medical profession as a whole finds itself caught in a wrenching transition. Its centuries-old image as caregiver-healer and family decision maker endowed with superhuman wisdom on matters of health and illness is being stripped away. Several forces are contributing to this shift. These are likely to be ongoing themes for the foreseeable future.

For instance, the physician is now expected to be a superspecialist equipped with the latest high-technology hardware. Many patients and families now expect to learn what is wrong through the application of sophisticated imaging procedures and a battery of biochemical tests. They expect to experience relief from suffering by the use of lasers, invasive catheters, and substances that modify immune systems or destroy alien organisms. There are frequent complaints about the paucity of generalists, but most people want "modern" doctors who are up to date on the latest advances.

Furthermore, the rapidly changing face of corporate medicine has accustomed patients to develop an alliance (if indeed, they feel any at all) with the institution, health maintenance organization, or plan in which they receive care rather than with an individual physician. Such issues as continuity of care, accountability for services, quality control, and legal liability are no longer the sole concerns of the attending physician. Conditioned by a societal climate of fast and faceless food servers, bank machines, and cable television sales channels, patients (especially those under 35 years of age) now tend to view their health caregivers in the same mold.

The consumer movement itself has caused major attitudinal shifts. Physicians are no longer the undisputed authority in the decision-making process concerning care; the results of their other efforts are not accepted with unquestioning humility and are constantly monitored (with a variety of motives) by hospital administrators, regulatory authorities, and attorneys. Most recently, a call has emerged for all reimbursement for medical services to be tied closely to informed consent procedures so that the decision-making process remains firmly in the hands of the consumer (Kapp 1989).

Finally, it is no longer acceptable to claim that certain aspects of human suffering are not the province of psychiatric medicine. During the past two decades, we have witnessed a remarkable shift in the attitudes of both clinicians and investigators toward the problems of multiply handicapped children and the mentally retarded and toward the special stresses imposed on the development of minority-group youngsters. Now the time has come to focus more attention on the devastating impact of parental acquired immune deficiency syndrome;

of substance abuse; of the abortion conflict and concerns raised by the new reproductive technologies; of the tragedy of homelessness; and on the chronically ill child.

As funding for long-term projects aimed at prevention of psychiatric morbidity becomes more available (in part because newer methodologies now promise the prospect of carrying out replicable preventive pilot studies), more child and adolescent psychiatrists will be attracted to make major investments in working with these high-risk populations. Subsequently, the patient mix appearing both in private and in public clinical settings will begin to reflect this influence.

Cost-Containment Practices

Current modes of cost containment usually include one or some combination of the following: 1) assigning payment ceilings at a national or regional level for many types of services; 2) attaching dollar values for the care of specific disorders (diagnosis-related groups, or DRGs) or for specifically designated diagnostic and treatment procedures (current procedure terminologies, or CPTs), further weighted by determining the degree of skill, time, and complexity involved (resource-based value scales) in their administration; and 3) controlling access to services through the use of clinical "gatekeepers" and/or by a system of managed care.

Any medical specialty that finds itself removed from the mainstream of practice may also be the last to find its services adequately covered by this "bottom-line" system of reimbursement.

The Scientific Data-Base Explosion

Several prestigious academic leaders both individually and in committees and task forces have identified a spectrum of research priorities for the next decade (e.g., Detre 1989; Earls 1982a; Institute of Medicine 1989; Judd and Glick 1989; Kupfer and Tuma 1989; Rutter 1986a, 1986b; Shapiro 1989). One would expect differences among these recommendations. There are a few, but there is a surprising and gratifying degree of agreement.

It is beyond the purpose and scope of this chapter to provide the details of these plans and to attempt to present their rationale. These are contained in the referenced publications. However, there seems to be little controversy about the recommendations that child and adolescent psychiatry (together with appropriate collaborators in other disciplines) attract its best minds for the immediate future toward expanding our knowledge base in the following areas: 1) developmental neurosciences; 2) prevention and special populations; 3) epidemiology of child and adolescent disorders; 4) assessment, diagnosis, and treatment; 5) services and systems of care; and 6) behavioral and social sciences.

Recently, a special committee of the Institute of Medicine (1989) concluded its report entitled "Research on Children and Adolescents With Mental, Behavioral and Developmental Disorders" with the following statement:

> The committee shares with others in the field an excitement about the demonstrable progress occurring in many segments of child mental health research. . . . The nation would do well to capitalize on the momentum that has developed during the past two decades.
> The committee has called for a broad initiative that would promote research simultaneously in many areas of child mental health. It has done so in the belief that no single approach or small group of studies can claim preeminence. . . . (p. 11)

In his presidential address to the American Academy of Child and Adolescent Psychiatry, Wiener (1988) expressed the need for change:

> Finally, and I think most fundamental for our future, is a commitment to the progressive expansion of a scientific data base that will earn and deserve the respectful attention of our medical colleagues, our public officials, our foundations, and our professional competitors. (p. 10)

Special Characteristics of Child and Adolescent Psychiatric Practice

Much of what has been outlined so far applies in a general way to all of medical practice. There are some special characteristics of the field of child and adolescent psychiatry that may create added pressures for rapid change. First, although its research enterprise is showing signs of growth, the field still lags behind many other disciplines in its understanding of the epidemiology, genetic basis, pathophysiology, and pathogenesis of disorders. Second, clinical practice remains highly labor intensive. Relatively few biomedical procedures are employed. Third, major investments of time and energy must be made in diagnostic and management efforts that are "indirect" (not involving face-to-face patient contact)—that is, with families, schools, and community agencies.

These features represent a kind of "baggage" that child and adolescent psychiatry carries into the last decade of the 20th century. They signify that, for this specialty, a particularly vigorous effort will be required to make the changes that are expected of the medical profession by individual patients and by our collective society.

Perhaps this discussion can conclude on a more hopeful note, however. At this writing, there is reason to expect that the so-called cognitive specialties (in contrast to the procedure-based specialties) will enjoy a different reimbursement scale in the future as some form of resource-based value scale for determining allowable fees comes into common use.

Changes During the Next Decade

What are these changes? I believe they can be predicted because they follow logically from the forces now impacting on the field.

Attention to Issues of Concern to All Physicians

Although many shifts in both activity and identity have occurred during the past decade, they have not been sufficient to ensconce child and adolescent psychiatry firmly in the spectrum of medical specialties. A more vigorous commitment to contribute to the work of organized medicine at all levels should be forthcoming. Perhaps the harshest criticism of the specialty remains that of its tendency toward isolation (Guze 1983).

This sustained display of genuine identification with all physicians (e.g., through serving on major county medical society committees, through joining in efforts to negotiate needed changes in local or state ordinances adversely affecting practice, through donating time to local community health organizations) will erase the image of this specialty as being different and removed from the mainstream of medicine.

All of this should be combined with a consistent effort to bring nosology, office, and hospital practices and cross-referral patterns into conformity with conventional medical practice.

Not only may this contribute to desired attitudinal shifts among medical colleagues; eventually, it could lead to more robust streams of referral and a more constructive kind of collaboration, especially with primary care physicians.

Just as importantly, current problems surrounding third-party reimbursement for professional services might be alleviated, as insurance carriers will not find it necessary to make judgments that are based on wholly "alien" (to them) concepts about disease, disability, and their management (American Medical Association 1989; Earls 1982b; Parry-Jones 1989).

Subspecialization

Since child and adolescent psychiatry is already a subspecialty, perhaps the term *superspecialization* might be more apt here. In any event, as the universe of data and skills continues to grow, it becomes less and less realistic to expect any single clinician to acquire the necessary mastery. In 10 years, we will have evolved a matrix of practitioners, some of whom will focus their efforts on circumscribed developmental epochs (e.g., infancy, preschoolers, adolescents), while others focus on major disease entities (e.g., anxiety disorders, substance abuse); still others will work primarily with high-risk populations (e.g., offspring of psychotic or brain-impaired parents, children of divorce) (Detre 1989). In larger metropolitan areas and in major medical centers, this trend will be the norm.

A welcome corollary of this inevitable development will be the evolution of entity-specific treatment regimens. These will largely replace the pattern of generic and often diffuse management approaches now in use. Indeed, there will be a trend toward identifying discrete management profiles for each disorder. Already the American Academy of Child and Adolescent Psychiatry is encouraging many of its clinically oriented committees to promulgate "practice guidelines" where feasible for each disorder. A recent effort aimed at increasing standardization of care for patients with attention-deficit hyperactivity disorder displays careful and thorough thought (American Academy of Child and Adolescent Psychiatry 1989).

Academic Centers

As noted above (Institute of Medicine 1989; Shapiro 1989), the next decade will see the emergence of child and adolescent psychiatry as an intense focus of both basic and clinical investigation. The federal establishment has evolved a spectrum of priorities requiring attention and appears willing to underwrite most of the cost needed to pursue this enterprise. It will fall to the discipline to recruit and train the investigators who will be entrusted with this task.

Dictated by research priorities, we will see the emergence of teams and networks of investigators as child and adolescent psychiatrists join geneticists, neurobiologists, epidemiologists, social scientists, and others. In larger training centers, it will become standard practice to require some research training for all residents and fellows, thus increasing the critical mass of academicians available to pursue the research goals that have been identified by the National Institute of Mental Health, the Institute of Medicine, and the American Academy of Child and Adolescent Psychiatry. Because there will be a growing need for more subspecialized training than can be provided by some smaller training programs, there will be growth in the academic consortia or networks where various subspecialty skills can be used synergistically.

Prevention

Prevention has always represented an important focus for child and adolescent psychiatrists. The field was predicated on the belief that early identification and intervention with high-risk groups was the sine qua non activity. Unfortunately, enthusiasm has far outstripped capacity. But as a result of several recent developments, it is becoming more clear that the prevention of mental disorders in young people is now not only a compelling priority but, at least in part, an achievable one. An excellent overview of the most contributory research findings is available elsewhere (Shaffer 1989; Shaffer et al. 1990).

The combination of a national awareness, even alarm, about suicide rates, substance abuse, and teenage pregnancy and abortion plus the emergence of newer methodologies for measuring risk factors and designing realistic interventions now makes preventive work an attractive pursuit.

During the next decade, many more child and adolescent psychiatrists will apply this knowledge to a spectrum of high-risk populations. If funding sources can resist pressures for quick answers to questions that cannot always be resolved within grant cycles designed for treatment techniques, and if investigators can approach all new preventive projects with the conviction that these projects demand rigorous design, the 1990s may see the dawn of a major preventive focus for the field.

Patterns of Practice, Competition, and Recruitment

Although most authorities agree that the trend toward managed care cannot be reversed or even slowed, it seems evident at this writing that too many decisions about the appropriateness of a given psychiatric treatment recommendation depend on 1) the incentive of cost containment, 2) the belief system of the clinical manager, or 3) some combination of the first two. One solution to this problem being pursued by legislators and third-party payers is to press for the development of practice guidelines. The intent of these would be to outline generally agreed-on diagnostic and treatment procedures for all types of illness.

At this writing, there are several bills before Congress dealing with issues of practice guidelines. The role of medical specialty organizations in providing expertise for these has yet to be defined. At least one bill would provide funding to establish a federal "forum" with a permanent staff. Such a forum would bring together providers, consumers, and payers who together might promulgate guidelines (Brook 1989).

The importance of such a development for child and adolescent psychiatry cannot be overemphasized. It comes at a time when the field is poised to carry out a series of epidemiologic and treatment outcome studies that could lead to rational practice guidelines. This compelling need to generate the data base that would place clinical practice in the field on sounder scientific footing may result in significant lessening of "town-gown" tensions. The issues surrounding the managed care versus fee-for-service controversy are an excellent example of the futility of separating clinical practice from clinical investigation.

Another major practice-related concern has to do with competition from other mental health professionals. There is some difference of opinion among leaders as to the significance of this problem. Many believe that the large number of clinical psychologists, social workers, mental health counselors, and developmental pediatricians represents a formidable competitive force in the delivery of services. I do not. The problem for child and adolescent psychiatry that I have encountered is largely one of unavailability or sometimes even invisibility. Many referral sources have considered these practitioners too isolated and too difficult to communicate with and have resigned themselves to implementing services without their expertise.

Consider the following. An analysis of some of the survey data collected during the work of Project Future of the American Academy of Child and Adolescent Psychiatry (Philips et al. 1983) indicates that, far from not wanting or needing any child psychiatric services, most social and allied health agencies had given up attempting to recruit such collaborators because they were "too unavailable" or because they did not seem motivated to work with populations of multiproblem children in institutional settings.

Furthermore, even the most conservative epidemiologic studies (e.g., Earls 1982a; Graham 1978) confirm the assertion that between 10% and 15% of children and youth are sufficiently behaviorally disordered to require professional attention, and at least one-third of these merit the service of a child and adolescent psychiatrist. Quick calculation leaves us with a final figure of more than two million. Since there are less than 5,000 child and adolescent psychiatrists in the United States, this means a doctor-patient ratio of less than 1:40,000! Slash this figure in half and there still remains an overwhelming patient population to serve.

In addition, the most authoritative government-sponsored survey of the medical work force in the United States (U.S. Department of Health and Human Services 1980) confirms that child and adolescent psychiatry is the area in shortest supply, and that a tripling or quadrupling of the numbers would barely meet the need for service.

These facts seem to me to be inconsistent with any conclusion that the profession is beset by any serious threat of competition. Rather, they suggest that the problems are those of activity within the mainstream of medicine, and that there is both an "image" problem concerning what the field can contribute to patient care and a communication deficit with consumers, the media, and organized medicine. Although some definite progress is being made to correct these shortcomings, much remains to be done.

Conclusion

What will the typical child and adolescent psychiatrist look like in the year 2000? If the tasks outlined above are accomplished, there will be no typical individual. Growth means differentiation and more developmentally sophisticated levels of performance. The field is now poised to work toward these next goals.

References

American Academy of Child and Adolescent Psychiatry, Work Group on Quality Issues (Jaffe S, chair): Practice parameters for the assessment and treatment of attention-deficit hyperactivity disorder. Washington, DC, American Academy of Child and Adolescent Psychiatry, 1989

American Medical Association, Council on Long Range Planning and Development, in cooperation with the American Psychiatric Association: The Future of Psychiatry. Chicago, IL, American Medical Association, 1989

Brook RH: Practice guidelines and practicing medicine. JAMA 262:3027–3030, 1989

Chess S: Child and adolescent psychiatry comes of age: a fifty year perspective. J Am Acad Child Adolesc Psychiatry 27:1–7, 1988

Detre T: Some comments on the future of child psychiatry. Academic Medicine 13:189–195, 1989

Earls F: Epidemiology and child psychiatry: future prospects. Compr Psychiatry 23:75–84, 1982a

Earls F: The future of child psychiatry as a medical discipline. Am J Psychiatry 139:1158–1161, 1982b

Graham P: Epidemiologic perspectives on maladaptation in children: neurologic, familial and social factors. J Am Acad Child Adolesc Psychiatry 17:197–208, 1978

Guze SB: Child psychiatry: taking stock, in Childhood Psychopathology and Development. Edited by Guze SB, Earls FJ, Barrett JE. New York, Raven, 1983, pp 203–210

Institute of Medicine: Research on Children and Adolescents With Mental, Behavioral and Developmental Disorders. Washington, DC, National Academy Press, 1989

Judd L, Glick I: The National Institute of Mental Health: prospects and promises. Biol Psychiatry 26:545–546, 1989

Kapp MB: Enforcing patient preferences: linking payment for medical care to informed consent. JAMA 261:1935–1938, 1989

Kupfer DJ, Tuma AH: Comment on "The National Institute of Mental Health: prospects and promises." Biol Psychiatry 26:547–549, 1989

Parry-Jones WLI: Annotation: the history of child and adolescent psychiatry: its present day relevance. J Child Psychol Psychiatry 30:3–11, 1989

Philips I, Cohen RL, Enzer NB (eds): Child Psychiatry: A Plan for the Coming Decades. Washington, DC, American Academy of Child and Adolescent Psychiatry, 1983

Rutter M: Child psychiatry: looking 30 years ahead. J Child Psychol Psychiatry 27:803–840, 1986a

Rutter M: Child psychiatry: the interface between clinical and developmental research. Psychol Med 16:151–169, 1986b

Shaffer D: Prevention of psychiatric disorders in children and adolescents: a summary of findings and recommendations, in Project Prevention in Prevention of Mental Disorders, Alcohol and Other Drug Use in Children and Adolescents. Edited by Shaffer D, Philips I, Enzer NB. Rockville, MD, U.S. Department of Health and Human Services, 1989

Shaffer D, Philips I, Enzer NB (eds): Prevention of mental disorders in children and adolescents. Washington, DC, American Academy of Child and Adolescent Psychiatry and Office for Substance Abuse Prevention, U.S. Department of Health and Human Services, 1990

Shapiro T (chair): Report of the Work Group on Scientific Issues. Washington, DC, American Academy of Child and Adolescent Psychiatry, 1989

U.S. Department of Health and Human Services, Health Resources Administration: Report of the Graduate Medical Education National Advisory Committee to the Secretary, Vol 1: summary report. Washington, DC, U.S. Department of Health and Human Services, 1980

Wiener JM: The future of child and adolescent psychiatry: if not now, when? J Am Acad Child Adolesc Psychiatry 27:8–10, 1988

Section II

Assessment and Diagnosis

Chapter 4

Normal Growth and Development: An Overview

Melvin Lewis, M.B., B.S., F.R.C.Psych., D.C.H.

Human development starts with genetic potential and blossoms through the interaction between the individual and the caring others in the individual's environment. Certain species' characteristics may strongly influence the emergence and form of particular patterns of functioning. For example, the prolonged relative biological helplessness of the human infant is associated with characteristic patterns of attachment behavior, which presumably have great survival value for the relatively helpless infant. Further, functions that are closely tied to central nervous system (CNS) maturation (e.g., motor development) appear to be more robust and resistant to environmental influences compared with, for example, the capacity to develop relationships, which is exquisitely sensitive to environmental influences.

Consequently, CNS maturational events and associated behaviors (e.g., electroencephalographic changes and the associated shift from a perceptual mode to a symbolic-linguistic mode at about 17 months) appear to be relatively discontinuous compared with the relative continuity of, for example, the temperament of the individual ("easy," "slow to warm up," and "difficult" temperaments).

For convenience we tend to focus our studies on discrete elements within our defined disciplines (e.g., neuroscience, developmental psychology, psychoanalysis). Yet development is a complex phenomenon, and in the end the discrete elements must all be integrated into a theory of the whole person. It may be noted that as yet no completely successful single theory attains this goal.

At the same time, several general concepts are helpful in attempts to organize our understanding of the development of the child. Maturation is the sequential emergence and linear growth of specific capacities. Development is the totality of full blossoming and the multiple, interlocking uses of these functions and skills, brought about by interaction between the individual and the environment. In this way, development is the result of the mutual influences of endowment, maturation, environment, and experiential factors.

The concept of stages is particularly useful since it enables one to analyze behavior, just as classification in biology serves as a basis for subsequent analysis and understanding. The following are the criteria for stages:

1. A stage, or structure, is characterized as a whole and not just as the juxtaposition of parts. The concept of definable stages means behavioral characteristics that have some degree of stability and autonomy.
2. There is an invariant sequence, or constant order of succession, from one stage to another.
3. While multiple and interrelated lines of stage development are present, each line may also have its own projectory (from preparatory level to a level of more or less completion) and rate of development, giving rise at any given moment to a multileveled organism.
4. Each successive stage in normal development represents an advance from the previous stage.

5. Each later stage supersedes all earlier stages in that structures constructed at a given age become an integral part of structures that follow.
6. The change is qualitative and not just quantitative.
7. Each stage proceeds in the direction of increasing complexity of organization, from a state of relative globality to a state of increasing differentiation and integration.
8. Biogenetic, environmental, experiential, and psychological factors guarantee and facilitate the developmental process, including coping and adaptation.
9. There are presumed critical, or sensitive, periods during which conditions are ideal for the normal emergence and development of important functions, such as attachment, gender identity, and language.

Developmental stage theories imply the development of a mental structure. Thus the structural theories of Freud, Erikson, and Piaget postulated a genetically determined capacity for the development of patterns, or systems, of behavior so that the child acts on the environment from the very beginning. The continuing sequence of behavior patterns that then emerge (i.e., "stages") are qualitatively different from each other. The clinical implications for treatment that flow from structural theories are that some kind of reorganization within the child is required (e.g., resolution of intrapsychic conflict, alteration of the family homeostasis, and acquisition of new schema).

On the other hand, some theories of function and behavior do not appear to have a strong developmental point of view and rely instead on certain principles of reaction. Reactive theories postulate that the child's mind begins as a tabula rasa and that the child then reacts to the environment. Major examples of this type of theory include stimulus-response theory, learning theories, classical conditioning theory, and operant conditioning theory. The clinical implication for treatment that flows from reactive theories is that symptoms are regarded as learned behavior; that is, the symptom is the disorder and that through relearning or environmental change the symptom is removed and therefore the disease is cured.

Although we can agree that development is a complex process involving biological, psychological, and social factors, the study of development is usually approached for convenience along the lines of some of its major functional components (see Figure 4-1). The developmental lines discussed below include motor sequence, language development, cognitive development, moral thinking, attachment, psychosexual phases, relationships, and temperament.

Maturation and Motor Sequence

Gesell and Amatruda (1941/1964) observed that most children creep, can be pulled to their feet, and have a crude, prehensile release by the time they are 10 months old. Within the next 2 months, they can walk with help and can grasp a small pellet. By 2 years of age, they are running with ease, although not with great skill.

A steady increase in motor skills can be observed in most children. By age 3, a child can stand on one foot, dance, and jump, and also is more dexterous than previously and can build a tower of 10 cubes. Ambidexterity gives way to lateralization some time during the third year, although handedness may not be firmly established for several years. Leg, eye, and ear dominance also may not become firmly established until the seventh, eighth, or ninth year, respectively, or even later.[1]

Children become increasingly agile as they grow and develop during the period of early childhood (e.g., learning to skip on alternate feet). Perceptual-motor skills also improve at this time: a child at age 2 years can copy a circle and by age 3, a cross; by age 5 a child can copy a square and by age 7 years, a diamond. Memory also improves with brain maturation: by age 6 the child can count five digits forward and three digits backward. Between 6 and 11 years of age, the child not only learns new motor skills, such as balancing on a bicycle, but at some point, perhaps around the age of 9, does so with apparent ease—the skill has become an automatic,

---

[1]Laterality is a measurable, specialized, central function of a paired faculty such as eyes, ears, hands, and feet. Preference is the subjective, self-reported experience of an individual and need not be the same as objectively measured laterality. The preference of an individual may be related more to the acuity of the peripheral organ (e.g., the ear) than to anything else. Dominance is used to describe the concept of cerebral hemisphere specialization (e.g., information processing, language and speech lateralization). Hemispheric lateralization appears to proceed sequentially from gross and fine motor skills to sensorimotor skills to speech and language (Leong 1976). Handedness is commonly consolidated by about age 5, footedness by about age 7, eye preference by about age 7 or 8, and ear preference by about age 9 (Touwen 1980).

Age (years)	Brain	EEG (Metcalf)	Motor (Gesell)	Language (Lennenberg)	Drawing (DiLeo)	Attachment (Bowlby)	Cognitive (Piaget)	Psychosexual (Freud)	Psychosocial (Erikson)	Environment
0–1	Decrease in lower frequencies / Increase in myelination / Increase in higher frequencies	0	Grasping Sucking Rooting Tonic neck Moro	Discriminates sounds Differential crying Coos Consonants	Crayons to mouth	Reflexes Orienting Signaling (0–3 months) Differential social responses (3–8 months)	Sensorimotor	Oral	Basic trust	Mothering person
1-2		5 cps	Pincer grasp Walks alone	2 words						
2–3				2 sentences 200 words	O2	Proximity seeking (1–3)	Preoperational	Anal	Autonomy	Parents
3–4		8 cps	Improved mastery	Uses consonants	+3	Goal-directed partnership (aet 3)		Phallic	Initiative	
4–7			Uses scissors	Normal language	□5 △6 ◇7			Oedipal	Industry	School and peers
7–12		11 cps	Bicycle riding				Concrete-operational	Latency		
>12		10 cps	Special skills				Formal-operations	Adolescence	Identity	Peers and adults

Figure 4.1   **Temporal correspondence of developing functions.**

established, and unself-conscious act requiring no effort of concentration.

Language Development

The sequence of emergence of actual sounds is broadly the same in all children everywhere (Lewis 1963). Children vocalize and respond to sounds from birth, possibly even prenatally. The infant can be soothed specifically by the voice of his or her mother (primary caregiver) as early as the first few weeks. The early phonetic characteristics of discomfort cries of the infant appear to be the vocal manifestations of the infant's total reaction to discomfort, determined in part by the physiologic contraction of the facial muscles. By about the sixth week, the infant begins to utter repetitive strings of sound called *babbling*. In doing so, satisfaction is found in producing at will those sounds that at first have occurred involuntarily; skill is acquired in making sounds; and the sounds of others are imitated as near as possible. The nearer the approximation of the infant's sounds to those of the parents, the more marked will be the parents' approval and the greater will be the infant's incentive to repeat sounds. In this way, the phonetic pattern of the child's mother tongue is acquired. What is important here is that in these earliest weeks the frequency and variety of sounds already may be restricted through inadequate fostering by the caring adult.

The capacity to discriminate between different sounds is present in the newborn (Friedlander 1970). Almost from the beginning the infant seems to be programmed to move in rhythm to the human voice (Condon and Sander 1974) and will orient with eyes, head, and body to animate sound stimuli (Mills and Melhuish 1974). Subsequent language development correlates most closely with motor development, although the two functions are not necessarily causally related in any specific way. Crying, which is present during fetal life, soon becomes differentiated during the first few months into recognized cries related to hunger, discomfort, pain, pleasure, and other stimuli (Wolff 1969). As crying decreases, cooing increases; vowel sounds (e.g., "oo") begin to dominate. Consonants begin to appear at about 5 months of age and words at about 1 year of age, with a range of 8–18 months (Morley 1965). At the same time, by 1 year of age the infant discriminates between and responds to differences in language, depending on who is speaking and how that person is speaking (e.g., the intonation and the amount of repetition used). Vocabulary gradually increases to about 200 words by age 2. Nouns appear first, then verbs, adjectives, and adverbs. Pronouns appear by about age 2, and conjunctions after age 2½. By this time, too, the child's understanding of language has increased immensely. Play at this stage in effect represents the child's "inner language." Between ages 2 and 4, the child has acquired, or learned, most of the fundamental (as opposed to the academic) rules of grammar, although how this is done is not known.

Linguistic shifts occur continuously. For example, at about age 6 or 7, children shift from making syntagmatic responses to making paradigmatic responses (Francis 1972). Syntagmatic associations are response items that are in a grammatical class different from that of the stimulus; the words just "go together" (e.g., hot–bath, or apple–eat). Paradigmatic associations are response items that belong to the same grammatical class as the stimulus (e.g., hot–cold, or apple–pear). Also, prior to age 6 or 7, children link temporal succession to succession of enunciation. For example, a young child will interpret the sentence "The girl goes upstairs when the boy has parked the car" to mean that the girl goes upstairs first and the boy parks the car afterward (Ferreiro 1971). After age 6 or 7, the child is no longer tied to this concrete perception of sequence. Furthermore, sometime between ages 5 and 10, children become more conscious of the structure of the language they use (Nelson 1977).

Finally, the child is able to speak and understand language independently of the context in which it occurs. At about age 12, when the child is in the stage of logical operations, language becomes a means of knowing.

The theory of language development is in a state of flux. The child apparently has a built-in capacity to abstract various universal relationships and regularities in the particular language heard and uses this capacity to construct an operation by means of which the principles for the formulation of an infinite number of sentences can be applied. Such an operation for language is obviously far more economical and powerful than anything the child might accrue or learn from simple imitation. Moreover, the capacity for this operational work seems not only to be related to the child's general cognitive capacities but also to be an integral part of the child's uniquely human condition.

As the child develops and moves from stage to stage, the capacity develops to react to increasingly complex stimuli, starting with intonation and moving through articulation of specific sounds to special syntactical and semantic stimuli. In this way, the child learns a linguistic code. All children appear to follow the same sequence in the development of phonology, syntax, and semantics. Chomsky's (1957) theory of generative transformational grammar suggests that in some way, perhaps through "innate intellectual structures," the child develops a basic grammar that can generate an infinite number of sentences and an optional transformational grammar that transforms the basis of a sentence into its various forms (e.g., passive and interrogative).

Alternatively, these inner structures may derive from the sensorimotor schemas (Piaget 1954). Indeed, the formation of such schemas during the long sensorimotor stage may be essential for the subsequent emergence of language and linguistic competence. Language in this view is one expression of what Piaget called the *semiotic function* (Inhelder 1971). Early schemas of experience precede symbolic language, and language comprehension precedes language production; children understand words and sentences long before they can say them (Lovell and Dixon 1967).

There is no satisfactory psychoanalytic theory for language acquisition (Wolff 1967). The child begins to use language as a symbolic instrument, initially (and necessarily) through the help of the mothering person, who will be referred to throughout this chapter as the "mother." For example, the mother uses a word (e.g., "Dada" or "Mama," then "Daddy" or "Mommy") as a symbol, and in so doing she helps in the organization of the symbolizing process that is taking place within the infant. She does not create that process within the infant; she facilitates its development. Initially, of course, considerable overextension occurs; a child may call all men Daddy (or all four-legged animals doggie) until further accommodation of the concepts, or schemas, of Daddy (or doggie) occurs.

It is very likely that the mother's spoken words initially are experienced by the infant as tones and rhythms, rather than as words with meanings, and as such are part of the unprecedented kinesthetic, tactile, visual, auditory, olfactory, and gustatory bombardment that the infant tries to assimilate and organize into schemas. Eventually, the child's percept of, say, "mother" and the word "Mother," already linked, becomes better defined. In this sense, mothers are sensitive language teachers of their children (Moerk 1974). The sensitive timing, repetition, and associated pleasurable affects with which the mother uses words for labeling, shaping, and so on, serve to stimulate the development of language. (Curiously, mothers seem to talk more to their baby girls than to their baby boys [Halverson and Waldrop 1970].)

Reinforcement may be more important for phonetic and semantic development than for syntactic development (Brown and Hanlon 1970). The best stimulus for syntactic development appears to be a rich conversational interchange without any attempt to modify the child's utterances (Cazden 1966).

Children continue to learn phonology, syntax, and semantics throughout the school years. The utterances of young children appear to depend on the support of the nonlinguistic environment. For example, if one asks a young child a question "out of the blue," one often draws a blank (Bloom 1975). Young children tend to respond more readily when they are asked to talk about events that are in a more immediately perceived context (Brown and Bellugi 1964).

Cognitive Development

The beginning of thinking is in the body. The infant reacts to a sensory stimulus with a motor reaction: place a finger in the infant's hand, and the infant grasps; a nipple in the mouth will initiate sucking; looking is the response to a pattern placed in front of the eyes. This sensorimotor pattern is the earliest kind of thinking, and it starts with such innate patterns of behavior as grasping, sucking, looking, and gross body activity.

The basic element in Piaget's theory of the child's cognitive development is the *schema*, which consists of a pattern of behavior in response to a particular stimulus from the environment. However, the schema is more than just a response, because the child also acts on the environment. For example, the infant sucks in response to a nipple. The schema of sucking then becomes increasingly complex as the child reacts to and acts on a wider range of environmental stimuli. Thus when the thumb is put into the mouth, the schema of sucking evoked by a nipple is gradually broadened to include this new and similar but not identical stimulus, the thumb. The new object (the thumb) is said to be assimilated into the original schema. At the same time, sucking behavior has to be slightly

modified because the thumb is different in shape, taste, and other characteristics from the nipple. This act of modification, which Piaget called *accommodation*, results in a new equilibrium. These two processes, assimilation and accommodation, proceed in ever-increasing complexities.

Four major stages of development are described in Piaget's theory: 1) a sensorimotor stage (0–18 months); 2) a preoperational stage (18 months–7 years); 3) a stage of concrete operations (7–11 years); and 4) a stage of formal operations (11–15 years).

In the sensorimotor stage (0 to 18 months of age), there are six substages:

1. In the first month, the infant exercises a function, such as looking or grasping, simply because it exists.
2. During the next 3 to 4 months (from 1 to 4½ months of age), new schemas are acquired. They are usually centered on the infant's own body (e.g., his or her thumb), constituting primary circular reactions.
3. Sometime between 4½ months to 8 or 9 months of age, the infant tries to produce an effect upon the object he or she sees or grasps. That is, he or she now involves events or objects in the external environment (e.g., a rattle), constituting secondary circular reactions.
4. By 8 or 9 months to 11 or 11½ months of age, the infant begins to be aware of the existence of unperceived objects hidden, say, behind a pillow or in peek-a-boo games. This is also the time of so-called stranger anxiety. The mental image of the object has now achieved some degree of permanence in the infant's mind (i.e., object permanence).
5. In the first half of the second year (11 or 12 months to 18 months of age), the child explores more thoroughly an object and its spatial relationship, for example, by putting smaller objects into and taking them out of larger ones.
   a. The child initiates changes that produce variations in the event itself, for example, dropping bread and then toys from different heights or different positions.
   b. The child actively searches for novel events (i.e., tertiary circular reactions).
6. By the end of the second year (18 months to 2 years of age), the child shows some evidence of reasoning; mental trial and error replaces

trial and error in action. For example, the child uses one toy as an instrument to get another.

The use of toys and play for a child is essentially a form of thinking. External objects (play items) are organized in such a way as to represent the child's internal symbolization of events and fantasies. Piaget called this evocation of past events and fantasies in the present play *deferred imitation*, a characteristic of symbolic thought.

The preoperational stage, occurring roughly between the ages of 2 and 7, clearly reflects progress over the preceding stage of sensorimotor intelligence. Two substages are described: the substage of *symbolic activity* and make-believe play and the substage of *decentration*.

The substage of symbolic activity and make-believe play occurs between 2 and 4 years of age. One can see in this substage the development of symbolic thought and of representation. Language becomes increasingly important as the child learns to distinguish between actual objects and the labels used to represent them. As a result, the child gradually becomes able to reason symbolically rather than motorically (as was the case in the preceding sensorimotor period when the infant was limited to the pursuit of concrete goals through action).

However, despite these significant advances, there are striking cognitive limitations to preoperational thinking that distinguish it from the logical thought processes that will emerge in those subsequent stages of concrete and, ultimately, formal operations. Principally, the child's judgments are dominated by the child's perceptions of events, objects, and experiences. Further, the child can attend to only one perceptual dimension or attribute at a time. The concept of time is also not available to a child at this stage. Sequences and daily routines can be recognized (e.g., mealtime, playtime, sleep time, day and night, and Daddy's or Mommy's going and coming), but the child has no concept of an hour, a minute, a week, or a month.

The preoperational child also is extremely egocentric. By that, Piaget did not mean that the child is selfish per se. Rather, Piaget employed the term *egocentric* to refer to a certain cognitive limitation of the preoperational stage, namely, that the young child is conceptually unable to view events and experiences from any point of view but his or her own. The child is clearly the center of his or her own representational world. Similarly, the child is unable to differentiate clearly between the self and

the world, between the subjective realm of thoughts and feelings and the objective realm of external reality.

In addition, at the preoperational stage, the child's reasoning is neither inductive nor deductive, but what Piaget called *transductive*. That is, the young child tends to relate the particular to the particular in an alogical manner. Events may be viewed as related not because of any inherent cause-and-effect relationship but simply on the basis of spatial or temporal contiguity or juxtaposition. Furthermore, the child at this stage is unaware of and therefore unconcerned about possible logical contradictions.

The substage of decentration occurs between 4 and 7 years of age. In this substage, an increased accommodation to reality gradually takes over with progressive decentering from the child's own interests, perception, and points of view. The decentering comes about partly because of the child's increased social involvement (e.g., at school). Social interaction virtually demands that the child use language, and the child discovers that what he or she thinks is not necessarily the same as what the child's peers think. The child begins to recognize other points of view.

The stage of concrete operations is usually seen from 7 to 11 years of age. The child at this stage is no longer bound by the configuration perceived at a given moment. Two variables can now be taken into account at once (e.g., height and width). Piaget (1952) performed what is now a classic experiment. One form of Piaget's experiment is as follows. A child is first asked to make sure that the amount of water in two identical beakers is the same:

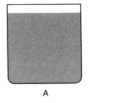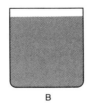

Water from one of the beakers is then transferred into a tall cylinder:

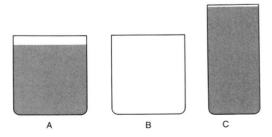

And the child is asked, "Is the amount of water in A the same as in C?"

A child who is in the preoperational stage will say "no," and then if asked why will say either that the water in the cylinder has more "because it's higher," or that the water in the beaker has more "because it's wider."

A child who is at the stage of concrete operations will be able to say, "Yes, the amount of water is the same," and if asked why will be able to say, "Because it's narrower (in the cylinder) and wider (in the beaker)."

The child has mastered what Piaget called the concept of *conservation*. The child acquires the concept of conservation not only for volume but also for number, class, length, weight, and area.

These types of conservation occur at different ages. The conservation of objects occurs quite early, usually by the end of the sensorimotor period. Quantity is conserved at age 6–8 years, and weight at 9–12 years. Probably the variation in age at which different conservations are achieved is related to how easily the property can be dissociated from the child's own action. As Piaget (1958) put it: "It is more difficult to . . . equalize . . . objects whose properties are less easy to dissociate from one's own action, such as weight, than to apply the same operation to properties which can be objectified more readily, such as length" (p. 249).

The age of 6 or 7 marks a key turning point in the child's thinking. After the age of 6 or 7, the child is no longer bound by his or her perception and can apply reasoning. It is the age at which the child starts first grade. It also corresponds in psychoanalytic theory to the time when the oedipal struggle is thought to be resolved and the superego consolidated. Feelings can be distanced, thought about, and put into context. The child also more readily can distinguish between fantasy and reality.

In short, the major advance in the concrete operations stage is that basic logical principles can be applied to the realm of concrete experiences and events without the child letting perceptions interfere. Gradually, logical thought processes become organized into an increasingly complex and integrated network through which the surrounding world is confronted and responded to systematically.

In the stage of formal operations, Piaget (1969) observed the following:

> The great novelty that characterizes adolescent thought and that starts around the age of 11 to 12, but probably does not reach its point of equilibrium until the age of 14 or 15, . . . consists in the possibility of manipulating ideas in themselves and no longer in merely manipulating objects. (p. 23)

The young adolescent can now use hypotheses, experiment, make deductions, and reason from the particular to the general. The adolescent is no longer tied to the environment. He or she in essence can now make theoretical statements independent of specific content and can apply this way of thinking to all kinds of data.

The result is a further release from the concrete world:

> The most distinctive property of formal thought is this reversal of direction between reality and possibility; instead of deriving a rudimentary type of theory from the empirical data, as is done in concrete inferences, formal thought begins with a theoretical synthesis implying that certain relations are necessary and this proceeds in the opposite direction. (Piaget 1958, p. 251)

Piaget provided a set of cognitive developmental norms that are useful to the clinician. For example, preschool children are often preoccupied with such super powerful and giant figures as dinosaurs and doll-figure heroes and heroines that represent the perceived powerful and idealized human figures in the child's life. This symbolic representation is evident in the symbolic play of young children. The clinician can use this information as a means of understanding the concerns, conflicts, wishes, and anxieties of a child, and may choose at a particular moment in psychotherapy to interpret to the child the meaning of play as gathered from the child's associations (e.g., verbalizations, activities) to this symbolic play. At the same time, Piaget's system offers an explanation of the preoperational child's difficulties in resolving emotional as well as intellectual problems. For such a child, fantasy and reality may be poorly differentiated, and affects may be more difficult to conceptualize (conserve).

The school-age child in the stage of concrete operations is trying to construct an orderly and lawful world and is becoming socialized. These processes can be seen in the child's use of rules in such games as checkers and Monopoly™, and in the child's acceptance of such symbols as paper money and the hierarchical implications in, for example, the game of checkers ("king").

Piaget's system is particularly helpful in school consultation for the child in the stage of concrete operations.

Moral Development

Moral behavior derives in part from the basic cultural rules governing social action that the child assimilates and internalizes. Moral development is the increase in the degree to which the internalization and accommodation of these basic cultural rules have occurred.

Fear of punishment is prominent in young children. Next to develop is an urge to confess. By age 12 or 13, most children seem to react directly to guilt and internal self-criticism when faced with the fact of their transgression, although this reaction often occurs at a much earlier age.

Piaget's view on the moral development of the child can be conceptualized in the context of the three major stages of cognitive development: 1) preoperational stage, 2) stage of concrete operations, and 3) stage of formal operations. In the preoperational stage—the morality of constraints—rules of behavior are viewed as natural laws handed down by the child's parents. Violation brings retribution or unquestioned punishment, and no account is taken of motives. In the stage of concrete operations, rules of behavior become a matter of mutual acceptance, with complete equality of treatment, but no account is taken of special circumstances. In the stage of formal operations—the morality of cooperation—rules can be constructed as required by the needs of the group so long as they can be agreed on. Motives are now taken into account, and circumstances may temper the administration of justice. As the child advances through these stages, progressive decentering occurs.

Building on Piaget's views, Kohlberg (1964) suggested three major levels of development of moral judgment (Table 4-1): 1) premorality (or preconventional morality), 2) morality of conventional role-conformity, and 3) morality of self-accepted moral principles.

Interestingly, Jurkovic (1980) noted that delinquents differ in their level of moral development just as they do in their personality and behavioral style: "Not only do they vary from one another in stages of moral development, but they also fluctuate in their own reasoning level on different moral problems" (p. 724).

Numerous criticisms have been made of Kohlberg's work. Certain of the stages, especially the later stages, have not been reliably replicated, and many believe that the descriptions of some of these stages are too politicized in favor of a liberal view-

Table 4-1. Kohlberg's three major levels of development of moral judgment

Level I: Premorality (or preconventional morality)
   a. Type 1. Punishment and obedience orientation (i.e., obedience to parents' superior force)
   b. Type 2. Naive instrumental hedonism (i.e., agreement to obey only in return for some reward)

Level II: Morality of conventional role-conformity
   a. Type 3. Good-boy morality of maintaining good relations, approval of others (i.e., conformity to rules in order to please and gain approval)
   b. Type 4. Authority-maintaining morality (i.e., adherence to rules for the sake of upholding social order)

Level III: Morality of self-accepted moral principles
   a. Type 5. Morality of social contract, of individual rights, and of, for example, democratically accepted law (with a reliance on a legalistic "social contract")
   b. Type 6. Morality of individual principles of conscience (There is voluntary compliance based on ethical principles; this level is probably not reached until early adolescence, and it may not be reached at all.)

point. Others think that the stages described are, in any event, bound by culture, the historical moment, middle-class status, and the male sex of the subjects. As a result of these criticisms, Kohlberg attempted some revisions. For example, Kohlberg (1978) and Colby (1978) subsequently identified two types of reasoning at each stage: type A emphasizes literal interpretation of the rules and roles of society, whereas type B is a more consolidated form and refers to the intent of normative standards. However, in general, Kohlberg essentially held to the same hierarchical sequence and idealized end point.

Gilligan (1982) offered a different view of moral development in which an expanding connection with and concern for others were thought to represent an alternative developmental pathway and goal. This alternative and equally valid pathway has been demonstrated more often in girls than in boys; that is, in general, girls seem to have "a greater sense of connection and concern with relationships more than with rules" (p. 202).

Attachment Behavior

Attachment is an affectional tie that one person forms to another person, binding them together in space and enduring over time. Attachment is discriminating and specific. One may be attached to more than one person, but there is usually a gradient in the strength of such multiple attachments (Schaffer and Emerson 1964). Attachment implies affect, predominantly affection or love.

Bonding implies a selective attachment (Cohen 1974) that is maintained even when there is no contact with the person with whom the bond exists.

Attachment behavior is behavior that promotes proximity to or contact with the specific figure or figures to whom the person is attached. Attachment behavior includes signals (crying, smiling, vocalizing), locomotions (looking, following, approaching), and contacts (clambering up, embracing, clinging). Sucking, clinging, following, crying, and smiling become incorporated by 8 or 9 months. Attachment behavior is strongest in toddlers; bonding is most secure in older children (Rutter 1976b).

Bowlby (1969) proposed that the biological function of the attachment behavior is to protect the infant from danger, especially the danger of attack by predators. The system may be activated by the hormonal state, environmental stimulus situation, and CNS excitation. The system is terminated in response to a specific terminating signal (e.g., attachment achieved) or by habituation. The attachment behavior system is in equilibrium with other important behavior systems—for example, exploratory behavior, which is elicited by stimuli that have novelty and complexity or change (and may draw the infant away from the mother).

At least 15 kinds of attachment behavior have been described (Ainsworth 1963), including differential crying, smiling, and vocalization; greeting responses, such as lifting of arms and hand clapping; crying when the mother leaves, scrambling over the mother, following the mother, clinging and kissing; and exploration away from the mother when the mother is a secure base, with rapid return to the mother as a haven of safety.

These attachment behaviors may vary in intensity. In certain pathologic states, such as infantile autism, they may all be absent.

Summary of Phases in the Development of Attachment

First phase: undiscriminating social responsiveness (0–3 months). From the beginning, the infant has some capacity to respond differentially to different stimuli and thus to discriminate them (see Table 4-2). Further, the range of stimuli to which

Table 4-2. First phase in the development of attachment

Primitive behaviors	Orienting behaviors	Signaling behaviors
Sucking Grasping	Visual fixation Visual tracking Listening Rooting Postural adjustment	Smiling Crying Vocalization

the infant is most responsive includes the range commonly emanating from human adults, including visual stimuli, auditory stimuli, and stimuli associated with feeding. Yet the infant does not initially discriminate among the persons presenting these stimuli.

When the infant does begin to discriminate between persons, this is done more readily through some modalities than others—for example, tactile-kinesthetic discrimination first, then auditory discrimination, and then visual discrimination at approximately 8 weeks.

Second phase: discriminating social responsiveness (3–7 months). The infant discriminates between familiar figures (mother and one or two others) and those who are relatively unfamiliar.

In the first subphase, there is discrimination and differential responses to figures close at hand (e.g., differential smiling, vocalization, and crying). In the second subphase, there is discrimination between figures at a distance (e.g., as evidenced by differential greeting and crying when a particular figure leaves the room).

Third phase: active initiative in seeking proximity and contact (7 months–3 years). At about 7 months, a striking increase occurs in the infant's initiative in promoting proximity and contact. Voluntary movements of the infant's hands and arms are now conspicuous in attachment behavior. Following, approaching, clinging, and similar behaviors become more significant. The infant is now attached.

In psychoanalytic theory, the infant at this stage is said to have an anaclitic (leaning on) type of object relation. In cognitive-developmental theory, the infant at this stage is said to be at the fourth subphase of sensorimotor development and to have acquired object permanence.

It is interesting to note here that Spitz (1965) talked of "organizers" as a concept to account for the factors that govern the process of transition from one level of development to the next: 1) the smiling response is the visible manifestation of a certain degree of organization in the psychic apparatus; 2) the second organizer is the 8-month anxiety, which marks a new stage in development; and 3) the third organizer is the achievement of the sign of negation and of the word no. In Spitz's view, this sign is the first abstraction, or symbol, formed by the child, usually at the beginning of the second year (around 15 months), when the infant turns his or her head away to refuse food (a response that has its origins in the rooting reflex).

Fourth phase: goal-directed partnership (3 years). The infant in the fourth phase infers something about the mother's "set goals" and attempts to alter her set goals to fit better with his or her goals in regard to contact, proximity, and interaction, provided the mother does not dissemble about what her set goals are (e.g., to leave the infant at nursery school).

Necessary Conditions for the Development of Attachment

The following conditions are prerequisites for the development of attachment: 1) "sufficient" interaction with the mother; 2) the ability of the infant to discriminate his or her mother or other attachment figure from other persons; and 3) the ability of the infant to have at least begun to conceive of a person as having a permanent and independent existence even when that person is not present to the infant's perception.

An infant's goal-corrected behavior probably becomes increasingly smooth and effective in parallel with the later stages of development of the concept of the object, which, according to Piaget, is completed at about 18 months. Piaget suggested that the concept of persons as permanent objects evolves in homologous stages but in advance of the development of things as permanent objects, presumably because an infant finds people the most interesting of objects.

Factors That Influence the Development of Attachment

Four factors influence the development of attachment. The first factor concerns sensitive phases in the development of infant-mother attachment. The sensitive phase during which attachments are most readily formed spans a period of months in the middle of the first year. It probably starts in the neonatal period. Provence and Lipton (1962) showed that infants kept in an institution until they are 8–24 months old find it difficult to become attached to a foster mother later, and that 24 months seems to be the upper limit of the sensitive phase for becoming attached for the first time. The second factor concerns infant-care practices, such as feeding practices. The third factor concerns maternal care, infant behavior, and the mother-infant interaction. The mother's contribution to attachment is affected by such factors as her hormonal state, her parity and experience, and her personality. The infant's contribution is affected by such factors as wakefulness and activity level, crying, temperament, genetic makeup, and organic makeup. The final factor influencing the development of attachment concerns maternal deprivation.

Strong attachments occur under the following five conditions:

1. When the interaction has a certain degree of intensity, as when a sensitive, responsive parent gives a great deal of attention to the child, talks with the child, and, especially, plays with the child (Stayton and Ainsworth 1973).
2. When the parent responds regularly and readily to the child's needs as signalled, say, by crying. The child is likely to become strongly attached to a parent who can recognize and respond to the child's signals.
3. When the number of caregivers is limited. The fewer the caregivers, the greater the attachment.
4. When the child's own contribution is strong—that is, when the child's needs and signals are strong.
5. When the child is in the early sensitive phase (of imprinting) (i.e., during first 2 years).

Lastly, several clinical types of attachment have been described, including secure, insecure-avoidant, insecure-resistant, and insecure-disorganized/disoriented (Main and Solomon 1986).

Clinically, attachment theory is useful as a basis for providing appropriate care of premature infants and very young children in a hospital, in deciding on adoption practices and child placement, and as a contribution toward understanding certain aspects of child abuse and delinquency.

Psychosexual Development

In psychoanalytic theory, the sexual aim of a young infant is said to be to obtain pleasure and relief from discomfort by the most immediate means possible. The infant draws pleasure from a wide variety of visual, tactile, kinesthetic, and auditory stimuli.

Oral Phase

By far the most sensitive and apparently the greatest source of pleasure appears to be in the region of the mouth. The object of the sexual instinct is apparently the body of the infant, seen in such "autoerotic" (self-stimulating) activities as mouthing and sucking. Questions have been raised about some of the viewpoints subsumed under the heading of orality (Sandler and Dare 1970). Moreover, Freud noted the following:

> The phylogenetic foundation has so much the upper hand over personal accidental experience that it makes no difference whether a child is really sucked at the breast or has been brought up on the bottle and never enjoyed the tenderness of a mother's care. In both cases the child's development takes the same path. (Freud 1940/1969, pp. 188–189)

Lastly, it is important to note that certain genetic factors and biological-orienting patterns are in operation prior to any psychological mechanisms. For example, the suck reflex is coordinated to the cyclic flow of breast milk (Dubignon and Campbell 1969), and by 6 days of age the infant can selectively orient himself or herself to smell, preferring mother's milk (MacFarlane 1975).

Anal Phase

As the infant develops and as speech and the capacity for symbol formation emerge, the child then begins to experience feelings about separateness and worth. A sense of autonomy develops, which has to be reconciled with ambivalent feelings; this process occurs at about the same time that new skills are acquired, only one of which is sphincter control.

During this process, acording to psychoanalytic theory, the anal mucosa is said to become "erotogenized" and may serve in part the aims of the ambivalent feelings just mentioned. Indeed, the young child may express his or her ambivalence in the (pleasurable) holding in and letting go of feses during bowel movements. However, this ambivalence may also be expressed in the controlling and clinging behavior seen in some 2- and 3-year-old children, suggesting that the alleged central role of the anal mucosa at this stage has probably been exaggerated, reflecting perhaps the pratices that prevailed at the time Freud made his observations.

Phallic-Oedipal Phase

When the child is between 3 and 6 years of age, behavior that is more clearly recognizable as "sexual" appears. The child at this stage is very much aware of the anatomical differences between the sexes and is curious about pregnancy, childbirth, and death. Sometimes this interest is represented in the play of the child. For example, play with toys that involve filling and emptying, opening and shutting, fitting in and throwing away, and the building up and knocking down of blocks, has been interpreted as representing a curiosity about the body and sexual functions.

Opportunities for the sequential development of play in childhood thus become as important for the sexual development of the child as they are for other purposes (e.g., problem solving, mastery of body skills, functional pleasure in play, coping with anxiety, facilitating relationships, and communication purposes). The child at this stage is said to experience intense sexual and aggressive urges toward both parents, but the aim is less well defined. Boys and girls may become absorbed by fairy-tale or television characters that serve to represent children's own fantasies. Such fantasies also emerge in the dreams of children.

Children of this age may also play at being mothers and fathers or doctors and nurses—working toward a partial fulfillment of their sexual aims, which at this time may be partially fused with their aggressive fantasies. Boys and girls may inflict pain on each other in keeping with their understanding of the sexual act as an act of violence. They may also be quite exhibitionistic and possessive, especially of the parent of the opposite sex. Hostility to the same-sex parent seems to be influenced by certain characteristic family patterns of relationships present in a particular society (Honigmann 1954).

Latency Phase

Between 6 and 12 years of age, during the elementary-school years, concepts of inevitability regarding birth, death, and sex differences become clarified, and the sense of time and the ability to differentiate between fantasy and reality become established. Defense mechanisms, which in general bar from consciousness certain unacceptable impulses and fantasies and at the same time provide some substitute gratification, are strengthened. The child consolidates earlier reactions, such as shame against exhibitionistic urges, disgust against messiness, and a sense of guilt that contains sexual and aggressive wishes. The child's play at this time is usually characterized by organization, whether in a board game or team game. Sex play, far from being dormant, continues actively, especially with voyeuristic tendencies and the urge to touch. The sex play often may be more discreet at this age (i.e., adults may see it less often), yet it may also be quite overt, with much interest and curiosity (Reese 1966). The object of the sexual instinct may be a peer, but the actual playmate may be of either sex.

Adolescence

When puberty comes, the young adolescent struggles to achieve body mastery, to control sexual and aggressive urges, to separtate from the family, to find new and appealing sexual relationships, and to achieve a sense of identity. In the course of this stuggle, the sexual behavior of the adolescent may range from an indiscriminate regression (toward expressions of earlier forms of the sexual drive, manifested in impulsive behavior, messiness, and alternating labile affects), to petting and mutual masturbation (which may be heterosexual or homosexual), and eventually to intercourse. Sometimes earlier aims and objects are temporarily gratified and used (e.g., in isolated acts of fellatio or in exhibitionistic behavior).

Ultimately, a mature primacy of the genital zone is established, with an appropriate object choice and an appropriate achievement of such new sexual aims as a love relationship, sexual intercourse, orgasm, discharge, and childbirth.

Rutter (1971, 1976a) reviewed the scientific literature on normal psychosexual development and concluded that Freud's description of the oral and anal stages is too narrow and somewhat misleading, that the oedipal situation is not universal, that Frued's description of the latency period is wrong in most respects, and that Freud's concept of an innate sex drive that has a quantifiable energy component is only a half-truth. Rutter noted that at present there is insufficient evidence to decide among the various psychological theories of sexual development.

Although it is true that the level of scientific reliability and validity in psychoanalytic research is generally low, clinical experience still has a very compelling, supporting quality. Interestingly, Freud too noted that the "artificial structure of hypothesis" that psychoanalysts use in their metapsychology may be "blown away" by the answers provided by biology (Freud 1920/1955, p. 60).

Relationships

In psychoanalytic theory, relationships are said to start with the virtual biological unity of the mother-infant couple. This period has been subdivided by some psychoanalysts (Mahler et al. 1975) into so-called autistic, symbiotic, and separation-individuation phases.

A prototypical early stage is said to be a part-object or need-fulfilling, anaclitic type of relationship based on the child's needs. This type of relationship generally ends when object constancy is achieved. Ambivalent relationships then develop, characterized by clinging behavior and attempts to dominate the love object.

A phallic-oedipal phase is said to follow, characterized by possessiveness of the parent of the opposite sex and jealousy of and rivalry with the parent of the same sex. In the postoedipal period, a lessening of drive urgency is said to occur, and a transference takes place from parents to other adults (e.g., teachers). Sublimation is seen. Disillusionment with the parents is another observable phenomenon.

In preadolescence, a return to early attitudes and behaviors, especially part-object, need-fulfilling, and ambivalent kinds, occurs.

Finally, in adolescence, a true interest is invested in persons outside the family.

Temperament

In the course of their clinical observations and research, Thomas and Chess (1977), in their New York Longitudinal Study, became fascinated with what they perceived as the individual styles that characterized each child—or rather, the peculiar shaping and reshaping of these styles as the child and his or her family developed. This phenomenon came to be known as the *temperament* of the child. Categories of behavior that are studied in the assessment of the temperament of an individual include 1) activity level, 2) rhythmicity (hunger, elimination, sleep-wake), 3) approach or withdrawal response, 4) adaptability to a change in the environment, 5) threshold of responsiveness, 6) intensity of any given reaction, 7) mood (quality, quantity), 8) degree of distractibility, and 9) persistence in the face of obstacles.

About 1 child in 10 was found to have a so-called "difficult" temperament, and about 1 in 6 was in a "slow-to-warm-up" group. About two-fifths of the children studied were found to have an "easy" temperament.

The New York Longitudinal Study showed, among other things, that the consistency of the interactional process between temperament and environment constituted a kind of continuity. This kind of continuity provided for a great deal of plasticity in development. Although this plasticity might make prediction uncertain, it also suggested that early parental errors and even specific emotional trauma to the child did not necessarily have fixed, inevitable consequences, and that therapeutic intervention could help at any stage of development. Indeed, it suggested that subsequent improved and positive experiences in themselves might have a therapeutic effect.

These ideas challenged some previously held views on the causes of various developmental and clinical phenomena. In particular, Thomas, Chess, and Birch (1968) added the important idea that the child, far from being a passive recipient or simply a responder to varous stimuli, was an active initiator and contributor to his or her own experience and development. They found too that this activity on the part of the child was determined to an extent by the child's temperament, and that the child's particular developmental characteristics contributed in important ways to some of the behavior disorders we see in children.

What was also new here was the notion of genotypical variations in style originating in the genotype of an individual and brought out and modified by the individual child's active interaction with the environment. In other words, here, as in breeds found in some other species, one could see a variety of strains among human beings (such as fearful, shy, and timid; or bold, outgoing, and aggressive), with each strain modified and capable of being shaped by experience, teaching, and learning.

A practical and central concept that Chess and Thomas (1977) devised to study and understand the child's struggle for mastery was the "goodness of fit" in the complex interactions over time between the child's temperament and the environment.

Temperament is not a theory of development; rather it is but one attribute of an individual—albeit an important one. Clinically, the concepts and findings of temperament studies are very useful in understanding and relieving certain parent-child problems.

Developmental Tasks

Finally, we may think about development in terms of its meaning for the individual from infancy through adolescence. Thus the developmental task of the very young infant is to achieve adaptation to the outside world. Sometime between 1½ and 3 years of age it becomes clear that a child is tackling several other developmental tasks. First, a fundamental task is to achieve greater physical independence. The maturation of the child's neuromuscular system is central to feelings of self-worth. The child makes a shift from a passive to an active position. Furthermore, the child now can think instead of act, using language with symbols and concepts. While the young child uses few words, mostly in the service of direct discharge of feelings (*primary process*), the child later uses language more independently of immediate need. Along with this development, definite attitudes toward people are formed, especially toward those who set limits. It is toward such persons that the child may behave in a negativistic manner. Thus the child may say, "I don't want to" and "No!" when a parent makes a request or sets a limit. It is as though the child is defining autonomy through oppositional behavior. However, in some instances, the behavior may be a manifestation of anxiety as the child struggles against a regressive pull. In other instances, the behavior may be a direct discharge of aggression against the parent, especially if the parent-child relationship is an ambivalent one.

Perhaps the crux of the school-age period of development is the child's move toward greater separation, independence, and autonomy at a time when he or she is still capable of being demanding, intrusive, and negativistic. The extent to which the child successfully emerges from this stage depends on many factors, including the degree to which the parents facilitate or hinder the child's progress.

Finally, at adolescence, at least four major groups of developmental tasks can be defined: 1) defining one's own self, 2) achieving separation and coming to terms with specific feelings about one's family, 3) developing love relationships, and 4) achieving mastery over one's impulses and body functions and capacities.

References

Ainsworth MDS: The development of infant-mother interaction among the Ganda, in Determinants of Infant Behavior, Vol 2. Edited by Foss BM. London, Methuen, 1963, pp 67–112

Bloom L: Language development review, in Review of Child Development Research, Vol 4. Edited by Horowitz FR. Chicago, IL, University of Chicago Press, 1975, pp 245–303

Bowlby J: Attachment and Loss, Vol 1: Attachment. New York, Basic Books, 1969

Brown R, Bellugi N: Three processes in the child's acquisition of syntax. Harvard Educational Review 34:133–151, 1964

Brown R, Hanlon C: Derivational complexity and order of acquisitions of speech, in Cognition and the Development of Language. Edited by Hayes JR. New York, John Wiley, 1970

Cazden C: Subcultural differences in child language: an interdisciplinary review. Merrill-Palmer Quarterly 12:185–219, 1966

Chomsky N: Syntactic Structures. The Hague, Mouton, 1957

Cohen LJ: The operational definition of human attachment. Psychol Bull 81:107–217, 1974

Colby A: Evolution of a moral-developmental theory, in Moral Development (New Directions for Child Development No 2). Edited by Damon W. San Francisco, CA, Jossey-Bass, 1978

Condon WS, Sander LW: Neonate movement is synchronized with adult speech: interactional participation and language acquisition. Science 183:99–101, 1974

Dubignon J, Campbell D: Sucking in the newborn during a feed. J Exp Child Psychol 7:282–298, 1969

Ferreiro E: Les relations temporelles dans la langue de l'enfant. Geneva, Droz, 1971

Francis H: Toward an explanation of paradigmatic-syntagmatic shift. Child Dev 43:949–959, 1972

Freud S: Beyond the pleasure principle (1920), in the Standard Edition of the Complete Psychological Works of Sigmund Freud, Vol 18. Translated and edited by Strachey J. London, Hogarth Press, 1955, p 60

Freud S: An outline of psycho-analysis (1940), in the Standard Edition of the Complete Psychological Works of Sigmund Freud, Vol 23. Translated and edited by Strachey J. London, Hogarth Press, 1969, pp 188–189

Friedlander BZ: Receptive language development in infancy: issues and problems. Merrill-Palmer Quarterly 16:7, 1970

Gesell AO, Amatruda CS: Developmental Diagnosis (1941), 11th Edition. New York, Paul Hoeber Medical Division, Harper & Row, 1964, pp 8–14

Gilligan C: In a Different Voice: Psychological Theory and Women's Development. Cambridge, MA, Harvard University Press, 1982

Halverson CF, Waldrop MF: Maternal behavior towards own and other preschool children: the problems of "ownness." Child Dev 41:839, 1970

Honigmann JJ: Culture as Personality. New York, Harper, 1954

Inhelder B: The sensory-motor origins of knowledge, in Early Childhood: The Development of Self-Regulatory Mechanisms. Edited by Walcher DN, Peters DL. New York, Academic, 1971, pp 141–155

Jurkovic GJ: The juvenile delinquent as a moral philosopher: a structural-developmental perspective. Psychol Bull 88:709–727, 1980

Kohlberg L: Development of moral character, in Review of Child Development Research, Vol 1. Edited by Hoffman ML, Hoffman LW. New York, Russell Sage Foundation, 1964, pp 400–404

Kohlberg L: Revisions in the theory and practice of moral development, in Moral Development (New Directions for Child Development No 2). Edited by Damon W. San Francisco, CA, Jossey-Bass, 1978, pp 83–87

Leong C: Lateralization in severely disabled readers in relation to functional cerebral development and synthesis of information, in The Neuropsychology of Learning Disorders. Edited by Knights RM, Baker DJ. Baltimore, MD, University Park Press, 1976, pp 221–231

Lewis M: Language, Thought and Personality in Infancy and Childhood. New York, Basic Books, 1963

Lovell K, Dixon EM: The growth of the control of grammar in imitation, comprehension and production. Journal of Child Psychology 8:31, 1967

MacFarlane JA: Olfaction in the development of social preference in the human neonate, in Parent-Infant Interaction (CIBA Foundation Symposium Ser No 33). Amsterdam, CIBA Foundation, 1975

Mahler MS, Pine F, Bergman A: The Psychological Birth of the Human Infant: Symbiosis and Individuation. New York, Basic Books, 1975

Main M, Solomon J: Discovery of an insecure, disorganized/disoriented attachment pattern: procedures, findings and implications for the classification of behavior, in Affective Development in Infancy. Edited by Yogman M, Brazleton TB. Norwood, NJ, Ablex Publishing, 1986

Mills M, Melhuish E: Recognition of mother's voice in early infancy. Nature 252:123–124, 1974

Moerk E: Changes in verbal child-mother interactions with increasing language skills of the child. J Psycholinguist Res 3:101–116, 1974

Morley ME: The Development and Disorders of Speech in Childhood, 2nd Edition. Edinburgh, E & S Livingston, 1965

Nelson KE: Aspects of language acquisition and use from 2 to age 20. Journal of the American Academy of Child Psychiatry 16:584–607, 1977

Piaget J (with Szeminska A): The Child's Conception of Number. Translated by Gattegno C, Hodgson FM. London, Routledge & Kegan Paul, 1952

Piaget J: Language and thought from a genetic point of view. Acta Psychol (Amst) 10:88–98, 1954

Piaget J: The Growth of Logical Thinking. New York, Basic Books, 1958

Piaget J: The intellectual development of the adolescent, in Adolescence: Psychosocial Perspectives. Edited by Caplan G, Lebovici S. New York, Basic Books, 1969, pp 22–26

Provence S, Lipton RC: Infants and Institutions. New York, International Universities Press, 1962

Reese HW: Attitudes toward the opposite sex in late childhood. Merrill-Palmer Quarterly 12:157–163, 1966

Rutter M: Normal psychosexual development. J Child Psychol Psychiatry 11:259–283, 1971

Rutter M: Other family influences, in Child Psychiatry. Edited by Rutter M, Hersov L. Oxford, UK, Blackwell, 1976a, pp 74–108

Rutter M: Separation, loss and family relationships, in Child Psychiatry. Edited by Rutter M, Hersov L. Oxford, UK, Blackwell, 1976b, pp 47–73

Sandler J, Dare C: The psychoanalytic concept of orality. J Psychosom Res 14:211–222, 1970

Schaffer HR, Emerson PE: Patterns of response to physical contact in early human development. J Child Psychol Psychiatry 5:1–13, 1964

Spitz R: The First Year of Life. New York, International Universities Press, 1965

Stayton DJ, Ainsworth MD: Individual differences in infant responses to brief, everyday separations as related to other infant and maternal behaviors. Developmental Psychology 9:226–235, 1973

Thomas A, Chess S: Temperament and Development. New York, Brunner/Mazel, 1977

Thomas A, Chess S, Birch H: Temperament and Behavior Disorders in Children. New York, New York University Press, 1968

Touwen BCL: Laterality, in Scientific Foundations of Developmental Psychiatry. Edited by Rutter M. London, Heinemann, 1980, pp 154–164

Wolff P: Cognitive consideration for a psychoanalytic theory of language acquisition, in Motives and Thought: Psychoanalytic Essays in Honor of David Rappaport. Edited by Holt R. New York, International Universities Press, 1967, pp 300–343

Wolff P: The natural history of crying and other vocalizations of early infancy, in Determinants of Infant Behavior. Edited by Foss BN. London, Methuen, 1969, p 81

Chapter 5

Concepts of Diagnostic Classification

David Shaffer, M.B., B.S., F.R.C.P., F.R.C.Psych.
Barbara Bettes, Ph.D.

odern psychiatric classification systems such as DSM-III-R (American Psychiatric Association 1987) and the 10th version of the International Classification of Diseases (ICD-10) (World Health Organization 1988) classify psychiatrically disturbed children in terms of their emotional symptoms and behaviors. This method makes no reference to underlying dynamics and implicitly rejects the proposition that symptoms are "surface" phenomena related nonspecifically to different subconscious mechanisms. With the exception of the highly qualified adjustment disorder diagnoses, DSM-III-R and ICD-10 pay little heed to environmental context. However, most sensible clinicians believe that a patient's environment and personal dynamics are important to understand in order to establish a clinical relationship and to draw up and implement a treatment plan. It is therefore reasonable to ask whether the behavioral descriptive approach is sufficient and whether it well serves clinicians and researchers.

In addressing these questions, there are three important considerations. First, when evaluating a patient and planning treatment, clinicians focus on the patient as an individual without reference to others. In the best clinical accounts, clinical features—which may include symptoms, family and social circumstances, and past history—are described with plentiful anecdote and example. This

also is the approach used in many single-case reports in the literature. However, to communicate in a way that allows one patient to be compared with another, this information has to be described within well-defined parameters. The parameters need not be confined to behavior; they may describe previous experience or even dynamics. No matter which parameter is chosen, however, individuals are described in terms of what they hold in common with others. Second, the major task of a classification system is to facilitate communication. To do this, it must be reliable. Different users evaluating similar patients should come to the same diagnostic conclusions. Reliability is likely to be greater if the classification system is based on clearly defined, observable or reportable phenomena (e.g., signs and symptoms) than if the system is based on features that require interpretation or inference (e.g., subconscious or cognitive processes). Third, for a behavioral descriptive classification system to be useful, as well as reliable, its categories must do more than describe the patient's current mental and behavioral state. Knowledge of the diagnosis should allow the professional to draw inferences about 1) likely etiology, 2) other clinical conditions commonly associated with the condition, 3) probable natural history, and 4) expected response to specified types of treatment.

A large body of research from clinical, epidemiologic, and natural history studies indicates that behavioral descriptive approaches work and that the nature of the child's symptoms holds the key to a lot more information than a current description of mental state (for examples of classic studies, see

This work was made possible by National Institute of Mental Health (NIMH) Research Training Grant T32MH16434 and NIMH Center Grant MH43878-01A1 to the Center to study youth depression, anxiety, and suicide.

Robins 1966; Rutter et al. 1970). For example, the two groups into which most child psychiatric patients fall—children with behavior that does not conform to social norms and is troublesome to others (the disruptive behavior or conduct disorders) and children who experience emotional distress from a combination of depressive and anxious feeling states—differ not only with respect to symptoms but also with respect to their demographics, past experiences, prognosis, and response to treatment.

Children with a disruptive or conduct disorder are predominantly boys, often from a disturbed home background where they received little supervision and harsh punishment. Many of these children have parents who are unhappily married, delinquent, or alcoholic. Many resist treatment, and the long-term prognosis for about half of these children will be poor, with childhood problems leading to adult sociopathy. By contrast, children with emotional (anxiety and affective) symptoms are as likely to be females as males, and their family circumstances and parenting experiences are generally no different from controls. Most will respond well to intervention and, with or without treatment, do well in the long term. Those children who go on to develop a psychiatric disorder as adults are likely to be anxious or depressed rather than sociopathic.

Uses and Problems in a Classification System

Uses

Communication. An accurate and "user-friendly" classification system helps communication among clinicians, researchers, and administrators. It provides a shorthand that allows communication of probable prognosis and treatment response.

Providing a structure for inquiry. An effective diagnostic system provides a structure for organized inquiry or research because it allows like to be compared with like. If a series of patients is to be followed, or if a new form of treatment is to be evaluated, the investigator using a systematic classification scheme will group similar patients together and contrast their prognosis with dissimilar ones. In the 1990s, this may seem obvious, but it has not been long since the literature consisted primarily of single-case reports, of treatment studies

that reported on mixed groups of children with quite heterogeneous symptom profiles, and of follow-up studies that included all children who had been hospitalized or seen in a clinic, regardless of their diagnostic characteristics.

Heuristic. Diagnostic categories that can be expressed in operational and reproducible terms—such as those in DSM-III (American Psychiatric Association 1980) and DSM-III-R—lend themselves to empirical study and have a potential for change and refinement. The category, even if it was first arrived at by consensus among experts rather than through empirical research, can be tested and, if faulty, can be changed. As an example, the DSM-III diagnosis of attention deficit without hyperactivity was designed for what was predicted would be a very small group of nonhyperactive inattentive children who would not be appropriately described by the designation attention-deficit hyperactivity disorder. When the diagnosis was first defined, little or nothing was known about such children, but its presence in the system stimulated research that validated its existence and led to elaborated clinical descriptions (Cantwell and Baker 1989; Lahey et al. 1987).

Problems Inherent in Diagnostic Systems

Labeling. Establishing a diagnosis is not an academic exercise; it is done in the interests of the patient, and it helps the clinician to determine the best treatment and to predict outcome. However, assigning a diagnosis is not a benign process and itself may lead to problems. Because advances in psychiatry have led to many more diagnosis-specific treatments, a wrong diagnosis may lead to inappropriate treatment. No matter how careful and sensitive the clinician is in relaying the implications of a diagnosis, qualifications and uncertainties may not be heard or heeded, and this may result in lower expectations or motivation or in an inappropriate restriction of educational or social opportunity. The fact that the diagnostic process is subject to error, misunderstanding, and abuse calls for the professional to be as careful as possible in conveying information to a child and family, to make sure that the communication has indeed been understood and to lay out specifically how the diagnosis should alter, if at all, any expectations for learning and behavior.

Validity. A diagnostic category may be invalid if it is based on incorrect information as, for example, when information is drawn from a biased sample or is otherwise carelessly or inappropriately collected. A category can also be nosologically invalid. Research on the concomitants of a diagnostic category is necessary to establish nosologic validity. The goal of a behavioral descriptive classification system is *not* to classify every variant of disorder that may be encountered by the clinician; such a classification system would be as limitless and meaningless as would a classification system for human beings that took account of every possible variation and combination of hair color, nose length, blood pressure, and clothing preference. Rather, the goal of a classification system is to establish distinct diagnostic categories that differ from one another not only in their symptoms or behaviors but also with respect to what may be more fundamental characteristics of a disorder. For example, it was assumed in DSM-III that, by designating separate categories for socialized and unsocialized conduct disorder, these conditions have distinctive origins, outcome, and associated features. There are many other instances in which subcategories are designated to reflect current usage but for which the etiology, natural history, and other information necessary to establish nosologic distinctiveness or discriminant validity are not available. Examples in DSM-III-R of such unproven categories include the distinctions between conduct disorder and oppositional defiant disorder, and differences between the various subtypes of anxiety disorders.

Reliability. As indicated above, a most important function of a classification system is its ability to communicate information. This will be affected by its reliability; that is, the way that different users applying the system to the same patient will select similar diagnostic categories.

Several factors affect reliability. One is the wording of criteria. Criteria that are phrased in specific, unambiguous language and that precisely state frequency, duration, and indicators of impairment are more likely to be used reliably than those that employ general or ambiguous terms such as *often*, *lengthy*, or *severe*. Another factor is criterion content. Symptoms or clinical phenomena that require interpretation or inference are prone to unreliable use. Categories that are differentiated from one another by quite small differences, as is the case with many of the subtypes, are open to unreliable use. A third factor is the structure of the system. Shorter lists of categories or criteria are easier to navigate correctly than are long ones; long lists encourage

users to select from only a part of the listing. The inclusion of parallel sections within the total system, as occurs with several of the child disorders in DSM-III, may lead to arbitrary use patterns. For example, avoidant disorder of childhood (in the child section) and social phobia disorder (in the general section) have very similar criteria.

Given these considerations, it may be no surprise that experimental comparisons between DSM-II (American Psychiatric Association 1968) and DSM-III found that, despite the inclusion of operationalized criteria, DSM-III was no more reliable than DSM-II (Mattison et al. 1979). The likely reason is that the positive effects of specific criteria were outweighed by the very much longer and more complex system in DSM-III.

Frequent revisions. It is a tribute to the powerful heuristic value of criterion-based classification systems that they appear to generate both debate and data, and as a result are subject to frequent revision. With each revision, new findings emerge that have direct implications for the existing classification scheme. Unfortunately, the process of revision is inconvenient; a revision may render diagnostic instruments obsolete and make studies adhering to one set of criteria difficult to compare with those adhering to a different set. Furthermore, each new revision requires an expensive educational effort for mental health professionals. The revisions to DSM-III in DSM-III-R were broadly criticized as cutting the ground from under established investigators and clinicians (Gift 1988; Zimmerman 1988).

Criterion-based Systems

DSM-III, DSM-III-R, and most recently ICD-10 RV (research version [World Health Organization 1988]) include a number of diagnostic categories that are defined with reference to sets of highly specific criteria. The use of specific criteria is not a new development in child psychiatry. Kanner's (1943) original description of early infantile autism, with its 11 features, is a classic example of a criterion-based diagnosis.

The nature and organization of criteria in DSM-III and in DSM-III-R vary a good deal. In some instances, a diagnosis requires the presence of symptoms defined at a single, very broad level. An example is the DSM-III version of conduct disorder that required "a repetitive and persistent pattern of conduct in which . . . the basic rights of others

. . . are violated" (p. 45), followed by certain examples and duration and exclusionary guidelines. In other instances, the requirement is that symptoms be drawn from specific subsets, each representing a broad construct. An example is the DSM-III-R criteria for autistic disorder, in which two of the described manifestations of impaired social interactions, and one each of impaired communication and a restricted repertoire of activities and interests, are necessary. In yet others, such as attention-deficit hyperactivity disorder in DSM-III-R, a single list of highly specific criteria is provided with no grouping into broader subsets.

The use of specific criteria brings with it certain predictable consequences. The main advantage is a greater clarity and precision that should increase the uniformity with which diagnoses are applied and ease the task of creating diagnostic instruments. However, a number of problems can arise in this approach.

Overspecificity. A very specific symptom description usually defines less behavior than does a more general one. This is a particular problem for child psychiatry where there are very marked age and quite marked sex differences in the manifestations of disorders. Highly specific criteria may be appropriate only for children of certain ages, or for boys or girls. For example, an inability to wait one's turn in line, or not speak out of turn (attention-deficit hyperactivity disorder in DSM-III-R), may be clinically significant in older children but is much less likely to be so in the very young. To compensate for this, the number of criteria has to be increased, in some instances to a number that cannot be easily remembered. Thus in DSM-III-R, there are 14 criteria for attention-deficit hyperactivity disorder, 16 for autistic disorder, and 9 for separation anxiety disorder. Even such long lists may not fully describe the universe of behaviors found in a given disorder, and this can give rise to the problem of false negatives.

Threshold problems. Rules have to be developed about the number of criteria necessary to constitute a diagnosis and about the parameters (e.g., duration, length) of the criteria themselves. There is rarely any empirical information that directs this process, and the threshold is usually arrived at by consensus among experts. Because it is difficult to envisage all clinical eventualities, a given threshold will sometimes not be met by a patient with a very small number of very serious symptoms, while a

different child with a sufficient number of minor symptoms may meet the criteria for the disorder but not capture the essence of the disorder.

Potential for instability. Very specific criteria may be highly sensitive to small changes in wording or to changes in threshold. A criterion revision may then result in large and unpredictable shifts in the prevalence of a disorder. For example, a number of impaired children who previously met DSM-III criteria for conduct disorder do not meet criteria for DSM-III-R conduct disorder (Piacentini et al. 1989). Conversely, a number of children who did not previously meet criteria for infantile autism in DSM-III do meet criteria for autistic disorder in DSM-III-R (Volkmar et al. 1988a).

Different Approaches to Classification

Historical Trends Toward Specificity and Complexity

In the 1920s, it was common for large public mental hospitals to employ their own diagnostic systems, consisting primarily of disorders found in such settings, that were mainly used locally. A particular hospital's listing could become more broadly circulated by professionals who moved on after receiving their training.

In a joint venture between the New York Academy of Medicine and the American Psychiatric Association's Committee on Statistics, a broadly accepted psychiatric diagnostic system was introduced as part of the "Standard Classified Nomenclature of Disease" in 1934. During World War II, the United States Army revised that list to cover conditions that were encountered in outpatient practice, and this formed the basis for the 1947 revision by the World Health Organization of the International Classification of Diseases (ICD-6). This revision was the first to include a section on mental disorders (although earlier editions had listed some psychiatric conditions as causes of death). In 1948 the same committee of the American Psychiatric Association set to work to revise that listing, the revision bearing fruit in 1952 with the first *Diagnostic and Statistical Manual of Mental Disorders* (DSM-I).

The field of child psychiatry was largely neglected in these early classification systems. The DSM-I system confined its listings to childhood schizophrenia and the adjustment disorders of infancy, childhood, and adolescence. Adjustment disorder of childhood was in turn subclassified into habit disturbance, conduct disturbance, and neurotic traits. The glossary that accompanied these categories consisted of only a few sentences. DSM-II was linked with and appeared at the same time as ICD-8 (World Health Organization 1969) (which included only one child category, psychiatric disorder of childhood). DSM-II provided a marginally more elaborate set of childhood disorder codes: behavior disorders, hyperkinetic reaction, and withdrawing and overanxious reactions. The behavior disorders were subdivided into three further categories: runaway, unsocialized aggressive, and group delinquent reactions. Etiologic assumptions are implicit, for all disorders were labeled "reactions," reflecting Adolf Meyer's (1957) view that mental disorders represented reactions of the personality to psychological, social, and biological factors (Spitzer 1980). The listings were accompanied by a brief glossary.

Two publications appeared in the late 1960s and 1970s that were to exert a significant influence on psychiatric nosology. The first was the proposal by Rutter et al. (1969) for a multiaxial classification system with a considerably expanded list of psychiatric disorders of childhood. The expanded list was eventually incorporated into ICD-9 (World Health Organization 1977) and was influential in providing the list of disorders that would be included in DSM-III. The proposal for a multiaxial classification would be adopted by DSM-III. The second publication was the proposal by Spitzer et al. (1978) for Research Diagnostic Criteria (RDC) for schizophrenia and the affective disorders. These were originally developed for a multicenter collaborative study of those disorders, but would form the model for the DSM-III systems.

It is apparent that there have been at least two tendencies as these systems have developed. First, there has been a trend toward much more elaborate and specific descriptions of disorders. DSM-III and DSM-III-R are both criterion based, offering little leeway for idiosyncratic application, while the accompanying texts in many respects resemble (and are used as) textbooks. Second, there has been considerable increase in the number of diagnostic categories specifically designated as applicable to children. DSM-I had 4, whereas DSM-III-R has 52 (including the developmental disorders on Axis II).

It is intended that DSM-IV, to be published in 1993, to coincide with the scheduled publication of ICD-10, should avoid many of the problems outlined earlier. Validity is to be increased by relying wherever possible on methodologically adequate data; disruption due to the introduction of a new system will be minimized by requiring strong evidence to support any change from DSM-III-R; thresholds will be examined empirically in specially designed field trials (Frances et al. 1989).

Dimensional Classification Systems

A different approach to classifying children's psychiatric disorders has been widely used during the past two decades. Although sometimes called an empirical approach, this may not be the best term, for as DSM and ICD acquire a firmer basis in research, they too are in fact becoming increasingly empirical.

Dimensional approaches apply statistical techniques such as factor analysis to symptom information (hence empirical because it is based on real data). The factors, or the patterns of symptom correlation that emerge, are then named (regrettably often with terms that can be confused with those used in other classification systems). Most often the symptom data will have been collected on symptom inventories completed by parents, by teachers, or by older children and adolescents, but the same procedure can be applied to symptom information collected by clinicians at interview. It is common practice for the analyses to be performed on homogeneous groups, such as all one sex or all roughly one age. This procedure will, in turn, yield factors that differ for different age and sex groups.

Statistical manipulation can also reveal more specific or narrower dimensions or factors. The dimensions do not describe patients but patterns of symptom aggregation, and most patients have high scores on several narrow factors and often on both major dimensions. A patient can be characterized by a profile of scores on the different "narrow" dimensions. Other statistical techniques such as cluster analysis can then be used to group together individuals with similar profiles.

Regardless of the child-adolescent population or the source of the symptom information, two principal groupings emerge from this procedure: one of disruptive behaviors, and a group composed of emotional and affective symptoms. These groups correspond broadly to the profiles provided at the start of this chapter. In the most widely used procedure that employs data collected on measures such as Achenbach's Child Behavior Checklist (Achenbach and Edelbrock 1983), these principal dimensions are named, respectively, the *externalizing* and *internalizing dimensions*.

The dimensional approach has been especially popular among researchers of child psychopathology. Possible reasons for this include the long tradition of using comprehensive symptom inventories, which lend themselves to dimensional analysis, in such research. Second, most disturbed children do not present with pathognomonic or bizarre symptoms that are never encountered among normal children. Child psychiatric symptoms are, in most cases, similar to normal behaviors, differing only in number, duration, or stage of development at which they occur. The dimensional approach is conceptually sympathetic to the notion of continuum.

The advantages of the dimensional approach include its nonreliance on clinical lore and case anecdotes that are typically used when a diagnostic system is first formulated and that may be subject to considerable bias. Furthermore, although the dimensional system uses cutoff points or thresholds to designate a "case," these points have a reference against the normal population rather than against an arbitrary number of criteria indicated by the DSM-III-R or ICD-10 RV manuals.

There are a number of problems with the dimensional approach, particularly its reliance on statistical distributions in determining "caseness." That is, caseness becomes a function of deviation from normal scores rather than impairment, which is the reference criterion used in everyday practice by clinicians and is implicit in the notion of a "mental disorder," which is the basis for the DSM and ICD systems. There is also little evidence to demonstrate that dimensional profiles are equal or superior to the categorical classification systems in predicting outcome or informing on antecedents. Another problem is that because factors or dimensions are usually age- and sex-specific, differences in factor structure exist for different age and sex groups. This makes it difficult to compare or even group different sex and age groups, because each will have a different symptom profile. Before accepting these differences, empirical research would be needed to show that corresponding factor profiles in girls and boys are related to the same antecedents and that a particular symptom profile at one age was predictive of the corresponding profile at a different age.

Nonbehavioral Classification: Multiaxial Systems

A limitation of a purely behavioral or symptomatic classification system is that clinical decisions and predictions are not usually based solely on symptomatic information. Clinical decisions and predictions also are influenced by the child's intellectual endowment, the child's personality or temperament, any associated physical illness, and the home environment. This information is collected routinely during the course of a clinical evaluation. It can be coded, and the codes can be organized using a multiaxial system.

A multiaxial system is an approach to organizing information in a systematic way. Various dimensions or axes are specified, rating rules are provided, and there is an expectation that some judgment or rating will be made for each of these dimensions.

The two principal advantages of a multiaxial approach are that it results in clinicians recording more relevant information that is more easily retrieved, and it encourages clinicians to review systematically the areas covered by the different axes. Thus in an experimental study (Rutter et al. 1975), it was found that when child psychiatrists were asked to rate the diagnoses of a mentally retarded child with psychiatric symptoms, they were much more likely to code both the psychiatric disorder and the intellectual deficit when offered a multiaxial framework than when simply given instructions to code all abnormalities present. Other studies have found that multiaxial systems offer similar advantages in the retention and organization of information (Mezzich and Mezzich 1985; Williams 1985). It is desirable that the user be able to code "no abnormality" on a given dimension if such is the case (Rutter and Shaffer 1980). The alternative, which is to apply a code *only* when there is an abnormality, leads to record review difficulties; the absence of information could indicate either that the dimension was never reviewed or that no abnormality was found.

DSM-III-R provides five axes. Axis I lists codes for clinical syndromes. Axis II lists codes for personality and developmental disorders. Axis III lists codes for physical disease. Axis IV codes the severity of a psychosocial stressor that has been present in the year prior to the evaluation. Axis V codes the degree of impairment that results from the psychiatric disorder. While most child psychiatrists and other professionals routinely use Axis I and Axis

II, only a small minority regularly make ratings on Axes IV and V (Setterberg et al., in press). This may be because many institutions do not require that Axes IV and V ratings be made, and they are not required for reimbursement purposes.

Some controversies that affect nonbehavioral and multiaxial classification systems are presented below, with particular reference to the multiaxial system described in DSM-III-R.

Axis I and II differentiation. Both Axis I and Axis II are used to code clinical psychiatric disorders, but the basis for assigning a diagnostic category to one rather than another is not clear, especially in the case of child psychiatric disorders. The DSM-III-R manual indicates that an Axis II condition should "generally begin in childhood or adolescence and persist in a stable form (without periods of remission or exacerbation) into adult life" (p. 16). However, this definition is not applied consistently. For example, some conditions that tend to improve over time, such as autism and learning disorders, are listed on Axis II, whereas such conditions as the disruptive and the gender identity disorders that fit the stated guidelines for Axis II are listed on Axis I.

Psychosocial factors. A number of different approaches have been used to code psychosocial circumstances and stresses on Axis IV. The approach taken by DSM-III and DSM-III-R is to list codes for the severity of psychosocial stressors considered to be relevant to the psychiatric disorder on Axis IV. The word *relevant* is ambiguous. It does not distinguish between stressors that have had a causal influence on the disorder and those that arise as a result of the disorder; in practice, that distinction is difficult to make. It may be difficult to recall the order of stressors and behavior or emotional problems accurately, because 1) most childhood disorders and many stressors are chronic, 2) distortions occur as part of a "search for meaning," and 3) the influence of subclinical premorbid states on an individual's functioning (which in turn may lead to stress) is difficult to reconstruct. However, differentiating between stressors with and without causal significance is important, for a disorder that clearly follows a stressor, such as a bereavement response, may have a better prognosis than one that arises spontaneously.

A second approach creates categories for different types of psychosocial stressors (Shaffer et al. 1991; van Goor Lambo et al. 1990). Two problems arise with this approach. First, if the stressors are described at a very general level, then the same stressor will be designated in a wide variety of cases and the coding has no discriminating value. Second, if stressors are described in more specific terms, then reliability falls to unacceptably low levels (Shaffer et al. 1991). A third approach is to use a continuous "psychosocial adversity index" (Rey et al. 1987; Shaffer et al. 1975) that groups psychosocial stressors together in a single weighted index of severity. A fourth approach that is being considered by the committee responsible for developing DSM-IV rates the adequacy of the child's psychosocial support from the family, school, and broader society (Schaffer et al. 1989). Although the expectation is that this will predict treatment compliance and natural history, the reliability and validity of this method have yet to be determined.

There have been attempts to classify other nonbehavioral dimensions than those listed above. These include Anna Freud's (1970) Hampstead Index, developed at the Hampstead Clinic to classify defense mechanisms and other psychoanalytic concepts, and the taxonomy proposed by the Group for the Advancement of Psychiatry (1974), which leans heavily on psychoanalytic theory, assumptions, and terminology. The Hampstead Index is extremely complex and has been designed to be applied to extensive analytic case records; thus it cannot readily be applied to a new case or to the same case after an initial evaluation.

Classification Issues in Specific Disorders

In this section, the method of classifying some of the common childhood disorders will be reviewed and specific classification problems will be identified. Each of the disorders to be reviewed is more fully discussed in later chapters in this volume.

Disruptive Disorders

In DSM-III-R, this category includes conduct disorder, oppositional defiant disorder, and attention-deficit hyperactivity disorder. These disorders share patterns of behavior that are generally unsanctioned and troublesome to others and that, in practice, often co-occur.

Three important nosologic questions arise in relation to these disorders. What is the nature of the relationship between them? Are there subtypes of conduct disorder? What is the status of attention deficit without hyperactivity (undifferentiated attention-deficit disorder in DSM-III-R)?

Co-occurrences. It has been estimated that as many as 78% of hyperactive children as defined by DSM-III also have features of antisocial behavior—hence the grouping in DSM-III-R of attention-deficit hyperactivity disorder with conduct and oppositional disorders under a broad general category of disruptive disorders (Loney and Milich 1982; Sandberg et al. 1980). All three disorders possess similar epidemiologic characteristics (Sandberg et al. 1980); each is more common in males than in females. They also have somewhat similar long-term prognoses, which regardless of the success of early treatment are generally poor. Despite these empirical findings, these disorders are regarded as two quite different disorders with different treatment implications (for attention-deficit hyperactivity disorder, most often psychopharmacologic; for conduct disorders, most often some form of parent training or other environmental manipulation).

There are a number of possible explanations for the frequent co-occurrence of attention-deficit hyperactivity disorder and conduct disorder. It is possible that the overlap is artificial; that is, that the characteristics used to define attention-deficit disorder in DSM-III (and in certain rating scales) include symptoms of conduct disorder and result in the spurious appearance of an association. Criteria for attention-deficit hyperactivity disorder were redrawn in DSM-III-R to avoid this problem, but it is not yet known whether the changes have reduced the association. A second possibility is that the definitional problems lie in the rater rather than in the rating system, and that terms such as *overactivity* and *inattention* are used loosely by parents, teachers, and (other) professionals alike to describe socially inappropriate, rather than simply excessive, activity (Shaffer and Greenhill 1979). Third, the co-occurrence of conduct disorder and hyperactivity may be a real phenomenon, and there may be a causal relationship between the two. For example, a hyperactive child reared in a stressful family with inadequate parental attention, who is subject to loose supervision and harsh, rejecting discipline (which hyperactivity readily elicits), will go on to develop a conduct disorder, whereas a nonhyperactive child born into the same type family will not. This theory would explain why only a minority of

children brought up under such conditions develop a conduct disorder.

The relationship between conduct disorder and oppositional defiant disorder is also unclear. Many young children who will go on to develop a conduct disorder pass through a stage during which their symptoms are characterized by marked interpersonal defiance and aggressiveness (the features of oppositional defiant disorder), although without major infringements of the law. It is therefore plausible that oppositional defiant disorder is nothing more than an early phase or aborted form of conduct disorder. Appropriately designed longitudinal and epidemiologic studies are needed to resolve this question.

Subtypes. A number of subtypes of conduct disorder have been proposed (Loeber and Schmaling 1985; Stewart and Behar 1983). These include the DSM-III subtypes of socialized (i.e., capable of forming friendships and experiencing remorse for their antisocial behavior) or unsocialized (i.e., having no close or loyal friendships and experiencing no guilt or remorse after performing an antisocial act); aggressive (with behavior such as fighting and bullying, robbery with confrontation) or nonaggressive; and antisocial behavior covert (carried out secretly to avoid discovery or confrontation) or overt (with fighting, open assault) (Loeber and Schmaling 1985). Other subtypes have been proposed; for example, those who commit offenses with others (so-called group delinquents), those whose disordered conduct occurs in a solitary setting, those whose main behavior disturbance is runaway behavior, and those whose conduct is associated with depression. Some subtypes depend on characteristics such as whether or not guilt is experienced; others, such as performing a crime with accomplices, have not been shown to predict outcome differentially (Robins 1966). The evidence for other proposals is either absent or is based on unrepresentative or biased samples. Because of the lack of convincing and consistent evidence, the status of these subdivisions remains in flux.

Attention-deficit disorder without hyperactivity. This DSM-III term now appears as undifferentiated attention-deficit disorder in DSM-III-R. Its history provides a good example of the heuristic value of organized classification systems. The entity was described speculatively, in the absence of research, to provide a category for children who have attentional problems but who are not hyperactive. Subsequent research (Lahey et al. 1987) revealed that there are indeed such children who are "sluggish" rather than overactive, daydream in class, appear to lack motivation, and frequently have an associated learning disorder. The appropriate placement of this category in DSM-IV is under consideration (Shaffer et al. 1989).

Anxiety Disorders

Child psychiatric patients with anxiety symptoms may fall into one of a number of categories, depending on the nature of their symptoms. These include overanxious disorder of childhood for children with a fear of new situations and performance anxiety; separation anxiety disorder for those with a fear of separation from important attachment figures; and avoidant disorder of childhood for children with marked social reticence and/or social withdrawal as a function of anxiety.

The classification of anxiety in children poses several problems. Of the greatest concern are the validity of the subdivisions, how comorbid depression should be classified, and duplication within the DSM-III-R system.

Validity of subdivisions. There are no published studies regarding the extent to which the different subtypes overlap. Further, no studies have been published about whether children with the different types differ from one another with respect to family history or background, response to treatment, or prognosis.

Comorbid depression. Children with anxiety symptoms frequently experience periods of depression. Indeed, anxiety and depression together is more common than depression alone (Anderson et al. 1987; Rutter et al. 1970). There is not yet sufficient research to inform us whether the combination of anxious and affective symptoms constitutes a distinctive diagnostic entity, whether anxiety predisposes to depression, or whether there are other reasons (Weissman et al. 1984) for the co-occurrence of these conditions.

Distinctions between child and adult anxiety disorders. There are marked similarities between two of the three anxiety disorders listed as usually having their onset in childhood (overanxious and avoidant disorders) and disorders listed under the general anxiety disorder section (generalized anxiety disorder and social phobia). This feature predisposes to unreliability, with some older children or young adolescents being diagnosed with a childhood onset condition, whereas others receive a general anxiety diagnosis. Research is needed to determine whether the childhood disorders develop into similar or different disorders in adulthood and to determine the extent to which they share common antecedents or other correlates.

Learning Difficulties

In DSM-III-R, learning disorders are grouped into a general category of academic skills disorders on Axis II. This general category includes separate categories for developmental arithmetic disorder, developmental expressive writing disorder, and developmental reading disorder. In practice, these disorders commonly co-occur. The major areas of controversy concern measurement and definition.

Academic achievement can be measured on standardized tests and, providing that the child has received a satisfactory education, is highly correlated with mental age. A learning disorder is held to be present when the child has been exposed to reasonable educational opportunities but performs significantly less well than would be expected from performance on tests of mental age. This discrepancy between mental age and performance age is an essential part of the definition, but many clinicians have experience with children who perform within expected levels on standardized achievement tests but who do not do well at school, and it has been suggested that these children also should be considered to have a learning disorder (Shaffer et al. 1989). The prevailing view is that the category should be retained solely for a cognitive phenomenon measurable on standard tests rather than for cases in which learning failure is due to ill-defined states, such as low achievement motivation.

Autism and Pervasive Developmental Disorder

The syndrome of autism is rare compared with most other child psychiatric conditions. It affects between 1 in 3,000 and 1 in 10,000 births (Gillberg 1984). Its cardinal features include onset before the age of 30 months; severe language abnormalities; social aloofness; a "need for sameness" shown by distress at a change in routine or when familiar arrangements or objects are moved; and bizarre stereotyped motor behaviors.

Some of the nosologic issues surrounding autism are the absence of pathognomonic features, its relationship to neurologic disorder, and its relationship to adult or "process" schizophrenia.

Pathognomonic features. None of the clinical features of the autistic syndrome are pathognomonic, and some or all may be found in children with developmental dysphasias or mental retardation (Wing and Gould 1979). Because it is difficult to draw precise boundaries between these conditions, DSM-III-R was set up so that the diagnosis could be made from a broad array of symptoms. One consequence of this is that a considerably wider range of children now meet criteria for the diagnosis (Volkmar et al 1988a). Some hold this to represent a "dilution" of what previously appeared to be a very specific disease concept (Shaffer et al. 1989).

Relationship to neurologic abnormality. There are some neurologic syndromes that nearly always are associated with autistic behavior, although they also feature a number of other clinical characteristics. In some instances, the basic abnormality is known, as is the case with Fragile X syndrome. In others, such as Rett's syndrome, it is not. The issue is whether once a well-defined syndrome has been identified, it should be singled out with a specific category or should continue to be classified within an undifferentiated category. Singling it out is likely to increase the frequency with which it is identified and may stimulate research in the area.

Distinction from schizophrenia. Historically, autism was viewed as a special manifestation of schizophrenia, and it is still sometimes referred to as *childhood psychosis* or *childhood schizophrenia*. However, there are a number of reasons for differentiating the two conditions (Gillberg 1984; Petty et al. 1984; Rutter 1972; Volkmar et al. 1988b). A family history of either autism or schizophrenia increases the risk for relatives of having the same condition, but not the other. Only a small number of autistic children will go on to develop schizophrenia in adulthood; similarly, a history of autism is extremely rare in adult schizophrenic patients. Sex ratios are different for the two disorders, and there is no evidence that antipsychotic drugs that are effective for adult schizophrenic patients have any utility for patients with autism. Thus, the terms childhood schizophrenia or psychosis are best avoided or confined to cases of early onset schizophrenia of the adult type.

Disorders of Infancy

The period of infancy may be one in which psychiatric disorders such as autism first become apparent. More speculatively, infancy may be a period when experiences will shape personality development or lead to later psychiatric disorders. The field of infant psychiatry is young, and many research observations made on infants have failed to predict clinically meaningful entities in later life. The existing classification systems recognize only two disorders of infancy: reactive attachment disorder of infancy and rumination disorder of infancy. The main nosologic questions are whether reactive attachment disorder is sufficiently well differentiated, and whether there is a basis for more elaborate categories.

Reactive attachment disorder is intended to code behaviors that may follow severe early neglect or abuse. Two types of behavior are regarded as possible consequences of this disorder: 1) social withdrawal, apathy, and unresponsiveness; and 2) indiscriminate sociability. The literature suggests that the former is most likely to be a response to neglect, the latter a response to frequent changes in the caregiving environment and in being reared by multiple caregivers (Tizard and Tizard 1971). The disorder as it appears in DSM-III-R is a departure from the behavioral descriptive rule because it includes a nonsymptomatic, presumed etiologic element as a necessary criterion: grossly pathogenic care. However, the inclusion of the parenting factor helps to distinguish those infants with similar patterns of behavior whose apathy stems from mental retardation or personality variables. The validity of this disorder has not been demonstrated. There have been no studies of the prevalence of reactive attachment disorder in cases of child abuse and neglect characterized by grossly abnormal care. Studies of attachment relationships in cases of child abuse or neglect indicate that, while maltreated children are more likely than nonmaltreated children to be insecurely attached, there is no attachment style characteristic of maltreated children (Gaensbauer and Harmon 1982; Schneider-Rosen et al. 1985). Furthermore, as many as 50% of children with nonorganic failure to thrive show features of secure attachment (Gordon and Jameson 1979).

Subthreshold Disorders: Adjustment Disorders

Adjustment disorders represent another class of disorders in which etiologic assumptions are made. Both DSM-III and DSM-III-R set a number of stringent requirements for the diagnosis to be assigned:

1. There should have been an identifiable stressor.
2. The maladaptive behavioral response to the stressor must occur within 3 months of exposure to the stressor.
3. The maladaptive behavioral response should not be an example of a nonspecific overreaction to stress or an exacerbation of a preexisting condition.
4. The maladaptive response should not last more than 6 months.
5. The features of the disorder should not meet threshold requirements for another similar Axis I diagnosis.

The nosologic concerns surrounding this group of diagnoses include how best to categorize the effects of chronic stress and the widespread misapplication of the diagnostic rules.

Research into the acute reactions of children to such stresses as the death of a relative, divorce, or hospitalization suggests that the 6-month duration criterion is appropriate, providing that all other environmental circumstances are satisfactory and that the stress has abated (Goodyer et al. 1987). However, in childhood and adolescence, it is not uncommon for an isolated stress event, such as the birth of a sibling or the death or divorce of a parent, to set in train further stresses that will endure; the disturbed behavior may persist for as long as the stress continues. Under these circumstances, the 6-month duration criterion is inappropriate, and it is important that the classification system accommodate this requirement.

Overuse and misuse. It is generally believed that the diagnosis of adjustment disorder is used more commonly for child patients than adults. It appears that many clinicians do not apply the strict and restrictive criteria listed above, leading to inaccurate and inappropriate usage (Setterberg et al., in press). Several factors seem to make this an often-inappropriate diagnosis of choice related to theoretical biases among clinicians. For example, many clinicians prefer a Meyerian "reactive" model of child psychopathology. Clinicians also hold a belief that adjustment disorder is a less stigmatizing diagnosis than other diagnoses that may apply. Finally, the criteria for adjustment disorders include a presumption of etiology, the notion of mildness (i.e., that the disorder does not meet diagnostic criteria for a regular Axis I diagnosis), and a prediction of a good prognosis. It could be that patients meeting any one—rather than all three—of these criteria are assigned the diagnosis.

Conclusion

The way psychopathology is classified exerts a profound influence on how clinical problems are evaluated and managed. Classification sets the direction of and the parameters for a good deal of academic and scholarly activity. It determines the adequacy of communication among parties involved in the diagnosis and treatment of children. The systems in use include many imperfections. Some categories have been formulated as informed guesses. Some are a compromise between established custom and new and not yet fully digested information. Others have stood the test of time. Although the introduction of frequent revisions may be disturbing and a nuisance, it is also a sign of the vitality of current classification systems and how actively they intersect with new knowledge and experience.

References

Achenbach TM, Edelbrock CS: Manual of the Child Behavior Checklist and Revised Child Behavior Profile. Burlington, VT, University of Vermont, Department of Psychiatry, 1983

American Psychiatric Association: Diagnostic and Statistical Manual of Mental Disorders. Washington, DC, American Psychiatric Association, 1952

American Psychiatric Association: Diagnostic and Statistical Manual of Mental Disorders, 2nd Edition. Washington, DC, American Psychiatric Association, 1968

American Psychiatric Association: Diagnostic and Statistical Manual of Mental Disorders, 3rd Edition. Washington, DC, American Psychiatric Association, 1980

American Psychiatric Association: Diagnostic and Statistical Manual of Mental Disorders, 3rd Edition, Revised. Washington, DC, American Psychiatric Association, 1987

Anderson JC, Williams S, McGee R, et al: DSM-III disorders in preadolescent children: prevalence in a large sample from the general population. Arch Gen Psychiatry 44:69–76, 1987

Cantwell DP, Baker L: Stability and natural history of DSM-III childhood diagnosis. J Am Acad Child Adolesc Psychiatry 28:691–700, 1989

Frances AJ, Widiger TA, Pincus HA: The development of DSM-IV. Arch Gen Psychiatry 46:373–375, 1989

Freud A: The symptomatology of childhood: a preliminary attempt at classification. Psychoanal Study Child 26:19–41, 1970

Gaensbauer TJ, Harmon RJ: Attachment behavior in abused/neglected and premature infants, in The Development of Attachment and Affiliative Systems. Edited by Emde RN, Harmon RJ. New York, Plenum, 1982, pp 263–279

Gift TE: Changing diagnostic criteria. Am J Psychiatry 145:1414–1415, 1988

Gillberg C: Infantile autism and other childhood psychoses in a Swedish urban region: epidemiological aspects. J Child Psychol Psychiatry 25:35–43, 1984

Goodyer IM, Kolvin I, Gatzanis S: The impact of recent undesirable life events on psychiatric disorders in childhood and adolescence. Br J Psychiatry 151:179–184, 1987

Gordon AH, Jameson JC: Infant mother attachment in patients with non-organic failure to thrive syndrome. Journal of the American Academy of Child Psychiatry 18:251–259, 1979

Group for the Advancement of Psychiatry: Psychopathological disorders in childhood: theoretical considerations and a proposed classification (Report No 62). New York, Group for the Advancement of Psychiatry, 1974

Kanner L: Autistic disturbance of affective contact. Nervous Child 2:217–250, 1943

Lahey BB, Schaughency EA, Hynd GW, et al: Attention deficit disorder with and without hyperactivity: comparison of behavioral characteristics of clinic-referred children. J Am Acad Child Adolesc Psychiatry 26:718–723, 1987

Loeber R, Schmaling KB: Evidence for overt and covert patterns of antisocial conduct problems: a meta-analysis. J Abnorm Child Psychol 13:337–352, 1985

Loney J, Milich R: Hyperactivity, inattention, and aggression in clinical practice, in Advances in Developmental and Behavioral Pediatrics, Vol 3. Edited by Wolraich M, Routh DK. Greenwich, CT, JAI Press, 1982, pp 113–147

Mattison R, Cantwell D, Russell AT, et al: A comparison of DSM-II and DSM-III in the diagnosis of childhood psychiatric disorders, II: interrater agreement. Arch Gen Psychiatry 36:1217–1222, 1979

Meyer A: Psychobiology: A Science of Man. Springfield, IL, Charles C Thomas, 1957

Mezzich AC, Mezzich JE: Perceived suitability and usefulness of DSM-III vs DSM-II in child psychopathology. Journal of the American Academy of Child Psychiatry 24:281–285, 1985

Petty LK, Ornitz EM, Michelman JD, et al: Autistic children who become schizophrenic. Arch Gen Psychiatry 41:129–135, 1984

Piacentini JC, Abikoff HA, Klein RG, et al: Teacher ratings of DSM-III-R disruptive behavior disorders: symptom and syndrome prevalence in a normative population. Paper presented at the annual meeting of the American Academy of Child and Adolescent Psychiatry, New York, October 1989

Rey JM, Plapp JM, Stewart G, et al: Reliability of the psychosocial axes of DSM-III in an adolescent population. Br J Psychiatry 150:228–234, 1987

Robins LN: Deviant Children Grown Up. Baltimore, MD, Williams & Wilkins, 1966

Rutter M: Childhood schizophrenia reconsidered. Journal of Autism and Childhood Schizophrenia 2:315–337, 1972

Rutter M, Shaffer D: DSM-III: a step forward or back in terms of the classification of child psychiatric disorders? Journal of the American Academy of Child Psychiatry 19:371–394, 1980

Rutter M, Lebovici S, Eisenberg L, et al: A triaxial classification of mental disorders in childhood. J Child Psychol Psychiatry 10:41–61, 1969

Rutter M, Graham P, Yule W: A Neuropsychiatric Study in Childhood. London, Heinemann/SIMP, 1970

Rutter ML, Shaffer D, Shepard M: A Multiaxial Classification of Child Psychiatric Disorders. Geneva, World Health Organization, 1975

Sandberg ST, Wieselberg M, Shaffer D: Hyperkinetic and conduct problem children in a primary school population: some epidemiological considerations. J Child Psychol Psychiatry 21:293–311, 1980

Schneider-Rosen K, Braunwald KG, Carlson V, et al: Current perspectives in attachment theory: illustration from the study of maltreated infants. Monogr Soc Res Child Dev 50(1-2, Serial No 209):194–210, 1985

Setterberg S, Ernst M, Rao U, et al: Child psychiatrists' views of DSM-III-R: a survey of usage and opinions. J Am Acad Child Adolesc Psychiatry (in press)

Shaffer D, Greenhill L: A critical note on the predictive validity of the hyperkinetic syndrome. J Child Psychol Psychiatry 20:61–72, 1979

Shaffer D, Chadwick O, Rutter M: Psychiatric outcome of localized head injury in children, in Outcome of Severe Damage to the Central Nervous System (CIBA Foundation Symposium Ser No 34). Edited by Porter R, Fitzsimons DW. Amsterdam, Elsevier, 1975, pp 191–213

Shaffer D, Campbell M, Cantwell D, et al: Child and adolescent psychiatric disorders in DSM-IV: issues facing the work group. J Am Acad Child Adolesc Psychiatry 28:830–835, 1989

Shaffer D, Gould M, Rutter R, et al: Reliability and validity of a psychosocial axis in patients with a child psychiatric disorder. J Am Acad Child Adolesc Psychiatry 30:109–115, 1991

Spitzer R: Introduction to DSM-III, in Diagnostic and Statistical Manual of Mental Disorders, Third Edition. Washington, DC, American Psychiatric Association, 1980

Spitzer R, Endicott J, Robins E: Research Diagnostic Criteria (RDC) for a selected group of functional disorders. New York, Biometrics Research, 1978

Standard Classified Nomenclature of Disease, 1st Edition. See Textbook and Guide to the Standard Nomenclature of Diseases and Operations. Chicago, IL, Physicians Record Company, 1934

Stewart MA, Behar D: Subtypes of aggressive conduct disorder. Acta Psychiatr Scand 68:178–185, 1983

Tizard J, Tizard B: The social development of two-year-old children in residential nurseries, in Origins of Human Social Relations. Edited by Schaffer HR. New York, Academic, 1971, pp 147–163

van Goor Lambo G, Orley J, Poustka F, et al: Classification of abnormal psychosocial situations: a preliminary report of a revision of a WHO scheme. J Child Psychol Psychiatry 31:229–241, 1990

Volkmar FR, Bregman J, Cohan DJ, et al: DSM-III and DSM-III-R diagnoses of autism. Am J Psychiatry 145:1404–1408, 1988a

Volkmar FR, Cohen DJ, Hoshino Y, et al: Phenomenology and classification of the childhood psychoses. Psychol Med 18:191–201, 1988b

Weissman MM, Leckman JF, Merikangas KR, et al: Depression and anxiety disorders in parents and children: results from the Yale Family Study. Arch Gen Psychiatry 41:845–852, 1984

Williams JB: The multiaxial system of DSM-III: where did it come from and where should it go? its origins and critiques. Arch Gen Psychiatry 42:175–180, 1985

Wing L, Gould J: Severe impairments of social interaction and associated abnormalities in children: epidemiology and classification. J Autism Dev Disord 9:11–29, 1979

World Health Organization: International Classification of Diseases, 6th Revision. Geneva, World Health Organization, 1947

World Health Organization: International Classification of Diseases, 8th Revision. Geneva, World Health Organization, 1969

World Health Organization: International Classification of Diseases, 9th Revision. Geneva, World Health Organization, 1977

World Health Organization: 1988 Draft of ICD-10 Chapter V: Categories F.00–F99: Mental, Behavioral and Developmental Disorders (Clinical Descriptions and Diagnostic Guidelines). Geneva, World Health Organization, 1988

Zimmerman M: Why are we rushing to publish DSM IV? Arch Gen Psychiatry 45:1135–1138, 1988

Chapter 6

Clinical Assessment in Infancy and Early Childhood

Stanley I. Greenspan, M.D.

Recent understanding of both normal and disturbed emotional functioning in infants and young children makes it possible to explore new comprehensive approaches to understanding early development and implementing patterns of assessment, treatment, and prevention. Descriptions of adaptive and maladaptive emotional milestones can be added to the well-known sensorimotor and cognitive milestones (Greenspan 1979, 1981, 1987, 1989). The importance of early assessment is indicated by studies of cumulative risk, which suggest that family and interactive patterns during infancy correlate with later cognitive and behavioral performance at age 4. For example, children with four or more infancy risk factors have a 24-fold increase in the probability of marginal IQ scores, in comparison to children with only one or two risk factors (Sameroff et al. 1987).

The following outline of approach to emotional assessment will include a guide that can be used for screening or as an outline for a comprehensive evaluation. Basic concepts relevant to assessment in infancy include 1) the importance of considering multiple lines of development (as compared with only physical or cognitive), 2) the components of a comprehensive approach, and 3) the sequence of normal and disturbed emotional development.

Multiple Lines of Development

The view of the infant as developing along multiple rather than single lines (i.e., physical, cognitive,

social-emotional, and familial) is perhaps self-evident; however, the implications of this approach are not always obvious. For example, babies who have been nutritionally compromised improve physically and gain weight more efficaciously when nutrition is provided together with adequate social interaction. An approach that focuses only on cognitive simulation to enliven a withdrawn baby may lead to further withdrawal if the infant has an undiagnosed sensory hypersensitivity. In contrast, a gradual soothing, individually tailored approach may be more effective.

Components of a Comprehensive Clinical Approach

A comprehensive clinical approach views infants in a context that includes not only multiple lines of development, but also the parents, other family members, and relevant variations in social structures, including the influence of poverty. A comprehensive approach would consider and work with, for example, the parents' predominant attitudes and feelings, family relationships, and other crucial contextual factors, such as the system of health and mental health services and relevant community structures. More isolated intervention strategies, while working to stimulate an infant's cognitive capacities, may limit involvement with parents to help only with issues such as food and housing or cognitive stimulation.

A comprehensive clinical approach must begin with the assessment of a number of conceptually consistent categories, as discussed below, that take into account multiple lines of development and deal with the full complexity of clinical phenomena.

Prenatal and Perinatal Variables

These variables, especially insults such as rubella, drug and alcohol use, and poor maternal nutrition, all have some impact on the infant's constitutional status and developmental tendencies. The prenatal variables include familial genetic patterns; mother's status during pregnancy, including nutrition, physical health and illness, personality functioning, mental health, and degree of stress; characteristics of familial and social support systems; characteristics of the pregnancy; and the delivery process, including complications, time in various stages, and infant's status after birth. The perinatal variables include maternal perceptions of her infant, maternal reports of the emerging daily routine, and observations of the infant and maternal-infant interaction.

Parent, Family, and Environmental Variables

These variables include evaluations of parents, other family members, and individuals who relate closely to the family along a number of dimensions. These assessments include each member's personality organization and developmental needs, child-rearing capacity, and family interaction patterns. Evaluations of the support system (extended family, friends, and community agencies) used or available to the family and of the total home environment (both animate and inanimate components) are also included. Of special importance is the capacity of the parents and family to calm and regulate the infant; reach out and foster attachment; perceive basic status of pleasure and discomfort; respond with balanced empathy (i.e., without either over-identification or isolation of feeling); perceive and respond flexibly and differently to the infant's cues; foster organized complex interactions; and support representational elaboration and differentiation.

Primary Caregiver and Caregiver-Infant/Child Relationship Variables

Evaluations in this area focus on the interaction between the infant and his or her important nur-

turing figures. Included are the status of the caregiver (e.g., teenage mother, single-parent family); the quality of shared attention, comfort, and regulation; the capacity for joint pleasure and intimacy; and the flexibility in tolerating tension and being able to return to a state of intimacy. Later, the capacities for reciprocal interaction to form complex emotional and behavioral patterns and to construct and differentiate mental representations are important.

Infant Variables: Physical, Neurologic, Physiologic, and Cognitive

These variables include the infant's genetic background and status immediately after birth, including the infant's general physical integrity (size, weight, general health), neurologic integrity, physiologic tendencies, rhythmic patterns, and levels of alertness and activity. Special attention should be paid to the infant's individual differences, including sensory hypo- or hyperreactivity, motor tone, motor planning, sensory processing (DeGangi et al., in press; Porges and Greenspan 1990), and cognitive level and style. Attention should also be paid to how these factors could foster or hinder the child's capacities to experience stimulation and regulate and organize experience; develop human relationships; interact in cause-and-effect reciprocal patterns; form complex behavioral and emotional and cognitive patterns; and construct representations to guide behavior, feelings, and thinking.

Infant Variables: Formation and Elaboration of Emotional Patterns and Human Relationships

This category involves the relationships between the infant and caregivers, which help the infant develop the capacity for a range of emotions (dependency to assertiveness) and relationship patterns, in the context of a sequence of organizational stages. These stages include the capacity for shared attention and engagement; purposeful interactions; complex and organized social and emotional patterns; construction of representations; and differentiation of internal representations along self versus nonself time and space dimensions (Greenspan 1981, 1989).

The Sequence of Adaptive and Maladaptive Emotional Development

The focus on the infant and his or her family from multiple aspects of development has made it possible to formulate developmental stages that focus on the infant's social and emotional functioning. These stages are based on an impressive number of studies of both normal and disturbed infant development.

Although there are no large-scale studies of disturbed affective patterns of infants and young children at different ages, there is extensive literature on the emotional development of presumed normal infants. Interestingly, during the past 15 years, there has been considerably greater documentation of normal emotional development in infants than probably in any other age group.

It is now well documented that the infant is capable, either at birth or shortly thereafter, of organizing experience in an adaptive fashion. He or she can respond to pleasure and displeasure (Lipsitt 1966); change behavior as a function of its consequences (Gewirtz 1965, 1969); form intimate bonds and make visual discriminations (Klaus and Kennell 1976; Meltzoff and Moore 1977); organize cycles and rhythms such as sleep-wake, alertness states (Sander 1962); evidence a variety of affects or affect proclivities (Ekman 1972; Izard 1978; Tomkins 1963a, 1963b); and demonstrate organized social responses in conjunction with increasing neurophysiologic organization (Emde et al. 1976). From the early months, the infant demonstrates a unique capacity to enter into complex social and affective interactions (Brazelton et al. 1974; Stern 1974a, 1974b, 1977). That the organization of experience broadens during the early months of life to reflect increases in the capacity to experience and tolerate a range of stimuli, including stable responses to social interactions and personal configurations, is also consistent with recent empirical data (Brazelton et al. 1974; Emde et al. 1976; Escalona 1968; Murphy and Moriarty 1976; Sander 1962; Sroufe 1979; Stern 1974a, 1974b).

Increasingly complex patterns continue to emerge as the infant further develops, as indicated by complex emotional responses such as surprise (Charlesworth 1969) and affiliation; wariness and fear (Ainsworth et al. 1974; Bowlby 1969; Sroufe and Waters 1977); exploration and refueling patterns (Mahler et al. 1975); behavior suggesting functional understanding of objects (Werner and

Kaplan 1963); and the eventual emergence of symbolic capacities (Bell 1970; Gouin-Decarie 1965; Piaget 1962/1972).

In addition to the studies on normal infant emotional development, important observations on disturbed development fill out the emerging picture of early emotional development. Interestingly, the study of psychopathology in infancy is a new area, even though the historical foundation for identifying disturbances in the early years of life is very impressive. Constitutional and maturational patterns that influenced the formation of early relationship patterns were already noted in the early 1900s, with descriptions of "babies of nervous inheritance who exhaust their mothers" and infants with "excessive nerve activity and a functionally immature" nervous system (Cameron 1919).

Winnicott (1931), who, as a pediatrician in the 1930s, began describing the environment's role in early relationship problems, was followed in the 1940s by investigators conducting the now well-known studies describing the severe developmental disturbances of infants brought up in institutions or in other situations of emotional deprivation (Backwin 1942; Bowlby 1951; Hunt 1941; Lowrey 1940; Spitz 1945). Spitz's films resulted in laws in the United States prohibiting care of infants in institutions.

Both the role of individual differences in the infant based on consitutional maturational and early interactional patterns and the "nervous" infants described by Rachford (1905) and Cameron (1919) again became a focus of inquiry, as evidenced by the observations of Burlingham and A. Freud (1942); by Bergman and Escalona's (1949) descriptions of infants with "unusual sensitivities"; by Murphy and Moriarty's (1976) description of patterns of vulnerability; by Thomas and Chess's (1977) temperament studies; by Cravioto and DeLicardie's (1973) descriptions of the role of infant individual differences in malnutrition; and by the impressive emerging empirical literature on infants (Brazelton et al. 1974; Emde et al. 1976; Gewirtz 1961; Lipsitt 1966; Rheingold 1966, 1969; Sander 1962; Stern 1974a, 1974b). More integrated approaches to understanding disturbances in infancy have been emphasized in descriptions of selected disorders and clinical case studies (Fraiberg 1979; Greenspan et al. 1987; Provence 1983).

To further understanding of both adaptive and disturbed infant functioning, an in-depth study of normal and disturbed developmental patterns in infancy was undertaken to develop a systematic comprehensive classification of adaptive and maladaptive infant and family patterns. Table 6-1 summarizes the observations of the adaptive and maladaptive infant and family patterns (Greenspan 1979, 1981, 1989).

The ability to monitor development progress with explicit guidelines facilitates the early identification of those infants, young children, and families who are either not progressing in an appropriate manner or who are progressing in a less-than-optimal way. For example, it is now possible to evaluate infants who continue to have difficulty regulating their state and developing the capacity for focused interest in their immediate environments, or who fail to develop a positive emotional interest in their caregivers. It is also possible to assess an infant's difficulty in learning cause-and-effect interactions and complex emotional and social patterns, or the infant's inability, by age 2 to 3, to create representations or symbols, and by ages 3 to 4, to differentiate these to guide emotions and behavior.

In exploring the factors that may be contributing to less-than-optimal patterns of development, the focus on multiple aspects of development offers many advantages. Some infants, for example, may evidence a motor delay because of familial patterns in which explorativeness and the practice of the motor system are discouraged. In other infants, there may be a maturational variation that, together with family patterns, is contributing to a motor lag. In still other cases, genetic or maturational factors may explain the delay completely. Even with a symptom as common as a motor lag, unless all aspects of all contributing factors are explored, it is likely that important contributing factors will go unrecognized. The focus on multiple aspects of development, in the context of clearly delineated developmental and emotional landmarks, opens the door to comprehensive assessment, diagnosis, and preventive intervention strategies. Such a comprehensive approach offers a developmental perspective on many of the severe disorders of early childhood, including autism and pervasive developmental disorder; mild-to-moderate disorders, such as conduct, anxiety, and attentional disorders; and

different forms of global lags in cognition (e.g., mental retardation), as well as any specific lags in receptive or expressive language, motor regulation, or sensory reactivity and processing (Greenspan 1989). A discussion of specific types of psychopathology, however, is beyond the scope of this chapter.

To facilitate screening and comprehensive evaluations, Table 6-2 provides a guide to emotional development in the context of sensorimotor, cognitive, and language development.

Conclusion

The framework presented here, both theoretical and practical, may also prove useful for guiding the comprehensive clinical evaluations that are indicated when an infant's emotional progress is lagging or shifting into a disordered configuration. The clinician may find it useful to use careful history taking, clinical interviews, observations of infant-caregiver and family interaction, and formal testing of sensorimotor and cognitive abilities to consider 1) if the infant and family have reached a certain emotional milestone (e.g., attachment, purposeful communication, representational capacities), and 2) if there are constrictions in the emotional domains engaged at that level. For either a deficit or a constriction, the clinician can determine the relative contributions of family, parent, infant-parent interaction, and infant constitutional-maturational factors.

In addition, determining overall developmental level and behavioral and emotional range at that level helps the clinician pinpoint the nature of the psychopathology (Greenspan 1981). Symptoms such as sleep problems, eating difficulties, or impulsive behavior may be part of an overall developmental lag or deficit or a more limited constriction in the range of emotional domains engaged in by the infant and family. In this way, the clinician can assess and treat emotional problems in infancy as part of a normative preventive developmental framework for emotional stages.

Table 6-1. **Developmental basis for psychopathology and adaptation in infancy and early childhood**

Stage-specific tasks and capacities	Capacities		Environment (caregiver)	
	Adaptive	Maladaptive (pathologic)	Adaptive	Maladaptive
Homeostasis (0–3 months) (self-regulation and interest in the world)	Internal regulation (harmony) and balanced interest in world	Unregulated (e.g., hyperexcitable); withdrawn (apathetic)	Invested, dedicated, protective, comforting, predictable; engaging and interesting	Unavailable, chaotic, dangerous, abusive; hypostimulating or hyperstimulating; dull
Attachment (2–7 months)	Rich, deep, multisensory emotional investment in animate world (especially with primary caregivers)	Total lack of, or nonaffective, shallow, impersonal, involvement (e.g., autistic patterns) in animate world	In love and woos infant to "fall in love"; affective multimodality pleasurable involvement	Emotionally distant, aloof, and/or impersonal (highly ambivalent)
Somatopsychologic differentiation (3–10 months) (purposeful, cause-and-effect signaling or communication)	Flexible, wide-ranging affective multisystem-contingent (reciprocal) interactions (especially with primary caregivers)	Behavior and affects random and/or chaotic, or narrow, rigid, and stereotyped	Reads and responds contingently to infant's communications across multiple sensory and affective systems	Ignores infant's communications (e.g., overly intrusive, preoccupied, or depressed) or misreads infant's communication (e.g., projection)
Behavioral organization initiative, and internalization (9–24 months)	Complex, organized, assertive, innovative, integrated behavioral and emotional patterns	Fragmented, stereotyped, and polarized behavior and emotions (e.g., withdrawn, compliant, hyperaggressive, or disorganized toddler)	Admiring of toddler's initiative and autonomy, yet available, tolerant, and firm; follows toddler's lead and helps toddler organize diverse behavioral and affective elements	Overly intrusive, controlling; fragmented, fearful (especially of toddler's autonomy); abruptly and prematurely "separates"
Representational capacity, differentiation, and consolidation (1½–4 years) (the use of ideas to guide language, pretend play, and behavior and eventually thinking and planning)	Formation and elaboration of internal representations (imagery); organization and differentiation of imagery pertaining to self and nonself; emergence of cognitive insight; stabilization of mood and gradual emergence of basic personality functions	No representational (symbolic) elaboration; behavior and affect concrete, shallow, and polarized; sense of self and other fragmented and undifferentiated or narrow and rigid; reality testing, impulse regulation, mood stabilization compromised or vulnerable (e.g., borderline psychotic and severe character problems)	Emotionally available to phase-appropriate regressions and dependency needs; reads, responds to, and encourages symbolic elaboration across emotional behavioral domains (e.g., love, pleasure, assertion) while fostering gradual reality orientation and internalization of limits	Fearful of or denies phase-appropriate needs; engages child only in concrete (nonsymbolic) models generally or in certain realms (e.g., around pleasure) and or misreads or responds noncontingently or nonrealistically to emerging communications (e.g., undermines reality orientation; overly permissive or punitive)

Table 6-1. (*Continued*)

Stage-specific tasks and capacities	Capacities		Environment (caregiver)	
	Adaptive	Maladaptive (pathologic)	Adaptive	Maladaptive
Capacity for limited extended representational systems and multiple extended representational systems (middle childhood through adolescence)	Enhanced and eventually optimal flexibility to conserve and transform complex and organized representations of experience in the context of expanded relationship patterns and phase-expected developmental tasks	Derivative representational capacities limited or defective, as are latency and adolescent relationships and coping capacities	Supports complex, phase- and age-appropriate experiential and interpersonal development (i.e., into triangular and posttriangular patterns)	Conflicted over child's age-appropriate propensities (e.g., competitiveness, pleasure orientation, growing competence, assertiveness, and self-sufficiency); becomes aloof or maintains symbiotic tie; withdraws from or overengages in competitive or pleasurable strivings

Source. Adapted from Greenspan 1981.

Table 6-2. Outline for the evaluation of the emotional development of infants and young children

General parenting patterns (by history and/or direct observation)

1. *Tends to engage his or her infant pleasurably* in a relationship (e.g., by looking, vocalizing, gentle touching), rather than tending to ignore his or her infant (e.g., by being depressed, aloof, preoccupied, withdrawn, indifferent). Yes/No/Unsure

2. *Tends to comfort his or her infant*, especially when the infant is upset (e.g., by relaxed, gentle, firm holding, rhythmic vocal or visual contact), rather than tending to make the infant more tense (by being overly worried, tense, or anxious, or mechanical or anxiously over- or understimulating). Yes/No/Unsure

3. *Tends to find appropriate levels of stimulation to interest his or her infant* in the world (e.g., by being interesting, alert, and responsive, including offering appropriate levels of sounds, sights, and touch—including the caregiver's face—and appropriate games and toys), rather than being hyperstimulating and intrusive (e.g., picking at and poking or shaking infant excessively to gain his or her attention). Yes/No/Unsure

4. *Tends to read and respond to his or her infant's emotional signals and needs in most emotional areas* (e.g., responds to the infant's desire for closeness as well as need to be assertive, explorative, and independent), rather than either misreading signals or only responding to one emotional need (e.g., can hug when baby reaches out, but hovers over baby and cannot encourage assertive exploration or vice versa). Yes/No/Unsure

5. *Tends to encourage his or her infant* to move forward in development, rather than to overprotect, "hold on," or infantalize. For example: Yes/No/Unsure
   a. Helps baby crawl, vocalize, and gesture by actively responding to infant's initiative and encouragement (rather than overanticipating infant's needs and doing everything for infant);
   b. Helps toddler make shift from proximal, physical dependency (e.g., being held) to feeling secure while being independent (e.g., keeps in verbal and visual contact with toddler as he or she builds a tower across the room);
   c. Helps 2- to 3-year-old child shift from motor discharge and gestural ways of relating to the use of "ideas" through encouraging pretend play (imagination) and language around emotional themes (e.g., gets down on floor and plays out dolls hugging each other or separating from each other, or soldiers fighting with each other);
   d. Helps 3- to 4-year-old take responsibility for behavior and deal with reality, rather than "giving in all the time."

Table 6-2.   (Continued)

General infant tendencies (all ages)

1. Is able to be calm and/or calm down and not be excessively irritable, clinging, active, or panicked.   Yes/No/Unsure
2. Is able to take an interest in sights, sounds, and people and is not excessively withdrawn, apathetic, or unresponsive.   Yes/No/Unsure
3. Is able to focus his or her attention and not be excessively distractible.   Yes/No/Unsure
4. Enjoys a range of sounds including high and low pitch, loud and soft, and different rhythms, and is not upset or confused by sounds.   Yes/No/Unsure
5. Enjoys various sights, including reasonably bright lights, visual designs, facial gestures, and moving objects, and is not upset or confused by various sights.   Yes/No/Unsure
6. Enjoys being touched (on face, arms, legs, stomach, trunk, and back), and bathed and clothed, and is not bothered by things touching his or her skin.   Yes/No/Unsure
7. Enjoys movements in space (e.g., being held and moved up and down, side to side), does not get upset with movement, and does not crave excessive movement.   Yes/No/Unsure
8. Enjoys a range of age-appropriate foods and is not bothered (e.g., with abdominal pains, skin rashes, or other symptoms) by any age-appropriate, healthy food as part of a balanced diet.   Yes/No/Unsure
9. Is comfortable and asymptomatic around household odors and materials and not bothered by any routine levels of household odors such as cleaning materials, paint, oil or gas fumes, pesticides, plastics, composite woods (e.g., plywood), synthetic fabrics (e.g., polyester), and so on.   Yes/No/Unsure

I. By 4 months
   Calms down and takes an interest in the world, and falls in love (as illustrated by a special interest and joy in the caregiver).
   A. Primary-emotional
      1. Responds to environment by brightening to *sights* (by alerting, calming, and focusing on objects rather than ignoring or becoming overexcited by bright lights or interesting objects).
      2. Responds to environment by brightening to *sounds* (same as above).
      3. Looks at person with great interest.
      4. Responds to social overtures with some vocalization, smile, or arm or leg movements.
   B. Emotional
      1. Looks at a person with a special joyful smile.
      2. Smiles joyfully when spoken to.
      3. Smiles joyfully in response to interesting facial expressions.
      4. Vocalizes back when spoken to.
      5. Maintains focused interest on caregiver (e.g., looking, listening, and showing some pleasure) for 1 minute or more.
      6. Calms down when comforted.
      7. Sleeps for intervals of 4 hours or more at night.
      8. Enjoys touch (e.g., stroking on arms, legs, stomach).
      9. Enjoys being cuddled and held firmly.
   C. Cognitive, sensory, or motor
      1. Cognitive
         a. Shows selective attention (special interest) in some sights or sounds.
         b. Coos with two or more different sounds.
         c. Enjoys moderate movement in space (up and down, side to side) and neither gets upset with gentle movement or craves excessive movement.
         d. Follows moving object or person easily.
         e. Turns head in the direction of a pleasant sound (rattle or voice).
      2. Sensory
         a. Holds and waves a small rattle.
         b. Keeps hands mostly open when quiet and alert.

Table 6-2.   (*Continued*)

    3. Motor
      a. Lifts head by leaning on elbows while on stomach.
      b. Holds head steady when sitting supported on caregiver's lap.

II. By 8 months
  Communicates intentionally (cause and effect) and begins to learn how people and things work.
  A. Primary-emotional
    1. Initiates simple interaction (e.g., expectantly looks for the caregiver to respond to facial expressions).
    2. Responds to gestures with gestures in return (e.g., when the caregiver goes to pick the child up, the child responds by raising arms and leaning forward).
  B. Emotional
    1. Initiates joy and pleasure (woos caregiver spontaneously).
    2. Initiates comforting (e.g., reaches up to be held).
    3. Responds to simple social games with pleasure, such as peek-a-boo or pat-a-cake, smiles or laughs when the caregiver does something silly like duck his or her head or pretend to sneeze.
    4. Shows assertiveness by reaching out for or going after an interesting toy that was taken away or put out of reach.
    5. Shows special interest in and cautiousness toward new people or unusual objects (e.g., usually examines from a distance before approaching).
  C. Cognitive, sensory, motor, or language
    1. Cognitive
      a. Focuses on toy, object, or person for 2 minutes or more.
      b. Explores a new toy (e.g., turns it to look at its different parts; mouths, shakes, and bangs toy on a surface).
      c. Likes to make things happen (bangs spoon on a pot, bangs two toys together, knocks down a stand-up toy).
      d. Follows an object as it goes out of sight (e.g., mother's face, food, or a toy that falls to the floor) and searches for it when out of sight (e.g., looking under a chair for a favorite ball).
    2. Sensory
      a. Reaches out and grasps an object or toy on a table while on the caregiver's lap.
      b. Picks up small objects like a Cheerio™ or raisin.
      c. Drinks from a cup or glass held by an adult.
    3. Motor
      a. Rolls back to stomach.
      b. Sits unsupported and plays from that position.
      c. Creeps or crawls.
      d. Pulls to stand in the crib or holding onto furniture.
    4. Language
      a. Imitates sounds (e.g., tongue click, fake cough, raspberry).
      b. Makes sounds from the front of mouth (da, ba, ma) and begins repeating them.

III. By 12 months
  Begins to develop a complex sense of self by organizing behavior and emotion.
  A. Primary-emotional
    1. Initiates complex interactions (e.g., hands parent toy to make it go, rolls a ball back and forth, uses gestures or vocalization to communicate the need for a desired object or food).
  B. Emotional
    1. Uses complex behavior to establish closeness (e.g., pulls the caregiver's leg *and* reaches up to be picked up).
    2. Asserts self through organized behavior, such as pointing and vocalizing at desired toy or exploring for desired objects or people.
    3. Responds to limits set by the caregiver's voice or gesture.
    4. Recovers from distress after 10–15 minutes.
    5. Seems to know how to get the caregiver to react (which actions make the caregiver laugh, which actions make him or her mad).

Table 6-2. *(Continued)*

    C. Cognitive, sensory, motor, or language
        1. Cognitive
           a. Plays on own in a focused, organized manner for 10 minutes or more.
           b. Copies simple gestures (waving bye-bye, shaking head "no").
           c. Uses hands and eyes more than mouth to examine a new object or toy.
           d. Looks at simple pictures in a book with the caregiver's help.
        2. Sensory
           a. Drops objects, such as blocks or toys, into a container.
           b. Feeds self small finger food.
           c. Chews small food like a Cheerio™ without choking.
        3. Motor
           a. Throws a ball forward.
           b. Walks holding onto furniture.
        4. Language
           a. Understands simple words, like *shoe*, or commands, like "give me a kiss."
           b. Uses sounds for specific objects, like "ba-ba" for bath, or "dup" for cup.
           c. Jabbers.

IV. By 18 months
Continues to develop a complex sense of self by intentional planning and exploration.
    A. Primary-emotional
        1. Shows intentional planning and exploration in interactions and play. For example, chooses a toy, finds mommy, and indicates with word or gesture that she is the play partner.
        2. Communicates needs and feelings from across the room as well as close up, in gesture or words, with touch or holding (e.g., can look at caregiver's admiring glance or hear reassuring word, smile happily, and return to organized play), or indicates interest in having caregiver join in play.
    B. Emotional
        1. Uses gestures and vocalizations to get parent's interest and a sense of closeness from across the room.
        2. Asks easily for help from adults with play activities, to get food, and so on.
        3. Balances a desire for independence and closeness (e.g., explores across the room and then comes back for a touch or cuddle).
        4. Shows assertiveness by organizing complex behavior to meet own needs (e.g., going to refrigerator, opening door, and pointing to food) or by refusing to comply with an adult or another child by saying "no" and doing something else.
        5. Protests or is angry, using voice and gestures, without having to cry, hit, or bite.
        6. Recovers from anger or upset within 15 minutes.
        7. Uses role playing as part of complex play (e.g., cooking with pots or washing dishes in play sink, driving toy fire engine with fire fighter's hat on).
    C. Cognitive, sensory, motor, or language
        1. Cognitive
           a. Searches for a desired object, such as a toy, in more than one place.
           b. Plays on own in a focused, organized manner for 15 minutes or more.
           c. Shows intentional planning and exploration by choosing a toy and then going to get it for play and exploration.
           d. Uses objects such as stuffed animals and toy telephones in play (e.g., putting animal to sleep, pretending to talk on the phone).
           e. Can imitate something seen a few minutes earlier.
        2. Sensory
           a. Recognizes many simple pictures in a favorite book.
           b. Recognizes pictures of familiar objects (e.g., a dog, a baby, a ball).
           c. Chews a variety of foods.
           d. Interested in puzzles and blocks, and tries to order them.
        3. Motor
           a. Walks with a sense of security.
           b. Tries to catch a ball rolled in his or her direction.
           c. Navigates well around furniture.

Table 6-2. **(Continued)**

    d. Scribbles with a pencil or crayon.

  4. Language

    a. Understands simple commands.

    b. Uses a variety of words to convey intentions and to label things.

V. By 2–2½ years

Creates new feelings and ideas.

  A. Primary

    1. Engages in pretend play (e.g., feeds doll and puts doll to sleep, has cars or trucks race).

    2. Uses words and/or gestures to express what is wanted.

  B. Emotional

    1. Uses words or gestures to get caregiver to participate in play (e.g., "come here," "hold dolly").

    2. Uses words to communicate desire for closeness (e.g., "hug").

    3. Uses simple repetitive play sequences to indicate interest in closeness (e.g., dolls being cuddled).

    4. Uses words for expressions of assertiveness ("Me want," "Give me").

    5. Uses simple repetitive play sequences to indicate interest in assertiveness (e.g., a truck race).

    6. Communicates anger with gesture, word, or wordlike sounds with insistence that caregiver comply.

    7. Recovers from anger or temper tantrum after 10 minutes.

  C. Cognitive, sensory, motor, or language

    1. Cognitive

      a. Plays in a focused, organized manner for 20 minutes or more.

      b. Searches for favorite toy where it was the day before.

      c. Engages in pretend play alone.

    2. Sensory

      a. Does simple shape puzzles with a few pieces.

      b. Plays with blocks with some order or design (builds a tower or lines up blocks in a train).

      c. Copies a circle.

    3. Motor

      a. Catches a large ball from a couple of feet away using arms and hands.

      b. Balances momentarily on one foot.

      c. Jumps with both feet off the ground.

      d. Walks up steps putting two feet on each step before going to the next.

      e. Runs.

    4. Language

      a. Uses simple two-word sentences ("Go bye-bye," "More milk").

      b. Understands simple questions ("Is Mommy home?").

VI. By 3–3½ years

Emotional thinking

  A. Primary

    1. Enjoys pretend play that conveys human dramas, which become more complex, so that one pretend sequence leads to another (e.g., instead of repetition where the doll goes to bed, gets up, goes to bed, the doll goes to bed, gets up, and then gets dressed; or the cars race, crash, and then go to get fixed).

    2. Knows what is real and what is not real (e.g., knows that cartoons are "pretend").

  B. Emotional

    1. Uses another person's help and some toys to play out complex pretend drama dealing with closeness, nurturing, or caregiving (taking care of a stuffed animal or doll that has fallen down and hurt itself).

    2. Uses another person's help and some toys to play out pretend drama dealing with assertiveness, exploration, or aggression (e.g., a truck race, monsters and soldiers fighting, a trip to grandma's house).

    3. Follows rules.

    4. Remains calm and focused for 30 minutes or more.

    5. Feels optimistic and confident.

Table 6-2. (*Continued*)

      6. Realizes how behavior, thoughts, and feelings can be related to consequences (if behaves nicely, makes caregiver pleased; if naughty, gets punished; if tries hard, learns to do something).

      7. Uses relationship between feelings, behavior, and consequences to be assertive (e.g., bargains, "eat broccoli later!").

      8. Interacts in socially appropriate way with adults.

      9. Interacts in socially appropriate way with peers.

  C. Cognitive, sensory, motor, or language

    1. Cognitive

      a. Plays in a focused, organized manner without another person for 20 minutes or more.

      b. Enjoys pretend play elements that are logically connected (e.g., "Dolly is spanked because she messed up").

    2. Sensory

      a. Puts pop beads together.

      b. Uses spatial designs that become more complex and have interrelated parts so that a block house has rooms or maybe furniture, or cars have different places to go, such as the store and the house or garage.

      c. Draws a person by putting indications of facial features or limbs on a circular shape.

    3. Motor

      a. Walks up stairs alternating feet.

      b. Catches a large ball using both hands.

      c. Kicks a ball.

    4. Language

      a. Uses sentences that become complex, with logical connecting words between phrases (e.g, "because" or "but" is used: "No like fish because icky").

      b. Asks "Why?," although not necessarily interested in the answer, and may repeat.

References

Ainsworth M, Bell SM, Stayton D: Infant-mother attachment and social development: socialization as a product of reciprocal responsiveness to signals, in The Integration of the Child Into a Social World. Edited by Richards M. Cambridge, UK, Cambridge University Press, 1974, pp 99–135

Backwin H: Loneliness in infants. Am J Dis Child 63:30, 1942

Bell S: The development of the concept of object as related to infant-mother attachment. Child Dev 41:291–311, 1970

Bergman P, Escalona SK: Unusual sensitivities in very young children. Psychoanal Study Child 3–4:333–352, 1949

Bowlby J: Maternal Care and Mental Health (WHO Monograph No 2). Geneva, World Health Organization, 1951

Bowlby J: Attachment and Loss. New York, Basic Books, 1969

Brazelton TB, Koslowski B, Main M: The origins of reciprocity: the early mother-infant interaction, in The Effect of the Infant on Its Care Giver. Edited by Lewis M, Rosenblum L. New York, John Wiley, 1974, pp 49–76

Burlingham D, Freud A: Young Children in Wartime. London, Allen & Unwin, 1942

Cameron HC: The Nervous Child. London, Oxford Medical Publications, 1919

Charlesworth WR: The role of surprise in cognitive development, in Studies in Cognitive Development: Essays in Honor of Jean Piaget. Edited by Elkind E, Flavell JH. London, Oxford University Press, 1969, pp 257–314

Cravioto J, DeLicardie E: Environmental correlates of severe clinical malnutrition and language development in survivors from kwashiorkor and marasmus, in Nutrition, the Nervous System and Behavior (PAHO Scientific Publication No 251). Washington, DC, PAHO, 1973

Ekman P: Universals and cultural differences in facial expressions of emotion. Nebr Symp Motiv, Vol 20, 1972

Emde RN, Gaensbauer TJ, Harmon RJ: Emotional Expression in Infancy: A Biobehavioral Study, Vol 37, 1976

Escalona SK: The Roots of Individuality. Chicago, IL, Aldine, 1968

Fraiberg S: Treatment modalities in an infant mental health program. Paper presented at "Clinical Approaches to Infants and Their Families," sponsored by the National Center for Clinical Infant Programs, Washington, DC, December 5–7, 1979

Gewirtz JL: A learning analysis of the effects of normal stimulation, privation and deprivation on the acquisition of social motivation and attachment, in Determinants of Infant Behavior, Vol 1. Edited by Foss BM. London, Methuen, 1961, pp 213–299

Gewirtz JL: The course of infant smiling in four child-rearing environments in Israel, in Determinants of Infant Behavior, Vol 3. Edited by Foss BM. London, Methuen, 1965, pp 205–260

Gewirtz JL: Levels of conceptual analysis in environment-infant interaction research. Merrill-Palmer Quarterly 15:9–47, 1969

Gouin-Decarie T: Intelligence and Affectivity in Early Childhood: An Experimental Study of Jean Piaget's Object Concept and Object Relations. New York, International Universities Press, 1965

Greenspan SI: Intelligence and Adaptation: An Integration of Psychoanalytic and Piagetian Developmental Psychology

(Psychological Issues No 47–48). New York, International Universities Press, 1979

Greenspan SI: Psychopathology and Adaptation in Infancy and Early Childhood: Principles of Clinical Diagnosis and Preventive Intervention (Clinical Infant Reports No 1). New York, International Universities Press, 1981

Greenspan SI: A model for comprehensive preventive intervention services for infants, young children and their families, in Infants in Multirisk Families. Edited by Wieder S, Lieberman AF, Nover RA, et al. New York, International Universities Press, 1987

Greenspan SI: The Development of the Ego. Madison, CT, International Universities Press, 1989

Hunt JM: Infants in an orphanage. Journal of Abnormal and Social Psychology 36:338, 1941

Izard C: On the development of emotions and emotion-cognition relationships in infancy, in The Development of Affect. Edited by Lewis M, Rosenblum L. New York, Plenum, 1978

Klaus MH, Kennell JH: Maternal-Infant Bonding: The Impact of Early Separation or Loss on Family Development. St. Louis, MO, CV Mosby, 1976

Lipsitt L: Learning processes of newborns. Merrill-Palmer Quarterly 12:45–71, 1966

Lowrey LG: Personality distortion and early institutional care. Am J Orthopsychiatry 10:576–585, 1940

Mahler MS, Pine F, Bergman A: The Psychological Birth of the Human Infant. New York, Basic Books, 1975

Meltzoff AN, Moore KM: Imitation of facial and manual gestures by human neonates. Science 198:75–78, 1977

Murphy LB, Moriarty AE: Vulnerability, Coping, and Growth. New Haven, CT, Yale University Press, 1976

Piaget J: The stages of the intellectual development of the child (1962), in Childhood Psychopathology. Edited by Harrison SI, McDermott JF. New York, International Universities Press, 1972, pp 157–166

Porges SW, Greenspan SI: Regulatory disordered infants: a common theme. Paper presented at the "RAUS Review Meeting on Methodological Issues in Controlled Studies on Effects of Prenatal Exposure to Drugs of Abuse," National Institute on Drug Abuse, Richmond, VA, June 8–9, 1990

Provence S: Infants and Parents: Clinical Case Reports (Clinical Infant Reports No 2). New York, International Universities Press, 1983

Rachford BK: Neurotic Disorders of Childhood. New York, EB Treat, 1905

Rheingold H: The development of social behavior in the human infant. Monogr Soc Res Child Dev 31:1, 1966

Rheingold H: Infancy, in International Encyclopedia of the Social Sciences. Edited by Sills D. New York, Macmillan, 1969

Sander LW: Issues in early mother-child interaction. Journal of the American Academy of Child Psychiatry 1:141–166, 1962

Spitz RA: Hospitalism. Psychoanal Study Child 1:53–74, 1945

Sroufe L: Socioemotional development, in Handbook of Infant Development. Edited by Osofsky J. New York, John Wiley, 1979

Sroufe L, Waters E: Attachment as an organizational construct. Child Dev 48:1184–1199, 1977

Stern DN: The goal and structure of mother-infant play. Journal of the American Academy of Child Psychiatry 13:402–421, 1974a

Stern DN: Mother and infant at play: the dyadic interaction involving facial, vocal, and gaze behaviors, in The Effect of the Infant on Its Caregiver. Edited by Lewis M, Rosenblum L. New York, John Wiley, 1974b, pp 187–213

Stern DN: The First Relationship: Infant and Mother. Cambridge, MA, Harvard University Press, 1977

Thomas A, Chess S: Temperament and Development. New York, Brunner/Mazel, 1977

Tomkins S: Affect, Imagery, Consciousness, Vol 1. New York, Springer, 1963a

Tomkins S: Affect, Imagery, Consciousness, Vol 2. New York, Springer, 1963b

Werner H, Kaplan B: Symbol Formation. New York, John Wiley, 1963

Winnicott DW: Clinical Notes on Disorders of Childhood. London, Heinemann, 1931

Chapter 7

The Clinical Interview of the Child

Clarice J. Kestenbaum, M.D.

The clinical interview always has been the sine qua non of the psychiatric evaluation. As Mackinnon and Michels (1971) observed in their book *The Psychiatric Interview in Clinical Practice*, a "clear understanding of the psychopathology and psychodynamics is the foundation of the psychiatric interview" (p. 1). In the assessment of an adult, the chief informant is the patient. Additional information may, of course, be requested from other physicians, hospital records, or psychological tests, but usually the skilled interviewer can obtain a psychiatric history and perform a mental status examination in one or two sessions if the adult is reasonably cooperative.

The task facing the child psychiatric interviewer, however, is far more complex. The interviewer first must take into account the child's age, cognitive level of development, and willingness to discuss problems. The examination of the child alone rarely, if ever, can serve as the only source of information sufficient to make a diagnosis; but the examiner can certainly form a valuable diagnostic impression. Information is needed that the child cannot supply: a developmental history (including genetic background), a broad understanding of the home environment, and some knowledge of the significant people in the child's life. A thorough assessment of the school and other aspects of the child's world often is needed for a comprehensive evaluation, including current or past events (e.g., the death of a parent, effects of divorce, or a traumatic event such as a fire or automobile accident) that may have a lasting impact on future development.

School reports as well as pediatric records (including a neurologic examination when indicated) may be sent to the diagnostician prior to the first visit. A psychological evaluation already may have been obtained or may be requested by the evaluator. Evaluation of family functioning is important. A family interview at some point in the evaluation process helps to determine the quality of the parent-child "fit"; for example, a depressed mother or alcoholic father and the effects of a disruptive home environment may become more apparent.

A more detailed discussion concerning history taking and the family interview is available elsewhere in this volume (see Leventhal and Conroy, Chapter 9; Sholevar, Chapter 10).

The clinical interview with the child should be considered as one piece of a puzzle that is ready to be assembled when all other data are gathered. In presenting a detailed method of approaching a child and the child's family from the initial telephone call to the final presentation of the findings, Gardner (1985) observed "that the initial interview and intensive evaluation should provide an in-depth understanding of the child's problems and also establish a good relationship or at least communication with the child and family members . . . without which the likelihood of a successful psychotherapy is minimal" (p. 371).

It is obvious that the evaluation process can take many weeks. The clinician who has the availability of the time and no concerns about third-party payers may see the child optimally four or five times before completing the evaluation. The interview technique depends on the orientation of the interviewer and is highly personal. I recall one senior psychiatrist's response to the question "What is the best way to learn interview technique?" "Twenty-five years of clinical experience," he answered. Child psychoanalysts such as Anna Freud (1946) and D. W.

Winnicott (1971) have made valuable contributions to our understanding of the process of child psychodynamic assessment. Good reviews of such techniques include Goodman and Sours' *The Child Mental Status Examination* (1967); Simmons' *Psychiatric Examination of Children* (1981); Greenspan's *The Clinical Interview of the Child* (1991); Coppollillo's *Psychodynamic Psychotherapy of Children: An Introduction to the Art and the Techniques* (1987); and Canino's "Taking a History" (1985).

In many cases, the clinical interview is performed under less-than-optimal circumstances. A court-referred adolescent or a child hospitalized on a pediatric ward may need an emergency consultation when other informants and data are not available.

Sometimes a single interview is all that the clinician is allowed even though a diagnostic impression must be formulated. Although structured interviews such as the Child Assessment Schedule (Hodges et al. 1982) and the Diagnostic Interview Schedule for Children (Costello et al. 1984) and semistructured interviews such as the Children's Version of the Schedule for Affective Disorders and Schizophrenia (Chambers et al. 1985) have been successfully designed for research purposes, they do not allow for the full range of feelings, personality organization, and coping mechanisms as does the free-range clinical interview. It was for these reasons that a semistructured clinical interview, the Mental Health Assessment Form (MHAF), was de-

---

Table 7-1.   Outline of the Mental Health Assessment Form

Part I—Mental status	Part II—Content of the interview
I. *Physical appearance*	VI. *Feeling states*
A. General attractiveness	A. Depression
B. Physical characteristics	B. Elation
C. Physical maturation	C. Mood disturbance (other)
D. Observable deviations in physical	D. Anger
characteristics	E. Anxiety
E. Grooming and dress	F. Irritability
F. Gender differentiation	G. Impulsivity
II. *Motoric behavior and speech*	VII. *Interpersonal relations*
A. Motor activity	A. The child's relationship to his or her family
B. Motor coordination	B. The child's relationship with other adult
C. Presence of unusual motoric patterns, habit	authority figures
patterns, and mannerisms	C. Relations with peers
D. Speech	D. Relationship to pets
III. *Relatedness during interview*	E. Modes of interaction with others
A. Quality of relatedness as judged by	F. Aggressive behavior
nonverbal behavior	G. Sexual behavior
B. Quality of relatedness as judged by verbal	VIII. *Symbolic representation (dreams and fantasies)*
behavior	A. Fantasy
C. Social interaction	B. Dreams
IV. *Affect*	IX. *Self-concept*
A. Inappropriate affect	A. Dissatisfaction with self
B. Constriction of affect	B. Comparison of self with peers
C. Elated affect	C. Comparison between self and ideal self
D. Depressed affect	X. *Conscience-moral judgment*
E. Labile affect	A. Deficit in development of conscience
F. Overanxious affect	B. Antisocial behavior
G. Angry affect	XI. *General level of adaptation*
H. Histrionic affect	A. Personality characteristics
V. *Language and thinking*	B. Defense mechanisms
A. Overall intelligence	C. Maladaptive solutions in dealing with anxiety
B. Cognitive functions	
C. External reality testing	
D. Use of language	
E. Thought process	
F. Attention span	

veloped by Kestenbaum and Bird (1978), providing a bridge between the structured questionnaire on the one hand and the open-ended clinical interview on the other. The MHAF may be used with children aged 6–12 years. (There is a supplement for adolescents.) It can be performed in a relatively brief period, 45 minutes, or extended for several sessions, depending on the clinical situation.

Cards or questionnaires are not used. The "structure" is in the mind of the examiner. The examiner needs to be familiar with child developmental principles and psychopathology, since the MHAF is intended for clinicians with a certain level of training and experience.

The interview itself involves an inquiry into all areas of a child's life and functioning, including specific questions about 1) the child in his or her family (a description of home and family life problems in family relationships); 2) the child in school (including relationship to teachers, peer relationships, sports, hobbies, homework); 3) fantasy life (quality and content of fantasies and dreams as well as problem-solving ability); and 4) personality organization (self-concept, overall mood, perceptions, coping mechanisms).

The MHAF consists of 189 items divided into two major sections (see Table 7-1). Part I is scored according to observable data and is primarily a mental status examination. It is subdivided into five major areas: physical appearance, motoric behavior and speech, relatedness during the interview, affect, and language and thinking. Part II scores information derived from the content of the interview. Both historical and developmental data elicited from the child during the interview are included. Part II also deals with the child's self-concepts and perceptions in his or her world. It is divided into six major areas: feeling states, interpersonal relations, symbolic representation (dreams and fantasies); self-concept, conscience-moral judgment, and general level of adaptation.

General level of adaptation includes positive attributes. These include personality characteristics such as skills or talents, interests (e.g., hobbies), perseverance ("stick-to-itiveness"), frustration tolerance, creativity, imagination, sense of humor, empathy, ability to cope with stress (e.g., actual events by history such as separations, hospitalizations, illness), and problem-solving ability (when given an imaginary situation).

The rater must use both clinical experience and theoretical knowledge to determine whether the particular item is to be scored within the expectable range, or the degree of deviance from age-group "norms."

There is a section at the end of the form for descriptive information.

The semistructured interview designed specifically for the MHAF interview can be geared toward younger or older children and takes into account degrees of cooperation and resistance.

Suggested questions are presented in an open-ended manner (see Table 7-2). The examiner is advised to follow the child's lead and not stay rigidly within a given framework. He or she may return at any time to topics that were brushed aside or ignored the first time around (Bird and Kestenbaum 1988).

Table 7-2.   Questions suggested for the semistructured interview

School
What grade are you in?
What is your best subject? Which is the worst?
Are you better in subjects in which you have to figure things out or ones that require memory?
Have you ever been held back in school?

Interpersonal relations (family)
Who lives at home with you?
Do you have brothers and sisters?
How do you all get along?
Who else is in your family?
When you have a problem, whom do you tell about it?
Does he/she help you with your problem?
Who is the closest person to you in your family?
Who gives you the most problems? Tell me about that.
How do you get along with your mother/father?
Who is your favorite?

(continued)

Table 7-2. *(Continued)*

Dependence-independence with family members
Do your parents tell you what to do or can you make some of your decisions?
What are the rules at home about going out alone or getting home, bringing friends home, etc.?
Have you ever been away from home at sleep-away camp or at a friend's home? How did you feel about being away?
What happens at home when you do something wrong or break the rules?

Interpersonal relationships: other adults
What kind of relationship do you have with other adults (grown-ups) outside the family (e.g., teachers, coach, minister, counselor)?
Is there someone you especially admire?
Which adults do you respect the least?

Interpersonal relations: peers
Do you have friends?
Are most of your friends about your age?
Do you have friends who are older? Younger?
Do you have a best friend?
How long has he/she been your best friend?
What sort of things do you do together?
Why did you pick him/her as your best friend?
How do you feel when something good (bad) happens to one of your friends?
Do you do what most kids want to do, or do they do what you want?
What happens when you can't get your own way?

Future plans
What would you like to be when you grow up?
Why do you think you would enjoy that?
Do you know any (name occupation choice)?
How good are your chances of becoming (occupation)?
What would you do if you couldn't be a (occupation)?
Have you ever had an after-school or summer job?
What did/do you do with the money you made/make?

Gender concepts and behavior
What are the advantages of being a boy (girl)?
What are the disadvantages?
Do you like being a boy/girl?
Suppose you could start all over again. Would you rather be a boy/girl?

Self-concept
If I asked your parents what they think about you, what would they say?
Suppose I asked your friends?
If you could change anything about yourself, what would you change?
How do you compare yourself with your friends (in sports, looks, intelligence, personality)?
Do you like the way you are? Do people like you?

Conscience
What was your best deed?
What is the worst thing you've ever done?
Did it get you into trouble?
How did you feel?
Did you ever take something that didn't belong to you? What?
What happened? How did you feel?
How do you feel when you do something you know is wrong?
Do you ever do it again?

Table 7-2.   (*Continued*)

Feeling states: general
How do you feel most of the time? (happy/sad)
How do you feel now compared with the way you usually feel?
What sort of things make you happy? Sad?
What things do you enjoy doing most of all?
What was the happiest time in your life?

Feeling states: anxiety
What things make you nervous?
What is the scariest thing that's ever happened to you?
What happens when you get scared like that?
When you are scared, does it bother you in other ways, like you can't sleep or get headaches?
Do you ever feel scared like that for no reason at all?
What does that feel like?

Feeling states: depression
What is the saddest thing that ever happened to you?
Do you ever feel sad even if there's no good reason? Tell me about that.
Do you ever think of dying? Have you ever thought of killing yourself? Have you ever tried to kill yourself?
When you feel sad like that, does it ever last many days in a row? How many days?
When you feel sad like that, does it bother you in other ways, like you can't sleep, appetite? Does that last many
    days in a row? How many days?
Did you ever feel the opposite, like you're on top of the world, for no reason at all? Tell me about it (duration,
    severity, other descriptive symptoms).

Feeling states: anger
What do you do when you really want something and you don't get your way?
Do you have a "short fuse" (lose your temper easily)?
What sort of things make you angry?
What do you do when you get very angry?
Do you ever get into fights? With whom?
(If yes) Do you fight alone or in a group?

Reality testing
Do you think there are people who can predict the future?
Do you believe in ESP? Have you had experiences like that? Some people, when they get very nervous, have funny
    experiences. Did it ever happen to you that you heard voices inside/outside your head? Were you fully awake?
    What did they say? (frequency, severity) What do you think that was?
Some kids have told me that they think their minds are controlled by something or someone else. Others believe
    someone is looking at them or talking about them when it really isn't so. Did something like that ever happen to
    you?

Fantasy
Do you have an active imagination?
When you're bored in school and looking out the window, what do you think about?
Make believe we just heard a loud noise outside the window. Can you make up a story about what happened?
Do you dream a lot?
How often do you dream?
Are most of your dreams good dreams or bad dreams?
Tell me about a dream that you remember.
Did you ever (do you) have a make-believe friend? Tell me about him/her.
Do you keep a diary of your secret thoughts?

Other
What do you think the future will be like?
What do you think happens to people after they die?
Do you play sports? Are you good in sports?
Do you have any hobbies?
Do you have any special talents (e.g., drawing, music)?

Interviewing the Younger Child (5–9 Years Old)

There is no "best way" to interview children. Various techniques are derived from practicing a variety of established approaches with numbers of children and adding new approaches that have proved helpful in establishing rapport with young children in a relatively brief time period (no checklists). What follows is a distillate of my clinical experience.

In most circumstances, one or both parents shall be interviewed before meeting with the child to ascertain the nature of the presenting problem, to obtain pertinent information, and to suggest ways of informing the child about the nature of the psychiatric examination. In those instances when the child refuses to leave the parent (usually a manifestation of separation anxiety), the parent is invited into the consultation room. Otherwise, the child is interviewed alone.

Most children spend a few minutes examining the strange surroundings, such as children's books, drawing materials, a dollhouse with simple furniture and little dolls, several hand puppets in full view, and a few standard games. An explanation may be given about the nature of the interview, with some reassurance if necessary.

The interview can begin by asking why the child has been brought to see me:

Marjorie (age 7): I don't know.
Dr. K: Did your mother explain that I am the kind of doctor who helps children with their feelings and troubles?
Marjorie: No.
Dr. K: Well, I am. Some children have the kind of troubles everyone can see. For instance, if there's a child in school who bullies other children, or yells or throws things in class or gets into fights. . . .
Marjorie: Billy's like that. He's always in the principal's office.
Dr. K: Yes, exactly. I might see someone like Billy to help him with his problem controlling himself. But I also see children who have problems no one can see—worries about their parents going away, bad dreams, sad feelings.

Marjorie said nothing but a solemn nod let me know my words made an impression.

After such an introductory statement, I shift gears and begin the interview with neutral questions about the child's home, family members, and pets. I might ask her to draw a floor plan of her house or apartment—her room, the distance from her parents'

room, the approximate distance to the school—and perhaps a rough sketch of her family. In 5 minutes I have already observed her enough to score (mentally) the first part of the MHAF: general attractiveness, motor activity and coordination, presence or absence of tics, quality of speech, and relatedness to me (usually determined by eye contact, shyness, withdrawal, and general affect). I can estimate her overall level of intelligence by her use of vocabulary and comprehension, her ability to follow directions, and her graphomotor skill in drawing. Of course, if there seems to be a problem in cognitive functioning, I will order a psychological examination if one had not already been obtained. I usually turn the conversation to the subject of favorite activities, friends, playdates, and "sleepovers."

In Marjorie's case, where her parents were concerned about school avoidance and somatic complaints, the child was not forthcoming about her worries and particularly avoided questions about school:

Dr. K: Marjorie, do you see that boy puppet over there? Reach in that bag and take out some of those people.
Marjorie: Those are finger puppets. (She took two puppets that represented children.)
Dr. K: I'll take these two (adult figures). Hi, I'm Mrs. Smith, your teacher. What are your names?
Marjorie (with a little prodding): Mary and Susie.
Dr. K (whispering to her): Which one knows all the right answers and which one has trouble? (Marjorie responds by pointing to each puppet.) All right, children. Today we'll have math. How much is 2 + 2? How do you spell cat?
Marjorie (answering for puppet figures): 4, but only Mary can spell cat. Susie can't read.
(After several minutes of simple questions, I introduced a third puppet: the good wizard.)
Dr. K: I am the wizard who can grant all your wishes. What would you want more than anything in the world, Susie?
Marjorie: To be smart.

In my experience, for a child with school problems, nothing so readily establishes the distinction between a learning disability and attention-deficit or conduct disorder as this kind of fantasy play. Further testing in Marjorie's case and appropriate academic intervention coupled with brief psychotherapy for herself and her family proved extremely helpful.

Other techniques with younger children are projective "make-believe" questions. For example, the same question brought forth very different responses from a dysthymic 8-year-old and a psychotic child of the same age:

> *Dr. K:* Billy, make believe you are looking out the window and you hear an enormous crash. What do you see?
> *Billy:* Two cars crash into each other.
> *Dr. K:* And then what happens?
> *Billy:* The ambulance comes.
> *Dr. K:* And then what?
> *Billy:* Nothing. Everyone is dead.

Most nondepressed children, unlike Billy, manage to get the passengers to a hospital where everyone is eventually saved. In response to the same question, Mark's was decidedly bizarre.

> *Mark:* A monster from outer space throws a bomb and the whole world is killed and all the people in it and you and me too and then he eats all the pieces up and ocean is all bloody and he drinks it and it's delicious.

Another projective technique is a variant of Winnicott's (1971) "squiggles" game: drawing a scribbled design and asking the child to use his or her imagination, to complete the drawing by turning it into anything he or she thinks of, and then to tell a story about the completed picture.

Asking for a description of a favorite television program is another useful maneuver. Does the child relate the story in a logical sequential fashion or are cognitive deficits demonstrated?

Overall mood can be elicited by the appearance of the "mood machine." Facing the child, I extend one arm, bent 90° at the elbow.

> *Dr. K:* William, pretend my arm is a pendulum and on one side we have "happiness," on the other side "sadness," and straight up is "neutral." (I swing my arm slowly.) Now, when my arm reaches the place that describes how you feel most of the time, yell "stop."

I then ask the child to describe the happiest and saddest events in his or her life. I often inquire about dreams and, when possible, ask the child to draw a picture of the dream. This can lead to inquiry about perceptual distortions, such as familiar objects taking on frightening aspects, illusions at night, hypnagogic phenomena, or hallucinations.

Eliciting feelings about family members should be done after rapport has been established. The parent with whom the child feels closest or safest can then be determined, as can the examiner's own impression of the "fairness" of discipline, any overly strict or punitive parenting, and any actual child

abuse. (Rarely will an abused child actually accuse the parent of physical or sexual abuse in the first session.)

Interviewing the Older Child (10–12 Years Old)

There is no explicit age cutoff point where the interviewer knows with certainty whether to begin with the version of the MHAF designed for younger children or shape questions according to the presumed cognitive level of the preadolescent or adolescent youngster. Some 10-year-olds do far better using techniques usually reserved for younger children; others conduct themselves like teenagers. A sensitive interviewer will know when to shift gears. In general, I begin with the chief complaint. Frequently, the older child also will deny having any problems.

> *William (age 10):* My parents said I had to come or I could not watch TV.
> *Dr. K:* Boy, they must really think there's a problem. What do you think about it?
> *William:* Nothing. Ask them!
> *Dr. K:* I did already, but you know, I'm not so interested in their opinion as I am yours. You know, the fact that they think there's a problem and even insist on your coming when you think there's no problem at all . . . well, even that's a problem! Besides, whatever you tell me is a one-way street. I want to hear all sides but I don't repeat back to them what you say. I like to form my own opinion.

Usually this type of opening is sufficient to establish some degree of rapport.

After inquiries about interests and school activities, children are asked to describe their friends (or enemies). Then they may be asked, for example, "If I asked your best friend about you, what would he (she) say?"

For preadolescents, self-esteem is very much connected to body image. "If there is anything you could change about yourself, what would it be?" (Most very young adolescents discuss their pimples, hair color, braces, or other unsightly blemishes. If the answer is "everything," depression is a major diagnostic consideration.)

It is important to obtain some idea about the development of empathy. Exploring feelings about animals is usually a useful approach. Inquire about family pets, their names, personality characteristics, and children's identifications with their pets.

Other questions probing for empathic feelings bring forth a variety of responses:

Dr. K: What would you do if a new girl appeared in class one day in the middle of the term?
Jill (age 11): Well, I'd go over to her and tell her my name and introduce her to my friends and show her where the bathroom is and all.
Dr. K: Why would you do that?
Jill: Well, I went to a new school once and I felt all scared and alone and so I'd know how she feels.
Billy (age 10, responding to the same question except that the newcomer is a boy): Well, I wouldn't hit him or anything . . . not on the first day.

Questions about superego or conscience formation usually bring a myriad of responses:

Dr. K: Let's suppose that a man is walking down the street in front of you and a $10.00 bill slips from his pocket and lands on the sidewalk. What would you do?
Arthur (age 11): I'd pick it up and call, "Hey mister, you dropped your money!" Maybe I'd get a reward.
Jim (age 10): I'd keep it. Finders keepers!
Martha (age 11): I'd run over and give it back.
Dr. K: What if he crossed the street and cars were coming?
Martha: I'd wait for the light to change and try to find him.
Dr. K: What if you couldn't?
Martha: Well, I'd take it to the police and ask if anyone lost $10.00.

Most children find the type of interview I have described reassuring and nonpressured. I usually try to end the session on an upbeat note with a statement such as "I think we can put our heads together and figure out what we want to do." If psychotherapy is indicated and the evaluating psychiatrist is not available for treatment, let the child know that as consultant you will find the right person to help with the problem. Always explain what the next step will be, whether it is further testing, a second interview, a family interview, or a visit with the parents alone.

Summing-up Session

When all information has been gathered and a diagnostic impression is formed, a treatment plan is formulated. Then an appointment is set up with the parents to discuss options.

Often several treatment modalities may be indicated: psychotherapy with parental counseling, psychoanalysis, pharmacologic intervention combined with therapy, family therapy, tutoring, or language and learning therapy. The recommendation could be a change of school, residential placement, or hospitalization. The parents need to feel comfortable discussing their finances and the range of possibilities so that the best arrangement can be instituted, taking individual circumstances into account. When acting as a consultant, one must be available for helping with the disposition and facilitating treatment, particularly in the event that the child or family is not satisfied with the referral. Setting the fee, establishing rules, discussing vacations, and the like take place during the summing-up session. Once a treatment plan has been selected, the child is invited to participate in the subsequent planning (for instance, the session time should not compete with a regular after-school activity) and discuss the reasons for the type of treatment offered.

Diamond (1988) discussed parental reluctance to accept treatment recommendations in an excellent chapter on general issues in clinical assessment, a reluctance that is usually reflected in whining, silent, or uncooperative children.

Conclusion

The semistructured interview described in this chapter is only one aspect of the total evaluation. It provides a reliable and comprehensive assessment of the signs and symptoms of psychiatric disorder as well as positive attributes and strengths. Moreover, such an interview is therapeutic in that a relationship is established from the outset, an important factor if further psychotherapy is the recommended intervention. Used together with the information based on physical examination, past history, and intellectual functioning, in addition to the problems reported by patients and their parents, it provides a valid psychiatric diagnosis that can result in an optimal psychotherapeutic intervention.

References

Bird H, Kestenbaum CJ: A semi-structured approach to clinical assessment, in Handbook of Clinical Assessment of Children and Adolescents. Edited by Kestenbaum CJ, Williams DT. New York, New York University Press, 1988, pp 19–30
Canino IA: Taking a history, in The Clinical Guide to Child

Psychiatry. Edited by Shaffer D, Erhardt AA, Greenhill LL. New York, Free Press, 1985, pp 393–408

Chambers WJ, Puig-Antich J, Hirsch M, et al: The assessment of affective disorders in children and adolescents by semi-structured interview: test-retest reliability of the K-SADS-P. Arch Gen Psychiatry 42:696–702, 1985

Coppollillo H: Psychodynamic Psychotherapy of Children: An Introduction to the Art and the Techniques. Madison, CT, International Universities Press, 1987

Costello AJ, Edelbrock CS, Dulcan M: Report on the NIMH Diagnostic Interview Schedule for Children (DISC). Washington, DC, National Institute of Mental Health, 1984

Diamond CB: General issues in the clinical assessment of children and adolescents, in Handbook of Clinical Assessment of Children and Adolescents. Edited by Kestenbaum CJ, Williams DT. New York, New York University Press, 1988, pp 43–55

Freud A: The Psycho-Analytic Treatment of Children. London, Imago, 1946

Gardner RA: The initial clinical evaluation of the child, in The Clinical Guide to Child Psychiatry. Edited by Shaffer D, Ehr-hardt AA, Greenhill LL. New York, Free Press, 1985, pp 371–392

Goodman JD, Sours JA: The Child Mental Status Examination. New York, Basic Books, 1967

Greenspan S: The Clinical Interview of the Child. Washington, DC, American Psychiatric Press, 1991

Hodges K, McKnew D, Cytryn L, et al: The Child Assessment Schedule (CAS) Diagnostic Interview: a report on reliability and validity. Journal of the American Academy of Child Psychiatry 21:468–473, 1982

Kestenbaum CJ, Bird HR: A reliability study of the Mental Health Assessment Form for school-age children. Journal of the American Academy of Child Psychiatry 17:338–347, 1978

Mackinnon R, Michels R: The Psychiatric Interview in Clinical Practice. Philadelphia, PA, WB Saunders, 1971

Simmons JK: Psychiatric Examination of Children, 3rd Edition. Philadelphia, PA, Lea & Febiger, 1981

Winnicott DW: Therapeutic Consultations in Child Psychiatry. New York, Basic Books, 1971

Chapter 8

The Clinical Interview of the Adolescent

John E. Schowalter, M.D.
Robert A. King, M.D.

The psychiatric evaluation of an adolescent is intended to obtain as full a picture as possible of the current difficulties in the overall context of the strengths and weaknesses of the adolescent and his or her family (Schowalter and Fisher 1982). Although formal psychological testing, structured instruments, laboratory data, or information gathered from school may be useful adjuncts, the heart of this clinical endeavor is the diagnostic interview with the adolescent and family.

The Prologue

It is important early on to clarify who is the moving force in seeking consultation and what is the adolescent's attitude toward the process. The adult patient, by seeking out a therapist, acknowledges, at least implicitly, a problem and a desire for assistance. In contrast, the primary-school–age child is most often simply brought by the parents. The adolescent's situation lies somewhere in between. Many adolescents take a cautious and ambiguous stance as to whether there is any problem for which help is wanted, or instead there is mere passive compliance with a parental initiative.

Several considerations must guide the clinician in deciding whether the first interview should be with the adolescent, the parents, or all together. Seeing the adolescent first underlines his or her active participation in the process and serves to allay anxiety that the doctor and parents will collude or gang up on the youngster. However, some adolescents will protest that this casts them in the role of being the problem or the patient, when in their view the difficulty lies instead with their parents or between family members. The clinician needs to make clear that he or she is not out to assign blame, but rather to help understand the difficulties the adolescent and the family have been confronting and to hear the views of all concerned. This usually requires both individual and family interviews. In most cases, the adolescent should be seen before the parents, but the parents may need to be seen first if they have difficulty in getting their child to come for the first appointment.

The parents also should be seen alone to hear their concerns, to assess their explicit and implicit reasons for seeking assistance at this time, and to obtain a developmental and family history. (Details of the family interview are discussed elsewhere in this volume [see Sholevar, Chapter 10].)

The interview with the parents also yields valuable data concerning their view of the role played by the adolescent and the symptomatology in the psychic economy of the parents as individuals, as a couple, and in the family as a whole.

It often is useful at some point in the evaluation to interview the adolescent and parents together. The clinician frames the meeting's purpose as a forum for family members to talk together; active structuring of this meeting may be needed to prevent the session from deteriorating into a "you hold him while I hit him" session in which the parents tell the doctor what is wrong with their child. Without the interviewer's active intervention, the adolescent may become very guarded or adversarial when seen with the parents. A family interview provides a useful opportunity to see how family members interact and to scrutinize overt and covert alliances and conflicts, shared family assumptions, coping patterns, and convergent and divergent areas of concern, as well as the family's ability to work together therapeutically and to make constructive use of the clinician.

Confidentiality

Adolescents generally are very sensitive to the extremity of some of their thoughts and actions. Many fear that this information might be divulged by the clinician to their parents or to other authority figures. It is important from the outset for the parents and the adolescent to know that therapist-patient interactions are confidential. The exception is when the therapist believes the patient or someone else is in danger. This rule should be spelled out at the beginning, not only for general clarity, but to emphasize that it is a generic and not a specific response to a particular patient or disclosure. Patients sometimes want the clinician to tell something to parents or others, "because you can say it much better than I can." Such a spokesperson role occasionally may be indicated, but should be preceded by a careful discussion and, if carried out, done in the adolescent's presence.

Developmental Issues and Interview Behavior

The clinician's approach to the interview with the adolescent is informed by an understanding of the developmental tasks and dynamics of adolescence and by the characteristic patterns used by adolescents to relate to adults and to manage their conflicts and anxiety (Meeks 1971; Mishne 1986). In the process of reworking and loosening dependent and libidinal ties to parents, adolescents turn, at times with a vengeance, to peers as objects of support and longing. Although some nonparental adults may be admired and turned to for guidance or identification, the adolescent's relationship with most adults is colored by a strong push toward autonomy and a great wariness of feeling vulnerable, dependent, or controlled. Even many adolescents who consciously want help approach a clinical evaluation with anxiety over revealing problems that they may regard as shameful weaknesses and with concerns over being criticized, controlled, over-

whelmed, or becoming regressively dependent. These apprehensions may take the form of bland denials of any difficulties or insistence that either "everything is OK," or "I can handle it by myself." Narcissistic vulnerability and difficulty tolerating ambivalence, internal conflicts, or painful feelings lead many adolescents to portray their problems as arising from outside, rather than from within themselves. Adolescents often externalize one side or another of their conflicted feelings. Thus a youngster may focus on bitter complaints of parental overprotectiveness, while ignoring inner insecurities or wishes to be taken care of. Many adolescents deal with anxiety, guilt, shame, and other painful affects by means of counterphobic maneuvers or reversal of affect. For example, frightened teenagers may pick fights rather than take flight, and it is not unusual for sad adolescents to feel primarily angry during an interview. The clinician must learn to look beyond the adolescent's surface behavior and develop a capacity to notice when the youngster "doth protest too much."

An unrealistic faith in the "omnipotence of thought" is also characteristic of many adolescents who want to believe that even long-standing maladaptive patterns can be overcome simply by having resolved to do things differently. Exploration of a problem area may thus be resisted with the sincere protestation, "Oh, I don't do that any more" (i.e., not since yesterday).

Adolescents' moods are labile, and their time perspective is short. Today's insoluble crisis, eternal passion, or irreversible decision may be forgotten by next week. Therefore, it is useful to be able to evaluate an adolescent over time to assess which issues are transient and which enduring. Of course, a propensity to frequent, albeit transient, upsets is in itself an important vulnerability to note.

Personal Issues for the Interviewer

Work with adolescents makes special demands on the clinician and is not to everyone's taste. Recall and comfort with one's own adolescence are an enormous advantage. Enjoying teenagers is a prime prerequisite, followed by tact, flexibility, and a sense of humor.

Schopenhauer once described friendship as "the art of distances." The same might be said of adolescent interviewing. Conveying a genuine and benign interest in the adolescent is essential. Condescension, aloofness, or excessive passivity in the interviewer is likely to be fatal. On the other hand, most adolescents will be frightened by overfamiliarity, seductiveness, or the clinician's failure to maintain an adult role. Adolescents' narcissism is exquisitely tender, and one must learn how to talk frankly, yet tactfully, about vulnerable areas in such a way that they do not feel they are being criticized. In the face of some adolescents' insistence that "you are either for me or against me," the clinician's task is to convey a genuine empathic interest in the adolescent's own view of the situation without collusively implying uncritical acceptance of that view. Clinicians who work with adolescents need a good measure of knowledge about their own adolescence and what they have made of that experience. Clinicians must also be aware of their feelings and biases about parenting. For example, at moments, the clinician may feel tempted to identify strongly with the patients' struggles against authority or feel a twinge of envy at their seeming freedom of sexual or aggressive expression; on the other hand, the clinician may find that certain adolescents or situations stir censorious or confrontational impulses or an identification with beleaguered or embattled parents. In short, the interviewer may feel either pressured to regress to an adolescent's viewpoint or propelled into a defensive parental stance.

The Interview

In the interview, the clinician is interested in several aspects of the presenting problem. What is the nature of the difficulty the adolescent is experiencing, and what areas of adaptive functioning are affected and to what degree? How does the adolescent think about the problem—as one lying entirely within, as a problem between himself or herself and others, or as a difficulty coming solely from without? Is the difficulty acute or long-standing? Which elements of the problem seem reactive and which appear related to intrapsychic conflict or character? Do the symptoms provide important secondary gains for the patient or family? If chronic medical illness or constitutionally based developmental difficulties (such as dyslexia) are present, what has the adolescent made of them?

Beyond the manifest problem, the clinician also wants to assess the adolescent's personality structure and level of psychosexual development. Of particular importance are such ego functions as the capacity to tolerate frustration or anxiety, the degree of psychological mindedness, the quality of mood regulation, and vulnerability to regression or impulsivity. This broader assessment of the adolescent's strengths and weaknesses is best accomplished in the course of reviewing how the adolescent is coping with the major adaptive tasks in the various realms of his or her life: school, family, and friends. It is important to inquire matter-of-factly about sadness, suicidality, eating habits, drug and alcohol use, and the presence of possible legal difficulties.

The degree to which one performs a formal, as opposed to an informal, mental status examination depends on variables such as the severity of the disorder, the reason for the evaluation, the time available, and the experience of the interviewer. A more formal approach is likely to be used when a disorder is severe, when precise documentation is required, or when there are concerns about the possibility of psychosis, dementia, or an organic brain syndrome. Basic areas to be covered in both formal and informal mental status examinations include the adolescent's general appearance, behavior, ability to relate, mood perceptions, thought content and coherence, memory, general information, intelligence, judgment, and insight.

To obtain a full picture, it is important not to limit the interview to areas of difficulty. The adolescent should know that the interviewer is interested in learning about him or her as a whole person, including areas of strength, enjoyment, and accomplishment. Adolescents may become defensive or blandly deny difficulties in the face of too-exclusive focus on pathology. The experienced and empathic diagnostician conveys a genuine interest in learning about the nature, quality, and depth of the young person's interests, hobbies, and recreations. Rather than demonstrating or feigning one's familiarity with the latest rock group, sports cars, or athletic team, it is preferable to let the adolescent teach one about his or her particular interests. In so doing, the adolescent is able to enjoy a sense of mastery and control and some sense of parity with the adult examiner. At the same time, the clinician is able to learn what blend of interests, identifications, sublimations, and direct instinctual and narcissistic gratifications animate the adolescent. The temptation to make early interpretations is best resisted. Even, perhaps especially, if accurate, they are more likely to scare the patient away than to impress him or her with the interviewer's sagacity.

A closely related area is that of values, ideals, and aspirations (Kernberg 1978). What are the adolescent's values and who are the adolescent's models for emulation or disidentification? Are these values congruent or in conflict with those of the patient's family, subculture, or larger society? What is the adolescent's sense of the future, and what aspirations, realistic or not, does the adolescent have for it?

The world of friends and peers is another related area for exploration. With whom does the patient "hang out"? What do they do for fun? How do they get along? Friends may be chosen on many grounds, including shared interests, admired virtues, or repudiated aspects of the adolescent's self. Friends may function as sources of support or admiration, as partners for sexual or aggressive exploitation, as collusive companions in regression or delinquency, as targets for projection, and so on. Asking the adolescent to tell one what a close friend is like provides an opportunity to learn how the adolescent thinks about people and relationships and to assess his or her capacity for empathy. Adolescents' own concerns are often more readily revealed in displacement: "I have a friend who is always. . . ." It is sometimes helpful to ask whether a friend is bothered by or involved with something the adolescent has denied but is likely involved in himself or herself.

The topic of peer friendships leads naturally to the topic of dating and sexual relationships. This is an area requiring tact and a good measure of rapport with the patient. Even so, one may not always receive a fully candid response during the diagnostic phase. Beyond the usual issues of privacy, this area of adolescents' lives is usually filled with concern and uncertainty, no matter how enlightened they may consider themselves to be. Does the teenager date, and is there anyone of either sex with whom he or she is close? What is the other person like, and what attracted each to the other? How has the relationship gone? Are there patterns in regard to the type of person found attractive and to the course of past relationships? When the patient has romantic daydreams (as we all do), what are they like? What is the script? Have any of the patient's relationships developed into sexual ones? Has the adolescent had other sexual experiences? Here one wants to be open to hear about possible episodes of sexual abuse and concerns about sexual

orientation. The goal goes beyond assessing the patient's popularity, experience, and ease with intimacy. Rather, the clinician is interested in the patient's "preconditions for loving" and the influences guiding object choice, as well as the extent to which recurrent anxiety, envy, ambivalence, sadomasochism, or issues of exploitation or narcissistic gratification interfere with the capacity for intimacy.

The Epilogue

Because of the adolescent's natural concern, it is important that at the end of the initial interview(s) the clinician summarize the findings. This should occur after the patient has been invited to add anything about which the interviewer has not asked and to say what he or she believes to be the best approach to be taken. Although this response may be quite different from what the clinician plans to propose, it is better to know areas of disagreement and resistance earlier than later.

Almost always, it is better first to share the recommendations and the reasons for them with the adolescent alone. An exception is when hospitalization is mandatory and parental support and quick action are required. Otherwise, it is useful to get the adolescent's reactions, to discuss any potential confidentiality questions, and to make any adjustments that seem indicated for the initial plan. The subsequent summarization for the parent or parents should be in the adolescent's presence.

References

Kernberg O: The diagnosis of borderline conditions in the adolescent. Adolesc Psychiatry 6:298–319, 1978

Meeks J: The Fragile Alliance. Baltimore, MD, Williams & Wilkins, 1971

Mishne JM: Clinical Work With Adolescents. New York, Free Press, 1986

Schowalter JE, Fisher SM: Special perspectives on treatment planning for adolescents, in Treatment Planning in Psychiatry. Edited by Lewis JM, Usdin G. Washington, DC, American Psychiatric Association, 1982, pp 337–376

Chapter 9

The Parent Interview

Bennett L. Leventhal, M.D.
Leslie M. Conroy, M.D.

The most commonly practiced procedure in all of medicine is the clinical interview. The capacity to perform this most critical clinical procedure is inherent to good practice, and in no other specialty is it more critical than in child and adolescent psychiatry. The clinical interview must be adapted to accommodate the examination of not only individuals who present with vastly different developmental capacities, but also the effective examinations of third parties who may be the sole source of information about the identified patient. One such third party is the parents of the child or adolescent patient. By providing information about the child and family, the parents enable the clinician to understand not only the child's behavior but also the functioning of the family, the individual, the environment, and the whole system in which the child exists (Group for the Advancement of Psychiatry 1957).

There would seem to be general agreement among clinicians that it is vitally important to be able to interview parents as part of the clinical process. However, there is some controversy, both theoretically and methodologically. On one hand, there is Freud (1909/1955), who spent a great deal of time and learned quite a bit about his famous patient, Little Hans, primarily from Hans' father. However, a rather different perspective is represented by some family therapists who view assessment and intervention with the child and parents as a simultaneous event and, consequently, may not even rely on the individual parent interview as part of their clinical process (Green 1982; Walsh 1983).

Rutter and Cox (1985) emphasized the impor-

tance of children's experiences in their family lives. They clearly identified not only the role of parents in modifying children's behaviors, but also the child's role in shaping parental behaviors. Additionally, they pointed out that there are different types of parenting, which interact in a unique way with a particular child's development, behaviors, and other characteristics, thus implying the necessity of interviewing parents in any evaluation or treatment process.

Given that parental interviewing is an important part of working with children and adolescents, we must be concerned about the utility of the information that is acquired. Does the parent interview provide a reliable account of the information necessary to formulate a diagnosis, establish a treatment plan, and monitor the treatment of a given child? When one thinks broadly about the notion of interviewing parents—that is, the use of structured interviews, unstructured interviews, and parent report scales—one recognizes that there is enormous variability in the quantity and quality and, hence, the reliability and validity of the information obtained. Indeed, studies have shown that parental reports of information are often temporarily distorted and that parents may deny a particular problem or are unable to recall pertinent past behavior (Chess et al. 1966). Mednick and Shaffer (1963) arrived at similar conclusions as a result of their studies of mothers' retrospective reports collected in a pediatric setting. Maternal interviews were compared with pediatric records, and the mothers' reports were found to be discrepant 21%–62% of the time for facts about discrete experiences, such as breast feeding, childhood illnesses, and the age of completion of toilet training.

Kashani et al. (1985) also found low agreement between parents and children on all DSM-III-R (American Psychiatric Association 1987) Axis I disorders. Interestingly, the patterns of disagreement were generally consistent in that children reported more anxiety and depressive symptoms, whereas parents stressed more externalizing symptoms, such as oppositional behavior and short attention span. The authors concluded that multiple sources of information might help the clinician arrive at a clearer clinical picture.

Weissman et al. (1987) reviewed numerous studies and identified discrepancies between parent and child reports on the nature, extent, and severity of children's symptoms. Irrespective of the interview setting, the diagnostic criteria, the method of interview, or the symptom scales, the authors found that children reported far more information about all their disorders. Indeed, Weissman et al. made the recommendation that, at least in certain types of studies, one should consider interviewing only the child if a choice had to be made.

In contrast to the foregoing, Orvaschel et al. (1981) found that parents were more accurate in providing factual time-related information. Using the Diagnostic Interview Schedule for Children (DISC; Costello et al. 1982) and the DISC-P (the Parents Interview of the DISC), Edelbrock et al. (1985) attempted to assess age differences in the reliability in interviews of children. Not surprisingly, they found that the reliability of a child's report increased with the child's age and with the presence of overt behaviors such as aggression and hyperactivity. The importance of parental collaboration was most evident in the results of structured parent interviews for younger children. In general, parents were felt to be more reliable than their children up until about the age of 10, after which time there was little or no difference in the parent and child reports.

Despite reported discrepancies, parents can and do provide essential information about a child's birth, development, medical history, and current functioning as well as symptomatology and the marital and family history. Diagnostic and clinical work with children is invariably "more than the classification of a child in a nosologic system based on the clinical observation and the description of the presenting signs and symptoms of deviant behavior" (Group for the Advancement of Psychiatry 1957, p. 322). Although so-called factual information about children and their functioning is important, other information that is not so concrete and not so obvious may be inconsistently collected, evaluated, and incorporated in the evaluation process. It is critical to remember that parental involvement and parental interviews are not just to provide this factual information. Instead, they are an integral part of developing the relationship between clinician, the patient, and the family. An alliance with the parents is very important in reaching a consensus about the nature of their problems and in developing and implementing a treatment plan (Simmons 1987).

Simmons (1987) warned the clinician to identify clearly "who is your patient." The child may be presented as the identified patient. However, careful discussion with the parents and the child, and examination of each parent, the marital couple, the family, the child's school, and the family's community, are necessary to assess the child and to develop an intervention plan. Thus most clinicians ultimately agree that the parent interview is but one component of an evaluation that, even if conducted in isolation, must be placed into the clinical context. Data gathered from the parents, as well as from other parties, may well be greatly affected by the attitude toward the referral as well as the child and other matters in the child's life. Furthermore, it would appear to be essential, in most clinical settings, to evaluate features such as parental temperament, personality organization, psychopathology, and other factors to place the data, which the parents provide, into a proper clinical context that also includes the child's role in the parents' struggles and unconscious and conscious wishes for the child, and so on (Greenspan 1991).

What, then, is the actual function of the parent interview? Certainly the gathering of information about the child's history and the child's present functioning is crucial. Equally important, however, is the opportunity for the clinician to develop an alliance. This alliance may be the key to sustaining an evaluation and treatment process and to fostering the child's relationship with the clinician. Developing an alliance with parents during the interview process is not simply a matter of collecting information; it is also important to give information. The clinician can, and should, identify strengths and weaknesses in the child and help the parents clarify what they already know. The clinician can also give information to the parents about normal child development and the clinical process. In this way, the parent interview becomes a two-way collaborative effort in the process of diagnosis and treatment of children.

Parent interviews come in a variety of shapes and forms. It is important for the clinician to identify the purpose of that interview beforehand. Some interviews are part of a diagnostic process, whereas others are a component of a treatment, be that treatment individual, family, or parent-oriented. Furthermore, some interviews take place under more casual circumstances, whereas others are in an acute setting, such as an emergency room or part of the inpatient, pediatric, or psychiatric consultation. Each comes with a different tone and has a separate set of goals.

The Components of an Interview

Irrespective of the setting or circumstances of the parent interview, each such interview has a set of discrete elements. For structured interviews using instruments, these elements are prescribed by the very nature of the instrument selected. However, some of the elements of the more traditional parent interview still apply.

Despite some assertions to the contrary, all good parent interviews are at least semistructured. Whether semistructured or fully structured, the structure is ultimately the responsibility of the interviewer. Thus all parent interviews require careful thought and planning. There are five components of each interview: preliminaries, prologue, the interview proper, closing, and the epilogue.

For any parent interview, the clinician must establish the goals for that particular interview and set a tentative agenda in advance. Such an agenda can then be followed through the course of the interview itself. Although it may seem a bit prosaic, one must remember that each interview begins with a beginning and that beginning sets the tone for the balance of the process.

Preliminaries

The preliminary phase is the planning for the interview process. The first tasks of this phase are to identify who is the patient and what is the purpose of the interview. This will, in turn, afford the clinician the opportunity to determine the type of interview to be conducted and the goals for the interview. For example, if the interview is to be diagnostic, then collecting information may be the most critical component of the interview; if the interview is a therapeutic interview, then the means of intervention and the goals of the treatment have to be clearly understood before the intervention is to begin. Once these have been determined, the clinician must ascertain that the amount of time and other conditions are suitable to meet the objectives of the interview.

Prologue

The prologue is the introductory phase of the parent interview. It begins with introductions, which must be respectful of the parental role and competence as well as the circumstances of the interview. Similarly, introductions must clearly identify the clinician and his or her role while also setting the ground rules regarding matters such as confidentiality. During this portion of the interview, it is useful to assess both the parents' and the doctor's expectations for the interview and to get some indications about parental defensiveness, shame, guilt, and embarrassment:

> It is never easy to think of a child as having these sorts of problems. You may even be embarrassed or scared. In spite of this, you have been able to come for help. Now, I would like to help you understand what's happening so we can make a plan to solve the problems facing both you and your child.

Interview Proper

The interview proper is the opportunity to establish an empathic relationship with the parents while collecting data and/or making the appropriate intervention. Even in a parent interview, this is the time to attend to the more traditional elements of the psychiatric evaluation. Transference, countertransference, resistance, defenses, strengths, weaknesses, and other similar matters as they specifically relate to the parents require careful assessment, while simultaneously attending to family matters such as family traditions, locus of control, discipline, family dynamics, communications, and other matters that are more commonly associated with parent and family function. At the same time, the interviewer must help the parents manage their anxiety and sense of responsibility for the child.

Closing

The closing portion of the parent interview is the clinician's opportunity to reassure the parents and reinforce their control and competence. It is also a time for answering questions that the parents may have and articulating the next step in the clinical process:

> At this point, there are several possibilities to explain the current situation. These are: 1 . . . 2 . . . 3 . . . 4. . . . I would like to suggest that we do the following to answer the remaining questions and establish a treatment plan. I realize that this may seem a bit overwhelming or confusing, so please, be sure that I have satisfactorily answered your questions before we proceed.

Epilogue

Finally, each clinician must allow some time to review the interview. By carefully reconsidering the data that have been acquired and the response to interventions, the validity of the plans and the next step can be reviewed, and planning for future activity in the case can be assessed before the report of the interview is generated. While this epilogue may be at the end, it may also be the beginning of further clinical activity with the parents and the child.

Source of Referral

It is always useful during the course of an interview to assess parental attitudes about the referral as well as the source of referral and why the parents have accepted the referral at the particular time of the evaluation. Such information may not only guide the process, but also helps identify those particular problems that are of acute interest to the patient as well as the family. For example, a family who is forced into an evaluation by an outside agency or the legal system may provide one particular perspective on an evaluation that is in sharp contrast to one that might be provided by a family for which there is an extensive history of psychiatric illness that is now being manifested by the child as the identified patient.

Impression of Parents

In addition to collecting information about the whys and wherefores of the referral, it is important to get at least a general impression of the parents, if not a detailed understanding of their own past, personality organization, and the established family patterns. This allows the clinician to develop a preliminary conceptual framework in which to place the child's and the parents' functioning in a family context. It is also important to gain some appreciation, not only of the parents' role in shaping the lives of children, but also of the capacity of children to shape the parental role (Rutter and Cox 1985).

> I want to be of help to *you* in determining why your child is having these problems. We will have to work together as we search for answers to your good questions and concerns.

Types of Interviews and Settings

Diagnostic Interview

In the diagnostic or history-taking interview, the information to be collected from parents is both factual and impressionistic. Because of the previously noted discrepancies between parental reports and actual occurrences (e.g., medical and school records, and records from previous evaluations or testing), it is important, whenever possible, to review additional sources of information. Several authors have offered detailed outlines of historical information to guide the interviewer (Canino 1985; French 1979). These and many other structured and unstructured interview schedules offer extensive outlines of variables such as pregnancies, labor and delivery, birth, infancy, medical history, and family history.

> A pediatric colleague completes the evaluation of a 10-year-old child with vague stomach pains before seeking a consultation by the child psychiatry C/L team. After reviewing the case with the consultants, the pediatrician might tell the parents, "There is nothing wrong with your son so I am asking the psychiatrist to see you. . . . It is very hard for you and your doctors to see your child in pain and not understand the cause. There are often multiple causes. The psychiatrist can help us solve this problem for your child."

Medical Consultation Setting

In medical consultation settings, the parents are important informants about the child's premorbid functioning and the impact of the child's illness on the child and the family. Even in this setting, it is important to identify who is the patient. This is particularly problematic as sometimes the consultee is not clear or may have an agenda that is completely different from that of the patient or the parents. Oftentimes, consultation requests are quite focused, and the parent interview must be targeted to deal with what might be perceived as confusion in this area. For example, an adolescent patient may be identified as noncompliant with the treatment when, in fact, the source of conflict originates out of ambivalent relationships between the primary treating physician and the parents' overparticipation and control of the medical treatment process. Thus the focus during the parent interview, while manifestly directed toward the child's medical care, may be more directly related to the parents' sense of control, frustration, and incompetence in the clinical situation:

> I realize that this has been a very difficult day for you and your daughter. Even though she is 15 years old and capable of using good judgment, she is now in a great deal of distress. As much as you might now wish to take her home and care for her at home, we must determine what will ensure her immediate safety.

Emergency Setting

In emergency settings, when the clinician is faced with the necessity of making relatively rapid decisions about assessment and treatment and, in particular, concerned with how to protect a child from danger, entirely different forms of parental interviews are necessary. Whether the risk of self-injury or injury to others is the question, or if the child is a possible victim of physical or sexual abuse, there is a change in the scope and direction of the parent interview. Clearly, in the emergency setting, the focus of the interview must be on the extent of risk of danger and the need to establish a safe and protective environment for the child. In such circumstances, extraordinary levels of defensiveness, anxiety, guilt, and avoidance of conflict may be present. In addition, because legal culpability for the events may be in question, careful attention to details such as evasiveness on the part of the parent must be monitored. Although alliance building and assessment of overall parent functioning are important, these can be dealt with in a more cursory fashion until fundamental safety issues and other acute matters are addressed.

> I have been appointed by the court to conduct an evaluation to determine what will be in the best interest of your child. This is a struggle between adults, and the sooner the adults resolve it the easier it will be for your child. As one of two parents, you are one of the two most important people in your child's life and in this evaluation process. Therefore, I need your assistance and cooperation. I would very much like to hear anything that you have to offer about your child. I will take whatever time is necessary to collect the necessary information to make recommendations to you and the court. Please feel free to tell me or give me whatever you feel is important.

Forensic Interviews (Including Custody Evaluations)

Custody evaluations and other forensic interviews find a particular tone set for the interview, a priori. In such a setting, parents and clinicians are often faced with profoundly adversarial relationships, which may focus not only on a marital struggle, but also on the different opinions regarding parenting (e.g., the parents', the lawyers', the courts'). Indeed, this process may, in and of itself, also contribute to a great deal of hostility and criticism about a particular parent's parenting and multiple accusations about the veracity of the history. Furthermore, there is often a great deal of defensiveness, if not outright fabrication, about the reporting of parental activities in the life of the child. As such, a parent interview in the forensic setting may leave the clinician feeling responsible to ascertain "absolute truth." This is virtually impossible. Instead, the clinician must stand outside the legal wrangling and focus on those consistent patterns of behavior that have existed over extended periods of time. Forensic interviews most often are repeated, and multiple sources of information are essential to get a reasonably clear, if not accurate, picture of the patterns of parental behavior as well as the child's behavior. In most forensic settings, the adversarial system leads to labeling of "winners" and "losers." Despite their best efforts, clinicians are often cast in this light as well. One must try not to cast oneself in this light, or take this attribution to heart either, nor take it as a measure of success or failure.

Other Settings

There are other settings in which child psychiatrists are asked to interview parents as part of the diagnostic or treatment process. Commonly, clinicians are asked to consult with pediatricians and other mental health professionals concerning psychopharmacologic interventions. A great deal of information prior to the consultation may be provided by the other professionals, and oftentimes the parents arrive in these settings with strong feelings that they are being criticized or that the situation is rapidly becoming hopeless. Still others approach the medication consultation with the notion that an ambrosia to treat their child finally and definitively may be imminently available. Such a setting necessitates not only careful gathering of history but also careful assessment of parental expectations. These expectations must be dealt with directly, along with providing detailed information about the treatment process. This means that the parents must be carefully and accurately informed about the types of medications to be used, the potential side effects and serious consequences related to these medications, and the real therapeutic potential. Since situations like these are often stressful and the information itself is critical, the parent interview in this case often takes on an instructive format, an instruction that must be carefully tested before the patient and family are sent on their way.

Conclusion

Fundamentally, the parent interview is a pedagogic process. It is an opportunity for the parents to teach the clinicians about themselves, their roles as parents, the child, and the family. It is also a time for the clinician to teach the parents about the clinical process and perhaps even about the parents themselves and their child. For all of this teaching to take place, each party must be open to the process. It is the interviewer's responsibility not only to ensure that his or her mind is open, but also to establish the same receptivity in the parents. Absent this, the parent interview will offer little reliable information and contribute little to the clinical enterprise.

Clarence Darrow once said that "the first half of our lives is ruined by our parents and the second half is ruined by our children" (see Peter 1977). The same can be said for the clincal process with children and parents. However, if we avoid ruin-

ation with the parents, then the work with the child will follow in due course.

References

American Psychiatric Association: Diagnostic and Statistical Manual of Mental Disorders, 3rd Edition, Revised. Washington, DC, American Psychiatric Association, 1987

Canino IA: Taking a history, in The Clinical Guide to Child Psychiatry. Edited by Shaffer D, Ehrhardt AA, Greenhill LL. New York, Free Press, 1985, pp 393–408

Chess S, Thomas A, Birch HG: Distortions in developmental reporting made by parents of behaviorally disturbed children. Journal of the American Academy of Child Psychiatry 5:226–234, 1966

Costello AJ, Edelbrock CS, Kalas R, et al: National Institute of Mental Health Diagnostic Interview Schedule for Children. Bethesda, MD, National Institute of Mental Health, 1982

Edelbrock C, Costello AJ, Dulcan MK, et al: Age differences in the reliability of the psychiatric interview of the child. Child Dev 56:265–275, 1985

French AP: Disturbed Children and Their Families: Innovations in Evaluation and Treatment. New York, Human Sciences Press, 1979

Freud S: Analysis of a phobia in a five-year-old boy (1909), in The Standard Edition of the Complete Psychological Works of Sigmund Freud, Vol 10. Translated and edited by Strachey J. London, Hogarth Press, 1955, pp 1–149

Green RJ: An overview of major contributions of family therapy, in Family Therapy: The Major Contributions. Edited by Green RJ, Framo JL. New York, International Universities Press, 1982, pp 1–35

Greenspan SI: The Clinical Interview of the Child. Washington, DC, American Psychiatric Press, 1991

Group for the Advancement of Psychiatry: The Diagnostic Process in Child Psychiatry (Report No 38). New York, Group for the Advancement of Psychiatry, 1957

Kashani JH, Orvaschel H, Burk JP, et al: Informant variance: the issue of parent-child disagreement. Journal of the American Academy of Child Psychiatry 24:437–441, 1985

Mednick SA, Shaffer JBP: Mothers' retrospective reports in child-rearing research. Am J Orthopsychiatry 33:457–461, 1963

Orvaschel H, Weissman MM, Padian N, et al: Assessing psychopathology in children of psychiatrically disturbed parents: a pilot study. Journal of the American Academy of Child Psychiatry 20:112–122, 1981

Peter LJ: Peter's Quotations. New York, Bantam, 1977, p 306

Rutter M, Cox A: Other family influences, in Child and Adolescent Psychiatry: Modern Approaches. Edited by Rutter M, Hersov L. London, Blackwell, 1985, pp 58–81

Simmons JE: Psychiatric Examination of Children. Philadelphia, PA, Lea & Febiger, 1987, pp 23–49, 157–169

Walsh F: Family therapy: a systemic orientation to treatment, in Handbook of Clinical Social Work. Edited by Rosenblatt A, Waldfogel D. San Francisco, CA, Jossey-Bass, 1983, pp 466–489

Weissman MM, Wickramaratne P, Warner V, et al: Assessing psychiatric disorders in children: discrepancies between mothers' and children's reports. Arch Gen Psychiatry 44:747–753, 1987

Chapter 10

The Family Interview

G. Pirooz Sholevar, M.D.

The diagnostic family interview is an invaluable tool to assist the child psychiatrist in the development of diagnostic and therapeutic goals. The multiple goals of the family interview may vary, depending on the clinician's theoretical orientation or the nature of the problem, and can shape the structure, form, and content of the session. The diagnostic interview can take place as the initial contact with the family, regardless of the nature of the presenting "problem"; it can be part of the comprehensive assessment of a symptomatic child or adult; or it can occur when therapeutic efforts of any type are partially or totally ineffective. It can occur in an outpatient or inpatient unit.

The assessment of the total family is important because a child is part of the family as an emotional unit rather than an autonomous psychological entity. In treating a patient, a child psychiatrist may fail to recognize how the problematic relationship between child and parents, or between parents and grandparents, contributes to the disorder and may therefore prescribe a prolonged and relatively ineffective course of individual or conjoint family therapy. A broader evaluation of the problems addressing multiple sets of variables can result in more successful treatment choices.

The family diagnostic interview is guided by the theoretical orientation of the clinician. A psychodynamic family therapist would pay special attention to traumatic events, developmental failures, and intrafamilial transference reactions, which may shape the contemporary interactions and identity of the family members in a decisive manner. The behavioral family therapist would focus on the antecedents and consequences of the problematic behavior and collect extensive data in this area. A communications orientation leads to an interest in the homeostatic mechanisms and rules maintaining the family transactions. A multigenerational family therapist would be most interested in the level of differentiation and the pathologic loyalty and indebtedness between the parents and their families of origin.

The goals of clinicians vary and may include 1) learning of family and individual variables that may play the decisive role in shaping the behavior of a problematic child; 2) assessing the adequacy of family functioning, structure, and development according to the family life cycle; and 3) conducting an initial family treatment session when the necessity of such a course has been recognized by the family or by the referral source.

The multiple goals stated above can influence the strategy of the clinician. In the first category, the clinician pays equal attention to the interpersonal, individual, and intrapsychic data. In the second category, the systematic exploration of the family structure is complemented by some interventions aimed at testing the flexibility of the family system and rules to determine if the most leverage and the least defensiveness can be gained in the individual or family treatment. In the third category, raising the positive expectancies of the family as a group may assume the first priority.

Stages of the Initial Family Session

The diagnostic family interview is commonly divided into the three segments of social stage, multidimensional inquiry into the presenting problem, and exploration of the structure and developmental phase of the family (Haley 1977; Minuchin 1974b).

In the social stage of the interview, the clinician acts as a host to the family according to the prevailing customs. The family is put at ease by engaging in mutual introductions, asking the family to introduce themselves by name, matching the names with family members, and inviting them to make themselves comfortable in the office. The family should be provided with adequate seating, preferably in a conversational living room arrangement, and with play material, table, and chairs for young children. Zilbach (1986) recommended that the clinician crouch down to establish eye-to-eye contact with young children when they enter the office and remember that some young children may be afraid of handshakes or physical touching. A few minutes may be spent in small talk, inquiring, for example, if the family had any difficulty finding the office or with transportation.

In the stage of multidimensional inquiry, the clinician asks the family to describe the problem that has prompted the clinical contact. Prior information about the family can be shared, which may exhibit the therapist's interest and style. The family members generally feel very comfortable with the initial part of this stage of evaluation because their statements are largely pre-rehearsed and allow them to present their "official" image to the clinician. The initial inquiry may be directed to the father, in recognition of the often tenuous nature of the father's relationship to the therapeutic setting, or to the mother as the person who may be most knowledgeable about the family life and problems. After hearing the views of one parent, the clinician should ask the other parent to express an account of the problem. The therapist should then inquire of the views of different family members on problematic areas in the family. It is preferable to elicit the views of the siblings of the identified patient about the problematic areas in the family before moving to the identified patient, because an early solicitation of the patient's views may increase defensiveness and further polarize the family.

The clinician should be prepared to encounter resistance from the family members against broadening the focus of the explorations and establishment of a true multidirectional partiality (Boszormenyi-Nagy 1972). Such resistances will become apparent by one or both parents demanding a solution for the presenting problem from the therapist, or by instructing the therapist on what to do (e.g., prescribe medication for a child's hyperactivity). Understanding such attempts as signs of a high level of family tension, the clinician should avoid confrontation with the parents and gently underline the importance of understanding everyone's viewpoint on family life as a necessary step for establishing a corrective course of action for the problems.

The family's manner of negotiating boundaries with the clinician as a member of the outside world may be exhibited by a readiness to include the therapist immediately in their conflicts, projections, and blaming. The emergence of an intense, negative transference to the therapist can give rise to countertransferential feelings, which should be used as a clue to the level of family health and pathology.

While listening to the family's presentation of the problem, the therapist should observe carefully the family's relatively unconstrained nonverbal behavior. The observation of any restless behavior in the children following a look at one of the parents and interruption, qualification, or negation of messages by one or multiple family members are the signals used to regulate family transactions and should provide the interviewer with useful clues on family structure to be tested in the next stage of the family interview. By the end of the second stage, each family member should have experienced a sense of participation in the interview and the opportunity for input in the evaluation. However, any excessive accommodation to some family members, particularly the autocratic and tyrannical ones, may undermine the potential trust of the scapegoated and peacemaking members, because they may assume an alliance between the therapist and the victimizers against the scapegoated victims.

Exploration of Family Structure

The observation of family interactions provides the clinician with valuable clues on different aspects of family structure: the level of differentiation, boundary formation, and boundary flexibility of different family subsystems and family members. The clinician is particularly interested in the functional adequacy of different family subsystems. The common family subsystems include the 1) marital-parental, 2) parent-child, and 3) sibling subsystems. Grandparental involvement, very common in certain ethnic and socioeconomic groups, would provide two additional subsystems of grandparent-parent and grandparent-grandchild.

In this stage of the family interview, the clinician devises active interventions or interpretations to test the adequacy of different family subsystems, such as the marital or parental subsystems. Generally, most clinically referred families reveal observable deficiencies in at least one of the family subsystems, such as the parent-child one, while proving adequate and resourceful in other ones, such as marital or sibling subsystems. Some family therapists may ask the members of such subsystems to discuss in the session a potentially conflictual subject, which will reveal their hidden disagreements, as well as their flexibility in family negotiation and compromise formation.

The strategy of broadening the focus of exploration extends the reach of the clinician beyond the problems of the identified patient to other functional and dysfunctional aspects of the family life. Depending on the level of tension in the family and the skill of the family therapist, the session may oscillate between two competing forces: the family pushing to return the discussion to the identified patient when the tension mounts and the therapist attempting to guide the discussion toward other family members and different family subsystems.

When a child psychiatrist attempts to broaden the problem, a major pitfall is an early focus on hidden or apparent marital problems. Generally, an early focus on marital difficulties is correlated with a high rate of dropout from treatment and negative therapeutic outcome due to heightened family tension. Additionally, the family may present the marital problems in an attempt to diffuse the therapeutic efforts directed at the identified child, without genuine motivation to deal with marital issues (Montalvo and Haley 1973).

The maintenance of the family's motivation to return for treatment is an important therapeutic goal. Therefore, at the time of heightened tension during the sessions, the therapist may choose to retreat from uncomfortable family topics until the tension is reduced.

In a family with a rigid structure, taking sides and confrontation in the first session may result in the interruption of the family evaluation. The clinician should always be aware of the unity of the family system as a natural group with strong ties of loyalty, common history, and rigid homeostatic rules dictating the behavior of each family member. A close and intricately functioning family can close ranks and readily extrude the therapist if the family's tolerance is exceeded, based on an incorrect assessment of the family's power or the therapist's status.

Specific Procedural Considerations

The multiple benefits of the family diagnostic interview include the recognition of subtle parental pathology, different aspects of individual and family dysfunction, and, most importantly, the presence of powerful dysfunctional interlocking relationships and loyalties. These can play a decisive role in reducing the adaptation of the family and production of symptoms in one or multiple family members.

For the initial family session, all members of the household and significant others should be invited; this includes young children, toddlers, and infants, who are an important source of diagnostic data about the family. The invitation should be extended in a matter-of-fact manner, emphasizing the importance of all family members' views for a full understanding of the problem. Simple statements such as "I'd like to meet you all, including the little ones" can readily communicate the clinician's goal. The success of the invitation is dependent on the conviction of the clinician about the importance of family interactional data. The clinician should avoid any lengthy phone discussion to justify the participation of all family members, because a prolonged explanation based on general assumptions can represent the therapist's lack of confidence. Once the family members recognize the importance of the family interview to the diagnostic process, they usually comply. The common parental fear about the "contamination" of younger children and "well siblings" by their exposure to the problems of the identified patient can yield readily to the clinician's reassurance. Other sources of fear in the family include the parents' fear of blame for the child's problems and the fear that the entire family may be pronounced "sick." The clinician can reduce the fears of the family by emphasizing the consultative nature of the family diagnostic interview, which does not imply any commitment to treatment on the part of the family. The refusal of an adolescent to attend a family diagnostic interview usually is indicative of the fear of the parents or the weakness of parental authority.

The family assessment can occur during one or multiple family sessions. The diagnostic interview preferably should be scheduled for 1½ hours to allow a systematic evaluation of the family in an unhurried fashion. One should be prepared for a high rate of cancellation for the initial family interview, with little hope of receiving remuneration for the cancelled session.

The assessment of family structure should include the determination of the characteristic constellations of family conflicts, patterns of control, clarity of parental authority and generational boundaries, expression of feelings, and family rigidity, including the brittleness of family defenses. Structural flexibility of the family includes the accessibility of alternative action patterns.

Assessment of family functioning should include the exploration of instrumental-adaptive functions of the family geared toward enhanced adaptation and problem resolution, as well as their affective-integrative function, addressing the expression of affect and provision of comfort. The lack of balance between these two sets of functions can result in an imbalanced family system with reduced adaptability. The elucidation of multigenerational dynamic and relational patterns may be an important factor, particularly with chronically and severely dysfunctional families.

The diagnostic family interview can be extended into interviews with family subgroups, such as parents, children, or with one child for exploration of other important information that may not be readily shared in a conjoint session. The intimate aspects of the parental relationship, such as their sexual functioning, can be explored in such an interview. The children may reveal phobias, food fads, or eating and elimination problems that may be too embarrassing for revelation in a diagnostic family session.

In the advanced stage of the initial interview, the impact of the clinician on the family may move the family beyond a rigid or stalemated position into a more flexible mode of family functioning characteristic of earlier stages of their family life. The early and ready occurrence of this phenomenon is indicative of flexibility in the family system and a favorable therapeutic outcome.

Additional guidelines for family assessment (Weber et al. 1985) include the following:

1. Establish structure in the interview to counter the common tendency of dysfunctional families toward chaos, a high level of blame, and "silencing" of their members. "Reframing," the restatement of a problem in a positive rather than a negative way, and diffusion of attacks by demonstration of a dyadic or triadic view of the problems are effective techniques to establish an empathic atmosphere.

2. Maintain objectivity, avoid side taking or premature closure of topics, and elicit the views of all family members.

3. Address the transactional patterns that are clearly burdensome to many family members and therefore more amenable to change (Gordon and Davidson 1981).

4. Understand role of different family members within the family unit. This is a significant factor. The roles of "scapegoat," "tyrant," "martyr," and "baby" are common in families with symptomatic children and adolescents.

5. Uncover the explicit and implicit rules that govern family interaction.

6. Determine the family's problem-solving behavior.

7. Understand the nature of boundaries, splits, alliances, and coalition formations in the family.

8. Assess the level of concordance between the developmental and chronological stages of the family.

9. Assess the concordance between the value system of the family and the surrounding community.

10. Help the families transcend the repetitive, immediate, and trivial problems and recognize the underlying patterns and major issues.

A significant goal of the family diagnostic interview is to help the family recognize and acknowledge its strengths as a family and the assets of family members, particularly the identified patient. The commonly observed emphasis of the family on negative attributes of the identified patient is only a manifestation of the family's negative view of itself as a family that is projected onto the identified patient. The recognition of the assets of the identified patient, which is usually resisted by the family as a whole, is generally followed by recognition of many assets and resources of the family, and enhancement of the family problem-solving capacity due to a heightened optimism and confidence.

The closing of the diagnostic family interview is an important component of the assessment. When the diagnostic family interview is part of an overall comprehensive evaluation, it is best to delay the therapeutic recommendation until the closing conference. Under other circumstances, the family diagnostic interview should be closed by highlighting the points of convergence among the problems of the identified patient, the information gathered from different family members, the transactional patterns in the family system, and the referral information. The clinician should attempt to integrate and summarize data, while highlighting the family's assets, positive attributes, and affectionate feelings for each other, which would enhance their optimism and confidence for undertaking a therapeutic endeavor. An experienced family therapist attempts to highlight the family's assets, knowing well that the family is aware of its conflictual interactions and relationships but barely cognizant of those assets that are the key to therapeutic success. An inexperienced family therapist tends to focus on family problems to reveal his or her observational acumen; this may inadvertently make the family feel severely disturbed and discouraged.

Family History

Significant experiences in the past may influence the family orientation and mythology, and directly or indirectly relate to the family problems. Such information includes the early death or suicide of a grandparent when a parent was very young, significant financial losses, or other events traumatic for the family. An overly solicitous father of a late-adolescent boy revealed that the year before his son's bar mitzvah, the son was involved in a serious accident requiring prolonged hospitalization and cancellation of the plans for his bar mitzvah. The paternal oversolicitousness toward the son was related to the impact of the accident, which was unknown to and irritating to the new stepmother.

The gradual unfolding of historical information in the family session is an important aspect of the family interview and generally reveals the affectively charged and dynamically significant past experiences of the family. This phenomenon of "living family history" (Ackerman 1958) exceeds the validity of the historical data obtained in a formal chronological, developmental history. The living family history may reveal past deprivations, successes, failures, hidden strengths, and weaknesses of the family that may be related to the current crisis (Sholevar 1985).

Most family therapists gather historical material as it arises in the family interview and occasionally probe specific issues in the past that appear likely to be related to current problems. The information can be gathered along chronological or analogical lines. Multigenerational family therapists gather such information within a multigenerational context. The revelation of family data may disclose that some of the current dysfunctions are a prolonged attempt at solving past problems, at times spanning many generations.

Family Life Cycle

The concept of the family life cycle proposes that family issues are different at various stages in a way analogous to the life cycle of individuals. This model describes a series of stages and their corresponding family tasks. The most commonly accepted models by Carter and McGoldrick (1980) and Zilbach (1988) describe the stages of coupling, becoming three with the arrival of the first child, and the family with young children. These stages are followed by a partial or more complete separation of the adolescent family members from the family, succeeded by the death of one spouse or partner, and continuing up until the death of the other partner. During different stages of the life cycle, the family structure is rearranged to facilitate the adaptation and mastery of family members. The concept of the family life spiral and its intergenerational dimension proposes overlapping issues in different generations. The family assumes a centripetal shape around birth and the early life of the children and a centrifugal shape as the children move into adolescence (Combrinck-Graham 1985). The family life-cycle models are used differentially by different family theorists, and they describe the emotional problems characteristic of periods of the life cycle that manifest themselves when the family becomes stagnant. The family crisis when adolescent children leave home is a common clinical problem (Duvall 1962; Haley 1973; Terkelson 1980; Zilbach 1988).

Establishment of a Therapeutic System and Joining Operations

Minuchin (1974a) has entitled the therapist's methods of creating a therapeutic system and positioning himself or herself as its leader as *joining operations*. The joining maneuvers are a prerequisite for subsequent family change and are necessary because the clinician encounters an organized family system. Such maneuvers include making contact with each family member in such a way that each feels heard, understood, and respected. Attention to the needs of younger, less articulate, or disruptive family members is an important aspect of joining. The accommodation by the therapist to the family system is necessary to "join" them. Mimesis is the accommodation of the therapist to the family's style, affective range, and tempo of communication. The therapist should accept the family's organization and experience the strength of its transactional pattern, the pain and pleasure of different family members, and the family's resistance to the interventions. The therapeutic challenge to the family should not endanger its return for the next session. Therefore, the initial joining maneuvers may be away from the therapeutic goal and in the service of the temporary alliance with the family members and rules.

The therapist's accommodation to the children and to their style of communication is an important but neglected area for many family therapists, who tend to be more responsive to the adult family members. Attention to children's communication, play, and art products can enhance their alliance with the clinician. Working with different segments of the family can be an important restructuring tool (Scharff and Scharff 1987; Zilbach 1986).

"Joining" is more related to the initial phase of the treatment and establishment of a family diagnosis in contrast to the restructuring methods that belong to the therapeutic phase proper.

Maintenance is a joining operation that refers to the accommodation techniques that provide planned support to the family structure. For example, the therapist may exhibit respect for a strong relationship between a mother and her children by making his or her contact with the children through the mother or by praising the complementarity between husband and wife where the husband defers to the wife's leadership. The maintenance operation may involve the active confirmation and support of the subsystems, such as the executive parental position.

Tracking is an accommodation technique by which the therapist follows the contents of the family's communication and encourages the members to continue with their expressions, asks clarifying questions, makes approving comments, and requests amplification of certain points. Tracking can

apply to the actions or verbal communication of the family.

Psychodynamic Family Data

In addition to attention to observable and conscious communications, the psychodynamically oriented family therapist is equally attentive to the manifestations of the unconscious life of the family. The unconscious is considered the repository of repressed object relations derived from past and present family experiences in response to the basic need for attachment to others. Special attention is paid to the creation of a "holding environment" in the treatment—a mode of functioning that contains the emerging family anxiety and therefore minimizes the need for projection and suppression. Two other important aspects of psychodynamic family therapy are attention to transference phenomena among family members and the clinician's own countertransference feelings. The emergence of a strong transference reaction toward the therapist in the diagnostic sessions is generally indicative of more severe psychopathology and possibly requires early transference interpretation. The therapeutic tool of countertransference feeling requires constant scrutiny and self-examination by the therapist to understand the nature of the family's communication (Scharff and Scharff 1987).

Psychodynamic family therapists are particularly allied with child and adolescent psychiatrists because of their mutual emphasis on the concordance between the developmental level of behavior in the patient and transactions in the family. Two special levels of arrest in relational development are excessive infantile dependency among family members and excessive oppositional and defiant behavior and power play. The goal of the treatment is to enhance cooperation, reciprocity, and tenderness characteristic of a more mature (genital) level of interaction and development among family members.

Family Interactional Diagnosis

The family diagnosis is a working hypothesis that encapsulates the clinician's observations of the family interactions, structure, and presenting problems. The dysfunctions in the above areas may be correlated with diagnosable disorders in a child or "primary relationship disorders" in the family, with no symptomatology in individual family members. The clinician's assessment places particular emphasis on the family as a whole and the course of the family in the future; this view contrasts with the family's approach, which is generally oriented toward the past and problems, particularly in an individual.

Minuchin (1974a) emphasized the following six major areas in family assessment:

1. The family structure, its preferred transactional pattern, and the available alternatives
2. The role of the symptoms in the maintenance of the family's preferred transactional pattern
3. The family system's flexibility and capacity for autonomous restructuring by reshuffling the system's alliances and coalitions to deal with stress
4. The family system's resonance and sensitivity to individual members' actions and feelings and their threshold for the activation of counterdeviation mechanisms
5. The family life context, including sources of support and stress in the family network
6. The family's developmental stage and its concordance with the family members' chronological stage

The interactional diagnosis is achieved by the process of gathering different classes of verbal and nonverbal information. The diagnosis has to be made after the therapist has entered and joined the family because the diagnosis cannot be made from outside. The therapeutic joining with the family would introduce alternative transactional patterns that are an important indicator of prognosis and therapeutic outcome.

Therapeutic Contract

The contracting phase is an important step prior to initiating formal family therapy. It refers to agreed-on issues and goals for treatment between the therapist and the family. In addition to accepting the family's wish for help with their presenting problem, the therapist recommends the broader goal of alteration in the family interactions underlying the problem, such as disciplin-

ing methods used with the children. Later on, the goals will expand to include the disagreement between the parents, such as in their views on child rearing or on other issues.

Many treatment failures are due to inadequate contracting between the family and the therapist. The problems of contracting include covert disagreement between the therapist and the family, within the family, or between the family and referral sources (e.g., the Department of Human Services or the court system).

Family Evaluation Scales

Family evaluation scales may augment the clinical interview by providing standardized, self-report data that can highlight the areas of family dysfunction. A comparison of family evaluation scales is available elsewhere (Forman and Hogan 1984; Touliatos et al. 1990). There are several commonly used scales.

The Beavers-Timberlawn Family Evaluation Scale (Lewis et al. 1976) is an observer-rated scale that addresses the structural dimensions of power hierarchy, parental coalition, family mythology, goal-directed negotiations, permeability, conflict, self-disclosure, and invasiveness. The controls and sanctions that are measured are 1) overt power and 2) responsibility.

The Family Adaptability Cohesion Evaluation Scale (Olson et al. 1982) is a self-report instrument that addresses the structural dimensions of systems feedback, negotiation, the family roles, boundaries, coalitions, space, decision making, and time. The controls and sanctions include assertiveness, control, discipline, rules, and independence.

The Family Assessment Device (Epstein and Bishop 1981) is based on McMaster's problem-centered model of family therapy. This self-report instrument assesses the structural dimensions of problem solving, communication, roles, and general functioning.

The Family Environment Scale (Moos and Moos 1980) measures social climates of all types of families, with subscales in such areas as family cohesion, expressiveness, conflict, independence, and achievement. It has been used widely in many research projects.

The Card Sorting Procedure (Reiss 1981) is an observer-rated instrument that addresses the structural dimensions of configuration, coordination, and closure.

References

Ackerman NW: The Psychodynamics of Family Life: Diagnosis and Treatment of Family Relationships. New York, Basic Books, 1958

Boszormenyi-Nagy I: Loyalty implications of the transference model in psychotherapy. Arch Gen Psychiatry 27:374–380, 1972

Carter E, McGoldrick M: The family life cycle and family therapy, in The Family Life Cycle. Edited by Carter EA, McGoldrick M. New York, Gardner Press, 1980, pp 3–20

Combrinck-Graham L: A model of family development. Fam Process 24:139–150, 1985

Duvall EM: Family Development. Chicago, IL, JB Lippincott, 1962

Epstein NB, Bishop DS: Problem-centered systems therapy of the family, in Handbook of Family Therapy. Edited by Gurman AS, Kniskern DP. New York, Brunner/Mazel, 1981, pp 444–482

Forman BD, Hogan BJ: Measures for evaluating total family functioning, Family Therapy 11:1–36, 1984

Gordon SB, Davidson N: Behavioral parent training, in Handbook of Family Therapy. Edited by Gurman AS, Kniskern DP. New York, Brunner/Mazel, 1981, pp 517–555

Haley J: Uncommon Therapy. Toronto, WW Norton, 1973

Haley J: Conducting the first interview, in Problem Solving Therapy. San Francisco, CA, Jossey-Bass, 1977, pp 9–47

Lewis JM, Beavers WR, Grossett JT, et al: No Single Thread. New York, Brunner/Mazel, 1976, pp 83–98

Minuchin S: Forming the therapeutic system, in Families and Family Therapy. Cambridge, MA, Harvard University Press, 1974a, pp 123–137

Minuchin S: The initial interview, in Families and Family Therapy. Cambridge, MA, Harvard University Press, 1974b, pp 206–239

Montalvo B, Haley J: In defense of child therapy. Fam Process 12:227–244, 1973

Moos R, Moos B: Family Environment Scale Manual. Palo Alto, CA, Consulting Psychologists' Press, 1980

Olson DH, McCubbin HI, Barnes H, et al: Faces II: Family Adaptability and Cohesion Evaluation Scales. St. Paul, MN, University of Minnesota, Family Social Science, 1982

Olson DH, McCubbin HI, Barnes H, et al: Family Inventories. St. Paul, MN, University of Minnesota, Family Social Science, 1985

Reiss D: The Family's Construction of Reality. Cambridge, MA, Harvard University Press, 1981

Scharff D, Scharff J: Object Relations Family Therapy. Northvale, NJ, Jason Aronson, 1987

Sholevar GP: Marital assessment, in Contemporary Marriage. Edited by Goldberg DC. Homewood, IL, Dorsey, 1985, pp 290–311

Terkelson KG: Toward a theory of the family life cycle, in The Family Life Cycle. Edited by Carter EA, McGoldrick M. New York, Gardner Press, 1980, pp 21–52

Touliatos J, Permutter BF, Straus MA: Handbook of Family Measurement Techniques. New York, Sage, 1990

Weber T, McKeever J, McDaniel SH: The beginner's guide to the problem-oriented first family interview. Fam Process 24:357–364, 1985

Zilbach JJ: Young Children in Family Therapy. New York, Brunner/Mazel, 1986

Zilbach JJ: The family life cycle, in Children in Families: Ecological and Treatment Perspectives. Edited by Combrinck-Graham L. New York, Guilford, 1988, pp 46–66

Chapter 11

Use of Rating Scales and Questionnaires

Anthony J. Costello, M.D.

Assessing the psychiatric characteristics of a child or adolescent has always been a difficult task, and the increasing understanding that has been reached in the last decade of the patterns of emotional and behavioral problems in children has not made this task any easier. Indeed, the contemporary need for greater precision in diagnosis and measurement of disorders, which has been driven by growing sophistication in the selection and specificity of treatments, and the demands of research have made it necessary to use increasingly elaborate measurement strategies. Although formal measurement procedures other than in the narrow field of attainment and ability testing have generally been seen as research tools, they are now increasingly being adopted by clinicians as aids to everyday practice. Both clinicians and researchers now need a good understanding of the choice of instruments available, their applications, and their limitations.

Standardized assessment introduces some of the principles of scientific method to the evaluation of the patient. The most fundamental principle is that the method can be replicated by others. This generally requires that a written description give sufficient information for a would-be user to apply the technique. Tests depending on specialized training that cannot be communicated in writing are suspect. Whenever such specialized training is needed, it leaves room for the possibility that something other than the techniques described in the instructions has to be learned and that what is being learned may be biased appraisal. Alternatively, it may be that the assessment strategy is so subjective that the user may drift away too easily from the required standard. Interviewing provides a very special problem, since it involves so many interpersonal skills. Generally, the difficulties of describing the subtleties of personal style, nonverbal communication, and other aspects of interviewing that are difficult to describe can be overcome by the use of instructional videotapes. With this teaching strategy, even the niceties of interviewing technique can be taught in a replicable fashion.

The instrument must have a performance demonstrably adequate for the application. The most immediate requirement is that the instrument should consistently produce the same result in those circumstances when the same result should be expected, regardless of who is administering the test, as long as the test instructions are being followed. In practical terms, this characteristic is generally measured by giving the same test twice to the same subject, preferably with a different test administrator. The measurement derived from comparing the two results is known as *test-retest reliability*; when two independent testers are used, it is a strenuous test of *interrater reliability*. It is important to remember that some characteristics of patients are likely to fluctuate markedly over time, and so one should not expect that exactly the same result will be obtained. If the characteristic is very transient, this may create practical problems. If the two tests are separated by a very short time interval, the subject's recollection of what he or she said on the first occasion may influence responses on the second administration as much as the subject's current state. If interrater reliability is being studied, this problem may sometimes be avoided by asking one rater to rate a videotape of the other rater's testing; but this introduces other problems because some of the differences between raters may arise from subject-rater interaction. Reliability is necessary but not sufficient evidence that a test is adequate.

A test may be reliable but not measure anything that is relevant to the problem being assessed. An instrument may be reliable, but not valid. However, a measure cannot be valid without also being reliable.

This leads to another property that must be demonstrated: the test must measure what it is supposed to measure. Sometimes validity is defined by the measurement itself. If a condition is defined by responses to a set of questions and these questions are asked by the instrument, then the instrument clearly has face validity. However, the demonstration of face validity is usually only an intermediate step toward other types of validation. Sometimes a simple external criterion that can be used to measure the test performance is available. In this way, Binet (Binet and Simon 1905) devised tests of ability that he could calibrate against a child's school performance. Unfortunately, it is rarely the case in psychiatry that simple external criteria of this sort are available to validate a test. More commonly it is necessary to rely on the relationship of test scores to a variety of other measures and to variables that have a predictable relationship with the characteristic being tested. This is the principle of construct validity. Obviously, construct validity is possible to use only if a theoretical structure that predicts the test's relationships to other measures is available.

For certain types of measurement, other psychometric characteristics, such as the internal consistency of items within the test, may be important. This is usually true of measures that attempt to quantify a characteristic on a single dimension (e.g., anxiety or depression). It cannot be applied to measures that assign an individual to a category, such as diagnostic instruments, although some measures that are derived from these instruments may be assessed by conventional psychometric qualities. Standardization, unlike the terms discussed so far, has no very precise meaning in the field of psychometrics. However, when standardized tests are referred to, it is usually implied that the tests' performance characteristics on a population sample that has been adequately defined are known.

Many tests are now used to identify individuals with particular characteristics. When this is the task required of a test, two other measures become important: sensitivity and specificity. Sensitivity is the proportion of true cases that the test selects. Specificity is the proportion of true cases among the group that the test identifies as cases. For screening purposes, it is most important to identify as many as possible of the cases in the sample, and sensitivity should be at a maximum. In defining a sample (e.g., for a drug study) or to describe other characteristics of a condition, the primary selection criterion is that no cases should be included that are not true cases, and then specificity becomes the most important requirement. In general, there is a trade-off between these two characteristics, so that instruments with high sensitivity tend to have low specificity, although this is not logically inevitable.

In deciding whether or not to use a standardized assessment procedure, some thought must be given to the relative utility of the procedure. Tests convey to the uninformed the impression of precision and authority, and it is tempting to bolster this impression by gathering together an impressive battery of procedures. However, it is often the case that many of these procedures add little or no information to that available from a core group, and the mere accumulation of tests does not promise superior precision. It should also be noted that many of the psychometric qualities discussed above remain unknown for many tests that are commonly used in psychiatry. Although this is regrettable, the absence of full information on performance should not necessarily deter a prospective user, for some information collected systematically may well be better than no systematic information at all.

There is a wide range of standardized instruments that can be used for psychiatric assessment of children and adolescents. The range is from broad-based symptomatic surveys, which can be used for preliminary evaluation or for screening purposes, to very detailed measures of specific symptomatology. There are also measures of environmental qualities that are relevant to the emotional status of a child, such as measures of family functioning or measures that can be used to assess the response of peers to the child. The range is too extensive to be reviewed adequately in the space available, so this chapter will be confined to a few examples of each category, and only the more popular and widely used instruments will be discussed.

Wide-Range Instruments

There have been many attempts to devise a checklist of child psychiatric symptoms that might be used to generate an overall measure of severity, to detect the presence of significant psychopathology, or to make at least a preliminary attempt at classifying the nature of the problem. Currently, the dominant instrument in the field is the Child Behavior Checklist, developed by Achenbach and Edelbrock (1983). Of the instruments currently available, this has provided by far the best performance data. A very large population sample has been used to generate normative data, so that the frequency distribution of each symptom and the total symptom score are well known, and if a study sample is considered similar to the standardization sample, then the statistical probability of unusual findings can be estimated. In addition, a rigorous factor analysis has established that responses can be grouped into two broad-band factors, which may be conveniently thought of as "internalizing" and "externalizing" problems; within these broad bands, several other factors have been established. Somewhat inconveniently, the factor structure is not stable across different age and sex groupings, and so to use the factor scores it is necessary to compare separately by each age and sex band. However, since the instrument covers the entire age range from 4 to 18 years old, this should not be surprising. The instrument is highly reliable and reasonably resistant to informant bias. It has been used as a screening instrument in two-stage epidemiologic studies with considerable success (Bird et al. 1987; E. J. Costello 1989) and provides useful epidemiologic information even as a single-stage procedure. Since the questionnaire takes only about 20 minutes to complete and is not very demanding of the informant's literacy, it has been used in many surveys where a more searching instrument would have been impossible to administer. It has even been used in translated versions for a number of cross-cultural studies, which now include comparisons from Holland (Achenbach et al. 1987a, 1987c, 1987d), Puerto Rico (Bird et al. 1989), and Thailand (Weisz et al. 1989), among other countries.

Parallel versions are available for teachers to complete and for self-report by youth above the age of 11 years. Not surprisingly, these instruments show the poor correspondence between informants that has been found with other studies that have compared information obtained from parent, teacher, and child (Rutter et al. 1970). For its purpose, the Child Behavior Checklist probably represents the best compromise available between extensive coverage and a reasonable length.

A more recent attempt to combine the symptom item pool of the Child Behavior Checklist with that of the Revised Behavior Problem Checklist (Quay 1983; Quay and Peterson, unpublished manuscript) and the Conners Parent Checklist (Conners 1973; Goyette et al. 1978), the two other leading contenders of this type of instrument, added surprisingly little (Achenbach et al. 1989). One disadvantage of instruments such as the Child Behavior Checklist is that the factor structure is inevitably most influenced by more commonly encountered problems and the size of the item pool corresponding to these problems. Syndromes that are rare, no matter how consistent their pattern, will not be reflected in the factors of the Child Behavior Checklist if standardization is performed on a representative sample. For example, autism, a condition afflicting only some 4 children in every 10,000 that has a reasonably consistent pattern of symptoms, does not emerge as a factor in the Child Behavior Checklist. Since a sample of about 100,000 would be needed for such a factor to emerge, this is not surprising, but it does limit the instrument's usefulness. Increasing the size of the item pool does not seem to make much difference to the factor structure. Despite this limitation, the instrument is still effective in identifying deviant children on the basis of the total symptom score, although the pattern of deviancy may not be recognizable from the checklist responses. A typology based on factor scores has been developed using cluster analysis but has not been widely used (Edelbrock and Achenbach 1980).

A preschool version of the Child Behavior Checklist is also available with a similar spread of items, modified to meet the needs of this age range on the basis of an epidemiologic survey (Achenbach et al. 1987b). The choice of instruments for this age range is much narrower. Until recently, the most widely used instrument was the Preschool Behavior Questionnaire (Behar 1977; Behar and Stringfield 1974), which is an adaptation of the Rutter A Scale (McGee et al. 1985; Rutter 1967), one of the earlier checklists devised solely for screening in a two-stage epidemiologic study. Although it is brief and thus easy for an informant to use, the Preschool Behavior Questionnaire has a much lower information content. It removes some items inapplicable to preschoolers and adds some that reflect symptoms more common in this age range, but it remains a very short scale that probably has less utility than the preschool version of the Child Behavior Checklist. Unfortunately, no direct comparisons of the two instruments are available. The only other noteworthy contenders for this age range are the exceedingly brief checklist, questionnaire, and interview devised by Richman and colleagues (McGuire and Richman 1986; Richman 1977; Richman and Graham 1971), which are nevertheless the basis for a study that provides the best information as yet on the outcome of behavior problems first evident in the preschool period (Richman et al. 1982).

A common problem is how to evaluate overall levels of functioning or disability, without reference to specific symptoms that may be so idiosyncratic that it seems impossible to compare one patient with another. The social competency scales of the several versions of the Child Behavior Checklist do not seem to have been widely used. Although they are simple, they may help to discriminate between children who have many symptoms but still function well and those who are functioning poorly. Another approach, based on a scale originally devised at the Menninger Clinic to evaluate progress and now incorporated into Axis V of DSM-III-R (American Psychiatric Association 1987), is to rate global functioning: the Children's Global Assessment Scale (Shaffer et al. 1983).

Diagnostic Instruments

The usual strategy when the checklist approach has been used has been to start with an attempt to identify common symptoms in childhood and then proceed to examine how these symptoms group empirically. The groupings derived in this way bear, as one would hope, some resemblance to syndromes defined by clinical experience, but the resemblance is a distant one, and data collected in this way, even if supplemented by additional questions, will usually only approximate to diagnoses based on criterial diagnostic systems, such as DSM-III (American Psychiatric Association 1980) or DSM-III-R. To make these diagnoses, it is necessary to collect all of the information required by the criteria. If all possible childhood psychiatric diagnoses are to be covered, a list of several hundred items must then be explored. It is a daunting task for clinical interviewers to collect this information consistently and comprehensively, and indeed, in practice, most clinicians explore a sequence of diagnostic hypotheses rather than systematically covering every possibility regardless of whether or not it is suggested by the presenting complaints. The failure of clinicians to ask about symptom-

atology comprehensively is one factor that has contributed to the variability of psychiatric diagnosis. Psychiatric diagnosis may also tend to be unreliable because different clinicians use different interpretations of the same criteria.

To overcome these difficulties, several standardized diagnostic interviews have been used. Although performance data are available for all of these instruments, they are at best sketchy by comparison with the data available for most checklists. In calling these interviews "standardized," one must exercise caution; the term really does not mean much more than that a standardized procedure for administration has been established. In some interviews, an attempt has been made to define the wording and presentation so precisely that one can expect that exactly the same material will be presented on a second administration. In this highly structured approach, when all the wording of the interview is written beforehand, the interviewer is given little latitude to exercise judgment, even if it appears from the informant's response that the question has not been understood. Examples of this approach are the Diagnostic Interview for Children and Adolescents (DICA) (Herjanic and Campbell 1977; Herjanic and Reich 1982) and the Diagnostic Interview Schedule for Children (DISC) (A. J. Costello, C. E. Edelbrock, M. K. Dulcan, et al., unpublished manuscript; Williams et al. 1989). In constructing these interviews, the authors have also made the assumption that answers to questions such as "Do you have trouble sleeping?" can be taken at face value. Diagnoses are then made by formal logical procedures or algorithms, which can be used in a computer program if the user prefers.

Such instruments tend to be very sensitive; few cases are missed, but some diagnoses that are made are false positives, which do not stand up to expert scrutiny. Specificity is lower, and strategies to improve specificity by appealing to the range of specific symptomatology that is revealed in the interview have not been very successful. Another problematic area is the reconciliation of information from parent and child, which typically has been collected independently in separate interviews. Both instruments have been used widely and have been revised to take into account the revisions of DSM-III-R; unfortunately, few performance data on the revisions have yet been made available. The DISC has undergone the most extensive revision, based on performance data from initial studies and subsequent epidemiologic surveys (Shaffer 1989). As yet it is too soon to be sure if what appear to be reasonable changes have actually improved the performance.

An alternative approach is to give the interviewer more latitude to exercise his or her judgment if the interviewee does not seem to understand the question. In semistructured interviews, suitable phrasing is suggested for questions, and the interviewer is encouraged to follow the examples; however, if the informant does not seem to understand, the interviewer is encouraged to adapt the question or rephrase it in words that are understood. Responses are coded on simple scales that permit the evaluation of each criterion needed for a diagnosis; but making a rating on the scale requires some knowledge of the diagnostic system and the relevant criteria. The Child Schedule for Affective Disorders and Schizophrenia (K-SADS) (Ambrosini et al. 1989; Chambers et al. 1985) is the most popular example in child psychiatry of this style of interviewing. The instrument is highly specific, but probably has low sensitivity. It has mainly been used to identify subjects for psychopharmacologic and other biological research, but has proved effective in very different settings from that for which it was originally developed (Apter et al. 1989). Since interviewers need extensive experience with the instrument and good clinical training, as in other semistructured interviews, the K-SADS is usually unsuitable for larger-scale epidemiologic studies. Performance data are based on the original interviewing procedure, in which the parent is first interviewed and then the child is interviewed by the same interviewer, who explores any discrepancies between the two informants in the interview. Such reconciliation of discrepant accounts also requires clinical judgment.

Among other diagnostic interviews that should be considered is the Interview Schedule for Children (Kovacs 1985), a semistructured interview that is unusual in that a follow-up version is available, thus overcoming the usual awkwardness inherent in asking the same questions all over again, which children often find pointless and boring. The Child Assessment Schedule (Hodges and Saunders 1989; Hodges et al. 1982) is a semistructured interview with good performance data that makes somewhat fewer demands on interviewers' clinical knowledge and has been used successfully by, for example, medical students. There are several detailed reviews of child psychiatric interviews that a potential user should consult (e.g., A. J. Costello 1991; Edelbrock and Costello 1988; Orvaschel 1989).

Specialized Assessments

Depression

Depression has received perhaps more attention than any other child psychiatric condition, and a bewildering variety of self-report measures, interviews, and rating scales are available. There are also a number of measures that address related constructs. Since interview data suggest that children commonly report more depressed feelings than their parents are aware of (Edelbrock et al. 1986), self-report measures are particularly important. Unfortunately, many of the measures, despite the face validity of the content, have proved more effective at discriminating behaviorally disturbed children from normal control subjects than at identifying depressed children among the behaviorally disturbed.

The most widely used of these instruments is the Children's Depression Inventory (Kovacs and Beck 1977), a 27-item scale derived from the adult Beck Depression Inventory (Beck et al. 1961). A short version is also available (Carlson and Cantwell 1979), but it has been less popular, probably because the Children's Depression Inventory is itself so simple to complete. The Beck Depression Inventory has been modified for adolescents (Chiles et al. 1980) and appears to be an effective instrument for this age range. Other scales modified from their adult counterparts have been somewhat less successful, as have several more elaborate scales devised specially for children. It seems possible that some of the constructs involved in the assessment of depression are difficult to communicate to children, perhaps because their sense of persistent affective states is less well developed than that of adults. This remains an area where much more research is still needed. More detailed reviews of these and other depression scales are available elsewhere (E. J. Costello and Angold 1988; Kazdin 1989, 1990).

The diagnosis of depression in studies where high specificity has been required has generally been made with the K-SADS (Chambers et al. 1985) or with the Interview Schedule for Children. Depression appears particularly difficult to diagnose adequately with highly structured interviews, although the more recent revision of the DISC (Shaffer 1989) shows improved performance in this respect. Other sources of information that can be assessed with standardized measure are clinicians' ratings, on the

Children's Depression Rating Scale (Poznanski et al. 1979, 1983, 1984), which has been adapted from the well-known Hamilton Rating Scale for Depression (Hamilton 1967). The Johns Hopkins Depression Scale (Joshi et al. 1990), an alternative rating scale that appears to have good diagnostic ability and that is much easier to use than lengthy interviews, has recently been developed. A teacher's version of the K-SADS, which includes a substantial amount of rating information, is also available in a preliminary form (Hoier and Kerr 1988). Peer observation appears to have significant utility. The Peer Nomination Inventory for Depression (Lefkowitz and Tesiny 1980), which is given to peers within the same group or classroom, shows good internal consistency, test-retest reliability, and interrater agreement. It correlates well with school performance, self-concept, and teachers' ratings, but probably measures longer-term characteristics of affective state than are generally included in a diagnosis of major depression.

Anxiety

In contrast to depression, research and clinical work in the field of anxiety have been relatively inadequately supplied with appropriate measures. No specific parent report inventories are available, although information from both checklist and interview studies suggests that parents are often unaware of the extent and severity of their child's anxiety, so the deficiency may be less critical to diagnosis. Of the broad-ranging diagnostic interviews, the Child Assessment Schedule (Hodges et al. 1982) has the strongest data supporting its ability to diagnose anxiety, although the Interview Schedule for Children has also proved successful (Last et al. 1987). A few self-report scales are available. The State-Trait Anxiety Inventory for Children (STAIC) (Spielberger 1973) was designed to make the useful differentiation between situational and trait anxiety, so that it might be expected to detect acute stress. Unfortunately, the data supporting this separation are somewhat confusing. State anxiety appears to have a higher test-retest reliability at 3 months than does trait anxiety. There are definite sex differences (Finch et al. 1974), but the test can be applied to children from grades 3 through 6. For older children, the relatively sophisticated adult alternative, on which standardization data are available for grades 9 through 16, can be used. The Children's Manifest Anxiety Scale (CMAS)

(Castenada et al. 1956) is also developed from an adult scale. It includes a brief lie scale. A revised version (Reynolds and Richman 1978) has good test-retest reliability and discriminates between normal and abnormal subjects, but appears insensitive to intercurrent stress and to treatment effects, and some items may also apply to depression. A parent version is available (Gittelman 1985), but as yet there is no information on its performance.

Two other scales deserve mention. One is the Visual Analogue Scale for Anxiety (Bernstein et al. 1986), a self-report instrument that allows the child to place a mark on a line to indicate his or her current anxiety. The line is defined by a calm face at one end and a nervous face at the other and by qualifying text. The strategy has been used in the past for the evaluation of anxiety in adults, and although it is often difficult to determine the quality that is being measured, treatment effects are probably more easily detected with this strategy than with any other instrument. It has some correlation with the trait anxiety subscale of the STAIC and with the revised Visual Analogue Scale for Anxiety (Bernstein et al. 1986). The Anxiety Rating for Children (Erbaugh 1984/1986) is a rating based on a semistructured interview with seven subscales rated by the clinician giving the interview. Although little information is yet available (Bernstein et al. 1986), it fills a notable gap in the evaluation of anxiety.

For the measurement of phobic conditions, the usual resort is a fear survey schedule. Two versions should be considered. The earliest, the Fear Survey Schedule for Children (Scherer and Nakamura 1968), is based on a similar schedule for adults and, although somewhat outdated, has the backing of a large research literature. The currently most effective schedule appears to be the Revised Fear Survey Schedule for Children (King et al. 1989; Ollendick 1983), which is sufficiently precise to discriminate even between separation anxiety and over-anxious disorder (Last et al. 1989). A further review of measures of anxiety is available elsewhere (Roberts et al. 1989).

Obsessive-Compulsive Disorder

Until recently, it was widely believed that obsessive-compulsive disorder was relatively uncommon in children and adolescents, and little attempt was made to explore the problem systematically in pediatric populations. Not surprisingly, the instrumentation has rested very heavily on established adult scales. The Leyton Obsessional Inventory (Cooper 1970) uses a card-sort procedure in which items are identified and then quantified for interference and resistance. Test-retest reliability is good, and changes in response to treatment can be demonstrated (Allen and Rach 1975). Although the adult form discriminates poorly between adolescent patients with obsessive-compulsive disorder and normal control subjects, a modified shorter version for children (Berg et al. 1986) discriminated adequately between adolescents with obsessive-compulsive disorder and control subjects, and moreover showed significant changes in response to treatment with clomipramine (Flament et al. 1985). A briefer form for epidemiologic surveys is available (Berg et al. 1989).

The Maudsley Obsessive Compulsive Questionnaire (Hodgson and Rachman 1977), developed for adults, also discriminates weakly between adolescents with obsessive-compulsive disorder and normal adolescents, and on only some of the scales (Clark and Bolton 1985). Rapoport and Elkins (unpublished) developed a global rating scale using a 15-point range with definitions tied to 3-point subranges. This scale provides a simple strategy for evaluating the patient, although it does not provide any guidelines on how to elicit the symptomatology. It is probably most useful for recording change at frequent time intervals, as in hospitalization, for which it was designed. Recently, Goodman et al. (1989a, 1989b) devised a flexible rating scale, the Yale-Brown Obsessive Compulsive Scale, that includes clinician ratings and patient reports, has good interrater reliability and validity, and is sensitive to treatment effects. This scale is probably the most comprehensive available and is closest to current diagnostic criteria. A children's version is available (Riddle et al. 1990). In view of the often-observed association of obsessive symptomatology with Tourette's syndrome, it is perhaps worth placing under this heading the Yale Global Tic Severity Scale (Leckman et al. 1989), which has considerable utility in assessing the response of this disabling symptom to medication.

Externalizing Disorders: Attention-Deficit Hyperactivity Disorder, Oppositional Defiant Disorder, and Conduct Disorder

Symptoms of the externalizing disorders are closely correlated, and it is desirable when any particular aspect of this group is being evaluated to do a complete review of all problems. The choice of informant remains somewhat problematic, although the issues in this area are somewhat different from those found in anxiety and depression. Whereas children and adolescents tend to report more anxiety and depression than their parents, for younger children the converse is generally true when the externalizing disorders are concerned. However, adolescents may well conceal from their parents some of their more problematic behaviors. The Conners Parent Rating Scale, which now contains 48 items (Goyette et al. 1978), is probably the most widely used instrument, although regrettably less research is available on the psychometric properties of the revision than for the original test. Despite its association with studies of attention-deficit hyperactivity disorder, this scale covers a wider range of symptoms, including many commonly associated with conduct disorder. It is sensitive to treatment effects (Pollard et al. 1983). An abbreviated symptom questionnaire containing the 10 most frequently endorsed items (Goyette et al. 1978) is a convenient measure for assessing change. A teacher's version of the Conners scale is also available (Goyette et al. 1978), which has proved hardy even when transplanted to Hong Kong (Luk and Leung 1989). A brief version of this has been used to select based on teachers' reports children who are hyperactive or aggressive (Loney and Milich 1982; Milich et al. 1980).

The Eyberg Child Behavior Inventory, another short (36-item) scale, is unusual in that performance data are available for the entire age range of 2–16. Not only does it have acceptable performance data (Eyberg and Robinson 1983; Robinson et al. 1980), but it is sensitive to treatment effects (Eyberg and Robinson 1982; Eyberg and Ross 1978; Packard et al. 1983; Webster-Stratten 1984). However, the brevity of the scale does not permit coverage of many significant behaviors. A more specific area still, but one that is occasionally problematic, is covered by the Children's Firesetting Interview (Kolko and Kazdin 1989b), and the risk of this behavior can also be assessed (Kolko and Kazdin 1989a).

The Self-Control Rating Scale (Kendall and Braswell 1982; Kendall and Wilcox 1979) assesses a more narrow range of behaviors associated with self-control, which may be helpful in planning interventions. For self-report of externalizing disorders, a much more limited range of specific instruments is available. There is a self-report version of the Eyberg inventory that has not been widely used although it appears promising. For adolescents, the instrument used in the National Youth Survey, the Self-Reported Delinquency Scale (Elliott and Ageton 1980; Elliott et al. 1985), covers a wide range of behaviors, mainly focusing on conduct problems, especially those that lead to adjudication of delinquency. Loeber et al. (1988) extended and modified this scale to apply to younger children. Although it can be argued that substance abuse covers a more specific area than conduct problems, it should be noted that covert behaviors of this type are more readily reported by children and adolescents themselves (Elliott and Ageton 1980; Williams and Gold 1972).

Identifying changes in rates of antisocial behavior is a more difficult task. Observation in settings where staff can observe for a significant part of the day is one solution, and instruments using the checklist approach can be applied. The Child Behavior Rating Form (Edelbrock 1985) has useful properties and has proved very effective as a measure of change and response to treatment in inpatient settings (Kolko 1988).

It is important to note that many conduct-disordered children do not show the full range of behaviors of which they are capable for some time after admission to a residential placement and, if well-designed behavioral contingencies are in place, may never show such behaviors in these settings. For children in homes or settings where staff are not available to observe on a daily basis, self-report is unsatisfactory; although children will acknowledge a tendency to misbehave, they may be reluctant to incriminate themselves over specific instances. For children living at home with their parents, the Parent Daily Report (Patterson et al. 1982) is an effective strategy. Parents are asked initially to identify symptoms of antisocial behavior. When the symptoms are identified, the parent is called by phone daily over a period of 7 days to report on the incidence of the behaviors in the previous 24-hour period. This strategy might well be used for other behaviors that typically fluctuate or occur episodically.

Pervasive Developmental Disorders

Scales for the assessment of pervasive developmental disorders have been heavily influenced by differing concepts of the diagnoses included under this heading, and the older instruments may include behaviors that are no longer considered central to the diagnostic concepts now current. Further-

more, it has to be remembered that whereas checklists dealing with current or recent psychopathology can usually be answered reliably, it is still doubtful if the parents' retrospective account is sufficiently accurate to determine, for example, the date of onset of specific symptoms, which is now critical to diagnosis.

The earliest instrument in the field was Rimland's Diagnostic Checklist for Behaviorally Disturbed Children (Rimland 1964). Although there is a fairly large standardization sample (Rimland 1971), the discriminant validity of the instrument is still open to question (DeMyer et al. 1971). The Behavior Rating Instrument for Autistic and Atypical Children (Ruttenburg et al. 1977; Wenar and Ruttenburg 1976) is more observationally based and has reasonable interrater reliability. It appears to be reasonably successful in discriminating autistic children, but is based on concepts that many in this field have repudiated. The most popular instruments currently available involve both checklists and observations. The Behavior Observation Scale for Autism (Freeman et al. 1978) includes observation in a standardized setting and is based on the premise that the behavior of autistic children is likely to fluctuate. Good interrater reliability is reported, but validity is still a problem (Parks 1983). The Childhood Autism Rating Scale (Schopler et al. 1980) is probably closest in content to current diagnostic criteria and has adequate interrater reliability and internal consistency, with some promising evidence for validity. It is another instrument that appears competent even when translated (Kurita et al. 1989). Although devised for children, it has proved useful for adolescents and adults as well (Garfin et al. 1988; Mesibov et al. 1989). Because children with pervasive developmental disorders often show uneven and idiosyncratic learning patterns, Schopler and Reichler (1979) developed the Psycho-Educational Profile to assess the uneven patterns of skills and learning that are so common in this group of children. It is more an assessment of developmental functioning than a diagnostic instrument, but it is particularly useful for development of treatment plans and educational programs and is probably more useful than conventional psychoeducational testing for this group of children.

Finally, from Rutter's colleagues comes an interview technique, the Autism Diagnostic Interview (Le Couteur et al. 1989) that, recognizing the difficulty of obtaining information on development by checklist or by highly structured interview, uses instead a semistructured approach with well-defined rating scales that the interviewer can use to record psychopathology. Initial data on the performance of this instrument are promising but have not yet been replicated. A parallel instrument, the Autism Diagnostic Observation Schedule (Lord et al. 1989), is available for recording observational data. Since both instruments take account of more recent thinking on diagnostic criteria, even though they are biased toward ICD-9 (World Health Organization 1977) and ICD-10 (World Health Organization 1987), they may be more helpful than their predecessors.

Although not a feature of pervasive developmental disorders, note should be made of the Kiddie Formal Thought Disorder Rating Scale (Caplan et al. 1989). Thought disorder in children has been difficult to evaluate, and this instrument, together with a semistructured interview, the Interview for Childhood Disorders and Schizophrenia (Russell et al. 1989), may be helpful in evaluating those rare children with adult-style schizophrenic features.

Eating Disorders

Eating disorders show a variety of symptomatology that has been somewhat difficult to codify into simple scales. One strategy is to concentrate on symptoms; another is to emphasize attitudes (e.g., a drive for thinness, body dissatisfaction, body distortion) that are commonly associated with eating disorders. Examples are the Eating Disorders Inventory (Garner et al. 1983) and the Eating Attitudes Test (Garner and Garfinkel 1979). An observational rating scale for eating disorders that is very useful for hospitalized patients is the Slade Anorexic Behavior Scale (Slade 1973). Two observers record the presence or absence of 22 behaviors that commonly occur in anorexia. Despite the fact that its value as a diagnostic scale is untested, it is useful as a measure of improvement, although, like all measures used in hospitalization, one must be wary of "honeymoon effects" (i.e., changes contingent on the admission itself). The Anorexic Attitudes Questionnaire (Goldberg et al. 1979) is another measure that can be used to assess severity and changes with treatment, although no data on normal subjects are available; it should not, however, be used as a diagnostic device. The most extensively used rating scale for the eating disorder patient is the Eating Attitudes Test (Garner and Garfinkel 1979), which in its current abbreviated version contains 26 items (originally it had 40). The test is effective in discriminating patients from control subjects, although it does not compare well with clinical diagnosis. The Eating Disorder Inventory (Garner et al. 1983), another self-report inventory, has broader coverage than other scales, with a number of subscales that tap psychological characteristics relevant to bulimia and anorexia.

Conclusion

This sampler of measures inevitably is incomplete, but it at least shows the wide range of measures now available. Although the performance data on many instruments are inadequate by the most rigorous standards, most if not all the data are sufficient to demonstrate that by the use of these and similar measures one can improve considerably on unstructured clinical impression. Research in child psychiatric disorders that does not make use of systematic measurement has little credibility today. The increasingly insistent demands from consumers, accreditation bodies, and third-party payers that clinicians demonstrate that their interventions are successful have started a trend for measurement to move into the clinical arena as well. Although this sometimes makes for more formal interactions with patients, it may in time foster a more honest and open relationship that depends less on beguiling but difficult-to-define "bedside manners" and more on a content that can be taught explicitly. The use of measurement to evaluate patients in clinical practice may also make it possible for individual clinicians to contribute more to the advancement of knowledge and to recover the value of the now-often-discounted individual case study.

References

Achenbach TM, Edelbrock C: Manual for the Child Behavior Checklist and Revised Child Behavior Profile. Burlington, VT, University of Vermont, Department of Psychiatry, 1983

Achenbach TM, Verhulst FC, Baron GD, et al: A comparison of syndromes derived from the Child Behavior Checklist for American and Dutch boys aged 6–11 and 12–16. J Child Psychol Psychiatry 28:437–453, 1987a

Achenbach TM, Edelbrock C, Howell CT: Empirically based assessment of the behavioral/emotional problems of 2- and 3-year-old children. J Abnorm Child Psychol 15:629–650, 1987b

Achenbach TM, Verhulst FC, Baron D, et al: Epidemiological comparisons of American and Dutch children, I: behavioral/emotional problems and competencies reported by parents for ages 4 to 16. J Am Acad Child Adolesc Psychiatry 26:317–325, 1987c

Achenbach TM, Verhulst FC, Edelbrock C, et al: Epidemiological comparison of American and Dutch children, II: behavioral/emotional problems reported by teachers for ages 6 to 11. J Am Acad Child Adolesc Psychiatry 26:326–332, 1987d

Achenbach TM, Conners CK, Quay HC, et al: Replication of empirically derived syndromes as a basis for taxonomy of child/adolescent psychopathology. J Abnorm Child Psychol 17:299–323, 1989

Allen JJ, Rach PH: Changes in obsessive-compulsive patients as measured by the Leyton Inventory before and after treatment with clomipramine. Scott Med J 20:41–45, 1975

Ambrosini PJ, Metz C, Prabucki K, et al: Videotape reliability of the third revised edition of the K-SADS. J Am Acad Child Adolesc Psychiatry 28:723–728, 1989

American Psychiatric Association: Diagnostic and Statistical Manual of Mental Disorders, 3rd Edition. Washington, DC, American Psychiatric Association, 1980

American Psychiatric Association: Diagnostic and Statistical Manual of Mental Disorders, 3rd Edition, Revised. Washington, DC, American Psychiatric Association, 1987

Apter A, Orvaschel H, Laseg M, et al: Psychometric properties of the K-SADS-P in an Israeli adolescent inpatient population. J Am Acad Child Adolesc Psychiatry 28:61–65, 1989

Beck A, Ward C, Mendelson M, et al: An inventory for measuring depression. Arch Gen Psychiatry 42:667–675, 1961

Behar L: The Preschool Behavior Questionnaire. J Abnorm Child Psychol 5:265–275, 1977

Behar L, Stringfield S: A behavior rating scale for the preschool child. Developmental Psychology 10:601–610, 1974

Berg CJ, Rapoport JL, Flament M: The Leyton Obsessional Inventory—Child Version. J Am Acad Child Adolesc Psychiatry 25:84–91, 1986

Berg CJ, Rapoport JL, Whitaker A, et al: Childhood obsessive compulsive disorder: a two-year follow-up of a community sample. J Am Acad Child Adolesc Psychiatry 28:528–533, 1989

Bernstein GA, Garfinkel BD, August GJ: Visual Analogue Scale for Anxiety, Revised. Presented at the annual meeting of the American Academy of Child and Adolescent Psychiatry, Los Angeles, CA, October 1986

Binet A, Simon Th: Méthodes nouvelles pour le diagnostic du niveau intellectuel des anormaux. Année Psychologique 11:191–244, 1905

Bird HR, Canino G, Ribera J, et al: Use of the child behavior checklist as a screening instrument for epidemiological research in child psychiatry: results of a pilot study. J Am Acad Child Adolesc Psychiatry 26:207–213, 1987

Bird HR, Gould MS, Yager T, et al: Risk factors for maladjustment in Puerto Rican children. J Am Acad Child Adolesc Psychiatry 28:847–850, 1989

Caplan R, Guthrie D, Fish B, et al: The Kiddie Formal Thought Disorder Rating Scale: clinical assessment, reliability and validity. J Am Acad Child Adolesc Psychiatry 28:408–416, 1989

Carlson GA, Cantwell DP: A survey of depressive symptoms in a child and adolescent psychiatric population. J Am Acad Child Adolesc Psychiatry 18:587–599, 1979

Castenada A, McCandless B, Palermo D: The children's form of the Manifest Anxiety Scale. Child Dev 27:317–326, 1956

Chambers W, Puig-Antich J, Hirsch M, et al: The assessment of affective disorders in children and adolescents by semistructured interview. Arch Gen Psychiatry 42:696–702, 1985

Chiles JA, Miller MI, Cox GB: Depression in an adolescent delinquent population. Arch Gen Psychiatry 37:1179–1184, 1980

Clark DA, Bolton D: An investigation of two self-report measures of obsessional phenomena in obsessive-compulsive adolescents: research note. J Child Psychol Psychiatry 26:429–437, 1985

Conners CK: Rating scales for use in drug studies with children. Psychopharmacol Bull (Special issue: Pharmacotherapy With Children), 1973, pp 24–84

Cooper J: The Leyton Obsessional Inventory. Psychol Med 1:48–64, 1970

Costello AJ: Structured interviewing, in Child Adolescent Psychiatry: A Comprehensive Textbook. Edited by Lewis M. Baltimore, MD, Williams & Wilkins, 1991

Costello EJ: Child psychiatric disorders and their correlates: a primary care pediatric sample. J Am Acad Child Adolesc Psychiatry 28:851–855, 1989

Costello EJ, Angold A: Scales to assess child adolescent depression: checklists, screens, and nets. J Am Acad Child Adolesc Psychiatry 27:726–737, 1988

DeMyer MK, Churchill DW, Pontius W, et al: A comparison of five diagnostic systems for childhood schizophrenia and infantile autism. Journal of Autism and Childhood Schizophrenia 1:175–189, 1971

Edelbrock C: Child Behavior Rating Form. Psychopharmacol Bull 21:835–838, 1985

Edelbrock C, Achenbach TM: A typology of child behavior profile patterns: distribution and correlates for disturbed children aged 6–16. J Abnorm Child Psychol 8:441–470, 1980

Edelbrock C, Costello AJ: Structured psychiatric interviews for children, in Assessment and Diagnosis in Child Psychopathology. Edited by Rutter M, Tuma AH, Lann IS. New York, Guilford Press, 1988, pp 87–112

Edelbrock C, Costello AJ, Dulcan MK, et al: Parent-child agreement on child psychiatric symptoms assessed via structured interview. J Child Psychol Psychiatry 27:181–190, 1986

Elliott DS, Ageton SS: Reconciling race and class differences in self reported and official estimates of delinquency. American Sociological Review 45:95–110, 1980

Elliott DS, Huizinga D, Ageton SS: Explaining Delinquency and Drug Use. Beverly Hills, CA, Sage, 1985

Erbaugh SE: Anxiety Rating for Children (1984). Cited in Bernstein GA, Garfinkel BD: School phobia: overlap of affective and anxiety disorders. Journal of the American Academy of Child Psychiatry 25:235–241, 1986

Eyberg SM, Robinson EA: Parent-child interaction training: effects on family functioning. Journal of Clinical Child Psychology 11:130–137, 1982

Eyberg SM, Robinson EA: Conduct problem behavior: standardization of a behavioral rating scale with adolescents. Journal of Clinical Child Psychology 12:347–354, 1983

Eyberg SM, Ross AW. Assessment of child behavior problems: the validation of a new inventory. Journal of Clinical Child Psychology 7:113–116, 1978

Finch AJ, Montgomery LE, Deardorff PA: Reliability of State-Trait anxiety with emotionally disturbed children. J Abnorm Child Psychol 2:67–69, 1974

Flament MF, Rapoport JL, Berg CJ, et al: Clomipramine treatment of childhood obsessive-compulsive disorder: a double-blind controlled study. Arch Gen Psychiatry 42:977–983, 1985

Freeman BJ, Ritvo ER, Guthrie D, et al: The Behavior Observation Scale for Autism: initial methodology, data analysis, and preliminary findings on 89 children. Journal of the American Academy of Child Psychiatry 17:576–588, 1978

Garfin DG, McCallon D, Cox R: Validity and reliability of the

Childhood Autism Rating Scale with autistic adolescents. J Autism Dev Disord 18:367–368, 1988

Garner DM, Garfinkel PE: The Eating Attitudes Test: an index of symptoms of anorexia nervosa. Psychol Med 9:273–279, 1979

Garner DM, Olmstead MP, Pollivy J: Development and validation of a multidimensional eating disorder inventory for anorexia nervosa and bulimia. International Journal of Eating Disorders 2:15–34, 1983

Gittelman R: Ratings for anxiety disorders. Psychopharmacol Bull 21:933–948, 1985

Goldberg SC, Halmi KA, Eckert ED: Attitudinal dimensions in anorexia nervosa. J Psychiatr Res 15:239–251, 1979

Goodman WK, Price LH, Rasmussen SA, et al: The Yale-Brown Obsessive Compulsive Scale, I: development, use and reliability. Arch Gen Psychiatry 46:1006–1011, 1989a

Goodman WK, Price LH, Rasmussen SA, et al: The Yale-Brown Obsessive Compulsive Scale, II: validity. Arch Gen Psychiatry 46:1012–1016, 1989b

Goyette CH, Conners CK, Ulrich RF: Normative data on Revised Conners Parent and Teacher Rating Scales. J Abnorm Child Psychol 6:221–236, 1978

Hamilton MA: Development of a rating scale for primary depressive illness. British Journal of Social and Clinical Psychology 6:278–296, 1967

Herjanic B, Campbell W: Differentiating psychiatrically disturbed children on the basis of a structured interview. J Abnorm Child Psychol 5:127–134, 1977

Herjanic B, Reich W: Development of a structured psychiatric interview for children: agreement between child and parent on individual symptoms. J Abnorm Child Psychol 10:307–324, 1982

Hodges K, Saunders W: Internal consistency of a diagnostic interview for children: the Child Assessment Schedules. J Abnorm Child Psychol 17:691–701, 1989

Hodges K, McKnew D, Cytryn L, et al: The Child Assessment Schedule (CAS) diagnostic interview: a report on reliability and validity. J Am Acad Child Psychiatry 21:468–473, 1982

Hodgson R, Rachman S: Obsessive compulsive complaints. Behav Res Ther 15:389–395, 1977

Hoier TS, Kerr MM: Extra-familial information sources in the study of childhood depression. J Am Acad Child Adolesc Psychiatry 27:21–33, 1988

Joshi PTJ, Capozzoli JA, Coyle JT: The Johns Hopkins Depression Scale: normative data and validation in child psychiatry patients. J Am Acad Child Adolesc Psychiatry 29:283–288, 1990

Kazdin AE: Childhood Depression. Newbury Park, CA, Sage, 1989

Kazdin AE: Childhood depression. J Child Psychol Psychiatry 31:121–160, 1990

Kendall PC, Braswell L: Cognitive-behavioral self-control therapy for children: a component analysis. J Consult Clin Psychol 50:672–689, 1982

Kendall PC, Wilcox LE: Self-control in children: development of a rating scale. J Consult Clin Psychol 47:1020–1029, 1979

King NJ, Ollier K, Iacuone R, et al: Fears of children and adolescents: a cross-sectional Australian study using the Revised-Fear Survey Schedule for Children. J Child Psychol Psychiatry 30:775–784, 1989

Kolko DJ: Daily ratings on a child psychiatric unit: psychometric evaluation of the Child Behavior Rating Form. J Am Acad Child Adolesc Psychiatry 27:126–132, 1988

Kolko DJ, Kazdin AE: Assessment of dimensions of childhood firesetting among patients and nonpatients: the Firesetting Risk Interview. J Abnorm Child Psychol 17:157–176, 1989a

Kolko DJ, Kazdin AE: The Children's Firesetting Interview with psychiatrically referred and non-referred children. J Abnorm Child Psychol 17:609–624, 1989b

Kovacs M: The Interview Schedule for Children (ISC). Psychopharmacol Bull 21:991–994, 1985

Kovacs M, Beck AT: An empirical clinical approach towards a definition of childhood depression, in Depression in Children: Diagnosis, Treatment and Conceptual Models. Edited by Schulterbrandt JG, Raskin A. New York, Raven, 1977, pp 1–26

Kurita H, Mikaye Y, Katsuno K: Reliability and validity of the Childhood Autism Rating Scale—Tokyo Version. J Autism Dev Disord 19:389–396, 1989

Last CG, Hersen M, Kazdin AE, et al: Comparison of DSM-III separation anxiety and overanxious disorders: demographic characteristics and patterns of comorbidity. J Am Acad Child Adolesc Psychiatry 26:527–531, 1987

Last CG, Francis G, Strauss CC: Assessing fears in anxiety-disordered children with the Revised Fear Survey Schedule for Children (FSSC-R). Journal of Clinical Child Psychology 18:137–141, 1989

Leckman JF, Riddle MA, Hardin MT, et al: The Yale Global Tic Severity Scale: initial testing of a clinician-rated scale of tic severity. J Am Acad Child Adolesc Psychiatry 28:566–573, 1989

Le Couteur A, Rutter M, Lord C, et al: Autism Diagnostic Interview: a standardized investigation-based instrument. J Autism Dev Disord 19:363–388, 1989

Lefkowitz MM, Tesiny EP: Assessment of childhood depression. J Consult Clin Psychol 48:43–50, 1980

Loeber R, Stouthamer-Loeber M, Van Kammen WB, et al: Development of a new measure for self-reported antisocial behavior for young children: prevalence and reliability. Paper presented at NATO Advanced Research Workshop on Self-Reported Methodology in Criminological Research, Noordwijkerhout, 1988

Loney J, Milich RS: Hyperactivity, inattention and aggression in clinical practice, in Advances in Behavioral Pediatrics, Vol 3. Edited by Wolraich M, Routh DK. Greenwich, CT, JAI Press, 1982, pp 113–148

Lord C, Rutter M, Goode S, et al: Autism Diagnostic Observation Schedule: a standardized observation of communicative and social behavior. J Autism Dev Disord 19:185–212, 1989

Luk SL, Leung PWL: Conners' Teacher's Rating Scale—a validity study in Hong Kong. J Child Psychol Psychiatry 30:785–793, 1989

McGee R, Williams S, Bradshaw J, et al: The Rutter Scale for completion by teachers: factor structure and relationships with cognitive abilities and family adversity for a sample of New Zealand children. J Child Psychol Psychiatry 26:727–739, 1985

McGuire J, Richman N: Screening for behavior problems in nurseries: the reliability and validity of the Preschool Behaviour Checklist. J Child Psychol Psychiatry 27:7–32, 1986

Mesibov GB, Schopler E, Schaffer E, et al: Use of the Childhood Autism Rating Scale with autistic adolescents and adults. J Am Acad Child Adolesc Psychiatry 28:538–541, 1989

Milich R, Roberts MA, Loney J, et al: Differentiating practice effects and statistical regression on the Conners Hyperkinesis Index. J Abnorm Child Psychol 8:549–552, 1980

Ollendick TH: Reliability and validity of the Revised Fear Survey Schedule for Children (FSSC-R). Behav Res Ther 21:685–692, 1983

Orvaschel H: Diagnostic interviews for children and adolescents, in Handbook of Child Psychiatric Diagnosis. Edited by Last CG, Hersen M. New York, John Wiley, 1989, pp 483–495

Packard T, Robinson EA, Grove DC: The effects of training procedures on the maintenance of parental relationship building skills. Journal of Clinical Psychology 12:181–186, 1983

Parks SL: The assessment of autistic children: a selective review of available instruments. J Autism Dev Disord 3:255–267, 1983

Patterson GR, Chamberlain P, Reed JB: A comparative evaluation of a parent training program. Behavior Therapy 13:638–650, 1982

Pollard S, Ward EM, Barkley RA: The effects of parent training and Ritalin on the parent-child interactions of hyperactive boys. Child and Family Therapy 5:51–69, 1983

Poznanski EO, Cook SC, Carroll BJ: A depression rating scale for children. Pediatrics 64:442–450, 1979

Poznanski EO, Cook SC, Carroll BJ, et al: Use of the Children's Depression Rating Scale in an inpatient psychiatric population. J Clin Psychiatry 44:200–203, 1983

Poznanski EO, Grossman JA, Buchsbaum Y, et al: Preliminary studies of the reliability and validity of the children's depression rating scale. Journal of the American Academy of Child Psychiatry 23:191–197, 1984

Quay HC: A dimensional approach to behavior disorder: the Revised Behavior Problem Checklist. School Psychology Review 12:244–249, 1983

Reynolds CR, Richman BO: What I Think and Feel: a revised measure of children's manifest anxiety. J Abnorm Child Psychol 6:271–280, 1978

Richman N: Is a behavior checklist for preschool children useful? in Epidemiological Approaches to Child Psychiatry. Edited by Graham PJ. London, Academic, 1977, pp 125–138

Richman N, Graham P: A Behavioral Screening Questionnaire for use with three year old children: preliminary findings. J Child Psychol Psychiatry 12:5–33, 1971

Richman N, Stevenson J, Graham P: Preschool to School: A Behavioural Study. London, Academic, 1982

Riddle MA, Hardin MT, King R, et al: Fluoxetine treatment of children and adolescents with Tourette's and obsessive compulsive disorders: preliminary clinical experience. J Am Acad Child Adolesc Psychiatry 29:45–48, 1990

Rimland B: Infantile Autism. New York, Appleton-Century-Crofts, 1964

Rimland B: The differentiation of childhood psychoses: an analysis of checklists for 2,218 psychotic children. Journal of Autism and Childhood Schizophrenia 1:161–174, 1971

Roberts N, Vargo B, Ferguson HB: Measurement of anxiety and depression in children and adolescents. Psychiatr Clin North Am 12:837–860, 1989

Robinson EA, Eyberg SM, Ross AW: The standardization of an inventory of child conduct problem behaviors. Journal of Clinical Child Psychology 9:22–28, 1980

Russell AT, Bott L, Sammons C: The phenomenology of schizophrenia occurring in childhood. J Am Acad Child Adolesc Psychiatry 28:399–407, 1989

Ruttenburg BA, Kalish BI, Wenar C, et al: Behavior Rating Instrument for Autistic and Other Atypical Children (BRIAC), Revised edition. Philadelphia, PA, Developmental Center for Autistic Children, 1977

Rutter M: A Children's Behaviour Questionnaire for completion by teachers: preliminary findings. J Child Psychol Psychiatry 8:1–11, 1967

Rutter M, Tizard J, Whitmore K: Education, Health and Behavior. London, Longmans, 1970

Scherer MW, Nakamura CY: A Fear Survey Schedule for Children (FSS-FC): a factor analytic comparison with manifest anxiety (CMAS). Behav Res Ther 6:173–182, 1968

Schopler E, Reichler RJ: Individualized Assessment and Treatment for Autistic and Developmentally Disabled Children. Baltimore, MD, University Park Press, 1979

Schopler E, Reichler RJ, DeVellis RF, et al: Toward objective classification of childhood autism: Childhood Autism Rating Scale (CARS). J Autism Dev Disord 10:91–103, 1980

Shaffer D: The Diagnostic Interview Schedule for Children (DISC-2): its development and administration. Paper presented at the annual meeting of the American Academy of Child and Adolescent Psychiatry, New York, October 1989

Shaffer D, Gould MS, Brasic J, et al: Children's Global Assessment Scale (CGAS). Arch Gen Psychiatry 40:1228–1231, 1983

Slade PD: A short anorexic behavior scale. Br J Psychiatry 122:83–85, 1973

Spielberger CD: Manual for the State-Trait Anxiety Inventory for Children. Palo Alto, CA, Consulting Psychologists Press, 1973

Webster-Stratten C: Randomized trial of two parent training programs for families with conduct-disordered children. J Consult Clin Psychol 52:666–678, 1984

Weisz JR, Suwanlert S, Chaiyasit W, et al: Epidemiology of behavioral and emotional problems among Thai and American children: teacher reports for ages 6–11. J Child Psychol Psychiatry 30:471–484, 1989

Wenar C, Ruttenburg BA: The use of BRIAC for evaluating therapeutic effectiveness. Journal of Childhood Schizophrenia 6:175–191, 1976

Williams JR, Gold M: From delinquent behavior to official delinquency. Social Problems 20:209–229, 1972

Williams S, McGee R, Anderson J, et al: The structure and correlates of self-reported symptoms in 11-year-old children. J Abnorm Child Psychol 17:55–71, 1989

World Health Organization: International Classification of Diseases, 9th Revision. Geneva, World Health Organization, 1977

World Health Organization: 1987 Draft of ICD-10 Chapter V: Mental, Behavioral and Developmental Disorders (Clinical Descriptions and Diagnostic Guidelines). Geneva, World Health Organization, 1987

Chapter 12

Psychological and Neuropsychological Testing

Rebecca E. Rieger, Ph.D.
Ida Sue Baron, Ph.D.

In this chapter, we will address the role, goals, methods, and usefulness of psychological and neuropsychological testing within the diagnostic and treatment process in child and adolescent psychiatry. The testing may enter the process at various points: it may generate a psychiatric consultation or referral; it may be elicited in the course of psychiatric study; or it may be solicited later in the treatment phase to document treatment responses and the nature and extent of treatment changes. Psychological evaluation can contribute to the psychiatric study by permitting observations not readily accessible from other sources of information, through the medium of specialized test instruments; by supplementing, confirming, or disconfirming formulations stemming from other sources (e.g., parent interviews, playroom interviews, school reports, and therapist reports); and by helping to clarify the interrelationship between symptomatology and more covert structural and dynamic factors influencing development, the emergence of symptoms, the course of a disorder, and responses to treatment.

The evolving changes in psychiatric practice regarding the expanding array of biological and psychological treatment choices, the growing emphasis on shortened hospital stays and treatment in the least restrictive setting, the increasing pressure from third-party payers, and legal challenges from patient advocates have generated concomitant changes and developments in the practice of psychological assessment (Wetzler and Katz 1989). There is an increasing demand for "targeted" or "focal" testing to answer limited (if difficult) questions in the most economical way—questions regarding differential diagnosis (e.g., schizophrenia versus bipolar mood disorder); risk factors like assaultiveness or suicidal danger; the possible presence of neurologic dysfunction; evidence of "treatability" within the available therapeutic modalities; and treatment responses to medication, milieu, and/or psychological intervention.

There are, however, referrals that require a broader or more intensive evaluation because they pose questions related to complex diagnostic issues and treatment outcomes. These referrals may, for example, revolve around the observation of recurrent emergency room visits and/or hospitalizations, noncompliance with treatment recommendations, and the effects of comorbidity (e.g., DSM-III-R [American Psychiatric Association 1987] dysthymic disorder with concomitant psychoactive substance abuse, or attention-deficit hyperactivity disorder with borderline personality disorder). The more comprehensive evaluation contributes both to understanding and to identifying dysfunction. The traditional psychological test battery (Lourie and Rieger 1974; Siegel 1987), labor intensive and time consuming though it is, permits a wide range of observations on overt and covert aspects of functioning in the context of normative comparisons and developmental expectations. The array of tests in a test battery also offers opportunities to note vulnerabilities and disabilities such as impaired visual-motor integrative skills and related learning disorders, and their impact on self-esteem, defensive operations, and personality formation. The greater concentration on the evaluation of cognitive processes and ego functioning in the more comprehensive assessment in addition permits finer discriminations between levels and severity of psychopathology (e.g., between borderline and psychotic modes of functioning), with treatment implications.

Decisions concerning the nature and scope of testing will depend largely on the purpose, locus, and implicit time constraints of the psychiatric referral. The psychological assessment process needs to address the referral questions, but *how* they are to be addressed should be at the discretion of the psychologist-clinician, since the range of available tests and specialized standardized questionnaires is very broad.

Tests differ in the degree of rigor with which they meet criteria of test construction. A discussion of test construction, criteria for reliability and validity, and normative applicability is available elsewhere (Anastasi 1988). Some have been deliberately and carefully crafted with respect to reliability, validity, and normative standards—that is, the measures have stability and reproducibility, including reliability of raters' scoring or judgments; they measure what they purport to measure; and they have been field tested on adequate numbers and representative segments of the populations for whom they were designed. This group of tests would include the principal intelligence tests (e.g., the Wechsler, Stanford-Binet, and McCarthy scales), neuropsychological inventories (e.g., Halstead-Reitan and Luria), specialized semistructured interviews (e.g., the Schedule for Affective Disorders and Schizophrenia), and self-report personality inventories (e.g., the Millon Adolescent Personality Inventory). Others evolved into tests that now meet reliability, validity, and normative criteria (e.g., the Minnesota Multiphasic Personality Inventory, the Bender Visual-Motor Gestalt Test, and the Rorschach). A third group, primarily within the "projective" tests, have various formalized scoring systems with evolving normative data (e.g., the Thematic Apperception Test) or represent new approaches to personality assessment with as-yet incomplete returns on their merits (e.g., the Apperceptive Personality Test).

Tests also differ in their structure, stimulus properties, and response restrictions or opportunities.

Structured, "objective," or psychometric tests elicit discrete, scorable answers to explicit verbal questions, questionnaire items, or responses to performance tasks and generally establish the subject's standing in comparison with a criterion group. The relatively unstructured, so-called projective tests are more open-ended in their response expectations and focus on the subject's more idiosyncratic, individual modes of response—how the subject tends to perceive, construe, interpret, and react to environmental and interpersonal stimuli and events. When structured tests are complex instruments like the major individually administered intelligence tests, which sample an array of cognitive operations, it is possible to observe distinctive individual subtest patterns and qualitative modes of response, in addition to noting the subject's overall standing in comparison with the peer age group, as summarized in the "IQ." Similarly, some projective tests have psychometric properties and can be scored to yield normative comparisons across an array of factors, including perceptual accuracy or reality testing, cognitive style, affect regulation, ego functioning, and object relatedness.

A basic assumption underlies all psychological testing: that the chosen test instrument is appropriate to the individual or group. It is therefore necessary for the clinical examiner to be aware of the subject's age or developmental stage, cultural and language milieu, demographic data indicating whether the subject shares the standardization criteria, and any discernible sensory or motor impairments that would invalidate or require alteration of the testing process. A knowledge of normal growth and development forms the context within which all assessment takes place; it is particularly relevant, however, with children and adolescents, in whom the nature, rate, and degree of change are so rapid.

The testing of children from ethnic minority groups has been the subject of considerable attention and controversy, revolving around several basic issues. Is failure to reflect or conform to majority norms indicative of disorder (i.e., is difference equivalent to inferiority)? Where test results are generally lower than the majority norms, are the test instruments discriminating in their demands and content? What are the relative advantages, weaknesses, and interpretive constraints in testing ethnic minority children? In recent years, there have been significant advances in the standardization of tests to include ethnic minorities in the standardization samples roughly equivalent to their representation in the most recent national census figures. Nevertheless, there continue to be legitimate criticisms of inadequate minority representation in some test content and standardization. Sattler (1988) offered a thoughtful discussion of the assessment of ethnic minority children. Where test results can point to deficiencies in the educational system, or to the effects of more general neglect or inequalities in the larger environment, they may be used constructively to generate appropriate changes and recommendations for remediation. At the very least, they can demonstrate problems facing ethnic minorities in areas where they are in competition with majority members.

In assessing the validity and representativeness of test findings, the examiner-clinician must be sensitive to the interpersonal, situational, and intrapsychic factors affecting the psychological evaluation. The examiner may influence test results by creating (or withholding) a facilitative climate of rapport and empathy to encourage maximal cooperation and effort on the part of the subject within the constraints of standard test administration. Additionally, the examiner's attitude and behavior may permit the subject to experience the inherently stressful testing situation as positive and growth-enhancing.

On the part of the subject, a basic issue will be that of trust, manifested in general and stage-specific ways. For the very young child, separation from the parent—the need to accompany a stranger in an unfamiliar setting—may be paramount in inhibiting or dominating test behavior, and it may require considerable examiner sensitivity, flexibility, and patience to gain the child's confidence. The latency-age, elementary-school child may interpret the testing as arising from his or her failure and parental authority disapproval and may perceive the examiner as a demanding and punitive object. In the adolescent, the issue of trust may revolve around feared invasion of privacy and the perception of the examiner as the agent of complaining parents or authority figures. The subject's concerns and fantasies will ultimately involve the *purpose* of the examination. The examiner's initial preparation of the subject, explanation of the implicit remedial and helpful goal of the process, and sympathetic confrontation of unrealistic understandings and anxieties will usually permit testing to go forward. When the examiner's efforts at reassurance are unsuccessful, the ensuing test results must be interpreted cautiously, weighing the role of situational and immediate interpersonal factors as against more enduring traits or psychopathologic states.

Within the limited scope of this chapter, discussion of psychological test instruments will necessarily be selective and incomplete and will generally pertain to tests in frequent use in clinical practice. Some tests, like the Rorschach, will receive disproportionate attention, to correct misconceptions about their properties and utility, not because of their greater importance or merit. In this chapter, psychological test instruments for children and adolescents will be classified under two major headings: 1) tests that have the assessment of the normality of maturational processes as their primary, if not exclusive, focus; and 2) tests that have the identification and diagnosis of deviations and pathology in development as their primary focus.

Tests Focusing on Normal Maturation and Development

The testing of infants, usually in relation to pediatric evaluations, is essentially the assessment of the normal maturation and development of the sensorimotor apparatus, early cognitive functioning, and beginning language acquisition. These occur within a social matrix but are largely reflective of biological processes that underlie the later emergence of the autonomous ego functions, unless the human or physical environment is significantly abnormal or unsupportive. The infant scales (e.g., the Bayley, Brazelton's Neonatal Behavior Assessment Scale, the Cattell, and the Gesell) can describe the current status of the baby in a variety of areas, in comparison with normative expectations, but they are generally lacking in predictive value beyond 2- to 3-month time intervals. In part, this relates to the intrinsic discontinuity between the early sensorimotor period and the later growth in ability to manipulate language and verbal concepts, and in part to the very rapid overall changes that occur.

As the child progresses from infancy through early childhood, there is an increasing repertoire of cognitive, affective, and behavioral capacities, and the nature and scope of assessment techniques broaden to include language development and manipulation, concept formation and reasoning, learning ability and social judgment, the realm of fantasy and play, and interpersonal relatedness.

Tests of Cognitive Development and Functioning

The testing of cognitive development and functioning is most usually in the domain of the intelligence tests, or supplementary neuropsychological tests where organic pathology is suspected. A vast literature exists about the nature of intelligence and the many ways it can be assessed (for a review, see Sattler 1988).

There is a widespread if not universal consensus that intelligence has genetic, environmental, and experiential components; that intelligence tests only sample the individual's capacities and skills, and that therefore the summary IQ does not represent a summation of all aspects of intelligence; that intelligence tests measure both a general factor and separate abilities; that while there may be individual differences, after the age of about 5 years the IQ tends to remain fairly stable for an individual (i.e., relative standing within the peer age group is not apt to change appreciably); and that the IQ is probably the best predictor of academic success (and of vocational achievement to a lesser extent) when testing is carried out in middle childhood. The original "intelligence quotient" was derived from the ratio of the individual's level of achievement (the "mental age") to the chronological age, with statistical adjustments for changes in the growth curve from middle adolescence. Present tests, including the newly restandardized Stanford-Binet, use the concept of the deviation IQ—where the individual falls in the normal distribution for his or her age group. Intelligence tests do not test innate ability or potential, but provide information about the individual's repertoire of cognitive knowledge and abilities at a particular point in time, and may be thought of as generalized achievement tests, sampling a wider range of acquired skills and concepts than the usual standardized, narrowly focused, school-related tests.

Intelligence tests vary in the chronological age periods or developmental phases that they serve in terms of normative data, appropriate content, and level of difficulty. Some, like the infant scales, have a very restricted age range. Others cover a wide life span (e.g., the Stanford-Binet Intelligence Scale, Fourth Edition, ages 2–23; the earlier Stanford-Binet, Form L-M, ages 2 through adult). The Wechsler scales serve a very wide range of ages (3–75) through three separate but similarly constructed scales (see below).

For the early childhood period, there are several well-standardized intelligence tests that yield IQs or analogous indices. The McCarthy Scales of Children's Abilities (McCarthy 1972) cover the age range of 2.5–8.5 and comprise a verbal scale, perceptual-performance scale, quantitative scale, memory scale, motor scale, and an overall general cognitive scale,

which yields a general cognitive index, essentially equivalent in its conception to an IQ measure. The McCarthy presents special opportunities to evaluate learning-disabled or otherwise exceptional children (Sattler 1978).

The Stanford-Binet Intelligence Scale—Fourth Edition (Thorndike et al. 1986) consists of 15 subtests (of which 8 start at age 2), covering the areas of verbal reasoning, abstract/visual reasoning, quantitative reasoning, and short-term memory. Raw scores for each subtest are converted into subtest scaled scores (mean ± SD, 50 ± 8), areas scores (100 ± 16), and a composite score (100 ± 16), the latter essentially equivalent to the Wechsler scales' deviation IQ. Factor analysis supports two factors at age 2–6: verbal comprehension and nonverbal reasoning/visualization. All of the subtests are judged to be either good or fair measures of the general intelligence "g" factor. Sattler (1988) concluded that despite some serious shortcomings, which he detailed, the test "is a potentially powerful tool for the assessment of the cognitive ability of young children, adolescents and young adults" (p. 290). Cronbach (1988) judged the McCarthy scales to be better for early ages.

The most widely used tests to assess intelligence and cognitive functioning are the three Wechsler scales, all derived from the Wechsler-Bellevue Intelligence Scale (Wechsler 1939). They are structured essentially the same, with a verbal scale, performance scale, and full scale, each having its own IQ, with a mean of 100 ± 15 points. Their strengths lie in good standardization, reliability, and validity, and in their multifactorial design, permitting assessment of both the general (g) factor and special ability clusters. The Wechsler scales all offer the examiner an array of observations about attention span, cognitive efficiency, cognitive style, emotional reactivity, and some interpersonal characteristics of the subject, as revealed in the testing interaction with the examiner. In addition, they have generated a substantial amount of research and reports from clinical practice, permitting enriched analyses and understandings of the test findings. Each Wechsler scale will be discussed further within the relevant developmental period.

The Wechsler Preschool and Primary Scale of Intelligence—Revised (WPPSI-R) (Wechsler 1989) has extended its range downward to age 3 and upward to age 7.3. It therefore covers the early childhood-preschool period and overlaps with the Wechsler Intelligence Scale for Children—Revised for the early grade-school period. The verbal scale consists of five subtests (information, comprehension, arithmetic, vocabulary, and similarities) and one optional subtest (sentences). The Performance Scale consists of five subtests (object assembly, geometric design, block design, mazes, and picture completion) and one optional subtest (animal pegs). The geometric design subtest is a recognition task for younger children and a drawing task for older ones. Although the overall test is quite lengthy and may strain the attention span of some young children, it permits the examiner a range of observations that can lead to diagnostic hypotheses concerning aspects of impaired functioning, which can lead to remedial planning.

The Kaufman Assessment Battery for Children (Kaufman and Kaufman 1983) is a fairly recent addition to the intelligence tests for preschoolers through grade school (ages 2.6–12.5). It consists of 16 subtests, within four scales: sequential processing scale, simultaneous processing scale, achievement scale, and nonverbal scale. The two processing scales combine in the mental processing composite, which serves as analogous to the IQ as a measure of intelligence. Since the mental processing composite does not include tests of verbal ability, it is weakened in estimating overall intellectual capacity. Although the test is useful to assess noncognitive abilities, it is flawed as a primary instrument for measuring intelligence in clinical evaluations.

The Columbia Mental Maturity Scale, Third Edition (Burgemeister et al. 1972) is an untimed test of reasoning ability that demands no verbal and minimal motor responses. It serves ages 3.6–9.11 and is particularly useful for children with sensory or motor deficits and those who have difficulty speaking. It is well standardized, has good reliability and validity, is relatively culture-free, and is a usable test of nonverbal intelligence. However, it tests the ability to form and manipulate concepts rather than general intelligence, and its scores are not interchangeable with those on the Wechsler scales or the Stanford-Binet.

The Goodenough-Harris Drawing Test (Goodenough and Harris 1963), a revision of the earlier Goodenough Draw-a-Man Test (1926), is meant to be a nonverbal measure of intellectual maturity, covering ages 3–15, but most appropriate up to age 10. It is well standardized and reliable, and discriminates maturational levels between ages 5 through 12, but it does not correlate highly with other intelligence tests. It can serve as a screening test of nonverbal intelligence, but it is not a measure of overall intelligence. It is also sensitive to psychological factors like self-concept and self-esteem (see further below) and is apt to underrate the IQs of emotionally disturbed children (Thompson and Finley 1963). Koppitz (1968) distinguished between developmental indicators and signs of emotional problems and related the emotional indicators to impaired school achievement. As a test involving perceptual-motor integration and a memory factor (the internalized body image), the drawings may also reveal neurologic dysfunction, evidenced in significant asymmetry, and marked disproportion and poor integration of body parts, beyond maturational expectations.

To test the intelligence of grade-school, latency-age children, the most respected and widely used test is the Wechsler Intelligence Scale for Children—Revised (WISC-R) (Wechsler 1974), covering ages 6.0–16.11, thus overlapping with both the WPPSI-R and the Wechsler Adult Intelligence Scale—Revised (WAIS-R) (discussed below). The WISC-R consists of 10 subtests and two supplementary ones, organized in a verbal scale (information, similarities, arithmetic, vocabulary, comprehension, and the optional digit span) and a performance scale (picture completion, picture arrangement, block design, object assembly, coding, and the optional mazes). The verbal scale, performance scale, and full scale IQs are all derived separately (the two supplementary subtests do not enter into the IQ calculations). Factor analysis yields three principal factors: verbal comprehension, perceptual organization, and freedom from distractibility, which is consonant with the two verbal and performance scales. The overlap with the WPPSI-R for the 6–7-year age interval permits a choice of instrument, but the WISC-R IQ tends to be lower, and in retesting it should not be considered a possible error of measurement unless the difference is substantial. Similarly, in the overlap with the WAIS-R for the 16–17-year age interval, the WAIS-R IQ tends to be higher. The Wechsler Intelligence Scale for Children—Third Edition (WISC-III) is scheduled for publication in 1991.

As noted above, the Stanford-Binet is also judged to be a very useful test of intelligence in the middle childhood period.

For the assessment of intelligence in adolescents, the most prominent tests are the Stanford-Binet, the WISC-R, and the Wechsler Adult Intelligence Scale—Revised (Wechsler 1981), which was standardized on two adolescent groups (16–17 and 18–19) as well as on adults to age 74. Unlike the WISC-R, the subtest scaled scores of the WAIS-R are based on a reference group of subjects in the standardization sample of 20- to 34-year-olds, and the three IQs (verbal, performance, and full scale) are listed in separate tables for each of the age groups. There are also tables giving age-corrected scaled scores to be used only for purposes of comparison and interpretation of the subtests, but not to derive the IQs. Standardization, reliability, and validity are all adequate. The highest reliability is among verbal subtests, and the full-scale IQ is more reliable than either verbal or performance IQs. However, the WAIS-R can yield substantial differences on retesting, and valid interpretation of changes needs other corroborative data (Sattler 1988).

Tests of Visual-Motor Integration and Maturation

In an assessment of normal development, tasks involving visual-motor integration and maturation are included in the major intelligence scales, among the performance subtests (e.g., block design, object assembly, and coding in the Wechsler scales; pattern analysis and copying in the Stanford-Binet). Additional tests that frequently appear in test batteries and measure visual-motor development are the Developmental Test of Visual-Motor Integration and the Bender Visual-Motor Gestalt Test.

The Developmental Test of Visual-Motor Integration was originally standardized in 1964 and was renormed in 1982 (Beery 1982). A brief copying test measuring perceptual-motor ability from ages 4 to 13, it has been found to correlate with developmental age and reading ability.

Bender (1938) introduced the Bender Visual-Motor Gestalt Test to assess perceptual-motor maturation and its functional or organic impairment. It was standardized for adolescents and adults by Pascal and Suttell (1951), who introduced a now widely accepted scoring system.

In 1963, Koppitz introduced a developmental scoring system for children ages 5.0–10.11 and published a 1975 follow-up volume reporting further research and application. She stressed that the Bender is best thought of as a test of visual-motor *integration*; that problems in copying the nine Bender figures may result from immaturity or impairment or in their integration; and that for the majority of school-age children who produce immature Bender results, it is the higher-level integrative function that is involved. Beyond age 10, the developmental scoring system reaches its ceiling; that is, for normal subjects, the test presents no problems, and

only markedly immature or impaired youngsters will obtain elevated scores. The absence of elevated scores cannot be interpreted as ruling out impairment. For adolescents, the Bender does not serve as a developmental index but can generate hypotheses about abnormalities in visual-motor functioning, possibly symptomatic of neurologic dysfunction. Canter (1976) developed the Background Interference Procedure to help discriminate Bender protocols of adolescents and adults with neurologic impairment from functionally disordered subjects and normal control subjects; it is now widely used.

Koppitz (1975) also developed a parallel set of scoring criteria for 12 emotional indicators that are not primarily related to age and maturation, as in the developmental scoring system. In clinical practice, the Bender test offers numerous opportunities for observation of behavior, management of motility, self-organization, and affective control. The instructions to copy the nine designs do not specify the size, arrangement on the page, overall use of space, consistency of approach, or accuracy of detail, permitting the expression of individual characteristics and the generation of hypotheses about personality and coping style, thus sharing some of the properties of a projective test (see below).

Tests of Academic Achievement

Although they are more often part of psychoeducational evaluations, tests of academic achievement are sometimes included in the clinical assessment of cognitive functioning to identify children and adolescents with learning disorders, or those exceptional children at both ends of the ability continuum, for purposes of educational placement and planning.

The Wide Range Achievement Test—Revised (Jastak and Wilkinson 1984), originally published in 1936 and periodically revised, is a brief, individually administered test of educational achievement consisting of reading, spelling, and arithmetic subtests at two levels: one for ages 5–11 years and one for ages 12 and up, thus covering the elementary, high school, and adult populations. The test is a useful screening instrument to assess word recognition, arithmetic, and spelling skills, but it does not offer information in the more complex achievement areas of reading comprehension and mathematical problem solving (Harrison 1988).

The Woodcock-Johnson Psycho-Educational Battery (Woodcock 1977) is widely used in school settings to assess cognitive ability, achievement, and interest level for ages 3 through adult. Sattler's (1988) review of the battery concluded that its tests of achievement are useful, but that its "Cognitive Ability Full Scale score should not be used as a replacement for other standardized measures of intelligence such as scores on the Wechsler Scales or Stanford-Binet Intelligence Scale: Fourth Edition" (p. 338).

Tests of Personality Development and Structure

The construct "personality" represents a multifaceted, complex integration of cognitive, affective, temperamental, and behavioral characteristics, coping patterns, defensive operations, mode of emotional expressiveness, self-concept, and repertoire of interpersonal relationships. It has probable constitutional, social, and experiential ingredients in a biopsychosocial model. There is good evidence that patterns are not invariant, that individuals may vary greatly in the degree to which they show continuity or discontinuity through the developmental stages, and that prediction of future personality structure, particularly from early developmental stages, is risky and likely invalid (Chess and Thomas 1984). Nevertheless, by definition, the terms *personality* and *personality structure* imply traits rather than states, and while changes occur over time, the individual maintains a recognizable and coherent evolving identity except under exceptional conditions or pathologic alterations. From a developmental perspective, personality tests can reflect maturational changes in the growing child and adolescent in the context of normative expectations, but valid tests must permit the individuality and complexity of the individual to emerge.

Among the tests of personality are some that present the subject with relatively ambiguous stimuli, are to various degrees unstructured and open-ended, and are popularly referred to as projective tests. Different from the psychoanalytic use of the term *projection*, which refers to a defensive disavowal of one's ego-dystonic feelings, the term *projective tests* derives from the projective hypothesis (Frank 1939; Murray 1938), that when faced with relatively ambiguous perceptual stimuli, one's own needs, interests, coping style, and personality organization will determine the pattern of responses.

Within this concept of a projective test of personality, the Rorschach Inkblot Test (Rorschach 1921) is probably the most widely used, with a vast lit-

erature of clinical and research data from the early 1920s to date. Herman Rorschach, a Swiss psychiatrist, designed it as a diagnostic test based on perception that he hoped would discriminate between schizophrenia and other forms of psychosis. Early in its history, studies began to appear documenting normative characteristics of other groups, including other clinical populations, normal adults, and children (Beck 1930; Hertz 1935, 1941).

Rorschach's premature death in 1921 interrupted his research and further development of his system of analyzing the formal elements of the response process; that is, to what elements of the 10 symmetrical inkblots the subject chose to respond: the location, form quality, color, shading, or inferred human movement. Interest in the content of each response burgeoned with the psychoanalytic movement, which looked to the Rorschach content as a royal road to unconscious and dynamic ideation. In the course of the last seven decades, five major systems of analyzing Rorschach protocols arose, all of which were sufficiently different from one another, making research on "The Rorschach" untenable. (For a historical review, see Exner 1986, pp. 6–14.) Research findings across systems were often either divergent or spuriously in agreement, since the underlying assumptions and methods were not comparable. The sixth and latest system—"A Comprehensive System" by Exner (1986)—was developed in an attempt to bring order, reliability, and enhanced validity to the Rorschach procedure and followed an exhaustive study of the different systems and research literature. It represents an integration, incorporating the strongest elements of each of the other systems in Exner's judgment, and it has launched renewed research interest, with constantly evolving normative information, modifications in interpretive strategies, and theoretical and clinical understanding of normal and pathologic personality structure and functioning.

Exner, and his principal collaborator, Weiner (Exner and Weiner 1982), conceived of the Rorschach test as basically a perceptual-cognitive task, in close accord with Herman Rorschach's original orientation: the focus is on how a person perceives, organizes, and construes his or her world, reflecting the individual's typical cognitive style and perceptual organization. Test responses are scored (coded) for location choice, determinants (i.e., form, color, shading, movement, or blends of the determinants), content categories, organizational activity, developmental level, form quality, and deviant verbalizations. These formal elements make up the first line of analysis: the structural summary. Most of these elements have relative stability over time, but some measures are less stable and reflect developmental stages; others vary over short time periods and may reflect transient situationally induced states rather than personality traits. Research data that document the relative stability-instability of different measures are presented.

The structural summary yields information about aspects of cognitive functioning such as accuracy of perception, conventional thinking, and degree of disordered ideation. It also informs about the quality and modulation of affect, stress tolerance, coping style (i.e., introversive, ambitent, or extratensive), degree of egocentrism, self- and other perception, and defensive operations. Norms for 1,390 nonpatient children (from age 5) and adolescents, and for 700 nonpatient adults were revised in 1989 and provide the context within which the data are evaluated, the norms representing not what is ideal or "normal," but what is common. Likewise, deviations from the norms do not necessarily imply pathology, a judgment that involves more complex assessment of the impact on overall personality functioning.

The second step in the Rorschach analysis is examination of the sequence of scores. In the sequence analysis, note is taken of consistency of approach, clustering of poor ("minus") responses, capacity to recovery (shift) from poor responses, variability in organizational activity, locations of "popular" and space responses, and pattern of the "special scores" (the indicators of disordered thinking, defensive operations, and aggressive or morbid ideation). Hypotheses are generated about stressors and sources of vulnerability to cognitive, affective, or behavioral dysfunction.

Examination of content and verbalizations is the third step in the analysis of the protocol. In the Exner system, content analysis is treated respectfully but gingerly in an attempt to avoid the pitfalls of unvalidated assumptions and interpretive excesses, yet to acknowledge the contribution of content to the understanding of personality. Exner (1989) stated that it is in the analysis of content that projection can be identified, principally in the movement responses (since the subject introduces an element not present in the static blot), in embellished responses (e.g., "an evil bat"), and to a lesser extent in the "minus" responses, where judgment is impaired.

The last step in the Rorschach assessment process is the integration of the complex data from the structural summary, sequence of scores, and content analysis to form a psychological portrait of the individual, including strengths, vulnerabilities, and potentials for behavior, with a view to responding to referral questions and formulating treatment recommendations where appropriate.

While the Rorschach is primarily a personality test, various indices of pathologic functioning have been derived from the structural summary data: the depression index and schizophrenic index, both recently revised; the suicide constellation; and the new hypervigilant index, coping deficit index, and obsessive-style index. They represent empirically derived but conceptually meaningful integrations of pathologic indicators, which have been validated against clinical populations. The suicide constellation is based on the protocols of 101 adults who effected suicide within 60 days of the administration of the Rorschach. The critical score of 8 yields few false positives and should alert the clinician to a high degree of suicidal risk. It is not, however, a valid measure for children below age 14; for middle adolescents, it is a useful warning or signal for further exploration. For older adolescents, the suicide constellation appears to have greater validity as a high-risk indicator. There is always the possibility of false negatives, and the absence of an elevated or pathologic index does *not* signify the absence of a disorder. The schizophrenia index is composed of significantly elevated scores on both distorted perceptions and disordered thinking, two prominent features of schizophrenia. The schizophrenia index can contribute to a diagnostic formulation that includes evidence of poor object relations and disturbances in affect tolerance and regulation. In older children and adolescents, Rorschach indicators of low self-esteem, painful self-concept, distressing and confused affects, and the presence of morbid content (i.e., elaborations about damage, death, or gloomy feelings) form the core of the depression index and are consistent with the conceptual understanding of depression (Exner and Weiner 1982, p. 134). There are no specific indices of other diagnostic categories, but Rorschach data can generate hypotheses or serve to confirm or disconfirm a diagnostic impression.

A parallel development to Exner's approach to Rorschach analysis stems from the greatly expanded interest in object-relational psychoanalytic theory, which focuses on the individual's evolving internal or mental self- and object representations and their synthesis to create a stable sense of self and a differentiation of self from others. In normal development, there is discernible growth of more differentiated, complex, and accurate representations of oneself and others, and the achieved level of maturity both influences and is reflected in the character of the individual's interpersonal relationships and ego functions. The Rorschach has proved to be a fruitful method for assessing object representations, with particular attention to the "concept of the object," which examines Rorschach human representations from a thematic or structural standpoint (Mayman 1967; Urist 1977). The most frequently used structural procedure was developed by Blatt and his colleagues (Blatt and Lerner 1983; Blatt et al., unpublished manuscript) based on developmental psychological principles. Blatt's "Concept of the Object" on the Rorschach scale was used with subjects from early adolescence (ages 11–12) to adult in a longitudinal study of normal development, and with adolescent inpatients (Blatt et al. 1976). An accumulating body of research explores the application of Blatt's scale and other object-relational approaches (e.g., analysis of primitive defenses) to issues of diagnosis and severity of psychiatric illness, particularly to the differentiation of neurotic, borderline, and psychotic levels of functioning in children, adolescents, and adults (Kwawer et al. 1980; Lerner and Lerner 1988).

The human figure drawings are also a source of information on the concept of the object, in the sense of self- and other representations, evaluated within normative maturational expectations. The concept may be expressed in structural elements, such as the size and relative size of figures, and omissions, exaggerations, or distortions of body parts. Content elements will also yield clues: the nature of the figures (e.g., ascribed age); degree of gender differentiation; realistic versus cartoon, fantasy, heroic, or debased; embellishments of clothing or "props" (e.g., weapons, crutches, mirrors); and the nature of expressed affect (e.g., angry or threatening, sad, happy or neutral). The human figure drawings can generate hypotheses about personality but have poor interrater reliability; although useful as a supplement in a test battery, they should not be used as primary evidence in personality evaluation.

Apperception Tests

Within a test battery, the Thematic Apperception Test (TAT) (Murray 1943) offers the best opportunity to observe the subject's self- and object representations in response to pictures that present multiple personal and interpersonal stimuli that vary in affective intensity and thematic material. The

subject is instructed to "make up a story," to tell what happened before, what is happening in the present, how the story will end, and what the characters are thinking and feeling.

Murray (1943) proposed analysis with respect to the subject's needs (i.e., inner states, conflicting needs), presses (i.e., environmental forces impinging on the individual), and outcome or resolution (i.e., the protagonist's activity or passivity, object relationships, superego development). Over the years, diverse scoring systems have arisen, none having attained universal acceptance. TAT responses can be analyzed and interpreted within the projective hypothesis (see above), since the pictures have a high degree of ambiguity, and the instructions invite and permit a wide range of responses—some expressing conscious ego-syntonic and ego-dystonic feelings and attitudes, others revealing more deliberately covert or unconscious reactions relating to the self in his or her world.

The analysis of content focuses on the identification figures; the protagonist's strivings, attitudes, and conflicts; the nature of environmental and internal obstacles and barriers; the concept of object relationships; and the prevailing affective tone. In addition, the formal aspects of communication may be observed: overall fluency, organization, consistency, complexity, and psychological mindedness, as well as evidence of idiosyncratic or manifestly disordered thinking. In the evaluation of dysfunction or pathology, the contribution of stage-relevant tasks, conflicts, and resolutions must be considered. With adolescents, these relate to the reworking of separation issues, attitudes toward parental authority, experimentation with individuation and the search for firm ego identity, management of heightened sexual pressures, growth of the capacity for dyadic love relationships, vocational goals, and future-mindedness. The TAT stories can cast light on vicissitudes in maturation by demonstrating any immature, avoidant, prematurely inflexible, inconsistent, chaotic, or unrealistic coping strategies.

In an effort to facilitate the identificatory process for black subjects, Thompson (1949) introduced his modification of the TAT with redrawn pictures to feature black figures (Riess et al. 1950).

The Children's Apperception Test (CAT) (Bellak and Bellak 1974) was developed for younger children (ages 3–10) in 1949. It consists of 10 cards depicting animals in ordinary human situations, since young children are apt to identify easily with animals and are likely to anthropomorphize, attributing human motivations and emotions to the animals. The CAT-H (Bellak and Bellak 1965) consists of human figures and situations that parallel those of the original CAT. The test is designed to address relevant developmental issues, particularly of the preschool and early elementary-school period, such as dependency, separation, regulation and control of body functions, oedipal fantasies and concerns, sibling rivalry, nocturnal fears, and anxiety over aggressive and libidinal urges.

The Michigan Picture Test (Hartwell et al. 1953), which appeared in the early 1950s and was revised in 1980 (Hutt 1980), is a variant of the TAT for grade-school children (ages 8–14) and features two sets of 12 pictures. It permits observation of stage-related issues concerning self-esteem, peer relations, learning and achievement, and superego development, as well as ongoing issues around dependency and family relationships. It can also reveal personality attributes such as coping style, affective tone, and modes of conflict resolution.

The Roberts Apperception Test for Children (Roberts and McArthur 1982), for ages 6–15, is a more recent story-telling instrument, with advantages over older apperception tests in that its stimuli are more modern in appearance and it offers a wider range of everyday interpersonal familial events. It has projective and psychometric properties and explicit guidelines for scoring, yielding information about areas such as conflict, anxiety, depression, aggression, punishment, dependency, and indices for ego functioning and aggression, and a level of projection scale. The clinician's overall global judgment may offer a more useful estimate of a subject's maladaptive functioning than specific areas (Mitchell 1985).

The Apperceptive Personality Test (Holmstrom et al. 1990) is a recently published, promising story-telling technique with both projective and psychometric approaches, based on research with late adolescents and adults. It yields information on clinical disorders, basic personality characteristics, and interpersonal attitudes. A strength of the test lies in the presentation of multiracial figures in the set of eight standard cards.

Tests Focusing on Psychopathology and Diagnosis

Self-report Personality Inventories

Self-report instruments permit subjects to express their own perspective on their experiences and internal emotional state in contrast to other more indirect and inferential approaches. To the degree that the subject is capable of self-reflection and is motivated to be truthful, such tests have manifest value. However, under conditions of reduced or impaired self-awareness, unreliable motivation, or deliberate efforts at misrepresentation, the self-reports have obvious limitations. Some tests have built-in "validity scales" to adjust for such test-taking patterns and problems. The well-established self-report instruments are, at minimum, useful as screening tests, which are cost-effective with respect to professional time, can generate hypotheses about personality functioning and psychopathology, or can lend support to hypotheses from other sources of information.

The Minnesota Multiphasic Personality Inventory (MMPI), revised and restandardized in 1989 as the MMPI-2 (Butcher et al. 1989), is the most widely used and exhaustively researched personality inventory. It was created in the early 1940s by psychologist Hathaway and psychiatrist McKinley (Hathaway and McKinley 1943) at the University of Minnesota Hospital to help in assessing adult psychiatric patients during routine workups, to determine the severity of their pathology, and to develop an objective way of estimating change in the course of psychotherapy or through other change agents. It is a self-administered, self-report inventory, consisting of 566 (567 in MMPI-2) affirmative statements to be answered true or false and is divided into 10 clinical and 3 validity scales. In the original MMPI, scale items were chosen empirically, solely on their ability to discriminate between psychiatric diagnostic groups, and between these clinical populations and a normal standardization sample. This normal sample was representative only of the age, sex, occupational, and racial distribution in Minnesota in the 1930 census. MMPI-2 has a greatly expanded and varied normative base, including members of ethnic minority groups.

The original clinical scales were named for the contemporary specific psychiatric syndromes, but in present use they are identified by their scale numbers: hypochondriasis (1-Hs), depression (2-D), hysteria (3-Hy), psychopathic deviate (4-Pd), paranoia (6-Pa), psychasthenia (7-Pt), schizophrenia (8-Sc), and hypomania (9-Ma). Two clinical scales—masculinity and femininity (5-Mf) and social introversion (0-Si)—were added later. Additional sets of critical items that were incorporated into "special" scales on the basis of extensive research identify specific problem areas. MMPI analysis is not based on individual clinical scales but on extensively researched 2- and 3-point code configurations.

Because the original MMPI was standardized on an adult population, it was found necessary to interpret adolescent protocols in the context of adolescent norms (Archer 1987) to avoid false positives, since a general elevation had been found on many of the clinical scales. An adolescent version of the MMPI-2, scheduled for publication in 1991, is slated to contain contemporary age-appropriate norms and content scales more specifically relevant to adolescent issues (e.g., peer influences, behavior problems, family dysfunction). In the interim, the MMPI-2 manual recommends using the original MMPI with adolescents. A set of interim guidelines for interpretation is available, incorporating the most current research findings (Williams 1989).

The Millon Clinical Multiaxial Inventory (Millon 1987), unlike the purely empirically derived MMPI, is an instrument reflecting both Millon's (1981) theory of personality structure and empirically derived content and interpretive guidelines. Millon was active in the development of the DSM-III (American Psychiatric Association 1980) Axis II criteria, and the Millon Clinical Multiaxial Inventory scales are designed to coordinate with the DSM-III-R personality disorders and Axis I clinical syndromes. The strength of this inventory lies in its capacity to reflect the presenting clinical symptomatology and underlying more-enduring personality patterns and the levels of pathological severity in both. The 175-item inventory combines ease of administration (requiring only an 8th-grade reading level), economy of time (about 25 minutes), and automated scoring that produces a profile report and a more comprehensive clinical interpretative report, contributing to its usefulness as a screening instrument.

The Millon Adolescent Personality Inventory, developed by Millon et al. (1977) for use with an adolescent population (13–18), was normed on a mixed sample of adolescents, both psychiatric outpatients and inpatients, and normal control subjects. It requires a 6th-grade reading level, and its 150 items yield 20 scales and two reliability and validity indices, designed to assess the adolescent's overall personality characteristics, including coping styles, expressed concerns, and behavioral patterns. The computer-generated clinical interpretive report ties in with DSM-III criteria of psychopathology, but the inventory also offers a guidance interpretive report for use by school guidance counselors to identify underachievers, students with "acting-out" tendencies, and students in other scholastic problem areas. Questions have been raised about aspects of validity and the applicability of the underlying theory to the relatively unsettled adolescent period (Brown 1985; Widiger 1985). However, if the Millon Adolescent Personality Inventory is integrated with other valid sources of information, it serves as a useful screening instrument for the adolescent population.

The Personality Inventory for Children (Lachar and Gdowski 1979), analogous in its construction to the MMPI, is a 600-item true-false questionnaire that is completed by parents about their children (ages 3–16). There are 16 scales that deal with behavioral, social, and emotional problems, among which are rationally derived scales for depression and anxiety, and empirically derived scales for hyperactivity, adjustment, and delinquency (Sylvester et al. 1987).

Sentence-Completion Tests

These are frequently included in test batteries for adolescents because they are economical in use of time and are usually well tolerated. They are semistructured, open-ended, self-administered brief tests designed to elicit information about a subject's feelings, conflicts, and concerns about the self and interpersonal relationships. They reveal primarily conscious attitudes, anxieties, and opinions, but also permit the examiner to note associative patterns, inconsistencies, emotional stressors, and interpersonal expectations. The most popular sentence-completion test is the Rotter (Rotter et al. 1954), consisting of 40 sentence stems scored on a 7-point scale reflecting the level of adjustment or maladjustment, and focusing on the degree of conflict. Another frequently used test, the Rohde (1957), purports to tap broader personality features relating to concepts akin to Murray's (1938) need-press paradigm.

Diagnosis-targeted Instruments

These instruments may include behavior rating scales, questionnaires, and structured and semistructured diagnostic interviews with children and/or their parents, in research and clinical use, with clearly defined objectives: to identify and classify (name) psychiatric disorders in accordance with external criteria, principally those of the DSM-III-R classification for children and adolescents. They can stand alone as preliminary screening instruments, or as change measures, with the establishment of baseline characteristics and subsequent indicators of treatment-related changes. They can also be included in a broader psychological evaluation to supplement, confirm, or disconfirm diagnostic formulations stemming from other test data. A discussion of their development, current research applications and revisions, and specific utility within the psychiatric diagnostic process is available elsewhere (see Costello, Chapter 11, this volume).

Neuropsychological Testing

Neuropsychological evaluation of psychiatric patients is typically requested when one, or a combination, of four basic questions arises. The first question is whether the observed behavior is primarily a consequence of cerebral processing dysfunction. If brain disorder is already documented, information is requested about the nature and extent of the disorder as manifested in the individual's behavior. The neuropsychological evaluation is thus requested to establish evidence of dysfunction not detected by more traditional neurodiagnostic procedures, by the clinical interview, or in routine psychological evaluation. For example, an aphasia may underlie a "thinking disorder"; head trauma may result in dramatic mood swings or memory change; severe obsessive-compulsive symptomatology may have an origin in a neurologic syndrome (i.e., Tourette's syndrome); or impoverished social behavior and suicidal thoughts may be symptomatic of underlying inability to interpret social cues (i.e., Asperger's syndrome) and be the culmination of a recognized pattern of social-emotional learning disability (Baron 1987; Rourke et al. 1989). Information may be requested about the child whose hallucinatory experiences are suspected symptoms of a convulsive disorder such as complex partial (temporal lobe) epilepsy.

A second question is whether the presenting clinical picture is a product of comorbidity—whether a contributing "organic" element confounds or contributes to the clinical presentation. Consideration of the overall pattern of neuropsychological functioning, obtained from diverse tests, is essential, as it is unlikely that a single test result will provide this answer. For example, documentation of impairment secondary to substance abuse might be found for an adolescent with a borderline personality disorder. Questions may arise about the interaction of a child's diagnosis of intractable convulsive disorder and a coexisting schizophrenic disorder, the impact of attention-deficit hyperactivity disorder on a conduct disorder, or how attention-deficit hyperactivity disorder and a learning disability interact with a depressive disorder.

A third question is whether data exist confirming that a child's development has been delayed or interfered with as a consequence of neurologic impairment. Neuropsychological data prove helpful when evaluating chronicity, for long-standing problems present with a different profile of functioning than acute or recent events. Patterns of effective and deficient learning, information processing, and retrieval across modalities (e.g., verbal and visual) are clarified by judicious selection of tests.

The fourth question is whether the neuropsychological evaluation can contribute to treatment recommendations or cognitive rehabilitation and, more particularly, monitor interval change consequent to a specific treatment regimen. More direct evidence about the cerebral bases for behavior can be obtained than would be possible with global psychological measures. Sometimes the profile of deficit can be so specific that the results highlight a necessary course of treatment or, in fact, underscore the intractable course to be expected given available treatment options. Delineation of strengths is equally important to elucidating dysfunction in the neuropsychological evaluation. An emphasis on weakness or abnormality of performance neglects the accumulation of data about preserved abilities. The neuropsychological process also allows for comparative function assessment over time. For example, baseline evaluation allows for serial evaluation of a new drug regimen.

The value of neuropsychological approaches to the study of psychopathology is that "they represent a technique, independent of the psychic symptoms, which is sufficiently sensitive to provide . . . [an] external criterion to the clinical syndromes of psychiatry. Thus, classification, and probably prognosis and therapeutic responses, can be externally evaluated and validated" (Flor-Henry 1983, p. 214). There are a variety of methodological approaches. Battery approach proponents may choose among a number of possibilities, the most recognized being the Halstead-Reitan Neuropsychological Test Battery for Children (Reitan 1955; Reitan and Davison 1974) and the Luria-Nebraska Neuropsychological Test Battery (Golden 1981). The limitations of giving identical tests to each child should be weighed against the research value of a well-validated, repeatable core group of tests. An eclectic clinical approach allows for individualized assessment. The clinician must depend on a solid neurologic and psychological base of experience and knowledge, incorporate reputable instruments (Lezak 1983), refer to normative data when appropriate, and utilize single-case analysis to tease apart behavioral variation. Such a philosophy, with the emphasis on quantifying qualitative behavioral observations, is exemplified by the "Boston Process Approach" (Milberg et al. 1986). Advocates of computer-assisted neuropsychology identify special problems of the neuropsychiatric population that computer applications address especially well (e.g., pharmacologic effects, attentional mechanisms, memory functioning) (Adams and Brown 1986). The available instrumentation (e.g., continuous performance tests) and bridging conceptual approaches are described in a voluminous literature.

Variability of cerebral organization makes it impossible to suggest that one particular test always implicates one specific brain region. Rather, one child's test score may support hypothesizing a particular focus of dysfunction, but the very same result for another child, in relation to the overall profile, could well support an entirely different conclusion. Inclusion of diverse tests, qualitative analyses of responses, and, on occasion, repetition of a test or function within a session (comparing the child with him- or herself over time) are effective procedures. Flexibility and extending testing beyond the bounds of standardized assessment rules (once the test can be scored reliably) often highlight the process the child employs, the shifts and responses that are distinctive and therefore potentially diagnostic and of therapeutic significance.

The evaluation of the child or adolescent will include behavior sampling in a number of broad areas, with the focus subsequently narrowed on an individual basis. A wide range of reputable tests is available to the clinician who must pare down and select tasks that allow for examination of specific behaviors of concern yet allow for the extended range of possibilities (Rudel 1988). As the child matures, the range and variety of behaviors that can be reliably assessed similarly grows.

The specific tests cited below in broad groupings are in no way intended to represent the full spectrum of available instruments for children and adolescents. Rather, they are intended to demonstrate the range and variety of functions that can be reliably assessed. An intelligence test will usually be included and examined for distinctive patterns of scaled score variability. However, one must not infer that unremarkable performance rules out the likelihood of cerebral dysfunction.

Executive functioning, as assessed with tests of conceptual flexibility, hypothesis generation, and mental shifting, is a major area of investigation with disturbing ramifications for prognosis if impaired. These tests give insight into the adaptability of the child; the child's responsiveness to social cues; and the ease with which new hypotheses can be planned or developed, effected, and tested. The Category Test and Trail Making Test (Reitan and Davison 1974), the Wisconsin Card Sorting Test (Heaton 1981), Raven's (1965) Progressive Matrices, the Stroop Color and Word Test (Flor-Henry and Golden 1978), and the similarities subtest of the WISC-R provide a variety of impressions about reasoning and cognitive flexibility.

Additionally, tasks subsumed under the heading of attention-concentration are being viewed in a new light. Denckla (1989) provided an operational framework for evaluating the interface of executive function with learning disabilities and attention-deficit hyperactivity disorder. She wrote of an increasing recognition of the need for even greater systematic, standardized assessment of executive functioning and finer discrimination of "attention," introducing the constructs of "initiate, sustain, inhibit, and shift," paired with tests best exemplifying each construct.

Receptive and expressive language tests determine the child's developmental progress and allow for an investigation of numerous skills essential for successful academic performance. The Aphasia Screening Test (Wheeler and Reitan 1962) can elicit language errors observed with neurologic deficit. Additionally helpful are tests assessing verbal fluency (Benton and Hamsher 1976); tests assessing auditory comprehension for lengthy and complex verbal commands, such as the Token Test for Children (DiSimoni 1978); tests assessing receptive language, such as the Peabody Picture Vocabulary Test (Dunn 1959); and tests requiring the child to exhibit written formulation (paragraph production), to read, to spell, to calculate, and in general to deal effectively with language symbols (achievement tests).

Learning and memory tests explore the child's capacity to integrate novel information and his or her facility in later retrieving incidentally acquired data. The Selective Reminding Test (Buschke 1973), California Verbal Learning Test (Delis et al. 1986), Rey-Osterreith Complex Figure Test (Osterreith and

Rey 1944; Waber and Holmes 1985), Hannay-Levin Continuous Recognition Memory Test (Hannay and Levin 1985), and tests of sentence and paragraph memory and design recall, are some examples of tasks that enable discrimination of verbal from non-verbal learning and recall.

Tests of the comparative efficiency of the two sides of the body generate judgments about lateralization of deficit and more specifically may identify specific cerebral regions as dysfunctional. Helpful are the Dynamometer Grip Strength and Tapping Test (Reitan and Davison 1974), the Grooved Pegboard (Reitan and Davison 1974) and Purdue Pegboard (Costa et al. 1963) dexterity tests, and the Tactual Performance Test (Heilbronner and Parsons 1989; Reitan and Davison 1974). The Reitan-Kløve Sensory-Perceptual Examination (Reitan and Davison 1974), which quantifies perception of tactile, auditory, and visual stimuli, is extremely valuable for confirming lateralized deficit. This screening may also offer useful data supporting impressions of attention-deficit hyperactivity disorder. This is true when a mild to moderate number of bilateral errors are observed together with susceptibility to poor performance on specific attention and concentration measures.

Tests of visual-perceptual, visual-motor, and visual-spatial integration include drawing tasks enabling assessments of graphomotor maturation, tests of visual-constructive integrative capacity, and tests of orientation and perceptual integrity. The Rey-Osterreith Complex Figure, WISC-R subtests of block design and puzzle assembly, and the test of line orientation (Benton et al. 1977) are helpful in exploring nonverbal efficiency. There is an increasing focus on exploring affective changes that accompany a variety of neurologic disorders and insults. Tests of affect recognition, perception of mood state, and face recognition exist and broaden the behaviors that can be clinically evaluated.

Integration of Psychological Test Findings

The nature of the psychiatric referral and the scope of the psychological examination will determine the timing and locus of the primary integrative process. When the psychologist is called on to contribute discrete, targeted, diagnostic data, the major integration will lie within the psychiatric diagnostic process, which will include developmental, social, and psychiatric history; clinical observation and in-terview; and note of treatment responses, past and present. But where the psychological evaluation is broader, and includes a variety of tests and behavioral observations, covering structural (i.e., constitutional, maturational, and instrumental) as well as dynamic (i.e., self- and other representational and relational) factors, the analytic, evaluative, and integrative process necessarily occurs also within the psychological assessment (Rothstein et al. 1988) and is reflected in the psychological report.

The testing situation itself, with its challenging and often anxiety-producing elements, permits observations of the relationship pattern with the examiner: issues of trust, dependency, narcissistic vulnerability, defensive structure, affect regulation, reality orientation, the transference paradigm, and some cues to the capacity for a therapeutic alliance. Within the testing procedures, the diversity of stimuli makes it possible to observe differential responses to tasks that are structured versus unstructured, cognitive versus affective, verbal versus manipulative-performance, simple versus complex, memory-dependent versus problem solving, timed versus untimed, and those that involve neutral and impersonal versus social and interpersonal subject matter.

Note will be taken of overall efficiency, the availability of conflict-free areas, the status of the autonomous ego functions (the maturational and developmental level of cognitive and language operations and instrumental achievement), the nature and level of self- and other representations, the nature and degree of affect tolerance and expression, and the areas of conflict and modes of defense and conflict resolution. In evaluating the pathologic aspects of functioning, critical areas will be: 1) the specificity or pervasiveness-severity of dysfunction (e.g., the cognitive-school difficulties, impulsive behavior and immature peer relations of the child with attention-deficit hyperactivity disorder versus the overall compromised functioning of the psychotic child); 2) the interaction between constitutional-structural vulnerabilities and impairments and maladaptive personality development (e.g., the relation of chronic, ongoing learning difficulties to symptoms of a narcissistic personality disorder, or the interaction of attention-deficit hyperactivity disorder and a conduct disorder or borderline personality); 3) the presence of ego weaknesses and vulnerability to cognitive disorganization and disordered thinking in the presence of intense affect (as in a borderline level of personality organization); and 4) the evidence of impediments to the formation of a therapeutic alliance, in the form of distrustful, pessimistic expectations of disappointment or harm from others.

Diagnostic formulations will be based on the presence of test data confirming symptoms of DSM-III-R Axis I and II disorders, as well as more dynamic understandings of evidence of underlying developmental factors, vulnerabilities, coping patterns, defensive structure, self-concept and self-esteem, interpersonal expectations, and environmental stressors.

Recommendations for treatment will derive from the source and primacy of symptoms, analyses of available resources and vulnerabilities, modes of personality functioning, and the complex nature of interactional effects.

In addition, treatment recommendations will include consideration of the chronicity and/or stability of the pathologic features and the demands inherent in different treatment modalities with respect to cooperation, participation, motivation, ego resources, and environmental and familial supports. For example, long-term, analytic therapy would require adequate ego strength, capacity for psychological-mindedness, discomfort with chronic disabling symptoms, motivation for change in the self, sufficient family stability, and a high degree of familial support for the treatment. Ultimately, treatment decisions will evolve from the overall integration of the results of the psychiatric study.

References

Adams KM, Brown GG: The role of the computer in neuropsychological assessment, in Neuropsychological Assessment of Neuropsychiatric Disorders. Edited by Grant I, Adams KM. New York, Oxford University Press, 1986, pp 87–99

American Psychiatric Association: Diagnostic and Statistical Manual of Mental Disorders, 3rd Edition. Washington, DC, American Psychiatric Association, 1980

American Psychiatric Association: Diagnostic and Statistical Manual of Mental Disorders, 3rd Edition, Revised. Washington, DC, American Psychiatric Association, 1987

Anastasi A: Psychological Testing, 6th Edition. New York, Macmillan, 1988

Archer RP: Using the MMPI With Adolescents. Hillsdale, NJ, Lawrence Erlbaum, 1987

Baron IS: The childhood presentation of social-emotional learning disabilities: on the continuum of Asperger's syndrome. J Clin Exp Neuropsychol 9:30, 1987

Beck SJ: The Rorschach Test in problem children. Am J Orthopsychiatry 1:501–509, 1930

Beery KE: Revised Administration, Scoring and Teaching Manual for the Developmental Test of Visual-Motor Integration. Cleveland, OH, Modern Curriculum Press, 1982

Bellak L, Bellak S: Children's Apperception Test (Human Figures). Larchmont, NY, CPS, 1965

Bellak L, Bellak S: Children's Apperception Test, Revised Edition. Larchmont, NY, CPS, 1974

Bender L: A Visual Motor Gestalt Test and Its Clinical Use. (Research Monogr No. 3). New York, American Orthopsychiatric Association, 1938

Benton AL, Hamsher K de S: Verbal fluency section, Multilingual Aphasia Examination. Iowa City, IA, University of Iowa, 1976

Benton AL, Varney NR, Hamsher K de S: Manual of Judgment of Line Orientation. Iowa City, IA, University of Iowa, 1977

Blatt S, Lerner H: Investigations in the psychoanalytic theory of object relations and object representations, in Empirical Studies of Psychoanalytic Theories, Vol 1. Edited by Masling J. Hillsdale, NJ, Analytic Press, 1983, pp 198–249

Blatt S, Brenneis C, Schimek J, et al: Normal development and psychopathological impairment of the Concept of the Object on the Rorschach. J Abnorm Psychol 4:364–373, 1976

Brown DT: Review of Millon Adolescent Personality Inventory, in The Ninth Mental Measurements Yearbook, Vol 1. Edited by Mitchell JV Jr. Lincoln, NE, University of Nebraska Press, 1985, pp 978–979

Burgemeister BB, Blum LH, Lorge I: Columbia Mental Maturity Scale, 3rd Edition. New York, Psychological Corporation, 1972

Buschke H: Selective reminding for analysis of memory and learning. Journal of Verbal Learning 12:543–550, 1973

Butcher JN, Dahlstrom WG, Graham JR, et al: Manual for the Restandardized Minnesota Multiphasic Personality Inventory: MMPI-2: An Administrative and Interpretive Guide. Minneapolis, MN, University of Minnesota Press, 1989

Canter A: The Canter Background Interference Procedure for the Bender-Gestalt Test: Manual for Administration, Scoring and Interpretation. Nashville, TN, Counselor Recordings and Tests, 1976

Chess S, Thomas A: Origins and Evolution of Behavior Disorders. New York, Brunner/Mazel, 1984, pp 269–272

Costa LD, Vaughan HG, Levita E, et al: The Purdue Pegboard as a predictor of the presence and laterality of cerebral lesions. Journal of Consulting Psychology 27:133–137, 1963

Cronbach L: Review of the Stanford-Binet Fourth Edition, in The Supplement to The Ninth Mental Measurements Yearbook. Edited by Conoley JC, Kramer JJ, Mitchell JV Jr, et al. Lincoln, NE, University of Nebraska Press, 1988, pp 200–203

Delis DC, Kramer JH, Kaplan E, et al: The California Verbal Learning Test. New York, Psychological Corporation, 1986

Denckla MB: Executive function, the overlap zone between attention deficit hyperactivity disorder and learning disabilities. International Pediatrics 4:155–160, 1989

DiSimoni F: The Token Test for Children Manual. Hingham, MA, Teaching Resources Corporation, 1978

Dunn LM: Manual for the Peabody Picture Vocabulary Test. Nashville, TN, American Guidance Service, 1959

Exner JE Jr: The Rorschach: A Comprehensive System, Vol 1, 2nd Edition. New York, John Wiley, 1986

Exner JE Jr: Searching for projection in the Rorschach. J Pers Assess 3:520–536, 1989

Exner JE Jr, Weiner I: The Rorschach: A Comprehensive System, Vol 3: Assessment of Children and Adolescents. New York, John Wiley, 1982

Flor-Henry P: Neuropsychological studies in patients with psychiatric disorders, in Neuropsychology of Human Emotion.

Edited by Helman KM, Satz P. New York, Guilford, 1983, pp 193–220

Flor-Henry P, Golden CJ: Manual for the Stroop Color and Word Test. Chicago, IL, Stoetling, 1978

Frank LK: Projective methods for the study of personality. J Psychol 8:389–413, 1939

Golden CJ: A standardized version of Luria's neuropsychological tests: a quantitative and qualitative approach to neuropsychological evaluation, in Handbook of Clinical Neuropsychology. Edited by Filskov SB, Boll TJ. New York, Wiley-Interscience, 1981, pp 608–642

Goodenough FL, Harris DB: Goodenough-Harris Drawing Test. New York, Psychological Corporation, 1963

Hannay HJ, Levin HS: Selective reminding test: an examination of the equivalence of four forms. J Clin Exp Neuropsychol 7:251–263, 1985

Harrison PL: Review of WRAT-R, in Supplement to the Ninth Mental Measurement Yearbook. Edited by Conoley JC, Kramer JJ, Mitchell JV Jr. Lincoln, NE, University of Nebraska Press, 1988, pp 88–89

Hartwell SW, Hutt ML, Andrew G, et al: The Michigan Picture Test: diagnostic and therapeutic possibilities of a new projective test for children. Am J Orthopsychiatry 21:124–137, 1953

Hathaway SR, McKinley JC: The Minnesota Multiphasic Personality Inventory. Minneapolis, MN, University of Minnesota Press, 1943

Heaton RK: A Manual for the Wisconsin Card Sorting Test. Odessa, FL, Psychological Assessment Resources, 1981

Heilbronner RL, Parsons OA: The clinical utility of the Tactual Performance Test (TPT): issues of lateralization and cognitive style. Clinical Neuropsychologist 3:260–264, 1989

Hertz MR: Rorschach norms for an adolescent group. Child Dev 6:69–75, 1935

Hertz MR: Evaluation of the Rorschach method and its application to normal childhood and adolescence. Character and Personality 10:151–162, 1941

Holmstrom RW, Silber DE, Karp SA: Development of the Apperceptive Personality Test. J Pers Assess 54:252–264, 1990

Hutt ML: Michigan Picture Test—Revised (MPT-R). San Antonio, TX, Psychological Corporation, 1980

Jastak S, Wilkinson GS: Wide Range Achievement Test—Revised. Wilmington, DE, Jastak Associates, 1984

Kaufman AS, Kaufman NL: Interpretive manual for the Kaufman Assessment Battery for Children. Circle Pines, MN, American Guidance Service, 1983

Koppitz EM: The Bender Gestalt Test for Young Children. New York, Grune & Stratton, 1963

Koppitz EM: Psychological Evaluation of Children's Human Figure Drawings. New York, Grune & Stratton, 1968

Koppitz EM: The Bender Gestalt Test for Young Children, Vol 2: Research and Applications (1963–1973). New York, Grune & Stratton, 1975

Kwawer JS, Lerner HD, Lerner PM, et al (eds): Borderline Phenomena and the Rorschach Test, Part IV: Children and Adolescents. New York, International Universities Press, 1980, pp 343–494

Lachar D, Gdowski CL: Actuarial Assessment of Child and Adolescent Personality: An Interpretive Guide for the Personality Inventory for Children Profile. Los Angeles, CA, Western Psychological Services, 1979

Lerner HD, Lerner PM (eds): Primitive Mental States and the Rorschach, Part IV: Primitive Mental States in Children and Adolescents. Madison, CT, International Universities Press, 1988, pp 559–680

Lezak MD: Neuropsychological Assessment, 2nd Edition. New York, Oxford University Press, 1983

Lourie RS, Rieger RE: The psychiatric and psychological evaluation of children, in American Handbook of Psychiatry, Vol 2, 2nd Edition. Edited by Caplan G. New York, Basic Books, 1974, pp 3–36

Mayman M: Object representations and object relationships in Rorschach responses. Journal of Projective Techniques and Personality Assessment 31:17–24, 1967

McCarthy D: Manual for the McCarthy Scales of Children's Abilities. San Antonio, TX, Psychological Corporation, 1972

Milberg WP, Hebben N, Kaplan E: The Boston Process Approach to neuropsychological assessment, in Neuropsychological Assessment of Neuropsychiatric Disorders. Edited by Grant I, Adams KM. New York, Oxford University Press, 1986, pp 65–86

Millon T: Disorders of Personality: DSM-III–Axis II. New York, Wiley-Interscience, 1981

Millon T: Manual for the MCMI-II, Second Edition. Minneapolis, MN, National Computer Systems, 1987

Millon T, Greene CJ, Meagher RB Jr: Millon Adolescent Personality Inventory. Minneapolis, MN, National Computer Systems, 1977

Mitchell JV Jr: The Ninth Mental Measurements Yearbook, Vol 1. Lincoln, NE, University of Nebraska Press, 1985

Murray HA: Explorations in Personality. New York, Oxford University Press, 1938

Murray HA: Thematic Apperception Test Manual. Cambridge, MA, Harvard University Press, 1943

Osterreith P, Rey A: Le test de copie d'une figure complexe. Archives de Psychologie 30:206–356, 1944

Pascal GR, Suttell BJ: The Bender Gestalt Test. New York, Grune & Stratton, 1951

Raven JC: The Coloured Progressive Matrices. London, HK Lewis, 1965

Reitan RM: An investigation of the validity of Halstead's measures of biological intelligence. Archives of Neurology and Psychiatry 73:28–35, 1955

Reitan RM, Davison LA: Clinical Neuropsychology: Current Status and Applications. Washington, DC, Winston, 1974

Riess BF, Schwartz EK, Cottingham A: An experimental critique of assumptions underlying the Negro version of the TAT. Journal of Abnormal and Social Psychology 45:700–709, 1950

Roberts GE, McArthur DS: Roberts Apperception Test for Children. Los Angeles, CA, Western Psychological Services, 1982

Rohde AR: The Sentence Completion Method: Its Diagnostic and Clinical Application to Mental Disorders. New York, Ronald, 1957

Rorschach H: Psychodiagnostik. Bern, Bircher, 1921 (Translated by Hans Huber Verlag 1942)

Rothstein A, Benjamin L, Crosby M, et al: Learning Disorders: An Integration of Neuropsychological and Psychoanalytic Considerations. Madison, CT, International Universities Press, 1988

Rotter JB, Rafferty JE, Lotsoff AB: The validity of the Rotter Incomplete Sentences Blank, High School Form. Journal of Consulting Psychology 18:105–111, 1954

Rourke BP, Young GC, Leenaars AA: A childhood learning disability that predisposes those afflicted to adolescent and adult depression and suicide risk. Journal of Learning Disabilities 22:169–175, 1989

Rudel RG: Assessment of Developmental Learning Disorders: A Neuropsychological Approach. New York, Basic Books, 1988

Sattler JM: Review of McCarthy Scales of Children's Abilities, in The Eighth Mental Measurements Yearbook. Edited by Buros OK. Highland Park, NJ, Gryphon Press, 1978, pp 311–313

Sattler JM: Assessment of Children, 3rd Edition. San Diego, CA, JM Sattler, 1988

Siegel MG: Psychological Testing from Early Childhood Through Adolescence: A Developmental and Psychodynamic Approach. Madison, CT, International Universities Press, 1987

Sylvester CE, Hyde TS, Reichler RJ: The Diagnostic Interview for Children and Personality Inventory for Children in studies of children at risk for anxiety disorders or depression. J Am Acad Child Adolesc Psychiatry 26:668–675, 1987

Thompson CE: The Thompson modification of the Thematic Apperception Test. Rorschach Research Exchange 13:469–478, 1949

Thompson JM, Finley CJ: The relationship between the Goodenough Draw-a-Man Test and the Stanford-Binet–Form L-M in children referred for school guidance services. California Journal of Educational Research 14:19–22, 1963

Thorndike R, Hagen E, Sattler J: Technical manual for Stanford-Binet Intelligence Scale, 4th Edition. Chicago, IL, Riverside, 1986

Urist J: The Rorschach test and the assessment of object relations. J Pers Assess 41: 3–9, 1977

Waber DP, Holmes JM: Assessing children's copy productions of the Rey-Osterrieth Complex Figure. J Clin Exp Neuropsychol 7:264–280, 1985

Wechsler D: The Measurement of Adult Intelligence. Baltimore, MD, Williams & Wilkins, 1939

Wechsler D: Wechsler Intelligence Scale for Children—Revised. New York, Psychological Corporation, 1974

Wechsler D: Wechsler Adult Intelligence Scale—Revised. San Antonio, TX, Psychological Corporation, 1981

Wechsler D: Wechsler Preschool and Primary Scale of Intelligence—Revised. San Antonio, TX, Psychological Corporation, 1989

Wetzler S, Katz MM: Contemporary Approaches to Psychological Assessment. New York, Brunner/Mazel, 1989

Wheeler L, Reitan RM: The presence and laterality of brain damage predicted from responses to a short aphasia screening test. Percept Mot Skills 15:783–799, 1962

Widiger TA: Review of the Millon Adolescent Personality Inventory, in The Ninth Mental Measurements Yearbook, Vol 1. Edited by Mitchell JV Jr. Lincoln, NE, University of Nebraska Press, 1985, pp 979–981

Williams CL: Use of the MMPI-2 with adolescents, in Topics in MMPI-2 Interpretation. Edited by Butcher JN, Graham JR. Minneapolis, MN, University of Minnesota, 1989

Woodcock RW: Woodcock-Johnson Psycho-Educational Battery: Technical Report. Allen, TX, DLM Teaching Resources, 1977

Chapter 13

Laboratory and Diagnostic Testing

Alan J. Zametkin, M.D.
Paul Andreason, M.D., M.S.
Markus J. P. Kruesi, M.D.

A wide array of laboratory measures are available to the clinician for the diagnosis and management of children with behavioral difficulties. Despite the rapid development of highly technical instrumentation for both imaging the brain and measuring esoteric endogenous and exogenous biologically active substances, the clinical history and interview still remain the crucial elements in evaluation and treatment of children and adolescents. A critique of the utility of all laboratory tests is beyond the scope of this chapter. It is hoped, however, that an appreciation will be provided for the utility of the more commonly considered measures as they apply to behavioral problems. Overviews of the role of the laboratory in psychiatry in general (Greden 1984; White and Barraclough 1989) explore issues such as sensitivity versus specificity in laboratory measures in general, and the utility of routine inpatient admission laboratory studies, a practice that rarely leads to change in initial diagnostic impression or management (Gabel and Hsu 1986). Much of common practice in child and adolescent psychiatry is in fact extrapolated from research in adult populations with few exceptions as outlined below. In this discussion, we will focus on the role of the laboratory in both evaluation and clinical management. We hope to clarify those laboratory measures or modalities that are critical, controversial, or noncontributory to dealing with common clinical problems.

The Role of the Laboratory in Evaluation

Dexamethasone Suppression Test (DST)

Dexamethasone is a long-acting glucocorticoid of which 1 mg is roughly equivalent to 25 mg of cortisol. Nonsuppression of cortisol secretion during the DST has been statistically correlated with the diagnosis of DSM-III-R major depression with melancholia (Khan 1987) or endogenous depression. However, the DST is not clinically useful in adults (Zimmerman et al. 1987), children (Doherty et al. 1986), or adolescents (Doherty et al. 1986; Klee and Garfinkel 1984). Although it may support a diagnosis of major depression with melancholia, it does not rule it out. The DST does not predict prognosis; it does not help in the choice of medication; and many false-positive results confound its interpretation. The DST does not effect the clinical management of major depression unless one is screening for Cushing's syndrome.

Thyroid Function Tests

Laboratory tests of thyroid function are useful in the evaluation of psychiatric symptoms, including anxiety, depression, mental retardation, dementia, restlessness, mental status change, and psychosis.

Tests include the serum thyroxin, triiodothyronine resin uptake (which truly measures the protein binding for thyroxin), the thyroid-stimulating hormone, and serum triiodothyronine levels. If in evaluating symptoms there are elements of the history or physical examination that lead a clinician to suspect that thyroid disease may be contributing to the disorder, screening thyroxin and triiodothyronine resin uptake should be done. If these screening examinations are abnormal or borderline normal, thyroid-stimulating hormone levels should be obtained. If preliminary studies are equivocal, a thyrotropin-releasing hormone stimulation test might be considered.

Depression in adolescents has been investigated using the thyrotropin-releasing hormone stimulation test; the test has not shown clinical utility in the diagnosis or treatment of depression (Khan 1987).

Electroencephalogram (EEG)

The *routine* use of the EEG in the evaluation of behavioral difficulties is not indicated, given the high prevalence of abnormal EEG findings in the general population (Kinsbourne 1985) and particularly for admission screening (Gabel and Hsu 1986). However, when the physical examination and history suggest gross motor seizures, absences, complex partial seizures, temporal lobe epilepsy, or dyscontrol syndromes, complete EEG and neurologic consultation should be obtained.

Catecholamine Assays

Clinically, catecholamine assays are used to investigate the suspicion of pheochromocytoma in the evaluation of anxiety when accompanied by abnormal or disturbed autonomic function. Homovanillic acid, vanillylmandelic acid, and metanephrines are measured in a 24-hour urine collection. It is not recommended that all patients with anxiety be screened for pheochromocytoma (Raj and Sheehan 1987). The large series of research studies measuring urinary and serum catecholamines in hyperactive children have no clinical application as yet (Zametkin and Rapoport 1987).

Enzyme Measurement

Monoamine oxidase (MAO), catechol-O-methyltransferase (COMT), dopamine beta-hydroxylase, and adenylate cyclase are commonly measured in research settings (Bowden et al. 1988) but have not thus far found a place in the clinical practice of child and adolescent psychiatry. Low dopamine beta-hydroxylase activity has been associated with undersocialized conduct disorders (Rogeness et al. 1984), but not in all studies (Pliszka et al. 1988).

The serum amylase level has been proposed as a useful indicator of vomiting activity in bulimic patients (Gwirtsman 1989).

Sexually Transmitted Disease

Children and adolescents with a history of sexual abuse or sexual activity who are being evaluated for symptoms of depression or changes in cognitive function should be evaluated for infection with the human immunodeficiency virus (HIV) and *Treponema pallidum*. Screening for *T. pallidum* is undertaken with the Venereal Disease Research Laboratory (VDRL) test. If this is positive, it should be followed with the fluorescent treponemal antibody absorption test (FTA-ABS). If the serum FTA-ABS is negative in the face of mental status changes and a positive VDRL, an infectious disease consultation with cerebrospinal fluid (CSF) FTA-ABS should be considered. Depression and changes in cognition have been described in HIV infection in children (Diederich et al. 1988). Children and adolescents considered at risk should be screened for HIV.

CSF Measures

Lumbar punctures to study CSF in child and adolescent psychiatric disorders occur in research centers (Kruesi 1989; Kruesi et al. 1985, 1990a). The marker of most immediate interest is the concentration of 5-hydroxyindoleacetic acid (5-HIAA), a serotonin metabolite. Lower concentrations have been associated with both self-directed and other-directed aggression in studies of adults (for a review, see Åsberg et al. 1987). Analogous inverse correlation between histories of aggression and CSF 5-HIAA concentration have been reported in children and adolescents (Kruesi 1989; Kruesi et al. 1990a). Follow-up studies in adults have suggested that low 5-HIAA concentrations may presage continued risk for aggression. The importance of these findings will be clarified over time. The prognostic import of low 5-HIAA concentrations in childhood psychiatric disorders needs to be documented.

Similarly, the treatment implications, if any, of an abnormal 5-HIAA have not yet been established.

Phenylketonuria is an inborn error of metabolism that is usually associated with mental retardation. Although phenylalanine-free diets decrease the cognitive and behavioral deficits, patients treated since infancy have an increased incidence of behavioral problems (Stevenson et al. 1979).

Toxicology

Drug screens for substances of abuse may be useful in new-onset psychosis or behavioral change in adolescents, as well as for monitoring compliance with drug abstinence as part of substance abuse treatment. Testing for drugs of abuse has been suggested for all psychiatric inpatient admissions (American Psychiatric Association 1989; Verbey et al. 1986a, 1986b).

Lead ingestion is a rare cause of behavioral difficulty; this environmental toxin can be measured.

Genetic Studies

Genetic etiologic risk for childhood psychopathology is supported by four types of data: 1) evidence for associations between specific chromosomal variants or abnormalities and psychopathology; 2) increased risk of the disorder among adopted-away offspring of affected individuals; 3) twin studies suggesting greater concordance for a particular disorder among monozygotic than among the genetically less similar dizygotic twins; and 4) family studies finding increased occurrence of certain disorders in at-risk family members (Leckman et al. 1987). Except for the presymptomatic identification of the Huntington's gene, little of the current revolution in molecular genetics has clinical application in child psychiatry, although "clinical medicine in the 21st century is almost certain to include wide-scale use of molecular genetic diagnostic tests" (Brandt et al. 1989, p. 3108). At present, karyotyping is probably the most common genetic assessment in child and adolescent psychiatry. Karyotyping to determine the chromosome number and morphology may be useful, particularly when abnormalities of sex chromosome number or properties are suspected.

In prepubertal children, one may not see the physical stigmata that cause a sex chromosome abnormality to be suspected. However, cognitive difficulties may increase the need for scrutiny. Available evidence suggests that an abnormal number of X chromosomes influences cognitive development and functioning (Walzer 1985). Patients with Turner's syndrome, 45 XO, have spatial-processing deficits (Walzer 1985). Klinefelter's syndrome—males with an additional X chromosome, 47 XXY—is associated with verbal cognitive deficits in most (Netley and Rovet 1982; Pennington et al. 1982; Ratcliffe et al. 1982a, 1982b; Walzer 1985; Walzer et al. 1978) but not all (Bender et al. 1986) reports of prospective studies. Dyslexia appears more frequently in Klinefelter's syndrome (Bender et al. 1986).

Increased numbers of Y chromosomes are also associated with increased risks of behavioral problems, notably impulsivity and immaturity (Ratcliffe and Field 1982).

Fragile X syndrome, so named because of the propensity for breakage under certain conditions, is the most common inherited form of mental retardation (Hagerman 1987) and carries with it an increased risk for psychopathology.

Potential benefits of childhood karyotyping may include 1) anticipation of future course (e.g., issues of decreased reproductive capability); 2) an "explanation" for parents to gather around; and 3) medical interventions. Preliminary experience with presymptomatic genetic testing for Huntington's disease suggests that when such testing is done along with supportive education, pretest counseling, psychological support, and regular follow-up, people who receive the test results cope well (Brandt et al. 1989).

Karyotyping can urge for certain medical interventions. Testosterone replacement for patients with Klinefelter's syndrome may lead to better social functioning (Nielsen et al. 1988) and, intriguingly, cessation of fire-setting behavior (Miller and Sulkes 1988). Although fertility is often diminished in persons with certain chromosomal abnormalities, case reports remind us not to view such conclusions as absolutes (Sheridan et al. 1989; Swapp et al. 1989).

Although Wilson's disease, a recessively inherited disorder of copper metabolism, is not diagnosable by genetic techniques, its identification is critical given that it is a treatable metabolic disorder that commonly presents in adolescence with incongruous behavior, personality change, cognitive impairment, anxiety, and depression (Dening and Berrios 1989). The laboratory fingerprint of Wilson's disease is characterized by low serum ceruloplasmin level, low total serum copper level, and raised urinary copper excretion.

Brain Imaging

All currently available imaging modalities—positron-emission tomography (PET), magnetic resonance imaging (MRI), computed tomography (CT), EEG spectral tomography, and cerebral blood flow—have been used in the investigation of clinical problems relevant to child psychiatry. CT has been the most extensively studied, being the first technique widely available. Studies of children with autism (Balottin et al. 1989; Campbell et al. 1982; Damasio et al. 1980; Gillberg and Svendsen 1983; Prior et al. 1984; Rosenbloom et al. 1984), retardation (Gillberg and Svendsen 1983; Moeschler et al. 1981), and attention-deficit disorder with hyperactivity (Nasrallah et al. 1986; Shaywitz et al. 1983) in general do not argue for routine use of imaging studies, despite significant findings with MRI in autism (Courchesne et al. 1988). Clinical indications do exist for the MRI or CT (with or without contrast), including signs of increased intracranial pressure, changing or degenerative neurologic signs, some craniofacial malformations, suspected syndromes, or inherited syndromes that include central nervous system structures. Although CT or MRI studies in psychosis in minors are rare (Reiss et al. 1983; Schulz et al. 1983; Woody et al. 1987), clinical practice (unsubstantiated by rigorous studies) suggests that CT or MRI be performed to rule out treatable intracranial disease (brain tumor).

No studies support the clinical usefulness of spectral topographic mapping with EEG (brain electrical activity mapping, or BEAM) in children or adolescents.

Except for presurgical screening in intractable epilepsy (Chugani, personal communication), the use of PET with either fluoro-2-deoxy-D-glucose to measure metabolism or $H_2^{15}O$ to measure blood flow has not found a niche outside the research setting. Clearly these techniques have all been applied to psychiatric disorders of childhood (Lou et al. 1984, 1989; Swedo et al. 1989), but as yet are not clinically indicated.

The Role of the Laboratory in Management

Tricyclic Antidepressants

Cardiac monitoring via electrocardiogram is an integral part of the treatment with tricyclic antidepressants of children and adolescents. Although some argue that the electrocardiogram need not be regularly assessed until patients reach 2.5–3.5 mg/kg, we would argue that without predrug baseline measures of cardiac function, any change noted at higher serum levels would be only in relation to a false baseline that may not represent the true unmedicated state.

Measurement of medication concentrations in blood or other body fluids is more of use in preventing toxicity than ensuring therapeutic benefit in pediatric psychopharmacology (Gualtieri et al. 1984). Concentration of tricyclic antidepressants can be helpful in avoiding toxicity (Puig-Antich et al. 1987; Ryan et al. 1986, 1987). Clomipramine is efficacious in ameliorating symptoms of obsessive-compulsive disorder in children and adolescents, but drug concentration is not predictive of response (Leonard et al. 1989).

Imipramine, amitriptyline, and nortriptyline serum levels are useful. Individual variation in the metabolism of these drugs often makes it necessary to monitor serum levels to provide an adequate dose or to avoid toxicity (Preskorn et al. 1989). Effective therapeutic levels of tricyclic antidepressants vary, depending on the pathologic entity being treated. However, antidepressant levels necessary for the relief of depression in children are comparable to those in adults (Geller et al. 1985; Morselli et al. 1983).

Nortriptyline and amitriptyline have been reported to have a "therapeutic window," or serum drug concentration range, in which optimal therapeutic response will be seen. There is often interlaboratory variation, but nortriptyline levels within 50–150 ng/ml are considered to be in this therapeutic range (American Psychiatric Association 1985). When using amitriptyline, combined amitriptyline plus nortriptyline levels in the range of 125–210 ng/ml seem to have the greatest therapeutic effect (Breyer-Pfaff et al. 1989).

Imipramine levels are reported as imipramine plus desipramine levels. Many laboratories report a therapeutic range of 150–300 ng/ml of the sum of serum values. However, the percentage of patients responding favorably increases when these levels approach 200–250 ng/ml, with possible impairment of therapeutic effect at levels of 250–300 ng/ml. Electrocardiogram changes also accompany plasma levels above 300 ng/ml (Morselli et al. 1983). Many studies show no increase in therapeutic response with imipramine plus desipramine levels higher than 250 ng/ml in adults (American Psychiatric Association 1985). Plasma levels that are effective for the treatment of enuresis and attention-deficit hyperactivity disorder may be lower than those needed for the treatment of depression. Plasma imipramine plus desipramine levels of 60–100 ng/ml (Morselli et al. 1983) seemed effective for enuresis.

Plasma levels of desmethylimipramine (desipramine) that are 125 ng/ml or greater increase the rate of therapeutic response in adults (American Psychiatric Association 1985). Only limited information is available about the usefulness of drug levels in other heterocyclic antidepressants.

Tricyclic antidepressants are used in the treatment of attention-deficit hyperactivity disorder, and blood levels may be of considerable value, although little relationship has been observed between blood level and response (Biederman et al. 1989). Tricyclic antidepressant levels should be drawn at least 5 days after dosage manipulation so that serum levels may reach steady state.

MAO Inhibitors

At this time, platelet MAO inhibition is seldom used clinically. However, this may not be true in the future because of its current use in research as a dosing standard with which to compare the relative efficacy of tricyclic antidepressants and MAO inhibitors. Platelet MAO inhibition may in the future help clinicians reach potentially effective doses with less uncertainty. Clinical response to phenelzine and isocarboxazid (but not necessarily tranylcypromine) correlates positively to platelet MAO inhibition in adults. In adult patients, 68% responded with platelet MAO inhibition of greater than 90% inhibition, but less than 44% of patients responded if the platelet inhibition was less than 80% (Robinson et al. 1978).

Lithium

Although lithium has been demonstrated to be effective in aggressive (Campbell et al. 1984) and bipolar children and adolescents, the therapeutic range of lithium concentration has not been definitely established and may be the same as in adults (Jefferson et al. 1987). Even without absolute certainty of the optimum lithium level in children and adolescents, monitoring is justified to avoid toxicity (Weller et al. 1987). Another justification for assay of medication concentration is documentation of

compliance. Saliva monitoring has been proposed as a noninvasive compliance check.

Patients that are to be treated with lithium should have baseline thyroid function tests, serum electrolytes (including blood urea nitrogen and creatinine), CBC, and a baseline electrocardiogram. Patients treated with lithium should have lithium levels checked twice weekly during stabilization and then monthly thereafter until stable.

Stimulants

Given the individual variability in blood levels of stimulants (Gualtieri et al. 1982), assays of stimulant blood levels are not clinically of use. Despite large number of studies on the effects of stimulants on hormones and catecholamine mutabilities, no laboratory measures are indicated for routine use of stimulants except baseline and follow-up liver function tests when using pemoline (Cylert).

Carbamazepine

Anticonvulsant medications such as carbamazepine are being used more commonly in children with behavioral difficulties. Before patients are started on carbamazepine, a complete blood count with platelets, reticulocyte count, and serum iron should be performed. After commencement of therapy, these measures should be repeated weekly for the first 3 months. Carbamazepine can cause aplastic anemia, agranulocytosis, leukopenia, and thrombocytopenia. The medication should be stopped if there is any sign of bone marrow suppression. Discontinuation guidelines in adults are available elsewhere (Post and Uhde 1988). Carbamazepine levels can be drawn, but have not been correlated to therapeutic response in psychiatric disorders. When carbamazepine is used to control partial complex seizures, the therapeutic level is generally 8–12 ng/ml.

References

American Psychiatric Association: Tricyclic antidepressants—blood-level measurements and clinical outcome: a Task Force report of the American Psychiatric Association. Am J Psychiatry 142:155–162, 1985

American Psychiatric Association: Diagnostic and Statistical Manual of Mental Disorders, 3rd Edition, Revised. Washington, DC, American Psychiatric Association, 1987

American Psychiatric Association: Treatments of Psychiatric Disorders: A Task Force Report of the American Psychiatric Association. Washington, DC, American Psychiatric Association, 1989

Åsberg M, Schalling D, Träskman-Bendz L, et al: Psychobiology of suicide, impulsivity, and related phenomena, in Psychopharmacology: The Third Generation of Progress. Edited by Meltzer HY. New York, Raven, 1987, pp 655–668

Balottin U, Bejor M, Cecchini A, et al: Infantile autism and computerized tomography brain-scan findings: specific versus nonspecific abnormalities. J Autism Dev Disord 19:110–117, 1989

Bender BG, Puck MH, Salbenblatt JA, et al: Dyslexia in 47, XXY boys identified at birth. Behav Genet 16:343–354, 1986

Biederman J, Baldessarini R, Wright V, et al: A double-blind placebo controlled study of desipramine in the treatment of ADD, II: serum drug levels and cardiovascular findings. J Am Acad Child Adolesc Psychiatry 28:903–911, 1989

Bowden CL, Deutsch CK, Swanson JM: Plasma dopamine β-hydroxylase and platelet monoamine oxidase in attention deficit disorder and conduct disorder. J Am Acad Child Adolesc Psychiatry 27:171–174, 1988

Brandt J, Quaid KA, Folstein SE, et al: Presymptomatic diagnosis of delayed-onset disease with linked DNA markers. JAMA 261:3108–3114, 1989

Breyer-Pfaff U, Giedke H, Gaertner H, et al: Validation of a therapeutic plasma level range in amitriptyline treatment of depression. J Clin Psychopharmacol 9:116–121, 1989

Campbell M, Rosenbloom S, Perry R, et al: Computerized axial tomography in young autistic children. Am J Psychiatry 139:510–512, 1982

Campbell M, Small AM, Green WH, et al: Behavioral efficacy of haloperidol and lithium carbonate: a comparison in hospitalized aggressive children with conduct disorder. Arch Gen Psychiatry 41:650–656, 1984

Courchesne E, Yeung-Courchesne R, Press G, et al: Hypoplasia of cerebellar vermal lobules VI and VII in autism. N Engl J Med 318:1349–1354, 1988

Damasio H, Maurer R, Damasio AR, et al: Computerized tomographic scan findings in patients with autistic behavior. Arch Neurol 37:504–510, 1980

Dening T, Berrios G: Wilson's disease: psychiatric symptoms in 195 cases. Arch Gen Psychiatry 46:1126–1134, 1989

Diederich N, Ackerman R, Jurgens R, et al: Early involvement of the nervous system by human immune deficiency virus (HIV): a study of 79 patients. Eur Neurol 28:93–103, 1988

Doherty MB, Madansky D, Kraft J, et al: Cortisol dynamics and test performance of the dexamethasone suppression test in 97 psychiatrically hospitalized children aged 3–16 years. Journal of the American Academy of Child Psychiatry 25:400–408, 1986

Gabel S, Hsu L: Routine laboratory tests in adolescent psychiatric inpatients: their value in making psychiatric diagnoses and in detecting medical disorders. Journal of the American Academy of Child Psychiatry 25:113–119, 1986

Geller B, Cooper TB, Chestnut EC: Serial monitoring and achievement of steady state nortriptyline plasma levels in depressed children and adolescents: preliminary data. J Clin Psychopharmacol 5:213–216, 1985

Gillberg C, Svendsen P: Childhood psychosis and computed tomographic brain scan findings. J Autism Dev Disord Vol 13:19–31, 1983

Greden JF: Laboratory tests in psychiatry, in Comprehensive Textbook of Psychiatry, Vol 4. Edited by Kaplan H, Sadock B. Baltimore, MD, Williams & Wilkins, 1984, pp 2028–2033

Gualtieri C, Wargin W, Kanoy R, et al: Clinical studies of methylphenidate serum levels in children and adults. Journal of the American Academy of Child Psychiatry 21:19–26, 1982

Gualtieri CT, Golden R, Evans RW, et al: Blood level measurement of psychoactive drugs in pediatric psychiatry. Ther Drug Monit 6:127–141, 1984

Gwirtsman H: Hyperamylasemia and its relationship to binge-purge episodes: development of a clinically relavant laboratory test. J Clin Psychiatry 50:196–204, 1989

Hagerman RJ: Fragile X syndrome. Curr Probl Pediatr 17:621–674, 1987

Jefferson JW, Greist JH, Ackerman DL, et al: Lithium Encyclopedia for Clinical Practice, 2nd Edition. Washington, DC, American Psychiatric Press, 1987

Khan AU: Biochemical profile of depressed adolescents. J Am Acad Child Adolesc Psychiatry 6:873–878, 1987

Kinsbourne M: Disorders of mental development, in Textbook of Child Neurology, 3rd Edition. Edited by Menkes JH. Philadelphia, PA, Lea & Febiger, 1985, pp 764–801

Klee S, Garfinkel B: Identification of depression in children and adolescents: the role of the dexamethasone suppression test. Journal of the American Academy of Child Psychiatry 23:410–415, 1984

Kruesi MJP: Cruelty to animals and CSF 5-HIAA. Psychiatry Res 28:115–116, 1989

Kruesi MJP, Linnoila M, Rapoport JL, et al: Carbohydrate craving, conduct disorder and low CSF 5-HIAA. Psychiatry Res 16:83–86, 1985

Kruesi MJP, Rapoport JL, Hamburger S, et al: CSF monoamine metabolites, aggression and impulsivity in disruptive behavior disorders of children and adolescents. Arch Gen Psychiatry 47:419–426, 1990a

Kruesi MJP, Lenane MC, Hibbs ED: Normal controls and biological reference values in child psychiatry: defining normal. J Am Acad Child Adolesc Psychiatry 29:449–552, 1990b

Leckman JF, Weissman MM, Pauls DL: Family-genetic studies and identification of valid diagnostic categories in adult and child psychiatry. Br J Psychiatry 151:39–44, 1987

Leonard H, Swedo S, Rapoport JL, et al: Treatment of childhood obsessive compulsive disorder with clomipramine and desmethylimipramine: a double-blind crossover comparison. Arch Gen Psychiatry 46:1088–1092, 1989

Lou H, Henriksen L, Bruhn P, et al: Focal cerebral hypoperfusion in children with dysphasia and/or attention deficit disorder. Arch Neurol 41:825–829, 1984

Lou H, Henriksen L, Bruhn P, et al: Striatal dysfunction in attention deficit and hyperkinetic disorder. Arch Neurol 46:48–52, 1989

Miller M, Sulkes S: Fire-setting behavior in individuals with Klinefelter syndrome. Pediatrics 82:115–116, 1988

Moeschler J, Bennett F, Comwell L, et al: Brief clinical and laboratory observations: use of the CT scan in the medical evaluation of the mentally retarded child. J Pediatr 98:63–65, 1981

Morselli P, Bianchetti G, Dugas M: Therapeutic drug monitoring of psychotropic drugs in children. Pediatric Pharmacology 3:149–156, 1983

Nasrallah H, Loney J, Olson S, et al: Cortical atrophy in young adults with a history of hyperactivity in childhood. Psychiatry Res 17:241–246, 1986

Netley C, Rovet J: Verbal deficits in children with 47,XXY and

47,XXX karyotypes: a descriptive and experimental study. Brain Lang 17:58–72, 1982

Nielsen J, Pelsen B, Sorenson K: Follow-up of 30 Klinefelter males treated with testosterone. Clin Genet 33:262–269, 1988

Pennington G, Bender B, Puck M, et al: Learning disabilities in children with sex chromosome anomalies. Child Dev 53:1182–1192, 1982

Pliszka S, Rogeness G, Renner P, et al: Plasma neurochemistry in juvenile offenders. J Am Acad Child Adolesc Psychiatry 27:588–594, 1988

Post R, Uhde T: Refractory manias and alternatives to lithium treatment, in Depression and Manias. Edited by Georgotas A, Cancro R. New York, Elsevier, 1988, pp 410–438

Preskorn S, Bupp S, Weller E, et al: Plasma levels of imipramine and metabolites in 68 hospitalized children. J Am Acad Child Adolesc Psychiatry 3:373–375, 1989

Prior M, Tress B, Hoffman W, et al: Computed tomographic study of children with classic autism. Arch Neurol 41:482–484, 1984

Puig-Antich J, Perel JM, Lupatkin W, et al: Imipramine in prepubertal major depressive disorders. Arch Gen Psychiatry 44:81–89, 1987

Raj A, Sheehan D: Medical evaluation of panic attacks. J Clin Psychiatry 48:309–313, 1987

Ratcliffe SG, Field MAS: Emotional disorder in XYY children: four case reports. J Child Psychol Psychiatry 23:401–406, 1982

Ratcliffe SG, Tierney I, Nshaho J, et al: The Edinburgh study of growth and development of children with sex chromosome abnormalities. Birth Defects 18:41–60, 1982a

Ratcliffe SG, Bancroft J, Axworthy D, et al: Klinefelter's syndrome in adolescence. Arch Dis Child 57:6–12, 1982b

Reiss D, Feinstein C, Weinberger DR, et al: Ventricular enlargement in child psychiatric patients: a controlled study with planimetric measurement. Am J Psychiatry 140:453–456, 1983

Robinson D, Nies A, Lewis R, et al: Clinical pharmacology of phenelzine. Arch Gen Psychiatry 35:629–635, 1978

Rogeness GA, Hernandez JM, Macadeo CA, et al: Clinical characteristics of emotionally disturbed boys with very low activities of dopamine betahydroxylase. Journal of the American Academy of Child Psychiatry 25:521–527, 1984

Rosenbloom S, Campbell M, George A, et al: High resolution CT scanning in infantile autism: a quantitative approach. Journal of the American Academy of Child Psychiatry 23:72–77, 1984

Ryan ND, Puig-Antich J, Cooper TB, et al: Imipramine in adolescent major depression: plasma level and clinical response. Acta Psychiatr Scand 73:275–278, 1986

Ryan ND, Puig-Antich J, Cooper TB, et al: Relative safety of single versus divided dose imipramine in adolescent major depression. J Am Acad Child Adolesc Psychiatry 26:400–406, 1987

Schulz S, Koller M, Kishore R, et al: Ventricular enlargement in teenage patients with schizophrenia spectrum disorder. Am J Psychiatry 140:1592–1595, 1983

Shaywitz B, Shaywitz S, Byrne T, et al: Attention deficit disorder: quantitative analysis of CT. Neurology 33:1500–1503, 1983

Sheridan R, Llerna J, Matkins S, et al: Fertility in a male with trisomy 21. J Med Genet 26:294–298, 1989

Stevenson J, Hawcroft J, Lobascher M, et al: Behavioral deviance in children with early treated phenylketonuria. Arch Dis Child 54:14–18, 1979

Swapp GH, Johnston AW, Watt JL, et al: A fertile woman with non-mosaic Turner's syndrome: case report and review of the literature. Br J Obstet Gynaecol 96:876–880, 1989

Swedo S, Schapiro M, Grady C, et al: Cerebral glucose metabolism in childhood-onset obsessive-compulsive disorder. Arch Gen Psychiatry 46:518–523, 1989

Verbey K, Martin D, Gold MS: Intrepretation of drug abuse testing: strengths and limitations of current methodology, in Psychiatric Medicine. Edited by Hall RCW. Jamaica, NY, Spectrum, 1986a

Verbey K, Gold MS, Mule JS: Laboratory testing in the diagnosis of marijuana intoxication and withdrawal. Psychiatric Annals 16:235, 1986b

Walzer S: X chromosome abnormalities and cognitive development: implications for understanding normal human development. J Child Psychol Psychiatry 26:177–184, 1985

Walzer S, et al: A method for the longitudinal study of behavioral development in infants and children: the early development of XXY children. J Child Psychol Psychiatry 19:213–229, 1978

Weller EB, Weller RA: Neuroendocrine changes in affectively ill children and adolescents. Endocrinol Metab Clin North Am 17:41–53, 1988

Weller EB, Weller RA, Fristad MA, et al: Saliva lithium monitoring in prepubertal children. J Am Acad Child Adolesc Psychiatry 26:173–175, 1987

White A, Barraclough B: Benefits and problems of routine laboratory investigations in adult psychiatric admissions. Br J Psychiatry 155:65–72, 1989

Woody R, Bolyard K, Eisenhauer G, et al: CT scan and MRI findings in a child with schizophrenia. J Child Neurol 2:105–110, 1987

Zametkin A, Rapoport J: Neurobiology of attention deficit disorder with hyperactivity: where have we come in 50 years? J Am Acad Child Adolesc Psychiatry 26:676–686, 1987

Zimmerman M, Coryell W, Pfohl B: Prognostic validity of the dexamethasone suppression test: result of a six-month prospective follow-up. Am J Psychiatry 144:212–214, 1987

Chapter 14

Diagnosis and Diagnostic Formulation

Theodore Shapiro, M.D.

Two sets of presuppositions provide the framework for diagnosis and diagnostic formulation. These include the decision of a professional group about the kind of categorization conventionally used to convey knowledge between peers and about the framework for research and therapeutic action that corresponds to the most recent knowledge and practice within a profession. The second presupposition concerns the goals and framework of parents and children who seek professional aid. The parents come to a child and adolescent psychiatrist, by and large, because something is awry in their child, and they cannot understand, control, maintain, or deal with the behaviors and suffering that accrue. They also believe that the child psychiatrist has a means of examining and discovering "what is wrong," with the hope that there is a biological, social, or psychological intervention that will remedy the discomfort or maladaptive behavior. Insofar as these two aims coincide, a formulation is constructed within the frame of reference used by the physician.

The child psychiatrist must make a diagnostic and dynamic formulation; that is, the data accumulated from the history, the other multiple sources of information, and the examination of the child must be tied together. Thus the way in which the formulation will be carried out has to serve two masters: one professional and the other the social contingencies of practicing child and adolescent psychiatry during a specific time. The child psychiatrist also must be considerate of a number of vantage points all at once to be comprehensive in the history gathering and examination of the child.

In the end, sufficient and appropriate data must be obtained so that the psychiatrist can bring together the disparate sources of information available into a coherent unifying presentation that will suit the family and help prescribe a direction for intervention. This task of formulation is especially crucial and demanding in child and adolescent psychiatry because of the many sources of information about the child or adolescent that are available. The psychiatrists must consider the following:

1. The role of the child as an organism and person with the disorder or possibly as symptom bearer in a family or community.
2. The biological and psychosocial immaturity of the child in the small brood of the human family and the fact that the youngster is brought by family or surrogates whose auxiliary function to the ego of that child changes with each stage of development.
3. That the embeddedness in a family network and protected developmental path are different for children than for adults.

In view of these issues, the clinician will be asked ultimately at which level his or her efforts will be dispatched. Is there a therapy available at an organismic level that is useful or a family or social intervention possible that can be exploited to answer an appeal for help that prompted consultation? If one does proceed with an intervention after assessment, an additional dynamic formulation must be added to the diagnostic formulation to help guide expectations and plans in a context of what is possible for this particular child and family (Group for the Advancement of Psychiatry 1974; Shapiro 1989).

The American Psychiatric Association and the American Academy of Child and Adolescent Psychiatry representing the profession have chosen an approach to diagnosis that is essentially based on cross-sectional categories describing specific syndromes for Axis I diagnoses in DSM-III-R (American Psychiatric Association 1987) and DSM-IV (American Psychiatric Association, in press; Cantwell 1988). The decision to use such an approach is based on the relative ease of empirical descriptive approaches, rather than elaborate theoretical structures that subsume other nomenclatures. On the other hand, this approach offers little guidance by which the clinician can organize ideas about etiologic or nosologic distinctions. Dimensional issues too, which are so vital to a developmental point of view of childhood, are excluded, diminishing similarities among children in the service of discriminant validity (Achenbach 1988; Nurcombe et al. 1989). Nonetheless, discrete syndromes have been described, with adequate validity that compare well to adult schemes, but with children we must also keep note of comorbidity and the developmental status of any child with any particular syndrome. In the service of these aims, the multiaxial formulation is essential to approximate a fuller description, as is the dynamic formulation. Employment of Axis II and Axis III permits us to bring into play clear developmental, biological, and medical disturbances most likely determined by the substrate providing a modifier for our Axis I diagnosis. Axis IV permits a similar consideration for social dimensions. Axis V gives some notion of chronicity by virtue of recording the highest level of functioning during the past year.

These formulations are based on a medical model that in its most mature stage presumes that diagnostics leads to therapeutics or that diagnostics and prognostics are tightly interwoven. The latter two facts are only partially so in child psychiatry and, for that matter, in general psychiatry, where we are struggling with more than the distinctiveness of diagnoses, but also attempting to determine whether these diagnoses carry continuing significance over the life span of the child (e.g., predictive validity, clear comorbidity). At any rate, in gathering the data from the early stages of history and observation, we then must arrive at a differential diagnosis and then determine whether the criteria for a specific disorder are fulfilled and if the exclusion criteria are present to arrive at one or another

Axis I or II diagnosis. This process permits us to incorporate information derived from both epidemiologic and biological research as well as follow-up research to arrive at professional concordance in the clinical setting. As noted, not all is said that can be about the case within this framework, and we need the additional power of a formulation based on other paradigms to establish whether the most central locus of problems is within the child, within the family, within society, or bound to the biological substrate that prompts the behaviors of the child. The completeness of both, a best bet diagnosis based on a clear differential diagnosis and a dynamic construction, should provide a whole formulation by which the second of the aims of history taking and examination is realized (i.e., to care for a patient and/or a patient's family arriving at the physician's office in need and/or in pain with wishes for some variety of relief or help).

Thus the aims of the diagnostic formulation and its corresponding dynamic formulation would be to permit the physician to act within the scope of a professional role using all the knowledge available to the field and providing a framework for action that is designed to intervene in the suffering and reduce the maladaptive impact of the disturbance that a childhood disorder creates in the family, in the school, and in the subjectivity of the patient.

Differential Diagnosis

As noted, there are many ways to approach diagnosis. DSM-III-R and DSM-IV cover a number of large categories that essentially pertain to four varieties of disorder and a subset of highly specific focal problems (Table 14-1). These are most basically disorders of conduct, emotion, development, and adjustment. We must add to these a number of disorders with more specialized symptom pic-

Table 14-1. Differential diagnostic decisions

Disorders of:
Conduct
Emotion
Development
Adjustment
Eating
Gender identity
Tics
Elimination
Speech
Other

Acute: Social upheaval/yes-no
Chronic: Reality disorganizing/preserving

tures: disorders of eating, gender identity, tics, elimination, speech, and others.

We begin our formulation by first making a yes-no query: Are the behaviors that are most prominent externalizing or internalizing? The differential in the behavioral line directed externally (alloplastic) essentially includes conduct disorders with symptoms of aggression, lying, stealing, and antisocial behavior, which may lead to interactions with the law in later life as in delinquency or minor disturbances or behavior within and outside the family pertaining to oppositional disorders and what have come to be known as status offenses. Behaviors such as running away, which would not be an offense under the law unless the individual were a minor, are represented in this area of conduct problem (Group for the Advancement of Psychiatry 1989).

Disorders of emotion (autoplastic) essentially pertain to anxiety disorders and depressive disorders. Most prominent among the childhood anxiety disorders would be a separation disturbance that is sometimes called the "shyness disorder" and in the past went under the old rubric of school reluctance or school phobia (Shapiro and Jegede 1973). Generalized anxiety disorder would be another consideration for diffusely anxious and phobic children; then, if the child fits categorically within the panic disorder group in late adolescence, this diagnosis could be registered.

Depression is somewhat of a newcomer to prepubertal children. It is certainly on the increase as far as our epidemiologic studies suggest (Kashani et al. 1987), and we can find children who fit criteria for major depressive disorder, once thought to be a third-decade illness. We also know much more about the tendency for recurrence in major depression and dysthymia of children (Kovacs et al. 1984). Other disturbances, such as anorexia nervosa and bulimia nervosa, may show associated depressive symptoms, and some suggest depression as the primary disorder. Although we are reluctant to make personality disorder diagnoses in young children, we do make clinical judgments about temperament, and we hear about the difficult child as an offshoot of one line of clinical investigation (Chess and Thomas 1987).

Developmental disorders constitute a large group of disorders including pervasive developmental disorders and autism, mental retardation, learning disabilities, and attention-deficit hyperactivity disorder as a special instance located on Axis I. All have specific features that earmark them as devel-opmentally significant because they assume persistence of certain capacities of younger children even though chronological age is advanced, and also show deviance insofar as the developmental profile of the disorders when taken together creates a formulation that suggests unevenness and maladaptiveness in the emergence of developmental competency. It should be noted that there is a large area of co-occurrence of conduct disorders and/or learning disabilities with attention-deficit hyperactivity disorder (Beitchman et al. 1986; Cantwell and Baker 1989). The clinician should keep in mind that comorbidity is prominent in childhood, and two Axis I or II diagnoses are not to be eschewed in the name of parsimony.

Disorders of adjustment represent a large group of Axis I diagnoses related to Axis IV severity. They should be short lived (less than 6 months) and must have clear precipitants. One can look at posttraumatic stress disorder as an adjustment disorder, but one that takes a larger toll on the individual's adaptive capacity with respect to immature status and the prolongation of symptoms beyond the adjustment period. We must look for *formes fruste* of these disorders too, and the special characteristics of these disorders in children may include flashbacks, visualizations, and so on. They may also include habitual replaying of games to master the original traumas (Pynoos and Nader 1989; Terr 1983).

In addition to these determinations in the differential diagnosis on Axis I, we would also like to see how acute or chronic these disorders are and, if so, whether they are reality disorganizing or reality preserving. These latter features give us another dimension that permits us to consider psychosis when it can be diagnosed, using the adult diagnostic schema as well as the childhood diagnostic program. Having arrived at a differential diagnosis, we now have options for prescription, but not all is told about the child from arriving at a diagnosis (Cantwell 1980, 1988). We need an additional formulation to pull together the data that have been gathered in the diagnostic process.

Formulation and Summary

Because children are developmentally immature and unable to fend for themselves biologically and psychosocially, the family or its surrogates are routinely consulted to provide information for the working formulation that will be a guide for action and convince the participant of the wisdom of the next step. This formulation must be organized in a way that can be useful for the clinician and can also be communicated to the parents, who decide on how recommendations are to be carried out. To make such a formulation, the physician is advised to subdivide the material available into psychosocial and developmental features that have been found during the examination (Table 14-2).

As the clinician catalogs the biological features of the material gathered, he or she considers familial factors, including disease and disorder in first-degree relatives, and a careful genetic history, as well as some of the important facts about developmental delays within the family that correlate with specific disorders. For example, Rutter and Folstein (1977) suggested that the heritable feature in autism may be language delay and deviance plus accidental perinatal stress factors. Family history of language delay should thus be highlighted in the biological background of a formulation. We know, for example, that hypoxia during the first trimester as evidenced by bleeding or other symptoms is of significance postnatally. We also know that chromosomal anomalies are relevant to developmental deviance. In fact, during the perinatal period itself, fetal distress and meconium staining are significant as are disturbances in the immediate postnatal period. Hyperbilirubinemia or intracranial bleeding and low birth weight warrant our attention for their impact on development. Anything that intrudes on brain integrity throughout the early life span—which could include toxic-metabolic states or infection such as meningitis, viral encephalitis, diabetic coma, or malnutrition—should alert us. These biological factors are significant for our etiologic inferences concerning biological insult and should be summarized for review in the formulation.

Social disturbances are pertinent to the increasing and widening cone of human contacts as the infant develops. Initially, the immediate caregiving nurturing environment is important, but this environment gradually increases as the child develops and begins to take in more and more people in the surroundings. This may include peers, both parents, surrogate caregivers, and ultimately, when the child begins school, teachers and a widening array of peers with whom interaction occurs. Finally, the community at large becomes the relevant world of the adolescent. Disturbances in each of these communities, objects of identification in early childhood, and, later, in early adolescence in school circumstances, crushes, heros, intrusions by family in incest, abuse, too rigorous or lax child-rearing, and drugs, may also take their toll on the child.

The social role of the child becomes very important as well in determining whether illness will ensue or whether the disorder is in the child or in the family (McDermott and Char 1974). The community may also become a toxigenic agent in minorities and in poverty, where schooling may be inferior or where delinquency and sociopathy reign. Nor should we miss the toxic effect of wealthy or charismatic parents.

The psychological intrapsychic vantage point may be addressed from data achieved in the interview of the child and from one's observations about family dynamics. It must be established whether symptoms presented appear to be meaningful to the child, represent symbolic transformations related to identifications, or are signs of maladaptive self-esteem regulation (Shapiro and Esman 1985). These three areas are easily tapped from the direct interview and from modification in the interview process utilizing special techniques, such as inquiries about figure drawings, symbolic play, squiggle games, and dreams.

The notion of acting out is a central dynamic proposition that attests to the idea that fantasies (either unknown or known to the child) determine overt behavior. These symbolic actions can be seen as externalizing conduct-disordered behaviors in children so disposed or as phobic anxiety behaviors, which also may partially result from identification with parents, siblings, or peers. The clinician's examination will lead to the determination of what kinds of conflict have been resolved in what kinds of behavior or symptoms. The stan-

Table 14-2.   Formulation and summary of features found during the examination

Biological
    Family
    Perinatal
    Injury
Social
    Family
    Peer
    Community
Psychological
    Conflict (intrapsychic)
    Identification
    Self-esteem regulation
Developmental
    Phase-stage–related behavior
    Reinforcing factors

dard diagnostic assessments that focus on simple differential diagnosis do not permit the elaboration of such formulations. Thus the nature of the net cast determines the fish caught: examiners who do not look will not find these features!

While these behaviors will be considered meaningful, we must also look at them from the vantage point of whether they are components of development that signify way stations in the progress of childhood. Since there are stages and phases of life where we expect certain behaviors as appropriate, we might have to expect symptoms to occur as some transient phenomena of the developmental course.

In fact, it is healthy if a child's attachment to the parent is secure, but we must then also expect separation anxiety at 10–18 months. However, it is maladaptive and inappropriate if separation anxiety occurs during school years as a symptom needing intervention. We also have to look at what sorts of reinforcing factors permit certain behaviors to arise or prevail at each developmental stage. For example, there are some parents who really do not use *any* disciplinary direct action to discipline their children for fear that any such action is overly aggressive and punitive. Frequently, such parents have had difficult and harsh rearing themselves. The notion that the developmental path will be traversed without parental guidance thus is another one of the factors that has to be taken into account in symptom formation in early childhood. Abusing parents have, themselves, frequently been abused.

Pulling together the biological, social, psychological, and developmental features of the history, contact with teachers and others, and examination of the child, we can present a coherent picture to the caregiver. The formulation may still lack coherence and be incomplete, however, despite its newfound orderliness. The dynamic formulation has traditionally been a feature of one point of view of psychiatry, namely, the psychoanalytic dynamic vantage. If we are to add this dimension to our formulation, we must apply a number of principles that would make the enterprise reasonable as a clinical part of the traditional formulation.

Dynamic Formulation

Clinically oriented dynamic formulations are conceptually related to models derived from Freudian psychoanalysis and the derivative dynamic and cognitive therapies (Shapiro 1989). Four fundamental notions are essential to this vantage point (Shapiro and Esman 1985):

Table 14-3.   The dynamic formulation

Summary paragraph
Nondynamic factors
Dynamic summary
Predictive responses

1. We assume the existence of unconscious mental function.
2. Observable symptoms and signs are driven by internalized conflicts that may be out of awareness.
3. Symptoms have meaning and significance to the child and are decipherable in terms of his or her life and experience.
4. There is a central need to displace internalized conflicts and maladaptive relationships onto the therapist as transferential behaviors.

The dynamic formulation includes a summary paragraph describing the complaints of the patient, diagnosis, and precipitating events (Table 14-3). Factors located in our description under biological features include genetics, social deprivation, traumatic facts, and other material from external sources of data that would contribute to making the current symptoms cohere.

The dynamic summary itself should be cast in a frame of reference that helps interpret presenting symptoms of the patient and his or her behavior. These integrative inferences are based on models of ego psychological factors, developmental lines (Anna Freud 1963), the separation-individuation model (Mahler et al. 1975), or any of the coherent dynamic schemas that seek to account for the meaning of behavior.

The dynamic formulation also includes predictive responses concerning therapeutic situation.

The following three vignettes of children at three stages of life are drawn from an article on dynamic formulation (Shapiro 1989).

Case 1

Sammy is 42 months old; he speaks at age level and in relevant sentences. He has no stereotypies, but seems withdrawn and unrelated. His play is restricted, and his graphomotor skills are poor. He meets criteria for pervasive developmental disorder not otherwise specified, having been markedly isolated in his earlier years and echolalic as he began to speak late at 2.5 years. Recently, he has shown increasing representational play, but has become hypervigilant, not permitting his mother to leave, clinging to her, and screaming as she tries to separate.

Sammy's developmental disorder involves his object constancy and his attachment to his mother. He has begun to differentiate and has passed through symbiosis and is attempting to maintain a stable representation of his mother. He is not yet able to do so. As his other developmental areas have improved, and his linguistic and cognitive skills emerge, his crisis in emotional removal becomes a central problem.

Therapeutically, one will have to anticipate modifications in treatment to include the mother and permit her to stay longer at his special school, until he can be given techniques to remain secure in his mother's absence. She and his father must be engaged in a continuing encounter to accept Sammy's developmental problems, help him to grow, and plan for special schooling. Their own despair and hope must be dealt with as they are helped to negotiate the real world for Sammy.

Commentary. The interplay of faulty cognition, attachment behavior, and object relations in a developmental disorder creates numerous problems. The clinician must be apprised of their interaction to help a child adapt to his or her surroundings and to permit parents to hope while realistically guiding the disabled child in a complex, specialized world. Even if one were to add new behavioral reinforcements, the meaning of the behaviors to parents adds new dimensions to the parents' worry, guilt, and even conflict. The best treatment involves approaching these issues.

Case 2

Jerry, a 7-year-old boy, was hitting his peers and had become a petty thief. These maladaptive behaviors were associated with talking back to his parents after 3 months in a new school. Academically, he could not yet read, but mathematics was at grade level. The diagnoses of conduct disorder (Axis I) and learning disability (Axis II) were established. There were no symptoms of anxiety, sadness, or other mental disturbances elicited.

The family had moved to a new school district a

year ago after the father was terminated from his former job. The father found a new position in a neighboring town, but there had been family discord and difficulty before the move. The mother was overwhelmed by Jerry's withdrawal and disciplinary problems. She also was burdened by having to care for Jerry's 4-year-old sister, who was born when he was almost 3 years old. He continually complained about diminished contact with his mother, who was busy with his sister, and responded sullenly to his father's eruptive and punitive interventions. His father had, in turn, been increasingly angry and demanding of the mother (Axis IV).

Developmentally, Jerry was a normal, full-term, spontaneous delivery with a paternal family history of learning difficulties. His mother was educated and sensitive, but easy to overwhelm. Developmental landmarks were on time, and although Jerry's response to his sister's birth seemed casual, he changed from an assertive and overactive boy to a withdrawn, eruptive, naughty child.

Jerry's current behavior is seen as an identification with the aggressor in a setting of experienced withdrawal of love by his mother, the object of his oedipal desires and his most steady internalized support. There is a strong regressive pull toward his sister's infantile behavior, while he also tries to compensate and reassert his masculine phallic role based on imitation of his father's violent assertive displays. The recurrent jeopardy of losing his mother's affection since his sister's birth was reexperienced when they moved, causing him to overidentify with his father's aggressiveness as he symbolically steals to undo his passive helplessness in not being able to learn and in trying to make friends.

Therapeutically, one would expect initial bravado and assertivenss with an insistent need to win. Jerry's move toward the therapist or tutor will be controlling and assertive until the underlying emotions can be elicited and confronted with permission for expression and until more regressive wishes are interpreted. He needs continuing support for his deficits in learning by resource room or tutorial contacts. Counseling for the parents should be entertained. They could be directed toward better toleration of his assertive behavior through seeing it as mock masculinity, and his regressive demands may be better tolerated as a plea for love at his sister's level.

Commentary. This case of a learning disabled, conduct-disordered child, if approached only from the standpoint of symptom clusters, might lead the clinician to some understanding of the social impact of the child's circumstance, only if Axis IV were considered. The stressors of the move, the father's eruptiveness, and the mother's irritability might turn our attention to the environment. However, in considering treatment, the parents' anger at the child, their inability to see his needs, and their focal attention to their own egocentric needs require work with them to interrupt their pattern of neglect and even mistreatment of Jerry. He could not be expected to show them the way, given his developing maladaptive internalized patterns, which only accentuate his "bad boy" image. On the other hand, the patterns are not so firmly internalized that one would treat the child first.

Case 3

Ron is an 8-year-old with impulsivity, excessive activity, and restlessness who has been diagnosed as having attention-deficit hyperactivity disorder. He seems to be insatiable in his wish to have things, constantly pleading with his mother to buy toys and wishing to take home toys of others. However, even when he does get some of the things requested, he tends to break them and to spoil events that he has longed for. He shows bravado with other children and assertiveness, which makes him unpopular, but sometimes he acts the clown in the classroom, seeking the attention of other children.

Ron has a high IQ despite his attentional problems and seems to have been able to compensate by learning quickly. He is either at or above age level on his achievement tests. He began to be treated this year with methylphenidate, but still has altercations with his mother and father, which end in screaming matches during which they tell him how he "spoils everything." Following each tearful encounter, he can be comforted and is remorseful.

His developmental history is marked by his mother's first trimester bleeding and by a bilirubin of 15 postnatally.

This child has achieved landmarks, with background difficulties in mastering his impulsiveness and distractibility. He too readily falls into a pattern with his parents in which his neediness for them and the things that they provide degenerates into accusations about his inability to enjoy things. The accusations are externally projected guilt representing a harsh superego serving inhibitions of forbidden wishes. He easily entered latency, permitting learning, but is constantly tormented by the need

to act out his guilt feelings by spoiling his good times to elicit the final comforting. The miscarried struggles between him and his father and mother, however, satisfying at some level, signify a maladaptive pattern stimulated from within and participated in by his parents.

In treatment, we will see a continuation of the oral hunger in settings of disappointments and frustration of need. He will also try to get the therapist to turn on him, fight with him, reprimand him, and hold him down in a continuing sadistic struggle that mimics his internal struggle with his superego. Although he compensates well for his impulsivity and although his medication helps, his problems with control continue because they are symbolically driven by conflict. Parental counseling could also help. A psychoeducational approach might lead to more capacity to sympathize.

Commentary. Children with attention-deficit hyperactivity disorder are more than drug-sensitive, attentionally deficient organisms. They also regress, arrest, and progress in a human environment. Moreover, the dynamic interaction with Ron's body and the tendency to symptom formation is relevant to management. As noted in the literature, these children need more than medicine: they need multimodal treatment.

Summary

As we read through these cases, it becomes quite apparent that the differential diagnosis and traditional clinical diagnostic formulation alone do not complete the descriptions of the child and his interactions with his body, his world, and his own inner life. We need the dynamic formulation as well to proceed therapeutically and to answer the questions about what in fact made the family come for help, what do they want from us, and what can we provide. Only with such an approach can the diagnostic formulation as a whole be utilized in the service of the informing interview with parents and the prospect of intervening appropriately and helpfully.

References

Achenbach TM: Integrating assessment and taxonomy, in Assessment and Diagnosis in Child Psychopathology. Edited by Rutter M, Tuma AH, Lann IS. New York, Guilford, 1988, pp 300–346

American Psychiatric Association: Diagnostic and Statistical Manual of Mental Disorders, 3rd Edition, Revised. Washington, DC, American Psychiatric Association, 1987

American Psychiatric Association: Diagnostic and Statistical Manual of Mental Disorders, 4th Edition, 1st Draft. Washington, DC, American Psychiatric Association, 1991

Beitchman J, Nair R, Clegg M, et al: Prevalence of psychiatric disorders in children with speech and language disorders. Journal of the American Academy of Child Psychiatry 25:528–535, 1986

Cantwell DP: The diagnostic process and diagnostic classification in child psychiatry: DSM-III. Journal of the American Academy of Child Psychiatry 19:345–355, 1980

Cantwell DP: DSM-III studies, in Assessment and Diagnosis in Child Psychopathology. Edited by Rutter M, Tuma AH, Lann IS. New York, Guilford, 1988, pp 3–36

Cantwell DP, Baker L: Stability and natural history of DSM-III childhood diagnoses. J Am Acad Child Adolesc Psychiatry 28:691–700, 1989

Chess S, Thomas A: Know Your Child. New York, Basic Books, 1987

Freud A: The concept of developmental lines, in The Psychoanalytic Study of the Child, Vol 18. New York, International Universities Press, 1963, pp 245–266

Group for the Advancement of Psychiatry: From Diagnosis to Treatment in Child Psychiatry. Northvale, NJ, Jason Aronson, 1974

Group for the Advancement of Psychiatry: How Old is Old Enough? Washington, DC, American Psychiatric Press, 1989

Kashani JH, Carlson GA, Beck NC, et al: Depression, depressive symptoms, and depressed mood among a community sample of adolescents. Am J Psychiatry 144:931–934, 1987

Kovacs M, Feinberg TL, Crouse-Novak M, et al: Depressive disorders in childhood, II: a longitudinal study of the risk for a subsequent major depression. Arch Gen Psychiatry 41:643–649, 1984

Mahler MS, Pine F, Bergman A: The Psychological Birth of the Human Infant. New York, Basic Books, 1975

McDermott J, Char WF: The undeclared war between child psychiatry and family therapy. Journal of the American Academy of Child Psychiatry 13:422–436, 1974

Nurcombe B, Seifer R, Scioli A: Is major depressive disorder in adolescence a distinct diagnostic entity? J Am Acad Child Adolesc Psychiatry 28:333–342, 1989

Pynoos R, Nader K: Children's memory and proximity to violence. J Am Acad Child Adolesc Psychiatry 28:236–241, 1989

Rutter M, Folstein S: Genetic influences and infantile autism. Nature 265:726–728, 1977

Shapiro T: The psychodynamic formulation in child and adolescent psychiatry. J Am Acad Child Adolesc Psychiatry 5:675–680, 1989

Shapiro T, Esman A: Psychotherapy with children and adolescents: still relevant in the 1980s? Psychiatr Clin North Am 8:909–921, 1985

Shapiro T, Jegede RO: School phobia: a babel of tongues. Journal of Autism and Childhood Schizophrenia 3:168–186, 1973

Terr L: Chowchilla revisited: the effects of psychic trauma four years after a school bus kidnapping. Am J Psychiatry 140:1543–1550, 1983

Chapter 15

Presentation of Findings and Recommendations

Hector R. Bird, M.D.

The postassessment or "informing" interview is a crucial aspect of the diagnostic process in child and adolescent psychiatry (Group for the Advancement of Psychiatry 1957). Its main purpose is to share the clinician's observations with the child's parents, to elaborate further on parental feelings and perceptions, and to discuss the clinician's recommendations so as to arrive collaboratively at a plan that will be helpful both to the child and to the child's family. It is generally the parents who have brought the child to treatment, and it is they who will need to implement the clinician's recommendations. If treatment is indicated, it is the parents who have to work out the practical arrangements to get their child to the clinician, as well as to subsidize the cost of treatment.

Parents generally approach this interview with a great deal of anxiety. The underlying emotion that generates their anxiety, and that parents bring with them into the office, is guilt. Quite often this guilt is externalized as anger toward their child and often toward the clinician. Parents view their child as their product (not entirely inaccurately); this leads them, however, to see their child's failings and difficulties as their own failure and to view their child's pathology as an affront to the adequacy of their parenting abilities. For many parents, the postassessment interview is the day of reckoning on which the "guilty" verdict will be passed by the all-knowing professional—the moment when all of their parental flaws and all of their mistakes and faulty child-rearing practices will be exposed. The parents generally arrive at the office on the defensive and anticipating an accusatory finger to be pointed at them, with a view of the clinician as their adversary. Thus the clinician's first task is to provide these anxious parents with reassurance and support.

One important way of providing support and reassurance to the parents is by conveying that regardless of the developmental, behavioral, or emotional difficulties, their child is basically a good person. While the parents may consider that they have "failed" in bringing up their child (and in some respects, this may indeed be true), it is important to make them feel that there are, equally, many things that they have done "right." This first step in the information-sharing process must heavily emphasize the child's observed assets: "Johnny is a very nice kid. He's . . . engaging . . . sensitive . . . well-related . . . witty . . . affectionate . . . has a great sense of humor. . . . There's a lot about him to be proud of." At this stage, one must be cautious to maintain a balance between the positive and the negative. To deny any kind of parental influence on the child's difficulties and to attribute everything to genetics or to temperament can be as detrimental as pointing the accusatory finger at the parents and placing the blame entirely on the way that they have brought up their child. The parents must be brought to the realization that they have as much to do with what are perceived as their child's positive characteristics as they may have to do with what are seen as their child's liabilities. If this is achieved, the parents will be more receptive to the information that is shared with them.

The informing interview should not be a lecture in which the clinician does all of the talking. The next step is to move into the problem areas and to summarize what has gone on from the onset of the consultative process: "When you first came to see me three weeks ago, your major concerns seemed to be that Johnny's work in school had gone downhill and that his teachers complained that he does not pay attention in class. . . . I wonder what your thoughts about this have been since we last met." It is important to share what has happened since the parents were last seen during the diagnostic process. How has their child reacted to the diagnostic interviews? What has the child's behavior been like? Has he or she given the parents any feedback about the meetings with the clinician? Have there been any observable changes in the child's behavior or emotional state?

It is also important that the parents understand that what is "wrong" with their child is not simply the maladaptive behavior that is manifested, but that these behaviors are closely linked to the child's emotions (Stevenson 1971). This understanding is often facilitated by an elaboration of those insights about their child, about themselves, and about the family interactions that may have been gained during the diagnostic process. It is thus crucial to de-emphasize how the child behaves and to emphasize how the child feels. Many parents require more than one session to explore their motivations, to relieve their guilt about having failed or their anger at their child, and, when treatment is indicated, to overcome the resistances to treatment that they may have.

Another important factor that serves to reassure the parents and to gain their confidence and alliance is for the clinician to be perceived as a reliable and competent professional whose observations and recommendations can be trusted (Adams 1982). From their brief contact during the diagnostic process, the parents may have developed fantasies about the clinician, some of which may already be transference reactions. When a recommendation for treatment is being made, it is pertinent to inquire somewhat in the line of, "I have a feeling that I can be helpful to your child, but I have known your child for only a few days and you have known her all her life. From what you have observed about me, do you think I am the kind of person that she will find helpful?" Although this is in many ways a "leading" type of inquiry, given that most par-

ents would find it difficult to reply: "No, you are not," this line of questioning opens up a dialogue and communicates to the parents that the clinician is not an all-powerful, all-knowing expert who will rescue their child. Rather, it conveys the fact that the clinician sees possible limitations to his or her capacities, as well as the need to have a good fit between the patient and the therapist.

To enhance communication with the parents, the clinician should avoid technical jargon and should provide observations and comments in lay terms. Even with highly educated parents, technical terms may not necessarily have the same meaning as they have for a trained professional. Greenspan (1981) recommended that the information about the child be addressed in a developmental context. It is easier for the parent to accept a statement like "Your child relates to others more like a 2-year-old would" than to say "There is a disturbance in the way that your child relates to other children" or "Your child is extremely immature in the way that he relates to others."

The clinician should try to limit the content of the interview(s) with the parents to those areas that will help the patient and to place limits on the extent to which either parent may try to capitalize on the occasion to discuss individual problems to the exclusion of the identified patient.

The post-diagnostic interview with parents whose child's prognosis is poor, such as an autistic child or a child with mental retardation, is particularly sensitive. Regardless of the diagnosis or of the prognosis that can be anticipated, it is obviously impossible for any clinician to predict the future unequivocally for an individual patient. It behooves the clinician to be well versed in the literature and in recent findings about the disorder at hand, so that a realistic appraisal of what or what not to expect can be communicated. The clinician should not feed into the parents' denial mechanisms by minimizing the severity of the psychopathology; by the same token, however, the parents cannot be allowed to leave the clinician's office in hopelessness and despair (Glenn 1984). Subsequent follow-up is indicated with such parents to help them share their future expectations. Prognosis is poor only when real outcome is much worse than the outcome that was anticipated. Outcome must be dissected into its component parts. If the child is intellectually dull and the parents' expectation is that their child will become a physician or a lawyer, then prognosis is extremely poor. If the parents can be led to tone down their level of expectation and can see their child as a productive member of society in a more menial task, then the prognostic statement can be more favorable.

The Issue of Confidentiality

Clearly, a child's family, and particularly the parents, constitute the most important source of social support. Very often, the clinician is hesitant to use this source of support to its fullest because of restricted conceptions of confidentiality that preclude discussion of children's problems with their parents. Such barriers often impair the clinician's ability to find the most effective approach to helping the patient (Barth 1986).

The child clinician's task is complicated because the therapeutic alliance has to be twofold. The therapeutic contract has to be negotiated with the child and with both parents. Particularly for those children whom one expects to have in treatment, a goal of the informing interview is to ensure that there is an alliance with the parents as well as with the child. The alliance with the parents will serve to maintain the child in treatment when resistance crops up. In an intact family, the clinician must emphasize the importance of sharing the results of the evaluation with both parents and must try to accommodate both parents in setting up the appointment(s). When there is a marital separation, the quality of the relationship between the parents will dictate whether separate appointments are needed. Even under those circumstances, it is desirable that both parents share the session with the clinician. A close observation of their interaction can provide the clinician with a firsthand view of circumstances that the child faces on a daily basis. As the senior members of the family and the ones who control the family resources, both parents are in fact in a position to sabotage the clinician's efforts and to act out any resistance to treatment. For this reason, their collaboration is essential.

From the very first contact, the clinician should inform the patient of the process that will be followed. The child and the family should know from the outset that the child will be interviewed individually, that there may be a family interview, and that after a number of sessions, the clinician has agreed to meet with the child's parents to convey to them the results of the evaluation and recommendations. The child should be conscious that the purpose of this informing interview is to share information so that his or her parents can be more

helpful and that it will not be a forum to manipulate the parents or to chide them on the patient's behalf.

The clinician can promise confidentiality within certain limits. The child must know from the outset the limitations to confidentiality. As a general rule, the clinician can promise confidentiality to a child with the proviso that any information that in the clinician's judgment is potentially self-destructive or destructive to others will be shared with those who can protect the child. In those instances, the clinician will specifically breach confidentialilty to protect the child and those around the child. Under the rubric of "self-destructive to others" are issues such as suicidality, antisocial behaviors, use of drugs and alcohol, and the like. To most children, these limitations to confidentiality are reassuring and promote a sense of safety in the situation, as well as confidence rather than mistrust in the clinician. Prior to meeting with the parents, the clinician should ask the patient for particular points of information that the patient wants kept confidential and should keep these confidential as long as the aforementioned proviso is kept. The clinician should also inquire from the patient whether there is any particular area on which the patient would like special emphasis to be placed in the meeting with the parents. This often promotes from an early stage a view of the clinician as a helping agent.

The issue of confidentiality is qualitatively different with younger children as compared with adolescents. Younger children find it difficult to conceive of events or circumstances that their parents either do not know or should not know about. It is usually not necessary to include younger children in the post-diagnostic interview, and most children will accept the fact that the clinician must meet with their parents in private.

Adolescence, however, is the second stage of separation-individuation, and whether or not it is acknowledged by the adolescent, the issue of privacy and confidentiality is of paramount importance, possibly of greater importance than it is with adult patients. Any real or imagined breach of the adolescent's confidence may irreversibly block the patient's capacity ever to trust this particular clinician. As a general rule, the adolescent should be given the option to be present at meetings with the parents for the purpose of presenting findings and making recommendations. Some adolescents will choose to be present; others will presumably not care. The choice, however, should be theirs, and the parents should have been advised at the outset that their child will be allowed to make this decision. Regardless of the adolescent's choice, prior to the informing interview, the clinician should specifically discuss with the adolescent what he or she is planning to tell the parents at the meeting. In this way, the adolescent can provide the clinician with specific feedback and can engage in some discussion about the points of information that will be shared with the parents. This discussion with the adolescent also has a therapeutic purpose in that it conveys to the adolescent the clinician's impressions and what the clinician will recommend, as well as the clinician's opinion that the adolescent is the central person in the entire process. This approach places the clinician and the patient on the same team.

In summary, the discussion with the family at this juncture can have therapeutic as well as prognostic implications. The informing interview is a critical aspect of the diagnostic process. If this interview is poorly handled, it can lead to premature closure of a process that is potentially beneficial and therapeutic to the child and to the child's family. When done thoughtfully and with sensitivity, it can serve to relieve parental anxiety and guilt, to provide alternative ways for the parents to look at and deal with their child's difficulties, and to establish an alliance between the clinician and the family.

References

Adams PL: A Primer of Child Psychotherapy, 2nd Edition. Boston, MA, Little, Brown, 1982

Barth RP: Social and Cognitive Treatment of Children and Adolescents. San Francisco, CA, Jossey-Bass, 1986

Glenn ML: On Diagnosis: A Systemic Approach. New York, Brunner/Mazel, 1984

Greenspan SI: The Clinical Interview of the Child. New York, McGraw-Hill, 1981

Group for the Advancement of Psychiatry: The Diagnostic Process in Child Psychiatry (Report No 38). New York, Group for the Advancement of Psychiatry, 1957

Stevenson I: The Diagnostic Interview, 2nd Edition. New York, Harper & Row, 1971

Section III

Developmental Disorders

Chapter 16

Mental Retardation

Ludwik S. Szymanski, M.D.
Lawrence C. Kaplan, M.D.

The ultimate objective of a physician is not only to cure illness, but to help the patient to achieve the best feasible quality of life and function as an individual and as a member of society. Probably this is nowhere more evident than in the treatment of persons who have mental retardation.

The current philosophy of care for retarded persons is best reflected in the Bill of Rights, adopted in 1968 by the International League of Societies for the Mentally Handicapped. Its main points are that retarded persons have

- The same basic rights as other citizens of the same age.
- The right to education and training to enable the development of potential to the fullest possible extent, no matter how severe the degree of disability.
- The right to live with own or foster family and to participate in all aspects of community life.
- The right to protection from exploitation, abuse, and degrading treatment.

Mental Retardation as a Psychosocial Phenomenon

The Nature and Definition of Mental Retardation

In comparison with other disorders encountered by physicians in general and psychiatrists in par-

ticular, mental retardation is unique in several respects (Szymanski and Crocker 1989). First, it is not a unitary entity with a defined cause, course, and pathognomonic features. It is a complex phenomenon characterized by a set of behaviors and behavioral deficits arbitrarily defined by society (and by professionals). It may have many causative factors and may run different courses. Second, social values and attitudes are at least as important as biological factors in all aspects of the outcome of mental retardation. Third, many professionals still adhere to various misconceptions about mental retardation, which often interfere with their functioning as clinicians in this field.

The earliest definitions of mental retardation were unidimensional, based on observable deficits in adaptive behaviors. Such definitions could change, depending on the expectations the society had of the individuals at a given age. A person who had little or no communication and no self-help skills (whom we would now call seriously or profoundly retarded) would be recognized in all cultures as exceptional. On the other hand, mildly retarded persons would not be very noticeable in settings where intellectual deficits would not be a major obstacle to adaptation and where simple but productive jobs could readily be found. After the introduction of psychometric tests to this country in 1908, mental retardation became defined primarily by low test scores (IQ). In 1959, a second dimension—deficits in adaptive behavior—was added to the definition of mental retardation (and was clarified in 1973) (Grossman 1983). This dimension is now included in all the official definitions of the

American Association on Mental Retardation (Grossman 1983) and in DSM-III-R (American Psychiatric Association 1987), which are essentially identical. The third criterion is onset (of retardation) before age 18 years. Some researchers have called for the return to a unidimensional definition based only on the IQ score (Zigler et al. 1984).

The nature of mental retardation is still controversial. According to one view (Ellis and Cavalier 1982), mentally retarded persons are deficient in at least one of the cognitive processes that are required for "intelligent behavior." Instead of focusing on discrete deficiencies, Detterman (1987) sees mental retardation as characterized by deficits in those abilities that are important in the functioning of the complex system of characteristics that together define human intelligence. A developmental approach (Zigler 1969; Zigler and Balla 1982) views the central problem in mental retardation as being the slower development of retarded persons and the lower ultimate level that they achieve, rather than a deficiency in basic cognitive processes. Whitman (1990) sees mental retardation as a "self-regulatory disorder" in that retarded persons are unable to generalize their knowledge outside of training situations. Szymanski et al. (1989) and Rubin (1989) conceptualize mental retardation as a final common pathway of a central nervous system dysfunction that may have varied causation.

The DSM-III-R criteria for mental retardation are given in Table 16-1. The DSM-III-R definition reflects only the current level of functioning, regardless of etiology and prognosis. Mental retardation is further subclassified by severity into mild, moderate, severe, and profound, according to the IQ level.

A person can be diagnosed as having mental retardation of higher or lower severity than the IQ alone would indicate, depending on the level of adaptive skills. Thus a person with an IQ of 68 might not be diagnosed as retarded if the person has basic academic skills, lives almost independently, and holds a regular job.

Epidemiology of Mental Retardation

Estimates of the prevalence of mental retardation have changed over the years, reflecting changes in the definition. The lowering of the cutoff IQ value in 1973 from 1 to 2 standard deviations below the mean, and the introduction of the diagnostic criterion of adaptive behavior, drastically lowered the estimated prevalence to about 1% of the general population. A recent review of epidemiologic studies (McLaren and Bryson 1987) found the estimated prevalence of mild mental retardation to be 3.7–5.9 per 1,000 of general population, and the estimated prevalence of moderate, severe, and profound retardation combined to be 3–4 per 1,000. The highest prevalence is in the 10–20-year age group, reflecting probably that mild mental retardation in many cases may become obvious only during school age, when the child is expected to achieve in academic learning. Mental retardation is also more prevalent in males, with an estimated ratio of 1.6:1.

Persons who have mental retardation often have associated disorders. In a review of existing studies, McLaren and Bryson (1987) estimated that seizure disorders occurred in 15%–30% of persons with mental retardation, motor handicaps (including cerebral palsy) occurred in 20%–30%, and sensory deficits occurred in 10%–20%. The prevalence of these disorders is proportional to the severity of retardation.

Evolution of Mental Retardation as a Psychosocial Phenomenon

Both mental retardation and mental illness are manifested by behaviors that deviate from norms for the particular sociocultural group and age. These conditions are often not understood, may be unpredictable, and evoke emotional reactions in others, including fear. Society's emotional responses to mentally ill and retarded persons led to mea-

---

Table 16-1. DSM-III-R diagnostic criteria for mental retardation

A. Significantly subaverage general intellectual functioning: an IQ of 70 or below on individually administered IQ test (for infants, a clinical judgment of significantly subaverage intellectual functioning, since available intelligence tests do not yield numerical IQ values).

B. Concurrent deficits or impairments in adaptive functioning, i.e., the person's effectiveness in meeting the standards expected for his or her age by his or her cultural group in areas such as social skills and responsibility, communication, daily living skills, personal independence, and self-sufficiency.

C. Onset before the age of 18.

Source. Reprinted with permission from American Psychiatric Association 1987.

sures such as isolating the afflicted individuals and shaped policies concerning their care. These, in turn, influenced the roles of professionals, including psychiatrists and other physicians. Table 16-2 summarizes the evolution of the attitudes toward mental retardation in modern times; detailed reviews are available elsewhere (Donaldson and Menolascino 1977; Kanner 1964).

Mental Retardation as a Biomedical Phenomenon

The Pathoetiology of Mental Retardation

It is helpful to consider mental retardation as a developmental and behavioral manifestation of variations in the form, function, and adaptation of the central nervous system (Kavanaugh 1988). The health professional must also consider the contribution of other organ systems, as well as the important effect of the environment on human beings, each of whom has unique responses to the various stresses and challenges of life.

With rapid advances in the prenatal and early postnatal detection of certain conditions, and with improvements in medical and educational supports, a number of clinical conditions traditionally associated with particular patterns of mental retardation appear to be quite different from their earlier descriptions (Lazar et al. 1982; Mayes et al. 1985). This underscores the importance of seeing mental retardation as a reflection of embryonic, perinatal, and postnatal influences, with the balance among these character-

Table 16-2.   Evolution of the attitudes toward mental retardation

Period	Society's attitudes	Psychiatrists' roles
Mid to late 19th century	Optimism, belief in education, "moral training" in special schools to return the person to society.	Psychiatrists in forefront of progress as leaders, educators, and diagnosticians. Precursor of the American Association on Mental Retardation founded in 1876 by psychiatrists.
End of 19th century to beginning of 20th century	Focus on neuropathology; retardation seen as incurable defect; therapeutic nihilism; protecting retarded persons from society.	Roles change to diagnostician, neuropathologist, and administrator.
Early to mid 20th century	Introduction of intelligence tests, which discover mildly retarded "morons"; assumption of link with antisocial behavior. Protecting society: custodial institutionalization, sterilization; "Tragic Interlude."	Psychiatrists become administrators; retarded persons seen as unable to benefit from psychiatric treatment (i.e., psychoanalytical therapy); early pioneers (e.g., Howard Potter) study, describe, and treat mental disorders in retarded persons.
Early second half of 20th century	Recognition of rights of retarded persons to public education, treatment, and life in community; the concept of normalization.	Studies on mental illness in retarded persons; psychiatrists become interested in this field, chiefly as psychopharmacologists, but also as therapists and diagnosticians.
Current period	Implementation of right of all handicapped children to education; deinstitutionalization and community living and working for adults.	Psychiatrists increasingly treat retarded people using all treatment modalities, and are accepted as team members.

Source.   Partly based on Donaldson and Menolascino (1977) and Kanner (1964).

izing the individual's actual clinical status (Kaplan 1985).

Three basic etiologic categories can assist the clinician in formulating diagnoses (Table 16-3):

1. Prenatal errors of morphogenesis of the central nervous system and/or other systems severe enough to alter normal development.
2. Alterations of the intrinsic biological environment of an individual such that the function of the central nervous system is also altered. (Such alterations may be established prenatally, but can evolve postnatally.)
3. Extraordinary extrinsic influences, resulting in a drastic change in mental function.

Errors in morphogenesis. In this group of conditions, embryonic development and fetal development are altered (Table 16-4) (Jones 1988; Jones and Rubinson 1983; Warkany et al. 1981). Approximately 4% of live-born infants are diagnosed as having major errors of morphogenesis seen in the first year of life. In a study by Holmes (1980), 2.4% of newborns had a major anomaly, and nearly 60% of these were associated with genetic or in utero causes.

Errors in morphogenesis may be due to malformations (failure of tissue to form normally from the time of conception), deformations (the alteration of normally forming tissues by abnormal mechanical forces), and disruptions (in utero injury or toxicity to tissues) (Cohen 1982). These events share the common theme of *prenatal* processes or events. They differ, however, in terms of the mechanisms by which form and function of the central nervous system are affected.

Malformations frequently occur as a direct effect

Table 16-3.   Etiologic categories of mental retardation

Errors of morphogenesis of the central nervous system
Malformation and malformation syndromes
In utero neurologic disease altering form and posture (deformations)
Disruption (injury) to developing central nervous system

Alterations in the intrinsic biological environment
Inborn errors of metabolism
Non-inborn changes in metabolism

Extraordinary extrinsic influences or events
Hypoxia
Trauma
Poisoning

of a single gene or chromosomal abnormality, but in fact the majority of these are either sporadic or multifactorial (Cohen 1982). Examples of multiple malformation syndromes include Brachmann-de Lange syndrome, Prader-Willi syndrome (Butler et al. 1986; Hawley et al. 1985; Kaplan et al. 1987), Pena-Shokeir syndrome (an autosomal recessive disorder involving severe mental retardation and upper motor neuron disease), and Down's syndrome (Hall 1986; Pueschel 1982). Implied in all of these examples is the concept that some signal or operator has directed a cascade of abnormal central nervous system growth and development, be it an identified gene or chromosome, or an unidentified stimulus that produces a recognizable pattern of abnormal morphogenesis. Myelodysplasia (spina bifida), which may be associated with mental retardation, represents a particularly striking example of a multiple malformation syndrome (Kaplan 1990). This condition, resulting from abnormal formation of the neural tube and its derivatives by the 28th day of gestation, presents in the newborn period as an open neural placode, the Arnold-Chiari II malformation (including hydrocephalus), brainstem abnormalities, and varying degrees of paralysis and bowel and bladder dysfunction. Despite the involvement of these multiple organ systems, the primary error of morphogenesis resides in the formation or differentiation of the early neural tube, its general effect being abnormal innervation of multiple organs.

Deformations are changes in the form or growth of tissues and organ systems that have been influenced by unusual mechanical forces (Dunn 1976). These deformations may be due to an abnormally shaped uterus compressing the developing calvarial bones and resulting in simple cosmetic changes in the shape of the head (plagiocephaly), or to abnormal fetal movement that may result in fixed contractures at birth, hip dislocation, or equinovarus deformity (club foot) (Clarren et al. 1979; Graham 1988). Rarely do deformations *cause* mental retardation per se, but identifying them is helpful since they may point to underlying congenital neurologic conditions that are associated with mental retardation.

Disruptions involve catastrophic gestational damage to the embryo or fetus, or possibly the steady "undoing" of formed and forming tissues and organ systems. This category of errors of morphogenesis includes the large and growing group of teratogens, chemicals or toxins that can disrupt

Table 16-4. Errors of central nervous system morphogenesis

Etiology	Example	Pathology	Diagnostic considerations	Degree of MR	Management considerations
Malformation					
Single gene recessive	Pena-Shokeir syndrome	Heterogeneous, muscle atrophy, abnormal spinal cord, cerebral dysgenesis	Neurogenic arthrogryposis, pulmonary hypoplasia, hypertelorism, phenotype overlaps with trisomy 18; autosomal recessive, decreased fetal movement	Severe to profound	Pulmonary insufficiency, seizures, swallowing difficulties; over half of cases autosomal recessive
	Seckel's syndrome	Microcephaly, cerebral dysgenesis	Severe short stature, prominent nose, hyperactivity common, severe microcephaly, autosomal recessive	Severe to profound	Generally stable; performance often exceeds clinical expectations
	Smith-Lemli-Opitz syndrome	Cerebral dysmorphogenesis; hypoplasia of frontal lobes, brain stem, cerebellum; irregular gyral patterns, heterotopias	Ptosis, anteverted nostrils, syndactyly 2nd and 3rd toes, hypospadias, cryptorchidism in males	Severe	Feeding difficulties, 20% of newborn survivors die in first year, irritability, significant management difficulties
Single gene dominant	Tuberous sclerosis	Glioma, angioma in cortex and white matter basal ganglia, periventricular mineralization, phakomata, fibrous angiomatous skin lesions, cystlike lesions in phalanges	Hamartomatous skin nodules, seizures, phakomata bone lesions	Unusual except with severe seizures	Seizures early in childhood, difficult to manage, occasional hypsarrhythmia, widely variable expression

(*continued*)

Table 16-4.   (Continued)

Etiology	Example	Pathology	Diagnostic considerations	Degree of MR	Management considerations
X-linked recessive	Menkes' syndrome	Cortical degeneration, gliosis, and atrophy; intracranial vascular elongation; tortuosity; sparse, stubby, "kinky" hair; defect in intestinal copper absorption	Progressive cerebral deterioration with seizures; twisted and fractured hair	Progresses to severe	Death usually by 3 years; hair normal at birth, loss of pigmentation by 6 weeks
	Fragile X[a] syndrome	Fragile site long-arm X chromosome (X_b 27); maternal carrier status important	MR, mild corrective tissue dysplasia, macro-orchidism, large-appearing ears	Mild to moderate in 80% of males	Gaze aversion common; hyperkinetic, emotionally labile; autistic behavior
Multifactorial	Neural tube defects	Includes hydrocephalus, Arnold-Chiari II malformation, spina bifida, neural tube closure defect by 18–28 days' gestation	Wide spectrum of clinical features, hydrocephalus typically progresses, ultrasound or CT helpful; degree of hydrocephalus difficult to correlate with cognitive outcome	Variable in mild hydrocephalus; cognitive function may be normal	Multidisciplinary attention needed in; orthopedic, urologic, neurosurgical, pediatric areas; habilitative potential often excellent
Sporadic or unknown	Brachmann-de Lange syndrome (Cornelia de Lange)	Unknown, cerebral dysgenesis, microcephaly	Synophrys, thin down-turning upper lip, hirsutism, micromelia, cardiac, renal genitourinary abnormalities	Variable; severe MR correlates with complexity of other congenital problems	Growth retardation common, seizures in 20%, coloboma and blindness may occur, some function loss

Table 16-4. (*Continued*)

Etiology	Example	Pathology	Diagnostic considerations	Degree of MR	Management considerations
	Williams' syndrome	Unknown, most cases sporadic	Prominent lips, stellate iris pattern, hoarse voice, supravalvular aortic stenosis, calcium metabolism problems	Average IQ 56 (41–80), expressive language delay	Often loquacious, personable; may develop spasticity later in life, hypotonia in infancy
Associated with chromosomal anomalies	Prader-Willi syndrome Labhart's syndrome	50% of cases associated with q11–q12 deletion of chromosome 15	Hypotonia, obesity, small hands and feet, hyperphagia common, narrow forehead, downward-slanted palpebral fissures	IQ range 20–80; often have behavioral problems, but not always	Evidence that dietary control and early intervention reduce behavioral problems; caloric intake less than typical for height
	Down's syndrome	Trisomy 21, D/G translocation	Microcephaly, brachycephaly, Brushfield spots, hypotonia, medial epicanthic folds, small ears, endocardial cushion defects	IQ range 25–50, occasionally higher	Extensive experience with early infant stimulation, Alzheimer's disease symptomalogy encountered frequently; Down's syndrome growth charts available
	Trisomy 18 syndrome	Trisomy 18	Microcephaly micrognathia, ventricular septal defect hypotonia, short sternum, high lethality	Profound	Mosaicism for extra chromosome 18 often associated with better outcome; 10% survival past first year

(*continued*)

Table 16-4. (*Continued*)

Etiology	Example	Pathology	Diagnostic considerations	Degree of MR	Management considerations
	Partial trisomy 14	Partial trisomy 14	Microcephaly micrognathia, ventricular septal defect hypotonia, may be lethal	Profound	Significant disability; motor impairment commonly seen
	Cri du chat syndrome	5p- (partial deletion chromosome 5)	"Cat-like" cry, microcephaly, downward-slanted palpebral fissures	Severe to profound	Diagnosis difficult in older individuals
	Angelman's syndrome	Unknown; some patients have deletions in q11–q12 region of chromosome 15	"Puppet-like" gait, paroxysmal laughter, cerebral palsy	Severe	Receptive skills often adequate for some communication; seizures
Deformations	Arthrogryposis secondary to CNS malfunction	CNS abnormality; diminished fetal movement leading to contractures at birth	Neuropathy and myopathy must be ruled out	Often none; related to degree of CNS abnormality	Contractures often improve after birth; physical therapy, occupational therapy critical; issues of body image
Disruptions	Porencephaly/ vascular	Vascular disruption of brain in utero	CT helpful	May be mild to severe	Motor impairment frequent
	Fetal alcohol syndrome and effects	Microgyria, CNS dysgenesis secondary to maternal alcohol use in pregnancy	Severity relates to amount and duration of exposure, small size, long philtrum, cardiac anomalies	Mild to severe, attention deficit common, hyperactivity	Careful developmental monitoring critical; social supports

Table 16-4. (*Continued*)

Etiology	Example	Pathology	Diagnostic considerations	Degree of MR	Management considerations
	Fetal warfarin syndrome	Bone and nasal pattern; CNS pattern including Dandy-Walker deformity secondary to 1st and/or 2nd trimester; maternal sodium warfarin (Coumadin) use in pregnancy, may be malformation if exposed in 1st trimester	Stippled mineralization of bone, rhizomelia, CNS malformation	Mild to moderate if CNS pattern occurs	Variable patterns; depends on degree of CNS involvement

Note. MR = mental retardation. CT = computed tomography. CNS = central nervous system.
[a]Represents an X-linked recessive disorder with a chromosomal marker.

normal morphogenesis (Shepard 1986). These include well-known substances such as alcohol, the largest cause of preventable mental retardation in the United States today; the anticoagulant sodium warfarin (Coumadin); and cocaine and crack, substances whose effects are largely unknown but appear to involve significant long-term effects even in the absence of distinct physical findings at birth (Kaplan 1985; Weiner et al. 1988; Zuckerman et al. 1989). Also included in the group of disruptions are certain viruses, particularly toxoplasmosis, rubella, and cytomegalovirus, and, less commonly, the effects of maternal hyperthermia and intrauterine vascular accidents involving either placenta or fetal cerebral blood vessels (Hoyme 1981; Nahmias 1974).

For all of the mechanisms of abnormal morphogenesis outlined, the effect on the developing central nervous system may follow an identifiable pattern or may be variable and depend on the extent, duration, and intensity of the abnormal genetic, environmental, and/or physical influences. It is these general categories that require careful consideration of family history and of drug and toxin use during the pregnancy. It is in these categories also that the clinician is likely to see patterns among children based both on their physical appearance and possibly on their developmental outcome. An example of this concept can be seen in males with the Fragile X syndrome in whom the sex-linked mode of inheritance often can be identified when taking a family history, but also in whom specific phenotypic features can be identified. In this example of a malformation syndrome, the possibility that the fragile site on the X chromosome in these affected individuals has a relationship to their mental retardation supports the idea of inheritance of a gene for mental retardation through the maternal X chromosome (Turner et al. 1986). A similar gene-chromosome behavioral-developmental association may also be true for the Angleman ("happy puppet") syndrome involving abnormalities in the molecular structure of chromosome 15 (Kaplan et al. 1987).

The identification of these general groups also permits the clinician to understand which conditions involving mental retardation may be preventable. Examples include the fetal alcohol syndrome, in which abstinence from alcohol is the prevention, and the fetal rubella syndrome, in which maternal immunity against the rubella virus is preventative (Hanshaw 1970).

These subgroup classifications do not define brain morphology or neurophysiologic function in any detail; however, as a group they imply that the infant at risk for mental retardation has experienced a static, nonprogressive alteration in the central nervous system that cannot be reversed or corrected. The child's development depends on the integrity of the brain; how that brain can support developmental growth and response to environmental pressures; and how the entire child, possibly challenged by other structural handicaps, can support and effect cerebral function.

Alterations of the intrinsic biological environment. As summarized in Table 16-5, there are several circumstances under which changes in the brain's biochemical environment lead to mental retardation. These include genetically determined enzyme deficiencies (Leroy 1983) such as phenylalanine hydroxylase deficiency, resulting in the mental retardation of phenylketonuria, or homocystinuria, which is associated with mental retardation as well as ophthalmologic and growth changes (Table 16-5) (Levy 1973; Scriver and Clow 1980). Precise diagnosis is important in these conditions because of the possibility of prevention or arrest of the mental retardation (Mercola and Cline 1980).

Another cause of mental retardation in an otherwise normal central nervous system is the cerebral edema encountered in Reye's syndrome, a hepatic encephalopathy (Shaywitz et al. 1980). Another is the potential injury to cortical tissue encountered in profound hypoglycemia.

Although the mechanisms of certain conditions are not understood, the natural history of children with certain clinical diagnoses still assists one in choosing a strategy to evaluate them. For example, Rett's syndrome presents the challenge of the female with loss of milestones within the first 2 years of life progressing to dementia, and with autism-like behavior, for which as yet no biochemical marker has been identified (Holm 1985). Nonetheless the abnormal movements seen in these children and their slow clinical deterioration suggest that the nature of this condition is neurodegenerative rather than, for example, related to a congenital, structural central nervous system abnormality.

Effects of extraordinary extrinsic influences. As illustrated in Table 16-6, a number of accidental and environmental factors may contribute to the pathogenesis of mental retardation.

Obvious examples include perinatal asphyxia, neonatal airway obstruction with profound hypoxemia, anesthetic complications, near-drownings, poisonings, and trauma. In each case, the specific circumstances, lost response, and environmental response interact to determine the final outcome (Seshia et al. 1983). While there are few data that precisely correlate specific clinical and historical factors with the degree of central nervous system and behavioral impairment, developmental prognosis can be built in part on the sense one has of both the duration of injury and the effectiveness of interventions.

Frequently, a child or an adult with mental retardation secondary to a catastrophic event presents with obvious upper motor neuron disease, especially secondary to profound hypoxia. One must not conclude, however, that mental retardation will always occur together with the obvious motor impairment. Many individuals with cerebral palsy, for example, are not mentally retarded.

Finally, while insults to an otherwise normal brain are usually static in nature and occur in the context of a single accident, the so-called plasticity of the human central nervous system contributes to the wide variability seen in the outcome of specific types of injury and should be taken into consideration in the evaluation process. This might explain, for example, why the child commencing a course of rehabilitation following head trauma may demonstrate recovery of some skills later on.

The Medical Evaluation of the Child With the Question of Mental Retardation

The algorithm in Figure 16-1 emphasizes the importance of a systematic approach in the identification and evaluation of mental retardation (Kaplan 1989).

Family and gestational histories. Maternal obstetrical history should include attention to miscarriages or infertility, drug and chemical exposure, and fetal movement in particular. Additional history of fetal distress or premature labor can also be helpful. Parents usually can accurately report diminished fetal activity or problems in the size of the fetus, and this should alert the clinician to review or request further prenatal obstetrical data. A family history of mental retardation may be very helpful, especially in males (fragile X syndrome). In obtaining a drug or alcohol history, it is useful

Table 16-5. Alterations in the intrinsic biological environment

Etiology	Example	Pathology	Diagnostic considerations	Degree of MR	Management considerations
Inborn errors of metabolism					
Auto recessive	Galactosemia	Disorder of carbohydrate metabolism, galactose-1-phosphate uridyl transferase	Normal at birth, failure to thrive, vomiting by 1st week, jaundice, hepatosplenomegaly, cataracts	Moderate MR, may be severe if untreated	Dietary restriction may reduce degree of disability, prenatal diagnosis possible
	Phenylketonuria	Disorder of amino acid metabolism, phenylalanine, hydroxylase	Normal at birth; vomiting, irritability 1st 2 months, developmental delay, seizures, microcephaly, spasticity	Severe to profound if untreated	Phenylalanine-restricted diet prevents MR; prenatal diagnosis possible; possible learning difficulties off diet
	Homocystinuria	Methionine metabolism defect	Normal at birth, 6–10-month onset of symptoms, seizures, delay glaucoma, lens dislocation, thromboembolism, cerebrovascular accidents	Moderate to severe	Dietary, cofactor therapy possible, may reduce degree of disability
	Niemann-Pick disease	Sphingomyelinase lipid metabolism	Different forms known, hepatosplenomegaly, cherry red macula, motor and cognitive deterioration after normal milestones	Profound MR possible	Some forms have no CNS involvement, others lethal
	Krabbe's disease	Galactocerebroside beta-galactosidase deficiency lipid metabolism	Elevated CNS protein spasticity, paresis, severity may vary, globoid cells seen	Wide variability in CNS function	Different forms, disability may vary
X-linked recessive	Hunter's syndrome (mucopolysaccharidosis II)	Iduronate sulfatase	Early onset, developmental delay, short stature, dysostosis	MR more severe than in Hurler's syndrome	Lethal disorder, quality of life critical, progressive disability

(continued)

Table 16-5. (*Continued*)

Etiology	Example	Pathology	Diagnostic considerations	Degree of MR	Management considerations
	X-linked ornithine carbarmyl transferase deficiency (Type II)	Urea cycle disorder, ornithine carbamyl phosphatase deficiency	Hyperammonemia in neonatal period	Severe to profound	Protein restriction; special medications reduce hyperammonemic crises; high lethality
Non-inborn change in metabolism	Hypoglycemia secondary to sepsis	Shock, hypermetabolism with glucose consumption	Profound hypoglycemia can result in seizures and CNS injury	Variable, may be severe depending on the degree and severity of hypoglycemia	Significant motor impairment; possible blindness reported; clinical variability may relate to degree of insult
	Cerebral edema secondary to hepatic encephalopathy (e.g., Reye's syndrome)	Possible CNS mitochondrial injury, direct cell injury, uncoupling of electron transport chain	Decreased cerebral blood flow may follow edema; brain-stem herniation infarction and necrosis secondary to compression	Variable	Motor impairment possible, delay usually global; variable outcome
	Cavernous venous thrombosis secondary to dehydration	Hypotension, decreased blood flow, stasis in cerebral blood vessels	Change in mental status at presentation or during rehydration; seizures, paralysis, coma	Variable	May have focal motor deficits; consider diagnosis with history of profound dehydration and altered mental state

Note. MR = mental retardation. CNS = central nervous system.

to ask about both the amount and the frequency of exposure.

General physical examination. The finding of three or more minor anomalies, phenotypic features that are obvious but not medically consequential, should alert the examiner to the possibility of a syndrome of abnormal morphogenesis. A finding of microcephaly in the newborn tells the examiner that brain growth and development were prenatally abnormal, raising the possibility of a malformation syndrome or of gestational disruption to the central nervous system. This finding should lead one to obtain a head ultrasound and cranial computed tomography (CT) scan, or a magnetic resonance image, if these are available. Abnormal scalp hair patterns are also often helpful in predicting cerebral dysgenesis, since these are laid down in response to the growth of brain and stretching of scalp (Smith and Gong 1973). Their abnormal appearance often implies problems of brain growth as early as the 18th week of gestation.

Midface asymmetry, especially undergrowth and abnormalities of the facial midline, may point to an underlying central nervous system malformation.

Table 16-6.   Extraordinary extrinsic influences

Etiology	Example	Pathology	Diagnostic considerations	Degree of MR	Management considerations
Hypoxia	Near-drowning	Hypoxia, cerebral edema, hypothermia	Long recovery phase common; prognosis dependent on status at scene of accident and onset of CPR	Wide variability dependent on water temperature, length of immersion, resuscitation	Rehabilitation may require counseling and support; parental guilt major concern; long recovery with uncertain deficits in some patients
	Neonatal asphyxia	Cerebral ischemia, hypoglycemia, acute renal failure	Obstetrical history helpful, initial arterial blood gas assists in predicting degree of hypoxia, profound hypotonia that persists longer than 72 hours worrisome; CT scan may show infarction or edema, seizures in first 24 hours common	Wide variability, may contribute greatly to causes of attention disorder; profound MR in severe cases	Motor disability common
	Obstructive airway epiglottitis, choanal atresia	Acute and complete blockage of airway resulting in hypoxia	Inability to ventilate similar to other conditions associated with hypoxia	Wide variability, may contribute to causes of attention-deficit disorder; often a cause of severe MR	Motor disability common
Trauma	Blunt head trauma, fractures	Hematoma, edema, tearing of brain tissue	History requires careful attention; exam often discloses other abuse; other potential causes of MR (e.g., lead) frequently seen	Variable	Parental involvement in therapy often limited; follow-up often requires social work

(continued)

Table 16-6. *(Continued)*

Etiology	Example	Pathology	Diagnostic considerations	Degree of MR	Management considerations
Poisoning	Acetaminophen	Severe hepato-toxicity, ex-hausts glutathione acidosis, shock, hepatic encephalopa-thy, hepatic failure, lethal	History, blood levels	Depends on oc-currence of CNS injury	Variable
	Tricyclic antide-pressants	Low toxic: thera-peutic ratio, arrhythmias, anticholinergic effects, sei-zures, coma; arrhythmias may lead to cardiac arrest	History, blood levels	Depends on oc-currence of CNS injury, usually sec-ondary to car-diopulmonary arrest	Variable
	Lead	Insidious effects in children typically due to pica (lead paint, solder, brass alloys) may be due to toxic doses, encephalopa-thy	Early effects: weight loss, vomiting, ab-dominal pain, headache, opaque flakes in gastrointes-tinal tract Late effects: sei-zures, MR, coma, in-creased intra-cranial pressure Lab: urinary coproporphy-rins, FEP, ur-ine Pb	Can be severe	Variable

Note. MR = mental retardation. CPR = cardiopulmonary resuscitation. CT = computed tomography. CNS = central nervous system. FEP = free erythrocyte protoporphyrin.

Close-set eyes (for measurement of which standard tables exist) often are encountered when a problem of the midline axis of the brain is present (Feingold and Bassert 1974). However, none of these findings is pathognomonic for the diagnosis of mental retardation. Rather, these are clues that mental retardation may occur, and its likelihood is greater when the dysgenesis is severe.

The neurologic examination or neurodevelopmental evaluation should include careful attention to the symmetry of movements, the pitch of the infant or child's cry, and response to stimuli (e.g., a bell or hand clapping). Often a high-pitched cry suggests long-standing prenatal insults. The child with irregular movements, extreme irritability, or hyperactive startle response may also be at risk for developmental disabilities. It should be pointed out, however, that failure to respond to sounds or visual stimuli may signal that the child is deaf or blind, but neither diagnosis implies mental retardation.

Laboratory investigations. A number of screen-

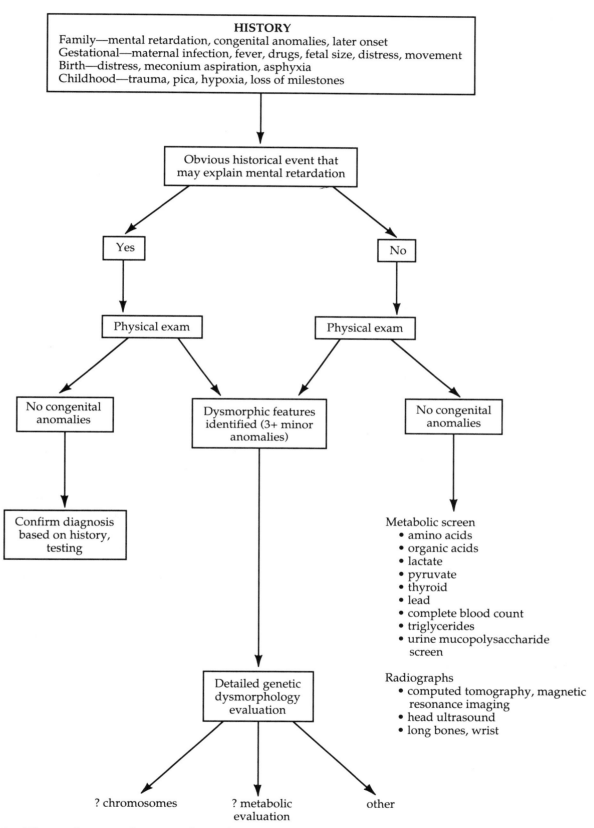

Figure 16-1.   Diagnostic approach to mental retardation for all ages.

ing studies are available. The urine amino acid screen is a chromatographic study that evaluates for elevated or decreased amino acids and some of their metabolites. Its importance is in identification of conditions that may be treated through diet (e.g., phenylketonuria) (Wilcken et al. 1980).

Another study is chromosome analysis, including, where indicated, the fragile X study. A dysmorphologist or geneticist may help in determining who should undergo these studies. When obtaining such tests, providing pertinent history and physical findings will help the laboratory determine which specific culture and staining methods need to be used (Ludman et al. 1984).

Serum levels of lactate, pyruvate, bicarbonate, and venous pH recently have become recognized as being helpful in identifying any inborn errors of metabolism, especially if the individual has been acidotic.

When there is suspicion of pica or significant lead exposure in the child with mental retardation, this laboratory study can be critical. Anemia may also be significant (Needleman 1989).

Cranial imaging includes head ultrasound (in infants whose anterior fontanel is open), cranial CT, and magnetic resonance imaging (MRI). The first of these is usually quite adequate in assessing brain dysmorphology. The MRI is particularly helpful in assessing gray and white matter differentiation, posterior fossa structures, and myelination. The CT scan has become the standard in the evaluation of ventricular enlargement and, when interpreted by an experienced specialist, defines much of what MRI can provide.

A number of mental retardation conditions for which laboratory studies can be helpful are indicated in specific clinical presentations. Examples of these include the hyperammonemia of urea-cycle disorders or biotinidase deficiency associated with seizures and developmental delay.

Psychiatry of Mental Retardation

Interface of Mental Retardation and Behavior

A most common misconception about retarded persons is the belief that they form a homogenous group with similar characteristics, behaviors, personality patterns, needs, and response to treatment. For example, mildly retarded persons are more similar to nonretarded persons than to se-

verely or profoundly retarded persons. Philips (1966) listed several of these misconceptions about mental retardation and behavior:

> That the maladaptive behavior of the retarded child is a function of his retardation, rather than of his interpersonal relationships; . . . that emotional disorder in the retarded is different in kind from that in a normal child; . . . that certain symptoms and specific maladaptive behavior patterns in a retarded child are the result of organic brain damage . . . (p. 112)

Szymanski and Crocker (1985, 1989) pointed out that if there is a personality feature characteristic of (but not unique for) a retarded person, it would be low self-image related to failures in life or to messages of rejection and failure received from significant persons and society.

Developmental Crises and Life-Course of Retarded Children and Adolescents

As their lives unfold, retarded children (and their families) face various challenges and developmental crises that are linked to the retardation, which may bring them to the attention of a psychiatrist.

Infancy and preschool age. Much of a retarded child's behavior and functioning at this stage will depend on whether there is a recognized etiology (e.g., Down's syndrome) or an associated handicap (e.g., congenital heart defect, sensory defect). Many of these conditions often require intensive treatment and hospitalization, often repeatedly. This creates a crisis of its own. Babies and young children who have an uncomplicated retardation may respond less readily to their parents, show fewer or delayed attachment behaviors, and appear to be less active (Buckhalt et al. 1978; Cicchetti and Sroufe 1978; Stone and Chesney 1978). In comparison with nonretarded infants of the same mental or chronological age, retarded infants tend to be more compliant and less vocally interactive (Hanzlik and Stevenson 1986). The delay in development of verbal communication is often an early complaint, and mothers may respond by adopting a communicative style that is directive and controlling. It is not clear to what degree this style may influence the child's communication (Mahoney 1988).

Early social interaction with peers also may be difficult for retarded children. They may have considerable communication difficulties, may lack age-expected self-care skills, and may be overtly rejected. Various disorders may be seen in this age group. At the Developmental Evaluation Center of the Children's Hospital in Boston, Massachusetts, of 100 children under 6 years of age, pervasive developmental disorder (not otherwise specified [NOS] or autistic disorder) was diagnosed in 45%, attention-deficit hyperactivity disorder in 12%, and posttraumatic stress disorder (following an abuse) in 8% (Szymanski 1989).

School age. At this period, learning academic skills and developing social skills and independence skills will be difficult for retarded children. Some mildly retarded children who have not yet been diagnosed are subjected to age-appropriate expectations that they cannot meet. As a result, they may develop behavioral problems, which may bring them to the attention of a psychiatrist. Many retarded children are placed in regular classes (mainstreamed) with nonretarded peers. The question whether mainstreaming is better than placement in separate special classes has not been definitely answered. Although the academic learning may be better in an integrated setting, social progress may be impaired because of poor acceptance by the peers (as well as by some teachers).

Most retarded children (except for very retarded ones) are quite aware of the difference between themselves and their peers and of the gap between what is expected of them and their actual performance. This awareness may have two effects. First, the child's low self-image further develops and becomes established. Second, various defense mechanisms are used, some of which may be maladaptive and may bring the child to a psychiatrist's attention (e.g., task avoidance, passivity, depression, aggressive acting out).

Adolescence. The most difficult developmental challenge at this period is the need for the child and for the family to accept the cognitive handicap as final (Szymanski and Crocker 1985, 1989). Paradoxically, less-retarded children may be more disadvantaged because they are more aware of their deficiencies and employ maladaptive defenses. The usual gap between physical puberty and emotional readiness for adult roles is even more accentuated, as most retarded youngsters have normal physical development. Realistic planning for the future is impeded by the uncertainty about their own abilities, low self-image, unwillingness to plan for a less than "normal" future, and lack of habilitation services. Developing mature peer and peer-group relationships is even more difficult. A latency-age

retarded child may be accommodated by normal peers in concrete play and interaction in peripheral and protected roles. However, it is much more difficult for retarded youngsters to participate in an adolescent group interaction that requires communication, cognitive, and abstraction skills.

The "sexual revolution" has not yet reached the mental retardation field, and old misconceptions and myths abound. These include the notions that retarded persons are uninhibited ("moral morons"), are unable to learn social mores, and are asexual or not interested in sexuality. Sexuality education may be very effective, providing that it focuses also on principles of appropriate relevant social behaviors and on the child's low self-esteem.

The defenses used during adolescence, as in earlier stages, may include passivity (withdrawal, task avoidance, regression) or acting out (aggressive behavior, delinquency, noncompliance). Unfortunately, these youngsters, in their quest for social acceptance, may be easy victims of sexual and other exploitation by their "normal" peers. Although various socially inappropriate behaviors may bring the child to psychiatric attention, it is essential to remember that such behaviors may also be symptoms of other mental disorders.

Parental Reactions and Adaptation to Child's Retardation

Initial reactions to the diagnosis. Children who are diagnosed at birth or in early infancy usually have severe retardation and an associated physical syndrome or handicap. The reaction to these children may be more intense, since the diagnosis is unexpected. The child's health problems may be overwhelming, and the parents may not have had the time to develop an attachment to the child. In the majority of these cases, the parents are told about the diagnosis by a physician, and the manner in which they are informed is crucial (Lynch and Staloch 1988). In particular, the physician should take adequate time for this informing conference, listen to the parents' concerns, express empathy and compassion but not pity or value judgments (e.g., "this child will devastate your family, you should institutionalize him"), and provide detailed and helpful information about available services and what the parents can do to promote the child's development. Above all, parents should never be told that nothing can be done for the child; such statements are untrue and destructive.

Traditionally, the parents were expected to have a depressive reaction to the birth of a retarded child. The retarded child might be seen as a loss of the ideal object: the expected normal child (Solnit and Stark 1961). However, it is also recognized that parental sadness is not necessarily a pathologic depression, but an adaptive reaction, a "chronic sorrow" (Olshansky 1962). Some studies have shown that there is no significant difference in the occurrence of psychopathology in parents of retarded and nonretarded infants (Harris and McHale 1989). Similarities have been drawn to the stage model of mourning (Klaus and Kennell 1976; Kubler-Ross 1969), in which the parents are expected to go through stages of adaptation such as shock, denial, anger, sadness, reorganization, and adaptation. More recent research suggests that such orderly schema may not always apply, and in some parents the various reactions may be intermixed, while in others the initial reactions may be generally negative, followed by denial and ending with adjustment (Mary 1990).

Family adaptation to child's retardation. Mild retardation unassociated with physical abnormalities is usually diagnosed later in life, often only when the child begins school. The parents usually are already aware of the child's developmental problems. Some parents, thinking that the child's developmental delay is caused by emotional problems, may have sought psychiatric consultation. These parents usually have developed an attachment to the child and also are aware of the child's strengths, which may attenuate their reaction to the diagnosis. Some families, however, may persist in denial and subject the child to continuous tests and unsuccessful therapies to cure the retardation.

Parental adjustment to a child's retardation is a multidimensional process that depends on many factors (Frey et al. 1989). Parents need adequate explanations for the child's condition and concrete help in finding the needed services. Their uncertainty about the child's future care is often the most stressful issue. Environmental factors, which are most important, include availability of medical, educational, and other services; access to understanding and helpful professionals; and a support network, such as parents' groups (e.g., Association for Retarded Citizens). While the earlier view was that a high rate of marital problems existed in these families, current clinical experience seems to be more positive (perhaps due to better available services for these children and families). Many families, in

fact, derive considerable and healthy gratification from their retarded child.

Family adaptation will, of course, be influenced by child-related factors, such as severity of the handicap and the need for medical care, communication level, and, in particular, behavioral and emotional difficulties that make the child's management difficult. The family adaptation is an ongoing process, as new challenges appear at each developmental stage.

Psychiatric Assessment of Retarded Persons

General principles. The diagnostic evaluation of retarded children and adolescents is similar to the evaluation of nonretarded ones in that it is based on a developmental approach and follows principles of sound psychiatric practice. Considering the multiplicity of cognitive and other deficiencies most retarded persons have, the assessment should be done within a framework of comprehensive understanding of biomedical and psychosocial problems of the patient. Past psychological, medical, neurologic, linguistic, and other evaluations should be reviewed and new ones requested, if needed. The diagnostician should be careful not to focus only on the questions of the caregivers that lead to the referral (both verbalized and "hidden" agendas), but should review the whole spectrum of the patient's functioning and problems (Szymanski 1977, 1980).

A detailed history is of paramount importance. Caregivers have a tendency to provide only the information that supports their concerns or professional beliefs. For example, those who are primarily behaviorally trained may focus on enumerating behaviors that are disturbing to the caregivers, such as "noncompliance" and "aggression" (as defined by them). However, this leaves open the question of whether the child has symptoms of depression, hallucinates, or even (if verbal) what the child thinks and feels about his or her own situation. Thus a detailed history is needed, describing what we call "external behaviors," observable to an outsider, as well as "internal behaviors" or emotions, which the patient may describe (if capable), or which are inferred from observable, "marker" behaviors. Also, it is necessary to obtain concrete descriptions of the actual behaviors, the situations in which they do and do not occur, and their evolution in time, and to correlate these with external events and treatments. This may require a systematic "review of systems" (functioning in all areas) to identify symptoms of defined mental disorders that may be present. The history is obtained from multiple sources, such as parents, teachers, and counselors, who observe the child in various settings.

Interviewing techniques. These techniques have been described elsewhere in detail (Szymanski 1977, 1980). The three crucial factors are 1) the interviewer's attitude (understanding of mental retardation, empathy but not pity, support without paternalism); 2) the interviewer's ability to adapt the communication style to the patient's communication skills; and 3) the interviewer's ability to set structure and limits and be directive, while still promoting spontaneous expression. Verbal interviewing techniques can be used with most patients, perhaps with the caregivers "translating" into the patient's communication level. The questions must be as neutral as possible, since retarded persons, fearing that they will make a mistake, tend to agree with clues in leading questions or, if given a choice of answers, select the last possibility they hear. It is essential to establish rather than assume that the patient understands the questions. For example, a mildly retarded patient's answer to the question "Do you hear a voice?" was, "Sure—I am not deaf." Retarded individuals often talk to themselves: this is usually similar to the young child's conversation with an imaginary friend and not necessarily evidence of psychosis. Nonverbal techniques such as play, drawings, and various activities are helpful. A visit to the patient's "natural environment" and unobtrusive behavioral observations may be crucial to the understanding of the clinical presentation.

Assessment of clinical data. The clinical data have to be understood in the context of the child's total clinical presentation, developmental and communication level, and education and experience. For example, a boy who is withdrawn and talks to himself may be hallucinating; may be rejected by his peers and feel depressed and lonely; may be trying to attract his teacher's attention; or may have an "imaginary friend," appropriate to his developmental, but not chronological, age. An "expanded diagnosis" should be produced to include, besides a formal diagnostic label, a review of the patient's strengths and liabilities, factors initiating and maintaining the problem, and a comprehensive treatment plan (Szymanski and Crocker 1989).

Mental Disorders in Retarded Persons

Epidemiology. Most of the epidemiologic studies of prevalence of mental disorders in retarded persons were done on selected populations. As a rule, they reflected a high prevalence of mental disorders in retarded children and adolescents: 60% (Chess and Hassibi 1970); 43% (Corbett et al. 1975); 87% (Philips and Williams 1975); and 74% (in mildly and moderately retarded children, Szymanski 1988). However, in two studies of unselected populations, the prevalence also was high: 61% in a retrospective study by Koller et al. (1983) and four to five times higher in retarded than in nonretarded children in the Isle of Wight study by Rutter et al. (1970). In summary, it is now generally agreed that virtually all types of mental disorders occur among retarded persons and that their prevalence is three to four times higher than in the general population.

Use of DSM-III-R with retarded persons. There is no evidence (nor reason to expect) that mental disorders in mentally retarded persons are different from those encountered in the general population (Philips 1966). The standard psychiatric nomenclature of DSM-III-R can be used even with significantly retarded and nonverbal persons, just as it is used with young children. In all cases, an effort should be made to fit the clinical presentation to a defined mental disorder rather than wrongly to assume that the behavioral symptoms are a part of mental retardation or represent a disorder unique to retarded persons.

Clinical Presentation of Major Mental Disorder in Retarded Persons

Mood disorders: depression. There is a remarkable similarity between the evolution of understanding of mood disorders in retarded persons (of any age) and in nonretarded children. In both cases, there were doubts whether depression could occur in these populations. One view held that retarded persons could not become depressed because they had no ability to realize their shortcomings and develop low self-esteem, whereas another view was that they were very much at risk for depression, because they had been, most probably, rejected by their mothers (Gardner 1967). In earlier studies of prevalence of mental disorders in retarded children and adolescents, depression was not mentioned (Chess and Hassibi 1970; Philips and Williams 1975). More recently, in a referred sample of mildly and moderately retarded children and adolescents, a mental disorder with significant components of depression was diagnosed in 14% (Szymanski 1988). Caregivers may overlook a depression in retarded persons, because their behavior may not be disturbing to others, and, in fact, they may be easier to manage (Szymanski and Biederman 1984; Szymanski and Crocker 1989).

Another obstacle to the diagnosis is the lack of language skills sufficient to reflect the traditional symptoms of depression (such as low self-image and hopelessness). However, of nine symptoms listed in the first group of DSM-III-R criteria for an episode of major depressive disorder (five are required for diagnosis), six can be observed by others and do not require that the patient be verbal: depressed or irritable mood, diminished interest in activities, significant weight loss or gain, insomnia or hypersomnia, any psychomotor agitation or retardation, and fatigue. Retarded persons with some language skills may provide information to satisfy other criteria, but they may be more concrete (e.g., may tell that they feel sick, rather than depressed) (Szymanski and Crocker 1989).

Many self-administered or informant-based rating scales have been developed to diagnose depression. Such instruments have been used with retarded persons, but they are not useful for a reliable diagnosis of depression in a specific individual (Reynolds and Baker 1988).

Mood disorders: manic and bipolar. Mania in retarded persons may be noticed more readily than depression, since the symptoms are disturbing to caregivers. There are no data on its prevalence among retarded children and adolescents. The symptoms have to be evaluated in the context of premorbid abilities and behavior. For example, a significantly retarded and nonverbal adolescent would not exhibit grandiosity, pressured speech, flight of ideas, and buying sprees, but one may notice insomnia, hyperactivity, distractibility, and irritability leading to aggression. Persons familiar with the individual will notice a mood change. The diagnosis may be difficult in the many retarded persons who are referred because of periodic disruptive behaviors. In some, these behaviors may represent a bipolar disorder; in others, they may be a reaction to periodic stresses, such as staff and school changes. In our clinic, the caregivers are requested to collect longitudinal data on major behavior and mood parameters, using simple rating instruments that are individualized for the patient.

Psychotic disorders. Children with a psychotic disorder may be first referred to the psychiatrist because of developmental delay, since psychosis may be associated with cognitive deficiencies (Russell and Tanguay 1981). The diagnosis of schizophrenia and other psychotic disorders in verbal, mildly retarded persons usually can be made in the same manner as in nonretarded persons, and the diagnosis of subtypes of schizophrenia is possible. In severely retarded persons, because of the lack of expressive language sufficient to manifest thought disorder, the diagnostician is limited to observable behavioral manifestations and to making a more general diagnosis of undifferentiated schizophrenia or psychotic disorder not otherwise specified (Heaton-Ward 1977; Reid 1972). A syndrome considered to be an early stage of childhood schizophrenia, and in which cognitive functioning may be compromised, has been described (Cantor 1988; Cantor et al. 1980, 1981, 1982). Infants or toddlers with this syndrome manifest sleep disturbance, hypotonia in the second year of life, social withdrawal, unusual behaviors (such as rocking), and fears. Some of them may have standard intelligence test scores within the mildly retarded range. However, since thought disorder may not yet be recognizable, the diagnosis of pervasive developmental disorder is typically used (in addition to retardation) (Kestenbaum et al. 1989). When these children reach late latency, symptoms of thought disorder are usually clear enough to permit a formal diagnosis of schizophrenia.

Results of most studies of epidemiology of psychotic disorders in retarded children are difficult to evaluate and compare because they use diverse methodologies and diagnostic criteria. In a study of 140 retarded children, psychotic disorder (including autism) was diagnosed in 13% (Corbett et al. 1975). In 256 children with combined mental retardation and emotional disorder, Menolascino (1969) diagnosed chronic brain syndrome with behavioral or psychotic reaction in 68%; however, the criteria for these diagnoses would not fit the currently accepted ones. Only 3% were seen as having "functional psychosis." In a sample of 52 mildly retarded children, Chess and Hassibi (1970) diagnosed psychosis in one. In 100 retarded children seen in a psychiatric clinic, Philips and Williams (1975) diagnosed disorders of "psychotic proportions" in 38, but these encompassed organic brain syndromes and autism as well as childhood schizophrenia. In a referred group of 60 children and adolescents, Reid (1980) diagnosed childhood psychosis in 8%. In our clinic, using DSM-III (American Psychiatric Association 1980) criteria, psychotic disorder was diagnosed in 3 of 413 retarded patients under 18 years of age. However, in 51 (12%), the diagnosis of atypical pervasive developmental disorder was made. In many of these, a diagnosis of psychosis was considered, but could not be made by DSM-III criteria.

Organic disorders. Psychiatrists have had a tendency to diagnose mental disorders in retarded persons as "organic." However, the fact that the child has mental retardation and perhaps an associated neurologic disorder (e.g., seizures) does not justify an automatic diagnosis of an organic disorder. DSM-III-R quite clearly requires that to use the "organic" diagnosis, not only the presence of the neuropathology but also its causative relationship to the behavioral manifestations must be proven (Lipowski 1980). This might be inferred from the nature of the clinical symptoms (e.g., if they are typical for a temporal lobe pathology, which has been demonstrated) and if there is a chronological correlation between the behavioral and neurologic findings.

Pervasive developmental disorders. Of children with this diagnosis, 75%–80% are also mentally retarded and are usually initially referred to developmental disabilities clinics because the first concern is with the developmental delay. The diagnoses of retardation and autism are not mutually exclusive. This question usually arises if the child manifests self-stimulatory behaviors, which are commonly labeled "autistic tendencies," and which are also seen in retarded children. The core symptoms of autistic disorder—qualitative impairment in reciprocal social relationships and in interpersonal communication—are not characteristic of uncomplicated mental retardation.

Stereotypic and self-abusive behaviors. These may occur as part of other mental disorder syndromes or independently; in either case, they may be the primary reason for psychiatric referral and the focus of treatment. Normal young children may engage in such behaviors (Werry et al. 1983), but in retarded and autistic persons, these behaviors may be of high intensity and persist into adult-

hood, including nonfunctional, repetitive behaviors (e.g., body rocking, head banging, and hand shaking). If there is tissue damage that requires medical treatment, the label of self-injurious behavior is used. These behaviors may lead to serious damage (e.g., retinal detachment and blindness due to head banging) and severely compromise the patient's adjustment. Stereotypies are estimated to occur in up to two-thirds of retarded persons, more often in the more severely retarded. They are also associated with disorders such as autism, blindness, and the Lesch-Nyhan syndrome (Harris, in press).

Treatment of Mental Disorders in Retarded Persons

Designing a treatment program. There are several special issues in the treatment of retarded children that have to be kept in mind. Retarded children usually are multihandicapped, since they have deficiencies in a number of areas that are interrelated and that have to be treated in concert. They are involved with many caregivers and professionals, who may have different views of the child, different expectations, and different complaints. Their cooperation and understanding of the treatment plan is essential. Last but not least, mental health professionals often do not understand the retarded child and limit themselves to symptomatic treatment of individual disruptive behaviors. Thus the following guidelines are important to the success of the treatment:

1. There should be a comprehensive diagnostic assessment.
2. The treatment program should be comprehensive, addressing all the patient's needs and not only the disruptive behaviors.
3. Causative factors (such as inappropriate school placement or inconsistent management by caregivers) should be addressed.
4. Psychiatric treatment approaches with the best benefit-risk ratio should be chosen, rather than those that are most convenient for the caregivers (such as quick symptom suppression with medications).
5. Target behaviors to measure the success of the treatment should be identified, and means of monitoring them should be established.
6. The caregivers should understand the treatment plan and should agree to it. They

should form a de facto interdisciplinary team with the clinician.

7. The adverse treatment effects should be regularly monitored, since the patients may not be able to report them.

8. Human rights and legal requirements (such as obtaining legal, informed consent for use of medications) should be respected.

General treatment measures. There are many measures that should be taken to enable retarded children to develop an optimal quality of life and to prevent psychosocial dysfunction (Szymanski 1987). These measures are particularly important with mildly and moderately retarded persons, who form the bulk of this population. Learning self-care and independence-related skills is essential. The right to appropriate public education in the least restricted environment (usually interpreted as community-based day school) and to related child- and family-oriented services is guaranteed by federal laws (Public Laws 94-142 and 99-457) and by many state laws. A most important goal of these measures is the facilitation of a sense of self-worth, leading to a positive self-image that may prevent development of learned helplessness, passivity, or maladaptive defenses. Thus even young children should be taught chores that they can perform and that help them feel that they are useful family members. Adolescents need prevocational, vocational, money management, and independent travel training. Appropriate and early sexuality education combined with an honest discussion of limitations, along with social skills training with opportunity to interact with appropriate peers, may prevent sexual acting out.

Psychotherapies. Retarded children and adolescents can benefit from various forms of psychotherapy as long as they have basic skills of verbal or nonverbal communication and find a willing and trained therapist. Principles of psychotherapy are the same as with nonretarded persons on the same developmental level. Details of the various therapeutic techniques helpful to retarded persons may be found elsewhere (Jakab 1970; Szymanski 1980). The goal is not, of course, to improve the child's intelligence but to ameliorate the psychopathology. An eclectic approach to therapy, utilizing reality-oriented cognitive techniques, behavior modification, role modeling, and, to a lesser degree, psychodynamic exploration, is needed. Besides individual psychotherapy, group psychotherapy and multiple family group psychotherapy may be most useful with retarded adolescents and young adults (Szymanski and Kiernan 1983; Szymanski and Rosefsky 1980).

Pharmacotherapy with retarded persons. *Use and misuse of psychotropic drugs.* There is a history of many years of irrational use of psychotropic drugs with retarded persons, particularly in institutions (see review by Rivinus 1980). These agents, usually antipsychotics, were often used to make the retarded persons more docile and easier to handle, even though their disruptive behaviors could actually represent a good adaptation to an understaffed facility and to the lack of any constructive programs and care. In the past two decades, a great deal of progress has occurred, partly due to improved general care and services for retarded persons and partly due to statutes and court decisions regulating the use of psychotropics with "incompetent" persons.

There is no evidence that psychotropic drugs have a unique effect on retarded persons. Therefore, usual principles of psychopharmacology apply equally to them. Common mistakes include overusage, the assumption that retarded persons form a homogeneous group, insufficient attention to comprehensive diagnostic assessment and treatment planning, and using medication as a substitute for services.

Principles of rational pharmacotherapy. The usual principles of treatment planning apply in particular to the rational use of psychoactive drugs. There is no special mystery to their use with retarded persons: the main difficulty is in diagnostic assessment (or rather making the expanded diagnosis). When the diagnosis is made, appropriate drugs may be used, whether the patient is retarded or not. The drugs should be used in the context of a comprehensive treatment program and not as a panacea. This is greatly facilitated if the psychiatrist functions as part of an interdisciplinary team, so that other professionals can become informed about the rationale for drug use and their collaboration on program development and collection of follow-up data can be secured. It has been shown that such collaboration in an interdisciplinary team in institutions may actually reduce the (unnecessary) use of drugs and improve their utilization when real indications exist (Findholt and Emmett 1990). These agents often work best in synergy with other treatment modalities. This is exemplified by the classic study of the use of haloperidol in combination with behavior modification with autistic children (Campbell et al. 1978).

The attitude of mental retardation professionals and of the general public is often antimedication. Statutes and regulations often equate drugs with aversive and intrusive measures, and some treatment programs pride themselves on being drug free, even when they have no such concerns about the use of physical punishment for minor problems (e.g., noncompliance). On the other hand, one can claim that retarded persons also have the right to the best available treatments, including drugs, that may improve their quality of life. The use of the drugs should be guided by the same principles as any medical treatment. Drugs are justified if they help to achieve the best possible quality of life for the patient (not necessarily the total elimination of all symptoms) and if the potential benefits well outweigh the potential adverse effects. As much as possible (and it should be possible in most, if not in all, cases), the drugs should be used for the treatment of a diagnosed mental disorder and not for objectionable single symptoms. Measures with fewer or no side effects should be tried first.

Follow-up on treatment effects. Since some retarded patients may not be able to report on sensations related to side effects, careful monitoring by the caregivers and the prescribing psychiatrists is essential. A list of target symptoms (or behaviors) to measure the effectiveness of the treatment should be prepared, preferably in the form of a simple rating scale, and baseline data should be obtained prior to onset of treatment. A similar list of potential side effects may also be prepared, and the caregivers should be taught to watch for their appearance. In some cases, pretreatment videotaping of a patient's behavior may be most helpful. This will help later to differentiate between relapse of the basic disorder and emergence of side effects. It also should be kept in mind that behavioral symptoms that may be confused with reemergence of the psychotic symptoms, including symptoms such as irritability, insomnia, and weight loss, may emerge when antipsychotics are abruptly discontinued (Gualtieri et al. 1986).

Roles of Psychiatrists in the Mental Retardation Field

The position statement on psychiatry and mental retardation, issued by the American Academy of Child and Adolescent Psychiatry (1988), lists four roles for psychiatrists in this field:

1. Provision of clinical services to retarded persons.
2. Prevention of mental disorders through early diagnosis, and provision of emotional supports to the child and the family.
3. Research.
4. Learning skills that are also useful in the practice of psychiatry in general.

The common theme of these roles is participation in an interdisciplinary developmental team (Cushna et al. 1980). The role of the modern psychiatrist on such a team is one of an equal member, not necessarily as a leader nor as an uninvolved consultant. Because of their roots in the biomedical and psychosocial aspects of medicine, psychiatrists can function in the unique role of a "synthesizer" who helps the team to integrate the contributions of various disciplines (West 1973). In particular, psychiatrists should not limit themselves to the role of medication specialist, even if other disciplines try to cast them in such a role. A psychiatric physician should not do a "medication review" (one of the common reasons for referring a retarded patient), but a "patient review," which focuses on all aspects of diagnosis and treatment. In summary, the field of mental retardation can be seen as an archetype for modern psychiatry anchored in biological and psychological medicine.

Prognosis in Mental Retardation

Two aspects of prognosis of mental retardation must be considered. The first is the prognosis of the underlying disorder or syndrome, such as phenylketonuria, congenital rubella, or hydrocephalus, each of which may have a certain course, depending on treatment, on complications, and on the natural history. The second aspect is the prognosis of the functional, "generic" mental retardation of unknown cause. The prognosis is defined here by the quality of life the retarded child ultimately will be able to achieve. Factors include, among others, the level of independence, self-care skills, social skills and opportunities, integration in society, opportunity to benefit from community resources, and opportunity and ability to lead a life as close as possible to what is considered normal in the particular culture. The latter is, in fact, the essence of the "normalization" philosophy (Wolfensberger 1972).

Developments in the past several decades have brought us closer to the normalization goal. Federal laws PL 94-142 of 1975 and PL 99-457 of 1987 have given disabled children and adolescents rights to public education and ancillary services, as well as to specialized services for their families. These may range from a few hours weekly of special tutoring to a full-time therapeutic residential school. The goal is a "least restrictive" placement, preferably in the community, to enable the child to live with the family. As a result, retarded children are now rarely, if at all, institutionalized (nor should they be). Retarded adults are trained for jobs in the competitive labor market or in sheltered settings (Kiernan and Stark 1986) and live with their families and in a variety of community settings (e.g., group homes, supervised apartments).

References

American Academy of Child and Adolescent Psychiatry, Committee on Mental Retardation and Developmental Disabilities: The roles and responsibilities of child and adolescent psychiatry in the field of developmental disabilities. American Academy of Child and Adolescent Psychiatry Newsletter, Winter 1988, p 7

American Psychiatric Association: Diagnostic and Statistical Manual of Mental Disorders, 3rd Edition. Washington, DC, American Psychiatric Association, 1980

American Psychiatric Association: Diagnostic and Statistical Manual of Mental Disorders, 3rd Edition, Revised. Washington, DC, American Psychiatric Association, 1987

Buckhalt J, Rutherford B, Goldberg K: Verbal and nonverbal interaction of mothers with their Down's syndrome and nonretarded infants. American Journal of Mental Deficiency 82:337–343, 1978

Butler MG, Meany FJ, Palmer CG: Clinical and cytogenetic survey of 39 individuals with Prader-Labhart-Willi Syndrome. Am J Med Genet 23:793–809, 1986

Campbell M, Anderson LT, Meier M, et al: A comparison of haloperidol, behavior therapy and their interaction in autistic children. Journal of the American Academy of Child Psychiatry 17:640–655, 1978

Cantor S: Childhood Schizophrenia. New York, Guilford, 1988

Cantor S, Trevenen C, Postuma R, et al: Is childhood schizophrenia a cholinergic disease? Arch Gen Psychiatry 37:658–667, 1980

Cantor S, Pearce J, Pezzot-Pearce T, et al: The group of hypotonic schizophrenics. Schizophr Bull 7:1–11, 1981

Cantor S, Evans J, Pearce J, et al: Childhood schizophrenia: present but not accounted for. Am J Psychiatry 139:758–762, 1982

Chess S, Hassibi M: Behavior deviations in mentally retarded children. Journal of the American Academy of Child Psychiatry 9:282–297, 1970

Cicchetti D, Sroufe A: An organizational view of affect: illus-
tration from the study of Down's syndrome infants, in The Development of Affect. Edited by Lewis M, Rosenblum LA. New York, Plenum, 1978

Clarren SK, Smith DW, Hansen JW: Helmet treatment for plagiocephaly and congenital muscular torticollis. J Pediatr 94:43–46, 1979

Cohen MM Jr: The Child With Multiple Birth Defects. New York, Raven, 1982

Corbett JA, Harris E, Robinson R: Epilepsy, in Mental Retardation and Developmental Disabilities, Vol 7. Edited by Wortis J. New York, Brunner/Mazel, 1975, pp 79–111

Cushna B, Szymanski LS, Tanguay PE: Professional roles and unmet manpower needs, in Emotional Disorders of Mentally Retarded Persons. Edited by Szymanski LS, Tanguay PE. Baltimore, MD, University Park Press, 1980, pp 3–17

Detterman DK: Theoretical notions of intelligence and mental retardation. American Journal of Mental Deficiency 92:2–11, 1987

Donaldson JY, Menolascino FJ: Past, current and future roles of child psychiatry in mental retardation. Journal of the American Academy of Child Psychiatry 3:352–374, 1977

Dunn PM: Congenital postural deformities. Br Med Bull 93:71–76, 1976

Ellis NR, Cavalier AR: Research perspectives in mental retardation, in Mental Retardation: the Developmental-Difference Controversy. Edited by Zigler E, Balla D. Hillsdale NJ, Erlbaum, 1982, pp 121–152

Feingold M, Bassert WH: Normal values. Birth Defects 10:1–5, 1974

Findholt NE, Emmett CG: Impact of interdisciplinary team review on psychotropic drug use with persons who have mental retardation. Ment Retard 1:41–46, 1990

Frey KS, Greenberg MT, Fewell RR: Stress and coping among parents of handicapped children: a multidimensional approach. Am J Ment Retard 94:240–249, 1989

Gardner WI: Occurrence of severe depressive reactions in the mentally retarded. Am J Psychiatry 124:142–144, 1967

Graham JM Jr: Smith's Recognizable Patterns of Human Deformation, Philadelphia, PA, WB Saunders, 1988

Grossman HJ (ed): Manual on Terminology and Classification in Mental Retardation. Washington, DC, American Association on Mental Deficiency, 1983

Grossman HJ (ed): Classification in Mental Retardation. Washington, DC, American Association on Mental Deficiency, 1983

Gualtieri CT, Schroeder SR, Hicks RE, et al: Tardive dyskinesia in young mentally retarded individuals. Arch Gen Psychiatry 43:335–340, 1986

Hall JG: Invited editorial comment: analysis of Pena-Shokeir phenotype. Am J Med Genet 25:99, 1986

Hanshaw GB: Developmental abnormalities associated with congenital CMV infection. Advances in Teratology 4:64–93, 1970

Hanzlik JR, Stevenson MB: Interaction of mothers with their infants who are mentally retarded, retarded with cerebral palsy, or nonretarded. American Journal of Mental Deficiency 90:513–520, 1986

Harris JC: Neurobiological factors in self-injurious behavior, in Assessment, Analysis and Treatment of Self-Injury. Edited by Luiselli JK, Matson J, Singh NN. New York, Springer-Verlag (in press)

Harris VS, McHale SM: Familiy life problems, daily caregiving activities, and the psychological well-being of mothers of mentally retarded children. Am J Ment Retard 94:231–239, 1989

Hawley PD, Jackson LG, Kurnit DM: Sixty-four patients with Brachmann-de Lange syndrome: a survey. Am J Med Genet 20:453–459, 1985

Heaton-Ward A: Psychosis in mental handicap. Br J Psychiatry 130:525–533, 1977

Holm VA: Rett's syndrome: a progressive developmental disability in girls. Developmental Behavioral Pediatrics 6:32–36, 1985

Holmes LB: Congenital malformations, in Manual of Neonatal Care. Edited by Doherty JP, Stark AR. Boston, MA, Little, Brown, 1980, pp 91–96

Hoyme EH, Higginbottom MC, Jones KL: Vascular etiology of disruptive structural defects in monozygotic twins. Pediatrics 67:288–291, 1981

Jakab I: Psychotherapy of the mentally retarded child, in Diminished People. Edited by Bernstein NR. Boston, Little, Brown, 1970

Jones KL: Smith's Recognizable Patterns of Human Malformation, 4th Edition. Philadelphia, PA, WB Saunders, 1988, pp 1–9

Jones KL, Rubinson LK: (1983) An approach to the child with structural defects. J Pediatr Orthop 4:238–244, 1983

Kanner L: Autistic disturbances of affective contact. Nervous Child 2:217–250, 1943

Kaplan LC: Congenital Dandy Walker malformation associated with first trimester warfarin: a case report and literature review. Teratology 32:333–336, 1985

Kaplan LC: Assessment and management of infants and children with multiple congenital anomalies, in Developmental Disabilities: Delivery of Medical Care for Children and Adults. Edited by Rubin IL, Crocker AC. Philadelphia, PA, Lea & Febiger, 1989, pp 97–116

Kaplan LC: Neural tube defects, in Manual of Neonatal Care. Edited by Cloherty JP, Start AR. Boston, MA, Little, Brown (in press)

Kaplan LC, Wharton R, Elias E, et al: Clinical heterogeneity associated with deletions in the long arm of chromosome #15: report of three new cases and their possible genetic significance. Am J Med Genet 28:45–53, 1987

Kavanaugh JF (ed): Understanding Mental Retardation. Baltimore, MD, Paul H Brookes, 1988

Kestenbaum CJ, Canino IA, Pleak RR: Schizophrenic disorders of childhood and adolescence, in American Psychiatric Press Review of Psychiatry, Vol 8. Edited by Tasman A, Hales RE, Frances AJ. Washington, DC, American Psychiatric Press, 1989, pp 242–261

Kiernan WE, Stark JA (eds): Pathways to Employment for Adults With Developmental Disabilities. Baltimore, MD, Paul H Brookes, 1986

Klaus MH, Kennell JH: Maternal-Infant Bonding. St. Louis, CV Mosby, 1976

Koller H, Richardson SW, Katz M, et al: Behavior disturbance since childhood among a 5-year birth cohort of all mentally retarded young adults in a city. American Journal of Mental Deficiency 87:386–395, 1983

Kubler-Ross E: On Death and Dying. New York, Macmillan, 1969

Lazar I, Darlington R, Murray H, et al: Lasting effects of early education: a report from the consortium for longitudinal studies. Monographs of the Society for Research in Child Development 47 (2–3, serial no 195), 1982

Leroy JG: Heredity, development, and behavior, in Developmental Behavioral Pediatrics. Edited by Levine MD, Carey WB, Crocker AC, et al. Philadelphia, PA, WB Saunders, 1983, pp 315–345

Levy HL: Genetic screening. Adv Hum Genet 4:1–3, 1973

Lipowski ZJ: A new look at organic brain syndromes. Am J Psychiatry 137:674–678, 1980

Ludman MD, Gilbert F, Hirschhorn K: Risk of recurrence of chromosome abnormalities. Pediatr Rev 6:141–142, 1984

Lynch EC, Staloch NH: Parental perceptions of physicians' communication in the informing process. Ment Retard 2:77–81, 1988

Mahoney G: Maternal communication style with mentally retarded children. Am J Ment Retard 92:352–359, 1988

Mary NL: Reactions of black, Hispanic and white mothers to having a child with handicaps. Ment Retard 28:1–5, 1990

Mayes LC, Kirk V, Haywood N, et al: Changing cognitive outcome in preterm infants with hyaline membrane disease. Am J Dis Child 139:20–24, 1985

McLaren J, Bryson SE: Review of recent epidemiological studies of mental retardation: prevalence, associated disorders, and etiology. Am J Ment Retard 92:243–254, 1987

Menolascino FJ: Emotional disturbances in mentally retarded children. Am J Psychiatry 126:168–179, 1969

Mercola KE, Cline MJ: The potentials of inserting new genetic information. N Engl J Med 303:1297–1300, 1980

Nahmias AJ: The TORCH complex. Hosp Pract [Off] 9:65–72, 1974

Needleman HL: The neurotoxic teratogenic and behavioral teratogenic effects of lead at low dose: a paradigm for transplacental toxicants. Prog Clin Biol Res 281:279–287, 1989

Olshansky L: Chronic sorrow: a response to having a mentally defective child. Social Casework 43:190–193, 1962

Philips I: Children, mental retardation and emotional disorder, in Prevention and Treatment of Mental Retardation. Edited by Philips I. New York, Basic Books, 1966, pp 111–122

Philips I, Williams N: Psychopathology and mental retardation: a study of 100 mentally retarded children, I: psychopathology. Am J Psychiatry 132:1265–1271, 1975

Pueschel SM: A Study of the Young Child With Down Syndrome. New York, Human Science Press, 1982

Reid AH: Psychosis in adult mental defectives. Br J Psychiatry 120:205–212, 1972

Reid AH: Psychiatric disorders in mentally handicapped children: a clinical and follow-up study. J Ment Defic Res 24:287–298, 1980

Reynolds MW, Baker JA: Assessment of depression in persons with mental retardation. Am J Ment Retard 93:93–103, 1988

Rivinus TM: Psychopharmacology and the mentally retarded patient, in Emotional Disorders of Mentally Retarded Persons. Edited by Szymanski LS, Tanguay PE. Baltimore, MD, University Park Press, 1980, pp 195–221

Russell AT, Tanguay PE: Mental illness and mental retardation: cause or coincidence? American Journal of Mental Deficiency 85:570–574, 1981

Rutter M, Graham P, Yule W: A Neuropsychiatric Study in Childhood. London, Spastics International Medical Publications, 1970

Scriver CL, Clow CL: Phenylketonuria: epitome of human biochemical genetics (2 parts). N Engl J Med 303:1336–1394, 1980

Seshia SS, Johnston R, Kasian G: Non-traumatic coma in childhood: clinical variables in prediction of outcome. Dev Med Child Neurol 25:493–501, 1983

Shaywitz BA, Rothstein P, Venes JL: Monitoring and management of increased intracranial pressure in Reyes syndrome: results in 29 patients. Pediatrics 66:198–204, 1980

Shepard TH: Catalog of Teratogenic Agents, 5th Edition. Baltimore, MD, Johns Hopkins University Press, 1986

Smith DW, Gong BT: Scalp hair patterning as a clue to early fetal brain development. J Pediatr 83:374–378, 1973

Solnit A, Stark M: Mourning and a birth of a defective child. Psychoanal Study Child 16:523–537, 1961

Stone NW, Chesney BH: Attachment behaviors in handicapped infants. Ment Retard 16:8–12, 1978

Szymanski LS: Psychiatric diagnostic evaluation of mentally retarded individuals. Journal of the American Academy of Child Psychiatry 16:67–87, 1977

Szymanski LS: Psychiatric diagnosis of retarded persons, in Emotional Disorders of Mentally Retarded Persons. Edited by Szymanski LS, Tanguay PE. Baltimore, MD, University Park Press, 1980, pp 61–81

Szymanski LS: Prevention of psychosocial dysfunction in persons with mental retardation. Ment Retard 25:215–218, 1987

Szymanski LS: Integrative approach to diagnosis of mental disorders in retarded persons, in Mental Retardation and Mental Health. Edited by Stark JA, Menolascino FJ, Albarelli MH, et al. New York, Springer-Verlag, 1988, pp 124–139

Szymanski LS: Psychiatric diagnoses in developmentally delayed young children. American Academy of Child and Adolescent Psychiatry Scientific Proceedings of the Annual Meeting 5:41–42, 1989

Szymanski LS, Biederman J: Depression and anorexia nervosa of persons with Down syndrome. American Journal of Mental Deficiency 89:246–251, 1984

Szymanski LS, Crocker AC: Mental retardation, in Comprehensive Textbook of Psychiatry, Vol IV. Edited by Kaplan HI, Sadock BJ. Baltimore, MD, Williams & Wilkins, 1985, pp 1635–1671

Szymanski LS, Crocker AC: Mental retardation, in Comprehensive Textbook of Psychiatry, Vol V. Edited by Kaplan HI, Sadock BJ. Baltimore, MD, Williams & Wilkins, 1989, pp 1728–1771

Szymanski LS, Kiernan WE: Multiple family group therapy with developmentally disabled adolescents and young adults. Int J Group Psychother 33:521–534, 1983

Szymanski LS, Rosefsky QB: Group psychotherapy with retarded persons, in Emotional Disorders of Mentally Retarded Persons. Edited by Szymanski LS, Tanguay PE. Baltimore, MD, University Park Press, 1980, pp 173–194

Szymanski LS, Rubin IL, Tarjan G: Mental retardation, in American Psychiatric Press Review of Psychiatry, Vol 8. Edited by Tasman A, Hales RE, Frances AJ. Washington, DC, American Psychiatric Press, 1989, pp 217–241

Turner G, et al: Conference report: Second International Workshop on Fragile X and X-Linked Mental Retardation. Am J Med Genet, Vol 23, No 11, 1986

Weiner L, Morse BA, Garrido T: FAS-FAE: focusing prevention on women at risk. Int J Addict 24:385–395, 1988

Werry JS, Carlielle J, Fitzpatrick J: Rhythmic motor activities (stereotypies) in children under five: etiology and prevalence. Journal of the American Academy of Child Psychiatry 22:329–336, 1983

West LJ: The future of psychiatric education. Am J Psychiatry 130:521–528, 1973

Whitman TL: Self-regulation and mental retardation. Am J Ment Retard 94:347–362, 1990

Wilcken B, Smith A, Brown DA: Urine screening for aminoacidopathies: is it beneficial? Results of a long-term followup of cases detected by screening one million babies. J Pediatr 97:492–496, 1980

Wolfensberger W: The Principle of Normalization in Human Services. Toronto, National Institute on Mental Retardation, 1972

Zigler E: Developmental vs difference theories of mental retardation and the problem of motivation. American Journal of Mental Deficiency 73:536–556, 1969

Zigler E, Balla D: Introduction: the developmental approach to mental retardation, in Mental Retardation: the Developmental-Difference Controversy. Edited by Zigler E, Balla D. Hillsdale, NJ, Erlbaum, 1982, pp 3–26

Zigler E, Balla D, Hodapp R: On the definition and classification of mental retardation. American Journal of Mental Deficiency 89:215–230, 1984

Zuckerman B, Frank DA, Hingson R, et al. Effects of maternal marijuana and cocaine use on fetal growth. N Engl J Med 23:762–768, 1989

Chapter 17

Autistic Disorder

Luke Y. Tsai, M.D.
Mohammad Ghaziuddin, M.D.

Definition and Diagnostic Criteria

Historical Background

Any discussion of autistic disorder must start with Kanner, who in 1943 described a group of 11 children with a previously unrecognized disorder. He noted a number of characteristic features in these children, such as an inability to develop relationships with people, extreme aloofness, a delay in speech development, noncommunicative use of speech, repeated simple patterns of play activities, and islets of ability. He described these children as having "come into the world with innate inability to form the usual, biologically provided affective contact with people" (Kanner 1943, p. 250). Despite all the variety of individual differences that appeared in the case descriptions, Kanner believed that only two features were of diagnostic significance: autistic aloneness and obsessive insistence on sameness. He adopted the term *early infantile autism* to describe this disorder and called attention to the fact that its symptoms were already evident in infancy.

During the next decade, clinicians in the United States and in Europe reported cases with similar features (Asperger 1944; Despert 1951; Van Krevelen 1952). However, controversy continued over the definition of the disorder because the name *autism* was ill-chosen. It led to confusion with Bleuler's (1911) use of the same term to describe schizophrenia in adults. This confusion led many clinicians to use terms such as *childhood schizophrenia, borderline psychosis, symbiotic psychosis,* and *infantile psy-chosis* as interchangeable diagnoses. Each label had its definition and roots in a particular view of the nature and causation of autism.

In an attempt to clarify the confusion, Eisenberg and Kanner (1956) reduced the essential symptoms to two: extreme self-isolation and preoccupation with the preservation of sameness. The peculiar abnormality of language was considered to be secondary to the disturbance of human relatedness, and hence not essential. They also expanded the age of onset to the first 2 years of life. Their efforts, however, were sometimes taken as a license to ignore age of onset as a necessary diagnostic criterion or to change the criteria altogether (Rutter 1978). For example, Schain and Yannet (1960) omitted preservation of sameness from their criteria; Creak et al. (1961) used nine diagnostic points to encompass all forms of childhood psychoses, including Kanner's (1943) infantile autism, within a single diagnosis (schizophrenic syndrome of childhood); and Ornitz and Ritvo (1968) emphasized disturbances of perception as a primary symptom that was not included by Kanner.

Rutter (1968) critically analyzed the existing empirical evidence and proposed that four essential characteristics of infantile autism stand out: 1) a lack of social interest and responsiveness; 2) impaired language, ranging from absence of speech to peculiar speech patterns; 3) bizarre motor behavior, ranging from rigid and limited play patterns to more complex ritualistic and compulsive behavior; and 4) early onset, before 30 months of age. These features presented in nearly all autistic children. There were many other specific features, but they were unevenly distributed. In 1978, the Professional Advisory Board of the National Society for Children and Adults with Autism further formulated a definition of the syndrome of autism. Autism was defined as a behavioral syndrome that manifested itself before 30 months of age and had the following essential features: 1) disturbances of developmental rates and sequences; 2) disturbances of responses to any sensory stimuli; 3) disturbances of speech, language, cognition, and nonverbal communication; and 4) disturbances of the capacity to relate appropriately to people, events, and objects (Ritvo and Freeman 1978). This definition and the definitions of Kanner (1943) and Rutter (1968) paved the way for two sets of criteria that are now widely used by clinicians all over the world: the International Classification of Diseases, 9th revision, Clinical Modification (ICD-9-CM) (U.S. Department of Health and Human Services 1980) and the Diagnostic and Statistical Manual of Mental Disorders, 3rd edition (DSM-III) (American Psychiatric Association 1980).

Although ICD-9-CM and DSM-III have similar definitions and diagnostic criteria for infantile autism, there are apparent differences in the concept of autism. In ICD-9-CM, infantile autism is classified as a subtype of "psychoses with origin specific to childhood," whereas in the DSM-III and DSM-III-R (American Psychiatric Association 1987) systems, infantile autism is viewed as a type of pervasive developmental disorder. Pervasive developmental disorders are defined as a group of severe, early developmental disorders characterized by delays and distortions in the development of social skills, cognition, and communication.

DSM-III-R Diagnostic Concept

In DSM-III, the pervasive developmental disorders include infantile autism (i.e., the onset of the disorder is before the age of 30 months), childhood onset pervasive developmental disorder (i.e., the disorder develops after the age of 30 months), atypical pervasive developmental disorder (i.e., autistic-like condition that cannot be classified as infantile autism or childhood onset pervasive developmental disorder), and residual infantile autism (i.e., a condition that no longer meets the full criteria of infantile autism but that was once diagnosed as such). Empirical data published after 1980, however, could not find any significant differences (except age of onset) between individuals with infantile autism and those with a diagnosis of childhood onset pervasive developmental disorder. Therefore, in DSM-III-R, childhood onset pervasive developmental disorder was dropped. In addition, it also was found to be difficult to differentiate between atypical pervasive developmental disorder and residual infantile autism. The DSM-III-R Pervasive Developmental Disorders Work Group, therefore, decided to take a combining approach and to include only two subcategories under pervasive developmental disorders: autistic disorder (roughly corresponding to infantile autism) and pervasive developmental disorder not otherwise specified (NOS). Although the concept of pervasive developmental disorders is retained in DSM-III-R, the diagnostic criteria for autistic disorder have been revised considerably (Table 17-1). The DSM-III criteria were descriptive, whereas the menu-like scheme of DSM-III-R criteria requires the presence of a minimum number of criteria in each of the three cardinal features described above. The revised criteria are much more concrete, observable, and operational than those in DSM-III. The revised criteria do not require raters to determine subjectively whether there is a "pervasive impairment" or a "gross deficit"; hence clinicians' hesitation to use the diagnosis of autistic disorder in older and higher functioning autistic individuals has been removed. DSM-III-R has broadened the diagnostic concept of autism from DSM-III, allowing for the gradation of behavior seen in autistic individuals. Thus it is not surprising that studies using DSM-III-R criteria have yielded higher prevalence rates of autistic disorder than those using DSM-III criteria for infantile autism (Factor et al. 1989; Hertzig et al. 1990; Spitzer and Siegel, personal communication; Volkmar et al. 1988).

ICD-10 and DSM-IV Diagnostic Concepts

The World Health Organization has planned to publish the 10th edition of the International Classification of Diseases (ICD-10). The draft of the ICD-10 (1987) shows that it has also adopted the diagnostic term of *pervasive developmental disorders*. In the ICD-10 system, these disorders include: 1) childhood autism, 2) atypical autism, 3) Asperger's syndrome, 4) Rett's syndrome, 5) childhood disintegrative disorder, 6) overactive disorders associated with mental retardation and stereotyped

Table 17-1. DSM-III-R diagnostic criteria for autistic disorder

At least eight of the following sixteen items are present, these to include at least two items from A, one from B, and one from C.

Note: Consider a criterion to be met *only* if the behavior is abnormal for the person's developmental level.

A. Qualitative impairment in reciprocal social interaction as manifested by the following:

(The examples within parentheses are arranged so that those first mentioned are more likely to apply to younger or more handicapped—and, in the later ones, to older or less handicapped—persons with this disorder.)

1. Marked lack of awareness of the existence or feelings of others (e.g., treats a person as if he or she were a piece of furniture; does not notice another person's distress; apparently has no concept of the need of others for privacy)
2. No or abnormal seeking of comfort at times of distress (e.g., does not come for comfort even when ill, hurt, or tired; seeks comfort in a stereotyped way, e.g., says "cheese, cheese, cheese" whenever hurt)
3. No or impaired imitation (e.g., does not wave bye-bye; does not copy mother's domestic activities; mechanical imitation of others' actions out of context)
4. No or abnormal social play (e.g., does not actively participate in simple games; prefers solitary play activities; involves other children in play only as "mechanical aids")
5. Gross impairment in ability to make peer friendships (e.g., no interest in making peer friendships; despite interest in making friends, demonstrates lack of understanding of conventions of social interaction, for example, reads phone book to uninterested peer)

B. Qualitative impairment in verbal and nonverbal communication, and in imaginative activity, as manifested by the following:

(The numbered items are arranged so that those first listed are more likely to apply to younger or more handicapped—and, in the later ones, to older or less handicapped—persons with this disorder.)

1. No mode of communication, such as communicative babbling, facial expression, gesture, mime, or spoken language
2. Markedly abnormal nonverbal communication, as in the use of eye-to-eye gaze, facial expression, body posture, or gestures to initiate or modulate social interaction (e.g., does not anticipate being held, stiffens when held, does not look at the person or smile when making a social approach, does not greet parents or visitors, has a fixed stare in social situations)
3. Absence of imaginative activity, such as playacting of adult roles, fantasy characters, or animals; lack of interest in stories about imaginary events
4. Marked abnormalities in the production of speech, including volume, pitch, stress, rate, rhythm, and intonation (e.g., monotonous tone, questionlike melody, or high pitch)
5. Marked abnormalities in the form or content of speech, including stereotyped and repetitive use of speech (e.g., immediate echolalia or mechanical repetition of television commercial); use of "you" when "I" is meant (e.g., using "You want cookie" to mean "I want a cookie"); idiosyncratic use of words or phrases (e.g., "Go on green riding" to mean "I want to go on the swing"); or frequent irrelevant remarks (e.g., starts talking about train schedules during a conversation about sports)
6. Marked impairment in the ability to initiate or sustain a conversation with others, despite adequate speech (e.g., indulging in lengthy monologues on one subject regardless of interjections from others)

C. Markedly restricted repertoire of activities and interests, as manifested by the following:

1. Stereotyped body movements, e.g., hand-flicking or -twisting, spinning, head-banging, complex whole-body movements
2. Persistent preoccupation with parts of objects (e.g., sniffing or smelling objects, repetitive feeling of texture of materials, spinning wheels of toy cars) or attachment to unusual objects (e.g., insists on carrying around a piece of string)
3. Marked distress over changes in trivial aspects of environment, e.g., when a vase is moved from usual position
4. Unreasonable insistence on following routines in precise detail, e.g., insisting that exactly the same route always be followed when shopping

(continued)

Table 17-1.   (*Continued*)

5. Markedly restricted range of interests and a preoccupation with one narrow interest, e.g., interested only in lining up objects, in amassing facts about meteorology, or in pretending to be a fantasy character

D. Onset during infancy or childhood.

Specify if childhood onset (after 36 months of age).

Source.   Reprinted with permission from American Psychiatric Association 1987.

movements, 7) other pervasive disorders, and 8) unspecified pervasive disorder. The ICD-10 definition of pervasive developmental disorders emphasizes that "childhood autism" is a distinct subgroup of these disorders. The ICD-10 draft defines childhood autism as

> a type of pervasive developmental disorder that is defined by the presence of abnormal and/or impaired development that is manifest before the age of three years; and by the characteristic type of abnormal functioning in all three areas of social interaction, communication, and restricted, repetitive behavior. (p. 191)

ICD-10 also offers operational diagnostic criteria for childhood autism. It is obvious that the concept of pervasive developmental disorders in ICD-10 is a "splitters" approach. This approach believes in the taxonomic validity of each subtype and aims to facilitate research in the subclassification of these disorders. It should be pointed out here that the ICD-10 diagnostic criteria for pervasive developmental disorders are not based on any systematically collected data. Therefore, it is expected that the new criteria will not satisfy everyone and will, no doubt, also be revised when improved understanding and further knowledge are gained. Nonetheless, it is hoped that refinement of the criteria would not only assure more reliable diagnosis but also provide further support to the taxonomic validity of the various pervasive developmental disorders.

The United States is under a treaty obligation with the World Health Organization to maintain a coding system consist with the ICD. The American Psychiatric Association has already appointed several committees to develop DSM-IV and intends to publish it in 1993. It is quite certain that DSM-IV will retain the concept that autistic disorder is a subtype of pervasive developmental disorders. However, it is uncertain at the present time which approach (i.e., lumpers or splitters) DSM-IV will take to subclassify these disorders. We agree that

DSM-IV should continue the use of pervasive developmental disorders as the major diagnostic category. However, for several reasons, the subclassification of pervasive developmental disorders should best follow what is currently being proposed by ICD-10 except that the diagnostic term *autistic disorder* should be used in DSM-IV instead of *childhood autism* because this disorder does not occur only in children.

Clinical Findings

Because the information is based on research done over the past four decades, various diagnostic systems were used for collection of data. We have, therefore, used the general term *autism* to describe infantile autism, childhood onset pervasive developmental disorder, and autistic disorder.

Age at Onset

Kanner (1943) described the syndrome as beginning shortly after birth. Subsequent observations by other workers, however, have found that in perhaps one-third of the autistic children, parents reported a clinical picture indistinguishable from Kanner's original autism, which arose after a period of apparently normal development (up to 2 years of age). Whether early development in these children had been truly normal in all aspects is hard to decide. Subtle signs occurring during the first 2 years of life may have been forgotten, overlooked, or denied by the parents because of difficulty in recall, anxiety, or lack of knowledge of normal child development.

A few investigators have reported the onset of typically autistic behavior beginning in the third to fifth year of life. In Rutter and Lockyer's (1967) series of 63 autistic children, 4 had an onset between the ages of 3 and 5½ years. Lotter (1966) found similar histories among the autistic children identified in his survey: a "setback in development" occurred in 3 of 32 children between the ages of 3 and 4½ years. Little is known about these cases in terms of etiology and outcome. In the ICD-10 classification, such cases will be described as having atypical autism.

Deficits in Social Behavior

Social deficits were considered by Kanner (1943) to be central to the pathogenesis of autism. In infancy, autistic babies tend to avoid eye contact and to demonstrate little conventional interest in the human voice. They do not assume an anticipatory posture or put up their arms to be picked up in the way that children who are not autistic do. They are indifferent to affection and seldom show facial responsiveness. As a result, parents often suspect that the child is deaf. In the more intelligent autistic individuals, lack of social responsiveness may not be obvious until well into the second year of life.

In early childhood, autistic children continue to show deviation in eye contact, but they may enjoy a tickle or may passively accept physical contact, such as lap sitting. They do not develop attachment behavior, and there is a relative failure to bond. They generally do not follow their parents about the house. The majority of them do not show normal separation or stranger anxiety. Adults usually are treated as interchangeable, so that they may approach a stranger almost as readily as they do their parents. There is a lack of interest in being with or playing with other children, or they may even actively avoid other children.

In middle childhood, greater awareness of the attachment to parents and other familiar adults may develop. However, serious social difficulties continue. These children show a disinterest in playing group games, and there is an inability to form peer relationships. Some of the least handicapped may become passively involved in other children's games or physical play. However, this apparent sociability is usually superficial.

As autistic children grow older, they may become affectionate and friendly with their parents and siblings. However, they seldom initiate social contacts and show an apparent lack of positive interest in people. Some of the less severely impaired autistic individuals may have a desire for friendships. But a lack of response to other people's interests and emotions and a lack of appreciation of humor often result in the autistic youngster's saying or doing socially inappropriate things that usually prevent the development of friendships.

Problem of Communication

Impairment in nonverbal communication. Autistic infants show their needs through crying and screaming. In early childhood, they may develop the concrete gesture of pulling adults by the hand to the object that is wanted. This is often done without a socially appropriate facial expression. Nodding and shaking of the head are seldom seen either as a substitute for or as an accompaniment of speech. They generally do not participate in imitative games. These children are less likely than other normal children to copy or follow their parents' activity.

In middle and late childhood, they use gestures infrequently, even when they understand other people's gestures fairly well. A small number of autistic children do develop the stage of imitative play, but this tends to be stereotyped and repetitive actions of their own experience.

Generally speaking, autistic children are able to show their emotions of joy, fear, or anger, but they tend to show only the extreme of emotions. Facial expressions that ordinarily reinforce meaning are usually absent. Some autistic people appear wooden and expressionless much of the time.

Impairment in understanding of speech. Comprehension of speech is impaired to a varying degree. Severely retarded autistic persons may never develop any awareness of the meaning of speech. Children who are less severely impaired may follow simple instructions if given in an immediate present context or with the aid of gestures. When impairment is mild, only the comprehension of subtle or abstract meanings may be affected. Humor and idiomatic expressions can be confusing for even the brightest autistic person.

Impairment in speech development. Many autistic persons have an impaired amount or pattern of babble in their first year. Nearly half of Kanner's subjects were still mute by age 5 (Eisenberg and Kanner 1956). About half of autistic patients remain mute all their lives (Ricks and Wing 1976). When speech has developed, it usually exhibits many abnormalities. Meaningless, immediate or delayed echolalia may be the only kind of speech that is acquired in some autistic individuals. However, while the echolalic speech may be produced quite accurately, the child often has little or no comprehension of the meaning. When echolalia is extreme, distorted syntax and fragmented speech patterns result. Other autistic persons may develop appropriate use of phrases copied from others. This is often accompanied by pronoun reversal in the early stages of language development.

Often the mechanical production of speech is impaired. The speech may be like that of a robot, characterized by a monotonous, flat delivery with little lability, change of emphasis, or emotional expression. Some children may use speech primarily for self-stimulatory purposes. Such speech tends to be repetitive in nature, with words, phrases, or sounds being produced over and over without any apparent relation to the environment or ongoing activity (Lovaas et al. 1977). Problems of pronunciation are common in young autistic children, but these tend to diminish with increasing age. There may be a marked contrast between clearly enunciated echolalic speech and poorly pronounced spontaneous speech. There may be chanting or singsong speech, with odd prolongation of sounds, syllables, and words. A questionlike intonation may be used for propositional statements. Odd respiratory rhythms may produce staccato speech in some autistic individuals.

Immature and abnormal grammatical constructions are often present in the spontaneous speech of autistic persons. Words and phrases may be used idiosyncratically, or phrases may be telegraphic and distorted. Words of similar sound or related meaning may be muddled. Autistic persons may label objects by their use or else coin words of their own. Prepositions, conjunctions, and pronouns often are dropped from phrases or are used incorrectly.

When functional speech develops, it tends not to be used in the usual way for social communication. Usually autistic people rely on stereotyped phrases and repetition when they talk. Their speech almost always fails to convey imagination, abstraction, or subtle emotion. They are generally poor in talking about anything outside the immediate context. They tend to talk excessively about their special interests, and the same pieces of information tend to recur whenever the same subject is raised. The most advanced autistic persons may be able to exchange concrete pieces of information that interest them, but once the conversation departs from this level, they become lost and may withdraw from social contact. In general, the ordinary to-and-fro chatter of a reciprocal interaction is lacking. Thus

they give the impression of talking "to" someone rather than "with" someone.

Unusual Patterns of Behavior

Autistic children's unusual responses to their environment may take several forms. All of the items of behavior mentioned here are common in autistic children, but a single child seldom shows all the features at one time.

Resistance to change. Autistic children are disturbed by changes in the familiar environment, and tantrums may follow even a minor change of everyday routine. Many autistic children line up toys or objects and become very distressed if these are disturbed. The behavior is twice as common in retarded autistic children as in autistic youngsters with normal intelligence (Bartak and Rutter 1976). Almost all autistic children show a resistance to learning or practicing a new activity.

Ritualistic or compulsive behaviors. Ritualistic or compulsive behaviors usually involve rigid routines (e.g., insistence on eating particular foods) or stereotyped, repetitive motor acts, such as hand clapping or finger mannerisms (e.g., twisting, flicking movements carried out near the face). Some children develop preoccupations, such as spending a great deal of time memorizing weather information, state capitals, or birth dates of family members. In adolescence, some of these behaviors may develop into obsessional symptoms (e.g., repeatedly asking the same question, which must be answered in a specific manner) and compulsive behaviors (e.g., compulsive touching of certain objects). Ritualistic or compulsive behaviors are more often displayed by normally intelligent autistic persons than by retarded autistic persons (Bartak and Rutter 1976).

Abnormal attachments. Many autistic children develop intense attachments to odd objects (e.g., pipe cleaners, small plastic toys). The child may carry the object at all times and protest or throw tantrums if it is removed; if the object is not eventually returned to the child, a new object is frequently chosen.

Unusual responses to sensory experiences. There may be a fascination with lights, patterns, sounds, spinning objects, and tactile sensations. Objects often are manipulated without regard for their usual functions. Thus young autistic children may perseveringly line up, stack, or twirl objects. They may repetitively flush toilets or turn on and off light switches. There may be a continuing preoccupation with certain features of objects, such as their texture, taste, smell, color, or shape. There often is either an underresponsiveness or an overresponsiveness to sensory stimuli. Thus they may be suspected of being deaf, near-sighted, or blind. Autistic children may actively avoid gentle physical contact, but react with intense pleasure to rough games. Some autistic children may follow extreme food fads.

Disturbance of Motility

The typical motor milestones may be delayed, but they are often within normal range. Young autistic children usually have difficulties with motor imitation, especially when they have to learn by watching and when the movements have to be reversed in direction. Many young autistic children are markedly overactive, but they tend to become underactive in adolescence. The autistic child often displays grimacing, hand flapping or twisting, toe walking, lunging, jumping, darting or pacing, body rocking and swaying, and head rolling or banging. These movements do not appear to be involuntary. In some cases they may appear intermittently, whereas in other cases they are continuously present. They are usually interrupted by episodes of immobility and odd posturing, with head bowed and arms flexed at the elbow. Many children exhibit body-tensing movements when they are excited about or absorbed in some sensory experience, such as watching a spinning toy.

Intelligence and Cognitive Deficits

Most autistic children are mentally retarded (Rutter 1978). About 40%–60% of autistic children have an IQ below 50; only 20%–30% have an IQ of 70 or more. Because a significant number of autistic children either are without functional speech or are untestable, the validity of testing intelligence in autistic children is questionable. Several observations argue against the notion that autism masks the intellectual potential of autistic children. First, Hingtgen and Churchill (1971) showed that low IQ scores are not a function of poor motivation, be-

cause even when motivation was greatly increased through operant techniques, intellectual performance still remained well below normal. Second, both short-term (Alpern and Kimberlin 1970) and long-term (Lockyer and Rutter 1969) studies have shown that autistic children who fail to score on IQ tests do so because they are severely retarded, not because of an unwillingness to attempt the tasks. Third, a number of autistic children had major improvements in autism during the follow-up period, but there was no change in IQ (Lockyer and Rutter 1969). Fourth, follow-up studies have shown that retardation present at the time of initial diagnosis tends to persist (Freeman et al. 1985).

Although both low IQ and high IQ autistic children are similar in terms of the main symptoms associated with autism, those with a low IQ show a more severely impaired social development and are more likely to display deviant social responses, such as touching or smelling people, stereotypies, and self-injury (Bartak and Rutter 1976). A third of mentally retarded autistic youngsters develop seizure disorders; this condition is less prevalent in those of normal intelligence (Rutter 1978). The prognosis is both worse and different for low-IQ autistic persons (Rutter 1970). Because the difference in outcome according to IQ is so marked, it is essential to obtain an accurate assessment of intelligence during the initial evaluation of every autistic child.

Earlier studies (Creak et al. 1961) suggested that the retardation accompanying autism is differentiated from general retardation by islets of normal or near-normal intellectual function, revealed particularly on performance tests or in special abilities of the idiot savant kind. Kanner (1943) noted the excellent rote memories of autistic children. The most common areas of special skill tend to be musical, mechanical, and mathematical abilities. Rutter and Lockyer (1967) noted that, in contrast to a clinic control group matched for IQ, autistic children were generally superior on the subtests requiring manipulative or visual-spatial skills or immediate memory, whereas they did poorly on tasks demanding symbolic or abstract thought and sequential logic. Other studies have shown that cognition in autistic children is impaired, most particularly in capacity for imitation, comprehension of spoken words and gestures, flexibility, inventiveness, rule formation and application, and information utilization. The impairment is both more severe and more extensive than in nonautistic children of comparable IQ (for review, see Werry 1979).

On the other hand, mentally retarded autistic children tend to have a wider cognitive deficit that involves general difficulties in sequencing and feature extraction, whereas in the normally intelligent autistic children, the deficits mainly affect verbal and coding skills (Rutter 1977).

Associated Features

The affective expression of autistic persons may be flattened, excessive, or inappropriate to the situation. Their mood often is labile. Sobbing, crying, or screaming may be unexplained or inconsolable. Hysterical laughing and giggling may occur for no obvious reason. Real dangers, such as moving vehicles or heights, may not be appreciated by a young autistic child, but the same child may be terrified of harmless objects or situations, such as a stuffed animal or visiting a relative's house. Peculiar habits, such as hair pulling or biting parts of the body, are sometimes present, particularly in mentally retarded autistic children. Lack of dizziness after spinning has often been observed, and some autistic children love to spin themselves for long periods. Epilepsy has been noted in between one-fourth and one-third of autistic persons. Several reports have suggested that many autistic individuals develop first seizures in adolescence (Deykin and MacMahon 1979; Rutter 1984). Recently, Volkmar and Nelson (1990) reported that risk for developing seizures in the autistic subjects is highest during early childhood.

Differential Diagnosis

Autism should be distinguished from the following conditions, some of which are described in detail in Chapter 18, this volume.

Asperger's Syndrome

Asperger's syndrome is a syndrome described by Asperger (1944) as an abnormal personality trait that is not evident until the third year of life. The main features are a lack of social intuition, leading to naive and tactless behavior and difficulty with social relationships; a normal intelligence but with poor coordination and visual-spatial perception; and obsessive preoccupation or circumscribed interest patterns. Wing (1981) reported that the picture described by Asperger could be seen in some adults who were clearly classic autistic as children but who had made progress in language and other skills, suggesting that Asperger's syndrome be considered as a mild form of autism. ICD-10, however, considers Asperger's syndrome as a distinct disorder that can be differentiated from autism.

Rett's Syndrome

Children with Rett's syndrome develop "autistic features" during the rapid developmental regression stage (usually appears at 1–2 years of age). The features include no sustained interest in persons or objects; stereotypic responses to environmental stimuli; absent or very limited interpersonal contact; manifestation of great anxiety and apparent fear when confronted with an unfamiliar situation, or even without evident stimulation; loss of already acquired elements of language; stereotypic hand movements, such as hand-washing movements in front of the mouth or chest and rubbing motions of the hands; and repetitive blows on the teeth, grabbing of the tongue, and other movements (Hagberg et al. 1983). However, the clinical course is quite different from that of autism, with Rett's syndrome progressing from relatively normal development up to about 6 months of age to various forms of progressive neurologic impairment, a progression not seen in autism.

Disintegrative Disorders

Disintegrative disorders are a group of childhood disorders that roughly fit Heller's (1930) account of dementia infantilis: a progressive intellectual deterioration with, ultimately, the appearance of neurologic signs. In these conditions, development usually appears normal or near-normal up to the age of 3 or 4 years, at which time there is a profound regression and behavioral disintegration. There is a loss of speech and language, social skills, and interest in objects. Interpersonal relationships are impaired. There is development of stereotypies and mannerisms. Sometimes these disorders develop after some clear-cut organic brain disease. More often there are no clinical signs of neurologic damage, but the subsequent course and postmortem studies often reveal some kind of organic cortical degeneration (Rutter 1977). The patterns of symptomatology differ in crucial aspects from those of autism.

General Mental Retardation

In general mental retardation, there are often behavioral abnormalities similar to those seen in autism. Wing (1975) found that about one-fourth of the severely retarded children in one area of London demonstrated a lack of affect, resistance to change, stereotypies, and bizarre responses to sensory input, but few could be called classically autistic. Furthermore, in general mental retardation, generalized delays in development occur across many areas. Some children, especially those with Down's syndrome, are quite sociable and can communicate in gesture and mime. Moreover, there are studies in which autistic children were found to be different from matched groups of children with mental retardation. The autistic children made less use of meaning in their memory processes, were impaired in their use of concepts, and were limited in their abilities of coding and categorizing (Hermelin and O'Connor 1970; Schopler 1966).

Developmental Language Disorder, Receptive Type

Children with a developmental language disorder, receptive type, may show some autistic behavior, especially before age 5 (Wing 1969). They may develop disturbances in relating and social responses, but they do not manifest the perceptual disturbances (e.g., sensory hyperreactivity or hyporeactivity) that are characteristic of autistic children (Ornitz and Ritvo 1976). Children with this type of lauguage disorder are much more likely to be able to relate to others by nonverbal gestures and expressions. When they do acquire speech, they also demonstrate communicative intent and emotion, characteristics that are not present in verbal autistic children. Furthermore, children with a receptive language disorder have some imaginative play, which is markedly deficient in autistic children (Bartak et al. 1975). Cantwell et al. (1989) reported an interim follow-up study of a group of "higher functioning" boys with autism and a control group of boys with severe receptive developmental language disorder. They noted that in middle childhood very few of the autistic boys had good language skills at follow-up, whereas nearly half of the language-disorder group were communicating well, a striking difference in view of the initial general similarity.

Courchesne et al. (1989) studied event-related brain potential in nonretarded autistic children, in children with a receptive developmental language disorder, and in normal children. Their findings suggest that higher functioning autism may be differentiated from receptive developmental language disorder using quantitative neurophysiologic measures.

Obsessive-Compulsive Disorder

Bartak and Rutter (1976) noted that about 68% of the normally intelligent autistic children had shown rituals. About 80% of these children also had "quasi-obsessive" behaviors. Difficult adaptation to new situations was found in about 74% of these children. Although Mesibov and Shea (1980) described ritualistic and compulsive behaviors as most intense during middle childhood and as tending to decrease during adolescence and adulthood, Rumsey et al. (1985a) reported that stereotyped, repetitive movements were highly prevalent (78%) and were directly observable among the higher functioning autistic men they studied. The movement most frequently observed involved the hands or arms with individual finger movement, rotating movements or whole-body rocking, and pacing.

Some of these obsessive and/or compulsive symptoms have obvious similarities to those seen in obsessive-compulsive disorder. It is conceivable that in some higher functioning autistic persons, quasi-obsessive behaviors reflect true symptoms of a coexisting obsessive-compulsive disorder. Because of difficulties in communicating with other people, as well as in showing appropriate affect, autistic individuals do not seem to resist their compulsions, to complain about the compulsive acts, or to manifest distress. This raises the possibility that clinicians may hesitate to diagnose superimposed obsessive-compulsive disorder in persons with autism.

Tourette's Syndrome

Compulsive and ritualistic behaviors (e.g., keeping objects neatly arranged and routines unchanged, compulsive touching of people and things nearby, compulsive shouting and swearing, echoing of words, sounds, and actions) that can occur in the syndrome of Gilles de la Tourette (or the syndrome of chronic multiple tics) resemble some phenomena occurring in autism. Sometimes separating symptoms of Tourette's syndrome from the symptoms of autism can be difficult. However, the examination of the total behavior pattern and developmental history should make the diagnosis clear. The individuals with Tourette's syndrome are aware of their disorder. They are frightened and are distressed because they do not feel that they can control it. They usually do not have significantly delayed and deviant language and speech development, and their tics often have a waxing and waning pattern.

However, some studies have described the development of Tourette's syndrome in autistic individuals (Barabas and Matthews 1983; Burd et al. 1987; Realmuto and Main 1982). One of us (L.Y.T.) has also seen a few such cases. It is unclear how frequently the two disorders might occur coincidentally. It is also uncertain how this finding might be linked to the etiology of the two disorders. This remains one of many areas requiring further investigation.

Schizophrenia

One well-established finding is that autistic children almost never develop a thought disorder with delusions and hallucinations. Only a few well-diagnosed autistic children have been reported to have developed schizophrenia during follow-up periods (Petty et al. 1984). However, a study by Howells and Guirguis (1984) demonstrated that whether an autistic child develops schizophrenia in adulthood may depend on which set of diagnostic criteria is used. Rutter and Schopler (1987) also questioned what weight to attach to these reports, as the systematic studies of autistic individuals have not found this transition. They suspect that the "supposed autism-to-schizophrenia change reflects a broader concept of autism or of schizophrenia or a difference in the interpretation of the odd thinking that is quite common in older autistic individuals" (p. 176).

Most autistic individuals do manifest prodromal or residual symptoms of schizophrenia (e.g., social isolation, impairment in role functioning or grooming, inappropriate affect.) Many higher functioning autistic persons exhibit illogical thinking, incoherence, and poverty in content of speech. Their lack of nonverbal communication may be seen as exhibiting blunt affect. The inappropriate laughing or weeping of an autistic person due to inability to comprehend the meaning of events may be interpreted as labile or abnormal affect. Some higher functioning verbal autistic persons have strange beliefs (e.g., that there is no air in other states), idiosyncratic interests (e.g., spending enormous amounts of time studying dinosaurs), or sensory experiences (e.g., seeing other people's faces in the air when alone in the room) bordering on delusions or hallucinations. These symptoms, however, are qualitatively different than those shown in schizophrenic patients. These "schizophrenic symptoms" may be caused by underdevelopment of cognitive and language-speech functions in autistic individuals, whereas the schizophrenic symptoms in schizophrenic patients are a deviance of previously relatively normal cognitive and language-speech development. Autistic persons tend to answer yes to questions they do not quite understand or tend to interpret meanings of words literally. Often autistic persons may talk or laugh to themselves while looking at something an observer cannot identify, or have some funny thoughts that they do not know how to share with the observer. This tends to be interpreted as listening to voices or seeing visions. Some autistic adolescents or adults continue to have childish fantasies of being an inanimate object, an animal, or a character of a fairy tale, which may be mistaken for delusions; the tendency of others to make irrelevant remarks or to talk excessively on their favorite topics may lead to a mistaken diagnosis of thought disorder.

Nevertheless, individuals with schizophrenia can be differentiated from higher functioning autistic persons on the basis of such factors as age of onset, developmental history, clinical features, and family history. Almost all autistic persons have an onset before 5 years of age, whereas the onset of schizophrenia in childhood is most often during the preadolescent or adolescent period. Eggers (1978) reported that the early development in slightly half the schizophrenic children was unremarkable. Although there is no evidence that schizophrenic children diagnosed by DSM-III-R criteria manifest severe developmental deficits, all autistic persons, including those with a higher functioning disorder, have a history of pervasive developmental disorder. There is an increased incidence of schizophrenia in the families of children with schizophrenia, but not of autism (Kolvin et al. 1971). A study of patterns involving intellectual functioning (Wechsler Intelligence Scale for Children, revised factor scores [Wechsler 1974]) by Asarnow et al. (1987) found that schizophrenic and autistic children did not differ significantly on the verbal and perceptual organization factors, but that the schizophrenic children had significantly lower scores on the freedom-from-distraction factor (including attention, short-term memory, visual-motor coordination, speed of responding, and mental arithmetic) than the nonretarded (higher functioning) autistic children. The only subtest on which the autistic children scored significantly lower than did the schizophrenic children was the comprehension subtest.

Elective Mutism

In elective mutism, the child refuses to speak in almost all social situations, despite the ability to comprehend spoken language and to speak. The child may communicate by gestures, nodding or shaking the head, or, in some cases, by monosyllabic or short, monotone utterances. The same child may talk normally at home with family members. Autistic children retain their characteristic language abnormalities in all situations. In any case, the whole pattern of behavior is markedly different in the two conditions.

Congenital Peripheral Blindness or Partial Sightedness

Children with congenital peripheral blindness or partial sightedness may show self-stimulation and stereotyped movements like those seen in autism. Blind children, however, usually develop an interest in their environment and do not have disturbances in relating with other people.

Psychosocial Deprivation

Although psychosocial deprivation is commonly mentioned as a possible cause of autism, no data from systematic studies have yet been presented to support such a view. On the other hand, there are reports of children who had been deprived over several years, resulting in severe retardation of all aspects of development, who then made rapid strides in development when they were rescued and put in a caring and stimulating environment. They showed no evidence of autism (Wing 1976). Thus a careful history and observation of a rapid response to environmental stimulation should differentiate this condition from autism.

Epidemiology

Prevalence

Epidemiologic studies in North America, Asia, and Europe have estimated the prevalence of autism to be between 2 and 13 per 10,000 children (Lotter 1966; Ritvo et al. 1989a; Steffenburg and Gillberg 1986; Sugiyama and Abe 1989; Treffert 1970; Wing and Gould 1979). At the moment, DSM-III-R suggests the prevalence of autistic disorder to be 2 to 4 per 10,000 children, and 10 to 15 children in every 10,000 for pervasive developmental disorder NOS.

It is not clear whether prevalence rates of autism in cities differ from those in rural districts. Treffert (1970) reported that there was no statistically significant difference between the rural and urban prevalence rates. However, some studies have found higher rates in urban areas (Hoshino et al. 1982; Steffenburg and Gillberg 1986).

Sex Ratio

All studies of autism have shown a predominance of boys over girls. Ratios from three to four boys to one girl have consistently been reported (for a review, see Tsai 1986). In addition, several recent studies have found that autistic girls tend to suffer a greater degree of morbidity; that is, a greater proportion of autistic females are more often severely impaired than are autistic males (Tsai 1986). The findings indicate that there are significant sex differences in the occurrence and the severity of autism.

Socioeconomic Class

Kanner (1943) originally observed that families of his patients were predominantly of an upper socioeconomic status. However, later population studies (Schopler et al. 1979; Tsai et al. 1982; Wing 1980) did not support Kanner's idea. As pointed out by Tsai et al. (1982), most of the studies showing high socioeconomic class bias were conducted before 1970, and those showing no bias were carried out after that date. When the possible effects of parental educational and occupational achievements and patterns of referral were controlled, autistic persons were found in all socioeconomic classes.

Etiology

Genetic Factors

Some genetic syndromes are associated with some cases of autism. These include phenylketonuria (Knoblock and Pasamanick 1975) and fragile X syndrome. Some investigators have found a high prevalence of fragile X syndrome in persons with autism (Blomquist et al. 1985), whereas others have failed to replicate this finding (Payton et al. 1989).

Several studies have shown that between 2% to 6% of the siblings of autistic children suffer from the same condition (Ritvo et al. 1989b; Rutter 1967; Tsai et al. 1981). When this estimated sibling incidence is compared with the general population risk, the rate of autism in siblings is 50 times higher. Folstein and Rutter (1977) studied 21 same-sex autistic twin pairs and found that 4 of the 11 (36%) monozygotic twin pairs were concordant for autism, as compared with none of 10 dizygotic twins. Discordance was usually associated with definite or suggestive evidence of organic brain dysfunction in the affected twin. The authors suggested that autism may develop on the basis of a combination of genetic predisposition and biological impairment. Ritvo et al. (1985) reported a study involving 281 families enrolled in the UCLA Registry for Genetic Studies in Autism. They included (by parental report) 22 sets of monozygotic twins, all concordant for autism; 18 sets of dizygotic twins, 2 sets of whom were concordant for autism; and 46 sets of nontwin siblings concordant for autism. Based on these preliminary findings, the authors suggested that a subgroup of autistic persons may develop this syndrome by way of a recessive gene transmission. Their suggestion, however, is based on a highly selected group of subjects.

Twenty-one pairs (11 monozygotic and 10 dizygotic) of twins and one set of identical triplets were found in the Nordic countries (Denmark, Finland, Iceland, Norway, and Sweden) (Steffenburg et al. 1989). The concordance for autism by pair was 91% in the monozygotic and 0% in the dizygotic pairs. In most of the pairs discordant for autism, the autistic twin had more perinatal stress. The authors concluded that their results lend support for the notion that autism has a hereditary component and that perinatal complication is a contributory factor in some cases.

Based on the findings from their twin study, Folstein and Rutter (1977) suggested that autism is one manifestation of an underlying genetic liability to cognitive dysfunction; that is, a cognitive disorder in its mildest form may present as learning disabilities and in its most severe form as autism. To date, family studies of autism seem to provide some support to such a hypothesis. The sibling data show that between 6% and 24% of the siblings of autistic probands have cognitive disorders (including autism, mental retardation, learning disability) and/or speech-language disorders (August et al. 1981; Freeman et al. 1986; Piven et al. 1990a).

The data available to date show that there is reasonable evidence for speculating that in a subgroup of autistic individuals, genetic factors may play a major contributory role.

Congenital Factors

Results of numerous studies show that many autistic children suffer from organic brain disorders (for a review, see Fish and Ritvo 1979). A wide variety of neurologic disorders have been reported: cerebral palsy, congenital rubella, toxoplasmosis, tuberous sclerosis, cytomegalovirus infection, lead encephalopathy, meningitis, encephalitis, severe brain hemorrhage, many types of epilepsy, and others. Many of these neurologic or congenital disorders derive from unfavorable prenatal, perinatal, and neonatal complications. It has been suggested that pre- or perinatal insults to the brain are the biological causation of autism for individuals whose autistic symptoms are manifested from birth, and postnatal cerebral infections or injuries have been suggested as the etiology for those whose autism is manifested after a period of apparent normal development. Several investigators report that pre-, peri-, and neonatal complications appear with increased frequency in the histories of autistic patients. These include increased maternal age, first- and fourth- or later born children, bleeding after the first trimester, use of medication, and meconium in amniotic fluid (for review, see Tsai 1987).

It seems in some instances that unfavorable pre-, peri-, and neonatal factors may be associated with autism. However, because of the lack of uniformity in applying diagnostic criteria for autism as well as to the selection of obstetric complications, these findings should be received with caution. Also, the data reviewed here do not indicate a unifying pathologic process in autism.

Immunological Studies

Chess (1977) reported an increased frequency of autism in individuals with congenital rubella. Deykin and MacMahon (1979) found that autism was associated with prenatal rubella or influenza infection in about 5% of cases. The presence of other infectious agents during pregnancy also was found to be low for the autistic children and their normal siblings in other studies (Mason-Brothers et al. 1987).

Young et al. (1977) studied the cerebrospinal fluid (CSF) immunoglobulin levels in 15 autistic children and found no abnormalities of glucose, protein cells, or folate, concluding that the hypothesis of slow virus playing a role in autism could not be supported.

Several studies have suggested the possibility of an immune defect in autistic disorder. In an attempt to diagnose prenatal rubella retrospectively, Stubbs (1976) gave rubella vaccine challenge to 15 autistic children and 8 control subjects matched for age. The rubella vaccine challenge did not differentiate autistic children from the control subjects. However, 5 of the 13 autistic children had undetectable hemagglutination-inhibition antibody titers despite previous vaccine, whereas all control subjects had detectable titers. Stubbs speculated that these autistic children might have an altered immune response or an immune defect.

Warren et al. (1986) reported finding several immune-system abnormalities in 31 autistic patients. In a further study of the activity of the natural killer cell (a large granular lymphocyte and a likely part of basic defense mechanism against virus-infected cells and malignancy), the authors found that about 40% of their autistic subjects had significantly reduced natural killer cell activity (Warren et al. 1987).

Based on the observation that reactivity to human myelin basic protein had been implicated in a number of central nervous system disorders such as multiple sclerosis, the Guillain-Barré syndrome, and acute disseminated encephalomyelitis, Weizman et al. (1982) investigated the cell-mediated immune response to human myelin basic protein using the macrophage migration inhibition factor test in 17 autistic patients and 11 control subjects with other mental disorders. Of the 17 autistic subjects, 13 (76%) exhibited inhibition of macrophage migration, whereas none of the control subjects was found to have such a response. The results were thus interpreted to suggest that a cell-mediated autoimmune response to brain antigen existed in some autistic individuals.

Westall and Root-Bernstein (1983), however, called for attention to be paid to the serotonin-binding sites in future studies of autism. This suggestion seemed to gain some support from Todd and Ciaranello (1985), who reported that about one-third of the autistic children in their study had an unusual antibody circulating in their blood and spinal fluid. This antibody appeared to attack the receptor for serotonin. In a further study, Todd et al. (1988, p. 647) concluded that "if antibody-mediated autoantigen recognition is important in, or related to, established infantile autism, only a few antigens are involved."

All these findings seem to suggest that depressed immune function, autoimmune mechanism, or faulty immune regulation may be associated with the etiology of autism. However, the exact cause-effect relationship remains unsettled. Clearly, more extensive studies are needed.

Neurologic Factors

Neurologic abnormalities have been reported in 30%–75% of several series of autistic patients (DeMyer et al. 1973; Gittelman and Birch 1967; Tsai et al. 1981). These include abnormalities of hypotonia or hypertonia, disturbance of body schema, clumsiness, choreiform movements, pathologic reflexes, myoclonic jerking, drooling, abnormal posture and gait, dystonic posturing of hands and fingers, tremor, ankle clonus, emotional facial paralysis, and strabismus. These are all signs of dysfunction in the basal ganglia, particularly the neostriatum, and closely related structures of the mesial aspects of the frontal lobe or limbic system.

Based on the analogy to signs and conditions seen in adults with certain forms of brain damage, Damasio and Maurer (1978) proposed that autism results from dysfunction in a system of bilateral central nervous system structures that include the ring of mesolimbic cortex located in the mesial frontal and temporal lobes, the neostriatum, and the anterior and medial nuclear groups of the thalamus. They suggested that such dysfunction might involve macroscopic or microscopic cerebral changes consequent to a variety of causes, such as perinatal viral infection, insult to the periventricular watershed area, or genetically determined neurochemical abnormalities. This hypothesis, although plausible, needs to be verified.

Neuroanatomical Factors

Neuropathologic studies. Very few neuropathologic studies have been done in autistic people. Postmortem brain studies of seven cases revealed negative findings (Darby 1976; Williams et al. 1980), but a few positive findings also have been reported (Ritvo et al. 1986). The findings include major cellular and structural changes in the amygdala, cerebellum, and hippocampus. Because these studies examined only limited brain structures of few subjects, the meaning of these findings is not clear. Nevertheless, these findings provide some direction (i.e., posterior cerebral fossa) for in vivo neuroanatomical imaging studies of autism.

Computed tomography (CT) scan studies. CT studies have identified gross abnormalities (e.g., porencephalic cyst) in a minority of autistic patients (Damasio et al. 1980; Gillberg and Svendsen 1983). However, CT studies remain contradictory and inconsistent. Some studies showing abnormalities such as reversed hemispheric asymmetry (Hier et al. 1979) and ventricular enlargement (Rosenbloom et al. 1984) have been challenged by others that fail to observe such findings (Creasey et al. 1986; Prior et al. 1984; Rumsey et al. 1988).

Magnetic resonance imaging (MRI) studies. MRI is rapidly replacing CT as the method of choice of obtaining detailed anatomical information about the brain. Because many autistic subjects require sedation to remain still for scanning, only a few head MRI studies have been carried out. Minshew et al. (1986) found that the cerebellum and fourth ventricle were normal in all 10 autistic patients with IQs of 70 or greater. However, three of the six patients with IQs of 70–85 had other abnormalities.

Gaffney et al. (1987a, 1987b) studied the head MRI of 14 autistic patients aged 4–22 years with IQs of 60 or greater. Six of the 14 patients had brain lesions seen on the MRI scans, but there was no single, circumscribed lesion common to all the autistic patients. Midsagittal MRI scans showed the fourth ventricle to be significantly larger and the entire brain stem to be significantly smaller in the autistic group, compared with the control group. In the coronal scans, the cerebella of the autistic patients were proportionally smaller and the fourth ventricles proportionally larger. Piven et al. (1990b) found cerebral cortical malformations in 7 of 13 high functioning autistic males. Courchesne et al. (1988) reported cerebellar hypoplasia in a group of 18 autistic patients, compared with the normal control subjects. However, Garber et al. (1989) found that the measurements of the midsagittal area and the volume of the fourth ventricle did not differ between 15 autistic persons and 15 normal control subjects. The finding of abnormalities of the cerebellum is consistent with microscopic postmortem findings described above. Although the link between the cerebellar abnormalities and autism has yet to be determined, MRI technology has provided an exciting new avenue for future in vivo studies of the brain.

Positron-emission tomography studies. Rumsey et al. (1985b) reported substantially elevated utilization of glucose throughout many parts of the brain of 10 autistic men, as compared with control subjects. More recently, Heh et al. (1989) reported no significant differences in mean cerebella glucose metabolism between seven adult autistic patients and eight age-matched control subjects, although all mean glucose rates of the autistic patients were either equal to or greater than those of the control subjects. Although the meaning of these findings remains to be determined, it appears that positron emission tomography should become increasingly important for researchers studying autism.

Neurophysiologic Factors

There are two rather disparate neurophysiologic hypotheses of autism. The first, which considers a primary cortical dysfunction in autism, emphasizes the autistic symptoms of language and communication and assumes an underlying specific cognitive disorder that is presumably of cortical origin. More specifically, this hypothesis considers that autism results from a disorder of hemispheric lateralization; that is, that the neural substrates in the left hemisphere necessary for sequential forms of information processing fail to develop (Prior 1979).

A second hypothesis proposes a primary brainstem dysfunction in autism. This hypothesis has been developed through observation of the impaired ability of autistic children in modulating their own responses to sensory input and consequently their own motor output (Ornirtz 1974, 1983). This hypothesis suggests a rostrally directed sequence of pathophysiologic influences originating in the brain stem and diencephalic structures, particularly the reticular formation of pontine and midbrain, substantia nigra, and the nonspecific nuclei of the thalamus (Ornitz 1985).

The cortical dysfunction hypothesis of autism has received some support from the fact that a significant proportion of autistic persons have electroencephalographic abnormalities (Ritvo et al. 1970; Tsai and Tsai 1984; Waldo et al. 1978). In general, these abnormalities tend to involve bilateral brain hemispheres and are characterized by focal or diffused spike, slow wave, or slow dysrhythmic patterns. The type of abnormality does not appear to be specific.

The sleep electroencephalographic studies in autistic children (Tanguay et al. 1976) have found that the eye movements of autistic children were more like those of normal infants than like those of age-matched control subjects. Computerized quantitative electroencephalographic studies indicate an abnormal pattern of cerebral lateralization in autistic individuals (Cantor et al. 1986). Maturational deviation has also been indicated in several auditory evoked-response studies of autistic children (Fein et al. 1981; Lelord et al. 1973; Tanguay et al. 1982). These findings may indicate a defective integration between the visual and auditory pathways in autistic children.

Several studies suggest that autistic people may have a diminished or altered capacity for selectively channeling information for further internal attention and processing, as well as differential hemispheric involvement in the attentional deficits (Courchesne et al. 1987; Dawson et al. 1988).

The hypothesis of brain-stem dysfunction in autism is supported to a limited extent by autonomic responses studies (Hutt et al. 1975), vestibular nystagmus studies (for review, see Ornitz 1985), and auditory brain-stem evoked-potential studies (Novick et al. 1980; Rumsey et al. 1984; Tanguay et al. 1982).

Biochemical Factors

The results obtained from neuropathologic and brain imaging studies strongly suggest that the cerebral defect in autism is microscopic or functional, without major gross neuroanatomical pathology. Thus it is necessary to examine the neurochemical correlates in autism.

Serotonin. Serotonergic activity in the brain has been linked to body temperature, pain, sensory perception, sleep, sexual behavior, motor function, neuroendocrine regulation, appetite, learning, memory, and immune response (for a review, see Young et al. 1982). Many studies have consistently reported that about one-third of autistic individuals have hyperserotonemia (for a review, see Anderson et al. 1987). There are three possible explanations for the hyperserotonemia: 1) enhanced platelet uptake, storage, or platelet volume, 2) increased synthesis, and 3) decreased catabolism.

Geller et al. (1988) reported no significant difference in platelet volumes between autistic patients and control subjects. Nor did the platelet volumes and blood serotonin concentration correlate.

Although previous studies found that the platelets' handling of serotonin (5-hydroxytryptamine [5-HT]) appeared to be normal in autism (Anderson et al. 1985; Boullin et al. 1982), other work has indicated that the role of the platelets may need to be reexamined (Katsui et al. 1986; Rotman et al. 1980). Furthermore, the autistic probands and their first-degree relatives have strong familial resemblance. There is positive correlation of both platelet-rich plasma 5-HT and platelet-poor (free) plasma 5-HT between the autistic probands and their first-degree relatives (Cook et al. 1988; Kuperman et al. 1985; Wright et al. 1989).

The studies of 5-HT synthesis in autism have been conflicting. Several studies have not found any difference between autistic and normal subjects (see Minderaa et al. 1987).

The occurrence of hyperserotonemia in autistic persons does not appear to be the result of decreased catabolism of serotonin. No consistent correlations have been found yet between blood serotonin level and any autistic behaviors or symptoms. Moreover, hyperserotonemia has also been found in some children who are severely retarded. Clearly, the mechanism and importance of hyperserotonemia in autism remains unclear.

Dopamine. The brain dopaminergic system is considered to affect several functions and behaviors, including cognition, motor function, eating and drinking behaviors, sexual behavior, neuroendocrine regulation, and selective attention. Campbell (1977) reported that neuroleptics, which are dopamine receptor–blocking agents, modulate several symptoms involving the motor system (e.g., hyperactivity, stereotypies, aggression, and self-injury) and made autistic children more compliant and receptive to special education procedures. On the other hand, dopamine agonists, such as stimulants, cause a worsening of preexisting stereotypies, aggression, and hyperactivity in autistic children (Young et al. 1982).

Studies of dopamine in autism have focused on the measurement of homovanillic acid (HVA), the main metabolite of dopamine. Cohen et al. (1974) found that the autistic children did not differ from other diagnostic groups in CSF level of HVA. However, the CSF level of HVA was found to be higher in the more severely impaired children, especially those with greater locomotor activity and more severe stereotypies. Leckman et al. (1980) also failed to find a difference in CSF HVA between "child psychosis (largely autism)" and "perceptual cognitive disorder" diagnostic groups. Gillberg and Svennerholm (1987) found elevated CSF HVA in autistic subjects. Two studies found no difference for plasma HVA between the autistic children and control subjects (Launay et al.1987; Minderaa et al. 1989). However, HVA concentrations have not been shown to correlate with any autistic behaviors or symptoms.

Epinephrine and norepinephrine. Epinephrine and norepinephrine are often discussed concurrently because of their similar effects on behavior. They are associated with cardiovascular function, respiratory function, appetite, activity level, arousal, attention, anxiety, response to stress, movement, sleep, memory, and learning (Young et al. 1982).

Plasma norepinephrine has been reported to be elevated in autistic subjects (Lake et al. 1977), but in platelets both epinephrine and norepinephrine were significantly lower in the autistic group as compared with the control group (Launay et al. 1987).

No difference in CSF MHPG (3-methoxy-4-hydroxyphenylglycol) between autistic persons and control subjects has been found (Young et al. 1982).

As it is believed that the catecholamine and indoleamine systems may be in dynamic balance and that disturbances in one or both systems may be involved in adult schizophrenia, it is well worth pursuing the studies of catecholamine in autism.

Dopamine beta-hydroxylase. Conflicting results have been reported on the study of dopamine beta-hydroxylase, the enzyme that controls the coversion of dopamine to norepinephrine. Goldstein et al. (1976) and Lake et al. (1977) found a decreased dopamine beta-hydroxylase activity in autistic patients as compared with control subjects, whereas Young et al. (1980) found no difference. The real meaning of blood dopamine beta-hydroxylase activity is unclear, since normal human beings also exhibit a wide range of this activity without evident effect.

Catechol-O-methyltransferase (COMT) and monoamine oxidase. Two metabolic enzymes, COMT and monoamine oxidase, may change norepinephrine activity. Giller et al. (1980) found no difference in COMT activity in cultured fibroblasts and in red blood cells between autistic children and control subjects. Monoamine oxidase activity also appeared to be normal in autistic patients (Young et al. 1982).

Peptides. Trygstad et al. (1980) described a number of different urinary peptides' profile patterns, each said to be characteristic of a different behavioral abnormality. The characteristic profile for autism was initially shown in 20 patients, with a variation of +30% for each peak. However, in an attempt to replicate such a finding from 69 urine samples obtained from three groups of young male adults (autistic, mentally handicapped, and normal), no consistent patterns of urinary chromatographic profile were identified (Couteur et al. 1988).

Nevertheless, the findings are intriguing, and further study may develop patterns with high specificity that may be used as diagnostic markers. Any isolation and identification of any factors present in the chromatographic fractions may also contribute to the understanding of the pathogenesis of autism.

Brain opioids. An endorphin hypothesis was proposed based on the analogy between opiate addiction and autism (Kalat 1978) and the similarity between opiate-induced psychosocial distortion in animals and clinical manifestations of autism (Panksepp 1979). Findings so far are quite preliminary, and it appears that the actual identity of the brain opioids needs to be ascertained so that the cause-effect mechanism can be established.

Other Biomedical Factors

A number of other abnormal biomedical measures in autistic persons have been reported. Sankar (1971) reported significantly lower blood adenosine triphosphatase activity in assays of red blood cells from autistic children. Katz and Liebman (1970) found an elevated CSF creatine phosphokinase activity in some autistic children, as well as in children with meningitis, a finding suggesting that autistic children with an increased CSF creatine phosphokinase activity may represent a subgroup of children whose autism is due to brain insult from infection. On the whole, the significance of these findings is far from clear, but these studies merit further exploration.

Psychogenic Factors

Kanner's (1943) original description of autism, as well as a number of subsequent reports by other workers, had suggested that parents of autistic children were highly intelligent, were preoccupied with abstractions, had limited interest in people, and were emotionally cold. Some studies reported findings of disturbances in family dynamics (Reiser 1963a, 1963b), unconscious parental hostility and rejection (Bettelheim 1967), parental perplexity, and lack of parent-child communicative clarity (Goldfarb et al. 1972). These investigators suggested that autism might be a response to these parental personality characteristics, to deviant parent-child interactions, or to severe early stress of various kinds. However, findings that support these psychogenic hypotheses have come from samples that did not make any distinction between autism and schizophrenia in childhood, from projective tests, and from selected family observations. Similar techniques and other well-controlled studies have produced largely negative findings (Ornitz and Ritvo 1976). There are good grounds for concluding that no psychological or social factors can cause autistic disorder.

Summary of Etiology

So far, no specific cause or causes have been identified. Neurobiological investigations in autism have found various abnormalities. However, no single measure of the abnormalities has been consistently found, and the etiologic implications of the findings are far from clear. This may be due to the possibility that autistic disorder is a behavioral syndrome that may include several different but distinct conditions. If this is the case, it is anticipated that future studies will determine a range of biological etiologies for the subgroups making up the autistic syndrome.

Treatment

Emphasis is now placed on treatments to promote the autistic child's more normal social and linguistic developments and on minimizing the child's maladaptive behaviors (e.g., hyperactivity, stereotypies, self-injury, aggressiveness), which interfere with or are incompatible with the child's functioning and learning. There has been an increasing focus on identifying and treating preschool autistic children through special education programs in highly structured environments and on working closely with the family members of autistic children to help them cope better with the problems faced at home. Educational treatment should be intensive and sustained. Educational remedies should emphasize acquisition of self-care, social, and job skills.

Extensive research in behavior therapy since the 1960s has shown that many autistic children can be taught special skills in the areas of social adaptation and cognitive and motor skills. Their maladaptive behavior can also be ameliorated significantly. Lovaas et al. (1976) reviewed the principles involved in behavior therapy with autistic children. A few points are emphasized here. First, behavior therapy programs should be designed for individual children because autistic children vary greatly in their handicaps and family circumstances. Some treatment approaches that work in certain cases may not work in others. Second, autistic children are handicapped in generalizing from one situation to another, so that the skills they have learned in a hospital or school tend not to transfer to the home or other settings. It is crucial in treatment to plan the approach specifically to ensure that the changes of the child's clinical state are being carefully monitored, that the problems in each setting are dealt with, and that steps are taken to encourage generalization of behavior changes. Third, because one of the treatment goals is to promote the child's social development, long-term residential treatment is a definite drawback. A home-based approach, which trains parents and local special education teachers to carry out behavior therapies, has been instrumental in achieving maximum results (Hemsley et al. 1978).

Pharmacotherapy does not alter the natural history or course of autism. It can be helpful, however, in controlling specific symptoms, such as hyperactivity, withdrawal, stereotypies, self-injury, aggressiveness, and sleep disorders. This subject has been reviewed by Campbell et al. (1984). Low-potency neuroleptics, such as chlorpromazine, have little if any therapeutic effect because they yield excessive sedation, even at low doses. On the other hand, haloperidol, a high-potency neuroleptic, has demonstrated both short-term and long-term efficacy in 40 young autistic children (ages 2.6–7.2 years) in doses ranging from 0.5 to 4.0 mg/day. At these dosages, haloperidol was significantly superior to placebo in reducing symptoms of withdrawal and stereotypies in these children who were 4.5–7.2 years of age. The combination of haloperidol and contingent reinforcement was found to be most effective in facilitating the acquisition of imitative speech. Long-term studies of haloperidol by Campbell et al. (1983a) have shown that the effect remains from 6 months to 2.5 years. At optimal doses, no untoward effects were noted. Above optimal doses or during dose regulation, excessive sedation was most common, followed by acute dystonic reaction. All drug-related movements ceased anywhere from 16 days to 9 months later. Campbell et al. (1983b) recommended that the dosage increments be gradual and made on a regular basis. The emergence of untoward effects may necessitate dosage reduction or administration of diphenhydramine (Benadryl). Furthermore, the haloperidol should be discontinued about every 6 months to determine whether the child needs further drug treatment.

Fenfluramine (an antiserotonergic anorectic) was initially reported as showing positive effects, but subsequent data from a multicenter study failed to show any positive effect (Campbell et al. 1988).

Recently, naltrexone, an opiate antagonist, has been given to a small group of autistic children and has shown positive effects on social relatedness and self-injury (Campbell et al. 1989). These findings, however, require replication in a larger sample of subjects using a double-blind, placebo-controlled research design.

So far no single treatment modality can alter the course of autism. To achieve significant goals of treatment of autistic children, comprehensive treatment programs, which include behavior modification and special education in a highly structured environment, are required. Pharmacotherapy may frequently be useful to control behaviors that are not responsive to behavior modification and special education techniques.

Clinical Course and Prognosis

The general picture of autism is of a disorder with a chronic course. Although social, conceptual, linguistic, and obsessive difficulties frequently persist, they do so in forms that are rather different from those shown in early years. A small number of autistic children (7 of 64) in Rutter and Lockyer's (1967) study showed a progressive deterioration in adolescence, characterized by a general intellectual decline. Between 7% and 28% of autistic children who had shown no clinical evidence of neurologic disorder in early childhood developed seizures for the first time in adolescence or early adult life. The seizures were usually major in type but tended to occur infrequently (Rutter 1977).

During adolescence, hyperactivity is often replaced by marked underactivity and lack of initiative and drive. Some autistic persons may have increased anxiety and tension. There may be inappropriate sexual curiosity that may lead to socially embarrassing behavior, such as masturbation in public or self-exposure.

In an extensive review of follow-up studies of psychotic children, Lotter (1978) found that between 5% and 17% of the autistic children had a good outcome as assessed from a judgment of overall social adjustment; that is, they had a normal or near-normal social life and demonstrated satisfactory functioning at school or work. But even those with a good adjustment generally continued to have difficulties in relationships and some oddities of behavior. Between one-sixth and one-fourth of the autistic persons had an intermediate outcome; that is, they had some degree of independence and only minor problems in behavior, but they still needed supervision and could not hold a job. Between 61% and 74% had a generally poor outcome, remaining severely handicapped and unable to lead any kind of independent life. Between 39% and 74% of the autistic persons were placed in institutions. These studies, however, followed the autistic persons up to the age of about 30 years only. Obviously, placement depends on age and on local patterns of available services. The effect of age in institutional placement is evident in the study of Rutter and Lockyer (1967); at the first follow-up, 44% were so placed; the proportion had risen to 54% 6 years later. Nonetheless, the program for the Treatment and Education of Autistic and Related Communication Handicapped Children (Division TEACHC) of the University of North Carolina has demonstrated that when community service is available and provides adequate educational and vocational training, only a minority (i.e., 8%) of the autistic individuals are placed in institutions (Schopler et al. 1982).

Three factors were consistently found to be related to outcome: IQ, the presence or absence of speech, and the severity of the disorder. IQ alone predicts best only those with poor outcome. A high nonverbal score with no subsequent language is of no predictive value, whereas if language subsequently does develop, the nonverbal score is a useful guide to later general IQ scores (Rutter 1970). One additional factor, work-school status, was found to be the best predictor of academic or work performance at follow-up (DeMyer et al. 1973). Four other variables have been reported to be significantly associated with outcome (although the correlations are less strong than in the previous three variables): amount of time spent in school, rating of social maturity, rating of social behavior, and developmental milestones.

Conflicting findings have been reported on a number of variables in relation to outcome: sex, brain dysfunction or damage, and the category "untestable" child. Factors that were unrelated to outcome included birth weight, perinatal complications, age of onset, history of a period of normal development before onset, late development of seizures, socioeconomic class, broken home, family mental illness, and type of treatment.

Research Issues

The inconsistent findings of previous neurobiological investigations may arise from a number of factors. These include the use of different diagnostic criteria for patient selection, failure to control developmental factors (many studies included both children and adults), lack of suitable control groups (most studies used normal rather than mentally retarded control subjects and hence failed to control for concomitant mental retardation that existed in a majority of the autistic subjects), failure to control for concomitant medical disorders (particularly central nervous system pathologies), and use of medications that may significantly affect a subject's neurochemical or neurophysiologic responses. Nevertheless, the lack of consistent and specific findings can also be viewed as supportive evidence of many different subgroups within the autistic syndrome. Future neurobiological research in the field of autism should focus on the question of specificity and selectivity within each of the subgroups.

References

Alpern GD, Kimberlin CC: Short intelligence test ranging from infancy levels through childhood levels for use with the retarded. American Journal of Mental Deficiency 75:65–71, 1970

American Psychiatric Association: Diagnostic and Statistical Manual of Mental Disorders, 3rd Edition. Washington, DC, American Psychiatric Association, 1980

American Psychiatric Association: Diagnostic and Statistical Manual of Mental Disorders, 3rd Edition, Revised. Washington, DC, American Psychiatric Association, 1987

Anderson GM, Schlicht KR, Cohen DJ: Two-dimensional high-performance liquid chromatographic determination of 5-hydroxyindoleacetic acid and homovanillic acid in urine. Anal Biochem 144:27–31, 1985

Anderson GM, Freedman DX, Cohen DJ, et al: Whole blood serotonin in autistic and normal subjects. J Child Psychol Psychiatry 28:885–900, 1987

Asarnow RF, Tanguay PE, Bott L, et al: Patterns of intellectual functioning in non-retarded autistic and schizophrenic children. J Child Psychol Psychiatry 28:273–280, 1987

Asperger H: Die autistischen psychopathen im kindesalter. Archiv für Psychiatrie und Nervenkrankheiten 117:76–136, 1944

August GJ, Stewart MA, Tsai L: The incidence of cognitive disabilities in the siblings of autistic children. Br J Psychiatry 138:416–422, 1981

Barabas G, Matthews WS: Coincident infantile autism and Tourette syndrome: a case report. Journal of Developmental Pediatrics 4:280–281, 1983

Bartak L, Rutter M: Differences between mentally retarded and normally intelligent autistic children. Journal of Autism and Childhood Schizophrenia 6:109–120, 1976

Bartak L, Rutter M, Cox A: A comparative study of infantile autism and specific developmental receptive language disorder, I: the children. Br J Psychiatry 126:127–145, 1975

Bettelheim B: The Empty Fortress: Infantile Autism and the Birth of the Self. New York, Free Press, 1967

Bleuler E: Dementia Praecox Oder Gruppe der Schizophrenien (1911). Translated by Zinkin J. New York, International Universities Press, 1950

Bloomquist HK, Bohman M, Edvinsson SO, et al: Frequency of fragile X syndrome in infantile autism. Clin Genet 27:113–117, 1985

Boullin D, Freeman BJ, Geller E, et al: Toward the resolution of conflicting findings. J Autism Dev Disord 12:97–98, 1982

Burd L, Fisher WW, Kerbeshian J, et al: Is development of Tourette Disorder a marker for improvement in patients with autism and other pervasive developmental disorders? J Am Acad Child Adolesc Psychiatry 26:162–165, 1987

Campbell M: Treatment of childhood and adolescent schizophrenia, in Psychopharmacology in Childhood and Adolescence. Edited by Wiener JM. New York, Basic Books, 1977, pp 101–118

Campbell M, Perry R, Bennett WG, et al: Long-term therapeutic efficacy and drug-related abnormal movements: a prospective study of haloperidol in autistic children. Psychopharmacol Bull 19:80–83, 1983a

Campbell M, Grega DM, Green WH, et al: Neuroleptic-induced dyskinesia in children. Clin Neuropharmacol 6:207–222, 1983b

Campbell M, Anderson LT, Deutsch SI, et al: Psychopharmacological treatment of children with the syndrome of autism. Pediatr Ann 13:309–316, 1984

Campbell M, Adams P, Small AM, et al: Efficacy and safety of fenfluramine in autistic children. J Am Acad Child Adolesc Psychiatry 4:434–439, 1988

Campbell M, Overall JE, Small AM, et al: Naltrexone in autistic children: an open dose range tolerance trial. J Am Acad Child Adolesc Psychiatry 28:200–206, 1989

Cantor DS, Thatcher RW, Hrybyk M, et al: Computerized EEG analyses of autistic children. J Autism Dev Disord 16:169–187, 1986

Cantwell DP, Baker L, Rutter M, et al: Infantile autism and developmental dysphasia: a comparative follow-up into middle childhood. J Autism Dev Disord 19:19–31, 1989

Chess S: Follow-up report on autism in congenital rubella. J Autism Dev Disord 7:69–81, 1977

Cohen DJ, Shaywitz BA, Johnson WK, et al: Biogenic amines in autistic and atypical children: cerebrospinal fluid measure of homovanillic acid and 5-hydroxyindole acetic acid. Arch Gen Psychiatry 31:845–853, 1974

Cook EH, Leventhal BL, Freedman DX: Free serotonin in plasma: autistic children and their first-degree relatives. Biol Psychiatry 24:488–491, 1988

Courchesne E: A neurophysiological view of autism, in Neurobiological Issues in Autism. Edited by Schopler E, Mesibov GB. New York, Plenum, 1987, pp 285–324

Courchesne E, Yeung-Courchesne BA, Press GA, et al: Hypoplasia of cerebellar vermal lobules VI and VII in autism. N Engl J Med 318:1349–1354, 1988

Courchesne E, Lincoln AJ, Yeung-Courchesne R, et al: Pathophysiologic findings in nonretarded autism and receptive developmental language disorder. J Autism Dev Disord 19:1–17, 1989

Couteur AL, Trygstad O, Evered C, et al: Infantile autism and urinary excretion of peptides and protein-associated peptide complexes. J Autism Dev Disord 18:181–190, 1988

Creak M, Cameron K, Cowie V, et al: Schizophrenic syndrome in childhood. Br Med J 2:889–890, 1961

Creasey H, Rumsey J, Schwartz M, et al: Brain morphometry in autistic men as measured by volumetric computed tomography. Arch Neurol 43:669–672, 1986

Damasio AR, Maurer RG: A neurological model for childhood autism. Arch Neurol 35:777–786, 1978

Damasio H, Maurer RG, Damasio AR, et al: Computerized tomographic scan findings in patients with autistic behavior. Arch Neurol 37:504–510, 1980

Darby JC: Neuropathologic aspects of psychosis in children. Journal of Autism and Childhood Schizophrenia 6:339–352, 1976

Dawson G, Finley C, Phillips S, et al: Reduced P3 amplitude of the event-related brain potential: relationship to language ability in autism. J Autism Dev Disord 18:493–504, 1988

DeMyer M, Barton S, DeMyer W, et al: Prognosis in autism: a follow-up study. Journal of Autism and Childhood Schizophrenia 3:199–246, 1973

Despert JL: Some considerations relating to the genesis of autistic behavior in children. Am J Orthopsychiatry 21:335–350, 1951

Deykin E, MacMahon B: The incidence of seizures among children with autistic symptoms. Am J Psychiatry 126:1310–1312, 1979

Eggers C: Course and prognosis of childhood schizophrenia. Journal of Autism and Childhood Schizophrenia 8:21–36, 1978

Eisenberg L, Kanner L: Early infantile autism 1943–55. Am J Orthopsychiatry 26:556–566, 1956

Factor DC, Freeman NL, Kardash A: A comparison of DSM-III and DSM-III-R criteria for autism. J Autism Dev Disord 19:637–640, 1989

Fein D, Skoff B, Mirsky AF: Clinical correlates of brainstem dysfunction in autistic children. J Autism Dev Disord 11:303–315, 1981

Fish B, Ritvo ER: Psychoses of childhood, in Basic Handbook of Child Psychiatry. Edited by Noshpitz JD. New York, Basic Books, 1979, pp 249–304

Folstein S, Rutter M: Infantile autism: a genetic study of 21 twin pairs. J Child Psychol Psychiatry 18:297–321, 1977

Freeman BJ, Ritvo ER, Needleman R, et al: The stability of cognitive and linguistic parameters in autism: a five-year prospective study. Journal of the American Academy of Child Psychiatry 24:459–464, 1985

Freeman BJ, Ritvo ER, Yokota A, et al: Autism, forme fruste: psychometric assessments of first-degree relatives, in Biological Psychiatry. Edited by Shagass C, Perris C, Struwe G, et al. New York, Elsevier Science, 1986, pp 1487–1488

Gaffney G, Tsai L, Kuperman S, et al: Cerebellar structure in autism. Am J Dis Child 141:1330–1332, 1987a

Gaffney G, Kuperman S, Tsai L, et al: Midsagittal magnetic resonance of autism. Br J Psychiatry 151:831–833, 1987b

Garber HJ, Ritvo ER, Chiu LC, et al: A magnetic resonance imaging study of autism: normal fourth ventricle size and absence of pathology. Am J Psychiatry 146:532–534, 1989

Geller E, Yuwiler A, Freeman BJ, et al: Platelet size, number, and serotonin content in blood of autistic, childhood schizophrenic, and normal children. J Autism Dev Disord 18:119–126, 1988

Gillberg C, Svendsen P: Childhood psychosis and computed tomographic brain scan findings. J Autism Dev Disord 13:19–32, 1983

Gillberg C, Svennerholm L: CSF monoamines in autistic syndromes and other pervasive developmental disorders of early childhood. Br J Psychiatry 151:89–94, 1987

Giller EL Jr, Young JG, Breakfield XO, et al: Monoamine oxidase and catechol-O-methyltransferase activities in cultured fibroblasts and blood cells from children with autism and the Gilles de la Tourette syndrome. Psychological Research 2:187–197, 1980

Gittelman M, Birch G: Childhood schizophrenia: intellect, neurologic status, perinatal risk, prognosis and family pathology. Arch Gen Psychiatry 17:16–25, 1967

Goldfarb W, Levy DM, Meyers DI: The mother speaks to her schizophrenic child: language in childhood schizophrenia. Psychiatry 35:217–226, 1972

Goldstein M, Mahanand P, Lee J, et al: Dopamine-beta-hydroxylase and endogenous total 5-hydroxyindole levels in autistic patients and controls, in The Autistic Syndrome. Edited by Coleman M. Amsterdam, Elsevier North-Holland, 1976, pp 57–63

Hagberg BA, Aicardi J, Dias K, et al: A progressive syndrome of autism, dementia, ataxia, and loss of purposeful hand use in girls: Rett's syndrome: report of 35 cases. Ann Neurol 14:471–479, 1983

Heh CWC, Smith R, Wu J, et al: Positron emission tomography of the cerebellum in autism. Am J Psychiatry 146:242–245, 1989

Heller T: Dementia infantilis (1930). Translated by Hulse WC. J Neur Ment Dis 119:471–477, 1954

Hemsley R, Howlin P, Berger M, et al: Treating autistic children in a family context, in Autism: A Reappraisal of Concepts and Treatment. Edited by Rutter M, Schopler E. New York, Plenum, 1978, pp 371–421

Hermelin B, O'Connor N: Psychological Experiments with Autistic Children. Oxford, UK, Pergamon, 1970

Hertzig ME, Snow ME, New E, et al: DSM-III and DSM-III-R diagnosis of autism and pervasive developmental disorder in nursery school children. J Am Acad Child Adolesc Psychiatry 29:123–126, 1990

Hier DE, LeMay M, Rosenberger PB: Autism and unfavorable left-right asymmetrics of the brain. J Autism Dev Disord 9:153–159, 1979

Hingtgen JN, Churchill DW: Differential effects of behavior modification in four mute autistic boys, in Infantile Autism. Edited by Churchill DW, Alpern CD, DeMyer M. Springfield, IL, Charles C Thomas, 1971, pp 185–199

Hoshino Y, Kumashiro H, Yshima Y, et al: The epidemiological study of autism in Fukushima-Ken. Folia Psychiatrica Neurological Japonica 36:115–124, 1982

Howells JG, Guirguis WR: Childhood schizophrenia 20 years later. Arch Gen Psychiatry 41:123–128, 1984

Kalat JW: Speculations on similarities between autism and opiate addiction. Journal of Autism and Childhood Schizophrenia 8:477–479, 1978

Kanner L: Autistic disturbances of affective contact. Nervous Child 2:217–250, 1943

Katsui T, Okuda M, Usuda S, et al: Kinetics of H-serotonin uptake by platelets in infantile autism and developmental language disorder (including five pairs of twins). J Autism Dev Disord 16:69–76, 1986

Katz RM, Liebman W: Creatine phosphokinase activity in central nervous system disorders and infections. Am J Dis Child 120:543–546, 1970

Knoblock H, Pasamanick B: Some etiologic and prognostic factors in early infantile autism and psychosis. Pediatrics 55:182–191, 1975

Kolvin I, Ounsted C, Humphrey M, et al: Six studies in the childhood psychoses. Br J Psychiatry 118:381–419, 1971

Kuperman S, Beeghly JH, Burns TL, et al: Serotonin relationships of autistic probands and their first-degree relatives. Journal of the American Academy of Child Psychiatry 24:189–190, 1985

Lake CR, Ziegler MG, Murphy DL: Increased norepinephrine levels and decreased dopamine-beta-hydroxylase activity in primary autism. Arch Gen Psychiatry 34:553–556, 1977

Launay JM, Bursztejn C, Ferrari P, et al: Catecholamine metabolism in infantile autism: a controlled study of 22 autistic children. J Autism Dev Disord 17:333–347, 1987

Leckman JF, Cohen DJ, Shaywitz BA, et al: CSF monoamine metabolites in child and adult psychiatric patients. Arch Gen Psychiatry 37:677–681, 1980

Lelord G, Laffont F, Jusseaume P, et al: Comparative study of conditioning of averaged evoked responses by coupling sound and light in normal and autistic children. Psychophysiology 10:415–425, 1973

Lockyer L, Rutter M: A five to fifteen year follow-up study of infantile psychosis, III: psychological aspects. Br J Psychiatry 115:865–882, 1969

Lotter V: Epidemiology of autistic conditions in young children, I: prevalence. Soc Psychiatry 1:124–137, 1966

Lotter V: Follow-up studies, in Autism: A Reappraisal of Concepts and Treatment. Edited by Rutter M, Schopler E. New York, Plenum, 1978, pp 475–495

Lovaas OI, Schreibman L, Koegel RL: A behavior modification approach to the treatment of autistic children, in Psychopathology and Child Development. Edited by Schopler E, Reichler RJ. New York, Plenum, 1976, pp 291–310

Lovaas OL, Varni J, Koegel RL, et al: Some observations on the non-extinguishability of children's speech. Child Dev 48:1121–1127, 1977

Mason-Brothers A, Ritvo E, Guze B, et al: Pre-, peri-, and postnatal factors in 181 autistic patients from single and multiple incidence families. J Am Acad Child Adolesc Psychiatry 26:39–42, 1987

Mesibov GB, Shea V: Social and interpersonal problems of autistic adolescents and adults. Paper presented at the meeting of the Southeastern Psychological Association, Washington, DC, March 1980

Minderaa RB, Anderson GM, Volkmar FR, et al: Urinary 5-hydroxyindoleacetic acid and whole blood serotonin and tryptophan in autistic and normal subjects. Biol Psychiatry 22:933–940, 1987

Minderaa RB, Anderson GM, Volkmar FR, et al: Neurochemical study of dopamine functioning in autistic and normal subjects. J Am Acad Child Adolesc Psychiatry 28:190–194, 1989

Minshew NJ, Payton JB, Wolf GL, et al: ^{1}H NMR imaging of autistics: implication for neurobiology. Ann Neurol 20:417, 1986

Novick B, Vaughn HG Jr, Kurtzberg D, et al: An electrophysiologic indication of auditory processing defects in autism. Psychiatry Res 3:107–114, 1980

Ornitz EM: The modulation of sensory input and motor output in autistic children. J Autism Dev Disord 4:197–215, 1974

Ornitz EM: The functional neuroanatomy of infantile autism. Int J Neurosci 19:85–124, 1983

Ornitz EM: Neurophysiology of infantile autism. Journal of the American Academy of Child Psychiatry 24:251–262, 1985

Ornitz EM, Ritvo ER: Perceptual inconstancy in early infantile autism. Arch Gen Psychiatry 18:76–98, 1968

Ornitz EM, Ritvo ER: The syndrome of autism: a critical review. Am J Psychiatry 133:609–621, 1976

Panksepp J: A neurochemical theory of autism. Trends Neurosci 2:174–177, 1979

Payton JB, Steele MW, Wenger SL, et al: The fragile X marker and autism in perspective. J Am Acad Child Adolesc Psychiatry 28:417–421, 1989

Petty LK, Ornitz EM, Michelman JD, et al: Autistic children who become schizophrenic. Arch Gen Psychiatry 41:129–135, 1984

Piven J, Gayle J, Chase G, et al: A family history of neuropsychiatric disorders in adult siblings of autistic individuals. J Am Acad Child Adolesc Psychiatry 29:177–183, 1990a

Piven J, Berthier ML, Starkstein SE, et al: Magnetic resonance imaging evidence for a defect of cerebral cortical development in autism. Am J Psychiatry 147:734–739, 1990b

Prior MR: Cognitive abilities and disabilities in infantile autism: a review. J Abnorm Child Psychol 7:357–380, 1979

Prior MR, Tress B, Hoffman WL, et al: Computed tomographic study of children with classic autism. Arch Neurol 41:482–484, 1984

Realmuto GM, Main B: Coincidence of Tourette's disorder and infantile autism. J Autism Dev Disord 12:367–372, 1982

Reiser DE: Psychosis of infancy and early childhood, as manifested by children with atypical development, I. N Engl J Med 269:790–798, 1963a

Reiser DE: Psychosis of infancy and early childhood, as manifested by children with atypical development, II. N Engl J Med 269:844–850, 1963b

Ricks DM, Wing L: Language communication and the use of symbols, in Early Childhood Autism. Edited by Wing L. Oxford, UK, Pergamon, 1976, pp 93–134

Ritvo ER, Freeman BJ: Current research in the syndrome of

autism: introduction—The National Society of Autistic Children's definition of the syndrome of autism. Journal of the American Academy of Child Psychiatry 17:565–575, 1978

Ritvo ER, Ornitz EM, Walter RD, et al: Correlation of psychiatric diagnoses and EEG findings: a double-blind study of 184 hospitalized children. Am J Psychiatry 126:988–996, 1970

Ritvo ER, Freeman BJ, Mason-Brothers A, et al: Concordance for the syndrome of autism in 40 pairs of afflicted twins. Am J Psychiatry 142:74–77, 1985

Ritvo ER, Freeman BJ, Scheibel AB, et al: Lower Purkinje cell counts in the cerebella of four autistic subjects: initial findings of the UCLA-NSAC autopsy research report. Am J Psychiatry 143:862–866, 1986

Ritvo ER, Freeman BJ, Pingree C, et al: The UCLA-University of Utah epidemiologic survey of autism: prevalence. Am J Psychiatry 146:194–196, 1989a

Ritvo ER, Jorde LB, Mason-Brothers A, et al: The UCLA-University of Utah epidemiologic survey of autism: recurrence risk estimate and genetic counseling. Am J Psychiatry 146:1032–1036, 1989b

Rosenbloom S, Campbell M, George AE, et al: High resolution CT scanning in infantile autism: a quantitative approach. Journal of the American Academy of Child Psychiatry 1:72–77, 1984

Rotman A, Caplan R, Szekeley GA: Platelet uptake of serotonin in psychotic children. Psychopharmacology (Berlin) 67:245–248, 1980

Rumsey JM, Grimes AM, Pikus AM, et al: Auditory brainstem responses in pervasive developmental disorders. Biol Psychiatry 19:1403–1418, 1984

Rumsey JM, Rapoport JL, Sceery WR: Autistic children as adults: psychiatric, social and behavioral outcomes. Journal of the American Academy of Child Psychiatry 24:465–473, 1985a

Rumsey JM, Duara R, Grady C, et al: Brain metabolism in autism: resting cerebral glucose utilization rates measured with positron emission tomography. Arch Gen Psychiatry 42:448–455, 1985b

Rumsey JM, Creasy H, Stepanek JS, et al: Hemispheric asymmetries, fourth ventricular size, and cerebellar morphology in autism. J Autism Dev Disord 18:127–137, 1988

Rutter M: Psychotic disorders in early childhood. Br J Psychiatry Spec Publ No I, 1967, pp 133–158

Rutter M: Concepts of autism: a review of research. J Child Psychol Psychiatry 9:1–25, 1968

Rutter M: Autistic children: infancy to adulthood. Seminars in Psychiatry 2:435–450, 1970

Rutter M: Infantile autism and other child psychoses, in Child Psychiatry: Modern Approaches. Edited by Rutter M, Hersov L. Oxford, UK, Blackwell, 1977, pp 717–747

Rutter M: Diagnosis and definition, in Autism: A Reappraisal of Concepts and Treatment. Edited by Rutter M, Schopler E. New York, Plenum, 1978, pp 1–25

Rutter M: Autistic children growing up. Dev Med Child Neurol 26:122–129, 1984

Rutter M, Lockyer L: A five to fifteen year follow-up study of infantile psychosis: description of sample. Br J Psychiatry 113:1169–1182, 1967

Rutter M, Schopler E: Autism and pervasive developmental disorders: concept and diagnostic issues. J Autism Dev Disord 17:159–186, 1987

Sankar DV: Studies on blood platelets, blood enzymes, and leukocyte chromosome breakage in childhood schizophrenia. Behavioral Neuropsychiatry 2:2–10, 1971

Schain RJ, Yannet H: Infantile autism: an analysis of 50 cases and a consideration of certain relevant neurophysiologic concepts. J Pediatr 57:560–567, 1960

Schopler E: Visual versus tactual receptor preference in normal and schizophrenic children. J Abnorm Psychol 71:108–114, 1966

Schopler E, Andrews CE, Strupp K: Do autistic children come from upper-middle class parents? J Autism Dev Disord 9:139–152, 1979

Schopler E, Mesibov GB, Baker A: Evaluation of treatment for autistic children and their parents. Journal of the American Academy of Child Psychiatry 21:262–267, 1982

Steffenburg S, Gillberg C: Autism and autistic-like conditions in Swedish rural and urban area: a population study. Br J Psychiatry 149:81–87, 1986

Steffenburg S, Gillberg C, Hellgren L, et al: A twin study of autism in Denmark, Finland, Iceland, Norway and Sweden. J Child Psychol Psychiatry 30:405–416, 1989

Stubbs EG: Autistic children exhibit undetectable hemagglutination-inhibition antibody titers despite previous rubella vaccination. Journal of Autism and Childhood Schizophrenia 6:269–274, 1976

Sugiyama T, Abe T: The prevalence of autism in Nagoya, Japan: a total population study. J Autism Dev Disord 19:87–96, 1989

Tanguay PE, Ornitz EM, Forsythe AB, et al: Rapid eye movement (REM) activity in normal and autistic children during REM sleep. Journal of Autism and Childhood Schizophrenia 6:275–288, 1976

Tanguay PE, Edwards RM, Buchwald J, et al: Auditory brainstem evoked responses in autistic children. Arch Gen Psychiatry 39:174–180, 1982

Todd RD, Ciaranello RD: Demonstration of inter- and intraspecies differences in serotonin binding sites by antibodies from an autistic child. Proc Natl Acad Sci USA 82:612–616, 1985

Todd RD, Hickok JM, Anderson GM, et al: Antibrain antibodies in infantile autism. Biol Psychiatry 23:644–647, 1988

Treffert DA: Epidemiology of infantile autism. Arch Gen Psychiatry 22:431–438, 1970

Trygstad OE, Reichelt KL, Foss I, et al: Patterns of peptides and protein-associated peptide complexes in psychiatric disorders. Br J Psychiatry 136:59–72, 1980

Tsai LY: Infantile autism and schizophrenia in childhood, in The Medical Basis of Psychiatry. Edited by Winokur G, Clayton P. Philadelphia, PA, WB Saunders, 1986, pp 331–351

Tsai LY: Pre-, peri-, and neonatal factors in autism, in Neurobiological Issues in Autism. Edited by Schopler E, Mesibov GB. New York, Plenum, 1987, pp 179–189

Tsai LY, Tsai MC: Using EEG diagnosis to subtype autistic syndrome. Paper presented at the International Conference on the National Society for Children and Adults with Autism. San Antonio, TX, July 1984

Tsai LY, Stewart MA, August G: Implication of sex differences in the familial transmission of infantile autism. J Autism Dev Disord 11:165–173, 1981

Tsai L, Stewart MA, Faust M, et al: Social class distribution of fathers and children enrolled in the Iowa autism program. J Autism Dev Disord 12:211–222, 1982

U.S. Department of Health and Human Services: International Classification of Diseases: Clinical Modification, 9th Revision. Washington, DC, U.S. Department of Health and Human Services, 1980

Van Krevelen DA: Early infantile autism. Acta Paedopsychiatria 91:81–97, 1952

Volkmar FR, Nelson DS: Seizure disorders in autism. J Am Acad Child Adolesc Psychiatry 29:127–129, 1990

Volkmar FR, Bregman J, Cohen DJ, et al: DSM-III and DSM-III-R diagnosis of autism. Am J Psychiatry 145:1404–1408, 1988

Waldo MC, Cohen DJ, Caparulo BK, et al: EEG profiles of neuropsychiatrically disturbed children. Journal of the American Academy of Child Psychiatry 17:656–670, 1978

Warren RP, Margaretten NC, Pace NC, et al: Immune abnormalities in patients with autism. J Autism Dev Disord 16:189–197, 1986

Warren RP, Foster A, Margaretten NC: Reduced natural killer cell activity in autism. J Am Acad Child Adolesc Psychiatry 26:333–335, 1987

Wechsler D: Wechsler Intelligence Scale for Children—Revised. New York, Psychological Corporation, 1974

Weizman A, Weizman R, Szekely GA, et al: Abnormal immune response to brain tissue antigen in the syndrome of autism. Am J Psychiatry 139:1462–1465, 1982

Werry JS: The childhood psychoses, in Psychopathological Disorders of Childhood, 2nd Edition. Edited by Quay HC, Werry JS. New York, John Wiley, 1979, pp 43–89

Westall FC, Root-Bernstein RS: Suggested connection between autism serotonin, and myelin basic protein. Am J Psychiatry 140:1260–1261, 1983

Williams RS, Hauser SL, Purpura DP, et al: Autism and mental retardation. Arch Neurol 37:749–753, 1980

Wing L: The handicaps of autistic children: a comparative study. J Child Psychol Psychiatry 10:1–40, 1969

Wing L: A study of language impairments in severely retarded children, in Language, Cognitive Deficits and Retardation. Edited by O'Conner N. London, Butterworths, 1975, pp 87–112

Wing L: Diagnosis, clinical description and prognosis, in Early Childhood Autism. Edited by Wing L. Oxford, UK, Pergamon, 1976, pp 15–64

Wing L: Childhood autism and social class: a question of selection. Br J Psychiatry 137:410–417, 1980

Wing L: Asperger's syndrome: a clinical account. Psychol Med 11:115–129, 1981

Wing L, Gould J: Severe impairments of social interaction and associated abnormalities in children: epidemiology and classification. J Autism Dev Disord 9:11–29, 1979

World Health Organization: International Classification of Diseases, 10th Edition, draft version. Geneva, World Health Organization, 1987

Wright HH, Carpenter R, Brennan W, et al: Elevated blood serotonin in autistic probands and their first degree relatives. J Autism Dev Disord 19:397–407, 1989

Young JG, Caparulo BK, Shaywitz BA, et al: Childhood autism: cerebrospinal fluid examination and immunoglobulin levels. Journal of Child Psychiatry 16:174–179, 1977

Young JG, Kyprie RM, Ross NT, et al: Serum dopamine-beta-hydroxylase activity: clinical applications in child psychiatry. J Autism Dev Disord 10:1–14, 1980

Young JG, Kavanagh ME, Anderson GM, et al: Clinical neurochemistry of autism and associated disorders. J Autism Dev Disord 12:147–165, 1982

Chapter 18

Other Pervasive Developmental Disorders

Luke Y. Tsai, M.D.

As described in the previous chapter, in the DSM-III (American Psychiatric Association 1980) classification of pervasive developmental disorders (PDDs), in addition to the infantile autism subcategory, there were two other subgroups: childhood onset PDD and atypical PDD. Since the publication of DSM-III, reports suggest that other developmental disorders such as Asperger's syndrome (Wing 1981), Rett's syndrome (Gillberg 1987), and disintegrative psychosis (Rutter 1985) should also be considered as separate subgroups of PDDs. However, the DSM-III-R (American Psychiatric Association 1987) Work Group on PDDs decided to use PDD not otherwise specified (NOS) as a single remainder category for all subtypes of PDDs except autistic disorder, which was considered as the same disorder as infantile autism. The DSM-III-R system (American Psychiatric Association) suggests that PDDNOS

> should be used when there is a qualitative impairment in the development of reciprocal social interaction and of verbal and nonverbal communication skills, but the criteria are not met for Autistic Disorder, Schizophrenia, or Schizotypal or Schizoid Personality Disorder. Some people with this diagnosis will exhibit a markedly restricted repertoire of activities and interests, but others will not. (p. 39)

However, the DSM-III-R scheme has not offered specific diagnostic criteria for PDDNOS.

The rationale for the DSM-III-R Work Group to adopt PDDNOS was based on the following two opinions: 1) the subgroups of PDDs could not be reliably distinguished from autistic disorder, and 2) the subgroups of PDDs did not differ from au-

tistic disorder on either etiologic variables or clinical course. The Work Group did not feel there was sufficient evidence for the taxonomic validity of the other subgroups of PDDs to justify the establishment of separate diagnostic categories (Waterhouse et al., unpublished manuscript). However, this decision has given rise to a number of significant controversies. Some discussions have centered around the diagnostic validity of PDDNOS; others have focused on the concern that further research of the taxonomic validity of the subtypes of PDDs other than autistic disorder would become virtually impossible because all these different groups are being bundled together in a way such that they all will lose crucial diagnostic distinctions (Tsai, in press). Thus the World Health Organization's (1987) ICD-10 scheme (which is scheduled to be published in 1993) proposes that the PDDs be subdivided into the following subcategories: 1) childhood autism, 2) atypical autism, 3) Asperger's syndrome, 4) Rett's syndrome, 5) other childhood disintegrative disorder, 6) overactive disorders associated with mental retardation and stereotyped movements, 7) other pervasive disorders, and 8) unspecified pervasive disorder. In this chapter, I will focus on the following four subgroups of PDDs: atypical autism, Asperger's syndrome, Rett's syndrome, and other childhood disintegrative disorder. There are two reasons for such an approach. First, in each of the four subgroups, there are new empirical data supporting the diagnostic validity. Second, it is highly possible that the DSM-IV (American Psychiatric Association 1991) classification will also consider these disorders as separate subtypes of

PDDs as the ICD-10 draft does. This chapter can be a supplement to the DSM-IV in terms of a source of information.

Atypical Autism

Definition and Diagnostic Criteria

In DSM-III, atypical PDD was used to classify those individuals who shared many, although not all, of the features of infantile autism and childhood onset PDD. In the ICD-10 draft classification, atypical autism is defined as a subtype of PDDs that differs from autism in terms of either age of onset or of failing to fulfill all three sets of diagnostic criteria for childhood autism. Thus atypical autism contains both childhood onset PDD and atypical PDD of DSM-III. The ICD-10 draft system also includes research diagnostic criteria (Table 18-1).

There has not been any systematic study specifically based on the DSM-III-R definition and criteria for PDDNOS. Therefore, as a single diagnostic entity, very little is known about PDDNOS except that it is "more common than Autistic Disorder in the general population" (American Psychiatric Association 1987, p. 34). Therefore the information on atypical autism presented in this chapter is derived mainly from studies that used DSM-III diagnostic criteria for atypical PDD as well as childhood onset PDD.

Clinical Findings

In the study of Prior et al. (1975), the "non-Kanner's" group of subjects, referring to Kanner (1943), could be considered as having atypical autism. In

Table 18-1.   ICD-10 research diagnostic criteria for atypical autism

A. Presence of abnormal/impaired development at or after age three years.
B. Qualitative impairments in reciprocal social interaction or communication, or restricted, repetitive, and stereotyped patterns of behavior, interests, and criteria (criteria for autism except that it is not necessary to meet the criteria in terms of number of areas of abnormality).
C. A failure to meet the diagnostic criteria for autism.

Source.   Reprinted with permission from World Health Organization (1987).

general, as compared with the "Kanner's" group, the non-Kanner's group had less severe symptoms across dimensions of socialization, communication, and repetitive activities, and a later age of onset.

Dahl et al. (1986) studied 390 children under 72 months of age; 24 were considered as having childhood onset PDD. They had impairment in human relationships, bizarre motor behavior, and confused and bizarre thinking. On the measures of cognitive functioning, these children showed a wide spread between the various sector means. There were no islets of intelligence. In general, the childhood onset PDD group was noted as more heterogeneous; many of these children showed clinical characteristics similar to those seen in children with infantile autism. Sparrow et al. (1986) reported similar findings in a follow-up study of 11 "atypical" and 14 normal children. The atypical and normal groups had similar cognitive measures; that is, both groups fell into the average to high-average range. However, poorer motor development and relatively impaired socialization and communication behaviors were much more characteristic of atypical children than of their similar-aged normal peers. The atypical children had a tenuous, brittle, and shallow manner of relating to others; major difficulties interacting with similar-aged peers; high levels of anxiety; perseveration; and fascination with odd or idiosyncratic substances or objects.

Levine and Demb (1987) reported a study of 18 preschoolers (14 boys) who had atypical PDD. In this group of children, only about one-third (35%) had normal or borderline IQs. More than two-thirds had a history of abnormal language or speech development. Receptive language was markedly impaired. None of the children had normal expressive language. Of these children, 94% showed unusual language or speech, including echolalia, perseveration, abnormal vocal quality (monotone, whisper, screaming), unintelligibility, idiosyncratic language (stereotyped, gibberish, cursing), excessive jargon, actively withholding speech, pronoun reversal, and hyperverbalization. These children tended to blend material from their personal experience into their communication when it did not fit in with the external context of the conversation. However, only six (33%) failed to use language for meaningful communication. It was also noted that these children had conflictual (e.g., manipulative or provocative behavior or negativism) and inappropriate (e.g., clinging, avoidance, or hitting and biting) relationships with parents, other adults, or children. Almost all of the children were noted or reported to have ritualistic or manneristic behaviors. Of these children, 88% were overactive with decreased attention span. Most of these children had excessive anxiety or were reported to have unusual or extreme fears (e.g., of the moon, water, the doorbell). They tended to exhibit inappropriate, flat, or labile affect. These children often were oppositional and, occasionally, were angry and aggressive. More than two-thirds of the children had fine and gross motor delays. The age of onset of these children's disorder was less than 30 months in at least 15 of the 18 cases.

Rescorla (1988) studied 204 boys between the ages of 3 and 5. Of this sample, 24% were considered to have a diagnosis of infantile autism, and 15% as having "autistic-like disorder." Many autistic-like children appeared to be highly anxious and tense, often expressing their confusions and preoccupations in repetitive and stereotypic verbalizations. Although they also had severe impairments in social relatedness, deviant and/or delayed language development, and bizarre and stereotypic behavior, these children had some age-appropriate cognitive skills, more social relatedness, and a greater ability to communicate than the children with infantile autism.

Differential Diagnosis

In Asperger's syndrome, there should not be a delay in cognitive and language development. In atypical autism, there is delayed as well as deviant development in cognition and language.

The observation of "thought disorders" in children with atypical PDD could support the view that this disorder is a variant of schizophrenia in childhood. Several points argue against such a notion. First, there is no deterioration from a previous level of functioning in these children. Second, there is no clear evidence of delusions or hallucinations in any of the children. Third, there is no evidence of family history of schizophrenia or other types of psychoses in these children.

Epidemiology

Prevalence. Atypical autism appears to occur most often in profoundly retarded people. It also has been noted in individuals with a severe specific developmental disorder of receptive language, some of whom show social, emotional, and/or behavioral symptoms that overlap with childhood autism. Levine and Demb (1987) reported that there were three times more children with atypical PDD than children with infantile autism during the time of their study.

In an epidemiologic study of children in the former London borough of Camberwell, Wing and Gould (1979) identified 74 children who had the "autistic triad"; that is, they had qualitative impairments in social interaction, communication, and a restricted range of imaginative activities. Of these children, 17 met the classic description of infantile autism. Another 57 were considered to have "atypical autism," thus yielding a prevalence rate of 16 per 10,000. Among the retarded, atypical autism was about three times more common than "classic autism."

Burd et al. (1987) reported results from an administrative survey of PDD cases in North Dakota. They identified a prevalence rate of 1.99 per 10,000 for atypical PDD.

These rather different prevalence rates of atypical autism readily illustrate the problem caused by imprecise definition, as well as the lack of reliable explicit diagnostic criteria for atypical autism.

Sex ratio. The disorder appears to be considerably more common in boys than in girls, with ratios ranging from 5:1 to 2:1 (Dahl et al. 1986; Sparrow et al. 1986). It is apparent that different definition and diagnostic criteria used by these studies produced somewhat different sex ratios.

Social class. The families of children with childhood onset PDD were somewhat better educated and of higher socioeconomic status (i.e., 50% from Class I and II) than the families in the other diagnostic groups. Levine and Demb (1987) also noted that the educational level of the atypical PDD group tended to be higher than that of other clinic patients. The significance of the finding is not clear; it requires further study using a large-scale sample.

Etiology

About 4.2% of the children with childhood onset PDD (Dahl et al. 1986) had evidence of neurologic disturbance (i.e., congenital central nervous system malformation). More than two-thirds of the children in the study of Levine and Demb (1987) had histories of medically complicated pregnancies and/or perinatal complications. About 44% had neurologic signs, including increased reflexes, lax ligaments, positive Babinski responses, hypotonia, poor cerebellar functioning, cataracts, macrocephaly, decreased strength, or drooling.

Available information appears to indicate that atypical autism has a great heterogeneity in terms of etiology. Thus it is expected that numerous etiologic factors would be identified in future research in this area.

Treatment

The treatment for persons with atypical autism is similar to that for those with autistic disorder and autism. However, it should be pointed out that special education systems in most states of this country do not have an educational category specifically for students with atypical autism. Many students with such a diagnosis are being placed in programs for students with other disorders, such as mental retardation, emotional disturbance, or behavior disorder. Hence these students with atypical autism fail to receive any programming that attends to their unique educational needs. It is important to work closely with school personnel to ensure the needed educational services for students with atypical autism.

Prognosis

For the moment there are no data on adults with atypical PDD. It is not clear whether these individuals would show significant improvement with longer educational and other treatments. More prolonged follow-up is needed to find out the final outcome of individuals with atypical autism.

Research Issues

Individuals with atypical autism may be more common than those with childhood autism, although they are less frequently studied. The validity of this diagnostic entity and its relationship to childhood autism and other PDDs remain unclear. It is not clear that atypical autism can be described as constituting a distinct diagnostic group. Existing data seem to indicate great heterogeneity, and there may be a need to divide it further into smaller groups in the future. Hence, the development of more ex-

plicit diagnostic criteria is an important topic of future research.

Asperger's Syndrome

Definition and Diagnostic Criteria

Asperger's syndrome was first described in 1944 by Hans Asperger, a Viennese child psychiatrist. Asperger regarded the syndrome he described as a personality disorder, and he used the term *autistic psychopathy*. According to Asperger's observation, individuals with Asperger's syndrome usually began to speak at approximately the same time as in normal children. A full command of grammar was acquired sooner or later. There might be difficulty in using pronouns correctly. The content of speech was usually abnormal and pedantic and consisted of lengthy disquisitions on favorite subjects. Often a word or phrase was repeated over and over again in a stereotyped fashion. Other features he described were the impairment of a two-way social interaction; totally ignoring demands of the environment; repetitive and stereotyped play; and isolated areas of interests. Asperger believed that the condition was never recognized in infancy and that those with the syndrome had excellent logical abstract thinking and were capable of originality and creativity in chosen fields.

Wing (1981) observed that half of her sample of 34 cases had been slow to talk, that careful questioning often elicited a history of a lack of communication behaviors in infancy, and that the apparent originality and special abilities were best explained by reliance on rote memory skills. Wing suggested that Asperger's syndrome be considered as a part of the "autistic continuum." She believes that Asperger's syndrome could be a mild variant of autism in relatively bright children. This view of Asperger's syndrome has received support from several prominent researchers in the field of autism research (e.g., Rutter and Schopler 1987; Szatmari et al. 1989).

Rutter (personal communication) recently reassessed this issue and wrote to the DSM-IV Work Group on PDDs, stating, "My own clinical research has been concerned with Asperger's syndrome, and I do think that there might be enough valid data at this point to support this as a valid subtype." He continued: "Our data suggest that children with autism and Asperger's syndrome differ on both early history and outcome. It is this difference on outcome, it seems to me, that would justify the specification of an Asperger's syndrome subgroup in ICD-10."

Neither Asperger nor Wing has offered detailed specific diagnostic criteria for Asperger's syndrome, and they both refer to partial or spectrum cases. Both DSM-III and DSM-III-R consider Asperger's syndrome a mild variant of autism and hence offer no specific definition and diagnostic criteria for it. The ICD-10 draft considers Asperger's syndrome as a distinct subtype of PDDs and defines it as a disorder characterized by the same type of qualitative impairment of reciprocal social interaction and restricted, stereotyped, repetitive repertoire of interests and activities that typify autism. There is no general delay or retardation in language or in cognitive development.

For research purposes, the ICD-10 draft also offers research diagnostic criteria for Asperger's syndrome (Table 18-2). Specifically, the ICD-10 classification emphasizes "a lack of any clinically significant general delay in language development" (p. 127), whereas other investigators allow for delay in language development as one of the

Table 18-2.   ICD-10 research diagnostic criteria for Asperger's syndrome

A. A lack of any clinically significant general delay in language or cognitive development. Diagnosis requires that single words should have developed by two years of age or earlier and that communicative phrases be used by three years of age or earlier. Self-help skills, adaptive behavior, and curiosity about the environment during the first three years should be at a level consistent with normal intellectual development. However, motor milestones may be somewhat delayed and motor clumsiness is usual (although not a necessary diagnostic feature). Isolated special skills, often related to abnormal preoccupations, are common, but are not required for diagnosis.
B. Qualitative impairments in reciprocal social interaction (criteria for autism).
C. Restricted, repetitive, and stereotyped patterns of behavior, interests, and activities (criteria for autism).
D. The disorder is not attributable to the other varieties of pervasive developmental disorder; schizotypal disorder; simple schizophrenia; reactive and disinhibited attachment disorder of childhood; obsessional personality disorder; obsessive-compulsive disorder.

Source.   Reprinted with permission from World Health Organization (1987).

inclusion criteria for Asperger's syndrome. Nonetheless, there is general agreement on the clinical features of the syndrome.

The following information on Asperger's syndrome must be received cautiously because it is derived from studies using diagnostic criteria that cannot ensure complete separation of Asperger's syndrome and autism. In fact, Gillberg (1989) admitted that "despite the diagnostic criteria used, it could be merely my own clinical notion that Asperger's syndrome seemed to be a more appropriate label in some cases and infantile autism in others" (p. 529).

Clinical Findings

Individuals with Asperger's syndrome usually like to be with other people and like to talk. Their conversation is often described as being stilted, gauche, thought disordered, or centering on idiosyncratic interests that preoccupy them. They have markedly impaired nonverbal expression. They are interested in human relationships but are unable to carry through social interactions with sufficient success to make relationships easy. Most of them are markedly clumsy.

Szatmari et al. (1989) noted that children with Asperger's syndrome more frequently approached others only to have their needs met, had a very clumsy social approach, engaged in one-sided social interactions, and had difficulty sensing or were detached from the feelings of others. Limited use of facial expression and gestures to communicate was a common characteristic of children with Asperger's syndrome. There were impairments in nonverbal communication. These children were often noted to talk too much or too little. They frequently showed abnormalities in inflection (either flat and monotonous or else exaggerated) and would repeat inappropriate phrases out of context. They also tended to have odd speech.

On the standardized neurocognitive measures, the children with Asperger's syndrome showed significant impairments on both verbal IQ (about 86) and performance IQ (about 88) subtests (Szatmari et al. 1990). Children with Asperger's syndrome performed quite well on tests requiring good rote memory, but they had deficits in tests depending on abstract concepts or sequencing in time (Wing 1981).

Differential Diagnosis

The differential diagnosis between autistic disorder/childhood autism and Asperger's syndrome may or may not be made easily, depending on how the two conditions are defined. The ICD-10 definition of Asperger's syndrome emphasizes a lack of general delay in language development. This point alone should distinguish individuals with Asperger's syndrome from those with autistic disorder. In addition, individuals with Asperger's syndrome and persons with autistic disorder differ in their ability to decode nonverbal social information and in their use of vocal intonation to communicate effectively (Szatmari et al. 1989).

The diagnosis of schizophrenia is extremely rare in childhood. In general, individuals with schizophrenia have fairly normal developmental history. Usually there is rather clear deterioration of daily functioning. Other features such as thought disorder, delusions, and hallucinations are also present in schizophrenia. Persons with Asperger's syndrome usually have early onset but make steady progress. There are no delusions or hallucinations. Also, there is no increased incidence of schizophrenia or other psychoses in family members.

Epidemiology

Prevalence. In the epidemiologic study carried out by Wing and Gould (1979), there was a prevalence rate of 0.6 per 10,000 for children with a combination of Asperger's syndrome and mild mental retardation. There was an additional 1.1 per 10,000 children who had been "autistic" in early life but who later in life showed features of Asperger's syndrome.

In a Swedish epidemiologic study (Gillberg and Gillberg 1989), among children with normal intelligence, rates of 10–26 per 10,000 are considered as minimum figures. Another 0.4 per 10,000 Swedish teenagers had the combination of Asperger's syndrome and mild mental retardation.

Sex ratio. Boys outnumber girls in all the studies of Asperger's syndrome. At the present time, the ratio has ranged from 3.8 to 10.5 boys to every girl (Szatmari et al. 1990; Wing 1981).

Social class. There seems to be a trend toward greater prevalence in higher social class. Wing (1981), however, also pointed out that the parents from the higher social class tended to have special interest in Asperger's syndrome, and hence would make effort to seek further information or service from the special clinics.

Etiology

Birth factors. Nearly half of those seen by Wing (1981) had a history of pre-, peri-, or postnatal complications, such as anoxia at birth. Szatmari et al. (1989) found that complications during pregnancy or the neonatal period in the Asperger's syndrome cases were about the same as those in the control group.

Genetic factors. Asperger (1944) considered the syndrome to be genetically related. He reported that the characteristics tended to occur in families, especially in the fathers, of those with the syndrome. Wing (1981) noted that 5 of 16 fathers and 2 of 24 mothers had behavior resembling that found in Asperger's syndrome.

The 28 cases of Asperger's syndrome in the study of Szatmari et al. (1989) came from 26 families. These included two children with Asperger's syndrome who were identical twins and another pair who were brothers. A fifth child with Asperger's syndrome had a retarded autistic brother; another subject had a sister diagnosed as schizophrenic. For the moment, the evidence for genetic factors is only suggestive.

Neurologic factors. No consistent or particular neurologic factors have been identified.

Neurophysiologic factors. In the series of Gillberg (1989), 5 of the 20 boys with Asperger's syndrome had a prolonged brain-stem transmission time (I-V interval) on auditory brain-stem response examination. Six of the 21 children had abnormal electroencephalograms (EEGs) in the waking state.

Neuroanatomical factors. Three of the 18 children with Asperger's syndrome studied by Gillberg (1989) had slight or moderate atrophy of the brain (internal, frontal-general, and occipital, respectively).

Summary of etiology. There have been too few studies of Asperger's syndrome to find specific etiologic associations. There is some evidence suggestive of neurobiological involvement.

Treatment

The treatment of individuals with Asperger's syndrome requires intervention at multiple levels.

Psychological. Family counseling should be provided to parents and should include a careful explanation of the disorder, realistic expectation of the child, and resources for obtaining support. Individual cognitive psychotherapy and group social skill training may be helpful to older children, adolescents, and adults.

Education. Working with the staff at the child's school is important, particularly helping them to recognize the need for special educational services. Tests measuring comprehension and abstract problem-solving skills are needed to elucidate fully the type of learning disability seen in these children. Treatment of both the learning disability and social skill deficits can often be accomplished by using cognitive-behavioral techniques. Early application of special motor skills training may be helpful for some clumsy individuals and may prevent further development of motor deficiency. Early application of occupational therapy may provide some skills that can be applied to vocational training. Vocational training should begin as early as possible.

Pharmacological. Medication can be useful if symptoms of attention deficit, anxiety, depression, or obsessive-compulsive behaviors become significant handicaps. I have had successful experience with stimulants (e.g., methylphenidate [Ritalin]), antidepressants (e.g., fluoxetine [Prozac]), and medications for obsessive-compulsive disorder (e.g., clomipramine [Anafranil]) in treating these conditions in individuals with Asperger's syndrome.

Clinical Course and Prognosis

Szatmari et al. (1989) reported that individuals with Asperger's syndrome seemed to improve with maturity, even into adulthood. Asperger (1944) also described the outcome of children with the syndrome to be "good." However, Wing (1981) described the outcome of persons with Asperger's syndrome as being rather poor. The ICD-10 Work Group also believes that there is a strong tendency for the abnormalities to persist into adolescence and adult life, and it seems that they represent individual characteristics that are not greatly affected by environmental influences. Psychotic episodes occasionally occur in early adult life.

Research Issues

It is quite obvious that much more research is needed to substantiate the diagnostic validity of Asperger's syndrome. I support the idea of adopting Asperger's syndrome as a subgroup of PDDs. It is hoped that future data collection based on such a concept will provide further information for a final study of taxonomy of Asperger's syndrome.

Rett's Syndrome

Definition and Diagnostic Criteria

Rett's syndrome was originally described by Rett (1966), who reported (in German) his findings in 22 patients. However, it did not gain wide recognition until 1983, when a series of 35 cases from a pool of French-Portuguese-Swedish patients was reported in English (Haas 1988).

The diagnostic criteria contain three categories: necessary criteria, supportive criteria, and exclusive criteria. The necessary criteria include apparent normal prenatal and perinatal period; apparent normal psychomotor development through the first 6 months (in some cases, development may appear to be normal for up to 18 months); normal head circumference at birth; deceleration of head growth between ages 5 months and 4 years; loss of acquired purposeful hand skills between ages 6 and 30 months; development of stereotypic hand movements, such as hand wringing or squeezing, clapping or tapping, with mouthing and "washing"/rubbing automatisms appearing after purposeful hand skills are lost; development of severely impaired expressive and receptive language; presence of apparent severe psychomotor retardation; appearance of gait apraxia and truncal apraxia-ataxia between ages 1 and 4 years; temporal social withdrawal; and diagnosis tentative until 2–5 years of age (Hagberg et al. 1985; Trevathan and Moser 1988).

The supportive criteria of Rett's syndrome include breathing dysfunction, such as periodic apnea during wakefulness, intermittent hyperventilation, breath-holding spells, and forced expulsion of air or saliva; EEG abnormalities; seizures; spasticity, often with associated development of muscle wasting; dystonia; peripheral vasomotor disturbances; scoliosis; growth retardation; and hypotrophic small feet. Although most patients with Rett's syndrome display many of the supportive criteria, diagnosis is possible in the absence of all the supportive criteria, especially in young patients.

The exclusion criteria of Rett's syndrome include evidence of intrauterine growth retardation; organomegaly or other signs of storage disease; retinopathy at birth; evidence of perinatally acquired brain damage; existence of identifiable metabolic or other progressive neurologic disorder; and acquired neurologic disorders resulting from severe infections or head trauma. The presence of one or more of the exclusion criteria excludes the diagnosis of Rett's syndrome, regardless of whether all of the necessary criteria have been met in an individual patient.

Differential Diagnosis

In the very first stage (at 1–2 years) of infantile neuronal ceroid lipofuscinosis (INCL), there is rapid regression with loss of acquired fine motor skills, learned words, and communication. It is very difficult to separate INCL from Rett's syndrome. However, careful observation will note transient drop spells, loss of head control, and irregular myoclonias in INCL. For accurate diagnosis of INCL, a biopsy with characteristic electron microscopic findings of "snowball" aggregate is necessary. After 3 years of age, a clinical differentiation becomes possible because of the presence of visual failure, rapid deterioration of head control, hyperexcitability, and trunk-limb extension tonus in INCL (Hagberg and Witt-Engerstrom 1990).

In the past, children with Rett's syndrome were frequently regarded as autistic (see Olsson and Rett 1987). Several independent studies of behavioral observations have demonstrated qualitative and quantitative differences between Rett's syndrome patients and persons with autism. The following are behaviors that were observed only in the Rett's syndrome patients and in no case of autism: slow movements plus hypoactivity; uniform stereotypic movements of hands with a broad-base stance; stereotypic "washing movements" of hands; stereotypic wetting of hands with saliva; stereotypic bringing together of hands; consistent, isolated stretching and flexing of the middle finger joints; episodic hyperventilation via mouth; and no chewing. Among behavior that is characteristic of autism, the following five traits were not seen in the Rett's syndrome patients: predominant rejection of caressing and tenderness; conspicuous physical hyperactivity in terms of continuous grabbing and concomitant locomobility; excessive attachment to certain objects; rotation of small objects; and stereotypic playing habits. Thus the authors demonstrated that Rett's syndrome and autism could be differentiated based on behavioral observations.

Other variables such as etiology, outcome, and response to treatment have not yet been studied systematically. Nonetheless, with increasing awareness of Rett's syndrome and its characteristic developmental profile (i.e., by 3–4 years of age), children with Rett's syndrome should have demonstrated the typical clinical features of Rett's syndrome and should be easily distinguishable from those with autism (Trevathan and Naidu 1988).

Differential diagnosis between Rett's syndrome and disintegrative disorder will be discussed below in the section on differential diagnosis of disintegrative disorder.

Epidemiology

Prevalence. The estimated prevalence is at least 1:10,000–15,000. Today, Rett's syndrome is known to exist in all races and probably in all countries. There are more than 1,500 recognized cases of Rett's syndrome worldwide. The many pathognomonic examples of its clinical expression have convinced clinicians of the existence of this unique syndrome (see Kerr and Stephenson 1985).

Sex ratio. Initially, Rett's syndrome was considered as a disorder only of females. There are only a few cases of males suspected of having Rett's syndrome.

Social class. Rett's syndrome is known to exist in all classes of families. There is no evidence suggestive of bias toward any social class.

Clinical Findings

It is essential to know that Rett's syndrome is a progressive neurologic disorder and that there is variability of clinical presentation that depends on patient age and stage of the disease. Hagberg and Witt-Engerstrom (1986) proposed a four-stage model: 1) early-onset stagnation stage is present between

6 months to 1½ years of age; 2) rapid developmental regression stage usually appears at 1–2 years of age; 3) pseudostationary stage usually occurs at 3–4 years of age, but can be delayed, and persists for many years or even decades; and 4) late motor deterioration stage often occurs during school age or early adolescence.

During the stagnation stage, there is deceleration of head growth, development of hypotonia, and loss of interest in play activity.

Many investigators reported that "autistic features" developed during the rapid developmental regression stage. The features include no sustained interest in persons or objects; stereotypic responses to environmental stimuli; absent or very limited interpersonal contact; manifestation of great anxiety and apparent fear when confronted with an unfamiliar situation, or even without evident stimulation; loss of already acquired elements of language; stereotypic hand movements, including especially "hand-washing" movements in front of the mouth or chest and rubbing motions of the hands; and repetitive blows on the teeth, grabbing of the tongue, and other movements. In addition, most patients develop seizures. Complex partial, atypical absence, generalized tonic or tonic-clonic, atonic, and/or myoclonic seizures occur in up to 80% of patients. After age 2 years, the EEG is typically abnormal, usually with a slow, poorly organized waking background. Some patients exhibit self-abusive behavior, such as chewing fingers and slapping the face (Trevathan and Moser 1988).

During the pseudostationary stage, most patients develop respiratory dysfunction, bruxism, truncal ataxia or apraxia with an unusual jerky quality, and early scoliosis. Many patients also have episodes of apnea during wakefulness. However, respiratory patterns are usually regular during sleep. The Rett's syndrome bruxism is an episodic creaking sound similar to that of a slowly uncorked wine bottle. Truncal ataxia sometimes presents at rest and can be exacerbated by physical stress. Neuromotor functions begin slowly, but steadily, to decline in most patients; however, 15%–20% of patients in this stage remain ambulatory (Hagberg 1989).

Most patients in the late motor deterioration stage present with tetraparetic weakness, muscle wasting, limb distortion, and severe scoliosis. The combination of lower motor neuron and basal ganglia dysfunction forces the patients into a wheelchair-dependent life. However, epilepsy in many Rett's syndrome patients spontaneously improves when they reach adulthood.

Etiology

Genetic factors. Because of the absence of males with the syndrome, it is unlikely that this syndrome is an acquired disease. The fact that probably less than 1% of Rett's syndrome cases are familial speaks in favor of a spontaneous mutation as the most common cause of Rett's syndrome. There is a report of a 100% concordance in eight sets of monozygotic twins and 0% concordance in six dizygotic twin pairs (Hagberg 1989). The available genetic data seem to suggest that Rett's syndrome is genetically determined and is consistent with the dominant X-linked mutation hypothesis with early spontaneous abortion of male fetuses.

Neuropathologic factors. Hagberg (1989) reported that mild gliosis was observed with no evidence of storage. Underpigmentation was observed in certain nigral structures; however, a normal number of nigral neurons were revealed with fewer melanin granules per neuron. The neuromelanin substructure was considered normal.

From the nine autopsy cases reported by Jellinger et al. (1988), there were consistent moderate diffuse cortical atrophy, underpigmentation of the zona compacta nigrae, decreased immunoreaction for prolactin and growth hormone in pituitary gland, increased beta-endorphins in thalamus and cerebellum, and general brain shrinkage with increasing age.

Neuroanatomical factors. Computed tomography scans have been reported as either normal or giving an appearance of cortical atrophy with enlarged sulci, suggesting the preferential involvement of gray matter. A magnetic resonance imaging study found frontal atrophy, corpus callosum hypoplasia, and widening of prepontine cistern and narrowing of the brain stem (see Nihei and Naitoh 1990).

Neurophysiologic factors. The EEG is abnormal in the majority of cases after age 2 years, although no specific abnormality has been described (Trevathan and Naidu 1988). During the second decade of life, paroxysmal abnormalities are less prominent, but the slow and somewhat poorly organized background abnormalities persist.

Neurochemistry. Nomura et al. (1987) believe that Rett's syndrome is a developmental monoamine deficiency disorder. Recently, Chatterjee et al. (1990) did two blind studies on the plasma glycosphingolipids in patients with Rett's syndrome, in patients with other developmental disorders, and in normal individuals from Baltimore, Maryland; Vienna, Austria; and Rostock, East Germany. An unusual glycosphingolipid was found in 70% of the patients with Rett's syndrome and in approximately 10% of the patients with other disorders. However, this glycosphingolipid was absent from the plasma of normal control subjects.

At the present time, there is no clear evidence that any biochemical abnormalities cause Rett's syndrome.

Summary of etiology. At present, it is unknown whether Rett's syndrome is a homogeneous disease or represents a heterogeneous group of conditions. Nonetheless, the data on concordance for Rett's syndrome in monozygotic twins and on discordance in dizygotic twins seem to indicate that Rett's syndrome is a genetically determined neurodegenerative disorder.

Treatment

Treating patients with Rett's syndrome requires that the child psychiatrist collaborate with allied disciplines and community agencies. The treatment plan will involve many levels.

Psychological. Family counseling should be provided to parents for careful explanation of the disorder and its prognosis, realistic expectation of the child, and resources for obtaining support. The child psychiatrist should pay special attention to the parents' level of emotional maturity and ability to accept the diagnosis and adjust to the problem. The parents should be given ongoing appraisals of the child's progress. Long-term counseling should also be planned. If the parents can no longer keep the child at home, the child psychiatrist should also help the parents select an alternative arrangement.

Education. The child psychiatrist should help parents to obtain special education (including pre-vocational and vocational training) and related services (e.g., physical therapy, special transportation to school) for their child with Rett's syndrome, as-

sist the parents in developing an individual educational plan for the child, and provide medical and psychiatric consultation to the classroom teacher.

Medical. Appropriate anticonvulsants should be given to children who develop epilepsy, which is common during the stagnation stage. Several investigators have reported that carbamazepine seems to be the most effective single anticonvulsant, especially in patients with a predominance of complex partial seizures (Trevathan and Naidu 1988). The medication should be carefully monitored. Most patients become wheelchair-bound during the late motor deterioration stage. General treatment should be directed toward correction of malnutrition, anemia, and electrolyte disturbances that may be caused by the patient's immobilized status. Exercises and physical therapy should be given to prevent muscle weakness and wasting. The skin over the coccyx and ischial tuberosities must be inspected daily.

Prognosis

Sudden, unexpected death of Rett's syndrome patients is not uncommon. However, the majority of Rett's syndrome patients survive at least into their 40s (Hagberg 1989).

Research Issues

There are few reports of males with Rett's syndrome. Further case studies are needed to investigate the genetic and metabolic etiologies of the syndrome.

Other Childhood Disintegrative Disorder

Definition and Diagnostic Criteria

Heller (1930) reported 28 cases of dementia in young children who had been entirely normal in development up to the age of 3 or 4 years. The term *dementia infantilis* was used to describe the disorder and is recognized as a syndrome (Heller's syndrome) in textbooks of pediatric neurology and child psychiatry.

Rutter et al. (1969) used the term *disintegrative*

psychosis of childhood to describe children with Heller's syndrome. The authors argued that most children with Heller's syndrome, after the initial process of disintegration, had remained static. Some even made small advances in social behavior by means of educational treatment. Only in a few cases was there progressive loss of intellectual capacity as seen in the various types of degenerative neurologic disorders. The diagnostic category of disintegrative psychosis of childhood has since been included in ICD-9, and it roughly follows Heller's account of dementia infantilis.

Disintegrative psychosis, however, was not included in either the DSM-III or DSM-III-R classifications of PDDs because it is viewed as a disorder that apparently is a nonspecific organic brain syndrome that consists of a dementia plus other behavioral abnormalities, such as rapid loss of language and social skills. This view has been criticized by Rutter (1985) as "an unjustified inference" because "there are well-reported cases of children with a clear cut clinical picture of disintegrative psychosis but without any unambiguous evidence of brain disease or damage" (p. 56). The ICD-10 draft classification uses the term *other childhood disintegrative disorder* as the diagnostic category and has defined the disorder as a type of PDD with a period of definitely normal development prior to the onset of the disorder; a definite phase of loss of previously acquired skills that extends across at least several areas of development; and the onset of characteristic abnormalities of social, communicative and behavioral functioning.

The draft of ICD-10 includes research diagnostic criteria for other childhood disintegrative disorder (Table 18-3). It is likely that this diagnostic category is rather heterogeneous and may include cases with disintegrative psychosis, Heller's syndrome (or dementia infantilis), and symbiotic psychosis. For the moment it seems highly desirable to retain it as a separate category so that the conditions can be identified for further study of the relationship between these conditions and other PDDs.

Clinical Findings

Individuals with disintegrative disorder demonstrate quite remarkable consistency in their clinical features. Characteristically, their general development usually is normal or near normal up to the age of 3 or 4 years. In most instances, without any obvious antecedent illness, these children become

Table 18-3. ICD-10 research diagnostic criteria for other childhood disintegrative disorder

A. An apparently normal development up to the age of at least two years. The presence of normal age-appropriate skills in communication, social relationships, play, and adaptive behavior at age two years or later is required for diagnosis.
B. A definite loss of previously acquired skills at about the time of onset of the disorder. The diagnosis requires a clinically significant loss of skills (and not just a failure to use them in certain situations) in at least two out of the following five areas:
  (1) expressive and/or receptive language;
  (2) play;
  (3) social skills and/or adaptive behavior;
  (4) bowel and/or bladder control;
  (5) motor skills.
C. Qualitatively abnormal social functioning. Diagnosis requires the demonstrable presence of abnormalities in any two of the following four groups:
  (1) qualitative impairments in reciprocal social interaction (of the type defined for autism);
  (2) qualitative impairment in communication (of the type defined for autism);
  (3) restricted, repetitive, and stereotyped patterns of behavior, interests, and activities including motor stereotypies and mannerisms;
  (4) a general loss of interest in objects and in the environment generally.
D. The disorder is not attributable to the other varieties of pervasive developmental disorder; acquired aphasia with epilepsy; elective mutism; schizophrenia; Rett's syndrome.

Source. Reprinted with permission from World Health Organization (1987).

anxious, irritable, negativistic, and disobedient, having frequent outbursts of temper without provocation and throwing their toys. In some cases, the disorder develops after measles, encephalitis, or some other clear-cut brain disease that damages the central nervous system (Rutter 1985). Over the course of a few months, these children have a complete loss of speech and language. There is impoverishment of comprehension of language as well as of cognitive function. They lose their social skills, and their interpersonal relationships are impaired. These children become disinterested in the environment. They also develop motor restlessness and stereotyped repetitive movements and mannerisms with grimacing and tics. During this regressive period, the children become incontinent and need to be fed. Functionally, all these children are severely mentally retarded, but in some cases there is retention of "islands" of relatively good abilities in some areas. General physical and neurologic examination usually reveals no abnormal physical signs. After the regression phase, the children are stable for many years. However, they are overactive with poor attention span, isolation, and obsessive behavior. Their comprehension of language is rather limited, as is their expressive language. However, they generally have relatively good motor abilities.

Differential Diagnosis

Millichap (1987) suggested that Rett's syndrome be regarded as a type of Heller's dementia (i.e., disintegrative disorders). Although both Rett's syndrome patients and most individuals with disintegrative disorder have a phase of deterioration or disintegration, only Rett's syndrome patients develop severe, lower motor neuron and basal ganglia dysfunction.

Epidemiology

Prevalence. Up to now, no detailed, large-scale epidemiologic studies have been carried out, so the exact prevalence of disintegrative disorder is unknown. It apparently is rare. The 10 cases identified in Volkmar and Cohen's (1989) study represent 6% of the larger sample of autistic individuals (also a rare group of people).

Sex ratio. There were eight boys and two girls in Evans-Jones and Rosenbloom's (1978) study. All 10 cases with disintegrative disorder in Volkmar and Cohen's (1989) study were males. It is clear that males predominate in disintegrative disorder.

Social class. This disorder does not seem to occur more frequently in any particular socioeconomic group.

Etiology

Stress factors. Evans-Jones and Rosenbloom (1978) reported that the deterioration often seemed to follow some life events, such as "sister's marriage," "mother's hospital admission," "birth of sibling," and so on. However, Rutter (1985) commented that these events were no more than the usual stresses that all children are subjected to at one time or another.

Birth complication factors. Evans-Jones and Rosenbloom (1978) reported no significant perinatal history in their series of cases. Volkmar and Cohen (1989) identified 10 cases who met ICD-10 draft criteria for disintegrative disorder. In 7 of the 10 cases, the pregnancy, labor, and delivery were unremarkable. In 2 cases, there was a history of threatened miscarriage, and in one case, general anesthesia was used for maternal surgery.

Genetic factors. Evans-Jones and Rosenbloom (1978) did not find any significant family history in their study. There was no preponderance of any particular socioeconomic group in their series of patients. Chromosome studies have not identified any abnormality (Volkmar and Cohen 1989).

Neuropathologic factors. Malamud (1959) reported a postmortem study that showed clear-cut evidence of cerebral degenerative disease suggestive of late infantile forms of cerebral lipoidosis. Creak (1963) also noted lipoidosis in two cases with disintegrative psychosis. Computed tomography scans were performed in 5 of the 10 patients of Volkmar and Cohen (1989) and were all normal.

Neurophysiologic factors. Evans-Jones and Rosenbloom (1978) studied 10 children with disintegrative psychosis. Abnormal EEGs were noted in 5 patients; however, there was no constant pattern. The EEGs of the patients in Hill and Rosenbloom's series (1986) were all normal. In Volkmar and Cohen's study (1989), EEGs were normal in 6 of the 10 cases, borderline in 2, and clearly abnormal in 2.

Summary of etiology. The form and course of the disintegrative disorders suggest there is an underlying basic neurologic dysfunction, but currently the etiology remains unknown in most of the cases.

Treatment

Psychological. Once the diagnosis is established, family counseling should be provided and aimed at relieving parents' guilt and minimizing the ambivalent feelings of the family members.

Educational. Educational and behavioral treatments are essential for controlling and minimizing aberrant behaviors as well as maximizing the potentials.

Medical. Children with disintegrative disorder require more general health care, including frequent clinic visits, proper diet and nutrition, prevention of infections, dental care, and physical fitness. Close neurologic monitoring and medical follow-up are essential in epileptic individuals receiving anticonvulsants. Medications such as haloperidol, benzodiazepines, and anticonvulsants have been used to modify behavior, but generally have not been effective. Psychotropic, antidepressant, and psychoactive medications should not be used to control "overactive behavior," "noisiness," "aggression," and "agitation" in persons with disintegrative disorder. However, these medications should be used to treat their concomitant psychiatric disorder.

Clinical Course and Prognosis

There is a strikingly uniform 6–9 months' duration of progressive loss of abilities. This is followed by a plateau and then a limited improvement. Hill and Rosenbloom (1986) reported a follow-up study of nine individuals with disintegrative psychosis followed for 11–16 years. Eight continued to fulfill the criteria necessary for a diagnosis of disintegrative psychosis. Two of the nine children developed grand mal seizures. However, none of the patients had shown continuing regression when reviewed 11–16 years later.

The prognosis of disintegrative disorder is usually very poor. In the cases with neurolipoidoses and leukodystrophies, there is progressive deterioration leading to death. In the other instances, the children remain without speech and are severely mentally retarded. They will remain wholly dependent individuals.

Research Issues

Future research should examine the prevalence of disintegrative disorder as well as compare its clinical course with that of late-onset autism. Any data that show significant differences between the two conditions will provide strong support of the taxonomic validity of disintegrative disorder.

References

American Psychiatric Association: Diagnostic and Statistical Manual of Mental Disorders, 3rd Edition. Washington, DC, American Psychiatric Association, 1980

American Psychiatric Association: Diagnostic and Statistical Manual of Mental Disorders, 3rd Edition, Revised. Washington, DC, American Psychiatric Association, 1987

American Psychiatric Association: Diagnostic and Statistical Manual of Mental Disorders, 4th Edition, First Draft. Washington, DC, American Psychiatric Association, 1991

Asperger H: Die autistischen psychopathen im kindesalter. Archiv für Psychiatrie und Nervenkrankheiten 117:76–136, 1944

Burd L, Fisher W, Kerbeshian J: A prevalence study of pervasive developmental disorders in North Dakota. Journal of the American Academy of Child Psychiatry 26:700–703, 1987

Chatterjee S, Ghosh N, Goh KM, et al: Glycosphingolipids in patients with the Rett syndrome. Brain Dev 23:85–87, 1990

Creak EM: Childhood psychosis: a review of 100 cases. Br J Psychiatry 109:84–89, 1963

Dahl EK, Cohen DJ, Provence S: Clinical and multivariate approaches to the nosology of pervasive developmental disorders. Journal of the American Academy of Child Psychiatry 25:170–180, 1986

Evans-Jones LG, Rosenbloom L: Disintegrative psychosis in childhood. Dev Med Child Neurol 20:462–470, 1978

Gillberg C: Autistic syndrome in Rett syndrome: the first two years according to mother reports. Brain Dev 9:499–501, 1987

Gillberg C: Asperger syndrome in 23 swedish children. Dev Med Child Neurol 31:520–531, 1989

Gillberg IC, Gillberg C: Asperger syndrome—some epidemiological considerations: a research note. J Child Psychol Psychiatry 30:631–638, 1989

Haas RH: The history and challenge of Rett syndrome. J Child Neurol 3(suppl):S3–S5, 1988

Hagberg BA: Rett syndrome: clinical peculiarities, diagnostic approach, and possible cause. Pediatr Neurol 5:75–83, 1989

Hagberg BA, Witt-Engerstrom I: Rett syndrome: a suggested staging system for describing impairment profile with increasing age toward adolescence. Am J Med Genet 24:47–59, 1986

Hagberg B, Witt-Engerstrom I: Early stage of the Rett syndrome and infantile neuronal ceroid lipofuscinosis: a difficult differential diagnosis. Brain Dev 12:20–22, 1990

Hagberg B, Goutieres F, Hanefeld F, et al: Rett syndrome: criteria for inclusion and exclusion. Brain Dev 7:372–373, 1985

Heller T: Uber Dementia infantalis. Zeitschrift für Kinderforschung 37:661–667, 1930. Reprinted in Howells JG (ed): Modern Perspectives in International Child Psychiatry. Edinburgh, Oliver & Boyd, 1979

Hill AE, Rosenbloom L: Disintegrative psychosis of childhood: teenage follow-up. Dev Med Child Neurol 28:34–40, 1986

Jellinger K, Armstrong D, Zoghbi HY, et al: Neuropathology of Rett syndrome. Acta Neuropathol (Berl) 76:142–158, 1988

Kanner L: Autistic disturbances of affective contact. Nervous Child 2:217–250, 1943

Kerr AM, Stephenson JBP: Rett's syndrome in the west of Scotland. Br Med J 291:579–582, 1985

Levine JM, Demb HB: Characteristics of preschool children diagnosed as having an atypical pervasive developmental disorder. J Dev Behav Pediatr 8:77–82, 1987

Malamud N: Heller's disease and childhood schizophrenia. Am J Psychiatry 116:215–218, 1959

Millichap JG: Rett syndrome: a variant of Heller's Dementia? Lancet 1:440, 1987

Nihei K, Naitoh H: Cranial computed tomographic and magnetic resonance imaging studies on the Rett syndrome. Brain Dev 12:101–105, 1990

Nomura Y, Honda K, Segawa M: Pathophysiology of Rett syndrome. Brain Dev 9:506–513, 1987

Olsson B, Rett A: Autism and Rett syndrome: behavioural investigations and differential diagnosis. Dev Med Child Neurol 29:429–441, 1987

Prior M, Perry D, Gajzago C: Kanner's syndrome or early onset psychosis: a taxonomic analysis of 142 cases. Journal of Autism and Childhood Schizophrenia 5:71–80, 1975

Rescorla L: Cluster analytic identification of autistic preschoolers. J Autism Dev Disord 18:475–492, 1988

Rett A: Ueber ein Cerebral-Atrophisches Syndrome bei Hyperammonamie. Vienna, Bruder Hollinek, 1966

Rutter M: Infantile autism and other pervasive developmental disorder, in Child and Adolescent Psychiatry. Edited by Rutter M, Hersov L. London, Blackwell, 1985, pp 545–566

Rutter M, Schopler E: Autism and pervasive developmental disorders: concepts and diagnostic issues. J Autism Dev Disord 17:159–186, 1987

Rutter M, Lebovici S, Eisenberg L, et al: A triaxial classification of mental disorder in childhood. J Child Psychol Psychiatry 10:41–61, 1969

Sparrow SS, Rescorla LA, Provence S, et al: Follow-up of "atypical" children: a brief report. Journal of the American Academy of Child Psychiatry 25:181–185, 1986

Szatmari P, Bremner R, Nagy J: Asperger's syndrome: a review of clinical features. Can J Psychiatry 34:554–560, 1989

Szatmari P, Tuff L, Finlayson MAJ, et al: Asperger's syndrome and autism: neurocognitive aspects. J Am Acad Child Adolesc Psychiatry 29:130–136, 1990

Trevathan E, Moser HW: Diagnostic criteria for Rett syndrome. Ann Neurol 23:425–428, 1988

Trevathan E, Naidu: The clinical recognition and differential diagnosis of Rett syndrome. J Child Neurol 3(suppl):S6–S16, 1988

Tsai LY: High-functioning autistic disorder: diagnostic issue, in High Functioning Individuals With Autism. Edited by Schopler E, Mesibov GB. New York, Plenum (in press)

Volkmar FR, Cohen DJ: Disintegrative disorder or "late onset" autism. J Child Psychol Psychiatry 30:717–724, 1989

Wing L: Asperger's syndrome: a clinical account. Psychol Med 11:115–129, 1981

Wing L, Gould J: Severe impairments of social interaction and association abnormalities in children: epidemiology and classification. J Autism Dev Disord 9:11–30, 1979

World Health Organization: International Classification of Diseases, 10th Edition, Draft Version. Geneva, World Health Organization, 1987

Chapter 19

Developmental Disorders of Language and Learning

Carl Feinstein, M.D.
Ann Aldershof, Sc.B., Ph.D.

The presence of a language disorder or a learning disability can have a major adverse impact on the development of children and adolescents. Furthermore, the high prevalence and multiple adverse consequences of these disabilities constitute a major public health and public policy concern. U.S. Department of Education data for the 1985–1986 school year revealed that 4.73% of all students in the United States were diagnosed as learning disabled and were served under Public Law 94-142 (Silver 1989). The U.S. Interagency Committee on Learning Disabilities estimated the actual prevalence rate of learning disabilities in United States students to be 5%–10% (Silver 1989). The prevalence rate for language disorders is similar, ranging from 6% to 15%, depending on the age of the population (Beitchman et al. 1986; Silva 1987).

Although much of the available literature treats language and learning disabilities as two different entities, this distinction is somewhat arbitrary. Follow-up of preschool language-disordered children reveals that many are later diagnosed as learning disabled during the school-age years (Aram and Hall 1989; Baker and Cantwell 1987; Silva 1987; Stevenson et al. 1985). Conversely, many children di-

agnosed at school age as learning disabled are found to have an underlying language disorder (Fundudis et al. 1979; Silva 1987; Stevenson and Richman 1978). Finally, numerous specific cognitive deficits occur in various combinations in both learning-disabled and language-disordered children (Mattis et al. 1975; Morris et al. 1986; Nussbaum et al. 1986).

According to DSM-III-R (American Psychiatric Association 1987), both language and learning disorders occur more frequently in boys than in girls, at a ratio of 3 or 4 to 1. However, when girls have these problems, the impairment and psychosocial consequences are at least as serious as they are for boys (Baker and Cantwell 1987). There are accumulating data indicating that the total number of children with language and learning problems is increasing, due to subtle central nervous system sequelae in some high-risk infants and children with serious childhood illnesses, whose lives have been spared by advances in medical technology (Duane 1979; Waber 1989).

The child and adolescent psychiatrist plays a critical role in the assessment and treatment of language- and learning-disabled children. A substantial body of research documents both that these disabilities persist over many years, and that children with these conditions have a greatly increased risk for psychiatric disorder (Beitchman et al. 1986; Cantwell and Baker 1977; Rutter 1987). Effective treatment of language- or learning-disabled children, as well as secondary prevention of psychiatric disorder, requires coordinated multidisciplinary inter-

This work was supported by Child and Adolescent Mental Health Academic Award 1K07MH00766 from the National Institute of Mental Health. Additional support was provided by Program Project NS 20489 from the National Institute of Neurologic Diseases and Strokes, U.S. Public Health Service.

vention (Silver and Hagin 1989). This includes cognitive and educational remediation, psychotherapeutic approaches, and measures to strengthen the family's ability to support the child's optimal development. Effective participation by the child and adolescent psychiatrist in this multidisciplinary setting requires a working familiarity with the concepts and procedures of pediatric neurology, speech and language pathology, neuropsychological assessment, and special education programming. Yet despite the involvement of these many disciplines, there are major gaps in current knowledge regarding phenomenology, classification, pathogenesis, and natural history of language and learning disabilities. The various causal relationships of language and learning disabilities to psychiatric disorders are difficult to elucidate, and the outcome of different intervention programs is unclear and insufficiently documented.

Language and speech disorders and learning disabilities (academic skills disorders) are classified as developmental disorders and are included in DSM-III-R Axis II as specific developmental disorders. According to DSM-III-R, specific developmental disorders "are characterized by inadequate development of specific academic, language, speech, and motor skills . . . that are not due to demonstrable physical or neurologic disorders, a Pervasive Developmental Disorder, Mental Retardation, or deficient educational opportunities" (American Psychiatric Association 1987, pp 39–40). When more than one specific developmental disorder is present, all are diagnosed, even when one is thought to be caused by another. The DSM-III-R classification of specific developmental disorders is best viewed as the current nosologic status of these conditions, rather than as a fully worked out nosology (Shaffer et al. 1989).

Developmental Language Disorders

Definition

Developmental language disorders are defined by DSM-III-R as impairments in the production or understanding of language, which is not the result of intellectual, sensory, or emotional disorders (American Psychiatric Association 1987, p. 47). Other specific exclusion criteria are pervasive developmental disorder, hearing defect, or neurologic disorder. DSM-III-R delineates two separate de-

velopmental language disorders: developmental receptive language disorder and developmental expressive language disorder. Additionally, it includes the diagnostic category of developmental articulation disorder, which is, theoretically, a disorder of motor speech rather than language. The DSM-III-R diagnostic criteria for the developmental language disorders are given in Table 19-1.

This classification scheme is comprehensive in that it covers the sending and receiving dimensions of communication. However, it does not address the individual components of linguistic functioning, such as phonology, morphology, syntax, semantics, or pragmatics, that are actually impaired in these disorders. Proper understanding of these linguistic components is required to interpret formalized assessment approaches meaningfully. Here, the definition of language disorders provided by the American Speech-Language-Hearing Association (1982) applies:

> A language disorder is the impairment or deviant development of comprehension and/or use of a spoken, written, and/or other symbol system. The disorder may involve (1) the form of language (phonologic, morphologic, and syntactic systems), (2) the content of language (semantic system), and/or (3) the function (use) of language in communication (pragmatic system) in any combination. The subsystems of language currently are thought to be phonology, morphology, syntax, semantics, and pragmatics. (p. 949)

History

The concept of developmental language disorder has evolved in the past century as the result of contributions from many disciplines. Significant early advances came from neurologists who recognized similarities between childhood language disorders and adult aphasias and coined the term *congenital aphasia* (Landau et al. 1960). This idea was modified by developmentalists who argued that delayed or deviant language development in young children had different implications for brain pathophysiology than the loss of previously acquired functions (Rapin and Allen 1988). This, in turn, led to new neurologically based terms and concepts to account for childhood language problems, such as *developmental dysphasia* (Benton 1978; Zangwill 1987). By the mid-1900s, speech and language pathologists suggested that a variety of receptive auditory processing deficits were implicated in childhood language disorders (Rees 1973; Tallal and Piercy

Table 19-1. DSM-III-R diagnostic criteria for developmental language disorders

Developmental receptive language disorder

A. The score obtained from a standardized measure of receptive language is substantially below that obtained from a standardized measure of nonverbal intellectual capacity (as determined by an individually administered IQ test).

B. The disturbance in A significantly interferes with academic achievement or activities of daily living requiring the comprehension of verbal (or sign) language. This may be manifested in more severe cases by an inability to understand simple words or sentences. In less severe cases, there may be difficulty in understanding only certain types of words, such as spatial terms, or an inability to comprehend longer or more complex statements.

C. Not due to pervasive developmental disorder, defect in hearing acuity, or a neurologic disorder (aphasia).

Developmental expressive language disorder

A. The score obtained from a standardized measure of expressive language is substantially below that obtained from a standardized measure of nonverbal intellectual capacity (as determined by an individually administered IQ test).

B. The disturbance in A significantly interferes with academic achievement or activities of daily living requiring the expression of verbal (or sign) language. This may be evidenced in severe cases by use of a markedly limited vocabulary, by speaking only in simple sentences, or by speaking only in the present tense. In less severe cases, there may be hesitations or errors in recalling certain words, or errors in the production of long or complex sentences.

C. Not due to a pervasive developmental disorder, defect in hearing acuity, or a neurologic disorder (aphasia).

Developmental articulation disorder

A. Consistent failure to use developmentally expected speech sounds. For example, in a three-year-old, failure to articulate p, b, and t, and in a six-year-old, failure to articulate r, sh, th, f, z, and l.

B. Not due to a pervasive developmental disorder, mental retardation, defect in hearing acuity, disorders of the oral speech mechanism, or a neurologic disorder.

Source. Reprinted with permission from the American Psychiatric Association (1987).

1978; Wiig and Semel 1976), which led to new terminology, such as *congenital auditory imperception* (Worster-Drought and Allen 1929), and *congenital auditory agnosia* (Karlin 1951). More recently, interest has shifted to determining types of develop-

mental language disorder in children empirically by studying differential patterns of delays and deficits in large groups of children with diverse language problems (Aram and Nation 1975; Wolfus et al. 1980).

Etiology and Pathogenesis

The etiology of developmental language disorders is generally believed to be biological, resulting from genetic and perinatal factors (Rapin 1988; Taylor and Fletcher 1983; Vohr et al. 1988). Increasing evidence from pedigree research supports the hypothesis of a genetic component in at least some types of language disorder (Tallal et al. 1989; Tomblin 1989).

Two very general but somewhat contradictory models of developmental pathogenesis for developmental language disorder are current in clinical psychiatry. The first views childhood language problems as nonspecific developmental delays in language, presumably resulting from early brain insult (Ingram 1976; Rutter 1982). This model, which has exerted the greatest influence on DSM-III-R, is relatively less concerned with the specific phenomenology of linguistic deficits or with neurolinguistically based subtyping. The second model, which has substantial multidisciplinary support, focuses on specific syndromes of neurocognitive deficits, auditory processing problems, and linguistic impairment found in children with developmental language disorder (Heywood and Canavan 1987; Rapin and Allen 1988; Tallal and Piercy 1978).

Numerous studies have found abnormalities in brain structure or function in at least some children with language deficits (Gordon 1987; Heywood and Canavan 1987; Taylor and Fletcher 1983). However, there is a wide range of views as to what constitutes evidence of a neurologic abnormality in given cases. Some consider the presence of language defects to be prima facie evidence of cortical dysfunction (Eisenson 1968). Some cite increased rates of neurologic "soft signs" (Denckla 1977; Shaffer et al. 1983), whereas others insist on "hard" findings from the sensorimotor neurologic examination as the only basis for evidence of neuropathology (Taylor and Fletcher 1983). Clearly, studies of neurologic etiology depend on the standard of evidence for neurologic impairment. Brain visualization and neurophysiologic techniques provide additional supportive, but not conclusive, evidence for a neurologic etiology. A variety of abnormalities have been reported in language-disordered children. These include computed tomography findings of abnormal brain morphology, nonspecific electroencephalographic abnormalities, and abnormal brain-stem auditory evoked responses (Lou et al. 1984; Piggott and Anderson 1983; Taylor and Fletcher 1983). However, whether these nonspecific neurologic findings indicate delayed neurologic maturation or specific, permanent neurologic deficit is still unclear (Bishop and Edmundson 1987; Rapin 1988).

Clinical Presentation and Diagnosis

Many children with developmental language disorders are first referred for a speech-language or psychological evaluation, finding their way to the child psychiatrist only if emotional or behavioral problems occur. The linguistic phenomena that lead to these referrals are quite variable, depending on the type of linguistic deficit and the age of the child. For toddlers and preschoolers, primary considerations include whether the child speaks at all, the number of words in the child's spoken vocabulary and their intelligibility, whether the child understands simple directions, and the child's ability to name objects. For school-age children, problems in the comprehension, formulation, and spoken expression of the syntactically and semantically more complex material required to function successfully at school are more common causes of referral. For teenagers, the issue is more likely to be the ability to formulate or comprehend abstract ideas, complex instructions, or metaphoric expressions in spoken or written language. Given both the dramatic changes in language capacities in very young children and the greatly increased complexity of the phenomena being evaluated, it is not surprising that nonspecialist clinicians are more likely to suspect a language disorder in the very young child than in the older child, unless the deficits for the older child are quite profound.

Children with receptive developmental language disorders show deficits in expression as well as in comprehension of language. As a result, this form of language disorder is more socially disabling and severe (D. Cohen et al. 1979). In its most severe form, specific receptive developmental language disorder involves an inability to comprehend even simple sentences, which may stem from a deficit in integrating auditory symbols (Richardson 1989). Children with expressive developmental language

disorders generally have good understanding of language but difficulty using it to communicate. Very young children with this disorder may have no speech at all. Other children will tend to use developmentally earlier forms of language; to speak in shorter, more telegraphic sentences; and to rely heavily on contextual cues and nonverbal communication. These children tend to make syntactic or semantic errors in sentence construction. Word finding difficulties may result in circumlocutions, reliance on jargon, or word substitutions (Richardson 1989). These problems result in speech that appears awkward, incoherent, or unintelligible. Adolescents with developmental language disorders may have special difficulty with the appropriate uses of language. For example, they may fail to tailor their communication to the listener's needs and status.

Language Assessment by the Psychiatrist

In view of the high comorbidity of language deficits and psychiatric disorders, the child psychiatrist should routinely take a careful history of language development and assess the current level of linguistic functioning. A useful preliminary evaluation can be done in the context of the clinical interview and mental status examination, prior to any referral for specialized language evaluations. Specific areas that the clinician should observe include inner language, comprehension, production, phonation, and pragmatics (Rutter 1987).

Inner language refers to the use of symbolization in the child's thought and can be most easily evaluated in younger children by observing play behavior for evidence of symbolic play, such as using a block for a truck (Rutter 1987). Language comprehension should be evaluated in terms of the child's ability to follow commands without gestures, to answer questions both relevant to the situation and out of context, to follow conversation, to understand abstract language, and to draw inferences. Language production involves an assessment of the amount of speech produced, fluency, and intelligibility. Additionally, specific components of the content to be evaluated are morphology (use of inflectional endings and functor words), syntax (word order, use of pronouns, and verb tense), and semantics (range of vocabulary). Phonation refers to the quality of the child's voice and includes pitch, volume, quality, intonation, and prosody (melody of speech). Pragmatic language involves the child's ability to use language for effective communication. This is evaluated by observing the child's ability to take into account the perspective of his or her conversational partner. It includes the child's adherence to social conventions for eye contact, gestures, and both verbal and nonverbal cues. It further involves the child's ability to sustain conversation, maintain a shared topic, and take turns in a dialogue. Finally, an assessment should be made of the age-appropriate comprehension and use of idiomatic expressions and metaphoric language.

Formal Cognitive and Linguistic Assessment

The assessment of cognitive abilities requires psychometric testing, which should not be limited to an intelligence test. Although an overall measure of intelligence is essential, it will not provide the specificity nor sensitivity to detect or delineate many linguistic deficits. Table 19-2 provides a list of linguistic and psychological tests.

Diagnosis

The diagnostic reasoning process involves two steps. First, a discrepancy between language skills and intelligence must be established. Then, each of the factors mentioned as exclusionary criteria is assessed to eliminate it as an explanation for the discrepancy. Developmental language disorders share symptoms with a number of other disorders, making a complete multidisciplinary assessment essential to establishing the diagnosis. Diagnoses to be ruled out include hearing impairment, mental deficiency, autism, developmental articulation disorder, and childhood aphasia. Traditionally, children with low scores on both verbal and nonverbal intelligence tests have been labeled mentally retarded. However, research suggests that developmental language disorders occur in mentally retarded individuals (D. Cohen et al. 1986; Rondal 1987). These children should receive both diagnoses if language function is impaired beyond what can be accounted for by the retardation.

Generally, the dramatic social deficits of infantile autism usefully distinguish it from developmental language disorder. However, children with severe combined receptive-expressive language impairment may also show grossly impaired communicative abilities, motoric stereotypies, so-cial awkwardness, resistance to change, and other symptoms (D. Cohen et al. 1979). Nevertheless, these children show greater awareness of affect and engage more in reciprocal social interaction and symbolic play than do autistic children (Allen et al. 1988). The quality of the language-disordered child's speech differs from that of the autistic child's speech in that the latter's is most commonly characterized by echolalia, perseveration, poor pragmatics, or lack of emotional inflection.

Developmental articulation disorder should be diagnosed in cases where the unintelligibility of the speech derives from poor articulation rather than from semantic or syntactic errors (Richardson 1989). Childhood aphasia is the appropriate diagnosis for children whose language is lost or diminished as the result of acquired neuropathology, trauma, or seizure disorder. This condition is not common in childhood, when most speech loss is transient (Dennis and Whitaker 1976).

Relationship to Psychiatric Disorder

A wide range of emotional and behavioral disorders have been described in children and adolescents with developmental language disorders. These may be emotional reactions to the linguistic deficit, symptoms of concomitant psychiatric disorders, or manifestations of a common underlying neurologic substrate (Cantwell and Baker 1977). Younger children have been noted to show signs of impulsivity, inattentiveness, aggressivity, lack of self-confidence, low frustration tolerance, anxiety, and social immaturity (Cantwell and Baker 1987; Love and Thompson 1988; Rutter 1977). Emotional problems often occur in adolescence when socialization skills are language based (Shapiro 1985) and include anxiety, compulsiveness, withdrawal, aggressiveness, and rigidity (Bergman 1987).

The incidence of psychopathology (diagnosed using DSM-III-R) seen in speech and language clinics is reported to be approximately 50% (Butler et al. 1973; Cantwell and Baker 1987; Stevenson and Richman 1978). Conversely, studies of psychiatric populations suggest that approximately half of the children seen in psychiatric settings have language disorders, which are often too subtle to be detected without specialized evaluations (Chess and Rosenberg 1974; N. Cohen et al. 1989; Gualtieri et al. 1983).

Table 19-2.   Linguistic and psychological tests

Test	Ages	Functions assessed
Language tests		
Batteries		
Sequenced Inventory of Communication Development (SICD)	0-4–4-0	Sound discrimination, auditory memory, receptive and expressive language
Test of Early Language Development (TELD)	3-0–7-11	Receptive and expressive language; oral and pointing responses
Test of Language Development (TOLD)	4-0–9-0	Auditory discrimination and memory, receptive and expressive language; oral and pointing responses
Test of Adolescent Language (TOAL)	11-0–17-5	Receptive and expressive language; oral and written responses
Clinical Evaluation of Language Function (CELF)	5-0–17-0	Screening test for auditory memory, receptive and expressive language; oral responses
Tests of specific functions		
Peabody Picture Vocabulary Test (PPVT)	1-9–18-0	Receptive auditory vocabulary; pointing to pictures
Token Test	3-0–12-0	Receptive auditory syntax; following verbal instructions
Goldman-Fristoe-Woodcock Auditory Selective Attention Test	3-0–12-0	Auditory memory; pointing to pictures
Goldman-Fristoe-Woodcock Test of Auditory Discrimination	3-0 to adult	Auditory discrimination of words; pointing to pictures
Expressive One Word Vocabulary Test (EOWVT)	3-0–12-0	Expressive vocabulary; picture naming
Arizona Articulation Proficiency Scale	3-0–11-0	Speech articulation; picture naming
Neuropsychological tests		
Batteries		
Halstead-Reitan Neuropsychologic Battery (HRNB)	9-0–14-0	Sensory-perceptual and sensorimotor skills; sustained attention, abstraction, concept formation
and Reitan-Indiana Neuropsychological Battery	5-0–8-0	
Tests of specific functions		
Beery-Buktenica Visual Motor Integration Test	1-9–15-11	Visual-motor perception test; copying geometric figures
Raven's Progressive Matrices	6-0 to adult	Nonverbal reasoning; choosing picture that best completes pattern or series
Leiter International Performance Scale	2-0–18-0	Nonverbal measure of perception, discrimination, and reasoning; moving blocks
Wisconsin Card Sorting Test (WCST)	8-0 to adult	Concept formation; flexibility in thinking, reasoning

(continued)

Table 19-2. (Continued)

Test	Ages	Functions assessed
General intelligence tests		
Bayley Scales of Infant Development	0-2–2-6	Psychomotor and mental development
Cattell Infant Intelligence Scale	0-3–2-6	Mental development
Batteries		
Kaufman Assessment Battery for Children (K-ABC)	2-6–12-5	Sequential and simultaneous processing, factual knowledge, and nonverbal reasoning
Wechsler Preschool and Primary Scale of Intelligence (WPPSI), and	4-0–6-0	Verbal and nonverbal intelligence
Wechsler Intelligence Scale for Children—Revised (WISC-R)	6-0–16-11	
Stanford-Binet Intelligence Scale	2-0–18-0	Verbal skills; nonverbal reasoning, memory
Educational achievement test batteries		
Wide Range Achievement Test (WRAT)	5-0–18-0	Reading, writing, spelling
Peabody Individual Achievement Test (PIAT)	5-0–18-0	Reading, math, spelling, general information
Woodcock-Johnson Psychoeducational Battery	3-0 to adult	Reading, spelling, writing, and all academic subjects

Treatment

There are two types of approaches to the remediation of language disorders. These are often used together. One approach is to focus on the deficient component of language and use various remedial techniques to increase skills (Hegde 1988). A second approach is to build on the child's strengths, effectively circumventing the language deficit (Schiefelbusch and Lloyd 1988). Interventions are designed to promote learning by bringing other modalities of input (e.g., visual) to bear and to increase the frequency of the child's effective communicative behaviors (Garcia and DeHaven 1974). Language therapy is increasingly designed to take place in relevant social environments where the focus is on functional language in transactional contexts (Schiefelbusch and Lloyd 1988).

Prognosis and Natural History

Most children with developmental language disorders speak by the time they are school age. However, more subtle but highly significant language deficits persist for many of these children. A 10-year systematic prospective study of children with developmental language disorders as preschoolers (Aram et al. 1984) found that only 30% of these children had a normal academic course. The rest had either repeated a grade or were in special education classes. Follow-up language testing of these children revealed that 62% had significantly below-average language scores. In language-disordered children, development of learning disability and psychiatric disorder are highly correlated (Baker and Cantwell 1987). Another follow-up study (Hall and Tomblin 1978) comparing children with developmental language disorders and those with articulation disorders found that the language-disorder group had more communication problems, academic difficulties, and behavior problems than did the articulation-disorder group. Indicators of poorer prognosis for language-disordered children include comprehension more impaired than expression (Gordon 1987), poor social skills (Rutter and Lord 1987), low IQ, psychopathology, and motor problems (Bashir et al. 1987).

Critical Review of Issues

Although significant progress has been made in the field of developmental language disorders, current concepts require further study to determine their validity and usefulness. In particular, there are major unsolved operational problems in making the diagnosis of developmental language disorder by simply identifying a discrepancy between measures of intelligence and measures of language functioning. While this discrepancy is typically established on the basis of test scores, there is lack of agreement in the field about which tests should be used for this purpose. There is also no consensus about which aspects of language are essential to the diagnosis. Similarly, controversy exists over how many linguistic capacities must be deficient and to what degree (Aram and Morris 1991). Unsolved issues exist concerning how large the discrepancy between language and nonverbal intelligence scores must be for diagnosis. Although one standard deviation has been traditionally used, this informal clinical practice has not been empirically validated. An important issue in test score interpretation is whether poor performance on language tasks represents a developmental delay as opposed to deviant or deficient language mechanisms. Although considerable individual variation exists in the attainment of language milestones, there is a paucity of clear guidelines as to how large a delay is pathologic. If language delay is part of a broader picture of developmental immaturity, it becomes particularly difficult to distinguish "normal variability" from neurologically based pathology (Beitchman 1985).

Most significantly, it is difficult to interpret the relationship between performance on language and other cognitive tests, because we lack a comprehensive, empirically validated neurologic model relating the many elements of cognitive and linguistic functioning. Even without resorting to strictly neurologic mechanisms, students of cognitive development point out that the acquisition of linguistic and that of cognitive functions are dynamically interrelated. Thus the meaning of a discrepancy between linguistic and other cognitive capacities is unclear. In fact, numerous studies suggest that many, if not all, children diagnosed as having developmental language disorder have other cognitive impairments, including attentional, memory, and conceptual deficits (Cromer 1987; Johnston and Smith 1989).

Developmental Articulation Disorders

Developmental articulation disorder describes the inability to produce certain speech sounds correctly at the appropriate age. As with the other developmental disorders, the symptoms must not be secondary to pervasive developmental disorder, mental retardation, impairment of the oral speech mechanism, or neurologic-sensory deficit. The DSM-III-R criteria for developmental articulation disorder are listed in Table 19-1. According to these criteria, the diagnosis is made by considering articulatory proficiency relative to age as well as the consistency of any deficit. As suggested by these diagnostic criteria, the primary clinical finding in a child who has developmental articulation disorder is decreased intelligibility of speech production in the context of normal sentence production and comprehension. Typically, the child's speech sounds immature. There is wide variation in the degree of intelligibility of children with this disorder. Many of these children have associated nonlinguistic findings, including neurologic soft signs, enuresis, developmental coordination disorder, and learning disabilities (Cantwell and Baker 1987). Approximately one-third of children with developmental articulation disorder have diagnosable psychiatric problems, commonly attention-deficit disorder or anxiety disorders (Baker and Cantwell 1982, 1985).

Developmental articulation disorders are estimated to affect 15% of children; 10% of children below age 8 and 5% of children above age 8 present with this condition (American Psychiatric Association 1987, p. 45). The disorder is more common in boys, affecting 6% of males and 3% of females. The etiology of developmental articulation disorders is unknown. Important contributing factors that have been suggested are mild hearing impairment, cognitive deficits, and faulty familial speech models (Winitz 1969). Defective auditory discrimination may impair language acquisition and may play an important role in articulation disorders (Locke 1980). Such auditory perceptual deficits could result from delayed maturation of neural substrates of the auditory system (Chase 1972). Treatment involves individual or group speech therapy, which is widely available in public school systems and reported to be quite effective (Johnson 1980). Spontaneous recovery often occurs by 8 years of age and may be hastened by the appropriate therapy. Poorer prognoses are mostly seen in children with co-occurring problems, such as stuttering or hypernasality (Johnson 1980).

Learning Disabilities

Definition

Learning disabilities are currently termed *academic skills disorder* by DSM-III-R and are defined as impairments in an academic area (i.e., reading, arithmetic, or expressive writing) that are not due to mental retardation, inadequate schooling, a vision or hearing defect, or a neurologic disorder. Each of the academic skills disorders has the same general definition, differing only in the specific capacity that is deficient. The criteria for each academic skills disorder are presented in Table 19-3. Several changes in the definition and diagnosis of academic skills disorders are being considered for DSM-IV (Shaffer et al. 1989). The name *academic skills disorders* may be changed to *learning disorders*. Two new diagnostic entities may be grouped within the learning disorders section: simple attention-deficit disorder and social skills learning disorder. Finally, the diagnostic criteria are being reexamined with regard to the role of psychological testing for delineating underlying cognitive impairments.

U.S. Public Law 94-142 (United States Congress 1975), a statute that profoundly affects referrals and programming for learning-disabled children, defines children with learning disorders in the following way:

> Those children who have a disorder in one or more of the basic psychological processes involved in understanding or in using language, spoken or written, which disorder may manifest itself in an imperfect ability to listen, think, speak, read, write, spell, or do math calculations. The term includes such conditions as perceptual handicaps, brain injury, minimal brain dysfunction, dyslexia, and developmental aphasia. The term does not include children having learning problems which are primarily the result of visual, hearing, or motor handicaps, of mental retardation, of emotional disturbances, or of environmental, cultural, or economic disadvantage. (Silver 1989, p. 309)

There are significant differences between the American Psychiatric Association (1987) definition and Public Law 94-142. Public Law 94-142 includes only children of normal intelligence,

Table 19-3.   DSM-III-R diagnostic criteria for specific developmental academic disorders

Developmental reading disorder
A. Reading achievement, as measured by a standardized, individually administered test, is markedly below the expected level, given the person's schooling and intellectual capacity (as determined by an individually administered IQ test).
B. The disturbance in A significantly interferes with academic achievement or activities of daily living requiring reading skills.
C. Not due to a defect in visual or hearing acuity or a neurologic disorder.

Developmental expressive writing disorder
A. Writing skills, as measured by a standardized, individually administered test, are markedly below the expected level, given the person's schooling and intellectual capacity (as determined by an individually administered IQ test).
B. The disturbance in A significantly interferes with academic achievement or activities of daily living requiring the composition of written texts (spelling words and expressing thoughts in grammatically correct sentences and organized paragraphs).
C. Not due to a defect in visual or hearing acuity or a neurologic disorder.

Developmental arithmetic disorder
A. Arithmetic skills, as measured by a standardized, individually administered test, are markedly below the expected level, given the person's schooling and intellectual capacity (as determined by an individually administered IQ test).
B. The disturbance in A significantly interferes with academic achievement or activities of daily living requiring arithmetic skills.
C. Not due to a defect in visual or hearing acuity or a neurologic disorder.

Source.   Reprinted with permission from the American Psychiatric Association (1987).

whereas the DSM-III-R definition allows for mentally retarded children with uneven cognitive profiles. The DSM-III-R definition excludes children whose learning problem is due to a neurologic disorder, whereas Public Law 94-142 encompasses brain injury and dysfunction.

History

Case studies of learning-disabled children appeared as early as 1896 with an article by Morgan. An early theoretical explanation for learning disabilities was offered by Orton (1928), who proposed that the problem was a lack of cerebral dominance. In the 1950s, Cruickshank (1967) studied a group of children with perceptual disabilities, attention deficit, poor motor coordination, and impulsivity. Because of their behavioral similarity to brain-damaged children, these children were described as having "minimal brain damage," despite the absence of any clear evidence of frank neurologic problems.

By the early 1960s, the concept of brain damage gave way to the notion of brain dysfunction or immaturity. Clements and Peters (1962) coined the term *minimal brain dysfunction* to describe a syndrome with a variety of features, including specific learning deficits, perceptual-motor problems, incoordination, hyperkinesis, impulsivity, equivocal neurologic signs, and abnormal electroencephalogram (EEG). Concurrently, the term *specific learning disability* was applied to describe the same population of children (Farnham-Diggory 1978). While these formulations implied an organic component, traditional sensorimotor neurologic examinations tended to be nonrevealing. During the 1970s, attention was focused on the attentional deficits in children thought to have minimal brain dysfunction. However, it became increasingly clear that use of stimulant medication significantly reduced hyperactivity and improved attention, but had no effect on specific learning problems (Gittelman 1983; Silver 1986). Neurologists became increasingly involved with this population, who were believed to have underlying brain dysfunction. However, the motor and sensory neurologic examinations did not adequately address the higher cortical functions presumed to be impaired in the learning disabled (Kinsbourne 1973). Despite the evident discontinuity between what is measured in the neurologic examination and the cognitive problems manifested in learning disabilities, the inability to identify "hard" neurologic signs in many learning-disabled children continues to impede progress in establishing the role of the central nervous system in learning disorders. Increasingly, neuropsychological and linguistic tests are being thought of as extensions of the neurologic examination, aiding in the identification of possible neurologic abnormalities in referred children.

Etiology and Pathogenesis

The etiology of developmental learning disorders is unknown but presumed to include a variety of neurocortical deficits, areas of neurologic dysfunction resulting in various disruptions of cognitive processing. It is likely that there are subtypes of each one of the "academic skills disorders," each reflecting a different etiology (Hynd et al. 1988; Lyon 1983; Morris 1988; Nussbaum et al. 1986). For example, cognitive deficits may result from either visual-spatial or linguistic processing problems, each of which presumably has a different neuroanatomical substrate.

Neurologic abnormalities in regions associated with language function (i.e., left hemisphere, particularly the peri-Sylvian region) have been reported and suggest a neurologic substrate in reading disorders. Specifically, Galaburda et al. (1985) described cortical ectopias and dysplasias in the left hemispheres, particularly in the peri-Sylvian area, of reading-disabled children. Another neuroanatomical anomaly reported in dyslexic children is the lack of increased size of the planum temporale area of the left hemisphere (Haslam et al. 1981; Rumsey et al. 1986) normally seen in most people. Electrophysiologic evidence from electroencephalographic and brain electrical activity mapping (Duffy et al. 1980) studies revealed differences in left hemisphere functioning of dyslexic children during various linguistic tasks. Similarly, a study of regional cerebral blood flow during a semantic classification task revealed that dyslexic subjects had larger asymmetries (left greater than right) than control subjects during performance of this task (Rumsey et al. 1987). In some cases, these postulated neurologic deficits may be genetically based, suggested by results of studies of family history (Shepherd et al. 1989), twin concordance rates (Vandenburg et al. 1986), and chromosome linkages (Smith et al. 1983).

Clinical Presentation

Clinically, learning-disabled children present with poor achievement in the academic area(s) of their disorder relative to their intelligence. Children with developmental reading disorder have poor reading ability often combined with spelling problems, poor writing, speech delay, or dyspraxia. Symptoms vary with IQ level; children with higher IQs show fewer neurologic signs and fewer symptoms of motor and language disorders (Shepherd et al. 1989). In general, many learning-disabled children have difficulty with active information processing (Torgeson 1982), which may manifest as difficulty in developing strategies for organizing, prioritizing, rehearsing, or presenting information, especially when it is linguistically based. In many cases, by the time a child is referred for evaluation, he or she is not only doing poorly in academic performance but is also lacking in the basic learning skills that are necessary to comprehend or master the more advanced material.

Often, a negative emotional cycle develops in which poor self-esteem, anxiety, alienation, or rebellion further interfere with the child's ability to participate effectively in school. As is the case with developmental language disorder, the rate of concurrent psychiatric disorder is high in learning-disabled children and adolescents (Glosser and Koppell 1987; Hunt and Cohen 1984; McConaughy and Ritter 1986). Attention-deficit disorders are reported to occur in 20% of the learning-disabled population (Halperin et al. 1984; Shaywitz and Shaywitz 1989). In fact, it is quite common that children who are ultimately diagnosed as learning disabled present initially with emotional or behavioral problems. Relative or absolute failure in school, a major developmental arena for the child and adolescent, is a major risk factor for psychiatric disorder (Offord and Waters 1983; Rutter and Giller 1983).

Diagnosis

Technically, the DSM-based diagnosis of a specific academic disorder is not predicated on school performance, but rather on standardized educational achievement testing. Thus, from the most narrow perspective, a psychiatric assessment is not required when a child with obvious academic difficulties is referred for evaluation. From the point of view of the public educational system (U.S. Public Law 94-142), a psychiatric evaluation is indicated only when it is necessary to address the exclusionary criteria of emotional disturbance as a causative factor. However, in view of the high rate of emotional or behavioral problems in learning-disabled children, the child and adolescent psychiatrist must remain vigilant to the possibility that youngsters referred for psychiatric evaluation of emotional or behavioral problems might also have an undiscovered learning disability.

As with developmental language disorders, the diagnosis of developmental academic disorder is made by first establishing a discrepancy between the academic skill and intelligence and then eliminating all other explanations for the discrepancy. Establishing this discrepancy involves a comparison between recent scores on scholastic achieve-

ment tests and a standardized intelligence test. Table 19-2 provides further information about these tests. The second part of the diagnostic procedure is concerned with differential diagnosis. Conditions often resulting in poor academic performance and precluding the diagnosis of specific developmental academic disorder include mental retardation, sensory impairment, neurologic damage or disease, psychiatric disturbance, and inadequate schooling.

Treatment

A wide variety of therapies have been used with learning-disabled children, but few have been subjected to well-controlled efficacy studies (Watson et al. 1982). Direct treatment approaches to dyslexia generally fall into two categories: those addressing underlying perceptual deficits and those addressing presumed underlying phonetic deficits (Gittelman 1983). More general approaches have also been taken, such as enhancing the child's attention or motivation for academic tasks. Attentional enhancement has been primarily pharmacologic, whereas motivational enhancement has relied on behavioral techniques (Gittelman 1983). A broad theoretical treatment issue in learning-disabled children, as in language-disordered children, is whether the goal should be to remediate deficiencies directly or to circumvent them by exploiting other cognitive strengths (Kirby 1980). By law, learning-disabled children must receive specialized instructions in the least restrictive setting, which often translates into resource-room placement for a portion of the school day.

Natural History

Since U.S. Public Law 94-142 mandating individualized educational programming has had such an impact on the education of learning-disabled children, it is difficult to distinguish between the natural longitudinal course of learning-disabled children and the effects of educational intervention. Although few longitudinal studies have been done on children with developmental arithmetic or expressive writing disorders, more work has been done in the area of developmental reading disorders. One study (Watson et al. 1982) found that 25% of children with mild reading disorders, and 5% of those with severe disorders early in elementary school, read at grade level by the end of school.

Critical Issues

There has been significant difficulty operationalizing the definition and diagnosis of learning disabilities. Controversies and unresolved methodological problems abound regarding how test results should be interpreted. Some clinicians (McCarthy 1975) contend, as does DSM-III-R, that the critical diagnostic issue is the difference between scores on intelligence tests and achievement tests; others (Sattler 1982) propose that the degree of scatter in test scores is the best indicator of learning disabilities.

The distinction in DSM-III-R between the types of specific academic developmental disorder, while useful for providing descriptions of clinical symptoms, does not capture the complexity or heterogeneity of learning disabilities and may not be sufficient to guide remediation efforts. Research suggests that each of the DSM-III-R subgroups is actually a heterogeneous disorder; children in each of these groups share the specific academic difficulty but may differ significantly in their underlying cognitive difficulty (Hooper and Willis 1989). For example, Boder (1973) described three subgroups of dyslexic individuals: "dysphonetic" (deficits in word analysis), "dyseidetic" (deficits in visual discrimination and visual memory), and a combined group. Research into this issue of heterogeneity has involved searching for new subgroups by subjecting the results of achievement and neuropsychological tests to multivariate analysis (Morris et al. 1986). For example, using this method, Petrauskas and Rourke (1979) found three subgroups of learning-disabled children: those with verbal deficits, those with problems in sequencing information, and those with difficulties in concept formation.

Summary

Developmental language disorders and learning disabilities are a heterogeneous set of disturbances seen in significant numbers of children and adolescents. They constitute a major vulnerability factor for psychiatric disorder and are comorbid conditions in many youngsters with psychiatric disorder. Because of these considerations, a careful assessment of language and learning skills should be a component of all psychiatric evaluations of children and adolescents. Treatment planning must address these deficits in communication and academic skills as well as the Axis I disorder and associated family problems. Untreated problems in these important domains of human functioning are likely to undermine both therapeutic efforts and ongoing successful psychosocial adaptation.

References

Allen DA, Rapin I, Wiznitzer M: Communication disorders of preschool children: the physicians responsibility. J Dev Behav Pediatr 9:164–170, 1988

American Psychiatric Association: Diagnostic and Statistical Manual of Mental Disorders, 3rd Edition, Revised. Washington, DC, American Psychiatric Association, 1987

American Speech-Language-Hearing Association: Definition: communication disorders and variations. ASHA 24:949, 1982

Aram DM, Hall NE: Longitudinal follow-up of children with pre-school communication disorders: treatment implications. School Psychology Review 18:487–501, 1989

Aram DM, Morris R: Validity of discrepancy criteria for identifying children with developmental language disorder (abstract). J Clin Exp Neuropsychol, Vol 13, No 1, 1991

Aram DM, Nation JE: Patterns of language behavior in children with developmental language disorders. J Speech Hear Res 18:229–241, 1975

Aram DM, Ekelman BL, Nation JE: Preschoolers with language disorders: 10 years later. J Speech Hear Res 27:232–244, 1984

Baker L, Cantwell D: Psychiatric disorder in children with different types of communication disorders. J Commun Disord 15:113–126, 1982

Baker L, Cantwell D: Psychiatric and learning disorders in children with speech and language disorders: a critical review. Advances in Learning and Behavior Disorders 4:1–28, 1985

Baker L, Cantwell DP: A prospective psychiatric follow-up of children with speech/language disorders. J Am Acad Child Adolesc Psychiatry 26:546–553, 1987

Bashir AS, Wiig EH, Abrams JC: Language disorders in childhood and adolescence: implications for learning and socialization. Pediatr Ann 16:145–156, 1987

Beitchman JH: Speech and language impairment and psychiatric risk: toward a model of neurodevelopmental immaturity. Psychiatr Clin North Am 8:721–725, 1985

Beitchman JH, Nair R, Clegg M, et al: Prevalence of psychiatric disorders in children with speech and language disorders. Journal of the American Academy of Child Psychiatry 25:528–535, 1986

Benton AL: The cognitive functioning of children with developmental dysphasia, in Developmental Dysphasia. Edited by Wyke MA. London, Academic, 1978

Bergman MM: Social grace or disgrace: adolescent social skills and learning disability subtypes. Reading, Writing, and Learning Disorders 3:161–166, 1987

Bishop DVM, Edmundson A: Specific language impairment as a maturational lag: evidence from longitudinal data on language and motor development. Dev Med Child Neurol 29:442–459, 1987

Boder E: Developmental dyslexia: a diagnostic approach based on three atypical reading-spelling patterns. Dev Med Child Neurol 15:663–687, 1973

Butler NR, Peckham C, Sheridan M: Speech defects in children aged seven years: a national study. Br Med J 1:253–257, 1973

Cantwell DP, Baker L: Psychiatric disorder in children with speech and language retardation: a critical review. Arch Gen Psychiatry 34:583–591, 1977

Cantwell D, Baker L: Developmental Speech and Language Disorders. New York, Guilford, 1987

Chase RA: Neurological aspects of language disorders in children, in Principles of Childhood Language Disabilities. Edited by Irwin JV, Marge M. Englewood Cliffs, NJ, Prentice-Hall, 1972

Chess S, Rosenberg M: Clinical differentiation among children with initial language complaints. Journal of Autism and Childhood Schizophrenia 4:99–109, 1974

Clements S, Peters J: Minimal brain dysfunctions in the school-age child. Arch Gen Psychiatry 6:185–197, 1962

Cohen D, Caparulo B, Shaywitz BA: Primary childhood aphasia and childhood autism: clinical, biological and conceptual observations. Journal of the American Academy of Child Psychiatry 4:604–645, 1979

Cohen D, Paul R, Volkmar FR: Issues in the classification of pervasive and other developmental disorders: toward DSM-IV. Journal of the American Academy of Child Psychiatry 25:213–220, 1986

Cohen NJ, Davine M, Meloche-Kelly M: Prevalence of unsuspected language disorders in a child psychiatric population. J Am Acad Child Adolesc Psychiatry 28:107–111, 1989

Cromer R: Language acquisition, language disorder, and cognitive development, in Language Development and Disorders. Edited by Yule W, Rutter M. Philadelphia, PA, JB Lippincott, 1987, pp 171–178

Cruickshank WM: The Brain-Injured Child in Home, School and Community. Syracuse, NY, Syracuse University Press, 1967

Denckla MB: Minimal brain dysfunction and dyslexia: beyond diagnosis by exclusion, in Topics in Child Neurology. Edited by Blaw ME, Rapin I, Kinsbourne M. New York, Spectrum, 1977

Dennis M, Whitaker HA: Language acquisition following hemidecortication: linguistic superiority of the left over the right hemisphere. Brain Lang 3:404–433, 1976

Duane DD: Toward a definition of dyslexia: a summary of views. Bulletin of the Orton Society 29:56–64, 1979

Duffy FH, Denckla MB, Bartels PH, et al: Dyslexia: regional differences in brain electrical activity by topographic mapping. Ann Neurol 7:412–420, 1980

Eisenson J: Developmental aphasia (dyslogia): a postulation of a unitary concept of the disorder. Cortex 4:184–200, 1968

Farnham-Diggory S: Learning Disabilities. Cambridge, MA, Harvard University Press, 1978, pp 1–27

Fundudis T, Kolvin I, Gardside RF: Speech Retarded and Deaf Children: Their Psychological Development. London, Academic, 1979

Galaburda A, Kemper T: Cytoarchitectonic abnormalities in developmental dyslexia: a case study. Ann Neurol 6:94–100, 1979

Galaburda AM, Sherman GR, Rosen GD, et al: Developmental dyslexia: four consecutive patients with cortical anomalies. Ann Neurol 18:222–233, 1985

Garcia E, DeHaven E: Use of operant techniques in the establishment and generalization of language: a review and analysis. American Journal of Mental Deficiency 79:169–178, 1974

Gittelman R: Treatment of reading disorders, in Developmental Neuropsychiatry. Edited by Rutter M. New York, Guilford, 1983, pp 520–541

Glosser B, Koppell S: Emotional-behavioral patterns in children with learning disabilities: lateralized hemispheric differences. Journal of Learning Disabilities 20:365–369, 1987

Gordon N: Developmental disorders of speech and language, in Language Development and Disorders. Edited by Yule W, Rutter M. Philadelphia, PA, JB Lippincott, 1987, pp 189–205

Gualtieri CT, Koriath U, vanBourgondien M, et al: Language disorders in children referred for psychiatric services. Journal of the American Academy of Child Psychiatry 22:165–171, 1983

Hall KH, Tomblin JB: A follow-up study of children with articulation and language disorders. J Speech Hear Disord 43:227–241, 1978

Halperin JM, Gittelman R, Klein DF, et al: Reading disabled hyperactive children: a distinct subgroup of attention deficit disorder with hyperactivity. J Abnorm Child Psychol 12:1–14, 1984

Haslam RHA, Dalby JT, Johns RD, et al: Cerebral asymmetry in developmental dyslexia. Arch Neurol 38:679–682, 1981

Hegde MN: Principles of management and remediation, in Handbook of Speech-Language Pathology and Audiology. Edited by Lass NJ, McReynolds LV, Northern JL, et al. Philadelphia, PA, BC Decker, 1988, pp 377–394

Heywood CA, Canavan AGM: Developmental neuropsychological correlates of language, in Language Development and Disorders. Edited by Yule W, Rutter M. Philadelphia, PA, JB Lippincott, 1987, pp 146–158

Hooper SR, Willis WG: Learning Disabilities Subtyping: Neuropsychological Foundations, Conceptual Models, and Issues in Clinical Differentiation. New York, Springer-Verlag, 1989

Hunt RD, Cohen DJ: Psychiatric aspects of learning disabilities. Pediatr Clin North Am 31:471–497, 1984

Hynd GW, Connor RT, Nieves N: Learning disability subtypes: perspectives and methodological issues in clinical assessment, in Assessment Issues in Child Neuropsychology. Edited by Tramontana MG, Hooper SR. New York, Plenum, 1988, pp 281–312

Ingram TTS: Speech disorders in childhood, in Foundations of Language Development, Vol 2. Edited by Lenneberg H, Lenneberg E. New York, Academic, 1976, pp 199–261

Johnson JP: Nature and Treatment of Articulation Disorders. Springfield, IL, Charles C Thomas, 1980

Johnston JR, Smith LB: Dimensional thinking in language impaired children. J Speech Hear Res 32:33–38, 1989

Karlin IW: Congenital verbal auditory agnosia. Pediatrics 7:60–69, 1951

Kinsbourne M: School problems. Pediatrics 52:697, 1973

Kirby JR: Individual differences and cognitive processes: instructional application and methodologic difficulties, in Cognition, Development, and Instruction. Edited by Kirby JR, Biggs JB. New York, Academic, 1980

Landau W, Goldstein R, Kleffner F: Congenital aphasia: a clinico-pathologic study. Neurology 10:915–921, 1960

Locke J: The inference of phoneme perception in the phonologically disordered child: a rationale, some criteria, the conventional tests. J Speech Hear Disord 45:431–444, 1980

Lou HC, Hennkson L, Bruhn P: Focal cerebral hypoperfusion in children with dysphasia and/or attention deficit disorder. Arch Neurol 41:825–829, 1984

Love AJ, Thompson MGG: Language disorders and attention deficit disorders in young children referred for psychiatric services: analysis of prevalence and a conceptual synthesis. Am J Orthopsychiatry 58:52–64, 1988

Lyon GR: Learning disabled readers: identification of subgroups, in Progress in Learning Disabilities. Edited by Myklebust HR. New York, Grune & Stratton, 1983

Mattis S, French J, Rapin I: Dyslexia in children and young adults: three independent neuropsychological syndromes. Dev Med Child Neurol 17:150, 1975

McCarthy JM: Children with learning disabilities, in The Application of Child Development Research to Exceptional Children. Edited by Gallager J. Reston, VA, The Council for Exceptional Children, 1975

McConaughy SH, Ritter DR: Social competence and behavioral problems of learning-disabled boys aged 6–11. Journal of Learning Disabilities 19:39–45, 1986

Morgan WP: A case of congenital word-blindness. Br Med J 2:1378, 1896

Morris RD: Classification of learning disabilities: old problems and new approaches. J Consult Clin Psychol 56:789–794, 1988

Morris R, Blashfield R, Satz P: Developmental classification of reading-disabled children. J Clin Exp Neuropsychol 8:371–392, 1986

Nussbaum NL, Bigler ED, Koch W: Neuropsychologically derived subgroups of learning-disabled children: personality/behavioral dimensions. Journal of Research and Development in Education 19:57–67, 1986

Offord DR, Waters BG: Socialization and its failure, in Developmental-Behavioral Pediatrics. Edited by Levine MD, Carey WB, Crocker AC, et al. Philadelphia, PA, WB Saunders, 1983

Orton ST: Word blindness in school children. Archives of Neurology and Psychiatry 14:581–615, 1928

Petrauskas R, Rourke B: Identification of subgroups of retarded readers: a neuropsychological multivariate approach. Journal of Clinical Neuropsychology 1:17–23, 1979

Piggott LR, Anderson TA: Brainstem auditory evoked responses in children with central language disturbance. Journal of the American Academy of Child Psychiatry 22:535–540, 1983

Rapin I: Disorders of higher cerebral function in preschool children. American Journal of the Disabled Child 142:1119–1124, 1988

Rapin I, Allen DA: Syndromes in developmental dysphasia and adult aphasia, in Language, Communication, and the Brain. Edited by Plum F. New York, Plenum, 1988, pp 57–75

Rees N: Auditory processing factors in language disorders. J Speech Hear Disord 38:304–315, 1973

Richardson SO: Developmental language disorder, in Comprehensive Textbook of Psychiatry V, Vol 2. Edited by Kaplan HI, Sadock BJ. Baltimore, MD, Williams & Wilkins, 1989, pp 1812–1817

Rondal J: Language development and mental retardation, in Language Development and Disorders. Edited by Yule W, Rutter M. Philadelphia, PA, JB Lippincott, 1987

Rumsey JM, Dorwart R, Vermness M, et al: Magnetic resonance imaging of brain anatomy in severe developmental dyslexia. Arch Neurol 43:1045–1046, 1986

Rumsey JM, Berman KF, Denckla MB, et al: Regional cerebral blood flow in severe developmental dyslexia. Arch Neurol 44:1144–1150, 1987

Rutter M: Speech delay, in Child Psychiatry: Modern Approaches. Edited by Rutter M, Hersov L. Oxford, UK, Blackwell Scientific, 1977, pp 688–716

Rutter M: Syndromes attributed to "minimal brain dysfunction" in childhood. Am J Psychiatry 131:21–33, 1982

Rutter M: Assessment objectives and principles, in Language Development and Disorders. Edited by Yule W, Rutter M. Philadelphia, PA, JB Lippincott, 1987, pp 295–311

Rutter M, Giller H: Juvenile Delinquency: Trends and Perspectives. New York, Penguin, 1983

Rutter M, Lord C: Language disorders associated with psychiatric disturbance, in Language Development and Disorders. Edited by Yule W, Rutter M. Philadelphia, PA, JB Lippincott, 1987

Sattler J: Assessment of Children's Intelligence and Special Abilities, 2nd Edition. Boston, MA, Allyn and Bacon, 1982

Sattler J: Assessment of Children. San Diego, CA, Jerome M Sattler, 1988

Schiefelbusch RL, Lloyd LL: Language Perspectives: Acquisition, Retardation and Intervention. Austin, TX, Pro-Ed, 1988

Shaffer D, O'Connor PA, Shafer SQ, et al: Neurological "soft signs": their origins and significance for behavior, in Developmental Neuropsychiatry. Edited by Rutter M. New York, Guilford, 1983

Shaffer D, Campbell M, Cantwell D, et al: Child and adolescent psychiatric disorders in DSM-IV: issues facing the work group. J Am Acad Child Adolesc Psychiatry 28:830–835, 1989

Shapiro T: Adolescent language: its use for diagnosis, group identity, values, and treatment. Paper presented to the American Society for Adolescent Psychiatry, Evanston, IL, 1985

Shaywitz BA, Shaywitz SE: Learning disabilities and attention disorders, in Pediatric Neurology, Vol 2. Edited by Swaimar KF. St. Louis, MO, CV Mosby, 1989

Shepherd MJ, Charnow DA, Silver LB: Developmental reading disorder, in Comprehensive Textbook of Psychiatry V, Vol 2. Edited by Kaplan HI, Sadock BJ. Baltimore, MD, Williams & Wilkins, 1989, pp 1790–1796

Silva PA: Epidemiology, longitudinal course and some associated factors: an update, in Language Development and Disorders. Edited by Yule W, Rutter M. Philadelphia, PA, JB Lippincott, 1987, pp 1–15

Silver AA, Hagin RA: Prevention of learning disorders, in Prevention of Mental Disorders, Alcohol and Other Drug Use in Children and Adolescents. Edited by Shaffer D, Silverman M, Anthony V. Washington, DC, Office of Substance Abuse Prevention (Monogr No 2), U.S. Department of Health and Human Services, 1989, pp 413–442

Silver LB: The "magic cure": a review of the current controversial approaches for treating learning disabilities. American Journal of the Disabled Child 140:1045–1052, 1986

Silver LB: Learning disabilities: introduction. J Am Acad Child Adolesc Psychiatry 28:309–313, 1989

Smith SD, Kimberling WJ, Pennington BF, et al: Specific reading disability: identification of an inherited form through linkage analysis. Science 219:1345–1347, 1983

Stevenson J, Richman N: Behavior, language and development in three-year-old children. Journal of Autism and Childhood Schizophrenia 8:299–313, 1978

Stevenson J, Richman N, Graham P: Behavior problems and language abilities at three years and behavioral deviance at eight years. J Child Psychol Psychiatry 26:215–230, 1985

Tallal P, Piercy M: Defects of Auditory Perception in Children With Developmental Dysphasia. London, Academic, 1978

Tallal P, Ross R, Curtiss S: Familial aggregation in specific language impairment. J Speech Hear Disord 54:167–173, 1989

Taylor HG, Fletcher JM: Biological foundations of "specific developmental disorders": methods, findings, and future directions. Journal of Clinical Child Psychology 12:46–65, 1983

Tomblin JB: Familial concentration of developmental language impairment. J Speech Hear Disord 54:287–295, 1989

Torgeson JK: The learning disabled child as an inactive learner: educational implications. Topics in Learning Disabilities 2:45–52, 1982

United States Congress: Public Law 94-142, "Education for All Handicapped Children Act of 1975." Washington, DC, U.S. Government Printing Office, 1975

Vandenburg SG, Singer SM, Pauls DL: The Heredity of Behavior Disorders in Adults and Children. New York, Plenum, 1986

Vohr BR, Coll CG, Oh W: Language development of low-birth-weight infants at two years. Dev Med Child Neurol 30:608–615, 1988

Waber D: Learning disabilities in children with cancer. Paper presented at educators' symposium, Dana Farber Cancer Institute, Boston, MA, 1989

Watson BU, Watson CS, Fredd R: Follow-up studies of specific reading disability. Journal of the American Academy of Child Psychiatry 21:376–382, 1982

Wiig EH, Semel EM: Language disabilities in children and adolescents. Columbus, OH, Charles E Merrill, 1976

Winitz H: Articulatory Acquisition and Behavior. Englewood Cliffs, NJ, Prentice-Hall, 1969

Wolfus B, Moskovitch M, Kinsbourne M: Subgroups of developmental language impairment. Brain Lang 10:152–171, 1980

Worster-Drought C, Allen IM: Congenital auditory imperception (congenital word deafness): with report of a case. Journal of Neurology and Psychopathology 9:193–208, 1929

Zangwill OL: The concept of developmental dysphasia, in Developmental Dysphasia. Edited by Wyke MA. London, Academic, 1987

Section IV

Schizophrenic and Affective Disorders

Chapter 20

Schizophrenic and Psychotic Disorders

Magda Campbell, M.D.
Elizabeth Kay Spencer, M.D.
Sharon C. Kowalik, M.D., Ph.D.
L. Erlenmeyer-Kimling, Ph.D.

Schizophrenia in children and adolescents is a disorder characterized by the same symptoms of psychosis as in adults; according to DSM-III-R (American Psychiatric Association 1987), there are hallucinations, delusions, and affective and thought disturbance during the active phase. DSM-III-R requires the duration of illness to be at least 6 months; this period may include prodromal or residual symptoms. However, while "functioning below the highest level previously achieved" (American Psychiatric Association 1987, p. 187) is a criterion for adults, in children or adolescents "failure to achieve the expected level of social development" is a diagnostic criterion (p. 187). The types of schizophrenia are catatonic, disorganized, paranoid, undifferentiated, and residual.

DSM (American Psychiatric Association 1952) listed schizophrenic reaction, childhood type; DSM-II (American Psychiatric Association 1968) listed schizophrenia, childhood type. In DSM-II, autism was classified under schizophrenia, childhood type. Childhood-type schizophrenia was ill defined and overinclusive. DSM-III (American Psychiatric Association 1980) used the same criteria for preadolescent children and adolescents as for adults. There is no comparison of DSM-III and DSM-III-R criteria for schizophrenia in either children or adolescents.

In adults, DSM-III-R criteria may be more restrictive (Fenton et al. 1988a).

Much of the literature on childhood onset schizophrenia prior to DSM-III suffers from methodological flaws: failing to use standardized, well-defined diagnostic criteria, and employing less-restrictive diagnostic criteria than applied to adult schizophrenic patients. The history of diagnosis and classification of schizophrenia in children has been reviewed elsewhere (Green et al. 1984; Howells and Guirguis 1984; Kestenbaum et al. 1989; Kydd and Werry 1982; Rutter 1972; Tanguay and Cantor 1986).

Diagnostic Criteria

DSM-III-R diagnostic criteria for schizophrenia are listed in Table 20-1. A review of the representative literature, consisting of 11 publications (Tables 20-2 and 20-3), indicates that preadolescent children display the same symptoms as do adolescents and adults diagnosed as schizophrenic. Although all of these studies are retrospective chart reviews, the diagnostic criteria employed in these studies are strict and fairly clearly specified. DSM-III criteria were employed in eight studies, Bleulerian criteria (Bleuler 1911) in one, Schneiderian first-rank symptoms (Schneider 1959) in one, and the same criteria as for schizophrenia in adults in one. Thus there is sufficient evidence that schizophrenia of childhood onset is not a discrete entity and should not

This work was supported in part by National Institute of Mental Health grants MH-32212, MH-40177, and IT 32 MH-18915 (Dr. Campbell) and 5 K07 MH-00763 (Dr. Spencer).

Table 20-1. DSM-III-R diagnostic criteria for schizophrenia

A. Presence of characteristic psychotic symptoms in the active phase: either 1, 2, or 3 for at least one week (unless the symptoms are successfully treated):
   1. Two of the following
      a) delusions
      b) prominent hallucinations (throughout the day for several days or several times a week for several weeks, each hallucinatory experience not being limited to a few brief moments)
      c) incoherence or marked loosening of associations
      d) catatonic behavior
      e) flat or grossly inappropriate affect
   2. Bizarre delusions (i.e., involving a phenomenon that the person's culture would regard as totally implausible, e.g., thought broadcasting, being controlled by a dead person)
   3. Prominent hallucinations [as defined in (1b) above] of a voice with content having no apparent relation to depression or elation, or a voice keeping up a running commentary on the person's behavior or thoughts, or two or more voices conversing with each other.
B. During the course of the disturbance, functioning in such areas as work, social relations, and self-care is markedly below the highest level achieved before onset of the disturbance (or, when the onset is in childhood or adolescence, failure to achieve expected level of social development).
C. Schizoaffective disorder and mood disorder with psychotic features have been ruled out, i.e., if a major depressive or manic syndrome has ever been present during an active phase of the disturbance, the total duration of all episodes of a mood syndrome has been brief relative to the total duration of the active and residual phases of the disturbance.
D. Continuous signs of the disturbance for at least six months. The six-month period must include an active phase (of at least one week, or less if symptoms have been successfully treated) during which there were psychotic symptoms characteristic of schizophrenia (symptoms in A), with or without a prodromal or residual phase, as defined below.
   Prodromal phase: A clear deterioration in functioning before the active phase of the disturbance that is not due to a disturbance in mood or to a Psychoactive Substance Use Disorder and that involves at least two of the symptoms listed below.
   Residual phase: Following the active phase of the disturbance, persistence of at least two of the symptoms noted below, these not being due to a disturbance in mood or to a psychoactive substance use disorder.
   Prodromal or Residual Symptoms:
   1. Marked social isolation or withdrawal
   2. Marked impairment in role functioning as wage-earner, student, or homemaker
   3. Markedly peculiar behavior (e.g., collecting garbage, talking to self in public, hoarding food)
   4. Marked impairment in personal hygiene and grooming
   5. Blunted or inappropriate affect
   6. Digressive, vague, overelaborate, or circumstantial speech, or poverty of speech, or poverty of content of speech
   7. Odd beliefs or magical thinking, influencing behavior and inconsistent with cultural norms, e.g., superstitiousness, belief in clairvoyance, telepathy, "sixth sense," "others can feel my feelings," overvalued ideas, ideas of reference
   8. Unusual perceptual experiences, e.g., recurrent illusions, sensing the presence of a force or person not actually present
   9. Marked lack of initiative, interests, or energy
   Examples: Six months of prodromal symptoms with one week of symptoms from A; no prodromal symptoms with six months of symptoms from A; no prodromal symptoms with one week of symptoms from A and six months of residual symptoms.
E. It cannot be established that an organic factor initiated and maintained the disturbance.
F. If there is a history of autistic disorder, the additional diagnosis of schizophrenia is made only if prominent delusions or hallucinations are also present.

Classification of course. The course of the disturbance is coded in the fifth digit:

   1-Subchronic. The time from the beginning of the disturbance, when the person first began to show signs of the disturbance (including prodromal, active, and residual phases) more or less continuously, is less than two years, but at least six months.
   2-Chronic. Same as above, but more than two years.

Table 20-1. (*Continued*)

3-Subchronic with Acute Exacerbation. Reemergence of prominent psychotic symptoms in a person with a subchronic course who has been in the residual phase of the disturbance.
4-Chronic with Acute Exacerbation. Reemergence of prominent psychotic symptoms in a person with a chronic course who has been in the residual phase of the disturbance.
5-In Remission. When a person with a history of schizophrenia is free of all signs of the disturbance (whether or not on medication), "in Remission" should be coded. Differentiating Schizophrenia in Remission from No Mental Disorder requires consideration of overall level of functioning, length of time since the last episode of disturbance, total duration of the disturbance, and whether prophylactic treatment is being given.
0-Unspecified.

Source. Reprinted with permission from American Psychiatric Association 1987.

be differentiated from schizophrenia of adults. Cantor et al. (1982) suggested that in very young children schizophrenia is displayed in a different manner than in adults, but this remains to be validated by data based on carefully designed prospective studies. As indicated below, the first psychotic episode in schizophrenic patients is usually in adolescence and reaches its peak incidence between the ages of 20 and 21 years; the symptoms in this age group are indistinguishable from those seen in adults. Systematized paranoid delusions represent the only exception: they are less common in adolescents than in adults.

Demographic and Other Characteristics and Clinical Findings

Demographic characteristics and clinical symptoms of a total of 273 patients, ages 4.75–15 years, reported in 11 representative studies, are summarized in Tables 20-2 and 20-3. The subjects were a mixture of inpatients and outpatients. In six reports, a retrospective chart review was employed.

Male to Female Ratio

Demographic characteristics include a male to female ratio ranging from 2.7:1 (Kolvin 1971a) to 1.14:1 (Kydd and Werry 1982) in the age group under 16. The exception is a report involving a sample of 16 schizophrenic children, in which the male to female ratio was reported to be 4.33:1 (Green and Padron-Gayol 1986).

Socioeconomic Status

There is a preponderance of patients in the lower socioeconomic classes, with the exception of one

study, in which 54% of the subjects belonged to socioeconomic status (SES) I and II (Russell et al. 1989). Another extreme is the report of Green et al. (1984): in the sample of 24 children none belonged to SES I or II. However, it should be noted that the sample sizes were small and may not have been representative because of the recruitment involved.

Intellectual Functioning

The IQs, when specified, seem to be on the lower side, ranging from 50 to 125 (Green and Padron-Gayol 1986; Green et al. 1984).

Clinical Symptoms

Of the clinical symptoms, hallucinations are the most frequently reported. Reports show that auditory hallucinations are present in about 80% (Russell et al. 1989) and in up to 93.8% of children who are 13 years of age or younger (Green and Padron-Gayol 1986). Visual hallucinations are reported in 30.3% (Kolvin 1971a) to 50% (Green and Padron-Gayol 1986) of cases; they are usually accompanied by auditory hallucinations. Tactile hallucinations are reported in a small percentage of schizophrenic children (Green and Padron-Gayol 1986; Green et al. 1984; Russell et al. 1989).

It should be noted that hallucinations in children are not necessarily a sign of schizophrenia: they are seen in a variety of conditions as well as in normal children. (For a review, see Pilowsky and Chambers 1986.)

Delusions are less frequent than hallucinations in this age group of schizophrenic children. Werry et al. (in press) found that delusions were infrequent; studies of others indicate that the frequency

Table 20-2. Demographic and onset characteristics of 273 patients reported in 11 representative studies

	Design	N	CA range[a]	M:F[b]	SES	IQ range	Patient status Inpatient	Patient status Outpatient	Age of onset	Premorbid personality	Type of Onset Acute	Insidious	Insidious with acute exacerbation	Subacute
Makita 1966	Retrospective chart review	32	?9–15	?	?	?	?		10–15					
Kolvin 1971a[c]		33		2.7:1	Excess of IV & V	Under 70: 16.6% Over 70: 83.4%			?		4	22	7	
Eggers 1978		57	7–13	1:1.28	?	Below avg.: 6 Average: 38 Above avg.: 13			7–14?	Deviant in 31	All?[d]			
Kydd and Werry 1982	Retrospective chart review	11(14)	9–15	1.14:1	IV & V: 10	Below avg.: 5 Average: 8 Above avg.: 2	X				5	4	0	6
Green et al. 1984	Retrospective chart review	24	6.7–11	1.66:1	IV & V: 20 III: 4	65–125	X		5–11		5	11	8	0
Green and Padron 1986	Retrospective chart review	16	5.7–12.6	4.33:1	?	Over 50 to 115 or higher	X		(5–6.11)[e] –10.11		5	6	5	0
Petty et al. 1984	Actual examination	3	8–12	3:0	?	78–87		X	8–13	Infantile autism	?	?	?	?
Volkmar et al. 1988	Retrospective chart review	14	7–14	2.5:1					7–14	86% odd	64%			
Watkins et al. 1988	Retrospective chart review	18	?	2.6:1			X	X	6–11.11	39% infantile autism		X?		
Russell et al. 1989	?	35	4.75– 13.25	2.1:1	V: 5 IV: 3 III: 8 II: 12 I: 7	76–114	X	X	3–11	26% developmental abnormalities				
Werry et al., in press	Follow-up: interview of 40%	30	18.3 (mean)	1:1	Upper-mid 43%; skilled 37%; lower 20%	23% less than 80		X	7–17	27% normal				

Note. SES = socioeconomic status.

[a]Chronological age range in years. [b]Ratio of males to females. [c]Also see Kolvin 1971b; Kolvin et al. 1971a, 1971b, 1971c. [d]All patients. [e]Only age range given was 5–6.11.

Table 20-3. Clinical symptoms of 273 patients reported in 11 representative studies

| | | | | | | Clinical symptoms (%) | | | | | |
| | | | | | | Hallucinations | | | | | |
	N	CA Range[a]	Comparisons/ controls	Instruments	Diagnostic criteria	Auditory	Visual	Tactile	Delusions	Affective disturbance	Thought disorder
Makita 1966	32	9–15	Autism COPDD		Schizophrenia in adults						60
Kolvin 1971a, 1971b Kolvin et al. 1971a & 1971b, 1971c	33	7–13	Autism		Schneiderian first-rank symptoms	81.8	30.3		57.6		
Eggers 1978	57	7–13	—		Bleulerian		93				
Kydd and Werry 1982	11(14)	9–15			DSM-III						
Green et al. 1984	24	6.7–11	Autism; conduct disorder	CBI ROS	DSM-III	79.2	37	8.3	54.2		100
Green and Pardon 1986	16	5.7–12.6	—		DSM-III	93.8	50	6.3	43.8		
Petty et al. 1984	3	8–12	—		DSM-III, except for deterioration in functioning	All[b]			All		All
Volkmar et al 1988	14	7–14	Autism COPDD schizoid disorder		DSM-III	79	36		All	86	79
Watkins et al. 1988	18			DSM-III Symptom Rating Scale; Achenbach CBC; DICA; videotape rated on CPRS-D	DSM-III		77			100	100
Russell et al. 1989	35	4.75–13.25		ICDS	DSM-III	80	37	—	63	74	40 (60)
Werry et al., in press	30	7–17	Bipolar disorder	SCID BPRS SANS SAPS	DSM-III-R	53	13	13	47	57	

Note. COPDD = Childhood onset pervasive developmental disorder. CBI = Children's Behavior Inventory. ROS = Rochester Research Obstetrical Scale. CBC = Child Behavioral Checklist. DICA = Diagnostic Interview for Children and Adolescents. CPRS-D = Children's Psychiatric Rating Scale—Developed. ICDS = Interview for Childhood Disorders and Schizophrenia. SCID = Structured Clinical Interview for DSM-III-R. BPRS = Brief Psychiatric Rating Scale. SANS = Schedule of Negative Symptoms. SAPS = Schedule of Positive Symptoms.
[a]Chronological age range in years.
[b]All subjects.

of delusions ranges from 43.8% (Green and Padron-Gayol 1986) to 63% (Russell et al. 1989). While some authors fail to specify the type of delusions, Russell et al. found that persecutory and somatic delusions were most common (20% each), whereas thought control and religious delusions were rare (3%) in children ages 4–13 years.

Affective disturbance was found to be common by Werry et al. (in press) and Watkins et al. (1988). Green et al. (1984) reported affective disturbance in 83.3%, Russell et al. (1989) in 74%, and Volkmar et al. (1988) in 70.7%.

Thought disorder in this age group of schizophrenic children was reported to be present in from 40% (Russell et al. 1989) to 100% (Green et al. 1984; Watkins et al. 1988) of cases. Several studies failed to specify the frequency of this symptom. The problems of assessing thought disorder in children have been addressed elsewhere (Arboleda and Holzman 1985; Caplan et al. 1989).

In the clinical experience of the senior author (M.C.), those children whose IQs are in the bright normal and superior range display symptoms and have clinical pictures that are indistinguishable from those seen in adults.

Deterioration in Functioning

For adults, the DSM-III-R criteria for schizophrenia require marked deterioration in functioning in the areas of work, social relations, and self-care. For children and adolescents, as indicated above, failure to achieve the expected level of social development is given as a criterion. Russell et al. (1989) reported that in their sample, ages 4–13 years, "all 35 subjects exhibited a marked deterioration from a previous level of functioning" (p. 402), verified by parents: the child either required psychiatric hospitalization or showed severe deterioration of behavior in school. All children met "strict" (p. 399) DSM-III criteria for schizophrenia. Green et al. (1984) reported a clear-cut deterioration in behavior with the onset of schizophrenia in all of their 24 subjects.

Duration of Illness

Concerning the duration of illness for "at least 6 months," 8 of the 11 publications listed in Tables 20-2 and 20-3 should meet this criterion, since they employed DSM-III criteria. However, only in 1 of the 8 studies is it specifically stated that all patients

showed evidence of schizophrenia, either acute or prodromal symptoms, for more than 6 months (Russell et al. 1989).

Type of Onset

As to the type of onset of illness, in the great majority of cases there were a variety of general, nonspecific behavioral symptoms prior to the onset of schizophrenia, or an insidious mode of onset. Of 17 hospitalized and carefully studied schizophrenic subjects, ages 7–13 years, 8 had an insidious onset, 8 had a "chronic" onset, and in only 1 was the onset acute (Asarnow and Ben-Meir 1988). Acute mode of onset is relatively rare in childhood.

In a comprehensive and critical review of the earlier literature, Offord and Cross (1969) found that "preschizophrenic" individuals in childhood show more antisocial and behavioral symptoms than children who do not grow up to be schizophrenic. Preschizophrenic children have poor peer relations and lower IQs and experience difficulties with academic work. Some of these reports were in agreement with the early findings of the Danish prospective studies of children born to schizophrenic mothers (Mednick and Schulsinger 1968). Schizotypal or schizoid personality disorders also were reported prior to manifestation of schizophrenia. In a comparison of 17 schizophrenic and 26 major depressive disorder children, all of whom were hospitalized, those with schizophrenia had lower IQs, more chronic dysfunctions, and poorer premorbid adjustment (Asarnow and Ben-Meir 1988). The latter included scale items of sociability-withdrawal, peer relationships, scholastic performance, school adaptation, and interests. Standardized diagnostic criteria were used; however, the premorbid adjustment ratings were done on the basis of the patient's school, medical, and prior evaluation records.

It has been suggested that a significant number of children who meet criteria for adult schizophrenia were diagnosed as having autistic disorder at preschool age (Cantor et al. 1982; Petty et al. 1984; Watkins et al. 1988). Of 17 hospitalized children who met DSM-III criteria for schizophrenia in interviews employing the Schedule for Affective Disorders and Schizophrenia for School-Age Children (Orvaschel et al. 1982), 4 (24%) were reported to have pervasive developmental disorder as a codiagnosis (Asarnow and Ben-Meir 1988). These children's full scale IQs ranged from 70 to 115 (mean

± SD, 89.71 ± 11.99). Others failed to confirm these findings (Green et al. 1984; Rutter, personal communication; Volkmar et al. 1988).

Russell et al. (1989) found that, prior to the onset of schizophrenia, 26% of the sample (9 of 35 children) displayed various symptoms seen in children who were diagnosed as having pervasive developmental disorder, without meeting all the criteria for the diagnosis of either autism or pervasive developmental disorder. The symptoms included echolalia and hand flapping. Kolvin (1971a) reported echolalia in 6% of schizophrenic (or late onset psychosis) children, whereas 49% had some developmental delay and 46% had speech delay. The retrospective diagnosis of autism prior to the onset of schizophrenia in a significant number of children could be a result of finding developmental delays and abnormalities and various behavioral symptoms (including social impairment) because the charts were reviewed retrospectively (Petty et al. 1984; Watkins et al. 1988). Of course, a failure to employ standardized diagnostic criteria in these patients may have contributed to or resulted in these unusual findings. Certainly these were not prospective studies of autistic children. Even though schizophrenia in a great percentage of cases can be preceded by a variety of developmental delays and symptoms, these symptoms usually do not meet strict criteria for autism.

Age of onset. Since the earliest reports on schizophrenia, it has been known that the condition seldom becomes manifest in children before 9 years of age (Bleuler 1911; Green et al. 1984; Kraepelin 1899; Makita 1966; Russell et al. 1989). In a large municipal acute-care hospital, the youngest schizophrenic child admitted over a period of 8 years was 5.7 years of age (Green and Padron-Gayol 1986). The youngest age at which a child developed schizophrenia, by history, was 5 years; this individual was a highly intelligent boy who, when hospitalized at the age of 8 years, was seen by the senior author (M.C.) and displayed a clinical picture of schizophrenia seen in adults (for details, see Green et al. 1984). Another child, a 10-year-old boy admitted to Bellevue Hospital, complained about fumes and poisoned food; he was fearful, paranoid and hostile; and he felt weak because "people with white skin are weak and with brown skin are strong." The doctor had "extragravitational power. . . . Everybody has gravity but you have extra," and the patient's entire body would tilt 45 degrees toward the examiner, indicating the doctor's power.

He would call the doctor "gravity girl." Everything had to do with magic, and people were coming from Mars.

In another sample of 35 schizophrenic children, a 4.9-year-old was the youngest; in the same sample, the youngest age of onset of symptoms was reported to be 3 years (Russell et al. 1989). It seems that symptoms do not vary during the prepubertal developmental period, but the hallucinations and delusions become more complex with age. As noted above, the same is true for children with superior IQs.

With the onset of puberty, there is a sharp increase in the frequency of schizophrenia as defined by DSM-III criteria, reaching its peak between the ages of 21 and 22 years in both sexes (Loranger 1984). However, schizophrenia in males starts at an earlier age than in females. In Loranger's study, the first psychotic episode between the ages of 5 to 14 years occurred in 10 males and in only 5 females, and between the ages of 15 and 19 years in 39 males and 23 females. Thus by the age of 19 years, 49% of males and only 28% of females had developed schizophrenia. In this sample consisting of 100 males and 100 females, the cumulative percentage of schizophrenia for males between 20 and 24 years was 74% and for females 49% (Loranger 1984). Bleuler (1911) cited Kraepelin's (1899) study involving 296 schizophrenic patients: 6% had onset of illness before the age of 15, 32.5% before 20, and 24.5% before 25 years of age. In a sample of 618 schizophrenics at Burgholzli, in only 4% of the sample was the age of onset before 15 years (6% of males and 4% of females); in 18% (21% of males and 16% of females) was the age of onset between 15 and 20 years; and in 22% was the age of onset 20 to 25 years (Bleuler 1911). Certainly both the earliest publications (Bleuler 1911; Kraepelin 1899) and more recent studies (Loranger 1984; Mirsky et al. 1985) are in agreement that schizophrenia is highly associated with adolescence.

Differential Diagnosis

As noted above, the DSM-III diagnostic criteria for schizophrenia with onset in childhood were the same as those for schizophrenia with onset in adolescence and adulthood. DSM-III-R introduced the modification that, rather than showing deterioration from a higher level of functioning, schizophrenic children and adolescents may fail to attain expected levels of function.

Pervasive Developmental Disorders

Despite historical controversy about the relationship of autism and schizophrenia with childhood onset, investigators have delineated characteristics that differentiate these clinical entities.

Children with pervasive developmental disorders present a clinical picture distinct from schizophrenia. Although many schizophrenic children have low average IQs, 75% of children with infantile autism function in the retarded range. Unlike schizophrenic disorders, autism and pervasive developmental disorders are not characterized by hallucinations and delusions. Schizophrenia is rarely, if ever, seen before 5 years of age, whereas autistic disorder can be recognized by 3 years of age in the vast majority of cases.

Schizophreniform Disorder, Brief Reactive Psychosis, and Psychotic Disorder Not Otherwise Specified

Children presenting with these psychotic disorders may appear to be schizophrenic, but fall short of DSM-III-R criteria for schizophrenia. Children with schizophreniform disorder have experienced duration of illness less than 6 months, and, with time, may attain the diagnosis of schizophrenia. Children diagnosed as having brief reactive psychosis experience psychotic symptoms for a few hours up to 1 month's duration, following a severe precipitating stress, and subsequently recover their premorbid level of functioning. It is emphasized, however, that schizophrenic children too may have the onset of psychosis in response to stress. Psychotic children whose symptomatology does not fall within specified diagnostic criteria are classified by DSM-III-R as having psychotic disorder not otherwise specified (NOS).

Personality Disorders

As noted in DSM-III-R, patients with schizotypal, borderline, schizoid, and paranoid personality disorders may experience transient psychotic symptoms. Comprehensive evaluation of the patient should focus on clarifying whether schizophrenic symptomatology is present.

Affective Disorders

Prepubertal children with major depressive disorders may experience hallucinations. Chambers et al. (1982) noted that 48% of prepubertal children with major depressive disorder reported hallucinations of any type, and that 36% reported complex auditory hallucinations. Delusions, however, are described as rare in major depressive disorder with onset in childhood (Puig-Antich et al. 1985).

In some cases, it may be difficult to distinguish bipolar affective disorder from schizophrenia in adolescence. Carlson and Strober (1978) conducted a retrospective review of the histories of six manic-depressive adolescent patients, all originally diagnosed as schizophrenic. Their first episodes of illness occurred at ages 12.8–16.6 years (mean 14.9), with a mean age of 19 years on follow-up. For these six patients, the authors determined 23 episodes of illness, 17 of mania, and 6 of depression, which were rediagnosed according to research criteria of Feighner et al. (1972) and Spitzer et al. (1978). None of the episodes met research diagnostic criteria for schizophrenia, but all did so for affective disorder. On follow-up, no patient's course suggested the evolution of schizophrenia.

These findings are similar to findings by others who have reevaluated patients originally diagnosed as schizophrenic. In a study of 26 patients (overall ages unspecified) with the admission diagnosis of acute schizophrenia, Taylor et al. (1974) found that rediagnosis according to research diagnostic criteria supported the diagnosis of schizophrenia in one and the diagnosis of mania in 13, for whom the mean age of onset of illness was 25.15 years.

In following up 40 patients older than 5 and younger than 17 years of age with nonorganic psychoses, Werry (personal communication, 1989) also described initial misdiagnosis of bipolar patients.

Organic Delusional Syndromes

Patients presenting with psychotic symptomatology also should be evaluated for organic etiologies. The differential diagnosis includes substance abuse; toxic or metabolic factors; central nervous system dysfunction, including seizure disorder or mass lesion; and infectious etiology, including acquired immune deficiency syndrome.

Epidemiology

Schizophrenia of prepubertal onset is rare. Some epidemiologic reports of psychiatric illness in prepubertal children have failed to identify schizophrenic patients among those studied. In the Isle of Wight study (Rutter et al. 1970), among 2,199 children aged 10 and 11 years screened, 126 children were found to have "some clinically significant psychiatric disorder" (p. 181). However, no children with "schizophrenia of later childhood and adult life" (p. 180) were identified. Similarly, no cases of schizophrenia between the ages of 2 to 12 years were found in the North Dakota prevalence study (Burd and Kerbeshian 1987). However, approximately a year after the completion of the North Dakota study, two children from the diagnostic pool seen in the office of the authors met DSM-III criteria for schizophrenia. The population of 2- to 12-year-olds in North Dakota was 110,723 at the time, so that, with these two subjects, the point prevalence rate of schizophrenia in North Dakota was 0.19 in 10,000 for this age group (Burd and Kerbeshian 1987). The prevalence of schizophrenia with onset in childhood was estimated to be 50 times less frequent than that of schizophrenia with onset in adulthood (Karno and Norquist 1989).

The point prevalence of adult schizophrenia ranges from 0.6 to 7.1 per 1,000 population (Karno and Norquist 1989; Torrey 1987). Higher prevalence rates have been reported in a specific area of Istria in Yugoslavia and in Ireland. Three months' prevalence rate of schizophrenia was 7.4/1,000 in Labin, Istria (Kulcar et al. 1971), and a lifetime prevalence of 8.3/1,000 was reported in Ireland (Walsh et al. 1980).

In a prospective longitudinal study, the Dunedin study in New Zealand, no case of schizophrenia was reported in a sample of 792 children at the age of 11 years (Anderson et al. 1987). This is an excellent study of a representative population, in which each subject is carefully evaluated, using a variety of measures, including the Diagnostic Interview Schedule for Children, Child Version, which is based on DSM-III criteria (Anderson et al. 1987).

Etiology

The etiology of schizophrenia remains unknown and the roles of genetic, neurobiological, and environmental and psychosocial influences remain controversial. A variety of etiologic models have been put forth, including a multifactorial model. Vulnerability and protective factors and stressful life events as well as their interactions have been studied. (For review, see Asarnow and Goldstein 1986; Cloninger 1989; Gottesman et al. 1987.) A genetic-environment interaction model is accepted by many investigators.

Genetics

Although there is no work as of this writing concerning the genetics of childhood onset schizophrenia, there is adequate evidence of the genetic influences in the etiology of adult schizophrenia (Kety 1983; Kety et al. 1968; Rosenthal et al. 1971). Increased prevalence of schizophrenia in family members has been demonstrated: in offspring (Bleuler 1978; Gottesman and Shields 1982; Mirsky et al. 1985) and in siblings (Gottesman and Shields 1972), as well as in adoption studies (Heston 1966; Kety et al. 1975) and in twin studies (Gottesman and Shields 1972, 1982), although there is some disagreement (Tienari 1963; Tienari et al. 1983). Whereas the risk of developing schizophrenia is not greater than 1% in the general population, it is 10%–15% if one parent is schizophrenic (Gottesman and Shields 1982). There is a threefold greater risk for illness in monozygotic cotwins when compared with dizygotic cotwins of schizophrenic twins (Gottesman and Shields 1972).

Of added interest is the work of Gottesman and Bertelsen (1989), who found in the Danish Identical and Fraternal Discordant Twin Study that the risk of schizophrenia in the offspring of the normal cotwins of schizophrenic identical twins was the same as in the offspring of the schizophrenic twin. By contrast, the offspring of the normal cotwins of schizophrenic fraternal twins had a schizophrenic risk much below the risk in the offspring of the schizophrenic twin. These results bring up the concept of unexpressed genotypes and suggest that there may be environmental events that trigger the development of schizophrenia. This may also explain childhood onset schizophrenia; in an individual who has the genetic predisposition, an environmental trigger, such as birth trauma, prematurity, low birth weight, or viral illness in utero or even in the first few years of life, may initiate the onset of schizophrenia in childhood. Further research in this area may reveal that certain insults in predisposed individuals are associated with adult onset schizophrenia, whereas others are of a magnitude to cause the appearance of this illness in childhood.

High-risk studies. High-risk studies began in the early 1950s with Fish's pioneering work (Fish et al. 1965); one of the main goals of this research was to differentiate antecedents or precursors of schizophrenia from abnormalities or deficits related to the illness itself (Asarnow and Goldstein 1986). The inclusion criteria for high-risk subjects have been described elsewhere (Asarnow and Goldstein 1986; Erlenmeyer-Kimling and Cornblatt 1987). Fish followed the offspring of 12 schizophrenic women from early infancy over a period of 30 years; 3 of the 12 developed schizophrenia. Abnormalities of neurologic and motor functioning, neurointegrative defects, attentional and information-processing impairment, disturbed social functioning, and somewhat lower IQs were reported at various developmental stages in children or adolescents at risk for schizophrenia, although not all findings were in agreement (Cornblatt and Erlenmeyer-Kimling 1985; Fish 1984; Fish et al. 1965; Marcus et al. 1987; Mednick and Schulsinger 1968; Mirsky and Silberman 1985; Parnas et al. 1982). (For a critical review, see Asarnow and Goldstein 1986; Erlenmeyer-Kimling and Cornblatt 1987.) Many of these high-risk studies will be expanded on later in this chapter.

Neurodevelopmental Model

This is another area in which very little research has been done concerning schizophrenia with childhood onset; most of the work has been with adults. A developmental approach is an intriguing way in which to view the etiology of schizophrenia (Murray et al. 1988; Weinberger 1987), and it can be conceptualized in at least two ways. One theory is that the brain develops normally but some insult, such as birth trauma or viral infection, occurs during the critical period of brain development. This insult may change the brain structure, with the subsequent development of schizophrenic behaviors. In support of this theory, several studies have suggested that the complications of pregnancy and/or low birth weight are associated with schizophrenia (Lane and Albee 1966; Pollin and Stabenau 1968). In further support of this, Marcus et al. (1985) found neurologic dysfunction in high-risk children with low-normal birth weights compared with low-risk children. Obstetrical complications have been implicated in schizophrenia (Foerster et al. 1988), and a relationship was reported

between obstetrical complications and enlarged ventricles in schizophrenic patients (Lewis et al. 1988; Schulsinger et al. 1984) and in subjects who are at high risk for the disorder (Schulsinger et al. 1984).

The second theory of the developmental model of schizophrenia assumes that the actual development of the fetal brain is defective in a way that may not be apparent in the younger years and that certain stresses during maturation may trigger the onset of the schizophrenic behavior. This hypothesis is particularly inviting in justifying certain etiologic factors such as viral or birth trauma or low birth weight, because, by suggesting that the individual's brain is more vulnerable than the normal brain, it can subsequently explain why so many persons who suffer from viral illnesses or birth trauma do not appear to develop schizophrenic behavior.

Cannon et al. (1989) hypothesized that there is a genetic predisposition to schizophrenia that is expressed, partially at least, as a disruption of fetal brain areas undergoing rapid development in the second trimester of intrauterine life. These neural developmental disruptions can result in an increased vulnerability to certain complications of pregnancy and delivery, and the combination of these factors may produce periventricular damage. Data from a subsample of the Danish high-risk project support this hypothesis (Cannon et al. 1989). Weinberger (1987) similarly discussed the possibility of a latent lesion in the brain, most likely found in the dorsolateral prefrontal cortex, that remains silent until it is unmasked by the neuromaturational changes of late adolescence or early adulthood. However, as has been pointed out by King (1988), such a model is difficult to accept completely considering childhood onset schizophrenia, although studies of event-related potentials as well as neuropsychologic tests in schizophrenic children suggest some dysfunction of the prefrontal cortex (Asarnow et al. 1986), which is one of the same areas that Weinberger associated with adult onset schizophrenia. King (1988) suggests that there may be either a more severe genetic load associated with childhood onset schizophrenia or a more severe amount of developmental damage or even more serious precipitating events. It may also represent a coexisting lesion not found in the adult type. Finally, the childhood variety of schizophrenia may have an entirely different lesion than the adult form of schizophrenia, but based on current neurophysiologic information, this seems less likely.

Computed Tomography

As of this writing, the only study that involves children is that of Reiss et al. (1983). This group studied computed tomography (CT) data of 20 psychiatric patients and 20 age- and sex-matched control patients whose ages ranged from 5 to 15 years (mean ages were 9.8 and 9.9 years, respectively). The authors reported significantly enlarged ventricles in the psychiatric patients. The two largest ventricle-brain ratios were for a schizotypal patient, who had no neurologic abnormality, and a schizophrenic patient, who had "abnormal EEG [electroencephalogram] or neuropsychological testing only" (p. 454). However, the psychiatric patients had a wide range of diagnoses (borderline personality, schizophrenia, pervasive developmental disorders, attention-deficit disorder, and Tourette's syndrome). Furthermore, only 7 of the patients had no neurologic abnormalities; the remaining 13 had some type of neurologic abnormality (neurologic diagnosis and/or EEG or neuropsychiatric abnormality). Benes et al. (1982) studied the CT scans of 11 adolescents and young adults with schizophrenia and found them not to differ from those of matched controls.

Neurologic-Physiologic Findings

Topographic electroencephalographic mapping. Much of this work has involved adult onset schizophrenia (Fenton et al. 1988b; Morihisa et al. 1983). Topographic electroencephalographic mapping has great potential in child psychiatry research, especially because of its potential contribution to the assessment of learning disabilities and attention-deficit disorders, both groups of which are often associated with schizophrenia.

Attentional/information-processing anomalies. This is a highly studied area of research. However, most of the studies involve children at risk for schizophrenia rather than children diagnosed as schizophrenic. Perceptual sensitivity has been shown to be impaired in high-risk children (Nuechterlein 1983; Rutschmann et al. 1977) but not in children of normal parents or children of parents with psychiatric disorders other than schizophrenia (Rutschmann et al. 1977), nor in hyperactive children (Nuechterlein 1983). A similar deficit also has been found among young adults with a profile from the Minnesota Multiphasic Personality Inventory (Hathaway and McKinley 1970) that shows schizotypal characteristics (Nuechterlein 1985). Erlenmeyer-Kimling et al. (1984) showed that the signal-noise discrimination during a continuous performance test at age 7–12 years was lower in high-risk children who showed clinical deviance (this deviance was not solely limited to schizophrenia) during late adolescence in the New York High-Risk Project.

Another test that has offered evidence for information-processing abnormalities among children of schizophrenic parents is the partial report span of apprehension procedure. This test has been found to differentiate a subset of foster children whose biological mothers were schizophrenic, from foster children who had no family history of schizophrenia and from children who served as controls (Asarnow et al. 1977). In addition, it was found that those children who showed the most impairment on this test tended to show some of the prodromal behaviors characteristic of children who develop schizophrenia as adults. Harvey et al. (1981) found serial recall in high-risk children to be deficient mainly for items that require active, effortful rehearsal to allow transfer to longer-term memory; this deficit was not found in the offspring of parents with unipolar or bipolar affective illness. Asarnow et al. (1986) studied 11 schizophrenic children, comparing them to normal children matched for IQ and to younger normal children with a mental age 4 years below the schizophrenic children. The data indicated that controlled attentional processes were impaired in the schizophrenic children. Event-related potential (ERP) values were most deviant in the frontal leads, although midline and lateralized deficits were detected at posterior recording sites and at vertex.

An abnormal P300 component of the long-latency ERP has been reported often in schizophrenia research; these studies have found that the P300 has a smaller amplitude in schizophrenic adults compared with normal adults (for a review, see Roth 1977). Few studies have examined the P300 potential in children with a diagnosis of childhood schizophrenia. Strandburg et al. (1984) found schizophrenic children to have a reduced amplitude for visual ERP late-positive components compared with age-matched controls. Erwin et al. (1986) examined a group of nine children (ages 10–13 years) who were diagnosed as having schizophrenia or schizotypal personality disorder, as well as nine age-matched normal children and nine younger normal children (ages 6–8 years) using an "odd-ball" P300 protocol. Their conclusions were that the schizophrenic children had smaller P300 responses to rare stimuli compared with the other groups, a finding which is similar to that of schizophrenic adults compared with normal adults (Roth 1977). However, in addition, they found that the clinical group had a positive deflection in the 300–400 milliseconds region for frequent as well as target and rare stimuli. High-risk children were evaluated by Friedman et al. (1982), and this group initially reported that, in analyses of a subset of the children under study, the high-risk children had auditory ERPs with smaller amplitude late-positive waves compared with children with normal parents. Subsequently, however, analyzing the auditory ERP data on the entire sample, including children of parents with affective disorder as well as the children of schizophrenic parents and parents without a history of psychiatric illness, Friedman et al. (1988) found no systematic differences among the three groups and thus no evidence suggesting waveform abnormalities in the high-risk children. These authors, however, found a significantly lower N100 amplitude to the frequent event in an oddball paradigm in the children of parents with affective disorder compared with the children at high risk for schizophrenia and the normal controls (Friedman et al. 1988).

High-risk children have been reported to exhibit a particular physiologic reaction to stress that is characterized by autonomic hyperresponsiveness followed by a rapid recovery and slow habituation, particularly in response to a loud, irritating noise stimulus (Mednick and Schulsinger 1968; Mednick et al. 1974). Subsequently, these authors reported these adolescent electrodermal characteristics to be predictive of later schizophrenic symptomatology among male, but not female, high-risk children (Mednick et al. 1978).

Other groups have attempted to duplicate these electrodermal findings. Prentky et al. (1981) found larger electrodermal responses to loud noises but were not able to replicate many of Mednick's other findings; Van Dyke et al. (1974) had findings similar to those of Prentky et al. (1981). Janes et al. (1978) did not find electrodermal differences between high-risk children and normal children, but they acknowledged that their protocol did not include an aversive stimulus that was comparable to the one used in Mednick's group. Both Erlenmeyer-Kimling et al. (1984) and Kugelmass et al. (1985) found no evidence of hyperresponsivity among high-risk children, and both groups also found an opposite cross-sectional difference (slower recovery after aversive noises). Electrodermal abnormalities have been considered to have positive prognostic value in adult schizophrenic patients. (For a review, see Dawson and Nuechterlein 1984.) However, clearly more work must be done with the high-risk studies, and preferably with studies involving schizophrenic children, to determine if autonomic anomalies play a similar role in childhood.

Fish was one of the first to report neurointegrative defects, such as pandysmaturation, in high-risk children (Fish 1957, 1977, 1984; Fish et al. 1965). In addition, Fish (1984) found evidence indicating that pandysmaturation may have been related to early adult schizophrenia in her sample of high-risk children. There are many other studies that document a variety of neurologic soft signs or motor dysfunctions; among the signs most frequently reported is impaired fine motor coordination (Erlenmeyer-Kimling et al. 1987; Hanson et al. 1976; Marcus 1974; Marcus et al. 1985; Rieder and Nichols 1979).

Biochemical Models

The few reports in children appear to have been done with schizophrenic patients as a control or comparison group rather than as the main focus of the study.

Weizman et al. (1988) studied plasma immunoreactive beta-endorphin levels in autistic, schizophrenic, and normal children. Their results suggest that untreated schizophrenic patients have beta-endorphin levels that do not significantly differ from those of normal children, although neuroleptic administration was associated with increases in beta-endorphin levels. Rogeness et al. (1988) examined the catecholamine metabolism and plasma dopamine beta-hydroxylase (pDBH) in 80 hospitalized boys who were diagnostically heterogeneous. Three of the four schizophrenic patients had pDBH levels of less than 6 μM/minute/liter (low pDBH group), and one was found to have a pDBH level greater than 15 μM/minute/liter (high pDBH group). The largest subgroup consisted of children diagnosed as having conduct disorder, undersocialized; 20 of these children were in the low pDBH group, whereas only 8 were in the high pDBH group; the difference was significant.

Treatment

There is little knowledge based on research regarding the effectiveness of various treatments for schizophrenic children and adolescents. In clinical practice, assessment of an individual child's strengths, weaknesses, and environmental resources is critical in treatment planning. Clinical judgment may suggest the use of combined modalities for an individual patient; individual psychotherapy, milieu therapy, group therapy, parent counseling, family therapy, special education, and psychopharmacology may be employed as deemed appropriate.

Psychotherapy

As described by Cantor and Kestenbaum (1986), individual psychotherapy may be used to promote ego-boundary development in preschool-age schizophrenic children and to strengthen reality testing and emerging identity and autonomy in school-age children. The therapist's roles include functioning as an auxiliary ego and facilitating the child's understanding of sensory perceptions. Similarly, for adolescent schizophrenic patients, individual or group psychotherapy can be beneficial in enhancing "self-regulation and the self-management of relationships," as well as education about the nature of the illness and its treatment (Steinberg 1985, p. 578).

Psychopharmacology

A review of the literature reveals that there are only a few reports as of this writing on the use of psychoactive drugs in either prepubertal or adolescent schizophrenic patients.

The methodologically best study was done in adolescent schizophrenic patients (Pool et al. 1976). These authors conducted a 4-week double-blind study of loxapine, haloperidol, and placebo in 75 newly admitted adolescents, ages 13–18 years, who were diagnosed as having acute schizophrenia or chronic schizophrenia with acute exacerbation. By random assignment, 26 patients received loxapine, 25 received haloperidol, and 24 received placebo. The average daily dose was 87.5 mg for loxapine and 9.8 mg for haloperidol. The following rating instruments were employed: Brief Psychiatric Rating Scale (BPRS) (Overall and Gorham 1962), Nurses'

Observation Scale for Inpatient Evaluation (NOSIE), (Honigfeld et al. 1966), and the Clinical Global Impressions (CGI) ("Addendum" 1973). Pool et al. concluded that both loxapine and haloperidol were superior to placebo for several rating items associated with schizophrenia. On the BPRS, loxapine significantly improved hallucinatory behavior and the factor thinking disorder at 2 weeks and hallucinatory behavior and disorientation and the factor excitement-disorientation at 4 weeks. Haloperidol showed only trends for hallucinatory behavior at 2 and 4 weeks. On the NOSIE, loxapine was found to be significantly better than placebo for manifest psychosis at 2 and 4 weeks, and it was significantly superior to haloperidol for social interest and manifest psychosis at 2 weeks. On the CGI, for patients with severe illness at baseline, there was a trend toward improvement by either drug compared with controls at 4 weeks. Of the side effects, parkinsonian muscle rigidity and sedation were most commonly associated with both drugs.

In a 4- to 6-week single-blind study, Realmuto et al. (1984) compared the high-potency neuroleptic thiothixene and the low-potency neuroleptic thioridazine for the treatment of 21 chronically ill inpatient schizophrenic adolescents, ages 11.75–18.75 years. Optimal dosage was 0.30 mg/kg for thiothixene (range, 4.8–42.6 mg; mean, 16.2 mg) and 3.3 mg/kg for thioridazine (range, 91–228 mg/day; mean, 178 mg/day). On the BPRS there was a significant reduction of symptoms ($P < .05$), although the patients remained impaired. Hallucinations, excitement, anxiety, and tension were reduced in the first 7 days of treatment. On the whole, thioridazine seemed more often to be associated with sedation than was thiothixene.

No conclusions can be made on the efficacy and safety of haloperidol (0.75–6.75 mg/day) and pimozide (1.0–9.0 mg/day) in the few prepubertal schizophrenic patients who were included in clinical trials involving larger samples of diagnostically heterogeneous patients (Debray et al. 1972; Naruse et al. 1982; Pangalila-Ratulangi 1973). Preliminary findings of a double-blind, placebo-controlled study of haloperidol suggest that prepubertal schizophrenic patients do respond to low doses (1.5–2.5 mg/day) (Spencer et al. 1990).

In their report of 15 schizophrenic patients, ages 10–15 years, Kydd and Werry (1982) noted that all the patients were medicated. They found that acute positive symptoms (delusions, hallucinations, thought disorder) showed greater improvement than did negative symptoms (withdrawal, blunted affect); they commented, however, that these observations may have occurred independently of medication.

Prognosis

Eggers (1978) conducted a follow-up study of 71 children, ages 7–13 years, diagnosed as schizophrenic and admitted between 1925 and 1961 to a West German university psychiatric service. Of the 71, 14 children were excluded from the follow-up study because of questions about the original diagnosis of schizophrenia. In this study, psychotic children were diagnosed as schizophrenic only if assessed as showing "schizophrenic symptoms as found in adult schizophrenia" (p. 22). The average length of follow-up was 15 years. On follow-up, 20% of the children had recovered completely; 30% were judged to have attained relatively good social adjustment; and 50% had moderate or poor remission. The 11 children with psychosis before age 10 all had poor outcome. Family incidence of psychiatric disorder and disturbed family environment were not found to influence prognosis. Premorbid personality development did have prognostic value in that children who appeared well adjusted prior to being ill showed greater likelihood of recovery. Above-average intelligence also predicted better outcome. A limitation of this study is the retrospective application of diagnostic criteria to patients first evaluated many years before.

Kydd and Werry (1982) reported on 15 schizophrenic patients, ages 10–15 years, who had been admitted as inpatients to a child psychiatric unit over a 10-year period. In this report, follow-up was conducted of 10 children who had first been seen at least 1 year previously. The follow-up interval ranged from 1 to 9 years (mean, 4.6 years). The children's diagnosis on admission had been made using Bleulerian/Schneiderian criteria. For follow-up, their presenting diagnoses were reassessed by DSM-III criteria, resulting in the diagnosis of schizophrenia in 11 and schizophreniform psychosis in 4; in the latter category, 3 patients had presented within the preceding year and hence were considered potentially schizophrenic. Factors associated with poor outcome were age under 14 at presentation, poor level of premorbid functioning, insidious onset, and disorganized subtype. All 3 children who were 15 years of age at presentation returned to their previous level of functioning. Factors associated with favorable outcome were affective symptoms and paranoid subtype.

Research Issues

The current understanding of the etiology and, particularly, the treatment of childhood and adolescent onset schizophrenia is very limited at best, and many opportunities for research exist in this field. Probably one of the reasons for a lack of research is the limited number of child schizophrenic subjects available for study. In addition, many procedures (e.g., CT, positron emission tomography) and psychoactive agents used relatively freely in adults are not used readily in children. Certainly much work needs to be done in the evaluation of treatment in this age group of schizophrenic patients. Carefully designed double-blind, placebo-controlled studies with descriptively homogeneous patients are needed. Of particular interest are some of the newer neuroleptics that have been reported to have fewer side effects, as well as the depot neuroleptics.

Research questions concerning the etiology of schizophrenia are also abundant. In addition to the continuation of the current high-risk studies, investigations of biochemical parameters such as dopamine metabolism (e.g., homovanillic acid in plasma) should be pursued. The recent development of magnetic resonance imaging, a technique that is safer than CT and that has the capacity for more detailed imaging, appears to offer research opportunities in this young schizophrenic population.

Prospective longitudinal studies of subjects diagnosed as schizophrenic in childhood should have the highest priority.

References

"Addendum—Children's ECDEU Battery." Schizophr Bull (special issue), 1973, p 202

American Psychiatric Association: Diagnostic and Statistical Manual of Mental Disorders. Washington, DC, American Psychiatric Association, 1952

American Psychiatric Association: Diagnostic and Statistical Manual of Mental Disorders, 2nd Edition. Washington, DC, American Psychiatric Association, 1968

American Psychiatric Association: Diagnostic and Statistical Manual of Mental Disorders, 3rd Edition. Washington, DC, American Psychiatric Association, 1980

American Psychiatric Association: Diagnostic and Statistical Manual of Mental Disorders, 3rd Edition, Revised. Washington, DC, American Psychiatric Association, 1987

Anderson JC, Williams S, McGee R, et al: DSM-III disorders

in preadolescent children. Arch Gen Psychiatry 44:69–76, 1987

Arboleda C, Holzman PS: Thought disorder in children at risk for psychosis. Arch Gen Psychiatry 42:1004–1013, 1985

Asarnow JR, Ben-Meir S: Children with schizophrenia spectrum and depressive disorders: a comparative study of premorbid adjustment, onset pattern and severity of impairment. J Child Psychol Psychiatry 29:477–488, 1988

Asarnow JR, Goldstein MJ: Schizophrenia during adolescence and early adulthood: a developmental perspective on risk research. Clinical Psychology Review 6:211–235, 1986

Asarnow RF, Steffy RA, MacCrimmon DJ, et al: An attentional assessment of foster children at risk for schizophrenia. J Abnorm Psychol 86:267–275, 1977

Asarnow R, Sherman T, Strandburg R: The search for the psychobiological substrate of childhood onset schizophrenia. Journal of the American Academy of Child Psychiatry 26:601–614, 1986

Benes F, Sunderland P, Jones BD, et al: Normal ventricles in young schizophrenics. Br J Psychiatry 141:90–93, 1982

Bleuler E: Dementia Praecox or the Group of Schizophrenias (1911). Translated by Zinkin J. New York, International Universities Press, 1950

Bleuler M: The Schizophrenic Disorders: Long-Term Patient and Family Studies. New Haven, CT, Yale University Press, 1978

Burd L, Kerbeshian J: A North Dakota prevalence study of schizophrenia presenting in childhood. J Am Acad Child Adolesc Psychiatry 26:347–350, 1987

Cannon TD, Mednick SA, Parnas J: Genetic and perinatal determinants of structural brain deficits in schizophrenia. Arch Gen Psychiatry 46:883–894, 1989

Cantor S, Kestenbaum C: Psychotherapy with schizophrenic children. Journal of the American Academy of Child Psychiatry 25:623–630, 1986

Cantor S, Evans J, Pearce J, et al: Childhood schizophrenia: present but not accounted for. Am J Psychiatry 139:758–762, 1982

Caplan R, Guthrie D, Fish B, et al: The Kiddie-formal thought disorder rating scale: clinical assessment, reliability, and validity. J Am Acad Child Adolesc Psychiatry 28:408–416, 1989

Carlson GA, Strober M: Manic-depressive illness in early adolescence. Journal of the American Academy of Child Psychiatry 17:138–153, 1978

Chambers WJ, Puig-Antich J, Tabrizi MA, et al: Psychotic symptoms in pre-pubertal major depressive disorder. Arch Gen Psychiatry 39:921–927, 1982

Cloninger CR: Schizophrenia: genetic etiological factors, in Comprehensive Textbook of Psychiatry V, Vol 1. Edited by Kaplan HI, Sadock BJ. Baltimore, MD, Williams & Wilkins, 1989, pp 732–744

Cornblatt B, Erlenmeyer-Kimling L: Global attentional deviance as a marker of risk for schizophrenia: specificity and predictive validity. J Abnorm Psychol 94:470–486, 1985

Dawson ME, Nuechterlein KH: Psychophysiological dysfunction in the developmental course of schizophrenic disorders. Schizophr Bull 10:204–232, 1984

Debray P, Messerschmitt P, Lonchap D, et al: The use of pimozide in child psychiatry. Nouvelle Presse Medicale I(43):2917–2918, 1972

Eggers C: Course and prognosis of childhood schizophrenia. Journal of Autism and Childhood Schizophrenia 8:21–36, 1978

Erlenmeyer-Kimling L, Cornblatt B: High-risk research in schizophrenia: a summary of what has been learned. J Psychiatr Res 21:401–411, 1987

Erlenmeyer-Kimling L, Friedman D, Marcuse Y, et al: The New York High-Risk Project, in Children at Risk for Schizophrenia: A Longitudinal Perspective. Edited by Watt NF, Anthony EJ, Wynne LC, et al. New York, Cambridge University Press, 1984, pp 169–189

Erwin RJ, Edwards R, Tanguay PE, et al: Abnormal P300 responses in schizophrenic children. Journal of the American Academy of Child Psychiatry 25:615–622, 1986

Feighner JP, Robins E, Guze SB, et al: Diagnostic criteria for use in psychiatric research. Arch Gen Psychiatry 26:57–63, 1972

Fenton WS, McGlashan TH, Heinssen RK: A comparison of DSM-III and DSM-III-R schizophrenia. Am J Psychiatry 145:1446–1449, 1988a

Fenton GW, Fenwick PBC, Armstrong GA, et al: Left hemisphere dysfunction and negative symptoms in schizophrenia: some EEG evidence. Schizophrenia Research 1:184–185, 1988b

Fish B: The detection of schizophrenia in infancy. J Nerv Ment Dis 125:1–24, 1957

Fish B: Neurobiological antecedents of schizophrenia in children: evidence for an inherited congenital neurointegrative defect. Arch Gen Psychiatry 34:1297–1313, 1977

Fish B: Characteristics and sequelae of the neurointegrative disorder in infants at risk for schizophrenia: 1952–1982, in Children at Risk for Schizophrenia: A Longitudinal Perspective. Edited by Watt N, Anthony EJ, Wynne LC, et al. New York, Cambridge University Press, 1984, pp 423–439

Fish B, Shapiro T, Halpern F, et al: The prediction of schizophrenia in infancy, III: a ten-year follow-up report of neurological and psychological development. Am J Psychiatry 121:768–775, 1965

Foerster A, Lewis S, Owen M, et al: Premorbid risk factors. Schizophrenia Research 1:121–122, 1988

Friedman D, Vaughan HG, Erlenmeyer-Kimling L: Cognitive brain potentials in children at risk for schizophrenia: preliminary findings. Schizophr Bull 8:514–531, 1982

Friedman D, Cornblatt B, Vaughan H, et al: Auditory event-related potentials in children at risk for schizophrenia: the complete initial sample. Psychiatry Res 26:203–221, 1988

Gottesman II, Bertelsen A: Confirming unexpressed genotypes for schizophrenia. Arch Gen Psychiatry 46:867–872, 1989

Gottesman II, Shields J: Schizophrenia and Genetics: A Twin Study Vantage Point. New York, Academic, 1972

Gottesman II, Shields J: Schizophrenia: The Epigenetic Puzzle. Cambridge, MA, Cambridge University Press, 1982

Gottesman II, McGuffin P, Farmer AE: Clinical genetics as clues to the "real" genetics of schizophrenia: a decade of modest gains while playing for time. Schizophr Bull 13:23–47, 1987

Green WH, Padron-Gayol M: Schizophrenic disorder in childhood: its relationship to DSM-III criteria, in Biological Psychiatry 1985. Edited by Shagass C, Josiassen RC, Bridger WH, et al. New York, Elsevier, 1986, pp 1484–1486

Green WH, Campbell M, Hardesty AS, et al: A comparison of schizophrenic and autistic children. Journal of the American Academy of Child Psychiatry 23:399–409, 1984

Hanson DR, Gottesman II, Heston LL: Some possible childhood indicators of adult schizophrenia inferred from children of schizophrenics. Br J Psychiatry 129:142–154, 1976

Harvey P, Winters K, Weintraub S, et al: Distractibility in children vulnerable to psychopathology. J Abnorm Psychol 90:298–304, 1981

Hathaway SR, McKinley JC: Minnesota Multiphasic Personality Inventory, Revised. Minneapolis, MN, University of Minnesota, 1970

Heston LL: Psychiatric disorders in foster home reared children of schizophrenic mothers. Br J Psychiatry 112:819–825, 1966

Honigfeld G, Gillis RD, Klett CJ: Nurses' Observation Scale for Inpatient Evaluation. Westwood, NJ, Behavior Arts Center, 1966

Howells JG, Guirguis WR: Childhood schizophrenia 20 years later. Arch Gen Psychiatry 41:123–128, 1984

Janes CL, Hesselbrock B, Stern J: Parental psychopathology, age and race as factors in electrodermal activity of children. Psychophysiology 13:24–34, 1978

Karno M, Norquist GS: Schizophrenia: epidemiology, in Comprehensive Textbook of Psychiatry V, Vol 1. Edited by Kaplan HI, Sadock BJ. Baltimore, MD, Williams & Wilkins, 1989, pp 699–705

Kestenbaum CJ, Canino IA, Pleak RR: Schizophrenic disorders in childhood and adolescence, in American Psychiatric Press Review of Psychiatry, Vol 8. Edited by Tasman A, Hales RE, Frances AJ. Washington, DC, American Psychiatric Press, 1989, pp 240–259

Kety SS: Mental illness in the biological and adoptive relatives of schizophrenic adoptees: findings relevant to genetic and environmental factors in etiology. Am J Psychiatry 140:720–727, 1983

Kety SS, Rosenthal D, Wender PH, et al: The types and prevalence of mental illness in the biological and adoptive families of adopted schizophrenics, in The Transmission of Schizophrenia. Edited by Rosenthal D, Kety SS. Oxford, UK, Pergamon, 1968, pp 345–362

Kety SS, Rosenthal D, Wender PH, et al: Mental illness in the biological and adoptive families of adopted individuals who have become schizophrenic, in Genetic Research in Psychiatry. Edited by Fieve RR, Rosenthal D, Brill H. Baltimore, MD, Johns Hopkins University Press, 1975, pp 147–165

King RA: Neurodevelopmental model of schizophrenia. Arch Gen Psychiatry 45:1051, 1988

Kolvin I: Psychoses in childhood: a comparative study, in Infantile Autism: Concepts, Characteristics and Treatment. Edited by Rutter M. Edinburgh, Churchill Livingstone, 1971a, pp 7–26

Kolvin I: Studies in the childhood psychoses, I: diagnostic criteria and classification. Br J Psychiatry 118:381–384, 1971b

Kolvin I, Ounsted C, Roth M: Cerebral dysfunction and childhood psychoses. Br J Psychiatry 118:407–413, 1971a

Kolvin I, Ounsted C, Humphrey M, et al: Studies in the childhood psychoses, II: the phenomenology of childhood psychoses. Br J Psychiatry 118:385–395, 1971b

Kolvin I, Ounsted C, Richardson LM, et al: Studies in the childhood psychoses, III: the family and social background in childhood psychoses. Br J Psychiatry 118:396–402, 1971c

Kraepelin E: Dementia Praecox and Paraphrenia (1899). Translated by Barclay RM (from the 8th German edition of the Textbook of Psychiatry). Edinburgh, Livingstone, 1919

Kugelmass S, Marcus J, Schmueli J: Psychophysiological reactivity in high-risk children. Schizophr Bull 14:66–73, 1985

Kulcar Z, Crocetti GM, Lemkau PV, et al: Selected aspects of the epidemiology of psychoses in Croatia, Yugoslavia, II: pilot studies of communities. Am J Epidemiol 94:118–125, 1971

Kydd RR, Werry JS: Schizophrenia in children under 16 years. J Autism Dev Disord 12:343–357, 1982

Lane EA, Albee GW: Comparative birth weights of schizophrenics and their siblings. J Psychol 65:227–231, 1966

Lewis S, Owen MJ, Murray RM: CT correlates of obstetric complications in schizophrenia. Schizophrenia Research 1:160–161, 1988

Loranger AW: Sex difference in age at onset of schizophrenia. Arch Gen Psychiatry 41:157–161, 1984

Makita K: The age of onset of childhood schizophrenia. Folia Psychiatrica Neurologica Japonica 20:111–121, 1966

Marcus J: Cerebral functioning in offspring of schizophrenics: a possible genetic factor. International Journal of Mental Health 3:57–73, 1974

Marcus J, Hans SL, Lewow E, et al: Neurological findings in high-risk children: childhood assessment and 5-year follow-up. Schizophr Bull 11:85–100, 1985

Marcus J, Hans SL, Nagler S, et al: Review of the NIMH Israeli Kibbutz-city study and the Jerusalem infant development study. Schizophr Bull 13:425–438, 1987

Mednick S, Schulsinger F: Some premorbid characteristics related to breakdown in children with schizophrenic mothers, in The Transmission of Schizophrenia. Edited by Rosenthal D, Kety SS. Oxford, UK, Pergamon, 1968, pp 267–291

Mednick SA, Schulsinger F, Higgins J, et al: Genetics, Environment, and Psychopathology. New York, Elsevier, 1974

Mednick SA, Schulsinger F, Teasdale TW, et al: Schizophrenia in high-risk children: sex differences in predisposing factors, in Cognitive Defects in the Development of Mental Illness. Edited by Serban G. New York, Brunner/Mazel, 1978, pp 169–197

Mednick SA, Machon RA, Huttunen MO, et al: Adult schizophrenia following prenatal exposure to an influenza epidemic. Arch Gen Psychiatry 45:189–192, 1988

Mirsky AF, Silberman EK (eds): Issue Theme: Israeli High-Risk Study. Schizophr Bull (special issue) 11:19–154, 1985

Mirsky AF, Silberman EK, Latz A, et al: Adult outcomes of high-risk children: differential effects of town and kibbutz rearing. Schizophr Bull 11:150–154, 1985

Morihisa JM, Duffy FH, Wyatt RJ: Brain electrical activity mapping (BEAM) in schizophrenic patients. Arch Gen Psychiatry 40:719–728, 1983

Murray RM, Lewis SW, Owen MJ, et al: The neurodevelopmental origins of dementia praecox, in Schizophrenia: The Major Issues. Edited by McGuffin P, Bebbington P. London, Heinemann, 1988, pp 90–106

Naruse H, Nagahata M, Nakane Y, et al: A multi-center double-blind trial of pimozide (Orap), haloperidol and placebo in children with behavioral disorders, using a crossover design. Acta Paedopsychiatrica 48:173–184, 1982

Nuechterlein KH: Signal detection in vigilance tasks and behavioral attributes among offspring of schizophrenic mothers and among hyperactive children. J Abnorm Psychol 92:4–28, 1983

Nuechterlein KH: Converging evidence for vigilance deficit as a vulnerability indicator for schizophrenic disorders, in Controversies in Schizophrenia: Changes and Constancies. Edited by Albert M. New York, Guilford, 1985, pp 175–198

Offord DR, Cross LA: Behavioral antecedents of adult schizophrenia: a review. Arch Gen Psychiatry 21:267–283, 1969

Orvaschel H, Puig-Antich J, Chambers W, et al: Retrospective assessment of child psychopathology with the Kiddie-SADS-E. Journal of the American Academy of Child Psychiatry 21:392–397, 1982

Overall JE, Gorham DR: The Brief Psychiatric Rating Scale. Psychol Rep 10:799–812, 1962

Pangalila-Ratulangi EA: Pilot evaluation of Orap (pimozide, R6238) in child psychiatry. Psychiatria Neurologia Neurochirurgia 76:17–27, 1973

Parnas J, Schulsinger F, Schulsinger H, et al: Behavioral precursors of schizophrenia spectrum. Arch Gen Psychiatry 39:658–664, 1982

Petty LK, Ornitz EM, Michelman JD, et al: Autistic children who become schizophrenic. Arch Gen Psychiatry 41:129–135, 1984

Pilowsky D, Chambers WJ (eds): Hallucinations in Childhood. Washington, DC, American Psychiatric Press, 1986

Pollin W, Stabenau JR: Biological, psychological and historical differences in a series of monozygotic twins discordant for schizophrenia, in The Transmission of Schizophrenia. Edited by Rosenthal D, Kety SS. Oxford, UK, Pergamon, 1968, pp 317–332

Pool D, Bloom W, Mielke DH, et al: A controlled evaluation of loxitane in seventy-five adolescent schizophrenic patients. Current Therapeutic Research 19:99–104, 1976

Prentky RA, Salzman LF, Klein RH: Habituation and conditioning of skin conductance responses in children at risk. Schizophr Bull 7:281–291, 1981

Puig-Antich J, Ryan N, Rabinovich H: Affective disorders in childhood and adolescence, in Diagnosis and Psychopharmacology of Childhood and Adolescent Disorders. Edited by Wiener J. New York, John Wiley, 1985, pp 113–150

Realmuto GM, Erickson WD, Yellin AM, et al: Clinical comparison of thiothixene and thioridazine in schizophrenic adolescent patients. Am J Psychiatry 141:440–442, 1984

Reiss D, Feinstein C, Weinberger DR, et al: Ventricular enlargement in child psychiatric patients: a controlled study with planimetric measurements. Am J Psychiatry 140:453–456, 1983

Rieder RO, Nichols PL: Offspring of schizophrenics, III. Arch Gen Psychiatry 36:665–674, 1979

Rogeness GA, Maas JW, Javors MA, et al: Diagnoses, catecholamine metabolism, and plasma dopamine-β-hydroxylase. J Am Acad Child Adolesc Psychiatry 27:121–125, 1988

Rosenthal D, Wender PH, Kety SS, et al: The adopted away offspring of schizophrenics. Am J Psychiatry 128:307–311, 1971

Roth WT: Late event-related potentials and psychopathology. Schizophr Bull 3:105–120, 1977

Russell AT, Bott L, Sammons C: The phenomenology of schizophrenia occurring in childhood. J Am Acad Child Adolesc Psychiatry 28:399–407, 1989

Rutschmann J, Cornblatt B, Erlenmeyer-Kimling L: Sustained attention in children at risk for schizophrenia: report on a continuous performance test. Arch Gen Psychiatry 34:571–575, 1977

Rutter M: Childhood schizophrenia reconsidered. Journal of Autism and Childhood Schizophrenia 2:315–337, 1972

Rutter M, Tizard J, Whitmore K (eds): Education, Health and Behavior. London, Longman, 1970

Schneider K: Clinical Psychopathology (English translation of 1950 edition). New York, Grune & Stratton, 1959

Schulsinger F, Parnas J, Petersen ET, et al: Cerebral ventricular size in the offspring of schizophrenic mothers: a preliminary study. Arch Gen Psychiatry 41:602–606, 1984

Spencer E, Padron-Gayol M, Kafantaris V, et al: Haloperidol in schizophrenic children, in Scientific Proceedings of the Annual Meeting of the American Academy of Child and Adolescent Psychiatry 6:64–65, 1990

Spitzer RL, Endicott J, Robins E: Research Diagnostic Criteria: rationale and reliability. Arch Gen Psychiatry 35:773–782, 1978

Steinberg D: Psychotic and other severe disorders in adolescence, in Child and Adolescent Psychiatry: Modern Approaches. Edited by Rutter M, Hersov L. Oxford, UK, Blackwell Scientific Publications, 1985, pp 567–583

Strandburg RJ, Marsh JT, Brown WS, et al: Event-related potential concomitants of information processing dysfunction in schizophrenic children. Electroencephalogr Clin Neurophysiol 57:236–253, 1984

Tanguay PE, Cantor SL: Schizophrenia in children. Journal of the American Academy of Child Psychiatry 25:591–594, 1986

Taylor MA, Gaztanaga P, Abrams R: Manic-depressive illness and acute schizophrenia: a clinical, family history and treatment-response study. Am J Psychiatry 131:678–682, 1974

Tienari P: Psychiatric illness in identical twins. Acta Psychiatr Scand 39 (suppl 171):1–195, 1963

Tienari P, Sorri A, Naarala M, et al: The Finnish adoptive family study: adopted-away offspring of schizophrenic mothers, in Psychosocial Intervention in Schizophrenia. Edited by Stierlin H, Wynne LC, Wirsching M. Berlin, Springer-Verlag, 1983, pp 21–34

Torrey EF: Prevalence studies in schizophrenia. Br J Psychiatry 150:598–608, 1987

Van Dyke JL, Rosenthal D, Rasmussen PV: Electrodermal functioning in adopted-away offspring of schizophrenics. J Psychiatr Res 10:199–215, 1974

Volkmar FR, Cohen DJ, Hoshino Y, et al: Phenomenology and classification of the childhood psychoses. Psychol Med 18:191–201, 1988

Walsh D, O'Hare A, Blake B, et al: The treated prevalence of mental illness in the Republic of Ireland: the Three County Case Register Study. Psychol Med 10:465–470, 1980

Watkins JM, Asarnow RF, Tanguay PE: Symptom development in childhood onset schizophrenia. J Child Psychol Psychiatry 29:865–878, 1988

Weinberger DR: Implications of normal brain development for the pathogenesis of schizophrenia. Arch Gen Psychiatry 44:660–669, 1987

Weizman R, Gil-ad I, Dick J, et al: Low plasma immunoreactive β-endorphin levels in autism. J Am Acad Child Adolesc Psychiatry 27:430–433, 1988

Werry JS, McClellan JM, Chard L: Childhood and adolescent schizophrenic, bipolar, and schizoaffective disorders: a clinical outcome study. J Am Acad Child Adolesc Psychiatry (in press)

Chapter 21

Mood Disorders in Children

Elizabeth Weller, M.D.
Ronald A. Weller, M.D.

Mood disorders in children have long been underdiagnosed in the United States because of the belief that a child's immature superego and personality structure would not allow the development or experience of a mood disorder (Koran 1975). However, detailed case descriptions of depressed youngsters suffering from sadness, irritability, changes in concentration, suicidal thoughts, hopelessness, changes in appetite and sleep, and other depressive symptoms have been reported for many years in the literature.

Both unipolar and bipolar disorders in children and adolescents have been described and treated in Europe for many years (Annell 1969a, 1969b; Frommer 1968). In 1971, the Union of European Pedopsychiatrists officially recognized and addressed the needs of depressed children and adolescents by declaring that depression is an important illness that comprises a significant proportion of mental disorders in children and adolescents. In 1975, the National Institute of Mental Health established a priority for children's mental health. At that time, a work group of researchers and clinicians studied the issue of depression in children. As a result of this work, a seminal book entitled *Depression in Childhood: Diagnosis, Treatment and Conceptual Models* was published (Schulterbrandt and Raskin 1977). This book should be read by all those interested in mood disorders in children and adolescents.

Although the 1970s will be known as the period when the existence of depression in children and adolescents was first officially recognized and ac-cepted, it was in the 1980s that interest in trying to diagnose bipolar disorder in children and adolescents accelerated.

Kraepelin (1921) felt bipolar disorders were rare but did occur in children and that there was a surge of new cases during adolescence. Some believed the behavior of normal children was so similar to hypomania that it was difficult to diagnose mania in children unless the condition was crystal clear in appearance.

It is difficult to diagnose depression and mania in children because children do not begin to use language as a vehicle for communicating information appropriately until around age 7 years. Even in the 1990s, verbal communication still is our best tool in diagnosing psychiatric disorders. Unfortunately, it has become common practice to use quick checklists or to talk only to parents about the child, instead of carefully evaluating the child and listening to what the child has to say. Without a direct evaluation of the child, one misses the core symptoms of mood disorders (e.g., feeling sad, having low self-esteem, feeling inadequate, having suicidal thoughts) and focuses only on the symptoms that motivate parents to bring the child to the clinic (e.g., irritability, getting in fights, other disruptive behaviors) (Cantwell and Carlson 1983; Weller and Weller 1984, 1986a, 1986b).

The 1970s and 1980s saw the development of new instruments to help diagnose psychiatric conditions in children and adolescents, including structured diagnostic interviews such as the Diagnostic Interview for Children and Adolescents (DICA) (Reich et al. 1982); semistructured interviews such as the Schedule for Affective Disorders and Schizophrenia for school-age children (K-SADS) (Chambers et al. 1985); and rating scales such as the Children's Depression Rating Scale—Revised (Poznanski et al. 1984) and the Mania Rating Scale (Young et al. 1978) adapted for children by Fristad et al. (1989). Another important development in the diagnosis of psychiatric disorders in children was the publication of the diagnostic criteria in DSM-III (American Psychiatric Association 1980) and DSM-III-R (American Psychiatric Association 1987), which have given us a common language so that we can communicate more clearly about psychiatric diagnoses. This has helped to reduce problems that arise when, for example, a child is diagnosed as manic in one center when in another he or she might be diagnosed as having schizophrenia. Unfortunately, with the severe shortage of well-trained child and adolescent psychiatrists (Graduate Medical Evaluation National Advisory Committee 1980), children may still be misdiagnosed. Many children are incorrectly diagnosed as having adjustment disorder with depressed mood for periods as long as 2 years. Also, children are being diagnosed as schizophrenic if they have heard voices telling them to kill themselves during a depressive episode.

Kashani and Eppright (Chapter 22, this volume) include a discussion of diagnostic criteria and include tables with DSM-III-R criteria for mood disorders. This chapter will focus on clinical presentation, differential diagnosis, epidemiology, etiology, assessment and treatment, prognosis, and research issues in prepubertal children.

Clinical Presentation

Infants

In their classic papers, Spitz (1946) and Bowlby (1951) described the mood of children who have been separated from their primary caregivers at an early age. Clinically, these children look depressed, cry a lot, react slowly to stimuli, exhibit retarded movements, and may have sleep and appetite disturbances. Spitz called this "anaclitic depression" because it appeared so similar to depression observed in adults. In institutionalized infants and toddlers, this same clinical picture has been called "hospitalism." As mentioned earlier, it is very difficult to make a completely informed diagnosis of depression in this age group because of poorly developed verbal communication.

Preschoolers

In somewhat older children, the clinical picture gets a little easier to decipher. Preschoolers with depression look very sad, have limited verbal communication, appear slowed down, and lack a "twinkle" in their eyes. As one of the parents of a depressed preschooler put it, "The bubble has gone out of her." In this age group, not gaining weight, not growing, and weepiness with "tummy aches" are also common symptoms.

School-Age Children

By the time children are 6 to 7 years old, their verbal repertoire makes them more accessible to be listened to and understood. Children 6–12 years old usually have no problem spontaneously admitting to symptoms such as poor mood ("low, down in the dumps" or "wanting to be nothing when I grow up"), trouble concentrating, poor performance in school, irritability, crying, and suicidal thoughts of which their parents are often not aware. It is not uncommon to see children who have attempted suicide to have even *that attempt* go unrecognized or be mistaken by their physicians or be attributed to "accident," because of the myth that children do not attempt suicide. In our experience, clearcut suicides in children before the age of 10 almost always have been labeled accidental deaths by the coroner. As a society, we have difficulty believing that children can be depressed and suicidal; we equate childhood with happiness, lack of worries, and no responsibilities.

Somatic symptoms may coexist with depressive symptoms in this age group, the most common being headaches and abdominal pain and discomfort. Such depressed children often are seen by the pediatrician or family physician, who conducts an extensive and expensive laboratory workup. At the end, the parents and child are told that "nothing is wrong" or "it is all in the head," with no recognition of or suggestion for treatment of the depression.

Differential Diagnosis

It is essential that a child be given a thorough physical checkup before making a diagnosis of a mood disorder. In the infant-toddler group, children who look sad, seem depressed or apathetic, and are not gaining weight should be evaluated for organic "failure to thrive." This would include ruling out central nervous system, hormonal, and gastrointestinal anomalies. In the absence of organic reasons for failure to thrive, etiologies such as neglect, abuse, and Münchausen's syndrome by proxy (i.e., parent fabricating psychiatric symptomatology in the child) should be considered. Hospitalization may be helpful in clarifying the diagnosis, as nonorganic failure-to-thrive children quickly improve in their affect and gain weight under the care of nurturing professionals. It is important to assess carefully the primary caregivers (usually mothers) of these children, who often suffer from undiagnosed depression, so they can be treated and then more effectively and safely care for their children. Similarly, in the depressed preschool child, it is also important to rule out a malignancy or child neglect and abuse (both physical and sexual) when considering the diagnosis of depression (Weller and Weller 1990).

In the school-age child, adjustment disorder with depressed mood (in response to a circumscribed noxious event in a child's life, such as divorce or sibling's birth) must be considered in the differential diagnosis. Children with adjustment disorder with depressed mood do not satisfy criteria for a major depressive episode but have depressive symptoms. Normal grief should also be in the differential; 37% of children who experience the death of a parent satisfy criteria for major depression in the 3 months after parental death (Weller and Weller 1990).

Dysthymia should also be included in the differential, although dysthymic children often *also* have a coexisting major depression (so-called double depression). Dysthymic children have a history of being cranky, unhappy, weepy, and apathetic for periods of time lasting as long as 1 year. Symptom-free periods are less than 2 months (American Psychiatric Association 1987).

Sometimes the schizophrenic prodrome in children starts with affective symptomatology. A positive family history of schizophrenia should alert the physician to this possibility. If the clinician is not sure whether to diagnose a child as schizophrenic or mood disordered, in the absence of long-term follow-up or past history of prior episodes (which are common circumstances in such children), the condition can be termed *undiagnosed* or the condition can be initially treated as a mood disorder, since mood disorders seem to have better prognoses than schizophrenic disorders (Akiskal and Weller 1989; Weller and Weller 1989).

Finally, anxiety disorders also should be considered in the differential diagnosis. There is a subgroup of affectively ill children who have concomitant anxiety disorders (separation anxiety, overanxious disorder). Successful treatment of mood disorders often in turn alleviates anxiety symptoms in these children.

In considering the diagnosis of mania in this age group, the possibility of attention-deficit hyperactivity disorder should always be carefully evaluated. Symptoms of both disorders can coexist. However, the symptoms of attention-deficit hyperactivity disorder may start as early as toddlerhood and continue in a chronic fashion. The situation gets worse as the child goes to school and problems with attention and inappropriate peer relationships become apparent.

Ongoing work by our group (Fristad et al., unpublished data) has attempted to develop a mania rating scale that would be useful in children. Initial work indicated that the Mania Rating Scale (Young et al. 1978) modified for use in children differentiated manic children from hyperactive children in the total score as well as in most individual items. However, Conners' (1973) hyperactivity questionnaire did not differentiate mania from attention-deficit disorder. To differentiate manic children from hyperactive children symptomatically, manic children often have later age of onset, push of speech, flight of ideas, punning, and clinging, as well as delusions and hallucinations. In a study of 10 prepubertal manic children (Varanka et al. 1988), all had psychotic symptoms. Psychotic symptoms are not typically present in attention-deficit hyperactivity disorder.

Another diagnosis that should be considered is conduct disorder. Most children with conduct disorder present with lying, stealing, and fighting. Manic symptomatology and psychotic symptoms are infrequent.

Childhood schizophrenia occurs in 1 in 10,000 of the population and should also be considered (J. R. Asarnow, personal communication). The exact prevalence of mania in children is not yet known. In adolescents and adults, schizophrenia is less common than mood disorders. This might also be true in children.

A literature review (Weller et al. 1986b) indicated that mania was underdiagnosed. Some children were misdiagnosed as having either schizophrenia, conduct disorder, or attention-deficit disorder, although they met DSM-III criteria for mania.

Epidemiology

Epidemiologic studies performed in different countries have yielded varying frequencies of depression. However, this does not mean that depression in Turkey (Polvan and Cebiroglu 1972) is less common than in Columbia, Missouri (Kashani et al. 1983). These apparently different rates can be attributed to several factors, such as different procedures for recruiting subjects as well as varying methods of study and assessment instruments.

Although the exact prevalence of depression in children is unknown, several studies provide useful information as to its occurrence. In the general population studied by Kashani et al. (1983), 2% of the children suffered from major depression. In preschoolers, the rate is less than 17% (Kashani and Carlson 1987). Of children admitted to pediatric hospitals for medical reasons, 7% suffer from depression (Kashani et al. 1981), as do 40% of children in pediatric neurology clinics presenting with headaches (Ling et al. 1970). Unfortunately, the shortage of trained mental health professionals as well as inappropriate use of rating scales to diagnose depression, such as the Children's Depression Inventory (Kovacs 1981), designed to measure severity of depression, has hampered efforts to provide depressed children optimal care.

To date, no epidemiologic study of mania in prepubertal children has been done. Although Kraepelin (1921) reported 0.4% of manic adults had an age of onset prior to age 10, modern epidemiologic studies will be needed to establish the prevalence of mania in prepubertal children.

Etiology

Multiple etiologies, such as genetic, biochemical, environmental, and intrapsychic factors, have been proposed as having a role in the genesis of depression.

Genetic Studies

Monozygotic twin adults have higher concordance rates for depression than dizygotic twin adults (Akiskal and Weller 1989). Also, studies of the biological and adoptive parents of adults suffering from depression show increased depression in the biological relatives compared with adoptive relatives. The same holds true for manic adults. Similar studies in depressed and manic children need to be done.

Biochemical

Several neurotransmitter systems have been implicated in depression, including the noradrenergic, serotonergic, cholinergic, and dopaminergic systems. It appears that one or more of these systems may be disturbed in a depressive episode. However attractive a biochemical hypothesis is in explaining the etiology of depression, much more work will be required before there is a full understanding of the biochemical abnormalities in such a complex organ as the human brain (Weller and Weller 1988).

Environmental

Environmental factors such as loss or stress may also be considered important etiologic variables. Since depression runs in families, often depressed children are living with and being cared for by a depressed parent (usually the mother). Depressed mothers' interactions with their children have been described as negative and belittling to the child. Also, when asked about their childhood, depressed adults report having very negative interactions with their parents.

Many other etiologic models have been suggested. It is apparent, however, that none of these models fully explains all cases of depression. The etiology at present should be considered multifactorial until further research provides additional information. A further discussion is provided by Kashani and Eppright (Chapter 22, this volume).

Assessment and Treatment

Before initiating treatment for a depressed child, a complete physical examination and laboratory tests to rule out medical conditions that mimic depression are necessary. These should include complete blood count with differential, electrolytes, liver function tests, thyroid function tests, blood urea nitrogen, creatinine, urinalysis, urine osmolality, and electrocardiogram, and, if clinically indicated, an electroencephalogram and computed tomography or magnetic resonance imaging scan should be done.

In preschoolers, play therapy or psychotherapy including family therapy may be used effectively. As of this writing, there are no double-blind, placebo-controlled studies that assess the effect of antidepressants in preschoolers. Because the condition appears infrequently (less than 1%) and is hard to diagnose in this age group, this is not surprising.

In preschool and school-age children, a thorough diagnostic evaluation should include interviews with the child together with the family, with the parents as a couple, with each parent separately, and with the child alone. Psychiatric information about the parents, their experiences while growing up, and the parenting they received, as well as a detailed three-generational family history of psychiatric disorders (particularly regarding mood disorders) may provide useful information. Structured diagnostic interviews (e.g., DICA-R, child and parent form) as well as semistructured interviews (e.g., K-SADS) can be used by the clinician to provide a complete review of possible psychiatric syndromes (Weller and Weller 1986a).

If psychotherapy is to be used for a depressed child, the clinician should take an active role. It gets "quite depressing" to sit and wait for a depressed child to talk. Engaging games such as the "Talking, Feeling, and Doing Game" are often helpful. Supportive therapy with the child and the family can be very productive, especially when it is accompanied by education about the illness. Do not blame the child or the family for having caused the depression. Many families are eager to cooperate when the depression is described in terms of an illness model. As the acute phase of the illness abates, they often are more open to considering family interactions that might be perceived as being stressful by the depressed child.

To date, the tricyclic antidepressants are the most often prescribed medications to treat depression (Weller et al. 1982). Because imipramine has been used for a long time to treat enuresis in children, many parents have heard of it and are less resistant to a 6-week trial with the understanding that it may be discontinued if ineffective. It is important to obtain consent from parents and assent from children prior to starting the medicine. Children often resist taking medications unless they understand

why the medication is necessary. Explanations that many children can understand include "to help you feel better, be less grouchy, sleep better, or eat better." Children do not like to appear different from their peers. Giving the medicine at home at bedtime may be a good choice; tricyclic antidepressants are equally efficacious whether given in divided doses or only at bedtime. Some advocate divided doses in prepubertal children to avoid extremes of high and low in plasma levels; further studies are needed, however, to prove this scientifically. Parents should be told that tricyclic antidepressants are not approved in children below the age of 12 years by the United States Food and Drug Administration.

There are two published double-blind, placebo-controlled studies of imipramine treatment of depression in prepubertal children. Puig-Antich et al. (1987) studied outpatient depressed prepubertal children. Plasma levels were measured but not controlled. Imipramine was not shown to be superior to placebo. However, when plasma imipramine levels were compared in responders and nonresponders, the responders had levels greater than 180 ng/ml. In another study, Preskorn et al. (1987) studied hospitalized depressed prepubertal children. The plasma levels were adjusted between 125 and 250 ng/ml. Those depressed children who had a nonsuppressed dexamethasone suppression test responded to imipramine but not to placebo. Children who had a negative test responded equally well to imipramine and placebo. Further double-blind, placebo-controlled studies on tricyclics are needed to assess these agents' efficacy in depressed children.

When starting a depressed outpatient child on imipramine, treatment should be initiated with small doses (e.g., 1–2 mg/kg/day) given orally and carefully increased (not to exceed 5 mg/kg/day) until therapeutic effects are achieved or intolerable side effects develop. Plasma level monitoring by a reliable laboratory, after the child has achieved a pharmacologic steady state (usually 5 days on the same dose), can be clinically helpful to assess adequacy of treatment and compliance. Low plasma tricyclic antidepressant levels can result from noncompliance or from rapid metabolism of the drug (Weller et al. 1982). High plasma levels can lead to an agitated toxic state and nonresponse (Preskorn et al. 1988). Electrocardiographic monitoring before increasing dosage, looking for prolongation of PR interval and QRS changes, is recommended.

Lithium carbonate has been recommended in the

treatment of bipolar illness (Campbell et al. 1989; Youngerman and Canino 1978). As of this writing, there are few studies and very few double-blind, placebo-controlled studies (DeLong and Aldershof 1987) proving the efficacy of lithium in prepubertal children. However, because lithium is effective in adults (Schou 1968) and in some adolescents with mania (Strober et al. 1990), it would seem logical to use it in manic children. When using lithium in children, parental consent should always be obtained. To be considered as adequate, lithium should be at therapeutic levels for at least 6 weeks. Weller et al. (1986a) described an easy way of starting children on lithium carbonate according to their weight so that therapeutic levels can be quickly achieved. Prior to starting on lithium, the blood workup for depression mentioned earlier, including urine osmolality and creatinine clearance, should be obtained. Because it is very difficult to collect a 24-hour urine sample in children (especially those with nocturnal enuresis), two 12-hour collections in the period the children are awake can be used.

Once a patient is stabilized and the lithium level is therapeutic (0.6–1.2 meq) and stable, the level can be assessed monthly to ensure safety and compliance. Children usually tolerate lithium better than do adults. Common side effects include enuresis (especially if there is preexisting history of enuresis), nausea (if given on empty stomach), and weight gain. A mild tremor frequently occurs but is usually tolerated by most children. Rarely, an acne-like rash may occur, but this also is tolerated by prepubertal children.

If use of lithium is to be long term, periodic assessment (every 6–12 months) of kidney and thyroid functions is recommended.

Lithium is also known to be deposited in bone. The significance of this is not known in adults. However, as children are still growing, the consequences of its deposition in bones should be studied further. No detrimental effects have been reported in children with long-term use (in some cases for as long as 15 years).

Prognosis

Several studies have shown that recurrence of depression is quite common in children (Kovacs et al. 1984). Also, dysthymic children have been reported to develop major depression (Kovacs et al. 1984). Approximately 80% of hospitalized de-

pressed children are rehospitalized within 2 years of discharge (Asarnow et al. 1988).

A positive family history for mood disorders is more frequent in depressed children than in depressed adults (Puig-Antich et al. 1988). This might mean depression in childhood is a more virulent illness and may have poorer prognosis.

Research Issues

Although little research was done on childhood mood disorders until the last decade, much progress has been made. A great deal more, however, remains to be studied.

The so-called cohort effect indicates that those persons who were born after 1940 are at increased risk for depression, mania, and schizoaffective disorders compared with those individuals born earlier (Gershorn et al. 1987; Klerman et al. 1985). If this effect continues, there may be a dramatic increase of depression and mania in children in years to come.

In designing future studies of depression and mania in children, children of mood-disordered adults with mania and depression should be studied prospectively. If mood disorders are detected early in these high-risk children, aggressive intervention may protect these children from developing the consequences of depression, such as low self-esteem, personality problems, and academic impairment.

Another way to study depression in children is to examine children who have experienced a tragic event, such as the death of a parent. If depression is due to actual or perceived loss, studying children who have experienced an actual loss may provide better insight into the role of loss or stress in the genesis of depression. If risk factors for children who will develop depression rather than normal grief can be identified, early intervention may be possible and depressive symptoms minimized (Weller and Weller 1990).

Another area to study more carefully is biological markers in high-risk populations (e.g., children of mood-disordered adults, grieving children with a family history of depression). If child and adolescent psychiatrists truly believe in early identification and prevention, it would be ideal to work on *trait* markers (which exist prior to an episode of illness) rather than *state* markers (which become abnormal during an episode of illness). However, true state markers also may be very helpful in clinical follow-up of identified cases (Weller and Weller 1988; Weller et al. 1985).

To understand and study mood disorders, one must realize that human beings are biological, psychological, and social entities. Environmental influences, including the most subtle psychological interactions, are mediated by the brain. Hence, abnormal mood or behavior may result directly from environmental influences *or* from the brain's inability to encode and interpret them properly (Puig-Antich 1986).

References

Akiskal HS, Weller EB: Mood disorders and suicide in children and adolescents, in Comprehensive Textbook of Psychiatry V, Vol 2. Edited by Kaplan HI, Sadock BJ. Baltimore, MD, Williams & Wilkins, 1989, pp 1981–1994

American Psychiatric Association: Diagnostic and Statistical Manual of Mental Disorders, 3rd Edition. Washington, DC, American Psychiatric Association, 1980

American Psychiatric Association: Diagnostic and Statistical Manual of Mental Disorders, 3rd Edition, Revised. Washington, DC, American Psychiatric Association, 1987

Annell AL: Lithium in the treatment of children and adolescents. Acta Psychiatr Scand Suppl 207:19–30, 1969a

Annell AL: Manic-depressive illness in children and effect of treatment with lithium carbonate. Acta Paedopsychiatry (Basel) 36:292–301, 1969b

Asarnow JR, Goldstein MJ, Carlson GA, et al: Childhood-onset depressive disorders: a follow-up study on rates of rehospitalization and out-of-home placement among child psychiatric inpatients. J Affective Disord 15:245–253, 1988

Bowlby J: Maternal Care and Mental Health, 2nd Edition. Geneva, World Health Organization, 1951

Campbell M, Cohen IR, Perry R, et al: Psychopharmacological treatment, in Handbook of Child Psychopathology, 2nd Edition. Edited by Ollendick TH, Hersen M. New York, Plenum, 1989, pp 473–498

Cantwell D, Carlson GA: Affective Disorders in Childhood and Adolescence. New York, SP Medical and Scientific Books, 1983

Chambers WJ, Puig-Antich J, Hirsch M, et al: The assessment of affective disorders in children and adolescents by semi-structured interview. Arch Gen Psychiatry 42:696–702, 1985

Conners CK: Rating scales for use in drug studies with children. J Psychosom Res (special issue), 1973, pp 24–29

DeLong GR, Aldershof AL: Long-term experience with lithium treatment in childhood correlation with clinical diagnosis. J Am Acad Child Adolesc Psychiatry 26:389–394, 1987

Fristad MA, Weller EB, Weller RA, et al: Assessing Mania in Prepubertal Children. Presented at poster session at the 36th annual meeting of the American Academy of Child and Adolescent Psychiatry, New York, October 1989

Frommer E: Depressive illness in childhood. Br J Psychiatry 2:117–123, 1968

Gershon ES, Hamovit JH, Guroff JJ, et al: Birth-cohort changes in manic and depressive disorders in relatives of bipolar and schizoaffective patients. Arch Gen Psychiatry 44:314–319, 1987

Graduate Medical Education National Advisory Committee: Report of the Graduate Medical Education National Advisory Committee to the Secretary, Department of Health and Human Services, Vol 1: Summary (USDHHS). Washington, DC, Health Resources Administration, Office of Graduate Medical Education, 1980

Kashani J, Carlson GA: Seriously depressed preschoolers. Am J Psychiatry 144:348–350, 1987

Kashani J, Barber G, Bolander F: Depression in hospitalized pediatric patients. J Am Acad Child Adolesc Psychiatry 20:123–134, 1981

Kashani J, McGee RO, Clarkson SE, et al: Depression in a sample of 9-year-old children. Arch Gen Psychiatry 40:1217–1223, 1983

Klerman GL, Lavori PW, Rice J, et al: Birth-cohort trends in rates of major depressive disorder among relatives of patients with affective disorder. Arch Gen Psychiatry 42:689–693, 1985

Koran LM: The reliability of clinical methods, data and judgements. N Engl J Med 293:642–646, 1975

Kovacs M: Rating scale to assess depression in school-aged children. Acta Pediatric Psychiatry 46:305–315, 1981

Kovacs M, Feinberg TL, Crouse-Novak M, et al: Depressive disorders in childhood, II: a longitudinal study of the risk for a subsequent major depression. Arch Gen Psychiatry 41:643–649, 1984

Kraepelin E: Manic Depressive Insanity and Paranoia. Edinburgh, Livingstone, 1921

Ling M, Oftedal C, Weinberg W: Depressive illness in childhood presenting as severe headache. Am J Dis Child 120:122–124, 1970

Polvan O, Cebiroglu R: Treatment with pharmacologic agents in childhood depressions, in Depressive States in Childhood and Adolescence. Edited by Annel AL. New York, John Wiley, 1972, pp 467–472

Poznanski EO, Grossman JA, Buchsbaum Y, et al: Preliminary studies of the reliability and validity of the Children's Depression Rating Scale. Journal of the American Academy of Child Psychiatry 23:191–197, 1984

Preskorn S, Weller E, Hughes C, et al: Depression in prepubertal children: dexamethasone nonsuppression predicts differential response to imipramine vs placebo. Psychopharmacol Bull 23:128–133, 1987

Preskorn S, Weller E, Hughes C, et al: Relationship of plasma imipramine levels to CNS toxicity in children (letter). Am J Psychiatry 145:897, 1988

Puig-Antich J: Biological markers: effects of age and puberty, in Depression in Young People; Developmental and Clinical Perspectives. Edited by Rutter M, Izard C, Read P. New York, Guilford, 1986, pp 341–381

Puig-Antich J, Perel JM, Lupatkin W, et al: Imipramine in prepubertal major depressive disorders. Arch Gen Psychiatry 44:81–89, 1987

Puig-Antich J, Goetz D, Davies M, et al: A controlled family history study of prepubertal major depressive disorder. Arch Gen Psychiatry 46:406–420, 1988

Reich W, Herjanic B, Welner Z, et al: Development of a structured psychiatric interview for children: agreement on diagnosis comparing child and parent interviews. J Abnorm Child Psychol 10:325–336, 1982

Schou M: Lithium in psychiatric therapy and prophylaxis. J Psychiatr Res 6:67–95, 1968

Schulterbrandt JG, Raskin A: Depression in Childhood: Diagnosis, Treatment, and Conceptual Models. New York, Raven, 1977

Spitz R: Anaclitic depression. Psychoanal Study Child 2:113–117, 1946

Strober M, Morrell W, Lampert C, et al: Relapse following discontinuation of lithium maintenance therapy in adolescents with bipolar I illness: a naturalistic study. Am J Psychiatry 147:457–461, 1990

Varanka TM, Weller RA, Weller EB, et al: Lithium treatment of manic episodes with psychotic features in prepubertal children. Am J Psychiatry 145:1557–1559, 1988

Weller EB, Weller RA: Current Perspectives on Major Depressive Disorders. Washington, DC, American Psychiatric Press, 1984

Weller EB, Weller RA: Assessing depression in prepubertal children. Hillside J Clin Psychiatry 8:193–201, 1986a

Weller EB, Weller RA: Clinical aspects of childhood depression. Pediatric Annals 15:843–847, 1986b

Weller EB, Weller RA: Neuroendocrine changes in affectively ill children and adolescents. Endocrinology of Neuropsychiatric Disorders 17:41–54, 1988

Weller EB, Weller RA: Pediatric management of depression. Pediatric Annals 18:104–113, 1989

Weller EB, Weller RA: Grief in children and adolescents, in Psychiatric Disorders in Children and Adolescents. Edited by Garfinkel B, Carlson G, Weller E. Philadelphia, PA, WB Saunders, 1990, pp 37–47

Weller EB, Weller RA, Preskorn SH, et al: Steady-state plasma imipramine levels in prepubertal depressed children. Am J Psychiatry 139:506–508, 1982

Weller EB, Weller RA, Fristad MA, et al: The dexamethasone suppression test in prepubertal depressed children. J Clin Psychiatry 46:511–513, 1985

Weller EB, Weller RA, Fristad MA: Lithium dosage guide for prepubertal children: a preliminary report. Journal of the American Academy of Child Psychiatry 25:92–95, 1986a

Weller RA, Weller EB, Tucker SG, et al: Mania in prepubertal children: has it been underdiagnosed? J Affective Disord 11:151–154, 1986b

Young RC, Biggs JT, Ziegler VE, et al: A rating scale for mania: reliability, validity and sensitivity. Br J Psychiatry 133:429–435, 1978

Youngerman J, Canino I: Lithium carbonate use in children and adolescents. Arch Gen Psychiatry 35:216–224, 1978

Chapter 22

Mood Disorders in Adolescents

Javad H. Kashani, M.D.
Thomas D. Eppright, M.D.

Definition

The term *mood* is defined in DSM-III-R (American Psychiatric Association 1987, p. 401) as "a pervasive and sustained emotion that, in the extreme, markedly colors [a] person's perception of the world." A *mood disorder* has been described as having as its "essential feature . . . a disturbance of mood, accompanied by a full or partial Manic or Depressive Syndrome, that is not due to any other physical or mental disorder" (p. 213). A *mood syndrome* (depressed or manic) comprises "a group of mood and associated symptoms 'hat occur together for a minimal duration of time" ,p. 213). It is postulated that these mood syndromes can develop as part of a mood disorder, as part of a nonmood psychotic disorder (e.g., schizoaffective disorder), or as part of an organic mental disorder (e.g., organic mood disorder). A *mood episode* (major depressive, manic, or hypomanic) is defined as "a mood syndrome that is not due to a known organic factor and is not part of a nonmood psychotic disorder (e.g., Schizophrenia, Schizoaffective Disorder, or Delusional Disorder)" (pp. 213–214). The word *affect*, as defined by Dorland (1985), is a "feeling of pleasantness or unpleasantness evoked by a stimulus; also the emotional complex associated with a mental state" (p. 37). The comparison between affect and mood, according to DSM-III (American Psychiatric Association 1980), is analogous to that between climate and weather, wherein affect is conceptualized as statelike and mood is described as traitlike.

Diagnostic Criteria and Clinical Findings

The major purposes of classification are communication, information organization and retrieval, description, prediction, and theoretical understanding (Carlson and Garber 1986).

The classification and diagnostic criteria for mood disorders in children and adolescents remain controversial. Carlson and Garber (1986) called for a clearer set of criteria for classifying childhood and adolescent psychiatric disorders. Cantwell and Baker (1988) noted that DSM-III quadrupled the number of childhood psychiatric disorders. They further remarked that DSM-III-R was comparable to DSM-III in that it served as a fountainhead of both concern about and stimulus for increased interest in the classification of childhood and adolescent psychiatric disorders.

The classification of mood disorders according to DSM-III-R is shown in Table 22-1. The DSM-III-R criteria for mood disorders in adolescents are comparable to the adult criteria. The diagnosis of major depressive episode closely resembles that for the adult criteria (see Table 22-2). The only difference is that while adults should have a depressed mood to satisfy the criteria, adolescents may exhibit an irritable mood.

The clinical picture of dysthymia (depressive neurosis) in adolescents differs somewhat from the adult criteria in that an irritable mood may be present in adolescents and children (in contrast to a depressed mood in adults) for most of the day,

Table 22-1. DSM-III-R classification of mood disorders

Bipolar disorders	Depressive disorders
Bipolar disorder	Major depression
Mixed	Single episode
Manic	Recurrent
Depressed	Dysthymia
Cyclothymia	Depressive disorder NOS
Bipolar disorder NOS	

Note. NOS = not otherwise specified.

more days than not, as indicated by either subjective account or observation by others, with a duration of 1 year in adolescents (compared with 2 years in adults) (see Table 22-3). There must also not be evidence of an unequivocal major depressive episode during the first year of the disturbance (2 years in adults).

The criteria for cyclothymia (a rare disorder with few published reports in adolescents) are identical to the adult criteria except that the duration of the disorder may be 1 year in adolescents, rather than 2 years (see Table 22-4).

Finally, the criteria for mania in adolescence are identical to the adult criteria (see Table 22-5).

Differential Diagnosis

A differential diagnosis for the mood disorders should be thorough and comprehensive. It is important that all organic causes that may precipitate affective-type symptoms be considered and excluded. Briefly, this is accomplished by obtaining a thorough medical history, performing an extensive physical examination, and ordering appropriate laboratory studies.

A mania-like syndrome may be present in various circumstances. Such a syndrome has been noted in some cases of organic mood syndromes, especially in conjunction with the use of drugs, such as amphetamines and steroids (American Psychiatric Association 1987). In some cases of depression, treated with either electroconvulsive therapy or antidepressant medications, manic-type symptoms may be precipitated. Certain subtypes of schizophrenia may mimic mania, especially paranoid type, when the prevailing symptomatology comprises psychotic delusions, hostility, and/or agitation (American Psychiatric Association 1987).

It has long been noted that children and adolescents with attention-deficit hyperactivity disorder exhibit symptoms resembling mania (i.e., mood lability, temper outbursts, and distractibility). However, approximately half of the attention-deficit hyperactivity disorder cases begin before the age of 4, whereas mania usually begins at a later age; additionally, elevated mood is usually absent in this disorder (American Psychiatric Association 1987).

Depressive symptomatology can be attributed to many factors. A few illnesses that can mimic depression include influenza, diabetes, and infectious mononucleosis (frequently seen in the adolescent population).

The illegal use of drugs and alcohol during adolescence is widespread, and one must continually be alert to the possible depressive effects of chronic alcohol use, marijuana, and even those drugs previously mentioned, such as cocaine and amphetamines (Wise and Rundell 1988).

Adolescents with the diagnosis of anorexia nervosa certainly may present with depressive-type symptoms (especially in light of the considerable amount of weight loss experienced), but may not be formally depressed, as their essential feature remains disturbance of body image (American Psychiatric Association 1987). In addition, catatonic schizophrenic patients who show signs of isolation and psychotic retardation may also appear to be depressed to the untrained observer (American Psychiatric Association 1987).

Somatization disorder can mirror depression closely, with anhedonia, fatigue, difficulty sleeping, psychomotor agitation or retardation, and anorexia frequently being seen (Hackett and Cassem 1987).

Some disorders can present as either mania or depression. Adolescents with anxiety-type symptoms can exhibit depressive symptoms with feelings of helplessness and impending disaster. Alternatively, they may appear to be manic with feelings of heightened perception and increased vigilance.

Lastly, an illness that is having a profound effect on both the psychiatric and medical populations, in both the adolescent and adult age groups, is acquired immune deficiency syndrome (AIDS). AIDS may present as a constellation of symptoms. It interfaces with depression simply by virtue of its characteristic weight loss and fatigue as well as its associated depressed affect. Manic-type symptoms also may be present in some AIDS patients (Belfer et al. 1988).

In summary, a differential diagnosis of adolescent mood disorders should include the aforementioned plus many more; still, the ability to properly diagnose adolescent disorders remains a challenge.

Table 22-2. DSM-III-R diagnostic criteria for major depressive episode

Note: A "Major Depressive Syndrome" is defined as criterion A below.

A. At least five of the following symptoms have been present during the same two-week period and represent a change from previous functioning; at least one of the symptoms is either (1) depressed mood, or (2) loss of interest or pleasure. (Do not include symptoms that are clearly due to a physical condition, mood-incongruent delusions or hallucinations, incoherence, or marked loosening of associations.)
   1. Depressed mood (or can be irritable mood in children and adolescents) most of the day, nearly every day, as indicated either by subjective account or observation by others
   2. Markedly diminished interest or pleasure in all, or almost all, activities most of the day, nearly every day (as indicated either by subjective account or observation by others of apathy most of the time)
   3. Significant weight loss or weight gain when not dieting (e.g., more than 5% of body weight in a month), or decrease or increase in appetite nearly every day (in children, consider failure to make expected weight gains)
   4. Insomnia or hypersomnia nearly every day
   5. Psychomotor agitation or retardation nearly every day (observable by others, not merely subjective feelings of restlessness or being slowed down)
   6. Fatigue or loss of energy nearly every day
   7. Feelings of worthlessness or excessive or inappropriate guilt (which may be delusional) nearly every day (not merely self-reproach or guilt about being sick)
   8. Diminished ability to think or concentrate, or indecisiveness, nearly every day (either by subjective account or as observed by others)
   9. Recurrent thoughts of death (not just fear of dying), recurrent suicidal ideation without a specific plan, or a suicide attempt or a specific plan for committing suicide
B. 1. It cannot be established that an organic factor initiated and maintained the disturbance
   2. The disturbance is not a normal reaction to the death of a loved one (uncomplicated bereavement)
      Note: Morbid preoccupation with worthlessness, suicidal ideation, marked functional impairment or psychomotor retardation, or prolonged duration suggest bereavement complicated by major depression.
C. At no time during the disturbance have there been delusions or hallucinations for as long as two weeks in the absence of prominent mood symptoms (i.e., before the mood symptoms developed or after they have remitted).
D. Not superimposed on schizophrenia, schizophreniform disorder, delusional disorder, or psychotic disorder NOS.

Major Depressive Episode codes: fifth-digit code numbers and criteria for severity of current state of bipolar disorder, depressed, or major depression:

1-Mild: Few, if any, symptoms in excess of those required to make the diagnosis, **and** symptoms result in only minor impairment in occupational functioning or in usual social activities or relationships with others.
2-Moderate: Symptoms or functional impairment between "mild" and "severe."
3-Severe, without Psychotic Features: Several symptoms in excess of those required to make the diagnosis, **and** symptoms markedly interfere with occupational functioning or with usual social activities or relationships with others.
4-With Psychotic Features: Delusions or hallucinations. If possible, **specify** whether the psychotic features are *mood-congruent* or *mood-incongruent*.
   Mood-congruent psychotic features: Delusions or hallucinations whose content is entirely consistent with the typical depressive themes of personal inadequacy, guilt, disease, death, nihilism, or deserved punishment.
   Mood-incongruent psychotic features: Delusions or hallucinations whose content does *not* involve typical depressive themes of personal inadequacy, guilt, disease, death, nihilism, or deserved punishment. Included here are such symptoms as persecutory delusions (not directly related to depressive themes), thought insertion, thought broadcasting, and delusions of control.
5-In Partial Remission: Intermediate between "In Full Remission" and "Mild," **and** no previous dysthymia. (If major depressive episode was superimposed on dysthymia, the diagnosis of dysthymia alone is given once the full criteria for a major depressive episode are no longer met.)
6-In Full Remission: During the past six months no significant signs or symptoms of the disturbance
0-Unspecified.
Specify **chronic** if current episode has lasted two consecutive years without a period of two months or longer during which there were no significant depressive symptoms.
Specify if current episode is **melancholic type.**

Source. Reprinted with permission from American Psychiatric Association 1987.

Table 22-3. DSM-III-R diagnostic criteria for dysthymia

A. Depressed mood (or can be irritable mood in children and adolescents) for most of the day, more days than not, as indicated either by subjective account or observation by others, for at least two years (one year for children and adolescents)

B. Presence, while depressed, of at least two of the following:
1. Poor appetite or overeating
2. Insomnia or hypersomnia
3. Low energy or fatigue
4. Low self-esteem
5. Poor concentration or difficulty making decisions
6. Feelings of hopelessness

C. During a two-year period (one year for children and adolescents) of the disturbance, never without the symptoms in A for more than two months at a time.

D. No evidence of an unequivocal major depressive episode during the first two years (one year for children and adolescents) of the disturbance
Note: There may have been a previous major depressive episode, provided there was a full remission (no significant signs or symptoms for six months) before development of the dysthymia. In addition, after these two years (one year in children or adolescents) of dysthymia, there may be superimposed episodes of major depression, in which case both diagnoses are given.

E. Has never had a manic episode or an unequivocal hypomanic episode.

F. Not superimposed on a chronic psychotic disorder, such as schizophrenia or delusional disorder.

G. It cannot be established that an organic factor initiated and maintained the disturbance, e.g., prolonged administration of an antihypertensive medication.

Specify primary or **secondary type:**
Primary type: the mood disturbance is not related to a preexisting, chronic, nonmood, Axis I or Axis III disorder, e.g., anorexia nervosa, somatization disorder, a psychoactive substance dependence disorder, an anxiety disorder, or rheumatoid arthritis.
Secondary type: the mood disturbance is apparently related to a preexisting, chronic, nonmood Axis I or Axis III disorder.

Specify early onset or **late onset:**
Early onset: onset of the disturbance before age 21.
Late onset: onset of the disturbance at age 21 or later.

Source. Reprinted with permission from American Psychiatric Association 1987.

Table 22-4. DSM-III-R diagnostic criteria for cyclothymia

A. For at least two years (one year for children and adolescents), presence of numerous hypomanic episodes (all of the criteria for a manic episode, except criterion C that indicates marked impairment) and numerous periods with depressed mood or loss of interest or pleasure that did not meet criterion A of major depressive episode.

B. During a two-year period (one year in children and adolescents) of the disturbance, never without hypomanic or depressive symptoms for more than two months at a time.

C. No clear evidence of a major depressive episode or manic episode during the first two years of the disturbance (or one year in children and adolescents).
Note: After this minimum period of cyclothymia, there may be superimposed manic or major depressive episodes, in which case the additional diagnosis of bipolar disorder or bipolar disorder NOS should be given.

D. Not superimposed on a chronic psychotic disorder, such as schizophrenia or delusional disorder.

E. It cannot be established that an organic factor initiated and maintained the disturbance, e.g., repeated intoxication from drugs or alcohol.

Source. Reprinted with permission from American Psychiatric Association 1987.

Epidemiology

Epidemiologic studies of mood disorders in adolescents remain limited (Carlson and Strober 1979). This may be because adolescence is traditionally considered a troubling time in which symptoms of turmoil are ordinary. Alternatively, some mental health professionals may be reluctant to "label" youths with psychiatric diagnoses that may follow them into adulthood. More accurate data are becoming available from several multicenter studies that are currently in progress.

Epidemiology means "the study of the relationships of the various factors determining the frequency and distribution of diseases in a human community" (Dorland 1985, p. 451). Some of the many factors that have been studied to date in mood disorders include age, social class, and sex.

In a study by Kashani et al. (1987), using structured interviews in a community adolescent sample, it was found that the prevalence of adolescent depression (between ages 14 and 16) was 4.7% for major depression and 3.3% for dysthymia. This was more than double the prevalence rate in school-

Table 22-5.   DSM-III-R diagnostic criteria for manic episode

Note: A "Manic Syndrome" is defined as including criteria A, B, and C below. A "Hypomanic Syndrome" is defined as including criteria A and B, but not C, i.e., no marked impairment.

A. A distinct period of abnormally and persistently elevated, expansive, or irritable mood.

B. During the period of mood disturbance, at least three of the following symptoms have persisted (four if the mood is only irritable) and have been present to a significant degree:

1. Inflated self-esteem or grandiosity
2. Decreased need for sleep, e.g., feels rested after only three hours of sleep
3. More talkative than usual or pressure to keep talking
4. Flight of ideas or subjective experience that thoughts are racing
5. Distractibility, i.e., attention too easily drawn to unimportant or irrelevant external stimuli
6. Increase in goal-directed activity (either socially, at work or school, or sexually) or psychomotor agitation
7. Excessive involvement in pleasurable activities which have a high potential for painful consequences, e.g., the person engages in unrestrained buying sprees, sexual indiscretions, or foolish business investments

C. Mood disturbance sufficiently severe to cause marked impairment in occupational functioning or in usual social activities or relationships with others, or to necessitate hospitalization to prevent harm to self or others.

D. At no time during the disturbance have there been delusions or hallucinations for as long as two weeks in the absence of prominent mood symptoms (i.e., before the mood symptoms developed or after they have remitted).

E. Not superimposed on schizophrenia, schizophreniform disorder, delusional disorder, or psychotic disorder NOS.

F. It cannot be established that an organic factor initiated and maintained the disturbance. **Note:** Somatic antidepressant treatment (e.g., drugs, ECT) that apparently precipitates a mood disturbance should not be considered an etiologic organic factor.

Manic episode codes: fifth-digit code numbers and criteria for severity of current state of bipolar disorder, manic or mixed:

1-Mild: Meets minimum symptom criteria for a manic episode (or almost meets symptom criteria if there has been a previous manic episode).

2-Moderate: Extreme increase in activity or impairment in judgment.

3-Severe, without psychotic features: Almost continual supervision required in order to prevent physical harm to self or others.

4-With Psychotic Features: Delusions, hallucinations, or catatonic symptoms. If possible, **specify** whether the psychotic features are *mood-congruent* or *mood-incongruent*.

Mood-congruent psychotic features: Delusions or hallucinations whose content is entirely consistent with the typical manic themes of inflated worth, power, knowledge, identity, or special relationship to a deity or famous person.

Mood-incongruent psychotic features: Either (*a*) or (*b*):

a) Delusions or hallucinations whose content does *not* involve the typical manic themes of inflated worth, power, knowledge, identity, or special relationship to a deity or famous person. Included are such symptoms as persecutory delusions (not directly related to grandiose ideas or themes), thought insertion, and delusions of being controlled.

b) Catatonic symptoms, e.g., stupor, mutism, negativism, posturing.

5-In Partial Remission: Full criteria were previously, but are not currently, met; some signs or symptoms of the disturbance have persisted.

6-In Full Remission: Full criteria were previously met, but there have been no significant signs or symptoms of the disturbance for at least six months.

0-Unspecified.

Source.   Reprinted with permission from American Psychiatric Association 1987.

age children (Kashani et al. 1983) and a higher rate than in preschoolers (Kashani and Carlson 1987). Kaplan et al. (1984) found that, by using a Beck (1976) cutoff score of 16, there was a point prevalence rate of 8.6% for major depression in their sample. Equally interesting, in the study by Kashani et al. (1987) and in another study by Rutter et al. (1976), almost one-half of the adolescents interviewed acknowledged having considerable misery and anguish.

Adolescents hospitalized for psychiatric disorders appear to have yet a greater rate of depressive disorders. Studies by Robbins et al. (1982) reported a diagnosis of major depressive disorder in 28% of the adolescents they screened. Strober et al. (1981) found a prevalence rate of 18.7%.

Studies have shown rates of depression in prepubertal children to be equal in both males and females. Studies by Kashani et al. (1987) and Rutter (1986b) show that the prevalence of both depressive symptoms and disorders increases with age, as does the girl-boy ratio. This phenomenon may center around social and biological factors (Rutter 1986a).

The epidemiology of bipolar mood disorder in adolescents has been coupled with that of adults. Studies have shown that many first hospitalizations for bipolar mood disorders occur during adolescence (Goodwin and Jamison 1990). The male to female ratio has been found to be roughly 1:1.2 (Hirschfeld and Goodwin 1988). The social class studies reveal a slight increase in the upper socioeconomic class (Weissman and Boyd 1983).

Kovacs et al. (1988) looked at comorbidity among youths with conduct disorder and found that 6 of 24 youths with a concomitant diagnosis of mood disorder and conduct disorder (25%) eventually developed some type of bipolar disorder. Therefore, with studies such as this, the diagnosis of a mood disorder certainly does not preclude the presence of other associated disorders (e.g., anxiety) (Kovacs et al. 1984).

Etiology: Theoretical Models

The literature to date on the etiology of childhood and adolescent mood disorders points to the premise that no one model can account for the entire cause. Indeed, a multiplicity of models may make varying contributions to a common pathway (Akiskal and McKinney 1975). In this section, the various approaches to the etiology and maintenance of adolescent mood disorders are reviewed. Areas to be explored include the biological, sleep architecture, psychodynamic, learned helplessness, cognitive distortion, social skills deficit, and family systems approaches. The most recent literature on the etiology of bipolar illness will also be reviewed.

Biological Formulation

Psychiatric researchers in recent years have commented on the idea that mood disorders may have a genetic predisposition. To date, studies have revealed a probable greater degree of penetrance in bipolar mood disorders and a lesser degree of genetic transmission in conditions such as reactive or neurotic depression (Hirschfeld and Goodwin 1988).

Most information on the genetic aspects of mood disorders has been ascertained from studies of twins. These studies have revealed a concordance rate of 65%–75% for major mood disorder in identical twins, compared with the 14%–19% rate in fraternal twins (Hirschfeld and Goodwin 1988).

Tsuang (1978) found an average monozygotic twin concordance rate of 76% for mood disorders. He also noted a rate of 19% for dyzygotic twins and a 67% concordance rate for monozygotic twins raised separately.

Studies by Puig-Antich (1980) allowed it to be postulated that major depression with occurrence in the prepubertal years may carry greater pathogenic loading than during adulthood.

Bipolar disorder. Studies to date indicate that bipolar disorder is prevalent in certain families. Hirshfield et al. (1986) found that 60%–65% of bipolar patients had family members with some history of major depression (bipolar or unipolar).

Neurotransmitter systems. Clinical observers have studied various biological phenomena associated with depression. Some of the neurotransmitters explored include norepinephrine, serotonin, gamma-aminobutyric acid, and dopamine, with the basic tenet being that the system involved is not functioning adequately. This was especially evident in the early studies of amines, in which Schildkraut (1965) and Bunney and Davis (1965) formulated the catecholamine hypothesis; that is, depression was thought to result from a deficiency of the catecholamines (norepinephrine), and mania from an excess.

Lastly, urinary metabolite research has focused on 3-methoxy-4-hydroxyphenylglycol (MHPG), the main metabolite of norepinephrine in the brain. Clinical evidence to date points to the fact that MHPG levels are decreased in depressed patients compared with controls and are even lower in bipolar patients (Hirschfeld and Goodwin 1988).

Neuroendocrine markers. Studies using a multiplicity of factors (e.g., radioimmunoassay and testing of cortisol levels) have demonstrated increased secretion of cortisol in some, but not all, depressed patients. Increased cortisol secretion is seen not only in depressed patients but also in bipolar and unipolar patients (Sachar 1975).

Weller et al. (1984) used the dexamethasone suppression test (DST) in six 12-year-old subjects with major depressive disorder; the authors reported 70% sensitivity and 93% specificity, but this study was performed without a normal or a nondepressed control group. A subsequent controlled study by Weller et al. (1985) revealed 94% sensitivity and 75% specificity using an 8:00 A.M. cortisol suppression index and a 4:00 P.M. DST. Alternatively, studies by Puig-Antich et al. (1989) revealed that 24-hour cortisol secretory patterns in a group of prepubertal children diagnosed with major depression (ill and recovered), normal control subjects, and nonaffected control subjects were all similar. They found cortisol hypersecretion only in a distinct subgroup of prepubertal children with major depressive disorder.

Studies indicate that united DST and cortisol suppression index may distinguish prepubertal depression from a normal control group and a group of psychiatric control subjects. To date, the specificity of this technique in differentiating prepubertal depressive subtypes has not been investigated.

Sleep Architecture

It has long been noted that polysomnography can reveal markers for major depressive disorder in adults. Lahmeyer et al. (1983) found reduced rapid eye movement (REM) latency in 13 depressive adolescents compared with 13 control subjects. Goetz and colleagues (cited by Ryan and Puig-Antich 1986) studied adolescents with endogenous and nonendogenous major depression during a depressive cycle versus normal control subjects (mean age 14.5 years). Sleep continuity disturbances were noted in the depressive adolescents during early adolescence; REM latency abnormalities characterized later adolescence.

Psychological Models

Psychoanalytic approaches to depression usually center around the classic works of Freud (1914/1956) and Abraham (1953), as well as the object-loss approach postulated by Spitz and Wolf (1946). Bibring (1965) felt that depression resulted when one was not able to achieve his or her ego ideals.

To date, no studies have satisfactorily linked the above factors to adolescent depression. What is helpful to clinicians is the understanding that these posits may provide toward the study of adolescent depression. Freud (1914/1956) reported that some adolescents with melancholias had what was felt to be a major depression with the loss of an ambivalently viewed object.

Learned Helplessness

Seligman (1975) formulated the idea of learned helplessness based on the premise that an individual, after exposure to some uncontrollable life events, may develop feelings of both helplessness and hopelessness.

Petti (1983) felt this theory may be an important factor in childhood depression, but this remains to be studied in adolescents.

Cognitive Distortion Model

Beck (1976) researched the cognitive aspects of depression. He postulated what has been labeled the cognitive triad, which centers around maladaptive cognitions involving one's self, one's worldly experiences, and future experiences. Usually these cognitive disturbers are based on adverse life events that occur during childhood and are eventually magnified over time. A depressed individual would perceive problems of daily living as significant stressors, eventually feeling hopeless with little control over future life events. To date, Emery et al. (1983) have been able to utilize cognitive therapy effectively in adolescents.

Social Skills Deficits

This view asserts that a decline in the type and magnitude of social activities may contribute to depression. Lewinsohn (1974) found that depressed persons 1) receive fewer positive reinforcements than do people who are not depressed, 2) extract fewer positive feedbacks from others, and 3) usually have less social competency than the nondepressed populace.

This theory is important since social skills acquisition and application are considerable during latency and adolescence: not acquiring these skills would be an additional risk factor for depression.

Family Systems Approach

The family systems approach to depression generally views depression as a behavior supported by numerous interacting systems.

Treatment in family systems concentrates on those aspects of the system that support or reinforce the depression. Minuchin (1974) researched two classes of symptoms. First is the system-maintained symptom, in which the individual as a member help support the depression. Second, this system postulates a role for the depressed individual's reinforcing the family system.

To date, research in family systems is limited. Because of the differences between children and adolescents, these two groups should be studied separately.

Treatment

Treatment approaches to adolescent mood disorders continue to be a very important topic in psychiatry. The two main approaches to treatment are the biological and psychological models.

Most psychotherapy studies have been anecdotal. Many clinicians believe this approach to be helpful; the degree of efficacy, however, is unknown (Ryan and Puig-Antich 1986). Some clinicians believe that the adolescent with mood disorder is especially aided by various combinations of therapy. This includes individual psychotherapy (e.g., cognitive, insight-oriented, supportive), as well as group or family therapy, tailored to the needs of the individual adolescent.

Looking at some of these approaches briefly, Beck's (1976) cognitive therapy has been primarily used in the adult population, but has been shown to be effective in an adolescent population as well. Wilkes and Rush (1988) use traditional cognitive therapy with its emphasis on "setting agendas, listing problem areas, the pursuit of cognition or 'ideas' during times of stress, logical analysis of cognition and scheduled homework assignments" (p. 385). They also use three other modalities: the therapeutic alliance, special attention to the adolescent's cognitive development, and the involvement of the family of origin in the assessment and treatment process. Wilkes and Rush address issues such as the power struggles that are frequently seen during therapy sessions with adolescents, and they tailor cognitive therapy to the adolescent's developmental level to maximize data acquisition and com-

munication. They also involve the family of origin to help understand the basic milieu from which an adolescent arises (e.g., rules, values, religious belief) (Wilkes and Rush 1988).

Bedrosian (1981) outlined strategies he incorporated when working with depressed adolescents. He advised investigators to

1. Shorten the traditional 50-minute session.
2. Emphasize the development of rapport and minimize potentially threatening situations.
3. Tolerate some areas of noncompliance, such as tardiness for sessions and reluctance to verbalize.
4. Maintain contact with family so that intervention is available when needed.
5. Respect the adolescent's privacy.
6. Create a collaborative atmosphere and try to reach the stated goals for each session.
7. Avoid demanding complex homework between sessions and limit assignments to concrete, behavioral tasks.

According to the family systems theory, the basic problems lie somewhere within the family dynamics. Treatment usually involves identifying and then correcting the family dynamic that perpetuates the disturbance. Research looking at this approach's effectiveness on mood disorders is just beginning, with some researchers advocating sequential analyses of the home milieu to validate its usefulness.

The social skills approach to treatment appears on the surface to have much merit, but research to date supporting its efficacy in adolescents is scanty. Controlled outcome studies utilizing this approach are not available. It is conceivable, however, that pharmacologic treatment combined with this approach may offer enhanced treatment efficacy.

Psychopharmacology

It is widely known that considerable numbers of child psychiatrists and various other physicians use antidepressants in the adolescent population, and uncontrolled studies have demonstrated favorable responses (Brumbach et al. 1977; Frommer 1967; Lucas et al. 1965; Weinberg et al. 1973). To date, however, few controlled studies have clearly shown efficacy in the use of antidepressant medication in the adolescent population. Kramer and Ferguine (1981) compared a placebo group with a group given amitriptyline (200 mg/day) for 6 weeks, with the results showing little qualitative difference between them (both groups showed some improvement). In a study by Puig-Antich et al. (1983), 39% of 30 adolescents with depression demonstrated improvement with the tricyclic imipramine. In this study, the mean daily dose used was 240 mg/day. Again, no placebo or control group was employed.

The biological approach to depression in adolescents still poses many unanswered questions. Among them, what is the role for "current" agents recently introduced (fluoxetine or bupropion), or even what is the efficacy of monoamine oxidase inhibitors? Also, what is the appropriate use of electroconvulsive therapy in treatment-resistant depression in this population?

The use of lithium carbonate in the adolescent population is another interesting area. Most studies indicate that lithium may have a role in the treatment of bipolar disorders in adults (Bunney et al. 1972; Goodwin et al. 1972; Persson 1972; Prien et al. 1974) as well as in adolescents. Studies to date indicate that the management of adolescent bipolar patients with lithium is comparable to that of young adults (Ryan and Puig-Antich 1986). Still, there are unresolved issues. For example, should medication be started after the first episode or after subsequent episodes? How long should adolescents be maintained on these medications? How can compliance be ensured or monitored in this impulsive patient population?

In closing, several issues remain concerning the biological treatment of mood disorders in adolescents. Questions include the role of carbamazepine and second-line agents (e.g., Depakene, benzodiazepines, and beta-blockers), each alone or in combination with lithium. We recommend continued trials in studying these treatment modalities.

Prognosis

The prognosis in mood disorders, if not treated, is frequently poor. Mood disorders, if not diagnosed and adequately treated in children and adolescents, are frequently complicated by subsequent drug and alcohol abuse, poor family and peer relations, deficient school achievement, and even suicide (Akiskal and Weller 1989).

Kovacs et al. (1984) studied the natural history and course of depressive disorders in children and adolescents of various ages. Their studies revealed that youth depression can have an extended duration. They found that children with adjustment disorder and depressed mood had no greater risk of developing depressive disorder than did the rest of the population. They also found that the duration of major depressive disorder in children roughly averaged 7½ months. In their study, 44% of depressed youth were in remission within 6 months of diagnosis and 92% recovered by 1½ years. Within 5 years of the first depressive episode, however, 72% suffered a recurrence (or a second episode). They found that dysthymic disorder lasted an average of 3 years in children and that 6½ years after the beginning of the symptoms 89% had recovered. Also, the younger the age at diagnosis of dysthymia, the longer was the course of the disturbance; many times patients with early onset dysthymia also had a major depressive episode during the course of their dysthymia.

Akiskal and Weller (1989) reported that adolescents diagnosed with depression are at an increased risk for other depressive episodes and bipolar illness. Some predictors of bipolar outcome in adolescent depression include acute onset, hypersomnic retarded depression, psychotic depression, postpartum onset, tricyclic hypomania, bipolar family history, loaded pedigree, and family history of mood disorders in consecutive generations.

Research Issues

Many facets of research in adolescent psychiatry remain to be explored. In summary, they include the following:

1. The evaluation of various medications in the treatment of mood disorders (e.g., use of fluoxetine, monoamine oxidase inhibitors, bupropion, trazodone) in depressive disorders
2. The use of clonazepam, valproic acid, and calcium-channel blockers in bipolar disorders
3. The role of electroconvulsive therapy in the treatment of mood disorders
4. The long-term side effects of lithium and carbamazepine in the adolescent population as these individuals progress to adulthood
5. The role of various psychotherapies in the treatment of adolescent mood disorders and their interaction with pharmacologic therapies
6. The long-term outlook for certain chronic psychiatric diseases (e.g., Does the dysthymic group respond differently to treatment over time than the major depressive group?) with

an emphasis on those with particularly poor progress

In closing, many questions remain. Certainly, however, today's unanswered questions are the foundations for tomorrow's research.

References

Abraham K: Notes on the psychoanalytic investigation and treatment of manic-depressive insanity and allied conditions, in Selected Papers of Karl Abraham. Translated by Bryan D, Strachey A. New York, Basic Books, 1953, pp 137–156

Akiskal HS, McKinney WT: Overview of recent research in depression. Arch Gen Psychiatry 32:285–305, 1975

Akiskal HS, Weller EB: Mood disorders and suicide in children and adolescents, in Comprehensive Textbook of Psychiatry V, Vol 2. Edited by Kaplan HI, Sadock BJ. Baltimore, MD, Williams & Wilkins, 1989, pp 1981–1994

American Psychiatric Association: Diagnostic and Statistical Manual of Mental Disorders, 3rd Edition. Washington, DC, American Psychiatric Association, 1980

American Psychiatric Association: Diagnostic and Statistical Manual of Mental Disorders, 3rd Edition, Revised. Washington, DC, American Psychiatric Association, 1987

Beck AT: Cognitive Therapy and the Emotional Disorders. New York, International Universities Press, 1976

Bedrosian RC: The application of cognitive therapy techniques with adolescents, in New Directions in Cognitive Therapy: A Casebook. Edited by Emery G, Holton SD, Bedrosian RC. New York, Guilford, 1981, pp 168–182

Belfer M, Krener P, Miller FB: AIDS in children and adolescents. J Am Acad Child Adolesc Psychiatry 27:147–151, 1988

Bibring E: The mechanism of depression, in Affective Disorders. Edited by Greenacre P. New York, International Universities Press, 1965, pp 13–48

Brumbach RA, Deitz-Schmidt SG, Weinberg WA: Depression in children referred to an educational diagnostic center. Journal of Diseases of the Nervous System 38:529–534, 1977

Bunney WE, Davis JM: Norepinephrine in depressive reactions. Arch Gen Psychiatry 13:483–494, 1965

Bunney WE, Goodwin FK, Davis JM, et al.: A behavioral-biochemical study of lithium in therapy. Am J Psychiatry 125:499–512, 1972

Cantwell D, Baker L: Issues in the classification of child and adolescent psychopathology. J Am Acad Child Adolesc Psychiatry 27:521–533, 1988

Carlson GA, Garber J: Developmental issues in the classification of depression in children, in Depression in Young People: Developmental and Clinical Perspectives. Edited by Rutter M, Izard CE, Read PB. New York, Guilford, 1986, pp 399–434

Carlson GA, Strober M: Affective disorder in adolescence: issues in misdiagnosis. J Clin Psychiatry 39:63–66, 1979

Dorland's Illustrated Medical Dictionary, 26th Edition. Philadelphia, PA, WB Saunders, 1985

Emery G, Bedrosian R, Garber J: Cognitive therapy and depressed children and adolescents, in Affective Disorders in Childhood and Adolescence: An Update. Edited by Cantwell DP, Carlson JA. Jamaica, NY, Spectrum, 1983, pp 445–471

Freud S: Mourning and melancholia (1914), in The Standard Edition of the Complete Psychological Works of Sigmund Freud, Vol 14. Translated and edited by Strachey J. London, Hogarth Press, 1956, pp 243–258

Frommer EA: Treatment of childhood depression with antidepressant drugs. Br Med J 1:729–732, 1967

Goodwin FK, Jamison KR: Manic-Depressive Illness. New York, Oxford University Press, 1990

Goodwin F, Murphy D, Dunner D, et al: Lithium response of unipolar versus bipolar depression. Am J Psychiatry 129:44–47, 1972

Hackett TP, Cassem NH (eds): Massachusetts General Hospital Handbook of General Hospital Psychiatry, 2nd Edition. Littleton, MA, PSG Publishing, 1987

Hirschfeld RMA, Goodwin FK: Mood disorders, in American Psychiatric Press Textbook of Psychiatry. Edited by Talbott JA, Hales RE, Yudofsky SC. Washington, DC, American Psychiatric Press, 1988, pp 403–441

Hirschfeld RMA, Klerman GL, Keller MB, et al: Personality of recovered patients with bipolar affective disorders. J Affective Disord 11:81–89, 1986

Kaplan SL, Hong GK, Weinhold C: Epidemiology of depressive symptomatology in adolescents. Journal of the American Academy of Child Psychiatry 23:91–98, 1984

Kashani JH, Carlson GA: Seriously depressed preschoolers. Am J Psychiatry 144:348–350, 1987

Kashani JH, McGee RO, Clarkson SE, et al: Depression in a sample of 9-year-old children. Arch Gen Psychiatry 40:1217–1223, 1983

Kashani JH, Carlson GA, Beck NC, et al: Depression, depressive symptoms and depressed mood among a community sample of adolescents. Am J Psychiatry 144:931–934, 1987

Kovacs M, Feinberg TL, Crouse-Novak M, et al: Depressive disorders in childhood, II: a longitudinal study of the risk for a subsequent major depression. Arch Gen Psychiatry 41:643–649, 1984

Kovacs M, Paulauskas S, Gatsonis C, et al: Depressive disorders in childhood, II: a longitudinal study of comorbidity with and risk for conduct disorders. J Affective Disord 15:205–217, 1988

Kramer AD, Ferguine RJ: Clinical effects of amitriptyline in adolescent depression. Journal of the American Academy of Child Psychiatry 20:636–644, 1981

Lahmeyer HW, Poznanski EO, Bellur SN: EEG sleep in depressed adolescents. Am J Psychiatry 140:1150–1153, 1983

Lewinsohn PM: A behavioral approach to depression, in The Psychology of Depression: Contemporary Theory and Research. Edited by Friedman RJ, Katz MM. New York, John Wiley, 1974, pp 157–178

Lucas AR, Kocket HJ, Grimm F: Amitriptyline in childhood depression. Journal of Diseases of the Nervous System 26:105–110, 1965

Minuchin S: Families and Family Therapy. Cambridge, MA, Harvard University Press, 1974

Persson G: Lithium prophylaxis in affective disorders. Acta Psychiatr Scand 48:462–479, 1972

Petti TA: Behavioral approaches in the treatment of depressed children, in Affective Disorders in Childhood and Adolescence: An Update. Edited by Cantwell DP, Carlson GA. Jamaica, NY, Spectrum, 1983, pp 417–443

Prien RF, Caffey EJ, Klett CJ: Factors associated with treatment success in lithium carbonate prophylaxis. Arch Gen Psychiatry 31:189–192, 1974

Puig-Antich J: Affective disorders in childhood. Psychiatr Clin North Am 3:403–424, 1980

Puig-Antich J, Cooper T, Ambrosini PJ, et al: Plasma level/clinical response relationship in major depressive disorder in adolescents. Paper presented at the annual meeting of the American Academy of Child Psychiatry, San Francisco, CA, October 1983

Puig-Antich J, Dahl R, Ryan N, et al: Cortisol secretion in prepubertal children with major depressive disorder. Arch Gen Psychiatry 46:801–809, 1989

Robbins DR, Alessi NE, Cook SC, et al: The use of the Research Diagnostic Criteria for depression in adolescent psychiatric inpatients. Journal of the American Academy of Child Psychiatry 21:251–255, 1982

Rutter M: Child psychiatry: the interface between clinical and developmental research. Psychol Med 16:151–169, 1986a

Rutter M: Depressive feelings, cognitions, and disorders: a research postscript, in Depression in Young People: Developmental and Clinical Perspectives. Edited by Rutter M, Izard CE, Read PB. New York, Guilford, 1986b, pp 491–519

Rutter M, Graham P, Chadwick OF, et al: Adolescent turmoil: fact or fiction? J Child Psychol Psychiatry 17:35–56, 1976

Ryan ND, Puig-Antich J: Affective illness in adolescence, in Psychiatry Update: American Psychiatric Association Annual Review, Vol 5. Edited by Frances AJ, Hales RE. Washington, DC, American Psychiatric Press, 1986, pp 420–450

Sachar EJ: Neuroendocrine abnormalities in depressive illness, in Topics of Psychoendocrinology. Edited by Sachar EJ. New York, Grune & Stratton, 1975, pp 135–156

Schildkraut JJ: The catecholamine hypothesis of affective disorders: a review of supporting evidence. Am J Psychiatry 122:509–522, 1965

Seligman MEP: Helplessness: On Depression, Development and Depth. San Francisco, CA, Freeman, 1975

Spitz RA, Wolf KM: Anaclitic depression: an inquiry into the genesis of psychiatric conditions in early childhood, II. Psychoanal Study Child 2:312–342, 1946

Strober M, Green J, Carlson G: Phenomenology and subtypes of major depressive disorder in adolescence. J Affective Disord 3:281–290, 1981

Tsuang MT: Genetic counseling for psychiatric patients and their families. Am J Psychiatry 135:1465–1475, 1978

Weinberg WA, Rutman J, Sullivan L, et al: Depression in children referred to an educational diagnostic center. J Pediatr 83:1065–1075, 1973

Weissman MM, Boyd JH: The epidemiology of affective disorders, rates and risk factors, in Psychiatry Update: The American Psychiatric Association Annual Review, Vol 2. Edited by Grinspoon L. Washington, DC, American Psychiatric Press, 1983, pp 406–428

Weller EB, Weller RA, Fristad MA, et al: The dexamethasone suppression test in hospitalized prepubertal depressed children. Am J Psychiatry 141:290–291, 1984

Weller RA, Weller EB, Fristad MA, et al: A comparison of the cortisol suppression index and the dexamethasone suppression test in prepubertal children. Am J Psychiatry 142:1370–1372, 1985

Wilkes TCR, Rush J: Adaptations of cognitive therapy for depressed adolescents. J Am Acad Child Adolesc Psychiatry 27:381–386, 1988

Wise M, Rundell J: Concise Guide to Consultation Psychiatry. Washington, DC, American Psychiatric Press, 1988

Section V

Disorders of Conduct and Behavior

Chapter 23

Attention-Deficit Hyperactivity Disorder

Laurence L. Greenhill, M.D.

Attention-deficit hyperactivity disorder (ADHD) has gradually assumed a central position in American child psychiatry. Compared with the other disruptive behavior disorders of childhood listed in DSM-III-R (American Psychiatric Association 1987), ADHD commands a lion's share of clinical meeting presentations, research reports, and journal entries. This is because ADHD disrupts the social and academic functioning of many school-age children and yet responds quickly, in most cases, to low doses of stimulant medication.

In this chapter, I will review the phenomenological basis of ADHD, its impact on academic and social functioning, and the status of available treatments. Because different studies use different diagnostic labels—either attention deficit disorder with hyperactivity (ADDH) from DSM-III (American Psychiatric Association 1980) or ADHD from DSM-III-R—I will typically use the more general term *attention-deficit disorder* (ADD) in this chapter.

Controversy

There has been a mounting public interest in ADD. Articles have appeared decrying the medicalization of the classroom (Schrag and Divoky 1975) and questioning the validity of the disorder. Others express upset by the wide range of prevalence estimates for ADD, which vary from 0.08% to 10% of the population (Kohn 1989). Another criticism is that any single ADD symptom listed in DSM-III-R can be found in children who are free of psychiatric disorder. Furthermore, ADD has been subject to a confusing number of name changes. In 1968, DSM-II (American Psychiatric Association 1968) called it the *hyperkinetic syndrome*. In 1971, other writers used the term *minimal brain dysfunction* (Wender 1971). By 1980, DSM-III had rejected minimal brain dysfunction (because of lack of any specific etiologic causation from brain damage) in favor of attention deficit disorder with hyperactivity (ADDH). DSM-III-R now calls the condition *attention-deficit hyperactivity disorder*. The diagnostic criteria for ADHD are given in Table 23-1.

Even as various experts struggled to refine the concept, clinicians forged ahead, dispensing stimulants (Safer and Krager 1988).

Epidemiology

As Cantwell (1982) pointed out, the prevalence reported for the ADD syndrome has depended on a number of factors, including the population studied, methods of investigation, and diagnostic criteria employed. One complicating issue is the high base rate of motor hyperactivity reported for normal children. Mothers reported overactivity in 57% of boys and 42% of girls (Lapouse and Monk 1953). First- and second-grade teachers found that 49% of boys and 24% of girls couldn't sit still, and a slightly lower percentage had attentional difficulties (Berry et al. 1985).

Screening with a single teacher rating form can produce higher prevalence rates for ADD. Trites et al. (1981) found that teachers scored 14.3% of 14,000 Ottawa school-age children above the cutoff score traditionally used for ADD children on the Conners Teacher Rating Scale (Conners 1969; Conners and Barkley 1990). Using an Abbreviated Conners Rat-

Table 23-1. DSM-III-R diagnostic criteria for attention-deficit hyperactivity disorder

Note: Consider a criterion met only if the behavior is considerably more frequent than that of most people of the same mental age.

A. A disturbance of at least six months during which at least eight of the following are present:

1. Often fidgets with hands or feet or squirms in seat (in adolescents, may be limited to subjective feelings of restlessness)
2. Has difficulty remaining seated when required to do so
3. Is easily distracted by extraneous stimuli
4. Has difficulty awaiting turn in games or group situations
5. Often blurts out answers to questions before they have been completed
6. Has difficulty following through on instructions from others (not due to oppositional behavior or failure of comprehension), e.g., fails to finish chores
7. Has difficulty sustaining attention in tasks or play activities
8. Often shifts from one uncompleted activity to another
9. Has difficulty playing quietly
10. Often talks excessively
11. Often interrupts or intrudes on others, e.g., butts into other children's games
12. Often does not seem to listen to what is being said to him or her
13. Often loses things necessary for tasks or activities at school or at home (e.g., toys, pencils, books, assignments)
14. Often engages in physically dangerous activities without considering possible consequences (not for the purpose of thrill seeking), e.g., runs into street without looking

Note: The above items are listed in descending order of discriminating power based on data from a national field trial of the DSM-III-R criteria for disruptive behavior disorders.

B. Onset before the age of seven.

C. Does not meet the criteria for a pervasive developmental disorder.

Criteria for severity of ADHD:

Mild: Few, if any, symptoms in excess of those required to make the diagnosis **and** only minimal or no impairment in school and social functioning.
Moderate: Symptoms or functional impairment intermediate between "mild" **and** "severe."
Severe: Many symptoms in excess of those required to make the diagnosis **and** significant and pervasive impairment in functioning at home/school and with peers.

ing Scale, Satin et al. (1985) identified 294 6–9-year-old boys (12%) as having ADD in a population of 1,884 boys; direct psychiatric interviews of a 92-member subsample established the accuracy of the DSM-III diagnosis with 91% sensitivity and 73% specificity.

In contrast, early epidemiologic studies yielded lower prevalence figures for ADD. The Isle of Wight study yielded only 2 ADD children from a population of 2,199 10–11-year-olds, using direct observation and structured diagnostic interview methods requiring agreement among different observers (Rutter et al. 1970). Prevalence figures from these studies have ranged from 1% to 1.5%, far below the 3%–5% quoted by American authors. Using multiple sources for diagnosis, Shapiro and Garfinkel (1986) found only 2.3% of a rural, nonreferred elementary-school population of 315 children met the inattentive-overactive signs of the ADDH disorder when screened using a combination of teacher rating scales, clinical interviews, and lab performance measures. British investigators have suggested that the ADD diagnostic label would have stronger construct validity if the afflicted child were restless in all situations, showing "cross-situational hyperactivity" (Sandberg et al. 1978). In contrast, both DSM-III and DSM-III-R require that overactivity, restlessness, and inattention be present in only one situation, usually school. In 1986, an editorial in *Lancet* entitled "Does Hyperactivity Matter?" (1986) suggested that the risk for adolescent and early-adult life psychopathology may not reside in being hyperactive but in other aspects of poor social and academic adjustment.

More recent epidemiologic surveys in Puerto Rico (Bird et al. 1988) and Canada (Offord et al. 1989) have given higher prevalence figures for ADD, averaging 10% of the population. The Puerto Rican study combined both clinical interviews with a Children's Global Assessment Scale (C-GAS) to include only those cases meeting clinical criteria who also were impaired (scores below 61); even with these restrictions, 9.5% of the population had ADD. Similarly, more recent British epidemiologic studies by American-trained researchers in London have found higher prevalence rates than were reported in the original Isle of Wight study when British patients are diagnosed using American criteria (Taylor 1986; Taylor et al. 1986a, 1986b).

The preponderance of males over females with ADD is an area of agreement across the various population studies, regardless of diagnostic criteria or survey method. Boys predominate in both epidemiologic and clinical samples, with boy-to-girl ratios ranging from 4:1 to 9:1 (Berry et al. 1985; Cantwell 1982). No clear explanation has emerged from any area of research to shed light on the relative vulnerability of males. Rather, rates of other central nervous system disorders predominate in preadolescent males, including learning disabilities, epilepsy, cerebral palsy, and psychiatric disorders in general.

Comorbidity

The heterogeneity of ADD may mean that it is not a spectrum disorder (Biederman et al. 1989c). Instead, it may be comorbid with a number of other childhood disorders (Biederman and Newcorn, unpublished manuscript). Three subtypes have been proposed, based on family-genetic data, including ADHD plus conduct disorder, ADHD plus major depression, and ADHD plus anxiety disorder. These subtypes may prove to have different natural histories as well as different responses to treatment (both behavioral and pharmacologic). It behooves the clinician to look for the comorbid condition in the ADD child and to consider the comorbid problem in formulating a treatment plan. For example, an ADD child comorbid for mood disorder may best be treated with a tricyclic antidepressant.

Higher rates of comorbidity are found in referred populations than in epidemiologic samples. For example, a survey of a Minnesota rural school system found that 2.3% of the sample had ADD, 3.6% had conduct disorder, and 3.3% had both disorders (Shapiro and Garfinkel 1986). Biederman et al. (1989c) compared 73 ADD children with 26 children with no mental disorder and confirmed that children referred for ADD were comorbid with diagnoses of major affective disorder, non-Tourette's syndrome tic disorder, or conduct disorder.

Clinical Description

Making the diagnosis of ADD depends more on taking a good behavioral history and less on a direct mental status examination of the child in the office. Under direct questioning, the child will often deny being symptomatic and not complain about any problem. The clinician must rely on reports from parents and teachers and use direct observations of the patient's behavior only if they are conducted in a social situation, such as a schoolroom. Even

after gathering a "classic" history of ADD, little chaos and mayhem may be seen in the first one-to-one exchange with the child. How can the clinician make a diagnosis if the disorder cannot be validated by direct observation in the interview?

The diagnostic decision and choice of treatment depend heavily on the clinician's experience working with other ADD children and common-sense clinical judgment. In addition, psychological reports can help by revealing attentional lapses during tedious repetitive tasks, such as the coding task of the Wechsler Intelligence Scale for Children—Revised (WISC-R) (Wechsler 1974). One clinical rule-of-thumb demands that the signs of the disorder must be present to a moderate degree in at least two of three settings (i.e., home, school, and clinician's office). The clinical descriptions of ADD and its functional impairment will vary across types of settings. Only a subsample of ADD children are constantly overactive in all environments and have "pervasive hyperactivity" (Shaffer and Greenhill 1979). These children score lower on standardized tests of intelligence and have increased cognitive deficits, worse overall disturbance, and greater attentional dysfunction than those with situational-based ADD (Sandberg et al. 1978). DSM-III-R does not distinguish between children with situational and pervasive ADHD.

Despite the changes in the American Psychiatric Association's manuals over the past 10 years, the syndrome has three key elements: a developmentally inappropriate level of motor hyperactivity, inattention in school, and impulsivity as regards rule-governed behavior (Barkley 1982; Carlson et al. 1986). The clinician's history-taking approach works best when the inquiry focuses on the positive signs of the disorder, exclusion criteria, severity measures, associated conditions, and family history. Such information can best be collected from both parents together.

The ADD child's behavioral traits often seem to be exaggerations of normal childhood activities. Signs of inattention and overactivity unpredictably interact with the environmental setting and are age-dependent. The younger the child, the more pervasive is the motor drivenness, and its appearance is less dependent on the setting. The young preschooler rapidly moves about the room, stimulus-driven to touch everything and manipulate each object in a haphazard manner. He climbs, jumps, and runs as if "driven by a motor" out of control. Birthday parties and peer-group get-togethers are quickly derailed by the ADHD child, who becomes wild, overactive, noisy, and unmanageable if the occasion is unstructured.

The school-age ADD boy may show a narrower range of impulsive and overactive behaviors, with large group settings required to bring out the most severe disturbances. In class, the inattentiveness predominates. There the ADD child appears to be daydreaming or preoccupied. The child squirms and moves restlessly about when seated. The in-attentiveness seriously interferes with academic performance, as revealed in the child's sloppy handwriting, careless errors, and messy papers. At home, parents find the ADD child "not listening," failing to follow through on even the most simple requests, and being unable to complete homework.

Past history of these children may indicate long-standing difficulties with impulse control, high levels of motor activity, and disruptiveness in groups. Activity levels in ADD children generally are higher, even during sleep (Porrino et al. 1983a). In gym class, levels may be lower, because ADDH children have trouble modulating their behavior downward (in academic class) or upward (during a soccer game) as the social setting demands. On the playground during recess, they may seem to be just as active as their playmates, yet other children often find that impulsivity and inattentiveness make them poor teammates (Whalen et al. 1979, 1987a, 1987b). Situations involving self-paced work (Whalen et al. 1979) exert the greatest stress.

DSM-III was based on a categorical scheme which dictates that a diagnosis could be made only if a child's misbehavior matched a pattern of a known disorder. DSM-III-R groups together a set of 14 unweighted operational descriptors of ADHD. These phrases can be used during the clinical evaluation as cues or inquiries. The items are listed in "descending order of discriminating power" (American Psychiatric Association 1987, p. 53). In DSM-III-R, a child needs to have 8 of 14 items endorsed if the diagnosis of ADHD is to be made. This type of approach has been dubbed polyethic, meaning that no single misbehavior can make the diagnosis. As a result, the diagnostic category is defined by determining if its members have the common characteristics or clinical features grouping them together (Carlson et al. 1986). The DSM-III-R "list" of ADHD behaviors was tested in a multicenter field trial. Compared to DSM-III, DSM-III-R increases the number of children labeled as hyperactive by about 25% (Lahey et al. 1990; Newcorn et al. 1989).

For purposes of clinical description, in this chapter I will highlight three cardinal signs of this disorder: hyperactivity, poor impulse control, and inattention.

Hyperactivity

Although teachers and clinicians may assume that developmentally inappropriate levels of activity are the pathognomonic sign of ADD, hyperactivity has been both emphasized and de-emphasized over the past decade (Carlson et al. 1986). The operational descriptor "acts as if 'driven by a motor'" in DSM-III (p. 44) was dropped from DSM-III-R's list of 14 symptoms. Yet the importance of the ADD child's high activity level has been supported by research in the past decade. ADD children, compared with normal control children, display higher activity levels, particularly when carrying out structured, in-seat activities (Abikoff and Gittelman 1985; Conners and Werry 1979). Naturalistic studies employing small, belt- or vest-mounted, solid-state, memory-activity monitors (Porrino et al. 1983b) also have shown that ADD children manifest significantly higher levels of activity in the classroom, at home, and while sleeping at night than do normal control children (Porrino et al. 1983a). Monitored activity levels fall to normal when the ADD children are treated with stimulants. The high levels of sleep activity in ADD children and the normalization of activity with stimulant treatment strengthen the syndrome's concurrent validity.

This higher-than-usual level of motility makes the ADD child appear to be driven, restless, and never tiring. Although some degree of hyperactivity is found normally in school-age boys (Lapouse and Monk 1953), the diagnosis of ADD should be limited to a developmentally inappropriate degree of gross motor activity in the school or home setting (American Psychiatric Association 1987). The child with ADHD seems to have the same difficulty sitting as does the patient with neuroleptic-induced akathisia. Therefore, sedentary activities such as sitting in school or church, taking rides in the car, or even going to the movies lead to high levels of noncompliance and restlessness. In the classroom, where children are asked to sit still, remain quiet, and work independently, ADD boys squirm in their chairs, hum, make noises, and tap on their desks. This disturbs other children. Hyperactive children also enjoy climbing and will climb along kitchen cabinets when their peers choose to walk on the floor.

DSM-III-R lists three symptoms to detect hyperactivity (1, 2, and 10 in Table 23-1).

Inattention

DSM-III-R attempts to operationalize inattention. To date, however, there is no standardized office procedure to measure attention in children. The inattention component is best determined by history. The clinician inquires about attentional problems by asking if the child has a short attention span, has difficulty concentrating, has an inability to modulate attention in response to externally imposed demand, has a problem in initiating tasks, or has trouble selectively attending to relevant stimuli while filtering out unnecessary noise (Carlson et al. 1986). Distractibility may not reflect a breakdown in filtering out unwanted input, but rather an active seeking out of more stimuli when the activity requiring attention produces boredom (Zentall and Meyer 1990).

When a child is inattentive, classwork is difficult to process. Goal-directed work cannot be completed without frequent refocusing from another person. More time is spent off the task and out of the seat. The child typically is oversolicitous with the teacher (calling out more often or trying to answer questions that are not understood). While other children complete their assignment sheets, tests, and workbook drills, the ADD child produces very little "product," even if he or she is the brightest child in the class. Teachers become frustrated when scanty, poor-quality work is produced by one of their brighter students.

At home, school-age ADD children often have trouble listening to adults. These children look away and do not make eye contact when talking to an adult. Asked to do chores, they forget what was asked of them and have difficulty carrying out multicommission commands. Following written instructions for constructing a model airplane requires effortful redirecting and maintenance of attention, from instruction sheet to the model and back again. Faced with a multistep instruction sheet, ADD boys may decide to slap together the model, based only on the picture on the box. As a result, important pieces are ignored or left out. In just such a manner, ADD children always seem to be rushed, too busy, or "on the way in a hurry" to some other activity. In other instances, they may start several activities at once and finish none of them.

Laboratory-based research studies have employed a number of procedures to monitor the task performance of children with ADD and have claimed that these laboratory measures can pick up attentional difficulties that otherwise would be seen only in a classroom. The best known is the Continuous Performance Test (CPT), which measures sustained attention (Cornblatt et al. 1988; Sykes et al. 1972; Weingartner et al. 1980). It requires the child to watch a computer screen continuously for 10–15 minutes. The child is instructed to pick out the correct "target" among a group of "nontarget" letters that flash on the screen and press a key as soon as the correct letter or combination of letters is seen. A wide range of modifications have been employed to avoid "floor and ceiling effects" (Cornblatt et al. 1988), including visually degrading the stimuli on the screen, playing movie sound tracks over earphones during the visual task, and even varying the time between stimuli, depending on the performance of the child. The CPT has been shown to be sensitive to drug effects (Garfinkel et al. 1986) and to dose of drug (Cornblatt et al. 1987; Rapport et al. 1985).

It should be cautioned that laboratory-based measures of attention do not always correlate with classroom performance. Any laboratory tool used in a 1-to-1 (1 child with 1 researcher) situation cannot easily recreate the demand set of the 1-to-30 environment found in a classroom (1 teacher to 30 students). Douglas (1983) wisely pointed out that sustained attention, which the CPT tracks, does not tap other important attentional functions required in complex tasks, such as self-regulation, the extent to which attention is self-directed and organized, the amount of effort that is invested, or whether the approach to a task involves a search strategy or is just simple exploration (Douglas 1983). In addition, recent research has downplayed the role of a sustained attentional deficit as the sole cognitive deficit in ADD (Solanto and Wender 1989; Swanson and Cantwell 1989).

Other laboratory measures have been used in research, and some find their way into a marketplace for practitioners. None of these tasks has been widely accepted for clinical work. One simple device tests motor steadiness; one group has been able to correlate diminishing error rates and the plasma levels of methylphenidate (Birmaher et al. 1989; Greenhill et al., unpublished manuscript). A rugged, portable CPT has been marketed with normative data to support its utility as a screening device (Gordon 1986; Gordon and Mettleman 1988; Gordon et al. 1989). The Paired-Associates Learning Task measures short-term memory and is also medication-sensitive, showing significant correlations with stimulant blood levels (Kupietz et al. 1982). The quality of performance on this test at various dosages of methylphenidate, for example, has been used as an argument for choosing lower doses to optimize cognitive performance in the classroom (Sprague and Sleator 1977).

These laboratory measures are not diagnostically specific. A study by Werry et al. (1987), however, reported no differences between children with ADHD, conduct disorder, or anxiety disorder on the CPT, suggesting that attentional dysfunction (as measured by the CPT) is a nonspecific correlate of child psychopathology in general (Werry et al. 1987).

Although DSM-III included a diagnostic category for children with inattentiveness but no hyperactivity (attention deficit disorder without hyperactivity or ADD-H), DSM-III-R does not include this disorder, because it failed to appear in the prepublication field trials.

DSM-III-R attempts to operationalize clinical expressions of inattention into a series of items that can be used as probes. By themselves, these items will not distinguish among normal children and children with a psychiatric disorder. To make the diagnosis of ADHD with some specificity, the clinician must obtain evidence that the deficit in organization, goal-directed activity, and sustained attention results in serious impairment in academic and social functioning. DSM-III-R lists six symptoms to detect inattention (3, 6, 7, 8, 12, and 13 in Table 23-1).

Impulsivity

Impulsivity means that the child acts without forethought of the consequences, appearing to be unaware of danger or the relationship between cause and effect. The ADD child has a willingness to "take dares" other children would not.

Complex academic tasks, which require individual initiation, self-monitoring, organization, and self-pacing, may best reveal the ADD child's impulsivity. In particular, behavior during homework may be the most distressing of the ADD child's "invisible handicap" (Taft, personal communication). Even bright children with this disorder report the rapid onset of boredom during homework and a strong feeling that "I work in school, so why should I have to continue this stuff at home?" In addition,

teachers may insist that the ADD child's uncompleted classwork be finished up at home, furthering burdening the child with the very tasks that the child finds most difficult. Secondary behavior patterns often develop around the homework struggle, particularly avoidance routines, such as "forgetting" assignments, leaving important books at school, and even dashing through the homework unconcerned about errors. Unsupervised, such a child will start three other activities and end up finishing neither the schoolwork nor the other projects. Parents quickly get discouraged, taking much of their leisure weekday evening hours to hover over the child while the child struggles with the homework.

During the early years, the ADD child's impulsivity may take the form of "stimulus drivenness," a robotlike behavior in which the child must pick up, touch, or manipulate every object in the room. This pressure drives toddlers from one toy to the next, disrupting all objects in their path; during school-age years, they constantly interrupt others and refuse to wait their turn in games. The thoughtless, unpremeditated quality of the hyperkinetic child's rule breaking often leads such children to get caught "holding the bag," while the real instigators are long gone. As a result, the ADHD child can land in trouble and be included with boys who have long histories of conduct problems.

Research studies have had the challenge of operationalizing an "impulsivity" dimension, a concept that is inferential at best. Measures have been constructed using a number of approaches, including direct observations of a child's self-control during interactions with adults and peers, inhibition of behavior (such as a "Draw-a-Line Slowly" task), and cognitive problem-solving measures (e.g., the Matching Familiar Figures Test [J. Kagan, unpublished test]) (Carlson et al. 1986). Direct observation studies have been most successful at tapping this impulsive dimension. These studies reveal that the ADD child interrupts more often, fails to wait for his or her turn in games, and ends up being disliked during peer nominations.

DSM-III-R lists five symptoms to detect impulsivity (4, 5, 9, 11, and 14 in Table 23-1).

Adolescent and Adult Outcomes

Adolescence for the child with ADHD is marked by academic problems in school. Approximately one-fourth of these patients will continue to show inattentiveness, restlessness, and hyperactivity by the age of 18 (Gittelman-Klein and Mannuzza 1987). Conduct problems appear during the end of the preadolescent period and may become severe in adolescence. The hyperactive boy with a "versatile" pattern of conduct disorder, including aggressivity, is at risk for being in trouble with the law in later years (Loeber 1988; Robins 1966). Treatment has been shown to be helpful within the first 3 years if medication and other therapies are combined (Satterfield et al. 1982), but long-term studies of those children treated with stimulants alone do not show an advantage in the academic area.

Adult outcome has been subject to some debate. Some of the early retrospective follow-up studies suggested that ADD predicted adult maladjustment and criminality. Careful prospective studies have found something different, at least in degree. Certain investigators (Weiss et al. 1979, 1985) have shown that most ADD children followed for 15 years or more do not have more trouble with the law or poorer jobs than control children, but the hyperactive sample has an attrition rate greater than 25%. A more recent prospective follow-up study (Mannuzza et al., unpublished manuscript), on the other hand, with only a 2% attrition rate, showed that 52% of the ADD children studied had no psychiatric diagnosis by age 18. As for the remaining 48%, approximately 25% of the ADD sample developed a diagnosis of conduct disorder by age 18, even though they had originally been selected not to have a diagnosis of conduct disorder at the beginning of the study (Gittelman-Klein and Mannuzza 1987).

A cautious approach to adult ADD disorders is justified. Wender et al. (1981), who have conducted a number of studies of ADD children grown up, insist on validating entrance criteria and ongoing measures by checking all reports with a "significant other" living in the home with the patient. This input is very valuable; the lack of such a close "rater" may explain the poor treatment response reported for stimulant-treated adult ADD populations (Gualtieri et al. 1985; Mattes et al. 1984). In any case, it has not been clear whether adults who had full ADD as children continue to have the same condition as adults. Are some of the "ADD children grown up" displaying a "residual" form of the disorder (say 6 out of 14 items in DSM-III-R)? Or do they just show the "adult equivalents" of childhood inattention that do not match the specific operational items in DSM-III-R? For example, should one use adult "equivalents" of the DSM-III-R items

for childhood ADHD: can't pay attention to one conversation at a cocktail party (inattention), gets many speeding tickets (impulsivity), or paces constantly while talking on the telephone (restlessness)? More work must be done; it would be best to recruit the "purest" sample possible, such as Zametkin et al. (1990) has done by interviewing fathers of ADD children who themselves had the condition in their childhood.

A number of factors complicate the treatment of adults with ADD for the clinician. Patients with substance abuse are aware that hyperactive adults are often treated with pemoline, methylphenidate, or even methamphetamine and will mimic the history and behavior to secure stimulant treatment. Second, patients with schizophrenia or schizotypal or borderline personality disorder can experience severe impulsivity and inattentiveness at a level necessary to fulfill some of the criteria of ADD. Stimulant treatment of such schizophrenia-spectrum patients will reliably induce or exacerbate a psychotic episode (Lieberman et al. 1987).

Evaluation Procedures and Differential Diagnosis

Children with ADD should receive a complete medical evaluation and examination. On occasion, a standard physical examination may reveal neurologic problems that completely explain the child's inattentiveness, restlessness, and impulsivity. In the sensory area, children with partial deafness or very poor vision may appear inattentive and restless to a teacher. Nonspecific signs found on a careful neurologic evaluation, on the other hand, probably contribute little to the evaluation of ADD children. These nonspecific signs, including minor physical anomalies, have been referred to as "soft neurologic signs" (Shaffer and Greenhill 1979). Soft signs present as asymmetries in reflex findings, minor choreoathetoid movements, an inability to carry out rapid alternating movements, and generally poor coordination. They are subject to intertest and interrater reliability problems. To date, their presence does not aid in making the diagnosis of ADD (Shaffer and Greenhill 1979). In fact, an epidemiologic study showed that these soft signs predict a higher-than-normal prevalence of anxiety disorders, not ADD (Shaffer et al. 1985).

There can be medical problems that may lead to a child who is overactive and inattentive. Severe language disorders will produce very aberrant behavior and, at times, are associated with motor hyperactivity and severe inattentiveness. Dermatologic conditions, such as eczema, and even pinworms may produce restlessness and disruptiveness in first graders and may appear to be a pure behavior disorder to the teacher. Even more rare, Sydenham's chorea will generate intense restlessness in children and requires careful workup and treatment. Finally, as many as 50%–60% of Tourette's syndrome patients, ages 6–18 years, may also have ADD (Cohen and Leckman 1989). Stimulants, which cause a release of catecholamines in the central nervous system, can exacerbate motor tics in these patients (Lowe et al. 1982), possibly by further intensifying the putative hyperdopaminergic state found in Tourette's syndrome. One recent study found that a 30 mg/day methylphenidate dose actually reduced the frequency of tics in four boys with ADD (Sverd et al. 1989), although Cohen and Leckman (1989) interpreted these findings with great caution and urged the clinician to find other means than stimulants to deal with the ADD in Tourette's syndrome. Clonidine has been used with greater safety in the treatment of both Tourette's syndrome and ADD.

The child's height and weight should be measured prior to any treatment, particularly if the child is to go onto stimulant medication, which may cause a temporary slowdown in weight gain. Other tests, such as computed tomography or magnetic resonance imaging, add no useful diagnostic or treatment information unless the neurologist suspects a space-occupying lesion in the child.

Age-appropriate overactivity may occur in children who show no impulsive or attentional problems. The high level of activity found in ADHD differs from other clinical states by its intense, non-goal-directed quality. Children who have a comorbid Axis I diagnosis of conduct disorder will have all the features of the ADHD syndrome, but their high propensity for aggressivity differs from the more typical hyperactive child's. The impulsivity of a conduct-disordered child has more of a calculating, premeditated quality not found in the reactive and impulsive misbehaviors of the hyperactive child.

Children with other psychiatric diagnoses may display the chaotic, stimulus-bound motor drivenness of the ADD child, yet be excluded from a formal hyperactive diagnosis. Severe and profoundly mentally retarded children may be quite hyperactive, but have been excluded by DSM-III-R. Schizophrenic children and those with affective disorders, manic type, display impulsivity, overactivity, and inattentiveness, but only secondary to the primary illness. DSM-III-R also excludes cases when the disorder's duration falls short of 6 months and appears after the age of 7 years, and where there is a clear psychosocial stressor.

Treatment

Before deciding on treatment, the clinician must first assess the severity of the behavior disorder. Environmental changes alone can greatly help those children with mild forms of ADD. Simple steps involve appropriate class placement in small, academic settings with a teacher who can deliver a good deal of structured supervision and close one-to-one attention. Parents can be counseled to establish a regular, consistent home routine for the child, as well as consistent responses to good behaviors (praise and attention) or to undesirable behaviors (ignore, take away reinforcer, or use time out). These techniques may be taught in a parent workshop or in individual office visits.

The child might be enrolled in a behavior modification program to reduce certain target impulsive behaviors. Parental counseling will also help the clinician evaluate the strengths of the parent-child relationship, relieve feelings of guilt in the parent, and help the parent to view the difficulties more objectively. For those children with moderate to severe disorder, the treatment plan should be supplemented with pharmacotherapy.

Pharmacotherapy

First and foremost, one should learn the parents' attitudes about the use of medications for their child's disorder. This should be approached directly, supporting the parents in a candid discussion about their fears and misconceptions. The child's history of medication treatments should also be gathered, looking particularly for previous medication trials, unfavorable experiences with psychotropic medications, and allergic reactions.

Time should be set aside to explain the treatment plan to both the parents and the child. Any plan that involves a behavioral plan at school or even a classroom change must be discussed carefully with the child. Children may not understand the need for a smaller class or the utility of a behavioral modification program without ample time for discussion. In addition, they may have strong feelings against being medicated, particularly if their parents are ambivalent. Often it is helpful to explain that the medication is a "crutch" that will enable them to do classwork when they want to, but does not control them (K. Minde, unpublished manuscript). Additionally, the patient may not want to take medication in school and will be able to discuss it openly. Methylphenidate-sustained release (SR-20) or pemoline, two long-acting stimulants, may help when dosing in school is not desirable. Some evidence exists that SR-20 may lose its effect for certain children when used as a maintenance medication (Fried et al. 1987), so close follow-up of these children is necessary.

Several different types of psychoactive preparations have proven useful for treating the hyperkinetic syndrome. More than 31 controlled studies involving more than 1,800 children have shown stimulants to be more effective than placebo (Barkley 1977). Stimulants have become the most common form of treatment for these children, inhibiting impulsivity and hyperactivity, while generally improving performance on attentional measures (Rapoport et al. 1980).

Psychostimulants. *Methylphenidate* (Ritalin) has become the most popular psychostimulant used in the United States. Methylphenidate is rapidly absorbed but enters the plasma in low concentrations, as low as 7–10 ng/ml, similar to the range for pituitary hormones (Gualtieri et al. 1982, 1984). These minute amounts are highly effective because methylphenidate's low plasma binding (15%) makes it highly available to cross the blood-brain barrier (Perel and Dayton 1976). The drug's main site of action is the central nervous system. The *d*-enantiomer appears to be more active than the *l*-enantiomer (Srinivas et al. 1987). The parent compound is reduced by esterases to ritalinic acid in the gastrointestinal tract, and then is oxidized (to *p*-hydroxymethylphenidate) and conjugated in the liver. Controlled treatment studies consistently have shown methylphenidate to be effective for the treatment of ADHD children.

Several reports (Abikoff and Gittelman 1985; Gittelman-Klein 1980; Pelham et al. 1985) have shown that double-blind ratings by parents, teachers, and professionals report that more than three-fourths of the children improved while treated with methylphenidate for at least 4 weeks. Even so, the reports of various observers do not often correlate highly with one another, perhaps because meth-

ylphenidate given in the morning may show improvement from the teacher, but not from the parent, who sees the child after the drug has worn off (Sandberg et al. 1978). Approximately 75% of methylphenidate-treated children are moderate to marked responders, showing a reduction in motor activity, an increase in time remaining seated, and much longer time on-task. These changes can be seen as early as 30 minutes after the child's very first dose of methylphenidate. The placebo response rate, on the other hand, is a meager 18% (Ullmann and Sleator 1986). School-age children increasingly are treated with this drug, as shown in epidemiologic surveys (Safer and Krager 1988; Schmidt 1988).

Response to methylphenidate is not age specific. Adolescents respond just as well as school-age children do (Varley 1983). Favorable reports have been given for methylphenidate treatment of adults with attentional problems (Wender et al. 1981; Wolkenberg 1987).

It is best to initiate drug treatment with the lowest possible dose of methylphenidate, such as 5 mg once in the morning, then advance to 5 mg twice a day (one pill each at 8:00 A.M. and at noon). Further increases are accomplished by raising the dose 5 mg per dose every 3 days. The final recommended maintenance doses may vary, a total daily dose of from 10 to 60 mg, and do not seem to be weight-dependent (Rapport and DuPaul 1986). If a favorable response occurs, it does so within the first 10 days of treatment. Plasma levels have not proven useful in clinical practice (Gualtieri et al. 1982) because of large interindividual variation, although other investigators have found that methylphenidate levels correlate with some experimental measures (Sebrechts et al. 1986).

Currently, methylphenidate is dispensed in 5 and 10 mg tablets; a liquid formulation has not been available. Sustained-release methylphenidate (20 mg) tablets, which peak at 4.7 hours and show a disappearance half-life of 8 hours, are now available (Birmaher et al. 1989; Pelham et al. 1987). This formulation avoids involvement of school personnel in medication administration, a prescribing pattern that is ideal for maintenance. Unfortunately, there is evidence that the sustained-release tablets may not be as effective as standard methylphenidate when used over 45-day treatment periods (Fried et al. 1987). This may be due to a mechanism akin to tachyphylaxis, or pharmacodynamic tolerance.

Methylphenidate's side effects include insomnia, anorexia, minor increases in systolic blood pressure, headaches, and stomachaches. There have been rare reports of hallicinosis, particularly in children with a past history of atypical psychosis. A past history of involuntary muscle movements (tics) or a family history of Tourette's syndrome is a contraindication to the use of methylphenidate, as it may "unmask" or exacerbate Tourette's syndrome (Denkla et al. 1976; El-Defrawi and Greenhill 1984; Golden 1974, 1977; Lowe et al. 1982). Growth slowdown can be seen with prolonged use of methylphenidate, although adults formerly treated with the drug do not differ in height from control individuals (Gittelman-Klein et al. 1987). Tolerance to methylphenidate may develop if treatment extends much past 1 year (Fried et al. 1987; Winsberg et al. 1987). This decrease in response should be treated with a switch to another psychostimulant.

Magnesium pemoline (Cylert) is a dopamine agonist that ameliorates the behavioral symptoms of ADD almost as well as methylphenidate does (Conners and Taylor 1980). Pemoline's relatively long 12-hour half-life means that once-a-day administration is possible. Since pemoline is a Class IV controlled drug, it may be prescribed using regular prescription blanks. Pemoline's ability to be given once per day makes it a good choice for hyperkinetic children who may be teased by classmates for taking pills in school, may have trouble with drug rebound, or may have difficulty with insomnia from late-afternoon stimulant doses. Others have cautioned that pemoline use is associated with choreoathetoid movements and a propensity to develop motor tics, even more than those seen with methylphenidate (Rapoport et al. 1982). A controlled study of 238 children revealed that pemoline exerts its strongest action by the third week and later (Page et al. 1974). Pemoline's dosage has been set by the manufacturer in pills or chewable tablets in multiples of the 18.75 mg lowest-dose tablet. Initiation of treatment requires a regimen of weekly dosage increases, either 18.75 or 37.5 mg, up to a total dose of 112.5 mg/day. Children often begin to show improvement at dose levels above 50 mg/day. Some irritability, insomnia, and anorexia may be seen in children on the drug; rare reports of elevated liver enzymes suggest that the clinician should conduct routine liver function tests and complete blood counts every 6 months.

Other drugs. Because approximately 20% of children do not respond to stimulants (Donnelly et al. 1989), other medications have been used in the treatment of ADHD. *Clonidine* (Catapres) is an im-

idazoline derivative that acts as an alpha-adrenergic agonist, affecting presynaptic receptors on norepinephrine neurons in the locus coeruleus. Research studies have employed clonidine in the treatment of narcotic withdrawal and Tourette's syndrome. It has been given to children with ADD in at least one controlled clinical study (Hunt et al. 1985) and seems promising as a drug for use in children with Tourette's syndrome who also have ADD. It is available as a small 0.1 mg pill or a skin-patch formulation. The skin patch must be watched carefully for allergic reactions. Dosing adjustments require starting at small doses, often half a pill (equivalent to 0.05 mg), or cutting the patch into smaller pieces. Because clonidine has not been approved for children, and because of its effect on blood pressure, children on this drug must have their blood pressure monitored on a regular basis.

Desipramine (Norpramin) has proven to be a very useful drug in the treatment of children with ADD. Recent controlled studies have shown it to be effective in treatment of this disorder for at least a 1-month period (Linnoila et al. 1979). One should consider this drug if the child has a comorbid condition on Axis I, such as a mixed picture of ADHD with either depression or conduct disorder (Biederman and Wright 1987; Donnelly et al. 1986). It is now administered in doses of up to 5 mg/kg/day (Biederman et al. 1989a). The total daily dose may be given as a single nighttime administration in adolescents (Ryan et al. 1987). A baseline electrocardiogram is recommended to establish pulse and blood pressure, PR interval (less than 200 milliseconds), and QRS complex of greater than 100 milliseconds. PR intervals over 100 milliseconds may constitute a mild conduction problem called incomplete intraventricular conduction defect of the right bundle branch type (Biederman et al. 1989b). Biederman et al. found 26.3% of their sample of ADD children had this defect when desipramine was titrated up to a total dose of 5 mg/kg/day. The blood pressure and pulse may go up as dosage is increased, so some clinicians have set limits for blood pressure (140/90 mm Hg) and for pulse (130 bpm). Sinus tachycardia, defined as ventricular pulse greater than 100 bpm, rose from a baseline of 17% in children on placebo to 35% when they were given the full desipramine dose (Biederman et al. 1989b). Electrocardiogram, blood pressure, and pulse should be checked at each 1 mg/kg dosage step. Desipramine has been used to treat those ADHD children who have severe side effects (mood changes, tics, increased hyperactivity) when treated with stimulants. A recent report of sudden death in three school-age children treated with desipramine ("Sudden Death in Children" 1990) has led to varying opinions about the risk of treatment (Popper and Elliot, in press; Riddle et al. 1991).

Carbamazepine (Tegretol) is an anticonvulsant that has been used to treat children with disruptive behavior disorders, although there are no indications for this application in the package insert. In addition, there have been no controlled studies of its efficacy in childhood behavior disorders. Its ability to cause leukopenia is well known, so the white blood cell count and absolute neutrophil count must be monitored on a monthly basis (absolute neutrophil count must be $\geq$ 1,500). There is one report of carbamazepine-induced mania in an adolescent.

Although monoamine oxidase inhibitors have been found to be very effective in the treatment of ADD (Zametkin and Rapoport 1987), impulsive youngsters and adolescents cannot be expected to control their diet, particularly when such desirable tyramine-rich foods (e.g., pizza) could cause hypertensive crises. In addition, ADD children on monoamine oxidase inhibitors might be given a stimulant pill by an unknowing but well-intentioned relative, and this could cause life-threatening hypertension.

Bupropion (Wellbutrin) is another antidepressant that has been reported to be effective in the treatment of ADD (Casat et al. 1989; Simeon et al. 1986). Bupropion is a dopamine agonist, similar to the putative action of stimulants. This medication was significantly more effective than placebo in reducing hyperactivity ratings on the Conners Teacher Questionnaire (Conners 1969; Goyette et al. 1979) in a controlled study of 30 ADD children (Casat et al. 1989) at a dose level of 6 mg/kg. Replication and comparisons with standard medications (e.g., methylphenidate, desipramine) are necessary before bupropion can be recommended for general use.

Lithium has been shown to be useful in the treatment of aggressive, hospitalized boys with conduct disorder (Campbell and Spencer 1988; Campbell et al. 1984), but reviews have shown no particular efficacy for the drug for those with ADHD (DeLong and Aldershof 1987). An early double-blind, controlled study comparing amphetamine with lithium carbonate in treatment-refractory boys with hyperkinetic syndrome showed a major advantage for the amphetamines (Greenhill et al. 1973). There is a need for controlled studies of lithium in the treatment of ADD children comorbid for conduct disorder.

Behavior Modification

The use of behavior modification to treat the hyperkinetic child has been advocated as an alternative to stimulants in the treatment of children with ADD. There are a number of reasons for this. Stimulants fail to work satisfactorily in up to 20% of cases; other stimulant-treated children develop limiting side effects, including insomnia, weight loss, severe behavioral "rebound," headaches, and, in rare cases, reduced white blood cell count. Some parents do not want their children on medication. A number of studies have shown that ADD children on maintenance medication alone fail to show long-term improvements in academic performance. For this reason, behavioral modification has become a frequently used modality in the treatment of ADD children. How does it fare in controlled studies?

Behavior modification has been compared to stimulant medication in a number of counterbalanced studies (Gittelman-Klein 1987). All active treatments proved to be more effective than placebo, giving strong evidence that behavioral modification can be as effective as medication for changing disruptive behavior in the classroom. On the other hand, behavior modification requires a large time commitment from the therapist to be effective, and this can be costly in comparison to time required to initiate and monitor a course of medication. The teacher also has to devote a great deal of time and effort to any behavior modification program, and this may not be practical when the rest of the class needs attention. In general, however, behavior modification is no more effective than stimulant treatment alone (Gittelman-Klein 1987).

Other Psychological Therapies

Psychotherapy has often been recommended for the hyperkinetic child, but there is little evidence to support its efficacy. More focused psychological interventions have included the "stop, look, and listen" refocusing approaches (Douglas et al. 1976, 1986) used to teach hyperkinetic children to sustain attention. A cognitive-behavioral approach has been assessed and found to be useful, but appears to be less effective than medications alone in controlled study comparisons (Abikoff and Gittelman 1985).

Tutoring and remediation may help some of the academic difficulties that occur in hyperactive children, but the training does not generalize into the behavioral area. A final approach involves parent education, and many clinicians have employed 10-week, 2-hour workshops to teach behavior modification management techniques to parent groups (DuPaul and Barkley 1990). As many as 70 regional chapters of the parent support group CHADD (Children with Hyperactive Attention Deficit Disorder) have formed. These groups provide a place for parents to share information on treatments, therapists, and educational programs.

General Rules for Successful Management

To provide for their many needs, hyperkinetic children are best handled by a multidisciplinary team, consisting of a medical doctor, a psychologist, a social worker, and an educational specialist. This can be provided by practitioners in separate offices, referring back and forth among colleagues or in group practice settings.

If medications are incorporated into the treatment plan, then certain approaches can be helpful. It is optimal to plan for an eventual once-a-day dosing regimen. Regular telephone contact with school personnel is absolutely necessary to collect information concerning the child's behavior and academic progress. Drug vacations should be used to evaluate the need for continuation. Tutoring may be necessary to teach children compensatory skills if learning difficulties are present. Children should be seen on a once-weekly to once-monthly schedule during treatment.

Conclusion

Children with ADD comprise a heterogenous group. The core problems of inattention, impulsivity, and overactivity are often complicated with comorbid conditions, including anxiety, depression, conduct disorder, and Tourette's syndrome. The combined disorder impairs functioning in school, at home, and with the peer group. Otherwise bright children prove to be nonproductive in school, outcasts from their peer group, and a disturbing presence to adults and other children. Over the years, ADD's description, taxonomy, and name have changed, with different components attaining prominence as its "core" deficit, such as hyperactivity or attention-deficit disorder. The lack of diagnostic certainty about the child's problem plus an effective but nondiagnostically specific medication treatment has led to controversy. Some groups fear that professionals may be suppressing childhood spontaneity with medication treatments instead of addressing problems in the educational system. Other professionals worry that children who are being withheld from medication by worried parents are being denied a necessary remedy. Until the etiology of the disorder is uncovered, ADD will remain a curious, unexplained disorder of childhood that responds, albeit temporarily, to a medication intervention.

References

Abikoff H, Gittelman R: Hyperactive children treated with stimulants. Arch Gen Psychiatry 42:953–961, 1985

American Psychiatric Association: Diagnostic and Statistical Manual of Mental Disorders, 2nd Edition. Washington, DC, American Psychiatric Association, 1968

American Psychiatric Association: Diagnostic and Statistical Manual of Mental Disorders. 3rd Edition. Washington, DC, American Psychiatric Association, 1980

American Psychiatric Association: Diagnostic and Statistical Manual of Mental Disorders, 3rd Edition, Revised. Washington, DC, American Psychiatric Association, 1987

Barkley RA: A review of stimulant drug research with hyperactive children. J Child Psychol Psychiatry 18:137–165, 1977

Barkley RA: Hyperactive Children: A Handbook for Diagnosis and Treatment. New York, Guilford, 1982

Berry CA, Shaywitz SE, Shaywitz BA: Girls with attention deficit disorder: a silent minority? A report on behavioral and cognitive characteristics. Pediatrics 76:801–809, 1985

Biederman J, Steingard R: Attention-deficit hyperactivity disorder in adolescents. Psychiatric Annals 19:587–596, 1989

Biederman J, Wright V: Desipramine in the treatment of children and adolescents with attention deficit disorder: a blind placebo study (abstract). Proceedings of the annual meeting of the American Academy of Child and Adolescent Psychiatry 3:53, 1987

Biederman J, Baldessarini RJ, Wright V, et al: A double-blind placebo controlled study of desipramine in the treatment of ADD, I: efficacy. J Am Acad Child Adolesc Psychiatry 28:777–784, 1989a

Biederman J, Baldessarini RJ, Wright V, et al: Double-blind placebo controlled study of desipramine in the treatment of ADD, II: serum drug levels and cardiovascular findings. J Am Acad Child Adolesc Psychiatry 28:903–911, 1989b

Biederman J, Faraone S, Keenan K, et al: Family genetic and psychosocial risk factors in attention deficit disorder (abstract). Biol Psychiatry 25:145A, 1989c

Bird H, Canino G, Rubio-Stipec M, et al: Estimates of the prevalence of childhood maladjustment in a community survey in Puerto Rico. Arch Gen Psychiatry 45:1120–1126, 1988

Birmaher BB, Greenhill LL, Cooper MA, et al: Sustained release methylphenidate: pharmacokinetic studies in ADDH males. J Am Acad Child Adolesc Psychiatry 28:768–772, 1989

Campbell M, Spencer K: Psychopharmacology in child and adolescent psychiatry: a review of the past five years. J Am Acad Child Adolesc Psychiatry 27:269–279, 1988

Campbell M, Small A, Green W, et al: Behavioral efficacy of haloperidol and lithium carbonate. Arch Gen Psychiatry 41:650–656, 1984

Cantwell D: The hyperkinetic syndrome, in Child Psychiatry: Modern Approaches. Edited by Rutter M, Hersov L. London, Blackwell Scientific, 1982, pp 524–555

Carlson C, Lahey BB, Neeper R: Direct assessment of the cognitive correlates of attention deficit disorders with and without hyperactivity. Journal of Psychopathology and Behavioral Assessment 8:69–86, 1986

Casat CD, Pleasants DZ, Schroeder DH, et al: Bupropion in children with attention deficit disorder. Psychopharmacol Bull 25:198–201, 1989

Cohen DJ, Leckman JF: Commentary. J Am Acad Child Adolesc Psychiatry 28:580–582, 1989

Conners CK: A teacher rating scale for use in drug studies with children. Am J Psychiatry 126:152–156, 1969

Conners CK, Barkley RA: Rating scales and checklists for child psychopharmacology. Psychopharmacol Bull 21:816–832, 1985

Conners CK, Taylor E: Pemoline, methylphenidate, and placebo in children with minimal brain dysfunction. Arch Gen Psychiatry 37:922–933, 1980

Conners CK, Werry JL: Pharmacotherapy of psychopathology in children, in Psychopathological Disorders of Childhood, 2nd Edition. Edited by Quay H, Werry JL. New York, John Wiley, 1979, pp 336–386

Cornblatt BA, Winters L, Maminski B, et al: Methylphenidate-SR: effect on sustained attention in ADDH males (abstract). Proceedings of the annual meeting of the American Academy of Child and Adolescent Psychiatry 3:47, 1987

Cornblatt BA, Risch JJ, Faris G, et al: The continuous performance test, identical pairs version (CPT-IP), I: new findings about sustained attention in normal families. Psychiatry Res 26:223–238, 1988

DeLong GR, Aldershof AL: Long-term experience with lithium treatment in childhood: correlation with diagnosis. J Am Acad Child Adolesc Psychiatry 26:389–395, 1987

Denkla MB, Bemporad JR, McKay MC: Tics following methylphenidate administration: a report of 20 cases. JAMA 235:1349–1351, 1976

Donnelly M, Zametkin A, Rapoport J, et al: Treatment of childhood hyperactivity with desipramine: plasma drug concentration, cardiovascular effects, plasma and urinary catecholamine levels and clinical response. Clin Pharmacol Ther 39:72–81, 1986

Donnelly M, Rapoport JL, Potter W, et al: Fenfluramine and dextroamphetamine treatment of childhood hyperactivity: clinical and biochemical findings. Arch Gen Psychiatry 46:205–212, 1989

Douglas VI: Attentional and cognitive problems, in Developmental Neuropsychiatry. Edited by Rutter M. New York, Guilford, 1983, pp 280–329

Douglas VI, Parry P, Marton P, et al: Assessment of a cognitive training program for hyperactive children. J Abnorm Child Psychol 4:389–410, 1976

Douglas VI, Barr RG, O'Neill ME, et al: Short-term effects of methylphenidate on the cognitive, learning and academic performance of children with attention deficit disorder in the laboratory and the classroom. J Child Psychol Psychiatry 27:191–211, 1986

DuPaul GJ, Barkley RA: Medication therapy, in Attention Deficit Hyperactivity Disorder: A Handbook for Diagnosis and Treatment. Edited by Barkley RA. New York, Guilford, 1990, pp 573–612

El-Defrawi MH, Greenhill L: Substituting stimulants in treating behavior disorders. Am J Psychiatry 141:610, 1984

Fried J, Greenhill LL, Torres D, et al: Sustained-release methylphenidate: long-term clinical efficacy in ADDH males. Scientific Proceedings of annual meeting of the American Academy of Child and Adolescent Psychiatry 3:47, 1987

Garfinkel BD, Brown WA, Klee SH, et al: Neuroendocrine and cognitive responses to amphetamine in adolescents with a history of attention deficit disorder. Journal of the American Academy of Child Psychiatry 25:503–510, 1986

Gittelman-Klein R: Diagnosis and drug treatment of childhood disorders: attention deficit disorder with hyperactivity, in Diagnosis and Drug Treatment of Psychiatric Disorders: Adults and Children. Edited by Klein DF, Gittelman-Klein R, Quitkin F, et al. Baltimore, MD, Williams & Wilkins, 1980, pp 590–756

Gittelman-Klein R: Pharmacotherapy of childhood hyperactivity: an update, in Psychopharmacology: The Third Generation of Progress. Edited by Meltzer HY. New York, Raven, 1987, pp 1215–1224

Gittelman-Klein R, Mannuzza S: Hyperactive boys almost grown up, III: methylphenidate effects on ultimate height. Arch Gen Psychiatry 45:1131–1134, 1987

Gittelman-Klein R, Landa B, Mattes JA, et al: Methylphenidate and growth in hyperactive children. Arch Gen Psychiatry 45:1127–1130, 1987

Golden GS: Gilles de la Tourette's syndrome following methylphenidate administration. Dev Med Child Neurol 16:76–78, 1974

Golden GS: The effect of central nervous system stimulants on Tourette's syndrome. Analysis of Neurology 2:69–70, 1977

Gordon M: Microprocessor-based assessment of attention deficit disorders. Psychopharmacol Bull 22:288–290, 1986

Gordon M, Mettelman BB: The assessment of attention, I: standardization and reliability of a behavior-based measure. J Clin Psychol 44:682–690, 1988

Gordon M, DiNiro D, Mettelman BB, et al: Observations of test behavior, quantitative scores, and teacher ratings. Journal of Psychoeducational Assessment 7:141–147, 1989

Goyette CH, Conners CK, Ulrich RF: Normative data on revised Conners parent and teacher rating scales. J Consult Clin Psychol 47:1020–1029, 1979

Greenhill LL, Rieder RO, Wender PH, et al: Lithium carbonate in the treatment of hyperactive children. Arch Gen Psychiatry 28:636–640, 1973

Gualtieri CT, Wargin W, Kanoy R, et al: Clinical studies of methylphenidate serum levels in children and adults. Journal of the American Academy of Child Psychiatry 21:19–26, 1982

Gualtieri CT, Hicks RE, Patrick K, et al: Clinical Correlates of Methylphenidate Blood Levels. New York, Raven, 1984

Gualtieri C, Ondrusek M, Finley C: Attention deficit disorder in adults. Clin Neuropharmacol 8:345–356, 1985

Hunt R, Minderaa R, Cohen D: Clonidine benefits children with attention deficit disorder and hyperactivity: report of a double-blind placebo-crossover therapeutic trial. J Am Acad Child Adolesc Psychiatry 24:617–629, 1985

Kohn A: Suffer the restless children. Atlantic Monthly 264:90–100, 1989

Kupietz SS, Winsberg BG, Sverd J: Learning ability and methylphenidate (Ritalin®) plasma concentration in hyperkinetic children. Journal of the American Academy of Child Psychiatry 21:27–30, 1982

Lahey BB, Loeber R, Stouthamer-Loeber M, et al: Comparison of DSM and DSM-III-R diagnosis for prepubertal children: changes in prevalence and validity. J Am Acad Child Adolesc Psychiatry 29:620–626, 1990

Lancet: Does hyperactivity matter? (editorial). Lancet 1:73, 1986

Lapouse R, Monk M: An epidemiologic study of behavioral characteristics in children. Am J Public Health 48:1134–1144, 1953

Lieberman JA, Kane JA, Sarantokos S, et al: Prediction of relapse in schizophrenia. Arch Gen Psychiatry 44:597–603, 1987

Linnoila M, Gualtieri CT, Jobson K, et al: Characteristics of the therapeutic response to imipramine in hyperactive children. Am J Psychiatry 136:1201–1203, 1979

Loeber R: Natural histories of conduct problems, delinquency, and associated substance abuse, in Advances in Clinical Child Psychology. Edited by Lahey BB, Kazdin A. New York, Raven, 1988

Lowe TL, Cohen DJ, Detlor J, et al: Stimulant medications precipitate Tourette's syndrome. JAMA 26:1729–1731, 1982

Mattes J, Boswell L, Oliver H: Methylphenidate effects on symptoms of attention deficit disorder in adults. Arch Gen Psychiatry 41:449–456, 1984

Newcorn JH, Halperin JM, Healey JM, et al: Are ADDH and ADHD the same or different? J Am Acad Child Adolesc Psychiatry 28:734–738, 1989

Nuechterlein KH: Signal detection in vigilance tasks and behavioral attributes among offspring of schizophrenic mothers and among hyperactive children. J Abnorm Psychol 92:4–28, 1983

Offord D, Boyle M, Racine Y: Ontario Child Health Study: correlates of disorder. J Am Acad Child Adolesc Psychiatry 28:856–861, 1989

Page JG, Bernstein JE, Janicki RS, et al: A multicenter trial of pemoline (Cylert) in childhood hyperkinesis, in Clinical Use of Stimulant Drugs in Children. Edited by Conners CK. The Hague, The Netherlands, Excerpta Medica, 1974, pp 98–125

Pelham WE, Bender ME, Caddell J, et al: Methylphenidate and children with attention deficit disorders. Arch Gen Psychiatry 42:948–952, 1985

Pelham WE, Sturges J, Hoza J, et al: Sustained release and standard methylphenidate effects on cognitive and social behavior in children with attention deficit disorder. Pediatrics 80:491–501, 1987

Perel JW, Dayton PG: Methylphenidate, in Psychotherapeutic Drugs, Part II. Edited by Usdin E, Forrest I. New York, Marcel Dekker, 1976, pp 1287–1316

Popper CW, Elliot GR: Sudden death and tricyclic antidepressants: clinical considerations for children. Journal of Child and Adolescent Psychopharmacology (in press)

Porrino LJ, Rapoport JL, Behar D, et al: A naturalistic assessment of the motor activity of hyperactive boys, I: comparison with normal controls. Arch Gen Psychiatry 40:681–687, 1983a

Porrino LJ, Rapoport LJ, Behar D, et al: A naturalistic assessment of the motor activity of hyperactive boys, II: stimulant drug effects. Arch Gen Psychiatry 40:688–697, 1983b

Rapoport JL, Buchsbaum MS, Weingartner H, et al: Dextroamphetamine: cognitive and behavioral effects in normal and hyperactive boys and normal men. Arch Gen Psychiatry 37:933–943, 1980

Rapoport J, Nee L, Mitchell S, et al: Hyperkinetic syndrome and Tourette syndrome, in Gilles de la Tourette Syndrome. Edited by Friedhoff AJ, Chase TN. New York, Raven, 1982, pp 423–426

Rapport MD, DuPaul GJ: Hyperactivity and methylphenidate: rate-dependent effects. Int Clin Psychopharmacol 1:45–52, 1986

Rapport MD, Stoner G, DuPaul GJ, et al: Methylphenidate in hyperactive children: differential effects of dose on academic learning, and social behavior. J Abnorm Child Psychol 13:227–244, 1985

Riddle MA, Nelson JC, Kleinman CS, et al: Case study: sudden death in children receiving Norpramin—a review of three reported cases and commentary. J Am Acad Child Adolesc Psychiatry 30:104–109, 1991

Robins L: Deviant Children Grown Up. Baltimore, MD, Williams & Wilkins, 1966

Rutter M, Tizard J, Whitehouse K: Education, Health and Behavior: Psychological and Medical Study of Childhood Development. New York, John Wiley, 1970

Ryan N, Puig-Antich J, Cooper T, et al: Relative safety of single vs divided dose imipramine in adolescent major depression. J Am Acad Child Adolesc Psychiatry 26:400–406, 1987

Safer DJ, Krager JM: A survey of medication treatment for hyperactive/inattentive students. JAMA 260:2256–2258, 1988

Sandberg ST, Rutter M, Taylor E: Hyperkinetic disorder in psychiatric clinic attenders. Dev Med Child Neurol 20:279–299, 1978

Satin M, Winsberg B, Monetti C, et al: A general population screen for attention deficit disorder with hyperactivity. J Am Acad Child Adolesc Psychiatry 24:756–764, 1985

Satterfield J, Hoppe C, Schell A: Prospective study of delinquency in 110 adolescent boys with attention deficit disorder and 88 normal adolescent boys. Am J Psychiatry 139:797–798, 1982

Schmidt WE: Sales of drug are soaring for treatment of hyperactivity. New York Times, April 27, 1988, C2

Schrag P, Divoky D: The Myth of the Hyperactive Child. New York, Pantheon, 1975

Sebrechts MM, Shaywitz SE, Shaywitz BA, et al: Components of attention, methylphenidate dosage, and blood levels in children with attention deficit disorder. J Pediatr 77:222–228, 1986

Shaffer D, Greenhill LL: A critical note on the predictive validity of the hyperactive syndrome. J Child Psychol Psychiatry 20:61–72, 1979

Shaffer D, Schonfeld I, O'Conner P, et al: Neurological soft signs. Arch Gen Psychiatry 42:329–335, 1985

Shapiro SK, Garfinkel HD: The prevalence of behavior disorders in children: the interdependence of Attention Deficit Disorder and Conduct Disorder. J Am Acad Child Adolesc Psychiatry 25:809–819, 1986

Simeon JG, Ferguson HB, Van Wyck Fleet J: Bupropion effects in attention deficit and conduct disorders. Can J Psychiatry 31:581–585, 1986

Solanto MV, Wender EH: Does methylphenidate constrict cognitive functioning? J Am Acad Child Adolesc Psychiatry 28:897–902, 1989

Sprague RL, Sleator EK: Methylphenidate in hyperkinetic children: differences in dose effects on learning and social behavior. Science 198:1274–1276, 1977

Srinivas NR, Quinn D, Hybbard JW, et al: Stereoselective disposition of methylphenidate in children with attention-deficit disorder. J Pharmacol Exp Ther 241:300–306, 1987

"Sudden Death in Children Treated With a Tricyclic Antidepressant." Med Lett Drugs Ther, June 1, 1990, pp 32, 53

Sverd J, Gadow K, Paolicelli L: Methylphenidate treatment of attention-deficit hyperactivity disorder in boys with Tourette's syndrome. J Am Acad Child Adolesc Psychiatry 28:574–579, 1989

Swanson J, Cantwell D: Cognitive toxicity of methylphenidate: evidence from reaction times study of memory scanning (abstract). Scientific Proceedings of the annual meeting of the American Academy of Child and Adolescent Psychiatry 5:49–50, 1989

Sykes DH, Douglas VI, Morgenstern G: The effect of methylphenidate (Ritalin) on sustained attention in hyperactive children. Psychopharmacologia 25:262–274, 1972

Taylor EA: Overactivity, hyperactivity, and hyperkinesia: problems and prevalence, in The Overactive Child. Edited by Taylor EA. London, SIMP/Blackwell, 1986, pp 1–18

Taylor E, Schachar R, Thorley G, et al: Conduct disorder and hyperactivity, I: separation of hyperactivity and antisocial conduct in British child psychiatric patients. Br J Psychiatry 149:760–767, 1986a

Taylor E, Everitt B, Thorley G, et al: Conduct disorder and hyperactivity, II: a cluster analytic approach to the identification of a behavioral syndrome. Br J Psychiatry 149:768–777, 1986b

Trites RL, Blouin AG, Ferguson HB, et al: The Conners Teacher Rating Scale: an epidemiological inter-rater reliability and follow-up investigation, in Psychosocial Aspects of Drug Treatment for Hyperactivity. Edited by Gadow K, Loney J. Boulder, CO, Westview Press, 1981

Ullmann RK, Sleator EK: Responders, nonresponders, and placebo responders among others during a treatment evaluation. Clin Pediatr (Phila) 25:594–599, 1986

Varley CK: Effects of methylphenidate in adolescents with attention deficit disorder. Journal of the American Academy of Child Psychiatry 22:351–354, 1983

Wechsler J: Wechsler Intelligence Scale for Children—Revised. New York, Psychological Corporation, 1974

Weingartner H, Rapoport JL, Buchsbaum MS, et al: Cognitive processes in normal and hyperactive children and their response to amphetamine treatment. J Abnorm Psychol 89:25–35, 1980

Weiss G, Hechtman L, Perlman T, et al: Hyperactives as young adults: a controlled prospective ten-year follow-up of 75 children. Arch Gen Psychiatry 36:675–681, 1979

Weiss G, Hechtman L, Milroy T, et al: Psychiatric status of hyperactives as adults: a controlled prospective 15-year follow-up of 63 hyperactive children. J Am Acad Child Adolesc Psychiatry 24:211–220, 1985

Wender PH: Minimal Brain Dysfunction in Children. New York, John Wiley, 1971

Wender P, Reimher F, Wood D: Attention deficit disorder in adults. Arch Gen Psychiatry 38:449–456, 1981

Werry JS, Elkind GS, Reeves JC: Attention deficit, conduct, oppositional, and anxiety disorders in children, III: laboratory differences. J Abnorm Child Psychol 15:409–428, 1987

Whalen CK, Henker B, Collins BE, et al: A social ecology of hyperactive boys: medication effects in structured classroom environments. J Appl Behav Anal 12:65–81, 1979

Whalen CK, Henker B, Castro J, et al: Peer perception of hyperactivity and medication effects. Child Dev 58:816–828, 1987a

Whalen CK, Henker B, Swanson JM, et al: Natural social behaviors in hyperactive children: dose effects of methylphenidate. J Consult Clin Psychol 55:187–193, 1987b

Winsberg BG, Matinsky S, Strauss J, et al: Is there dose-dependent tolerance associated with chronic methylphenidate therapy in hyperactive children: oral dose and plasma concentrations. Psychopharmacol Bull 23:107–110, 1987

Zametkin AJ: Cerebral glucose metabolism in adults with hyperactivity of childhood onset. N Engl J Med 323:1361–1366, 1990

Zametkin AJ, Rapoport JL: Neurobiology of attention deficit disorder with hyperactivity: where have we come in 50 years? J Am Acad Child Adolesc Psychiatry 26:676–686, 1987

Zentall SS, Meyer MJ: Self-regulation of stimulation of ADD-H children during reading and vigilance task performance. J Abnorm Child Psychol 15:519–536, 1987

Chapter 24

Oppositional Defiant Disorder

James Egan, M.D.

Definition

DSM-III-R (American Psychiatric Association 1987) categorizes three related yet discriminable entities under the heading of disruptive behavior disorders. Included in this group are conduct disorder, oppositional defiant disorder (ODD), and attention-deficit hyperactivity disorder. There are two major reasons for grouping these disorders. First, there is a high degree of covariance among them. Second, they all tend to cause more distress to others than to those who are afflicted with these disorders. The victims are more troubling than troubled.

ODD roughly correlates with passive-aggressive disorders in previous nomenclatures. The essential feature is noncompliance to authority figures. It usually is mostly directed to parents, but may progress to include even teachers and other authority figures.

Clinical Findings

These children tend to demonstrate their aggression by covert means in contrast to those children with conduct disorder. The violation of the rights of others is also less severe than in conduct disorder. The defiance of authority and the manifestation of underlying aggression are predominantly by passive means.

The clinical picture of ODD is quite variable and depends on the interaction of the child's temperament, age, prior experiences, and parental psychologies. DSM-III-R diagnostic criteria for ODD are given in Table 24-1. Early in childhood, the child may be fussy or colicky or difficult to quiet or soothe. The parent frequently perceives the child as difficult or "bad" and eventually anticipates unrewarding and noncompliant responses from the child. The inner experience of the child is one of helplessness, neediness, and frustration. The parent attempts to "gain control" by insisting on compliance by the child in some area of functioning, often around talking, eating, sleeping, or toileting. Where oppositional behaviors to these demands become prominent and severe, they frequently warrant the additional diagnosis of elective mutism (Paez and Hirsch 1988), an eating or sleeping disorder, or enuresis or encopresis. A type of learning difficulty with academic underachievement is frequently manifested in later childhood at which time the oppositional trends consolidate around school performance.

In general, no specific area of noncompliance in ODD is so dominant as to warrant an additional diagnosis. Rather, the behavioral manifestations are general and varied and change with circumstances and age. The symptoms are usually exaggerated manifestations of child-rearing problems common to most parents. Issues of keeping a tidy room, picking up after oneself, taking baths, not interrupting or talking back, doing homework, and practicing the piano provide adequate grist for the oppositional child's mill. The course is frequently a shifting one, with bursts of efforts at parental control and discipline with appropriate punishments and consequences. These are usually interspersed with some hollow threats and aborted punishments. The parents often lose control in response to the child's continued provocations. They

276

Table 24-1. DSM-III-R diagnostic criteria for oppositional defiant disorder

Note: Consider a criterion met only if the behavior is considerably more frequent than that of most people of the same mental age.

A. A disturbance of at least six months during which at least five of the following are present:
1. Often loses temper
2. Often argues with adults
3. Often actively defies or refuses adult requests or rules, e.g., refuses to do chores at home
4. Often deliberately does things that annoy other people, e.g., grabs other children's hats
5. Often blames others for his or her own mistakes
6. Is often touchy or easily annoyed by others
7. Is often angry and resentful
8. Is often spiteful or vindictive
9. Often swears or uses obscene language

Note: The above items are listed in descending order of discriminating power based on data from a national field trial of the DSM-III-R criteria for disruptive behavior disorders.

B. Does not meet the criteria for conduct disorder, and does not occur exclusively during the course of a psychotic disorder, dysthymia, or a major depressive, hypomanic, or manic episode.

Criteria for severity of oppositional defiant disorder:

Mild: Few, if any, symptoms in excess of those required to make the diagnosis **and** only minimal or no impairment in school and social functioning.
Moderate: Symptoms or functional impairment intermediate between "mild" and "severe."
Severe: Many symptoms in excess of those required to make the diagnosis **and** significant and pervasive impairment in functioning at home and school and with other adults and peers.

Source. Reprinted with permission from American Psychiatric Association 1987.

then regret this loss of verbal or physical control and, in a misguided effort at undoing, are excessively rewarding and gratifying following the explosive outburst.

Children with ODD frequently dawdle and procrastinate. They often "forget" or "fail to hear." A common clinical observation is that of school underachievement. They fail to do their work, forget to bring the work or assignments home, or turn them in late. Anxious parents frequently try to compensate for the child's "immaturity" or "poor organizational skills" by pressing harder, only to

have the child intensify his or her efforts, thereby appearing to be pseudodefective or pseudoimbecilic. Children with ODD often have previously been referred for a hearing evaluation, which turns out to be normal; it is often assumed that there must be a hearing impairment to account for the noncompliance. This is a manifestation of the success by which overt aggression has been disguised.

In general, these children continually provoke parents, siblings, and teachers, resulting in a variety of angry, punitive, and critical responses, during which the children argue, blame others, and lose their tempers. They often experience adaptive failure, especially at school; this, coupled with the chronic criticism they receive, often leads to low self-esteem. This is further supported by the fact that these children tend to feel unfairly picked on and feel that their behavior is reasonable and just given the unfair treatment they have received.

Differential Diagnosis

As previously noted, ODD is frequently found in association with conduct disorder and attention-deficit hyperactivity disorder. In fact, 75% of children with attention-deficit hyperactivity disorder have an associated behavior disorder, generally ODD, and conduct disorder. In some reports, as many as 40% of children with depression will show conduct disorder. Since all the features of ODD are subsumed in the conduct disorder diagnosis, one can presume that even more than 40% of depressed children are also oppositional. Thus, when evaluating any one of the disruptive behavior disorders, one must look carefully for the presence of the other two (Gilpin and Maltz 1980; Werry et al. 1987).

Mania or hypomania or other psychotic disorders also may present as ODD and thus need to be considered when making the diagnosis of ODD (Rey et al. 1988).

In some children with separation anxiety disorder, there is frequently an admixture of oppositional features. Clingy attachment merges into or possibly reflects oppositional defiance. In adolescents with separation anxiety disorder, oppositional defiant symptoms are often prominent.

Epidemiology

Disorders of behavior are by far the most common reasons for referral to child psychiatrists. In some studies, these disorders account for two-thirds of all referrals (Costello et al. 1985).

Recent studies have reported a prevalence of 6% for ODD in 11-year-olds in the general population. ODD is twice as common in boys as girls (Anderson et al. 1987; Cantwell 1989).

Etiology

Both developmental and learning theories offer theoretical models to explain the development of ODD. Each of these models offers a differing view as to the etiology and pathogenesis of ODD; as a result, certain treatment implications can be inferred from each.

Developmental theory would suggest that ODD is an example of a fixation at the stage of anal development, or of separation from the object of attachment. In this theory, ODD reflects a severe persistence of the "terrible two's." Negativism, defiance, and noncompliance would be viewed as maladaptive efforts to deal with the conflict between the wish for autonomy and separation and the wish for dependency. By being oppositional, one asserts independence and thereby makes a statement regarding one's separate autonomous standing, while unconsciously aware that the provocative noncompliance will elicit in the authority figure renewed efforts at gaining compliance, thereby affording the child additional attention and dependency gratification. ODD is thus conceptualized as a separation disorder. This is in keeping with the view initially proposed by David Levy (1955; see also Egan 1988, 1989).

From the perspective of learning theory comes a competing view of pathogenesis. In this model, the symptoms of ODD are understood to reflect the effects of negative reinforcement. In an attempt to achieve compliance, the parent or authority figure reminds, scolds, lectures, berates, physically punishes, or nags the child in the vain hope of diminishing the oppositional behavior. These negative reinforcers, however, increase the rate and intensity of noncompliant behaviors (Forehand et al. 1975; Wells and Egan 1988).

Treatment

In practice, one frequently treats ODD with a combination of behavioral parent training and individual and family dynamic psychotherapy.

References

American Psychiatric Association: Diagnostic and Statistical Manual of Mental Disorders, 3rd Edition, Revised. Washington, DC, American Psychiatric Association, 1987

Anderson JC, Williams S, Silva PA: DSM-III disorders in preadolescent children. Arch Gen Psychiatry 44:69–76, 1987

Cantwell DP: Oppositional defiant disorder, in Comprehensive Textbook of Psychiatry V, Vol 1. Edited by Kaplan HI, Sadock BJ. Baltimore, MD, Williams & Wilkins, 1989, pp 1842–1845

Costello EJ, Edelbrock CS, Costello AJ: Validity of the NIMH Diagnostic Interview Schedule for children: a comparison between psychiatric and pediatric referrals. J Abnorm Child Psychol Vol 13, 1985

Egan J: Etiology and treatment of borderline personality disorder in adolescents. Hosp Community Psychiatry 45:111, 1988

Egan J: Identity and borderline disorders in children and adolescents, in Comprehensive Textbook of Psychiatry V, Vol 1. Edited by Kaplan HI, Sadock BJ. Baltimore, MD, Williams & Wilkins, 1989, pp 1889–1894

Forehand R, King H, Peed S, et al: Mother-child interactions: comparison of a non-compliant clinic group and a non-clinic group. Behav Res Ther 13:79–84, 1975

Gilpin DC, Maltz P: The oppositional personality in childhood. Child Psychiatry Hum Dev 11:79–86, 1980

Levy DM: Oppositional syndromes and oppositional behavior, in Psychopathology of Childhood. Edited by Hoch PH, Zubin J. New York, Grune & Stratton, 1955, pp 204–226

Paez P, Hirsch M: Oppositional disorder and elective mutism, in Handbook of Clinical Assessment of Children and Adolescents. Edited by Kestenbaum CJ, Williams DT. New York, NYU Press, 1988, pp 800–812

Rey JM, Bashir MR, Schwarz M, et al: Oppositional disorder: fact or fiction? J Am Acad Child Adolesc Psychiatry 27:157–162, 1988

Wells KC, Egan J: Social learning and systems family therapy for childhood oppositional disorder: comparative treatment outcome. Compr Psychiatry 29:138–146, 1988

Werry JS, Elkind GS, Reeves JC: Attention deficit, conduct, oppositional, and anxiety disorders in children, III: laboratory differences. J Abnorm Child Psychol 15:133–143, 1987

Chapter 25

Conduct Disorder: Conceptual and Diagnostic Issues

Carl P. Malmquist, M.D.

A direct approach to defining conduct disorders occurs in DSM-III-R (American Psychiatric Association 1987). This operational approach allows clinicians to have an official reference for diagnostic purposes. It is important to keep in mind that DSM-III-R simply sets out a specific list of symptoms or signs for a psychiatric diagnosis. In practice, the term *conduct disorder* is used by clinicians and others who deal with children and adolescents to refer to a generic group of children whose antisocial behavior appears to be a problem. These children also are referred to by some as delinquents or predelinquents. Kazdin (1987) refers to conduct disorders when a pattern of antisocial behavior is present and, in addition, there is a significant impairment in everyday functioning at home or school, and the behaviors become unmanageable by significant others. The point is that the behavior in question is something beyond the level of fighting, lying, stealing, and so on that is accepted in the course of normal child development.

Different disciplines approach the behavior from their own perspectives. Developmental psychologists are more likely to classify such children by use of an axis of internalizing-externalizing behaviors. Correctional workers simply refer to delinquency, whether or not it has been legally adjudicated by a court. Psychodynamically oriented clinicians refer to acting-out behaviors that may or may not be from internalized conflicts.

Diagnostic Classification

The original DSM-III (American Psychiatric Association 1980) classification used a breakdown into four categories: undersocialized aggressive, undersocialized nonaggressive, socialized aggressive, and socialized nonaggressive. Clinicians and researchers began to raise questions about the validity of these subtypes. For example, how generalizable are these categories across different age groups or to different developmental periods? How do specific disturbances, such as persistent lying or fire-setting, fit into one of these groups? A prepubertal child with lying as a pervasive problem might have a plethora of accompanying symptoms, but two more would be needed before a diagnosis could be made. Epistemic questions arose, such as what knowledge was gained in describing a boy of 11 with striking symptoms of lying, truancy, and petty pilfering over a period of 6 months, by placing him in one of the four categories.

Questions about the meaning of "aggressive" arose that are still with us in DSM-III-R. If aggressive means overt physical aggression, lying would not qualify. However, some clinicians see lying as "passive aggressive" and would view such a child as an aggressive type. A legalistic flair is evident in viewing an aggressive child as one who engages in an activity that violates the basic rights of others (over a 6-month period) and would include not only violence against persons or property, but also theft while confronting a person. The problem was then to split out what was nonaggressive. Examples were disobedience to parents or school rules, running away from home, or engaging in persistent lying or stealing. These correspond to legal categories encountered in juvenile courts or correctional systems, where the categories are incorrigibility, absenting, or theft.

Determination of whether the child was socialized or undersocialized was to be based on the presence of "social bonding." For this dichotomy, instead of quasi-legal categories, a checklist of attachment behaviors was to be the determiner: peer group friendships within a 6-month period, extending out to others, feeling appropriate guilt, loyalty to companions, and showing concern for their welfare. Any two of this list would indicate an attachment as equivalent to being socialized; but only one item on the checklist would place the child in the undersocialized grouping.

DSM-III-R classifies conduct disorder behavior into three types: group, solitary aggressive, and undifferentiated types. Although DSM-III-R states that the categories largely correspond to empirical studies, the studies are primarily from correctional or juvenile court populations where juveniles are classified into lone perpetrators or group participants. The solitary aggressive type is noted to correspond to the old undersocialized aggressive type, with a predominance of aggressive physical behaviors. The group type is the approximate version of the socialized nonaggressive type, with conduct problems occurring mainly as a group activity. The undifferentiated type is not defined beyond referring to it as a residual group that has a mixture of clinical features that cannot be classified and do not fit the other two categories. Interestingly, DSM-III-R notes that the latter type may be far more prevalent than the other two types. When a nosology has a residual as its largest group, a large amount of work remains to derive a classification or to validate the categories.

In terms of diagnosis, DSM-III-R allows the clinician to pick out any 3 of 13 symptoms listed that have been present for 6 months or more. The combination allows for diverse symptom pictures to be present, yet all carry the same diagnosis of conduct disorder. Some may be overtly acting out with physically assaultive behavior accompanied by cruelty and by such acts as setting fires. Another may carry the same diagnosis and simply be a child who is absenting from home with minimal stealing and lying.

Clinical Findings

The clinical findings for a conduct disorder are based on the symptoms presented in Table 25-1. The symptoms may be viewed as representing the application of the concept of antisocial behavior to a developmental stage. Some of the behaviors are based on direct clinical observation or reports from those who have contact with the child over time. Note that the DSM-III-R approach is categorical, where certain symptoms presenting for 6 months or more give a diagnosis.

A noncategorical (dimensional) approach focuses on the degree to which the symptoms or characteristics are seen as significant. A dimensional approach allows a diagnosis apart from a categorical yes or no. It relies on correlations among several specific characteristics, perhaps symptoms but also problem areas, and then summarizes them by way of quantitative techniques. Data about a child may be obtained from diverse sources (e.g., parent questionnaires, child rating scales). When different factors or dimensions are isolated, diagnostic categories or topologies are constructed. In a factor-analytic study, the most common characteristics associated with conduct disorder were fighting, disobedience, temper tantrums, destructiveness, and uncooperativeness (Quay 1986). Cluster analytic studies have identified aggressive or delinquent types of behavior (Edelbrock and Achenbach 1980). A multivariate approach utilized a group of adjudicated delinquents to assess their integration level ("I-Level") based on the presumption that a higher level of integration of experiences, perceptions, and awareness becomes evident as a child matures. Different types of delinquency would reflect different levels of integration. Jesness and Wedge (1984) delineated nine subtypes: 1) undersocialized active, 2) undersocialized passive, 3) conformist, 4) group-oriented, 5) pragmatist, 6) autonomy-oriented, 7) introspective, 8) inhibited, and 9) adaptive. The subtypes suggest different backgrounds, attitudes, aptitudes, and predictions for antisocial behavior.

Applying a developmental perspective to clinical manifestations sees young children more in terms of overt aggressive displays. These may be manifested at home toward family members or at nursery schools. The aggression may be random or

Table 25-1. DSM-III-R diagnostic criteria for conduct disorder

A. A disturbance of conduct lasting at least six months, during which at least three of the following have been present:
1. Has stolen without confrontation of a victim on more than one occasion (including forgery)
2. Has run away from home overnight at least twice while living in parental or parental surrogate home (or once without returning)
3. Often lies (other than to avoid physical or sexual abuse)
4. Has deliberately engaged in fire setting
5. Is often truant from school (for older person, absent from work)
6. Has broken into someone else's house, building, or car
7. Has deliberately destroyed others' property (other than by fire setting)
8. Has been physically cruel to animals
9. Has forced someone into sexual activity with him or her
10. Has used a weapon in more than one fight
11. Often initiates physical fights
12. Has stolen with confrontation of a victim (e.g., mugging, purse snatching, extorting, armed robbery)
13. Has been physically cruel to people

Note: The above items are listed in descending order of discriminating power based on data from a national field trial of the DSM-III-R criteria for disruptive behavior disorders.

B. If 18 or older, does not meet criteria for antisocial personality disorder.

Criteria for severity of conduct disorder:

Mild: Few if any conduct problems in excess of those required to make the diagnosis, **and** conduct problems cause only minor harm to others.

Moderate: Number of conduct problems and effect on others intermediate between "mild" and "severe."

Severe: Many conduct problems in excess of those required to make the diagnosis, **or** conduct problems cause considerable harm to others, e.g., serious physical injury to victims, extensive vandalism or theft, prolonged absence from home.

generalized destructive behavior; a selective type, such as repeated striking out at a particular person; or in a particular activity, such as lighting matches. While temper tantrums are often described as typical of the 2–3-year-olds, the degree and frequency of these tantrums need to be kept in mind. Passive-aggressive traits such as oppositional behavior, with refusal to obey or comply, may be noticeable. It is apparent that some of these overt behaviors may also be present in other diagnoses, particularly in attention-deficit hyperactivity disorder (ADHD), in which motorically driven behavior, coupled with impulsivity, elicits secondary interactions from others and takes on features of a conduct disorder. Similarly, inattentiveness in the ADHD child may be interpreted as defiance.

By the time of elementary school age, when socialization should be progressing, more overt aggressive displays are in the offing for the conduct-disordered child. The more intelligent and verbal child may be learning to provoke and to spar verbally, but the conduct-disordered child is physically aggressive with peers. In the lower grades, this involves pushing and shoving; in the course of the elementary school years, this becomes fighting. If there are conflicts with parents, the anger may be acted out at home and at school. More specific behavior patterns emerge at this time. Stealing can become more conspicuous. This may involve taking money from parents. The next step is petty pilfering from the teacher or other children at school. If confronted by another child, fighting and stealing become entwined. Some stealing may be engaged in as a peer phenomenon, the origin of group stealing.

An alternative to fighting when accused of stealing is simply to deny it—in effect, a form of lying. Children with more pronounced antisociality can lie with bland denials that will serve them well in later court proceedings. Those with a more histrionic flare handle matters with scenes of dramatic denials. It is quite revealing to notice that, just a short time ago, it was believed that children under 7 years did not lie (Ekman 1989), which has recently figured in cases in which a child is alleged to have been sexually abused. Piaget (1932) is often cited as the source for believing a child under 7 does not really lie because the child cannot distinguish fantasy from reality. Yet the intrusion of fantasy and wishes into truth distortion is a process seen in many children throughout latency and into adulthood when they receive diagnoses of histrionic or borderline personality disorder when a more pathologic level of lying occurs. Persistent cheating at games or in schoolwork seems allied to patterns of lying in children.

More fragmented behavior may occur with or

without fighting. The school-age version of a temper tantrum is seen in noisy, disturbing classroom behavior. The child may also "fly off the handle" when confronted about such behavior. He or she may talk loudly in class or be indifferent to the focus of the class. More aggressive displays include pushing things over or stalking out of the room. Again, the difference between the silent sulker and the dramatic performer comes to the fore. The more manipulative and coercive child may also have learned how to use other people by threats or cajolery, such as demanding money from other children or threatening others to do their homework for them "or else." Truancy and running away from home now may enter the picture.

Children with a greater degree of disturbance begin to exhibit behaviors such as torturing animals, fire setting, and truancy. In the younger child, the fire setting may begin with playing with matches. By school age, this may progress to setting objects on fire in school or with a peer group. These acts have many components, and they can be associated with different types of psychopathology. This similarly holds for acts such as hanging animals, setting them on fire, and other kinds of sexualized or sadistic behaviors. To delineate the significance of these symptoms in a particular child requires a thorough diagnostic assessment.

By adolescence, there are diverse expressions of these antecedent aggressive behaviors. For some, aggression becomes the dominant motif. A turn toward group aggression is the bridge to joining gangs that engage in vandalistic, predatory, or self-aggrandizing behaviors. Complicating the picture is that some of the acts begin as an attempt to intimidate, but lead to more aggressive assaultive or sexual behavior because they were not confronted. The role of alcohol and substance abuse stands by itself, yet it should be noted that, during early adolescence, the use of chemicals may complicate and contribute to conduct disorders.

Differential Diagnosis

When a child has been engaging in behaviors consistent with a conduct disorder, a thorough history and direct evaluation of the patient, the family, and the current milieu are crucial. It is assumed that a physical and neurologic examination with appropriate laboratory work will be done if there are any suggestions of organicity. Some feel that a neurologic deficit is the substratum for a conduct dis-

order, even though abnormalities are not detectable. Some measures have been developed to assess antisocial behavior, either by self-report if an adolescent or by significant others for the younger child. Although none are in standardized usage, some of the common ones are the Adolescent Antisocial Self-Report Behavior Checklist (Kulik et al. 1968); the Eyberg Child Behavior Inventory (Eyberg and Robinson 1983), which investigates conduct problems in the 2–12 age range, and is completed by significant adults in a child's life; and the Family Interaction Coding System (Patterson 1982), which records daily behaviors in antisocial children as they interact with parents and siblings. There are several parent and teacher rating scales that rely on lists of characteristics with different factors or constellations of symptoms involving antisocial behavior being split out. The Child Behavior Checklist (Achenbach and Edelbrock 1983) is a typical instrument with which parents rate 118 items about their children. In addition, customary psychometric devices are often useful at different ages. When the child reaches adolescence, the Minnesota Multiphasic Personality Inventory (Hathaway and McKinley 1989) may be useful. Diagnostic interview systems such as the Schedule for Affective Disorders and Schizophrenia for School-Age Children (Chambers et al. 1985), the Diagnostic Interview for Children and Adolescents (Herjanic and Reich 1982), and the Child Assessment Schedule (Hodges et al. 1982) are also in use to help narrow down a diagnostic group. With thorough history, evaluation, and testing, differential diagnosis of conduct disorder in a child can be attained, as well as a determination of whether a specific conduct disorder predominates, such as lying, stealing, or fire setting.

Given a thorough assessment in this manner, the clinician is faced with assessing the most likely possibilities. Before considering more esoteric diagnoses, the clinician should consider the possibility that a child may be striving to cope with a disruptive environment.

A 10-year-old girl who had lived with her mother over the preceding 5 years following a parental divorce was described as usually quiet and acquiescent. However, when her mother began to date a man and he eventually moved into their home, a series of events began to occur. Lipstick writing on the walls in the home and at the school occurred, some of these with profanity. The girl began to avoid coming home after school and began to lie about her whereabouts. Fires in wastebaskets were reported, and the girl was referred for evaluation.

In such cases, some type of adjustment disorder must be ruled out. Similarly, in transitions from one developmental stage to another, antisocial behavior may occur. Some of this behavior can be understood in the context of transient threats to security or self-esteem. If not handled skillfully, however, it can progress to conduct disorder problems. A preadolescent male witnessing family violence over several years may begin to emulate such behaviors.

The desirability of thorough exploration of organic factors is seen when antisocial behavior is connected with some degree of retardation or central nervous system impairment. Possibilities are a variant form of seizure disorder, a head injury from high risk or provocative behavior, or central nervous system readiness to react in exaggerated responses with rage reactions as has been postulated for borderline personality disorder (Stone 1988).

Among other diagnoses needing consideration is ADHD, as noted earlier. Children with both conduct disorders and ADHD can present with learning disabilities. DSM-III-R requires the behaviors to continue over 6 months.

Another possibility is oppositional defiant disorder in which the challenging, angry, and provocative behavior spills over into antisocial acts. Often the analogy is made that oppositional behavior is to passive-aggressive personality disorder as antisocial behavior is to antisocial personality disorder.

There is a possibility of a mood disorder leading to antisocial behavior, but thorough and independent confirmation of the depression should be made before causally attributing antisocial behavior to a depression. Some of these children, particularly boys, present with emerging paranoid features that figure in the behavior of an assaultive or fire-setting type. Only when the natural history of these children is examined does the full clinical picture emerge. There is also an impression that some of the girls who engage in lying, stealing, or manipulative behavior are those who later emerge with diagnoses of borderline personality disorder.

Epidemiology

An immediate problem in obtaining a base rate on conduct disorders is the confusion in studies about what is being measured. Some studies focus on generalized antisocial behaviors; others use a sociological approach based on the prevalence of delinquency in subcultural settings; and yet others measure delinquencies reported from court populations based on a legal definition. All of these may overlap. Yet, unless clinicians are to rely on a sociological or legal grouping, an operational definition of conduct disorder is needed. In the absence of such a clinical foundation, we do not have a clinical disorder per se. The need for validated diagnostic categories thus becomes crucial for epidemiologic studies. For example, legal definitions will give the lowest base rates, and confidential self-report surveys will give the highest.

Robins (1981) referred to the problem of antisocial development in childhood as one that has the most serious consequences for society among childhood diagnoses. The problem is assessing an age group that has a high prevalence of antisocial behavior, yet that does not tell us the significance, if any, of the behavior. Court data are biased in terms of variables such as detection, apprehension, arrest, and processing steps. Social class variables also operate in terms of a well-known phenomenon of higher-socioeconomic-level children being more likely to be viewed as clinical problems in contrast to children on the lower socioeconomic level who are processed in court and correctional systems.

Figures on the incidence of antisocial behavior vary widely using different populations. A common range is 5%–25%. Urban versus rural, inner-city versus suburbs, and racial factors all operate as socioeconomic variables. There is also a diagnostic overlap problem that complicates epidemiologic findings. Gender differences contribute, with an estimate of at least five boys to one girl, although this gap may be narrowing.

Commonality of conduct disorder symptoms in other diagnoses needs emphasis. If we resolve symptom expressions of antisociality in some other diagnosis, what remains? Some argue that what remains is a sociological group, one not primarily clinical. Behavioral lists, such as stealing, fighting, fire setting, and truancy, and their relative incidence at different ages or developmental levels, can be compiled. These provide a developmental sociology or symptom list paralleling different developmental stages. While such behaviors are prevalent in children, it is difficult to ascribe clinical significance to them unless they are recurrent and pervasive. The approach is to say that if conduct disturbance symptoms are persistent and the child is suffering from them, we have a clinical problem. However, what if the child is not disturbed and suffering but others suffer, such as parents or the school? This is the cutting edge between conduct disorder symptoms that are internalized versus those that are enacted in the absence of inner conflict.

Etiology

It is difficult to discuss the etiology of a diagnostic category in which the validity of the diagnosis itself is in question. To talk about etiology means we presume a primary diagnosis of conduct disorder independent of other psychiatric diagnoses that could adequately explain the symptomology. A common description is that the etiology is multifactorial, which is equivalent to an acknowledgment that we do not know that any one etiology is explanatory. With conduct disorders we can only assess risk factors that heighten the probability for antisocial behaviors to emerge in a child. Such listings are associations that do not establish causality. Lacking knowledge of etiologic factors beyond listing risk factors, caution should be used in thinking that all that is needed to lower the incidence is to lower the risks. Such a conclusion does not follow, since we are not actually dealing with etiology but with a broad grouping of predisposing factors.

We know that personality characteristics in children that contribute to a conduct disorder involve traits or temperaments of mood instabilities, aggressivity, emotional lability, impulsivity, and maladaptive traits. It is often difficult to separate the contributions of these traits from the reactions to such traits by parents and others. Reference to organic factors and altered neurophysiologic functioning has been made. Evidence for antisocial behavior as correlated with these factors is equivocal since studies go in both directions. Some of these traits lead children into high-risk activities that, in turn, lead to trauma and injuries.

The relationship of these traits to genetic components has also been considered (DiLalla and Gottesman 1991). Recurrent questions arise about the impact of antisocial families in producing delinquent offspring. Is it genes, identification with the parent or sibling, mismatch between parents and offspring, or superego deficits in the parents that are played out? Since twin studies have shown a significant concordance of antisocial behavior among monozygotic compared with dizygotic twins, this needs to be considered (Christiansen 1974). Adoption studies of children separated from biological parents at birth tend to show more antisocial behavior occurring in the offspring when a biological parent also has antisocial behavior (Cadoret 1978). Such studies also show a cumulative factor from both loadings. Thus in a Stockholm adoption study based on 862 men born out of wedlock and adopted to nonrelatives at an early age, there was 1.9 times the risk of criminality if either biological parent had a history of criminality in the absence of alcohol abuse (Cloninger et al. 1982).

In terms of environmental variables, the etiologic factors for antisocial development include low family income, large family size, parental criminality, low intelligence, and family conflict, which encompassed unsatisfactory parental attitudes and discipline (West and Farrington 1973). West and Farrington predicted that boys with three of these loadings were in a high-risk category, and follow-up revealed 50% had become delinquent and 33% were recidivistic. The factors were seen as cumulative. Yet there were a high number of false negatives and low sensitivity, which points up the weaknesses in correlational studies. We also need to keep in mind the implications of false positives from the labeling effect.

More specific factors implicated in the child's environment can be summarized:

1. Prevalence of family conflict in the form of marital discord, divorce, or husband-wife beatings. (These settings also include inconsistency or inattention to the child's behavior, such as rules about bedtime, staying on the streets, and generally lax supervision.)
2. Psychopathology in the family; criminal behavior and alcoholism in the parents, especially when occurring in a father; and antisocial and aggressive behavior in the family as a heightened background factor.
3. Birth position, with middle children having a greater risk compared with first-born, youngest, or only children.
4. Large family size.
5. Social class, although this overlaps with many other factors, such as family stresses, poverty, and size of family.
6. Harsh or inconsistent disciplinary techniques where there may be a high incidence of child neglect or abuse (Widom 1989). (Other studies identify erratic or indulgent parental behaviors.)
7. The quality of schooling has been stressed.

Based on 12 different school settings, attendance, dropouts, delinquency rates, and academic performance were studied (Rutter 1981). Praise, emphasis on academics, a pleasant school environment, stress on individual responsibility, accessible teachers who were well-organized and focused on good behavior, and agreement among staff on academic matters and discipline were predictive of good student behavior. A subculture of antisocial behavior may be a contributory factor, even in the absence of the above variables. In practice, it is often difficult to untangle the general milieu in which a child is being reared—such as in a lower-socioeconomic-class area with a high incidence of delinquency, or the absence of father figures—from other etiologic agents.

Treatment

Given this large array of etiologic possibilities, along with questions about the diagnostic validity of conduct disorder, what can be recommended about treatment? Ideally, the treatment would be applied to the primary clinical disorder, such as oppositional defiant disorder or ADHD, as two frequently cited examples. If no other disorder appears in the course of a diagnostic assessment, a child may be reacting to an environmental situation. In many ways, conduct disorder is one of the most difficult disorders to treat because the clinician is seeking to validate some other diagnosis that is operating or to modify a noxious environment that is feeding into the behavior. It is obvious that no one treatment can be recommended in all cases. Individual selectivity and matching is the key.

Behavioral techniques often are used to control key behaviors. The goal is to alter the inadequate learning responses of the child, as part of the ground rules that have allowed antisocial behavior. In contrast, socialized behaviors are reinforced. Techniques vary from token economies to fostering problem-solving skills. Operant conditioning includes reinforcement or punishment techniques. An increasingly popular variation is cognitive therapy, where the maladaptive or self-defeating cognitions of the child are focused on in an effort to promote prosocial behavior.

Individual psychodynamic psychotherapy has its advocates and critics. Many fascinating case studies based on psychoanalytic approaches have been reported. The problem is the difficulty in applying this approach to the large numbers of children with these problems. There is also the problem of using such an approach if the behavior is not due to internalized conflict. Even if a child is motivated and can attach to the therapist, questions are raised about results in terms of changing behavior. A psychoanalytic approach focuses on the defenses that have been erected, such as acting out, to deal with the conflict promoting antisocial behavior. However, some of these children function at a primitive developmental level where they are impaired in forming and maintaining attachments and affects about others in more than a transient sense. Some argue that psychotherapy worsens delinquent behavior and should be avoided (Shaffer 1984).

Correctional systems have long used forms of group therapy for conduct problems. This may vary from a focus on conflicts to attempts at behavioral modification. Family therapy may be used when the conduct appears to stem from family stresses. While some family therapies focus on family structure and malfunctioning, others attempt to use a ''family management'' approach that rewards good behavior or promotes consistency in parenting and discipline. This approach is limited if the disturbed conduct is severe, such as fire setting or physically assaultive behaviors. The assumption throughout these therapies is that these are motivated individuals who will work on their problems and commit themselves to an ongoing program. In many cases, unfortunately, the assumption is not valid.

Residential treatment approaches include separate institutions, as well as child psychiatry units and day-care units. In times past, use of such facilities, including commitment to correctional facilities via juvenile courts, was one of the main treatment approaches employed with conduct-disordered children. Apart from the fact that health insurance programs now place limitations on the length of stay for hospitalization, it was questionable whether removing children from their environment resolved conduct disorder problems. If removal was effective, was it that, per se, which changed behavior, or was it whatever other treatment modality that was employed? Unless the decision was that the child should never return home, the same influences awaited the child on returning.

Psychopharmacology has its place, depending on the diagnosis. Psychostimulants may have a beneficial effect with ADHD children. There have been attempts to contain aggressive behavior by the use of neuroleptic medications such as haloperidol. Anticonvulsants have been tried. The results are equivocal, given the mixture of diagnoses. Lithium carbonate has similarly been tried. Such drug interventions need careful assessment in terms of the cost-benefit analysis, with assessments of side effects and long-term consequences of drug use being compared with the long-term clinical improvement.

Prognosis

Twenty-five years ago, Robins (1966) did a 30-year follow-up of antisocial children seen in a child guidance clinic. The antisocial boys showed a later arrest rate of 71%, and half of them had a pattern of repetitive arrests, with almost as many being imprisoned. The psychosocial pathology was striking, with half having drinking problems in adulthood and a pattern of failures in marriages and jobs. Kazdin (1987) summarized subsequent studies that confirm continuing problems and a dismal prognosis.

Besides diagnoses of antisocial personality, there is a higher incidence of alcohol and drug abuse and somatization and a greater risk of psychiatric hospitalization. Physical health is impaired, with higher mortality rates and high rates of hospitalization for physical problems. General criminal behavior is manifested with arrest records, convictions, serious offenses, and driving while intoxicated. Employment performance is marginal at best, with frequent job changes and dependence on financial assistance. There is a high rate of job dropout, low school achievement, divorce, remarriage, and separation. Caution is needed in using such follow-up data. Robins (1978) noted that, even with severe antisocial children, less than half become antisocial adults. Clinicians and those concerned about these children must bear in mind that those showing serious symptomatology in childhood, such as fire setting or compulsive stealing, are not all predestined to become antisocial. Labeling can be detrimental; even without treatment, at least half somehow extricate themselves from antisocial development. Many complex interrelated variables operate in a particular child, influencing the outcome and making prediction difficult.

Research Issues

An urgent issue is the clarification of conduct disorders as a primarily psychiatric diagnosis versus representing symptoms and signs of some other psychiatric diagnosis. This will require longitudinal follow-up for children who meet the current DSM-III-R and upcoming DSM-IV criteria to see what diagnoses, if any, these children have as adults. We know from existing studies that some of them will meet criteria for antisocial personalities as adults, but the majority do not. More specificity is needed for determining the significance of antisocial manifestations in young children.

Even with behavior such as fire setting, which is suggestive of a specific type of psychopathology, research indicates that the symptom is simply one among many conduct problems occurring in a disturbed home environment (Showers and Pickrell 1987). Investigation is needed to determine whether these children move through a sequence from a pediatric population to mental health clinics and then either to psychiatric hospitalization or to chronic antisociality. We also need to know much more about girls who engage in this behavior.

While the proliferation of checklists and symptom inventories goes on, no one of them has attained sufficient validity with conduct-disordered children. Many of these approaches fail to discriminate among diagnostic possibilities. Perhaps the focus on greater validity in the measures used in assessing these children and their families will have a future payoff. There is a need to determine why discrepancies exist among sources reporting on children's behavior, especially with respect to conduct disorders. Two factors need consideration: the discrepancy between parents and children (and between parents and children, and those who come from different perspectives, such as teachers and clinicians); and whether there is a significance to different symptoms of conduct disorder (Herjanic and Reich 1982). Kazdin (1987) pointed out how other areas in the lives of these children may be as important as their antisocial behavior, such as cognitive functioning, social skills, and academic performance. The in-depth study of these families and the role of life events are equally significant.

Earls (1989) proposed a preventive trial for conduct disorder, in view of its being one of the most important public health problems in psychiatry. The experiment would select children born of antisocial parents who are seen as being at risk to repeat the cycle of deviance portrayed in their parents. It would begin with infants, follow them to school age, and involve parents, children, and caregivers in a developmental center. The goal would be to increase the competence of the child in language and prosocial behavior, while decreasing his or her exposure to dysfunctional parenting and an impoverished environment. Assessment of success would be made at school age to see whether the incidence of conduct problems had been reduced from 50% (the morbid risk without intervention) to 25%. If so, it would be called a complete success. Such large-scale efforts to diminish risk factors in the vulnerable child, while increasing biological and social competence, need further assessment. Without such avenues, as professionals, we are likely to repeat our own past cycles of efforts whose success has not been much greater than no intervention. Our underlying hope is that the resilience of the child will come through in a sufficient number of cases.

References

Achenbach TM, Edelbrock CS: Manual for the Child Behavior Checklist and Revised Child Behavior Profile. Burlington, VT, University Associates in Psychiatry, 1983

American Psychiatric Association: Diagnostic and Statistical Manual of Mental Disorders, 3rd Edition. Washington, DC, American Psychiatric Association, 1980

American Psychiatric Association: Diagnostic and Statistical Manual of Mental Disorders, 3rd Edition, Revised. Washington, DC, American Psychiatric Association, 1987

Cadoret RJ: Psychopathology in adopted-away offspring in biological parents with antisocial behavior. Arch Gen Psychiatry 35:176–184, 1978

Chambers WJ, Puig-Antich J, Hirsch M, et al: The assessment of affective disorders in children and adolescents by semistructured interview: test-retest reliability of the K-SADS-P. Arch Gen Psychiatry 42:696–702, 1985

Christiansen KO: Seriousness of criminality and concordance among Danish twins, in Crime, Criminology and Public Policy. Edited by Hood R. London, Heinemann, 1974, pp 63–78

Cloninger CR, Sigvardsson S, Bohman M, et al: Predisposition to petty criminality in Swedish adoptees, II: cross-fostering analysis of gene-environment interaction. Arch Gen Psychiatry 39:1242–1247, 1982

DiLalla LF, Gottesman II: Biological and genetic contributors to violence—Widom's untold tale. Psychol Bull 109:125–129, 1991

Earls F: Epidemiology and child psychiatry: entering the second phase. Am J Orthopsychiatry 59:279–283, 1989

Edelbrock CS, Achenbach TM: A typology of child behavior profile patterns: distribution and correlates for disturbed children aged 6–16. J Abnorm Child Psychol 8:441–470, 1980

Ekman P: Why Kids Lie. New York, Charles Scribner, 1989

Eyberg SM, Robinson EA: Conduct problem behavior: standardization of a behavioral rating scale with adolescents. Journal of Clinical Child Psychology 12:347–354, 1983

Hathaway SR, McKinley JC: Minnesota Multiphasic Personality Inventory–2. Minneapolis, MN, University of Minnesota, 1989

Herjanic B, Reich W: Development of a structured psychiatric interview for children: agreement between child and parent on individual symptoms. J Abnorm Child Psychol 10:307–324, 1982

Hodges K, McKnew D, Sytryn L, et al: The Child Assessment Schedule (CAS) diagnostic interview: a report on reliability and validity. Journal of the American Academy of Child Psychiatry 21:468–473, 1982

Jesness CF, Wedge RF: Validity of a revised Jesness Inventory I–level classification with delinquents. J Consult Clin Psychol 52:997–1010, 1984

Kazdin AE: Conduct Disorders in Childhood and Adolescence. Newbury Park, CA, Sage, 1987

Kulik JA, Stein KB, Sarbin TR: Dimensions and patterns of adolescent behavior. J Consult Clin Psychol 48:1134–1144, 1968

Patterson GR: Coercive Family Process. Eugene, OR, Castalia, 1982

Piaget J: The Moral Judgment of the Child (1932). New York, Free Press, 1965

Quay HC: A critical analysis of DSM-III as a taxonomy of psychopathology in childhood and adolescence, in Contemporary Directions in Psychopathology. Edited by Millon T, Klerman G. New York, Guilford, 1986, pp 151–165

Robins LN: Deviant Children Grow Up. Baltimore, MD, Williams & Wilkins, 1966

Robins LN: Sturdy childhood predictors of adult antisocial behavior: replications from longitudinal studies. Psychol Med 8:611–622, 1978

Robins LN: Epidemiological approaches to natural history research: antisocial disorders in children. Journal of the American Academy of Child Psychiatry 20:566–580, 1981

Rutter M: Epidemiological/longitudinal studies in causal research in child psychiatry. Journal of the American Academy of Child Psychiatry 20:513–544, 1981

Shaffer D: Notes on psychotherapy research among children and adolescents. Journal of the American Academy of Child Psychiatry 23:552–561, 1984

Showers J, Pickrell E: Child firesetters: a study of three populations. Hosp Community Psychiatry 38:495–501, 1987

Stone M: Toward a psychobiological theory of borderline personality disorder. Dissociation 1:2–15, 1988

West DJ, Farrington DP: Who Becomes Delinquent? London, Heinemann, 1973

Widom CS: The cycle of violence. Science 244:160–166, 1989

Chapter 26

Conduct Disorder in Childhood

Robert L. Hendren, D.O.

Children and adolescents with a conduct disorder diagnosis are a varied group. This is due to the variety of factors associated with the expression of antisocial behavior. First, the classification of conduct disorder is a controversial and unsettled issue in mental health (Cantwell and Baker 1988). Depending on the constellation of symptoms, conduct disorder might include delinquent behavior, antisocial behavior, or aggressive behavior. Children with a diagnosis of conduct disorder may also be depressed, may have attention-deficit hyperactivity disorder, or may be psychotic. Second, the etiology of conduct disorder is complex and multifactorial, with biological, psychological, and social factors having varying degrees of importance. A comprehensive assessment and treatment program depends not only on the knowledge of developmental signs and symptoms, but also on a thorough exploration of the biopsychosocial factors underlying the etiology of this particular disorder.

The prevalence of conduct disorder is difficult to estimate because of the different definitions that have been used and the variations that occur in different age groups, between the sexes, and within a particular culture. DSM-III-R (American Psychiatric Association 1987) estimates the prevalence at approximately 9% for males and 2% for females under 18 years of age. The rates of specific behaviors that constitute most descriptions of conduct disorder are much higher. One survey among youths aged 13–18 found that 50% admitted to theft, 35% to assault, and 45% to property destruction; 60% admitted to more than one type of antisocial behavior, such as drug abuse, vandalism, and ag-

gressiveness (Feldman et al. 1983). If one considers all youth who regularly engage in some type of antisocial behavior at some period of time in their life, the prevalence of at least a mild form of the disorder is clearly great.

Diagnosis

DSM-III-R

The essential feature of conduct disorder, according to DSM-III-R (see Table 25-1 [Chapter 25, this volume]), is a persistent pattern of behavior that violates the basic rights of others and major age-appropriate societal norms or rules. Included are behaviors that range from acts of violence, stealing, and lying, to truancy, running away, and fire setting. Since the diagnoses in DSM-III-R are based on descriptions and not on etiology, individuals who meet the criteria for conduct disorder are often quite varied in their underlying psychopathology. The diagnosis also depends on the social context, so that individuals may be variably diagnosed in different settings. Thus individuals diagnosed as conduct disordered are a very heterogeneous group.

There are three subtypes of conduct disorder in DSM-III-R: 1) the group type, 2) the solitary aggressive type, and 3) the undifferentiated type. The central feature of the solitary aggressive type is aggressive physical behavior initiated by the individual with little attempt to conceal the antisocial behavior. The group type is characterized by antisocial behavior that occurs as part of a group activity with friends to whom the individual is loyal. The group type is believed to be more common than the solitary aggressive type. The undifferentiated type is a residual category for children or adolescents with a mixture of clinical features that cannot be classified as either group or solitary aggressive type. It is believed to be more common than either of the other two.

The research literature does not clearly support the validity or stability of the three subtypes of conduct disorder in DSM-III-R (Cantwell and Baker 1988, 1989). In a cluster analysis of disturbed children, Wolff (1971) found two separate groups of behaviorally disturbed children: aggressive-overactive and antisocial. Factor analytic studies by Achenbach and associates (Achenbach and Edelbrock 1978, 1981; Achenbach et al. 1987) found the categories of aggressive and nonaggressive antisocial to be the most distinct subgroups. In a review of the literature on delinquency, Rutter and Giller (1984) found that the categories of socialized and undersocialized are the most valid method of subgrouping. These two subtypes have differing associated features and outcomes, with the socialized subtype having a better long-term prognosis. However, at least one study found that group involvement is common in delinquent conduct, and there is no category of offense that is predominantly solitary (Emler et al. 1987). Adolescent girls were especially likely to commit offenses in the company of others. In a 4-year follow-up study, Cantwell and Baker (1989) found that the conduct disorder diagnoses were not stable. At follow-up, many of the children initially diagnosed as conduct disordered had other diagnoses, and a few were well at follow-up. Thus the research literature to date suggests that the subcategories of socialized-undersocialized and aggressive-nonaggressive may have some predictive validity depending on the population being studied, but these categories are far from validated.

Other Diagnostic Approaches

Other approaches to categorizing conduct disorder are similar to that of DSM-III-R in that there is an attempt to identify salient symptoms that yield reliable and clinically meaningful ways of grouping antisocial behavior (Kazdin 1987). Patterson (1982) found two meaningful symptom clusters in children whose primary symptom was either aggression or stealing. Family structure and response to treatment differed, with the group of children who steal being less responsive to treatment and having

a poorer prognosis. Children with characteristics of both types are more likely to have a history of child abuse.

Another method for the classification of antisocial behavior was based on an overt-covert distinction (Loeber and Schmaling 1985). Overt behaviors, such as physical and verbal aggression, are more direct; covert behaviors, such as stealing, fire setting, and truancy, are not as openly confrontational. Cluster analyses support the validity of these distinctions. Children with a mixture of the two appear to be at greater risk for future dysfunction.

The draft of ICD-10 (World Health Organization 1988) has yet another method for the subclassification of conduct disorder, which includes a number of "combination categories" that represent commonly co-occurring conditions. For example, there are categories for depressive conduct disorder and hyperkinetic conduct disorder. Subdivisions of conduct disorder include conduct disorder confined to the family context, unsocialized conduct disorder, socialized conduct disorder, and conduct disorder not otherwise specified (Cantwell and Baker 1988).

All of the classification systems proposed for antisocial behavior in childhood and adolescence contain some commonalities. Each approach identifies certain symptom clusters, such as aggression and delinquency, as important subcategories. However, neither the category of conduct disorder nor the subcategories have proved to have valid developmental and predictive significance.

Comorbidity

Many children and adolescents who meet the criteria for a diagnosis of conduct disorder have other coexisting psychiatric disorders that may have led to their antisocial behavior and will significantly influence their responsiveness to treatment and their long-term prognosis (Woolsten et al. 1989). For instance, depressionlike symptoms have been noted in some patients with conduct disorder (Jensen et al. 1988; Kovacs et al. 1988). Puig-Antich (1982) reported that conduct-disordered symptoms may start and stop with the onset and recovery from affective illness. Conduct disorder that is comorbid with depression is also found to run a variable course, which may or may not go away as the depression improves (Kovacs et al. 1988).

Children and adolescents with a diagnosis of conduct disorder are also found to have coexisting attention-deficit disorder with hyperactivity. Reeves et al. (1987) found that children with attention-deficit disorder with hyperactivity plus conduct disorder or oppositional disorder were very similar to children with attention-deficit disorder with hyperactivity alone on most demographic and clinical variables. This combination is associated with more severe physical aggression and antisocial behaviors than is found in children with a diagnosis of conduct disorder alone and represents a more serious form of conduct disorder (Walker et al. 1987). In addition, a significant number of children first diagnosed as having conduct disorder are found to have attention-deficit disorder with hyperactivity at follow-up (Cantwell and Baker 1989).

Some children and adolescents with a propensity toward the later development of schizophrenia may exhibit early antisocial behavior that would lead to their being diagnosed as having conduct disorder. There is a clear familial link between schizophrenia and antisocial behavior (Silverton et al. 1988). Some children who later develop schizophrenia are known to exhibit aggressive and antisocial behavior in the years preceding the onset of the schizophrenia (Offord and Cross 1969; Watt et al. 1983).

Disturbances in conduct are also found in children with Tourette's syndrome. One study has estimated that 10%–30% of cases of conduct disorder may be due to the presence of a Tourette's syndrome gene in children who are not economically disadvantaged (Comings and Comings 1987).

This overlap or comorbidity of disorders found in children and adolescents diagnosed as conduct disordered points out yet again the heterogeneity of this patient group. Clinicians and researchers working with this group must carefully examine all of the symptoms and background information to identify factors that accurately classify each child and adolescent.

Etiology

The etiology of conduct disorder is complex and multifactorial. Biological, psychological, and social factors interact, having varying degrees of importance. The eventual outcome of conduct disorder in marked aggressivity, delinquency, another psychiatric disorder, or healthy behavior depends on the interaction of each factor with the individual's development (Lewis et al. 1987). Delineation of some of the known biopsychosocial factors follows, but it should be kept in mind that it is the interaction

of these variables that leads to a complete understanding of the etiology of the disorder.

Biological

Characteristics of childhood temperament are considered to be genetic or constitutional in origin and to show some consistency across time (Thomas and Chess 1977). Children characterized as possessing a difficult temperament are more likely to show or develop behavioral problems (Rutter et al. 1964). The familial genetic factors that predispose a child to conduct disorder and delinquency also make it more likely that at least one parent will be antisocial (Lahey et al. 1988b; Mednick et al. 1984; Moffitt 1987). Children with a difficult temperament may interact with their family and environment in such a way that the initial behavioral disturbance becomes even more problematic (Patterson 1982).

It is a commonly held belief that hormonal changes have a direct influence on adolescent behavior. However, most scientific studies to date have failed to demonstrate this direct effect (Petersen 1985). At least a few studies have found that hormone levels correlate with emotional dispositions and aggressive attributes in boys. Susman et al. (1987) found that higher levels of androstenedione were related to higher levels of acting-out problems in boys. Olweus et al. (1988) found that high levels of testosterone caused boys to be more impatient and irritable, resulting in an increased propensity to engage in aggressive-destructive behavior. Disturbed serotonergic function has also been implicated in episodic aggression (Brown et al. 1988). Disturbed platelet monoamine oxidase has been reported in disruptive behavior disorders (Stoff et al. 1989).

Minor neurologic abnormalities are found in some children and adolescents with delinquency (Lewis et al. 1987). However, many of these neurologic abnormalities are associated with a variety of psychiatric disorders and may not relate exclusively to conduct disorder. For example, Satterfield et al. (1987) followed hyperactive children into adolescence and found that the nondelinquent hyperactive subjects had abnormal auditory-evoked response potentials, whereas the delinquent hyperactive subjects had normal maturational changes in these same measures. In addition, since delinquent children are known to have had more head and face trauma (Lewis et al. 1979), early neurologic signs may be the result of abuse or risk-taking behavior rather than due to constitutional abnormalities (Kazdin 1987).

Neuropsychological deficit has a clear association with delinquency. There is a consistent association between low IQ and delinquency that holds when assessed prospectively and is independent of social class (Moffitt et al. 1981). The functions most consistently cited as impaired across studies are verbal and executive (attention, concentration, abstraction, planning, inhibition of inappropriate responses, and sequencing) (Moffitt and Silva 1988).

Psychological

Cognitive factors. Delinquent and aggressive children are found to have distinctive cognitive and psychological profiles compared to children with other psychiatric disorders and normal control subjects. A group of delinquent males in a correctional facility displayed more immature modes of role-taking, logical cognition, and moral reasoning (Lee and Prentice 1988). When compared with low-aggressive boys, high-aggressive boys are found 1) to define social problems based on the perception that others are hostilely motivated adversaries, 2) to find fewer and less effective solutions, and 3) to generate fewer consequences for exhibiting aggression (Guerra and Slaby 1989). In addition, high-aggressive delinquents have been found less able to perceive the viewpoints of other people than were low-aggressive delinquents (Short and Simeonsson 1986). Discrepancies between verbal and performance IQs or between the "neurotic" and "psychotic" scale elevations on the Minnesota Multiphasic Personality Inventory (Hathaway and McKinley 1970) were found to predict continued behavior problems in a group of delinquent adolescents (Lindgren et al. 1986).

Family factors. Parental psychopathology and disturbed family functioning frequently are found in children who have or who eventually develop conduct disorder. Antisocial personality disorder, criminal behavior, and alcoholism, particularly in the father, are the stronger and more consistently reported family factors that increase the child's risk for conduct disorder (Robins 1966; Rutter and Giller 1984). In addition, mothers of children with a diagnosis of conduct disorder frequently demonstrate antisocial personality disorder, somatization disorder, or alcohol abuse (Lahey et al. 1988b). In this study by Lahey et al., this evidence of parental psychopathology was found among children with

conduct disorder, but not among children with attention-deficit disorder with hyperactivity.

It is a commonly held belief that children who are aggressive have parents who are themselves aggressive, especially toward the children. However, a critical review of the studies supporting this association (Widom 1989) concluded that there is a lack of convincing evidence that this linkage is simple or direct. Further refinement of the study of the association between parental and child violence reveals certain processes that transmit aggressiveness to children (McCord 1988). The messages that expressive behavior, including injurious actions, is normal and justified and that egocentrism is both normal and virtuous are examples of these processes.

Families of delinquent children and adolescents are generally found to be less warm and to have more conflict than families of nondelinquents (Hetherington et al. 1971). Family interactions are characterized as unsupportive and lacking in the ability to cope with transitions and stress (Tolan 1988). Families of delinquent children are also found to have less emphasis on personal growth dimensions, such as independence, achievement, and cultural and ethical interests, than families of nondelinquent children (LeFlore 1988). In addition, the mother-child dyad is characterized by more conflict (Forehand et al. 1987).

Families of conduct-disordered children and adolescents have a number of other characteristics in common that emerge from descriptive studies. Parental divorce is correlated with the development of conduct disorder in the children (Rutter 1971). However, this linkage is found between parental antisocial personality disorder, divorce, and conduct disorder, but not directly between divorce and conduct disorder (Lahey et al. 1988a). Also, it appears that whether or not the parents are separated, it is the extent of the parental discord that is associated with the high risk for childhood dysfunction (Heatherington et al. 1979). Other family variables related to conduct-disordered offspring include large family size and greater risk for conduct disorder in the middle child, especially when separated by several years from older brothers (Wadsworth 1979).

Social

Early antisocial behavior and peer group rejection are important factors found to precede delinquent behavior (Snyder et al. 1986). However, the predictive ability of deviant peer affiliation for delinquent outcome is related to the amount of parental supervision.

Low socioeconomic status is associated with a higher level of conduct disorder and delinquency (Rutter and Giller 1984). However, when factors associated with social class, such as family size, overcrowding, and supervision, are controlled, social class shows very little relationship to antisocial behavior (Wadsworth 1979).

Cultural variables also are associated with antisocial behavior. Culturally derived beliefs, such as acceptance of aggression, respect for authority, role of the parent, and the value of independence, are noted to be significant factors in the expression of aggression and antisocial behaviors (Ekblad 1988).

Assessment

The assessment of the signs, symptoms, and risk factors of conduct disorder in children and adolescents should include information from multiple sources. This includes current behavior as well as developmental signs and symptoms. Diagnostic interviews, rating scales, and the review of pertinent records from the school and clinics (health care, mental health, juvenile court) are useful ways to gather information.

The assessment is guided by a knowledge of the biopsychosocial model of etiology. Information about cognitive style, family structure and functioning, physical signs and symptoms, and the environment is gathered to supplement the presenting signs and symptoms. This information should include the presence or absence of symptoms necessary to make a diagnosis using DSM-III-R. However, as discussed previously, this diagnosis is not specific to one particular disorder, nor does it guide treatment or predict outcome. Additional biopsychosocial and developmental information may help to do this.

A number of rating scales are available to help identify disturbed behavior. The Child Behavior Checklist (Achenbach and Edelbrock 1983) is designed for teachers and parents to complete and yields a scale score on such symptom clusters as delinquency, aggression, hyperactivity, depression, and others. Self-report measures have proven effective in identifying antisocial behavior, especially in adolescents (Farrington 1984). Peer ratings of behavior and likability as well as those of teachers in elementary school reveal significant predic-

tive factors for delinquent behavior in adolescence (Tremblay et al. 1988).

One of the most important factors in the assessment of antisocial behavior in children and adolescents is the attitude of the clinician making the assessment. Clinical judgment is significantly affected by contextual factors, such as resource availability and agency setting, in the assessment of amenability to treatment (Mulvey and Reppucci 1988). The setting in which one works, as well as one's own biases, can in part determine the adequacy of the assessment and treatment recommendations. For this reason, it is important that the clinician has knowledge of the etiology, treatment approaches, resources, and outcome variables when approaching the assessment of a young person exhibiting antisocial behavior.

Current Treatments

Treatment of youth with conduct disorder occurs in a variety of settings, including short- and long-term inpatient psychiatric units, residential and day-treatment centers, correctional facilities, and outpatient settings. There also is a wide variability in treatment approaches. Behavior therapy, family therapy, individual and group therapy, parent management training, cognitive therapy, and pharmacotherapy are all used to a greater or lesser extent, depending on the treatment setting and the clinician's orientation. One of the major problems facing researchers in this area is the nonspecificity of the diagnosis of conduct disorder.

As previously discussed, children and adolescents exhibiting antisocial behavior vary widely in their psychopathology. Some may be significantly depressed; some may be psychotic; and others may have attention-deficit hyperactivity disorder. Others may not have any psychiatric disorder other than conduct disorder. Their behavior may be the result of their culture or a history of abuse or neglect. Most treatment reports do not differentiate the associated psychopathology. As a result, an approach believed successful with certain conduct-disordered patients in a particular setting cannot be generalized to all children and adolescents with a diagnosis of conduct disorder. Keeping this caveat in mind, the more successful approaches will be briefly described. Further descriptions of treatment modalities are found in Chapters 50–56 in this volume.

Problem-Solving Skills Training

Cognitive-behavioral approaches with conduct-disordered youth focus on modifying cognitive deficiencies (e.g., communication skills, problem-solving skills, impulse control, and anger management), believed to underlie antisocial behavior (Faulstich et al. 1988). Generally, these are step-by-step approaches to interpersonal situations that utilize modeling, rehearsal, role playing, and the development of an internal dialogue for self-evaluation (Kazdin 1987). The majority of the studies of this approach provide anecdotal information attesting to its success (Englander-Golden et al. 1989; Haggerty et al. 1989; Hains and Hains 1987). In a controlled study, Kazdin et al. (1989) randomly assigned 112 severely delinquent children to one of three treatments: problem-solving skills training, problem-solving skills training with therapeutic practice activities, or client-centered relationship therapy. Both of the problem-solving skills training interventions showed significantly greater reductions in antisocial behavior and greater increases in prosocial behavior than did relationship therapy. These effects were evident at the end of treatment and at 1-year follow-up.

Family-Focused Treatments

The earlier review of family functioning as an etiologic factor in the development of antisocial behavior identified the important role of dysfunctional family structure and interactions. Family therapy, using a wide variety of techniques, attempts to alter the family system. Many of the studies of the efficacy of family therapy in alleviating antisocial behavior in children rely on weak or questionable methodologies. However, in a review of the rather extensive literature, Tolan et al. (1986) found consistently positive results from family therapy. In many cases, family therapy was more effective than other therapeutic modalities. Behavioral, structural, strategic, and communication techniques appeared most effective. Future research needs to 1) delineate family systems' variables associated with childhood antisocial behavior, 2) verify particular techniques that are effective with particular family dysfunctions, and 3) evaluate the long-term effectiveness of family therapy compared with other treatment modalities.

Parent management training attempts to alter coercive parent-child interactions that foster anti-social behavior in the child (Patterson 1982). The major intervention is the direct training of parents to interact differently with their child, so that prosocial behavior is rewarded. Outcome studies of this technique demonstrate consistently positive results (Kazdin 1987; Kazdin et al. 1987). Outcome is affected by the duration of treatment, severity of family dysfunction, and social supports outside the home. Preliminary evidence suggests that aggressive, conduct-disordered children do better with this technique than do nonaggressive, conduct-disordered children (Patterson 1982). Further research is needed to delineate parent and child characteristics that respond best to parent management training. However, at this point, parent management training is one of the best researched and most promising treatment interventions for conduct-disordered children and adolescents.

Pharmacotherapy

Psychotropic drugs have not yet shown specific effectiveness in the treatment of conduct disorder. Several drugs are used to treat symptoms associated with conduct disorder. For instance, haloperidol was effective in reducing aggressiveness, temper tantrums, and explosiveness in behavior-disordered children (Werry and Aman 1975). Both haloperidol and lithium carbonate have been found to be effective in decreasing behavioral symptoms in treatment-resistant, hospitalized, conduct-disordered children (Campbell et al. 1984). Lithium was also effective in reducing aggressive and explosive behavior in a subgroup of behavior-disordered children who had symptoms of an affective disorder (DeLong and Aldershof 1987). A subgroup of behavior-disordered children with neurologic and medical disease in this same study also demonstrated decreases in rage and aggressive outbursts with lithium treatment. Propranolol has also proven to be effective in the treatment of aggressive behavior in children and adolescents with chronic brain dysfunction and in a few conduct-disordered youth refractory to other pharmacologic approaches (Kuperman and Stewart 1987).

Stimulant medication has been used for the treatment of conduct disorder, but the results do not provide definite conclusions about effectiveness because of equivocal findings or methodological problems. On the basis of their review, Rifkin et al. (1986) suggested a stimulant trial for conduct-disordered patients when other treatments have not been successful, especially when the patient has symptoms characteristic of attention-deficit disorder.

The number of studies examining the efficacy of antidepressants in the treatment of conduct-disorder is surprisingly small, considering the degree of comorbidity with depression. Puig-Antich (1982) found that conduct disorder symptoms abated after imipramine treatment in a group of boys with comorbid major depressive disorder and conduct disorder. Treatment with bupropion of boys with chronic conduct disorder and attention-deficit disorder resulted in improvements in behavior, affect, and anxiety (Simeon et al. 1986). Tricyclic antidepressants were found to result in improvements in behavior, mood, and cognition in an uncontrolled group of conduct-disordered preadolescents with comorbid depression, even when the depression was not initially evident (A. J. Schacht et al., submitted for publication). Further methodologically sound studies are necessary to delineate the subgroup of conduct-disordered youth who respond to antidepressants. Currently, it is worth considering a trial of antidepressant medication in children and early adolescents with conduct disorder who have not responded to nonpharmacologic interventions.

Prognosis

The clinical course of children with conduct disorder is variable, with mild forms showing improvement over time while the more severe forms tend to be chronic (American Psychiatric Association 1987). The difficulty in developing an agreed-on subclassification of conduct disorder (see above) has hindered outcome research, and researchers have developed their own subtypes to classify outcome. Aggressive conduct disorder is a commonly used subtype and carries a worse prognosis. Outcome studies of aggressive, conduct-disordered boys found that about half continued to have conduct disorder at follow-up 2 years later (Stewart and Kelso 1987). Persistence of conduct disorder was predicted by a variety of antisocial and aggressive symptoms, fire setting, early age of onset, family deviance, and inattention (Kelso and Stewart 1986). However, a history of violence in childhood is not necessarily predictive of adult violent crime. Lewis et al. (1989) found that the interaction of such intrinsic vulnerabilities as cognitive, psychiatric, and neurologic impairment and a history

of abuse or family violence was a better predictor of adult violent crime than was a history of violence.

Longer-term outcome studies (Robins 1966; Robins and Ratcliff 1979) found that 23%–41% of highly antisocial children became antisocial adults, and 17%–28% did not. Factors that predicted adult antisocial behavior included a variety of antisocial behaviors in childhood, drug use before age 15, placement out of the home, and growing up in extreme poverty (Robins and Ratcliff 1979). Death from uncertain causes and suicides were found to be the most frequent causes of death when young people with antisocial behavior were followed up (Rydelius 1988).

Early age of onset is the factor most consistently found to be associated with poor outcome (Tolan and Lorion 1988). Tolan (1987) found that a combination of demographic, individual, school, and family variables predicted age of onset. In a longitudinal study of high-risk children in Hawaii, certain factors were frequently found in adult males with a criminal record (Werner 1989). These included 1) having a younger sibling born less than 2 years after the subject, 2) being raised by an unmarried mother, 3) not having a father present during infancy and early childhood, 4) experiencing prolonged disruptions in family life, and 5) having a working mother without suitable caregivers during the first year of life.

Not all children exhibiting antisocial behavior go on to become antisocial adults. Results of the long-term follow-up study in Hawaii mentioned above found that "resilient" high-risk children who did not develop serious behavior disorders were more likely to be first-borns with high intelligence from smaller families with low discord (Werner 1989). A study of children from families judged to be at high risk of producing a delinquent child found that boys who demonstrated satisfactory social adjustment as men were characterized as neurotic at age 10, had few or no friends at age 8, and did not spend leisure time with their fathers (Farrington et al. 1988). It appeared that shyness acted as a protective factor against delinquency for nonaggressive boys, but it was found to be an aggravating factor for aggressive boys.

In summary, the most consistent factors that predict poor prognosis for antisocial behavior in children are early age of onset; antisocial acts across multiple settings, such as the home, school, and community; and a diversity of antisocial behaviors (Rutter and Giller 1984). Further research is needed to identify prognostic factors associated with disorders comorbid with conduct disorder, such as attention-deficit hyperactivity disorder, psychosis, and depression.

Prevention

Conduct disorder and the eventual outcome of this disorder appear to have a developmental etiology. Patterson et al. (1989) proposed that there is a reliable developmental sequence of experiences, starting with ineffective parenting practices, that leads to antisocial behavior. This is followed by academic failure and peer rejection, which, in turn, lead to depressed mood and involvement in a deviant peer group. Prevention efforts that intervene early in this sequence have greater success than those that intervene later. Parent training interventions have been successful when applied to younger antisocial children (Kazdin 1987). Academic skills training has also shown promise as an intervention with predelinquent children (Johnson and Breckenridge 1982), especially when there is an associated learning disability (Grande 1988; Meltzer et al. 1986). School-based interventions with the parent, teacher, and child have significantly decreased short- and long-term behavior problems at school and in the community (Bry 1982). Finally, community-based interventions that involve activity and skill training programs have shown some promise (Offord and Jones 1983), although they have not yet demonstrated broad-based and long-lasting results.

Research Issues

It is clear that more and better quality research is necessary. Greater specificity of diagnostic criteria will help delineate subcategories within the currently heterogeneous group of conduct-disordered youth. This should include comorbidity and etiologic factors, such as family dysfunction and cognitive and neurologic dysfunction, as well as cultural and environmental influences. Outcome studies will be more meaningful when a specific subclassification system delineates particular aspects of the disorder that make an individual more vulnerable or resilient. Greater diagnostic specificity will also be useful in assessing the effectiveness of various treatment interventions with particular symptom constellations. This exciting area for research has far-reaching implications not only for the prevention and treatment of serious mental disorders, but also for the healthy functioning of our society.

References

Achenbach T, Edelbrock CS: The classification of child psychopathology: a review and analysis of empirical efforts. Psychol Bull 85:1275–1301, 1978

Achenbach T, Edelbrock CS: Behavioral problems and competencies reported by parents of normal and disturbed children aged 4 through 16. Monogr Soc Res Child Dev 46 (serial no 188), 1981, pp 1–82

Achenbach T, Edelbrock CS: Manual for Child Behavior Checklist and Revised Behavior Profile. Burlington, VT, Department of Psychiatry, University of Vermont, 1983

Achenbach T, Verhulst FC, Baron GD, et al: A comparison of syndromes derived from the Child Behavior Checklist for American and Dutch boys aged 6–11 and 12–16. J Child Psychol Psychiatry 28:437–453, 1987

American Psychiatric Association: Diagnostic and Statistical Manual of Mental Disorders, 3rd Edition, Revised. Washington, DC, American Psychiatric Association, 1987

Brown CS, Kent TA, Bryant SG, et al: Blood platelet uptake of serotonin in episodic aggression. Psychiatry Res 27:5–12, 1988

Bry BH: Reducing the incidence of adolescent problems through preventive intervention: one and five year follow-up. Am J Community Psychol 10:265–276, 1982

Campbell M, Small AM, Green WH, et al: Behavioral efficacy of haloperidol and lithium carbonate. Arch Gen Psychiatry 41:650–656, 1984

Cantwell DP, Baker L: Issues in the classification of child and adolescent psychopathology. J Am Acad Child Adolesc Psychiatry 27:521–533, 1988

Cantwell DP, Baker L: Stability and natural history of DSM-III childhood diagnoses. J Am Acad Child Adolesc Psychiatry 28:691–700, 1989

Comings DE, Comings BG: A controlled study of Tourette Syndrome II conduct. Am J Hum Genet 41:742–760, 1987

DeLong GR, Aldershof AL: Long-term experience with lithium treatment in childhood: correlation with clinical diagnosis. J Am Acad Child Adolesc Psychiatry 26:389–394, 1987

Ekblad S: Influence of child-rearing on aggressive behavior in a transcultural perspective. Acta Psychiatr Scand Suppl 344:133–139, 1988

Emler N, Reicher S, Ross A: The social context of delinquent conduct. J Child Psychol Psychiatry 28:99–109, 1987

Englander-Golden P, Jackson JE, Crane K, et al: Communication skills and self-esteem in prevention of destructive behaviors. Adolescence 24:481–502, 1989

Farrington DP: Measuring the natural history of delinquency and crime, in Advances in the Behavioral Measurement of Children, Vol 1. Edited by Glow RA. Greenwich, CT, JAI Press, 1984

Farrington DP, Gallagher B, Morley L, et al: Are there any successful men from criminogenic backgrounds? Psychiatry 51:116–130, 1988

Faulstich ME, Moore JR, Roberts RW, et al: A behavioral perspective on conduct disorders. Psychiatry 51:398–416, 1988

Feldman RA, Caplinger TE, Wodarski JS: The St. Louis Conundrum: The Effective Treatment of Antisocial Youths. Englewood Cliffs, NJ, Prentice-Hall, 1983

Forehand R, Long N, Hedrick M: Family characteristics of adolescents who display overt and covert behavior problems. J Behav Ther Exp Psychiatry 18:325–328, 1987

Grande CG: Delinquency: the learning disabled student's reaction to academic school failure? Adolescence 23:209–219, 1988

Guerra NG, Slaby RG: Evaluative factors in social problem solving by aggressive boys. J Abnorm Child Psychol 17:277–289, 1989

Haggerty KP, Wells EA, Jenson JM, et al: Delinquents and drug use: a model program for community reintegration. Adolescence 24:439–456, 1989

Hains AA, Hains AH: The effects of a cognitive strategy intervention on the problem-solving abilities of delinquent youths. J Adolesc 10:399–413, 1987

Hathaway SR, McKinley JC: Minnesota Multiphasic Personality Inventory—Revised. Minneapolis, MN, University of Minnesota, 1970

Hetherington EM, Stovwie RJ, Ridberg EH: Patterns of family interaction and child-rearing attitudes related to three dimensions of juvenile delinquency. J Abnorm Psychol 78:160–176, 1971

Hetherington EM, Cox M, Cox R: Family intervention and the social, emotional, and cognitive development of children following divorce, in The Family: Setting Priorities. Edited by Vaughn V, Brazelton T. New York, Science and Medicine, 1979

Jensen JB, Burke N, Garfinkle BD: Depression and symptoms of attention deficit disorder with hyperactivity. J Am Acad Child Adolesc Psychiatry 27:742–747, 1988

Johnson DL, Breckenridge JN: The Houston parent-child development center and the primary prevention of behavior problems in young children. Am J Community Psychol 10:305–316, 1982

Kazdin AE: Conduct Disorders in Childhood and Adolescence (Developmental Clinical Psychology and Psychiatry Series Vol 9). Newbury Park, CA, Sage, 1987

Kazdin AE, Esveldt-Dawson K, French NH, et al: Effects of parent management training and problem-solving skills training combined in the treatment of antisocial child behavior. J Am Acad Child Adolesc Psychiatry 26:416–424, 1987

Kazdin AE, Bass D, Siegel T, et al: Cognitive-behavioral therapy and relationship therapy in the treatment of children referred for antisocial behavior. J Consult Clin Psychol 57:522–535, 1989

Kelso J, Stewart MA: Factors which predict the persistence of aggressive conduct disorder. J Child Psychol Psychiatry 27:77–86, 1986

Kovacs M, Paulauskas S, Gatsonis C, et al: Depressive disorders in childhood, III: a longitudinal study of comorbidity with and risk for conduct disorders. J Affective Disord 15:205–217, 1988

Kuperman S, Stewart M: Use of propranolol to decrease aggressive outbursts in younger patients. Psychosomatics 28:315–319, 1987

Lahey BB, Hartdagen SE, Frick PJ, et al: Conduct disorder: parsing the confounded relation to parental divorce and antisocial personality. J Abnorm Psychol 97:334–337, 1988a

Lahey BB, Piacentini JC, McBurnett K, et al: Psychopathology in the parents of children with conduct disorder and hyperactivity. J Am Acad Child Adolesc Psychiatry 27:163–170, 1988b

Lee M, Prentice NM: Interrelations of empathy, cognition, and moral reasoning with dimensions of juvenile delinquency. J Abnorm Child Psychol 16:127–139, 1988

LeFlore L: Delinquent youths and family. Adolescence 23:629–642, 1988

Lewis DO, Shanok SS, Balla DA: Perinatal difficulties, head and face trauma, and child abuse in the medical histories of seriously delinquent children. Am J Psychiatry 136:419–423, 1979

Lewis DO, Pincus JH, Lovely R, et al: Biopsychosocial character-istics of matched samples of delinquents and nondelinquents. J Am Acad Child Adolesc Psychiatry 26:744–752, 1987

Lewis DO, Lovely R, Yeager C, et al: Toward a theory of the genesis of violence: a follow-up study of delinquents. J Am Acad Child Adolesc Psychiatry 28:431–436, 1989

Lindgren SD, Harper DC, Richman LC, et al: "Mental imbalance" and the prediction of recurrent delinquent behavior. J Clin Psychol 42:821–825, 1986

Loeber R, Schmaling KB: Empirical evidence for overt and covert patterns of antisocial conduct problems: a meta-analysis. J Abnorm Child Psychol 13:315–335, 1985

McCord J: Parental behavior in the cycle of aggression. Psychiatry 51:14–23, 1988

Mednick SA, Gabrielli WF, Hutchings B: Genetic factors in criminal behavior: evidence from an adoption cohort. Science 224:891–893, 1984

Meltzer LJ, Roditi BN, Fenton T: Cognitive and learning profiles of delinquent and learning disabled adolescents. Adolescence 21:581–591, 1986

Moffitt TE: Parental mental disorder and offspring criminal behavior: an adoption study. Psychiatry: Interpersonal and Biological Processes 50:346–360, 1987

Moffitt TE, Silva PA: Neuropsychological deficit and self-reported delinquency in an unselected birth cohort. J Am Acad Child Adolesc Psychiatry 27:233–240, 1988

Moffitt TE, Gabrielli WF, Mednick SA: Socioeconomic status, I.Q., and delinquency. J Abnorm Psychol 90:152–156, 1981

Mulvey EP, Reppucci ND: The context of clinical judgement: the effect of resource availability on judgements of amenability to treatment in juvenile offenders. Am J Community Psychol 16:525–545, 1988

Offord DR, Cross LA: Behavioral antecedents of adult schizophrenia. Arch Gen Psychiatry 21:267–283, 1969

Offord DR, Jones MB: Skill development: a community intervention program for the prevention of antisocial behavior, in Childhood Psychopathology and Development. Edited by Guze SB, Earls FJ, Barrett JE. New York, Raven, 1983

Olweus D, Mattsson A, Schalling D, et al: Circulating testosterone levels and aggression in adolescent males: a causal analysis. Psychosom Med 50:261–272, 1988

Patterson GR: Coercive Family Process. Eugene, OR, Castalia, 1982

Patterson GR, DeBaryshe BD, Ramsey E: A developmental perspective on antisocial behavior. Am Psychol 44:329–335, 1989

Petersen AC: Pubertal development as a cause of disturbance: myths, realities, and unanswered questions. Genet Soc Gen Psychol Monogr 111:205–232, 1985

Puig-Antich J: Major depression and conduct disorder in prepuberty. Journal of the American Academy of Child Psychiatry 2:118–128, 1982

Reeves JC, Werry JS, Elkind GS, et al: Attention deficit, conduct, oppositional, and anxiety disorders in children, II: clinical characteristics. J Am Acad Child Adolesc Psychiatry 26:144–155, 1987

Rifkin A, Wortman R, Reardon G, et al: Psychotropic medication in adolescence: a review. J Clin Psychiatry 47:400–408, 1986

Robins LN: Deviant Children Grown Up. Baltimore, MD, Williams & Wilkins, 1966

Robins LN, Ratcliff KS: Risk factors in the continuation of childhood antisocial behavior into adulthood. International Journal of Mental Health 7:96–111, 1979

Rutter M: Parent-child separation: psychological effects on the child. J Child Psychol Psychiatry 12:233–260, 1971

Rutter M, Giller H: Juvenile Delinquency: Trends and Perspectives. New York, Penguin, 1984

Rutter M, Birch HG, Thomas A, et al: Temperamental characteristics in infancy and the later development of behavior disorders. Br J Psychiatry 110:651–661, 1964

Rydelius A: The development of antisocial behavior and sudden violent death. Acta Psychiatr Scand 77:398–403, 1988

Satterfield JH, Schell AM, Backs RW: Longitudinal study of AERP's in hyperactive and normal children: relationship to antisocial behavior. Electroencephalogr Clin Neurophysiol 67:531–536, 1987

Short RJ, Simeonsson RJ: Social cognition and aggression in delinquent adolescent males. Adolescence 21:159–176, 1986

Silverton L, Harrington ME, Mednick SA: Motor impairment and antisocial behavior in adolescent males at high risk for schizophrenia. J Abnorm Child Psychol 16:177–186, 1988

Simeon JG, Ferguson HB, Fleet JVW: Bupropion effects in attention deficit and conduct disorders. Can J Psychiatry 31:581–585, 1986

Snyder JJ, Dishian TJ, Patterson GR: Determinants and consequences of associating with deviant peers during preadolescence and adolescence. Journal of Early Adolescence 61:20–43, 1986

Stewart M, Kelso J: A two-year follow-up of boys with aggressive conduct disorder. Psychopathology 20:296–304, 1987

Stoff DM, Friedman E, Pollock L, et al: Elevated platelet MAO is related to impulsivity in disruptive behavior disorders. J Am Acad Child Adolesc Psychiatry 28:754–760, 1989

Susman EJ, Inoff-Germain G, Nottelmann ED, et al: Hormones, emotional dispositions, and aggressive attributes in young adolescents. Child Dev 58:1114–1134, 1987

Thomas A, Chess S: Temperament and Development. New York, Brunner/Mazel, 1977

Tolan PH: Implications of age of onset for delinquency risk. J Abnorm Child Psychol 15:47–63, 1987

Tolan PH: Socioeconomic, family, and social stress correlates of adolescent antisocial and delinquent behavior. J Abnorm Child Psychol 16:317–331, 1988

Tolan PH, Lorion RP: Multivariate approaches to the identification of delinquency proneness in adolescent males. Am J Community Psychol 16:547–561, 1988

Tolan PH, Cromwell RE, Brasswell M: Family therapy with delinquents: a critical review of the literature. Fam Process 25:619–650, 1986

Tremblay RE, LeBlanc M, Schwartzman AE: The pediatric power of first-grade peer and teacher ratings of behavior: sex differences in antisocial behavior and personality at adolescence. J Abnorm Child Psychol 16:571–583, 1988

Wadsworth M: Roots of Delinquency: Infancy, Adolescence, and Crime. New York, Barnes & Noble, 1979

Walker JL, Lahey BB, Hynd GW, et al: Comparison of specific patterns of antisocial behavior in children with conduct disorder with or without coexisting hyperactivity. J Consult Clin Psychol 55:910–913, 1987

Watt NF, Grubb TW, Erlenmeyer-Kimling L: Social, emotional, and intellectual behavior at school among children at high risk for schizophrenia. J Consult Clin Psychol 50:171–181, 1983

Werner EE: High risk children in young adulthood: a longitudinal study from birth to 32 years. Am J Orthopsychiatry 59:72–81, 1989

Werry JS, Aman MG: Methylphenidate and haloperidol in children: effects on attention, memory and activity. Arch Gen Psychiatry 32:790–795, 1975

Widom CS: Does violence beget violence? A critical examination of the literature. Psychol Bull 106:3–28, 1989

Wolff S: Dimensions and clusters of symptoms in disturbed children. Br J Psychiatry 118:421–427, 1971

Woolston JL, Rosenthal SL, Riddle MA, et al: Childhood comorbidity of anxiety/affective disorders and behavior disorders. J Am Acad Child Adolesc Psychiatry 28:707–713, 1989

World Health Organization: Mental, Behavioral, and Developmental Disorders: Clinical Descriptions and Diagnostic Guidelines (ICD-10, draft of Chapter V: Categories F.00–F99). Geneva, World Health Organization, 1988

Chapter 27

Adolescent Conduct and Antisocial Disorders

Dorothy Otnow Lewis, M.D.

The behavior of the antisocial adolescent is often so obnoxious that the clinician must overcome an initial inclination to dismiss the youngster as simply conduct disordered or delinquent and allow the juvenile justice system to take over. Almost every psychiatric disorder of childhood and adolescence can at some point present as a disorder of behavior. Since most diagnoses have better prognoses than conduct disorder and more specific treatment implications, it behooves the clinician to make every effort to rule out other diagnostic possibilities and restrain the impulse to throw the key away.

Definition and Diagnostic Criteria

The current definition of conduct disorder must be understood in the context of its history as a diagnostic category. According to DSM-II (American Psychiatric Association 1968), the diagnosis antisocial personality could be applied to children and adolescents as well as to adults. Individuals so designated were described as being "incapable of significant loyalty to individuals, groups, or social values. They are grossly selfish, callous, irresponsible, impulsive, and unable to feel guilt or to learn from experience and punishment" (p. 43). These unfortunate attributes were considered "life-long patterns, often recognizable by the time of adolescence or earlier" (p. 41).

Because of the apparent immutability of this condition, an alternative diagnosis, unsocialized aggressive reaction of childhood (or adolescence), was made available in DSM-II for those children and adolescents for whom there existed some hope of redemption, those whose characterological traits were not so firmly established as to preclude all change. Of note, the nouns and adjectives used to delineate youngsters with antisocial personality and unsocialized aggressive reaction in DSM-II were more judgmental than scientific and reflected clearly the attitude of many clinicians toward behaviorally disturbed children and adolescents.

DSM-III (American Psychiatric Association 1980) introduced the new category *conduct disorder*. Like its predecessor, unsocialized aggressive reaction, conduct disorder was used to designate behaviors ranging from relatively minor infractions of rules to violent acts. Heavily influenced by the work on delinquency of Jenkins and Hewitt (1944), Quay (1964a, 1964b, 1975), and Robins (1966), conduct disorder was divided into four different categories: aggressive and nonaggressive, and socialized and undersocialized. Those individuals classified as undersocialized and aggressive were described as lacking normal empathy and affection.

In an effort to eliminate clinical criteria based on moral judgments or on inferences regarding unconscious attitudes, DSM-III-R (American Psychiatric Association 1987) attempted to use exclusively behavioral data to make the diagnosis of conduct disorder. In DSM-III-R, conduct disorder is defined as a disturbance of behavior lasting at least 6 months in which the basic rights of others and/or the major age-appropriate norms and rules of society are violated. To receive the diagnosis, a child or adolescent needs to manifest only 3 of 13 problematic behaviors, ranging in severity from truancy and running away to rape and assault. There is no lower age limit before which the diagnosis cannot be made. The upper age limit is vague; a person 18 years old or older, not meeting criteria for antisocial personality disorder, may be diagnosed as having conduct disorder. In the interest of greater objectivity, the categories of aggressive-nonaggressive and socialized-undersocialized have been superceded by three categories: 1) solitary aggressive, 2) group type, and 3) undifferentiated. The severity of the disorder is rated on a 3-point scale consisting of mild, moderate, and severe.

Because the DSM-III-R criteria for conduct disorder are signs, not symptoms, no distinction is made between, for example, adolescents who frequently fight because they are paranoid and feel threatened, those who fight because of impulsivity and emotional lability secondary to organic impairment, and those who fight in response to teasing. Similarly, no distinction is made between those who stay away from school because voices tell them to and those who are truant because of frustration caused by a learning disability. Clearly, all of the 13 behavioral criteria for diagnosing conduct disorder occur at times as part of numerous other diagnoses, the common manifestations of which may be some form of antisocial behavior. Underlying disorders include mental retardation, the mood disorders, organic syndromes (e.g., attention-deficit hyperactivity disorder), and schizophrenia. The skillful clinician will be adept at discerning the underlying neuropsychiatric vulnerabilities that present on the surface as simply behavior problems. Therefore, the more experienced the clinician, the less frequently will conduct disorder be used as a diagnosis.

Clinical Findings

Psychiatric Vulnerabilities

The psychopathology underlying the antisocial behaviors of adolescents is rarely flamboyant. Rather, their psychiatric signs and symptoms most often place adolescents on the border of numerous different kinds of diagnoses. When these signs and symptoms fail to meet the full set of criteria for other established diagnoses, they tend to be over-

looked. Thus episodic psychotic, affective, or organic symptoms are often ignored, and adolescents with such symptoms are usually diagnosed simply according to their antisocial behaviors.

Another characteristic of conduct-disordered adolescents that contributes to the failure of clinicians to recognize other than characterological problems is the fact that most seriously delinquent juveniles would rather be considered "bad" than "nuts." They strive to deny or minimize symptoms of mental illness. One of the most common phenomena associated with aggressive attacks by behaviorally disturbed adolescents is the misperception that they have been insulted behind their backs, or that they have been looked at in a threatening way. Ironically, it is usually the most recurrently violent, paranoid, grandiose youngsters who manage to conceal their underlying disturbance with a boastful, ostensibly callous facade. When asked about attitudes toward the victim, the more paranoid the youngster, the more likely he or she is to respond, "I don't care," or "He deserved it." Thus the youngsters who are most seriously disturbed and out of touch with reality are also those most likely to be dismissed as severely sociopathic. Paranoia and adolescent bravado are often dismissed by the inexperienced examiner as manifestations of a lack of empathy.

Although few conduct-disordered adolescents will appear to be schizophrenic, many of those most repetitively antisocial will be found to have psychotic first- and second-degree relatives (Heston 1970, 1977). The identification of psychotic symptomatology in such youngsters is especially difficult during adolescence. Bender (1959) observed that many children who were identified as psychotic in childhood appeared to be simply antisocial in adolescence. It may be that the adolescent's reluctance to reveal symptoms, coupled with clinicians' greater tolerance for aberrant behaviors in adolescent patients, impedes the recognition of psychotic symptomatology in this age group.

Because they often frighten caregivers, many aggressive youngsters, previously diagnosed psychotic or brain damaged, are extruded from treatment centers, their symptomatology reinterpreted as merely characterological or a reflection of social disadvantage. Lewis and Shanok (1980) found that almost 60% of the first group of violent youngsters incarcerated on the secure unit of a correctional school in Connecticut had previously been treated in psychiatric hospitals and/or residential treatment centers. This finding provided an independent measure of the degree of psychopathology previously identified in this group of seriously antisocial youngsters.

The irritability and rage that often accompany episodic depression, especially when aggravated by alcohol or drug ingestion, can also present as a conduct disorder. Bipolar disorder, especially in its manic phase, may also present as episodic destructive behaviors or sporadic episodes of robbery and burglary. The tendency of manic adolescents to indulge in dangerous behaviors and to stay up all night is often interpreted as adolescent rebellion. The clinician must keep in mind the fact that adolescent turmoil is *not* the flamboyant condition it was once thought to be. In female delinquents, manic episodes are frequently manifested by sexual promiscuity and a heedlessness for the possible consequences of such behaviors.

Suicidal behaviors, both deliberate and unconscious, are frequent in the conduct-disordered adolescent population. Although these behaviors are not necessarily manifestations of depression, they still must be taken seriously. They are often expressions of extreme frustration, pain, anger, and, of course, impulsiveness. They should not be dismissed as manipulative behaviors. The death rate among seriously delinquent adolescents is approximately 50 times that of nondelinquent adolescents and is almost invariably violent in nature (i.e., suicide, homicide, or accidents) (Yeager and Lewis 1990).

Drug and alcohol abuse is common among conduct-disordered adolescents. It is not unusual to obtain a history of drug and alcohol abuse beginning at age 11 or 12 years. Children raised in some of the most emotionally and physically abusive households have sometimes started drinking as early as 8 years of age. There is a current tendency to send young substance abusers to substance abuse programs and to look no further for the causes of the substance abuse. Substance abuse is used by different children and adolescents for different reasons, including anxiety, depression, psychosis, hyperactivity, and attempts to self-medicate. A diagnosis of substance abuse alone in a conduct-disordered youngster sometimes reflects a failure to explore underlying symptomatology. This tendency to overlook psychopathology underlying substance abuse is lamentable, because the kinds of disorders in question (e.g., depression, psychosis) are often responsive to specific pharmacologic interventions. Since most drug programs look askance at the use of medication, the depressed or borderline psychotic adolescent in such a program is unlikely to receive the kind of medication that might diminish the perceived need for alcohol or drugs.

One of the psychiatric conditions that is most frequently overlooked in the conduct-disordered population, especially the violent population, is multiple personality. Although it is a disorder that begins very early in life, most cases have been in treatment many years before the condition is recognized. This disorder is probably far more common among episodically violent youngsters than we realize, since many violent youngsters have histories of having been physically and sexually abused, and the most extreme forms of abuse are associated with the development of multiple personality.

Many of the symptoms and signs of conduct disorder—such as episodic destructiveness, extreme moodiness, impaired memory for behaviors, wandering off and not returning home for hours or days, finding something in one's possession and denying knowledge of how it got there, and frequent lying (or apparent lying)—are also characteristic of adolescents with multiple personality. In the author's experience, the fact that we do not make the diagnosis more often has been more a reflection of our failure to consider it (or, worse, our belief that it does not exist) than a reflection of its rarity.

Neurologic Vulnerabilities

Few antisocial and conduct-disordered adolescents have obvious neurologic impairments or impairments that can be localized to a specific portion of the brain. However, the most seriously antisocial tend to have histories of having suffered from accidents, injuries, and illnesses that affect central nervous system functioning. Careful assessment will often reveal subtle indicators of central nervous system dysfunction. A medical history will frequently bring to light a history of symptoms such as frequent severe headaches, episodes of dizziness, and even episodes of blackouts (not necessarily under the influence of alcohol or drugs), about which the youngster never thought to complain (Lewis et al. 1976, 1982a, 1982b).

Attentional problems as well as problems with hyperactivity are frequent concomitants of behavior problems. Such youngsters often demonstrate a variety of minor neurologic problems such as inability to skip, poor fine motor coordination, and impaired short-term memory. These kinds of nonlocalized indicators of central nervous system dysfunction are many times dismissed by neurologic consultants as noncontributory to behavior problems. Their importance rests on the fact that children with such vulnerabilities also often have trouble modulating feelings and controlling behavior.

Few conduct-disordered adolescents suffer from epilepsy, although there is some evidence that psychomotor seizures (complex partial seizures) are more common in violent delinquents than in the general population (Lewis et al. 1982a). Psychomotor symptoms, such as impaired memory for nonviolent as well as violent behaviors, olfactory hallucinations, and vivid recurrent episodes of déjà vu, are fairly common findings in the aggressive delinquent population. Many seriously delinquent children (as well as many incarcerated adults) will be found to have equivocal or diffusely abnormal electroencephalograms. These kinds of signs and symptoms suggest that, in some conduct-disordered youngsters, abnormal electrical activity in the brain, possibly in the limbic system, may contribute to behavioral problems. As in the case of the psychoses, the signs and symptoms of conduct-disordered children place them on the border of several different kinds of neurologic diagnoses.

Cognitive Vulnerabilities

Although few conduct-disordered adolescents are severely retarded, their low-normal scores on standard intelligence tests (Hirschi and Hinderlang 1977; West 1982) once more place them on the border of a diagnosis with potential treatment implications. Because so many delinquent youngsters come from minority and socioeconomically disadvantaged backgrounds, there is a tendency among clinicians to dismiss low scores as evidence merely of cultural deprivation rather than as an indication of a need for remediation. Unfortunately, whatever the explanation for cognitive limitations, they do affect functioning. Poor judgment, impaired abstract reasoning, and difficulty planning ahead and anticipating consequences all contribute to behavioral problems.

In the conduct-disordered population, learning disabilities are important manifestations of cognitive dysfunction (Poremba 1975; Virkkunen and Nuutila 1976). It is likely that the language and reading problems characteristic of many delinquent youngsters impair their ability to put their thoughts, feelings, and attitudes into words rather than actions. For adolescents with these kinds of cognitive difficulties, school becomes a place of frustration rather than of gratification and learning. Without proper assistance, such children often drop out of school early. When left to their own devices on the streets, what was initially a relatively minor behavior problem often becomes frank delinquency. Because conduct-disordered children are often on the border of cognitive impairment or intellectual deficiency, they tend to receive neither the attention reserved for the severely impaired nor that afforded the intellectually gifted.

In summary, the clinical picture of conduct-disordered children and adolescents is that of a group of youngsters with a multiplicity of different kinds of neuropsychiatric and cognitive vulnerabilities that place them on the border of other diagnoses. Unfortunately, none of these vulnerabilities is obvious. However, if recognized, each has implications for treatment.

Differential Diagnosis

Conduct disorder is a common expression of numerous different conditions. Children and adolescents are generally limited in their abilities both to conceptualize and to convey in words how they are feeling, what they are thinking, and why they are acting the way they are. Any condition or combination of conditions that diminishes impulse control, jeopardizes reality testing, increases suspiciousness, and impairs judgment is likely to result in a disorder of conduct. At some stage in the evolution of neuropsychiatric conditions ranging from schizophrenia to encephalitis, antisocial, even aggressive behaviors, may occur. Therefore, the differential diagnosis of conduct disorder is almost as broad as are the fields of child psychiatry and child neurology.

In a way, conduct disorder is often a transitional designation used when underlying causes for aberrant behaviors have not yet been identified. Hence, the diagnosis of conduct disorder in psychiatry, at this point in our understanding, is analogous to the diagnosis of fever of unknown origin in internal medicine.

Epidemiology

The incidence and prevalence of conduct disorder are uncertain. Clearly, behaviors that are perfectly normal at age 5 years may be considered characteristic of conduct disorder in adolescence. Thus frequent temper tantrums during the preschool years (Goodenough 1931; McFarlane et al. 1954) are of far less concern than similar types of behaviors during adolescence.

Lefkowitz et al. (1977) reported that aggressive behaviors at 8 years of age were good predictors of aggression during adolescence. Similarly, West and Farrington (1973) found that 27% of 8- and 10-year-olds who, according to teachers and peers, demonstrated behavior problems went on to demonstrate repeatedly delinquent behaviors in adolescence. In contrast, fewer than 1% of nontroublesome 8- and 10-year-olds became recidivist delinquents. Despite these kinds of findings, it is essential to appreciate the fact that the majority of behaviorally disturbed children do not go on to become sociopathic adults (Robins 1966; Rutter and Giller 1984). Furthermore, although more than 30% of adolescents may come in conflict with the law in certain areas, only about 5% of this group will become recidivists (Wolfgang et al. 1972).

More alarming is the finding that "conduct disorders tend to be followed by a wide range of emotional, social and relationship problems in addition to antisocial behavior" (Rutter and Giller 1984, p. 60). Furthermore, even those behaviorally disordered children who are later diagnosed sociopathic also suffer from a multitude of other kinds of nonsociopathic psychiatric symptoms (Robins 1966).

There seems to be a demonstrable relationship in delinquents between degrees of early neuropsychiatric impairment, family pathology, and the severity of adult violent behaviors (Lewis et al. 1989). Thus data from a variety of different kinds of studies indicate strong linkages among serious conduct disorder, a variety of neuropsychiatric signs and symptoms, a history of abuse, and ongoing major problems in social adaptation.

Etiology

There is without a doubt an important relationship between the sociocultural environment in which a child is raised and the development of behavior problems. Clearly, there is more violent crime in the United States than in Great Britain. Similarly, violence is more common in socioeconomically disadvantaged inner-city neighborhoods than in suburban and rural settings.

Sociologists have suggested that crime is primarily the result of attempts of the disadvantaged to achieve status and material wealth through the only means available to them (Merton 1938, 1957). Others have theorized that certain kinds of antisocial behaviors are not abnormal; rather they are thought to reflect behaviors consistent with the values of delinquent subcultures (Cohen 1956). The influence of peers on the genesis of antisocial behaviors has also been stressed. However, newer evidence suggests that membership in delinquent groups may be more a reflection of the kind of youngster who tries to join the group. As Wilson and Herrnstein (1985) observed, the onset of antisocial behavior almost always precedes gang membership. In fact, Friedman et al. (1975) found that the most powerful predictor of gang membership was a youngster's violent behaviors prior to joining a gang. Thus the importance of peer influences and the notion of a subculture of violence deserve careful reexamination. To what extent does the family instability, social disorganization, poor physical health, and disproportionate amount of mental illness in certain socioeconomically disadvantaged neighborhoods contribute to adaptational problems? To what extent do especially vulnerable individuals gravitate to these kinds of environments? In short, seriously antisocial behavior cannot be regarded simply as the reflection of a characterological flaw or as a consciously chosen alternative life-style.

Biochemical Factors

Although little is known about the relationship of neurotransmitters to the etiology of antisocial behavior in humans, animal studies have revealed effects on behavior of such neurotransmitters as dopamine, norepinephrine, and serotonin (Alpert et al. 1981). Some of the most intriguing studies over the past decade suggest that there may indeed be an association between diminished amounts of serotonin in the central nervous system and impulsive aggressive behaviors (Coccaro et al. 1989).

Physiologic and Medical Perspectives

Studies comparing the different physiologic responses of delinquents and nondelinquents to aversive stimuli have led some investigators to conclude that antisocial individuals are born with an autonomic nervous system that recovers more slowly than normal from stressful stimuli (Hare 1970; Mednick 1981). These investigators theorize that such delinquency-prone youngsters receive little immediate reinforcement for the inhibition of antisocial acts and therefore are slower than others to learn to inhibit aggressive behaviors.

Others have studied the possible effects of hormones on behavior. In one of the first systematic studies of male aggression and testosterone, Persky et al. (1971) reported a positive correlation between self-assessed aggression and plasma levels of testosterone. Others, however, have been unable to replicate these findings (Kreuz and Rose 1972; Meyer-Bahlburg et al. 1974). In one of the only studies of hormonal activity in juvenile delinquents, Mattsson et al. (1980) found that incarcerated recidivist males had slightly higher testosterone levels than did normal male adolescents.

Clearly, males in our society are far more aggressive than females. Of note, studies of girls treated with cortisone replacement for adrenogenital syndrome suggest that these girls are more energetic and physically active than healthy girls (Ehrhardt 1975). There is also evidence that boys treated with cortisone for adrenogenital syndrome are more physically active and athletic than normal males.

Consistent with the findings suggesting an association between hormones and behavior, particularly aggressive behavior, are Dalton's (1984) reports of increased aggressive behavior premenstrually in certain samples of women.

Closely related to the physiologic findings are the results of studies indicating that delinquent youngsters have especially adverse medical histories (Lewis and Shanok 1977), trauma to the central nervous system being especially characteristic of aggressive delinquents (Lewis and Shanok 1979; Lewis et al. 1988). Clearly, any trauma affecting the central nervous system may affect neurotransmission, hormonal secretion, mood, activity level, emotional lability, and impulsivity.

Psychosis and Aggression

Much as we in the mental health professions might wish to minimize, if not entirely deny, any association between mental illness and violence, there is strong evidence that paranoid delusional thinking is associated with aggressive acts. Not only does paranoid ideation contribute to violence in psychiatric patients (Yesavage 1983a, 1983b, 1983c,

1983d), but these kinds of symptoms have also been reported to exist and to influence violent behaviors in certain seriously disturbed populations of offenders (Taylor 1985; Taylor and Gunn 1984). Clinical studies of the psychiatric status of aggressive delinquents (Lewis et al. 1979, 1988, 1989) suggest that the more violent the youngster, the more likely the youngster is to suffer from psychotic symptoms, particularly paranoid ideation, and these symptoms often contribute to a propensity to lash out at others in response to real and imagined threats.

A prospective study of youngsters evaluated psychiatrically prior to the commission of murder (Lewis et al. 1985) revealed that all had histories of psychotic symptoms of one sort or another (e.g., hallucinations, illogical thought processes). The most common symptom and the one most closely associated with their violent acts, however, was paranoid ideation and misperceptions.

One of the reasons why the psychotic symptoms of many recurrently aggressive youngsters are not recognized is that the symptoms tend to occur sporadically. Despite their episodic violent, sometimes bizarre behaviors and their occasional paranoid misperceptions and auditory hallucinations, these children and adolescents maintain fairly normal facades when not under extreme stress. Furthermore, as described above, they try to conceal their symptoms, preferring to be considered bad to being considered sick. Hence they are usually dismissed as simply being conduct disordered.

Genetic Perspectives

Reports in the 1960s suggested that genetic markers for sociopathic tendencies might exist. Several studies indicated a higher prevalence of the 47XYY abnormality in institutionalized populations than in the general population, especially in populations of violent offenders (Casey et al. 1966; Forssman and Hambert 1967; Nielson 1968) and in populations of mentally ill offenders (Casey et al. 1966; Jacobs et al. 1968). However, other studies have shown a low prevalence of the 47XYY complement of chromosomes in prison populations (Baker et al. 1970; Jacobs et al. 1971) and have indicated that the vast majority of individuals with this chromosomal constellation remain outside prisons and mental hospitals (Gerald 1976). There are studies, however, that suggest that dysfunctional households may determine whether or not an individual with certain genetic anomalies will manifest antisocial behaviors (Nielson 1970).

Studies of adopted-away offspring of criminal fathers (Hutchings and Mednick 1974) revealed that such children were more likely to become antisocial than were adopted-away children of noncriminal fathers. Those children at greatest risk were the biological children of criminal fathers adopted into antisocial households. Studies like these, which rely on registered parental criminality, must be interpreted with caution since they do not take into consideration the likelihood that parental criminality may simply be the most obvious manifestation of a variety of different kinds of neuropsychiatric disturbances that increase children's vulnerabilities to maladaptation.

At this time it seems extremely doubtful that a specific genetic factor for antisocial behavior exists. However, inherent vulnerabilities to any number of neuropsychiatric disorders, including mood disorders, epilepsy, the schizophrenias, and hyperactivity, diminish the child's ability to withstand certain kinds of environmental stressors and, in this way, may contribute to antisocial behaviors.

Parental Factors and Physical Abuse

Many investigators have recognized the contribution of parental psychopathology to children's disturbed behaviors (Guze 1976; Robins 1966). The parental diagnoses have tended to fall into two categories: sociopathy and alcoholism. More recent clinical and epidemiologic studies suggest that many of the parents of delinquents suffer from more serious psychiatric disorders, including psychoses, which are often overlooked because their more obvious antisocial and addictive behaviors mask other underlying psychopathology (Lewis et al. 1981).

Probably the most damaging aspects of parental behavior in terms of engendering conduct disorders are family violence and physical abuse. The histories of severely behaviorally disturbed aggressive children reveal, again and again, a pattern of physical and/or sexual abuse. Unfortunately, most of this abuse goes unrecognized and unreported and hence rarely elicits protection from the state. Once again, the conduct-disordered child is on the border of a potentially remediable situation: child abuse. One of the reasons that delinquency is relatively infrequent in children recognized by state agencies to have been abused (Widom 1989) is probably the fact that in such cases interventions

have often occurred. The overwhelming majority of child abuse in the delinquent population, however, is never brought to the attention of outside agencies.

How does parental brutality beget violence in adolescents? First, parental violence becomes a model of behavior. Second, it often results in central nervous system damage, which contributes to an adolescent's difficulty controlling impulses and functioning well at school or in the community. Finally, it engenders rage that is frequently displaced from the abusing parent onto other figures, such as teachers and peers.

The Interaction of Biopsychosocial Factors

Clearly, conduct disorder is not a single entity. Sometimes it is an early manifestation of what will later emerge as a well-established diagnostic entity, such as a bipolar mood disorder or a schizophrenic disorder. More often it will prove to be the behavioral result of the interaction of a variety of different neuropsychiatric vulnerabilities and an abusive, violent family environment.

Treatment

To date, there is no specific treatment modality that has been proven effective for conduct-disordered adolescents despite the numerous different kinds of approaches that have been tried. After a fairly comprehensive review of treatment modalities, Kazdin (1987) was forced to conclude that "no particular approach has been shown to ameliorate antisocial behavior" (p. 74).

It is not surprising that such is the case, since adolescents with a myriad of different kinds of vulnerabilities and combinations of vulnerabilities meet DSM-III-R criteria for conduct disorder. In fact, no single modality should be expected to "cure" any individual adolescent, much less cure most conduct-disordered adolescents. The multiplicity of needs must be identified and addressed if behavior is to improve. Despite the heterogeneous needs of behaviorally disordered adolescents, single modalities of treatment continue to be developed and tried.

One of the modalities that has received special attention in the recent past is parent management training. This treatment method is based on the theory that parents unwittingly encourage undesirable behaviors, in part by failing to attend to appropriate behaviors and in part by administering excessively harsh punishments for deviant behaviors. Therefore, parents of antisocial children are taught new ways of interacting with their offspring. They are helped to use positive reinforcement, to make use of mild punishments if necessary, and to develop ways of negotiating with their children (Patterson 1982). Studies of the effectiveness of this kind of parent training suggest that it may be quite useful in the case of motivated, relatively intact, relatively well-functioning families. Unfortunately, because it depends so heavily on parent participation, it is not useful for the great majority of multiproblem families in which parents themselves are too disturbed and disorganized to participate consistently.

Functional family therapy is another parent-oriented intervention. Based on systems theory and behavioral psychology, it focuses on the analysis of problems in terms of the functions they serve for the family as a whole as well as for the individual family member. Because families of behaviorally disturbed children tend to be defensive and nonsupportive, efforts are made in treatment to enhance direct communication and supportive interactions. This treatment, like parent management training, depends on a motivated, articulate clientele and thus, again, cannot be expected to be effective for the chaotic, multiproblem family that has difficulty keeping appointments, much less articulating problems.

A treatment modality that focuses on the child or adolescent is problem-solving skills training. This modality focuses on improving cognitive abilities and tries to help youngsters identify problems, recognize causal relationships, appreciate consequences, and find alternate ways of dealing with stressful situations.

In recognition of the fact that many families of conduct-disordered children are unwilling or unable to take advantage of institution-based programs, a variety of different kinds of community-based interventions have been developed (Hamparian 1987). Some have made use of college students (Seidman et al. 1980) and adult "buddies" (O'Donnell et al. 1979), who function as friends, advocates, and role models for conduct-disordered adolescents.

Although there have been attempts to treat conduct-disordered children and adolescents with specific medications such as dextroamphetamine, lithium carbonate, and haloperidol (Campbell et al. 1984; Platt et al. 1984; Tupin 1987), there is really no single type of medication that is especially useful. This is because of the diverse psychopathology underlying conduct disorder. On the other hand, medication chosen to address specific symptoms in individual adolescents can be an important aspect of treatment. Medications such as stimulants, antiepileptics, antidepressants, antipsychotics, and even beta-blockers may be useful adjuncts to an overall therapeutic program.

The treatment of conduct-disordered adolescents must be based on comprehensive clinical evaluations and must be multimodal if it is to be helpful. It must address the medical, psychodynamic, cognitive, educational, family, and environmental vulnerabilities of each adolescent. Furthermore, since the kinds of vulnerabilities characteristic of conduct-disordered adolescents are usually chronic, any effective treatment program must incorporate a plan for ongoing support systems. The finest multidisciplinary approach to treatment will fail if it is time limited to 2–4 years, and if it then returns the youngster to the chaotic environment from which he or she came without providing adequate medical, emotional, and educational supports.

Prognosis

When conduct disorder is considered to be a discrete entity, characterized by specific antisocial behaviors, its prognosis is grim. As mentioned, follow-up studies of conduct-disordered children and adolescents suggest that a sizable minority go on to commit antisocial acts in adulthood. What is more, the overall adult adjustment of seriously behaviorally disordered adolescents is often poor, as reflected in unstable marriages, unsatisfactory job histories, and numerous symptoms of psychopathology other than antisocial behaviors. Suicide and other forms of violent death are common outcomes.

On the other hand, in the author's experience, one can expect remarkably positive behavioral responses to individually tailored therapeutic interventions.

As Kazdin (1987) observed, "The breadth of dysfunctions of antisocial youths and their families makes the task of developing effective treatments demanding, if not close to impossible" (p. 95). Clinical experience suggests that only when a treatment program identifies and addresses each of the behaviorally disturbed child's vulnerabilities and needs can it hope to be successful. What is more, because the needs and vulnerabilities are chronic, programs must appreciate the need for ongoing support systems and continuity of care throughout adolescence if such multiply handicapped youngsters are to adapt appropriately to society.

Research Issues

Considering the extraordinary cost to society of antisocial behavior, remarkably little research has focused on its causes, treatment, or prevention. The reasons why so little scientific investigation has addressed these kinds of issues are, in themselves, important questions to be explored.

Since violent acts take such a great toll on society, the study of violent antisocial behavior deserves special emphasis. Research is needed to understand better the types of intrinsic vulnerabilities that decrease impulse control, intensify feeling states, and impair judgment and reality testing. These kinds of investigations should be conducted on different levels, from the molecular and biochemical to the clinical. Because the intrinsic vulnerabilities contributing to antisocial behaviors are so varied, research that increases our understanding of the etiology and treatment of most other psychiatric conditions (e.g., mood disorders, psychoses) will also be relevant to understanding violent behaviors in many individuals.

It is extremely unusual for a single intrinsic vulnerability, in and of itself, to cause violent behaviors. Although there have been occasional reports in the literature of the onset of violent behaviors secondary to the growth of specific brain tumors, for the most part, the ways in which intrinsic vulnerabilities will manifest themselves behaviorally depend on the individual's upbringing and on immediate environmental stressors or precipitants. Thus research on aggression must focus on environmental and experiential issues as well as on intrinsic characteristics. These kinds of studies should focus not only on individual family characteristics but also on social conditions and personal and cultural values.

Clearly, if we are to begin to understand the causes of violence and to diminish its impact, multidisciplinary collaborative research is needed. It is not enough to recognize the different kinds of factors associated with violent behaviors; it is necessary, rather, to elucidate the ways in which these biopsychosocial phenomena interact with one another to produce violence.

References

American Psychiatric Association: Diagnostic and Statistical Manual of Mental Disorders, 2nd Edition. Washington, DC, American Psychiatric Association, 1968

American Psychiatric Association: Diagnostic and Statistical Manual of Mental Disorders, 3rd Edition. Washington, DC, American Psychiatric Association, 1980

American Psychiatric Association: Diagnostic and Statistical Manual of Mental Disorders, 3rd Edition, Revised. Washington, DC, American Psychiatric Association, 1987

Alpert JE, Cohen DJ, Shaywitz BA, et al: Neurochemical and behavioral organization: disorders of attention, activity, and aggression, in Vulnerabilities to Delinquency. Edited by Lewis DO. New York, Spectrum, 1981, pp 109–174

Baker D, Telfer MA, Richardson CE, et al: Chromosome errors in men with antisocial behavior: comparison of selected men with "Klinefelter's syndrome" and XYY chromosome pattern. JAMA 214:869–878, 1970

Bender L: The concept of pseudopsychopathic schizophrenia in adolescents. Am J Orthopsychiatry 29:491–509, 1959

Campbell M, Small AM, Green WH, et al: Behavioral efficacy of haloperidol and lithium carbonate. Arch Gen Psychiatry 41:650–656, 1984

Casey LJ, Segall DR, Street K, et al: Sex chromosome abnormalities in two state hospitals for patients requiring special security. Nature 209:641–642, 1966

Coccaro EF, Siever LJ, Klar HM, et al: Serotonergic studies in patients with affective and personality disorders: correlates with suicidal and impulsive aggressive behavior. Arch Gen Psychiatry 46:587–599, 1989

Cohen AK: Delinquent Boys: The Culture of the Gang. New York, Free Press, 1956

Dalton K: The Premenstrual Syndrome and Progesterone Therapy, 2nd Edition. Chicago, IL, Yearbook Medical, 1984

Ehrhardt AA: Prenatal hormonal exposure and psychosexual differentiation, in Topics in Psychoendocrinology. Edited by Sachar EJ. New York, Grune & Stratton, 1975, pp 67–82

Forssman H, Hambert G: Chromosomes and antisocial behavior. Excerpta Criminologica 7:113–117, 1967

Friedman CJ, Mann F, Friedman AS: A profile of juvenile street gang members. Adolescence 40:563–607, 1975

Gerald PS: Current concepts in genetics: sex chromosome disorders. N Engl J Med 294:706, 1976

Goodenough FL: Anger in Young Children. Minneapolis, MN, University of Minnesota Press, 1931

Guze SB: Criminality and Psychiatric Disorders. New York, Oxford University Press, 1976

Hamparian DM: Control and treatment of juveniles committing violent offenses, in Clinical Treatment of the Violent Person. Edited by Roth LH. New York, Guilford, 1987, pp 156–177

Hare RD: Psychopathy: Theory and Research. New York, John Wiley, 1970

Heston LL: The genetics of schizophrenia and schizoid disease. Science 167:249–256, 1970

Heston LL: Schizophrenia. Hosp Pract [Off] 12:43–49, 1977

Hirschi T, Hinderlang MJ: Intelligence and delinquency: a revisionist view. American Sociological Review 42:571–587, 1977

Hutchings B, Mednick SA: Registered criminality in the adoptive and biological parents of registered male criminal adoptees, in Genetics, Environment and Psychopathology. Edited by Mednick SA, Schulsinger F, Higgins J, et al. Amsterdam, Elsevier North-Holland, 1974, pp 215–227

Jacobs PA, Price WH, Court Brown WM, et al: Chromosome studies on men in a maximum security hospital. Ann Hum Genet 31:339–358, 1968

Jacobs PA, Price WH, Richmond S, et al: Chromosome surveys in penal institutions and approved schools. J Med Genet 8:49–58, 1971

Jenkins RL, Hewitt L: Types of personality structure encountered in child guidance clinics. Am J Orthopsychiatry 14:84–94, 1944

Kazdin AE: Conduct Disorders in Childhood and Adolescence, Vol 9. Beverly Hills, CA, Sage, 1987

Kreuz LE, Rose RM: Assessment of aggressive behavior and plasma testosterone in a young criminal population. Psychosom Med 34:321–332, 1972

Lefkowitz MM, Eron LD, Walder LO, et al: Growing Up To Be Violent: A Longitudinal Study of Aggression. Oxford, UK, Pergamon, 1977

Lewis DO: Delinquency, psychomotor epileptic symptomatology, and paranoid ideation: a triad. Am J Psychiatry 133:1395–1398, 1976

Lewis DO, Shanok S: Medical histories of delinquent and nondelinquent children: an epidemiological study. Am J Psychiatry 134:1020–1025, 1977

Lewis DO, Shanok S: Perinatal difficulties, head and face trauma, and child abuse in the medical histories of seriously delinquent children. Am J Psychiatry 136:419–423, 1979

Lewis DO, Shanok S: The use of a correctional setting for follow-up care of psychiatrically disturbed adolescents. Am J Psychiatry 137:953–955, 1980

Lewis DO, Shanok S, Pincus J, et al: Violent juvenile delinquents: psychiatric, neurological, psychological, and abuse factors. Journal of the American Academy of Child Psychiatry 18:307–319, 1979

Lewis DO, Shanok SS, Balla DA: Parents of delinquents, in Vulnerabilities to Delinquency. Edited by Lewis DO. New York, Spectrum, 1981, pp 265–295

Lewis DO, Pincus JH, Shanok SS, et al: Psychomotor epilepsy and violence in an incarcerated adolescent population. Am J Psychiatry 139:882–887, 1982a

Lewis DO, Shanok SS, Pincus JH, et al: The medical assessment of seriously delinquent boys: a comparison of pediatric psychiatric, neurological and hospital record data. J Adolesc Health Care 3:160–164, 1982b

Lewis DO, Moy E, Jackson L, et al: Biopsychosocial characteristics of children who later murder: a prospective study. Am J Psychiatry 142:1161–1167, 1985

Lewis DO, Pincus JA, Bard B, et al: Neuropsychiatric, psychoeducational and family characteristics of 14 juveniles condemned to death in the United States. Am J Psychiatry 145:584–589, 1988

Lewis DO, Lovely R, Yeager C, et al: Toward a theory of the genesis of violence: a follow-up study of delinquents. J Am Acad Child Adolesc Psychiatry 28:431–438, 1989

MacFarlane JW, Allen L, Honzik MP: A Developmental Study of the Behavior Problems of Normal Children Between 21 Months and 14 Years. Berkeley, CA, University of California Press, 1954

Mattsson A, Schalling D, Olweus D, et al: Plasma testosterone, aggressive behavior, and personality dimensions in young male delinquents. Journal of the American Academy of Child Psychiatry 19:476–491, 1980

Mednick SA: The learning of morality: biosocial bases, in Vulnerabilities to Delinquency. Edited by Lewis DO. New York, Spectrum, 1981, pp 187–204

Merton RK: Social structure and anomie. American Sociological Review 3:672–682, 1938

Merton RK: Social Theory and Social Structure, Revised Edition. New York, Free Press, 1957

Meyer-Bahlburg HFL, Nat R, Boon DA, et al: Aggressiveness and testosterone measures in man. Psychosom Med 36:269–274, 1974

Morgan M: Effects of post-weaning environment on learning in the rat. Animal Behavior 21:429, 1973

Nielson J: The XYY syndrome in a mental hospital. British Journal of Criminology 8:186–203, 1968

Nielson J: Criminality among patients with Klinefelter's syndrome and XYY syndrome. Br J Psychiatry 117:365–369, 1970

O'Donnell CR, Lydgate T, Fo WS: The buddy system: review and follow-up. Child Behavior Therapy 1:161–169, 1979

Patterson GR: Coercive Family Processes. Eugene, OR, Castalia, 1982

Persky H, Smith KD, Basu GK: Relation of psychologic measures of aggression and hostility to testosterone production in man. Psychosom Med 33:265–277, 1971

Platt JE, Campbell M, Green WH, et al: Cognitive effects of lithium carbonate and haloperidol in treatment-resistant aggressive children. Arch Gen Psychiatry 41:657–662, 1984

Poremba C: Learning disabilities, youth and delinquency: programs for intervention, in Progress in Learning Disabilities, Vol 3. Edited by Myklebust HR. New York, Grune & Stratton, 1975, pp 123–149

Quay HC: Dimensions of personality in delinquent boys as inferred from the factor analysis of case history data. Child Dev 35:479–484, 1964a

Quay HC: Personality dimensions in delinquent males as inferred from the factor analysis of behavior ratings. Journal of Research on Crime and Delinquency 1:33–37, 1964b

Quay HC: Classification in the treatment of delinquency and antisocial behavior, in Issues on the Classification of Children, Vol 1. Edited by Hobbs N. San Francisco, CA, Jossey-Bass, 1975

Robins LN: Deviant Children Grown Up. Baltimore, MD, Williams & Wilkins, 1966

Rutter M, Giller H: Juvenile Delinquency: Trends and Perspectives. New York, Guilford, 1984

Seidman E, Rappaport J, Davidson WS: Adolescents in legal jeopardy: initial success and replication of an alternative to the criminal justice system, in Effective Correctional Treatment. Edited by Gendreau RP. Toronto, Butterworth, 1980

Taylor PJ: Motives for offending among violent and psychotic men. Br J Psychiatry 147:491–498, 1985

Taylor PJ, Gunn J: Violence and psychosis, I: risk of violence among psychotic men. British Medical Journal (Clinical Research) 288:1945–1949, 1984

Tupin JP: Psychopharmacology and aggression, in Clinical Treatment of the Violent Person. Edited by Loren HR. New York, Guilford, 1987, pp 79–94

Virkkunen N, Nuutila A: Specific reading retardation, hyperactive child syndrome and juvenile delinquency. Acta Psychiatr Scand 54:25–28, 1976

West DJ: Delinquency: Its Roots, Careers and Prospects. Cambridge, MA, Harvard University Press, 1982

West DJ, Farrington DP: Who Becomes Delinquent? London, Heinemann Educational, 1973

Widom CS: The cycle of violence. Science 244:160–166, 1989

Wilson J, Herrnstein RJ: Crime and Human Nature. New York, Simon & Schuster, 1985

Wolfgang ME, Figlio RM, Sellin T: Delinquency in a Birth Cohort: Studies in Crime and Justice. Chicago, IL, University of Chicago Press, 1972

Yeager CA, Lewis DO: Mortality in a group of formerly incarcerated juvenile delinquents. Am J Psychiatry 147:612–614, 1990

Yesavage JA: Bipolar illness: correlates of dangerous inpatient behavior. Br J Psychiatry 143:554–557, 1983a

Yesavage JA: Correlates of dangerous behavior by schizophrenics in hospital. J Psychiatr Res 18:225–231, 1983b

Yesavage JA: Dangerous behavior by Vietnam veterans with schizophrenia. Am J Psychiatry 140:1180–1183, 1983c

Yesavage JA: Inpatient violence and the schizophrenic patient: a study of brief psychiatric rating scale scores and patient behavior. Acta Psychiatr Scand 67:353–357, 1983d

Section VI

Anxiety Disorders

Chapter 28

Separation Anxiety, Overanxious, and Avoidant Disorders

Henrietta L. Leonard, M.D.
Judith L. Rapoport, M.D.

Definition

In DSM-III-R (American Psychiatric Association 1987), separation anxiety disorder (SAD) is characterized by excessive anxiety about being apart from the individuals to whom a child is most attached. Frequently there are excessive worries that harm may come to either a parent (or attachment figure) or the child, which would result in their separation.

Overanxious disorder (OAD) is characterized in DSM-III-R by unrealistic and excessive worries that make a child anxious and preoccupied. The child may spend large amounts of time being overly concerned and may require much reassurance.

Avoidant disorder of childhood or adolescence is characterized in DSM-III-R by excessive avoidance of unfamiliar people in children who do desire social involvement. The "shrinking" behavior must be severe enough so as to interfere in the children's peer relationships.

Diagnostic Criteria

A child with SAD experiences tremendous fears and worries about being apart from those most important to him or her ("attachment figures"), typically the mother or father. The individual must have had the symptoms for at least 2 weeks and have had the onset prior to the age of 18 years. The child must exhibit three of the nine symptoms listed in Table 28-1 to meet DSM-III-R diagnostic criteria.

OAD is defined as "excessive or unrealistic anxiety or worry for a period of six months or longer" (American Psychiatric Association 1987, p. 63). To meet DSM-III-R diagnostic criteria, an individual must have at least four of the seven symptoms listed in Table 28-2. Usually these worries focus on past or future events and/or issues of competency, which result in feelings of self-consciousness and inadequacy, tension, the need for reassurance, and/or somatic complaints. If the individual is 18 years or older, the diagnosis of generalized anxiety disorder precludes that of OAD. If another Axis I diagnosis is concurrent, those symptoms cannot entirely account for the symptoms attributed to OAD.

Avoidant disorder is defined as "excessive shrinking from contact with unfamiliar people, for a period of six months or longer, sufficiently severe to interfere with social functioning in peer relationships" (American Psychiatric Association 1987, p. 62). The individual seeks relationships with family members and familiar figures, and those are typically close and satisfying. Since "fear of strangers" is normal in the younger-aged group, one must be at least 2½ years old before the diagnosis can be considered. The diagnosis of avoidant *personality* disorder, which describes a persistent and pervasive pattern, precludes the diagnosis of avoidant disorder in childhood (Table 28-3).

Table 28-1.   DSM-III-R diagnostic criteria for separation anxiety disorder

A. Excessive anxiety concerning separation from those to whom the child is attached, as evidenced by at least three of the following:

1. Unrealistic and persistent worry about possible harm befalling major attachment figures or fear that they will leave and not return
2. Unrealistic and persistent worry that an untoward calamitous event will separate the child from a major attachment figure, e.g., the child will be lost, kidnapped, killed, or be the victim of an accident
3. Persistent reluctance or refusal to go to school in order to stay with major attachment figures or at home
4. Persistent reluctance or refusal to go to sleep without being near a major attachment figure or to go to sleep away from home
5. Persistent avoidance of being alone, including "clinging" to and "shadowing" major attachment figures
6. Repeated nightmares involving the theme of separation
7. Complaints of physical symptoms, e.g., headaches, stomachaches, nausea, or vomiting, on many school days or on other occasions when anticipating separation from major attachment figures
8. Recurrent signs or complaints of excessive distress in anticipation of separation from home or major attachment figures, e.g., temper tantrums or crying, pleading with parents not to leave
9. Recurrent signs of complaints of excessive distress when separated from home or major attachment figures, e.g., wants to return home, needs to call parents when they are absent or when child is away from home

B. Duration of disturbance of at least two weeks.

C. Onset before the age of 18.

D. Occurrence not exclusively during the course of a pervasive developmental disorder, schizophrenia, or any other psychotic disorder.

Source. Reprinted with permission from American Psychiatric Association 1987.

Clinical Findings

Separation Anxiety Disorder

In SAD, the underlying worries focus on fearing that harm may come to the attachment figure or the child; for example, worrying that someone might be a victim of an accident, murder, or kidnapping. Frequently, the manifestations of the underlying

Table 28-2.   DSM-III-R diagnostic criteria for overanxious disorder

A. Excessive or unrealistic anxiety or worry, for a period of six months or longer, as indicated by the frequent occurrence of at least four of the following:

1. Excessive or unrealistic worry about future events
2. Excessive or unrealistic concern about the appropriateness of past behavior
3. Excessive or unrealistic concern about competence in one or more areas, e.g., athletic, academic, social
4. Somatic complaints, such as headaches or stomachaches, for which no physical basis can be established
5. Marked self-consciousness
6. Excessive need for reassurance about a variety of concerns
7. Marked feelings of tension or inability to relax

B. If another Axis I disorder is present (e.g., separation anxiety disorder, phobic disorder, obsessive-compulsive disorder), the focus of the symptoms in A are [*sic*] not limited to it. For example, if separation anxiety disorder is present, the symptoms in A are not exclusively related to anxiety about separation. In addition, the disturbance does not occur only during the course of a psychotic disorder or a mood disorder.

C. If 18 or older, does not meet the criteria for generalized anxiety disorder.

D. Occurrence not exclusively during the course of a pervasive developmental disorder, schizophrenia, or any other psychotic disorder.

Source. Reprinted with permission from American Psychiatric Association 1987.

Table 28-3.   DSM-III-R diagnostic criteria for avoidant disorder of childhood or adolescence

A. Excessive shrinking from contact with unfamiliar people, for a period of six months or longer, sufficiently severe to interfere with social functioning in peer relationships.

B. Desire for social involvement with familiar people (family members and peers the person knows well), and generally warm and satisfying relations with family members and other familiar figures.

C. Age at least 2½ years.

D. The disturbance is not sufficiently pervasive and persistent to warrant the diagnosis of avoidant personality disorder.

Source. Reprinted with permission from American Psychiatric Association 1987.

fear of being separate include the reluctance to be apart (at school or at bedtime) or nightmares about separation. Often there are multiple somatic complaints (e.g., stomachaches, headaches). Until recently, there have been virtually no empirical investigations on this disorder.

Francis et al. (1987) studied the phenomenology of SAD in 45 children (5–16 years of age) and found that females and males were almost indistinguishable in the specific expression of their symptoms. However, age did distinguish both the specific symptomatology and the total number of symptoms. The youngest children and the adolescents had the largest number of specific symptoms in comparison with the middle-aged group. The young children (5–8 years old) were the most likely to worry about calamitous events befalling attachment figures and to exhibit school refusal. The middle-aged children (9–12 years old) were most likely to show excessive symptoms of withdrawal, apathy, sadness, or poor concentration. Adolescents (13–16 years old) were most likely to have school reluctance and somatic symptoms. Francis et al. emphasized the limits of using a clinic population and stressed the need for normative developmental data.

School Refusal

School refusal, itself not a separate DSM-III-R diagnostic category, is a frequently presenting childhood symptom commonly presumed to be the behavioral manifestation of a SAD. However, school refusal can stem from many different diagnoses, including SAD, OAD, simple phobia of school, depression, or conduct disorder. Reviews of school phobia are available elsewhere (Atkinson et al. 1985; Coolidge 1979; Last and Francis 1988).

Last et al. (1987e) compared children with school refusal who met DSM-III (American Psychiatric Association 1980) criteria for SAD to those with phobic disorder of school (simple or social) and found that these two groups were phenomenologically different. The authors emphasized that the symptom of having difficulty in attending school can result from the fear of being apart from one's attachment figure (SAD) or from excessive fear (phobia) about some aspect of the school (e.g., teacher, principal, classes, peers, activities) itself. The 48 children with SAD were younger (mean age, 9.4 years versus 14.3), more likely to be female (69% versus 37%), more likely to be from a lower socioeconomic group (68% versus 29%), and more likely to have a co-

existing DSM-III diagnosis (92% versus 63%) than the children with school phobia. Additionally, the mothers of the SAD children were four times more likely than the mothers of the school phobic children to have an affective disorder. Last et al. estimated that the rate of SAD was 2.5 times greater than that of school phobia based on the referral rate to the anxiety clinic in question. They concluded that the SAD children were more severely disturbed than the children with school phobia, because the SAD children almost always had a second diagnosis.

Bernstein and Garfinkel (1986) emphasized the overlap of affective and anxiety disorders in chronic school refusers. In their sample of 26 adolescents (15 males; mean age, 13.7 years) with school refusal, 18 (69%) met criteria for a depressive diagnosis and 16 (62%) met criteria for an anxiety diagnosis. The individuals with the most severe symptomatology were those with two coexisting diagnoses; 13 (50%) met both a depressive and an anxiety diagnosis concurrently. Bernstein and Garfinkel emphasized the difficulty in sometimes distinguishing severe anxiety from depression in this school refusal population.

Overanxious Disorder

OAD is characterized by excessive worrying about such things as future events, social acceptability, personal adequacy and competency, or meeting others' expectations. It is not uncommon for the individual to have somatic symptoms or trouble falling asleep because of the worrying. These children have been described as "overly mature," since they may attempt to carry out their tasks and responsibilities "perfectly" and seek reassurances for their worries and self-doubts. OAD children are described as being very sensitive to criticism and may easily have their feelings hurt. They may try to please others but subjectively believe that their actions are never good enough. These children are warm in their interactions and do enjoy the social contact, but they worry about their performance and their social acceptability.

Mattison and Bagnato's (1987) report supported the validity of the OAD diagnosis in boys 8–12 years old. They found that a clinically derived DSM-III diagnosis of OAD could be verified empirically on parent-rated (Child Behavior Checklist [Achenbach and Edelbrock 1983]) and self-rated (Revised Children's Manifest Anxiety Scale [Reynolds 1982]) scales.

In their study of OAD, Strauss et al. (1988b) found that the specific symptom expression varied by age. Fifty-five children from a clinic population were divided into a younger group (less than age 12 years) (*n* = 23; 56% female) and an older group (12 years or older) (*n* = 32; 62% female). The older children had more of the specific symptoms of OAD than did the younger children; specifically, 66% of the older group met five or more of the diagnostic characteristics, whereas only 35% of the younger group did (*P* < .05). Comorbidity distinguished the two groups. The older children were more likely than the younger children to have concurrent major depression (47% versus 17%, *P* < .05) or simple phobia (41% versus 9%, ns). The younger group was more likely to have concurrent diagnoses of SAD (70% versus 22%, *P* < .01) or attention-deficit disorder (35% versus 9%, *P* < .05). Interestingly, the prevalence of OAD was equal in this clinic sample across different ages. Sex ratio, socioeconomic status, and race did not distinguish between the older- and younger-aged groups. Nearly every child, regardless of age, endorsed the specific symptom of "unrealistic worry about future events." Strauss et al. emphasized the diagnostic.validity of the OAD diagnosis, but comorbidity is common.

Seeking to describe the demographic characteristics and the comorbidity of SAD and OAD empirically, Last et al. (1987c) reported on a large study of 91 children and adolescents evaluated in an anxiety disorder clinic using semistructured interviews (Interview Schedule for Children). Of 69 children, 22 (32%) met DSM-III criteria for SAD, 26 (38%) met criteria for OAD, and 21 (30%) met criteria for both SAD and OAD. Children with SAD were significantly younger (mean age, 9.1 years) than children with OAD (mean age, 13.4 years). Since the majority of SAD children were prepubertal (91%) and the OAD children pubertal (69%), Last et al. hypothesized that SAD may be a risk factor for the later development of OAD. Gender did not distinguish the SAD and the OAD groups. Of the SAD group, 75% were in the lower socioeconomic group (Hollingshead IV and V); 80% of the OAD children were in upper groups (I, II, and III). Comorbidity was common; one-third of the children in this study met DSM-III criteria for major depression. Children with OAD were significantly more likely than SAD patients to receive a diagnosis of an additional anxiety disorder, specifically simple phobia or panic

disorder. This parallels the findings in adults with generalized anxiety disorder who meet the additional diagnosis of panic disorder (Barlow et al. 1986). Although these data may reflect a referral bias, the authors concluded that the data support the DSM-III (and DSM-III-R) diagnostic categories of SAD and OAD.

Avoidant Disorder

Avoidant disorder of childhood is characterized by warm, satisfying relationships with family members but excessive shrinking of contact with strangers. This avoidance must be severe enough to interfere with peer functioning and have lasted at least 6 months. Avoidant disorder is more common in girls than boys. These children are typically shy and withdrawn, and they act timid or embarrassed when expected to meet people. When forced into social interaction, a child may cry, become quite anxious, or hide. Avoidant-disordered children have few relationships with friends, and consequently there is a delay of normal social relationships, which may become particularly obvious in adolescence. If a child is forced to face a new social situation, such as a new town or school, or dating pressures, the anxiety may be exacerbated. As a result of the individual's failure to establish satisfying peer relationships, frequently there are feelings of low self-confidence, depression, and isolation. No systematic study of the phenomenology or the diagnostic validity of avoidant disorder could be found. A persistent pattern for many years might qualify the individual for avoidant personality disorder; however, no data are available for the long-term outcome of children with avoidant disorder.

Comorbidity

Do the anxiety and other disorders commonly coexist, and do they follow the pattern that is seen in adults? As reported earlier in this chapter, Last et al. (1987c) noted some specific patterns of comorbidity of the anxiety disorders, particularly for the OAD group. Of the 26 with OAD, 15 (58%) met diagnostic criteria for at least one additional anxiety diagnosis, as compared with only 1 (4.5%) of the 22 in the SAD group. In the OAD group, 7 (26.9%) had simple phobia, 4 (15.4%) had panic disorder, 3 (11.5%) had avoidant disorder, and there were two cases (7.7%) each of social phobia, agoraphobia, and obsessive-compulsive disorder. Importantly, affective disorder (either major depression or dysthymic disorder) was the most common coexisting diagnosis, with 7 (31.8%) in the SAD group and 11 (42.3%) in the OAD group.

Last et al. (1987b) extended their comorbidity findings and reported on the diagnosis of 73 consecutive admissions to an outpatient anxiety disorder clinic for children and adolescents. The most common primary diagnoses were 24 (33%) with SAD, 11 (15%) with OAD, 11 (15%) with social phobia for school, 11 (15%) with major depression, 4 (5%) with simple phobia, 3 (4%) with agoraphobia, and 3 (4%) with obsessive-compulsive disorder. Children with a primary diagnosis of SAD were the least likely to meet criteria for a concurrent anxiety disorder; those with major depression were the most likely to receive a concurrent anxiety diagnosis. Of the children with primary SAD, 8 had OAD. OAD children were most likely to have social phobia (some for school) ($n = 4$, 36%), oppositional disorder ($n = 4$, 36%), or avoidant disorder ($n = 3$, 27%). The group with primary phobic disorder for school had several coexisting anxiety diagnoses, with 3 cases (27%) of nonpredominating social phobia and 2 cases (18%) each of OAD, simple phobia, major depression, and panic disorder. The most common concurrent secondary diagnoses for the major depression group (who were referred to an anxiety disorder clinic) were social phobia ($n = 6$, 55%) and OAD ($n = 5$, 45%). The majority of the patients referred to this anxiety disorder clinic had at least one diagnosis in addition to their primary diagnosis.

The high prevalence of comorbidity for the anxiety and depression disorders in children essentially parallels that which is found in anxious adults (Barlow et al. 1986). Gittelman and Klein (1984) postulated that SAD may be the childhood precursor of adult agoraphobia. Last et al. (1987b) noted that SAD was the most common diagnosis in this child clinic population, just as agoraphobia is one of the most common anxiety diagnoses in an adult clinic (Barlow et al. 1986). Last et al. discussed the possibility that OAD may be the childhood "equivalent" of generalized anxiety disorder seen in adults.

The relationship between anxiety and depression is complicated; clearly there is an association, yet it is not well understood. Four controlled studies have examined this relationship in the pediatric population. Hershberg et al. (1982) compared 14 anxious children with 28 depressed ones. The authors reported that the anxious children had some depressive symptoms and the depressed children had some symptoms of anxiety, but most of the time the patients did not meet criteria for the second diagnosis. Bernstein and Garfinkel (1986) reported that 50% of 26 chronic school refusers met DSM-III criteria for both depression and anxiety. Kolvin et al. (1984) stated that of 51 school phobic children, 45% were currently depressed. In Strauss et al.'s (1988a) population of 106 children and adolescents with an anxiety disorder, 28% met DSM-III criteria for major depression. Geller et al. (1985) found a similar relationship between anxiety and depression in a much younger age group. Of the 59 5- to 16-year-olds (36 prepubertal and 23 postpubertal) with major depression determined by structured interviews from the Kiddie Schedule for Affective Disorders and Schizophrenia (Chambers et al. 1985), 86% of the prepubertal group and 47% of the postpubertal group also met criteria for SAD. These findings from clinic patients have been extended to an epidemiologic population detailed later in this chapter (Anderson et al. 1987). Of the 59 children with an anxiety disorder (from a population of 792), 23 (39%) had an additional diagnosis of attention-deficit disorder ($n = 14$, 24%), conduct disorder ($n = 19$, 32%), or depression ($n = 10$, 17%).

Differential Diagnosis

Sometimes the anxiety disorders may resemble one another, and frequently several anxiety disorders coexist; yet the primary focus of the anxiety needs to be carefully delineated. In OAD, the anxiety is not specifically focused on separation, such as is true in SAD. In panic disorder, the anxiety is focused on the fear of having a panic attack, rather than on actually being separated from parental figures (as in SAD) or as a more diffuse general anxiety (as in OAD). Shy children are distinguished from those with avoidant disorder in that they eventually do warm up to unfamiliar people and have no impairment in peer relationships. SAD differs from avoidant disorder in that the fear is about being separated from parental figures and not of being with unfamiliar people. The OAD diagnosis cannot be made if the anxiety stems from an affective or psychotic disorder. All the symptoms of an adjustment disorder with anxious mood would be attributable to a *specific* psychosocial stressor.

Epidemiology

Orvaschel and Weissman (1986) reviewed the few existing pediatric psychiatric epidemiologic studies. Unfortunately, no large population studies could be found specifically assessing DSM-III (or DSM-III-R) diagnoses by structured interviews.

Anderson et al. (1987) screened 792 11-year-old New Zealand children for DSM-III diagnoses using the Diagnostic Interview Schedule for Children (Robins et al. 1979). The 1-year prevalence was 3.51% ± 0.2% (28 cases) for SAD and 2.9% ± 1.2% (23 cases) for OAD; there were no cases of avoidant disorder reported.

This prevalence changes in an older adolescent population, such that OAD was found to be more prevalent than SAD. Kashani and Orvaschel (1988) reported the 6-month prevalence rates for DSM-III diagnoses based on interviews with 150 community-based 14- to 16-year-olds using the Diagnostic Interview for Children and Adolescents (Herjanic and Reich 1982). Based on this interview, 26 (17.3%) met diagnostic criteria for an anxiety diagnosis. Of the 150 adolescents, 13 (8.7%) (7 boys) were identified as "cases" based on meeting DSM-III criteria and having significant functional impairment and needing treatment. Of the identified cases, 11 (7.3%) met criteria for OAD and 1 (0.7%) for SAD. Despite the limitations that this is a small community sample and that it makes the distinction between meeting criteria and that of requiring treatment, this study suggests that OAD may be more prevalent in the adolescent age population than had previously been thought.

Etiology

Traditionally, anxiety has been understood as a symptom resulting from unconscious internal conflicts stemming from the basic drives of sex and aggression (Freud 1920/1955). Anxiety exhibited later in life may represent early childhood conflicts. Bowlby (1973) emphasized the importance of the child's attachment to one person (mother or primary caregiver) and the fact that this attachment is instinctive. Mahler et al.'s (1975) theory of separation-individuation suggested that anxiety could result from the difficulty of mastering the fear of loss of mother by separation (and not being able to cope without her) and/or fear of fusion with mother (not being able to be autonomous). If the early issues of separation and autonomy are not successfully mastered, separation anxiety can continue into late childhood and adulthood.

Behavioral and biological theories have added to the psychodynamic formulation. Behavioral theories of anxiety suggest that stimuli evoke innate behaviors, from which complicated responses are "conditioned" or "learned." Types of conditioning include Pavlovian, operant, and modeling. These theoretical frameworks are important, as behavioral treatment plans are built on these foundations. Biological theories of anxiety are based on the fact that anxious patients appear to have an exaggerated central and autonomic nervous system arousal to the provoking stimuli, and that people differ in their physiologic response. These concepts are important in understanding the indications for and the efficacy of pharmacologic agents, which in part change the level of physiologic response. For example, D. F. Klein (1981) stated that psychoactive medications that are effective for panic attacks may raise the individual's "alarm threshold." What is common to all these different models is that anxiety usually is based on the fear of potential danger.

Many have noted that "anxious parents in anxious homes have raised anxious children." However, both genetic (Weissman et al. 1984) and environmental factors (Eisenberg 1958; Prince 1968) have been implicated in the transmission. Controlled studies looking at the relationship between parental psychopathology and anxiety disorders in children have sought to clarify these clinical observations. Research has focused on the risk factors for the childhood anxiety disorders using "top down" (looking at parents with known psychiatric diagnoses to see what disorders the children have) and "bottom up" (looking at the child as the identified patient and studying the parents' diagnoses). Additionally, the relationship between childhood and adult disorders is studied by obtaining childhood histories (retrospective recall) of adults with anxiety disorders, psychiatric diagnoses in parents of identified children, long-term follow-up of anxious children, measurements of biological "markers" in the anxiety disorders, and pharmacologic treatment responses (for a review, see Casat 1988).

In the top-down studies, Weissman et al. (1984) compared children of 133 adults with depression either with or without a coexisting anxiety disorder (agoraphobia, panic, or generalized anxiety disorder) with those of 82 control parents. An adult with depression and anxiety conferred the greatest risk for SAD in the child. There was a rate of 37% for SAD in the children of the parents with depression and panic, 11% in those with depression and agoraphobia, and 6% in those with depression and generalized anxiety disorder. In contrast, there were no cases of SAD in the children of normal control subjects or of depressed adults with no coexisting anxiety disorder. An anxiety disorder in an adult conferred an increased risk of major depression in the children; the reverse, however, was not true. Major depression without an anxiety diagnosis in the parent did not increase risk of anxiety disorder in the children. Weissman et al. concluded that there is a relationship between having both depression and an anxiety disorder in the parent and the diagnosis of that person's child(ren).

Turner et al. (1987) studied the relationship between parent and child psychopathology in 59 children from 7 to 12 years of age using a structured psychiatric interview (Anxiety Disorders Interview Schedule [DiNardo et al. 1983]). Sixteen children of a parent with an anxiety disorder (either agoraphobia or obsessive-compulsive disorder), 14 of a parent with dysthymic disorder, 13 of a parent with no identified psychiatric diagnosis, and 16 normal control children (no information obtained on psychiatric status of their parents) were studied. The children of parents with an anxiety disorder were twice as likely to have a DSM-III anxiety disorder diagnosis than were children of dysthymic parents, and were seven times more likely to have this disorder than were the two normal control groups of children. Additionally, the children having a parent with an anxiety disorder had more school difficulties, somatic complaints, solitary activities, and worries. Clearly, the offspring of patients with anxiety disorder appear to be at greater risk.

In a bottom-up design, Last et al. (1987d) reported the lifetime psychiatric diagnoses in 58 mothers of children with SAD and/or OAD as compared to 15 mothers of children with a psychiatric diagnosis other than anxiety or depression. The Diagnostic Interview Schedule for Children was used for the children and the Structured Clinical Interview for DSM-III was used for the mothers. Of the mothers of children with SAD and/or OAD, 54 (93%) had a lifetime anxiety diagnosis; this was significantly higher than the 6 (40%) found among the mothers of control children ($P < .005$). This study was the first to evaluate systematically the association between the child and parent diagnoses using the child as the identified patient. The authors cautioned that these data must be interpreted in light of the fact that this was a psychiatrically referred child clinic sample and that either genetic or environmental transmission may be implicated.

Klein (1964) reported that half of 32 hospitalized agoraphobic patients recalled marked separation anxiety in their childhood. Last et al. (1987a) examined whether mothers of anxious children retrospectively recalled having had a childhood anxiety disorder, and if so, was it the same diagnosis as that of their child's. Mothers of 64 children with SAD and/or OAD were compared with those of 33 children with a nonanxiety psychiatric diagnosis. Mothers of children with OAD ($n = 43$) had a significantly higher incidence of having had OAD themselves as a child (42%), as compared with mothers of controls (15%) and of SAD children (9%) ($P < .01$). Surprisingly, mothers of SAD children ($n = 38$) did not differ from the OAD mothers or the control mothers in their lifetime history of SAD. The authors suggested that there may be a specific relationship between OAD, but not SAD, in mothers and the same disorder in their children, although conclusions are limited because of the nature of retrospective recall. Longitudinal studies are needed to verify whether SAD may be the childhood equivalent or the precursor of adult panic disorder with agoraphobia.

Behavioral inhibition to the unfamiliar is a term describing the behavioral withdrawal from unfamiliar stimuli, such as people, situations, or toys (Kagan et al. 1984, 1987). It is hypothesized that this "irritable" response seen in children at 21 or 31 months of age may be continuous with that of shy and fearful toddlers and that of cautious, quiet, and introverted school-aged children. The opposite of shy, inhibited, introverted children are those who are sociable, uninhibited, outgoing, extroverted, or fearless in response to unfamiliar people, objects, or events (Rosenbaum et al. 1988). This is of theoretical interest as temperament characteristics could be understood as inherited response dispositions (Daniels and Plomin 1985; Goldsmith 1983). This concept is expanded to hypothesize that separation anxiety disorder may be a "temperamental quality" that predisposes one to school avoidance as a child and to panic disorder and agoraphobia as an adult (Rosenbaum et al. 1988). A follow-up study of these "inhibited children" found them to be at increased risk for overanxious, phobic, and multiple anxiety (two or more anxiety disorders per child) disorders later in childhood, suggesting that behavioral inhibition may be a risk factor for an anxiety disorder later in childhood (Biederman et al. 1990). Cloninger (1988) hypothesized that "the neural systems that modulate the activation, maintenance, and inhibition of behavioral responses to experience are regulated by different monoaminergic neurons with independently inherited neurophysiological properties" (p. 92). Behaviors result from "the interaction of multiple genetic and environmental factors [in the context of a] developmental perspective of multivariate dynamic systems," (p. 92) and there is not a "simple relationship between specific monoamines and specific behaviors" (p. 92). Clearly, the hereditability of temperament and its continuity require further systematic study.

Treatment

A complete diagnostic assessment of the child with an anxiety disorder would include seeing the child and parents, both individually and together, and considering whether important adults in the child's life and siblings should also be included. Reports from the school, from previous or current psychotherapists, and from the pediatrician may be important. While collecting a complete description of the current symptomatology, a developmental (both medical and psychological) history should be reviewed. A family assessment is important to evaluate possible problems of family discord, marital difficulties, difficulties of an individual family member, inappropriate roles or boundaries, or emotional or physical abuse. In general, a multi-treatment modality approach is often designed to integrate psychodynamic, behavioral, and psycho-pharmacologic treatments for both the child and the family.

Psychodynamic

Lewis (1986), Meares (1980), and Trautman (1986) reviewed the development of the psychodynamic theories of anxiety in children, starting with Freud's (1917/1963, 1920/1955, 1926/1959) theories about anxiety being a response to danger and a reaction to separation from the mother. For many children with SAD, OAD, and avoidant disorder, a psychodynamic approach focusing on understanding the underlying fears and worries is often the most appropriate. Generally, these children do well in individual psychotherapy and are able to master issues of separation, autonomy, self-esteem, and achieving age-appropriate behaviors. Parents are often an integral part of the treatment, as they are encouraged

both to understand the child's need for reassurance and to push toward increasing the child's age-appropriate independent behaviors and responsibilities. With the SAD child, evaluation of each parent's own issues about separation is critical, as parents may communicate their own fears and uncertainties about the child's safety and autonomy.

Psychopharmacologic

Virtually every class of psychopharmacologic medication, including the antipsychotics, antihistamines, antidepressants, anxiolytics, and stimulants, has been tried for the childhood anxiety disorders (see review by Gittelman and Koplewicz 1986). However, only a few controlled pharmacologic treatments of any of the childhood and adolescent anxiety disorders exist. The bulk of the literature consists of case reports and open trials reporting mostly on children with SAD and/or school phobia. There is no clinical evidence that antipsychotics, antihistamines, or stimulants have any therapeutic efficacy for anxiety disorders. Indeed, school phobia has been reported to *develop* in patients while on haloperidol and pimozide, and this entity has been labeled "neuroleptic separation anxiety disorder" (Linet 1985; Mikkelson et al. 1981).

The tricyclic antidepressant trials for SAD and/or school phobia have received the most attention and are the best substantiated. Gittelman-Klein and Klein (1971) reported the hallmark treatment study of school phobia in which imipramine was superior to placebo. Berney et al. (1981) reported that low-dose clomipramine (ranging from 40 mg/day for 9-year-olds to 75 mg/day for 14-year-olds) was not superior to placebo in a double-blind trial for school phobic children (mixed diagnostic group of SAD and phobia for schoolchildren). Neither of these two controlled studies excluded depressed children. Bernstein et al. (1987) compared imipramine, alprazolam, and placebo in a double-blind trial for a group of school phobic children (ages 7–17). Concurrent treatments consisted of individual psychotherapy and of returning the child to school. Preliminary findings of the first 25 children found that both medications were superior to placebo ($P < .05$). Symptoms decreased more with alprazolam (at 0.03 mg/kg) than with imipramine (3 mg/kg) on a specific scale, the Anxiety Rating for Children. These controlled studies suggest that imipramine and alprazolam may have a role in the treatment of SAD and school phobia.

Although the anxiolytics are frequently used for adults, their safety and efficacy in children still require further investigation. Behavioral disinhibition and pathologic agitation have been reported with these medications (Kraft et al. 1965). Physical dependence after chronic use is of great concern (Busto et al. 1986). There are no controlled trials of an anxiolytic for childhood anxiety, other than Bernstein et al.'s (1987) report on alprazolam for school phobia described above. Simeon and Ferguson (1987) reported an open trial of alprazolam (range, 0.50–1.5 mg/day) with 12 children having OAD and/or avoidant disorder. They concluded that the children clinically improved after 4 weeks of alprazolam in comparison to after 1 week of placebo, as measured on anxiety and depression rating scales. Alprazolam was well tolerated without impairment in cognition, electrocardiogram, or vital signs. Pfefferbaum et al. (1987) found alprazolam to be safe when used for anticipatory and acute anxiety in 13 pediatric cancer patients prior to painful procedures.

Buspirone, a nonbenzodiazepine anxiolytic, which is less sedating than the benzodiazepines and not habituating, has been used in adults for anxiety disorders. Kranzler (1988) reported that buspirone successfully treated the symptoms of OAD in a 13-year-old boy at dosages of 5 mg twice a day after 4 weeks. Because of the uncontrolled design of this study and the lack of long-term follow-up data, no definitive conclusions can be drawn; however, these findings may suggest some parallels in drug responsivity between children and adults.

Behavioral and Cognitive Therapy

In general, the behavioral therapy approach focuses on a child's actions and emphasizes treatment in the context of the family and the school, rather than focusing on intrapsychic conflicts. Cognitive therapy focuses on identifying self-defeating thoughts and teaches patients to restructure thoughts into a positive framework, which leads to assertive and adaptive actions. Although behavior therapy is frequently used and is generally accepted as an effective treatment modality, the literature consists mostly of open trials and case reports utilizing specific techniques. Wells and Vitulano (1984) and Carlson et al. (1986) have written excellent reviews of behavioral therapy treatment of the childhood anxiety disorders.

Most clinicians would agree that behavioral interventions are an important part of the treatment plan of returning to school a child with school refusal. In one of the few controlled systematic studies, Blagg and Yule (1984) reported on 66 patients with the diagnosis of school refusal. Behavioral treatment was used with 30 school refusers, who were then compared with 16 who received general inpatient psychiatric care and hospital school and to 20 who received psychotherapy and home tutoring. Random assignment to the treatment groups was not done. At 1-year follow-up, the group that had received the behavioral treatment was doing significantly better than either of the other two groups, as measured by a child's return to full-time school. The authors suggested that this finding argues for the efficacy of behavioral treatment for children with school refusal.

Mansdorf and Luken (1987) reported a comprehensive treatment strategy using an integrated cognitive and behavioral approach for the separation anxiety child with school phobia. They emphasized that both the assessment phase and the treatment phase must include the parents, the family, and the school as well as the child. The assessment phase consisted of a "cognitive evaluation" of the child (ascertaining what the meaning of attending school and separating from the parents was). The parents were evaluated as to how they perceive the child's difficulties and how they would be able to carry out a very structured, operant-control behavioral program. The school and home were assessed to determine what the consequences of the child not attending school were. The interventions consisted of "cognitive self-instruction" (teaching the child to use coping self-statements). The parents were taught to identify their own distorted beliefs concerning expectations of their child. The environmental restructuring involved setting up specific positive reinforcements for school attendance. Although this report consisted of only two cases, the comprehensive and unique framework merits attention.

Strauss (1988) reported a complete behavioral treatment strategy for OAD, although no empirical studies could be found for this disorder. Strauss described a four-step treatment approach. First, relaxation techniques with visual imagery were taught. Second, children learned to identify "positive self-statements," which consisted of eliminating beliefs that may have been contributing to their anxiety. Third, a token program, which rewarded a child when exercises were done correctly, was implemented. Fourth, "cognitive control" taught the child to reexperience and rework an anxiety-provoking experience by reexperiencing the situation through imagery and successfully terminating the scene with relaxation.

Operant-based programs have been the most commonly used for children with school phobia disorder (Ayllon et al. 1970) and for socially avoidant children (Clement and Milne 1967). In their review, Ollendick and Francis (1988) suggested that the operant-based treatments may not be as successful as the classical conditioning strategy, but without controlled studies it is impossible to determine. Cognitive restructuring based on changing the behavior and emotion by changing the pattern of thought shows promise, but needs further investigation.

Ross et al. (1971) used modeling and social reinforcement in the successful treatment of a 6-year-old boy with severe fear and avoidance of relationships. The strategy consisted of establishing generalized imitation, participant modeling, and social reinforcement of appropriate behaviors.

Rotheram-Borus (1989) emphasized that avoidant children have "defects" of affect (e.g., perception of it), cognitive processing (how self-negatives are generalized to an anxiety and/or how situations are perceived), and behavioral skills. She suggested that a cognitive-behavioral treatment strategy is most successful with this particular group and developed a very structured group therapy approach. First, children learn to identify affect by developing a vocabulary for feelings, learning how to assess their intensity, and acquiring techniques to control and express their feelings. The links between thoughts, feelings, and actions are identified. Second, cognitive processing is analyzed to see how self-negative thoughts may be generalized to produce anxiety and avoidance. Third, behaviors are analyzed to identify maladaptive and nonfunctional patterns, and then positive interactions are preached.

Numerous other behavioral techniques have been used for treating anxious children, including systematic desensitization, modeling, relaxation techniques, and imagery. No systematic, controlled studies could be found for these specific strategies. Interest now focuses on the integration of psychodynamic, pharmacologic, and behavioral therapy. A double-blind, controlled trial comparing the efficacy of behavioral therapy combined with placebo to that of behavioral therapy plus imipramine in nondepressed children with separation anxiety or

school phobia is ongoing (C. Last, personal communication). The challenge lies in designing and implementing an appropriate and integrated treatment plan.

Prognosis

Children with anxiety disorders display a spectrum of symptomatology, which may range from mild subjective distress and worrying to overwhelming anxiety that interferes in functioning. Without long-term follow-up data for these disorders, it is speculative to predict prognosis. Most likely, some children master their anxiety and have little residual impairment; others may have a chronic course characterized by exacerbations of their disorder over the childhood years and into adulthood. If the anxiety symptoms interfere with the normal developmental tasks of developing self-esteem and peer relationships, later stages may be affected, which may ultimately impact on interpersonal relationships. Additionally, children with ongoing somatic complaints may exhibit this pattern for years and end up with multiple medical evaluations. Longitudinal studies are indicated.

Compelling questions concern what childhood anxiety disorders are the "equivalents" of or precursors to those of adults. As was raised earlier in this chapter, is OAD the childhood equivalent of adult generalized anxiety disorder? Does SAD predispose an adult to agoraphobia with panic disorder? Do children who exhibit "behavioral inhibition to the unfamiliar" become introverted adolescents and adults?

Research Issues

Systematic studies are needed to assess the validity of the diagnostic entities of SAD, OAD, and avoidant disorder. The literature suggests that despite the frequent comorbidity of SAD and OAD, they are phenomenologically separate entities. No systematic study of avoidant disorder exists from which to draw a similar conclusion.

Are temperamental characteristics inherited, and if so, how are they modified by one's environment? Certainly, the research with behavioral inhibition is intriguing and suggests that early behavioral traits may predict later ones. The relationships between the childhood diagnoses of SAD, OAD, and avoidant disorder and the adult diagnoses of agoraphobia, generalized anxiety disorder, and social phobia or avoidant personality disorder, respectively, require further study.

The paucity of controlled studies for any of the treatment interventions (psychodynamic, behavioral, or pharmacologic) limits the clinician's choices in recommending interventions. With the increasing use of pharmacotherapy, the safety and efficacy of these medications require controlled studies.

References

Achenbach TM, Edelbrock C: Manual for the Child Behavior Checklist and the Revised Child Behavior Profile. Burlington, VT, Department of Psychiatry, University of Vermont, 1983

American Psychiatric Association: Diagnostic and Statistical Manual of Mental Disorders, 3rd Edition. Washington, DC, American Psychiatric Association, 1980

American Psychiatric Association: Diagnostic and Statistical Manual of Mental Disorders, 3rd Edition, Revised. Washington, DC, American Psychiatric Association, 1987

Anderson JC, Williams S, McGee R, et al: DSM-III disorders in preadolescent children. Arch Gen Psychiatry 44:69–76, 1987

Atkinson L, Quarrington B, Cyr JJ: School refusal: the heterogeneity of a concept. Am J Orthopsychiatry 55:83–101, 1985

Ayllon T, Smith D, Rogers M: Behavioral management of school phobia. J Behav Ther Exp Psychiatry 1:125–138, 1970

Barlow DH, DiNardo PA, Vermilyea JA, et al: Co-morbidity and depression among the anxiety disorders: issues in diagnosis and classification. J Nerv Ment Dis 174:63–72, 1986

Berney T, Kolvin I, Bhate SR, et al: School phobia: a therapeutic trial with clomipramine and short-term outcome. Br J Psychiatry 138:110–118, 1981

Bernstein GA, Garfinkel BD: School phobia: the overlap of affective and anxiety disorders. Journal of the American Academy of Child Psychiatry 25:235–241, 1986

Bernstein GA, Garfinkel BD, Borchardt C: Imipramine versus alprazolam for school phobia. Paper presented at the annual meeting of the American Academy of Child and Adolescent Psychiatry, Washington, DC, October 1987

Biederman J, Rosenbaum JF, Hirshfeld DR, et al: Psychiatric correlates of behavioral inhibition in young children of parents with and without psychiatric disorders. Arch Gen Psychiatry 47:21–26, 1990

Blagg NR, Yule W: The behavioral treatment of school refusal: a comparative study. Behav Res Ther 22:119–127, 1984

Bowlby J: Attachment and Loss, Vol 2: Separation, Anxiety and Anger. London, Hogarth, 1973

Busto U, Sellers EM, Naranjo CA: Withdrawal reaction after long-term therapeutic use of benzodiazepines. N Engl J Med 315:854–859, 1986

Carlson CL, Figueroa RG, Lahey BB: Behavior therapy for childhood anxiety disorders, in Anxiety Disorders of Childhood. Edited by Gittelman R. New York, Guilford, 1986, pp 204–232

Casat CD: Childhood anxiety disorders: a review of the possible relationship to adult panic disorder and agoraphobia. Journal of Anxiety Disorders 2:51–60, 1988

Chambers WJ, Puig-Antich J, Hirsch M, et al: The assessment of affective disorders in children and adolescents by semistructured interview. Arch Gen Psychiatry 42:696–702, 1985

Clement PW, Milne DC: Group play therapy and tangible reinforcers used to modify the behavior of 8-year-old boys. Behav Res Ther 5:301–312, 1967

Cloninger CR: A unified biosocial theory of personality and its role in the development of anxiety states: a reply to commentaries. Psychiatr Dev 2:83–120, 1988

Coolidge JC: School phobia, in Basic Handbook of Child Psychiatry, Vol 2. Edited by Noshpitz J. New York, Basic Books, 1979, pp 453–463

Daniels D, Plomin RL: Origins of individual differences in shyness. Developmental Psychology 21:118–121, 1985

DiNardo PA, O'Brien GT, Barlow DH, et al: Reliability of DSM-III anxiety disorder categories using a new structured interview. Arch Gen Psychiatry 40:1070–1074, 1983

Eisenberg L: School phobia: a study in the communication of anxiety. Am J Psychiatry 114:712–718, 1958

Francis G, Last C, Strauss C: Expression of separation anxiety disorder: the roles of age and gender. Child Psychiatry Hum Dev 18:82–89, 1987

Freud S: Introductory lectures on psychoanalysis, Lecture 25, anxiety (1917), in The Standard Edition of the Complete Psychological Works of Sigmund Freud, Vol 16. Translated and edited by Strachey J. London, Hogarth Press, 1963, pp 392–411

Freud S: Beyond the pleasure principle (1920), in The Standard Edition of the Complete Psychological Works of Sigmund Freud, Vol 18. Translated and edited by Strachey J. London, Hogarth Press, 1955, pp 1–64

Freud S: Inhibitions, symptoms and anxiety (1926), in The Standard Edition of the Complete Psychological Works of Sigmund Freud, Vol 20. Translated and edited by Strachey J. London, Hogarth Press, 1959, pp 75–175

Geller B, Chestnut EC, Miller MD, et al: Preliminary data on DSM-III associated features of major depressive disorder in children and adolescents. Am J Psychiatry 142:643–644, 1985

Gittelman R, Klein DF: Relationship between separation anxiety and panic and agoraphobic disorders. Psychopathology 17 (suppl 1):56–65, 1984

Gittelman R, Koplewicz S: Pharmacotherapy of childhood anxiety disorders, in Anxiety Disorders of Childhood. Edited by Gittelman R. New York, Guilford, 1986

Gittelman-Klein R, Klein DF: Controlled imipramine treatment of school phobia. Arch Gen Psychiatry 25:204–207, 1971

Goldsmith JJ: Genetic influences on personality from infancy to childhood. Child Dev 54:331–355, 1983

Herjanic B, Reich W: Development of a structured psychiatric interview for children: agreement on diagnoses comparing child and parent on individual symptoms. J Abnorm Child Psychol 10:307–324, 1982

Hershberg SG, Carlson GA, Cantwell DP, et al: Anxiety and depressive disorders in psychiatrically disturbed children. J Clin Psychiatry 43:358–361, 1982

Kagan J, Reznick JS, Clarke C, et al: Behavioral inhibition to the unfamiliar. Child Dev 55:2212–2225, 1984

Kagan J, Reznick JS, Snidman N: The physiology and psychology of behavioral inhibition in young children. Child Dev 58:1459–1473, 1987

Kashani JH, Orvaschel H: Anxiety disorders in mid-adolescence: a community sample. Am J Psychiatry 145:960–964, 1988

Klein DF: Delineation of two drug-responsive anxiety syndromes. Psychopharmacologia 5:397–408, 1964

Klein DF: Anxiety reconceptualized, in Anxiety: New Research and Changing Concepts. Edited by Klein DF, Rabkin JG. New York, Raven, 1981, pp 235–263

Kolvin I, Berney TP, Bhate SR: Classification and diagnosis of depression in school phobia. Br J Psychiatry 145:347–357, 1984

Kraft IA, Ardali C, Duffy JH, et al: A clinical study of chlordiazepoxide used in psychiatric disorders of children. International Journal of Neuropsychiatry 1:433–437, 1965

Kranzler H: Use of buspirone in an adolescent with overanxious disorder. J Am Acad Child Adolesc Psychiatry 27:789–790, 1988

Last CG, Francis G: School phobia, in Advances in Clinical Child Psychology, Vol 11. Edited by Lahey B, Kazdin A. New York, Plenum, 1988, pp 193–218

Last CG, Philips JE, Statfeld A: Childhood anxiety disorders in mothers and their children. Child Psychiatry Hum Dev 18:103–112, 1987a

Last CG, Strauss CC, Francis G: Comorbidity among childhood anxiety disorders. J Nerv Ment Dis 175:726–730, 1987b

Last CG, Hersen M, Kazdin AE, et al: Comparison of DSM-III separation anxiety and overanxious disorders: demographic characteristics and patterns of comorbidity. J Am Acad Child Adolesc Psychiatry 26:527–531, 1987c

Last CG, Herzen M, Kazdin AE, et al: Psychiatric illness in the mothers of anxious children. Am J Psychiatry 144:1580–1583, 1987d

Last CG, Francis G, Hersen M, et al: Separation anxiety and school phobia: a comparison using DSM-III criteria. Am J Psychiatry 144:653–657, 1987e

Lewis M: Principles of intensive individual psychoanalytic psychotherapy for childhood anxiety disorders, in Anxiety Disorders of Childhood. Edited by Gittelman R. New York, Guilford, 1986, pp 233–255

Linet LS: Tourette syndrome, pimozide, and school phobia: the neuroleptic separation anxiety syndrome. Am J Psychiatry 142:613–615, 1985

Mahler MS, Pine F, Bergman A: The Psychological Birth of the Human Infant: Symbiosis and Individuation. New York, Basic Books, 1975

Mansdorf IJ, Lukens E: Cognitive-behavioral psychotherapy for separation anxious children exhibiting school phobia. J Am Acad Child Adolesc Psychiatry 26:222–225, 1987

Mattison RE, Bagnato SJ: Empirical measurement of overanxious disorder in boys 8 to 12 years old. J Am Acad Child Adolesc Psychiatry 26:536–540, 1987

Meares R: A psychodynamic view of anxiety, in Handbook of Studies on Anxiety. Edited by Burrows GD, Davies B. Amsterdam/New York, Elsevier, 1980, pp 39–57

Mikkelsen EJ, Detlor J, Cohen DJ: School avoidance and school phobia triggered by haloperidol in patients with Tourette's disorder. Am J Psychiatry 138:1572–1576, 1981

Ollendick TH, Francis G: Behavioral assessment and treatment of childhood phobias. Behav Modif 12:165–204, 1988

Orvaschel H, Weissman MM: The epidemiology of anxiety disorders in children, in Childhood Anxiety Disorders. Edited by Gittelman R. New York, Guilford, 1986, pp 58–72

Pfefferbaum B, Overall JE, Boren HA, et al: Alprazolam in the treatment of anticipatory and acute situational anxiety in children with cancer. J Am Acad Child Adolesc Psychiatry 26:532–535, 1987

Prince GS: School phobia, in Foundations of Child Psychiatry. Edited by Miller E. London, Pergamon, 1968, pp 413–434

Reynolds CR: Convergent and divergent validity of the Revised Children's Manifest Anxiety Scale. Educational Psychol Measurement 42:1205–1212, 1982

Robins LN, Helzer J, Croughan J, et al: National Institute of Mental Health Diagnostic Interview for Children and Adolescents. Bethesda, MD, National Institute of Mental Health, 1979

Rosenbaum JF, Biederman J, Gersten M, et al: Behavioral inhibition in children of parents with panic disorder and agoraphobia. Arch Gen Psychiatry 45:463–470, 1988

Ross D, Ross S, Evans TA: The modification of extreme social withdrawal by modification with guided practice. J Behav Ther Exp Psychiatry 2:272–279, 1971

Rotheram-Borus M: Treatment of the avoidant child. Paper presented at the annual meeting of the American Academy of Child and Adolescent Psychiatry, New York, October 1989

Simeon JG, Ferguson HB: Alprazolam effects in children with anxiety disorders. Can J Psychiatry 32:570–574, 1987

Strauss CC: Behavioral assessment and treatment of overanxious disorder in children and adolescents. Behav Modif 12:234–251, 1988

Strauss CC, Last CG, Hersen M, et al: Association between anxiety and depression in children and adolescents with anxiety disorders. J Abnorm Child Psychol 16:57–68, 1988a

Strauss CC, Lease CA, Last CG, et al: Overanxious disorder: an examination of developmental differences. J Abnorm Child Psychol 16:433–443, 1988b

Trautman PD: Psychodynamic theories of anxiety and their application to children, in Anxiety Disorders of Childhood. Edited by Gittelman R. New York, Guilford, 1986, pp 168–187

Turner SM, Beidel DC, Costello A: Psychopathology in offspring of anxiety disorders patients. J Consult Clin Psychol 55:229–235, 1987

Weissman MM, Leckman JE, Merikangas KR, et al: Depression and anxiety disorders in parents and children: results from the Yale Family Study. Arch Gen Psychiatry 41:845–852, 1984

Wells K, Vitulano L: Anxiety disorders in children, in Behavioral Theories and Treatment of Anxiety. Edited by Turner SM. New York, Plenum, 1984, pp 413–433

Chapter 29

Obsessive-Compulsive Disorder

Henrietta L. Leonard, M.D.
Judith L. Rapoport, M.D.

Definition

Obsessive-compulsive disorder (OCD) is characterized in DSM-III-R (American Psychiatric Association 1987) by recurrent obsessions and/or compulsions that are distressful and/or interfere in one's life. Obsessions are defined as persistent thoughts, images, or impulses that are ego-dystonic, intrusive, and, for the most part, senseless. "Compulsions are repetitive, purposeful, and intentional behaviors that are performed in response to an obsession, according to certain rules, or in a stereotyped fashion" (American Psychiatric Association 1987, p. 245). Children and adolescents are diagnosed using unmodified DSM-III-R criteria.

Diagnostic Criteria

In OCD, a person may have either obsessions or compulsions, or both (Table 29-1). An individual typically attempts to ignore, suppress, or neutralize the intrusive obsessive thoughts. The person identifies that these thoughts are senseless and the product of his or her own mind and therefore are not "thought insertion." The specific content of the obsession cannot be related to another Axis I diagnosis, such as thoughts about food resulting from an eating disorder or guilty thoughts (ruminations) from depression. Generally, compulsions serve to neutralize or alleviate anxious discomfort or to prevent a dreaded event. The person recognizes that the behavior is excessive or unreasonable, although this may not always hold true for young children.

For the obsessions and compulsions to be severe enough to meet DSM-III-R diagnostic criteria for OCD, they must "cause marked distress, be time-consuming [take more than an hour a day], or significantly interfere with the person's normal routine, occupational functioning, or usual social activities or relationships with others" (American Psychiatric Association 1987, p. 245).

Clinical Findings

In the first report in the literature of childhood OCD, Janet (1903, p. 17) described a 5-year-old's obsessions as an "arduous rethinking of the obvious." He suggested that obsessional thoughts are like "mental tics." Kanner's child psychiatry textbook of 1935 reviewed the German literature and reported that the OCD children were raised with an "overdose of parental perfectionism." Berman (1942) reported several childhood OCD cases and commented on their similarity to adults with the illness. Despert's (1955) report of 68 patients with "obsessive-compulsive neurosis" noted that despite the distress caused by the symptoms, the patients were surprisingly secretive about their obsessions and compulsions. In his thorough description of a series of 49 pediatric cases, Adams (1973) noted the preponderance of boys and, in some cases, a very early age of onset.

At the National Institute of Mental Health (NIMH), 70 consecutive child and adolescent patients were prospectively examined (Swedo et al. 1989c). These 47 boys and 23 girls who met diagnostic criteria for primary severe OCD had a mean age of onset of

Table 29-1.   DSM-III-R diagnostic criteria for obsessive-compulsive disorder

A. Either obsessions or compulsions:

Obsessions: 1, 2, 3, and 4:

1. Recurrent and persistent ideas, thoughts, impulses, or images that are experienced, at least initially, as intrusive and senseless, e.g., a parent's having repeated impulses to kill a loved child, a religious person's having recurrent blasphemous thoughts.

2. The person attempts to ignore or suppress such thoughts or impulses or to neutralize them with some other thought or action.

3. The person recognizes that the obsessions are the product of his or her own mind, not imposed from without (as in thought insertion).

4. If another Axis I disorder is present, the content of the obsession is unrelated to it, e.g., the ideas, thoughts, impulses, or images are not about food in the presence of an eating disorder, about drugs in the presence of a psychoactive substance use disorder, or guilty thoughts in the presence of a major depression.

Compulsions: 1, 2, and 3:

1. Repetitive, purposeful, and intentional behaviors that are performed in response to an obsession, or according to certain rules or in a stereotyped fashion.

2. The behavior is designed to neutralize or to prevent discomfort or some dreaded event or situation; however, either the activity is not connected in a realistic way with what it is designed to neutralize or prevent, or it is clearly excessive.

3. The person recognizes that his or her behavior is excessive or unreasonable (this may not be true for young children; it may no longer be true for people whose obsessions have evolved into overvalued ideas).

B. The obsessions or compulsions cause marked distress, are time-consuming (take more than an hour a day), or significantly interfere with the person's normal routine, occupational functioning, or usual social activities or relationships with others.

Source. Reprinted with permission from American Psychiatric Association 1987.

10 years. Seven of the patients had had the onset of their illness prior to the age of 7 years. Boys had an earlier age of onset, around age 9 (prepubertal); girls were more likely to have theirs around age 11 (pubertal). Tourette's syndrome was an exclusionary criterion, so there were no patients with this diagnosis; however, 20% of the NIMH patients had had a simple motor or vocal tic at some time in their life.

The clinical presentation of childhood OCD is essentially identical to that seen in adults (Rapoport 1986). The most common presenting ritual symptom was excessive "cleaning" (hand washing, showering, bathing, or tooth brushing), which was seen in 85% of the patients (Swedo et al. 1989c). Repeating rituals, as characterized by going in/out doors, going up/down from chairs, restating phrases, and rereading, were reported by 51%. Checking behaviors, such as making sure that doors and windows were locked, that appliances were turned off, or that homework was done "right," were reported in 46%. Other common rituals included counting (18%), ordering/arranging (17%), and hoarding (11%). More unusual obsessions included scrupulosity (13%), the preoccupying fear that one might harm oneself or others (4%), or having a tune in the head (1%) (Swedo et al. 1989c). The majority of the obsessions and rituals revolved around an internal sense that "it didn't feel right" until the thought or action was completed. For example, a boy might have to retrace his steps from the car into the house in a very elaborate and specific manner (two steps forward, look to the sky, three steps backward, glance to the left, and think a good thought until it "felt right").

In the NIMH series, there were only 3 (4%) cases of "pure obsessives," and most patients had a combination of both obsessive thoughts and compulsive rituals. A subgroup of "pure compulsives" acknowledged their ritualistic behaviors but were unable to attribute them to any obsessive thought. Frequently, children disguised their rituals until they became so extreme as to be discovered. Although still meeting DSM-III-R diagnostic criteria because of interference from time expended and acknowledgment of futility, some of the very young children denied any anxiety or distress in association with their rituals. Almost all patients reported that their principal symptom changed over time and that their symptoms waxed and waned in severity.

The less severely ill patients, and those attempting to hide their symptoms, are difficult to recognize. Behaviors suggesting an OCD diagnosis include spending long, unproductive hours on homework; erasing test papers and homework excessively (until paper is torn); retracing over letters or words; or rereading paragraphs. For example, a girl might be unable to complete an assignment at school because she could not get beyond the first question because of redoing it so many times. A dramatic increase in laundry, an insistence on wearing clothes or using a towel only once, or toilets being stopped up from too much paper may indicate an obsession about germs. Other suspicious behaviors include long, rigid bedtime rituals; an exaggerated need for reassurance; requests for family members to repeat phrases; a preoccupying fear of harm coming to oneself or others; or a persistent fear that one has an illness. Hoarding of useless objects, such as empty juice cans, magazine subscription coupons, or garbage passed on a street, should be differentiated from normal childhood collecting of rocks, sticks, or other treasures.

Differential Diagnosis

Disorders of depression and anxiety (separation anxiety, overanxious, and generalized anxiety disorders) with obsessional features may initially resemble OCD. Obsessive rumination and brooding may be seen in a major depressive disorder, although they are apt to be more content-specific and not seen as senseless. The fear of harm coming to oneself or others can be typical of separation anxiety disorder, but in OCD this thought usually results in the performance of compulsive rituals. The excessive and unrealistic worry typical of overanxious disorder would not typically be accompanied by classic compulsive rituals. In avoidance due to a simple phobia, it would be uncommon for germs to be the primary object avoided; and the phobic person's fear decreases when not confronted with the stimuli, unlike that of OCD patients.

Although superficially resembling the stereotypies seen in autism, mental retardation, pervasive developmental disorders, and organic brain damage syndromes, OCD rituals differ because they are well organized, complex, and ego-dystonic. In addition, the clinical pictures and the accompanying symptoms can help to differentiate between stereotypies and compulsive rituals. The anorectic or bulimic patient's "obsessive" interest in calories, exercise, and food and "compulsive" avoidance, measuring, and monitoring of food may resemble OCD, but when considered in context, the differential diagnosis is clear. Some OCD patients have rituals about food, such as eating all the cold food first, eating vegetables first, or feeling very concerned as to how food is arranged on the plate.

There is no disturbance, however, of body image. Tourette's syndrome patients may have associated obsessive-compulsive symptomatology (Frankel et al. 1986). Generally, if an action is preceded by a specific cognition, then it is considered to be a compulsive ritual; however, some complex motor tics may be preceded by a sensation or thought. Sensory tics are not usually accompanied by anxiety. In some cases, it may be impossible to distinguish a complex motor tic from a compulsive ritual, especially in patients with both OCD and Tourette's syndrome. However, it is important to attempt to make the distinction, since each responds to different treatments.

Epidemiology

Initially, estimates of the incidence of childhood OCD were made from psychiatric clinic populations. Berman (1942) reported "obsessive-compulsive phenomena" in 6 of 2,800 (0.2%) patients; Hollingsworth et al. (1980) found 17 in 8,367 (0.2%) child and adolescent inpatient and outpatient records. Judd's (1965) retrospective chart review revealed 5 cases in 425 (1.2%) pediatric charts.

The Isle of Wight study, the first epidemiologic study, reported "mixed obsessional/anxiety disorders" in 7 of 2,199 (0.3%) 10- and 11-year-old children surveyed (Rutter et al. 1970). In a whole-population adolescent epidemiology study, Flament et al. (1988) reported a weighted point prevalence rate of 0.8% and lifetime prevalence of 1.9%. These figures suggest that OCD is a relatively common psychiatric disorder in adolescents. This is compatible with the estimated 2% prevalence in the general population (Karno et al. 1988) and the finding that at least one-third to one-half of adult OCD patients had their onset in childhood (Black 1978).

Etiology

The etiology of OCD is unknown, but it appears to be the result of a frontal lobe–limbic–basal ganglia dysfunction (Wise and Rapoport 1989). Neurotransmitter dysregulation and genetic susceptibility also play a role. The "serotonin hypothesis of OCD" is based on the results of treatment studies, which demonstrate that the serotonin reuptake blockers are specifically efficacious for the treatment of OCD (for a review, see Zohar and Insel 1987).

Evidence supporting these theories include neuroanatomical, neurophysiologic, and neuroimmunological associations and metabolic abnormalities. Numerous brain injuries resulting in basal ganglia damage have been reported to be related to the onset of OCD; for example, postencephalitic Parkinson's disease (von Economo 1931) and carbon monoxide poisoning (LaPlane et al. 1984). Neuroimaging studies report that adult OCD patients with a history of childhood onset of their illness have decreased caudate size (a principal structure in the basal ganglia) on computed tomography scans (Luxenberg et al. 1988) and abnormal patterns of regional glucose metabolism positron-emission tomography scans in comparison with a group of normal control subjects (Swedo et al. 1989a). Additionally, there is an increased incidence of OCD in pediatric patients with Sydenham's chorea (an autoimmune attack on the basal ganglia caused by a streptococcal infection) in comparison to "controls" with rheumatic fever (Swedo et al. 1989b). These results suggest both anatomical and physiologic differences. Further evidence for a frontal lobe–basal ganglia dysfunction comes from the neuropsychological testing of these patients (Cox et al. 1989).

A genetic basis for OCD is suggested by the familial links between Tourette's syndrome and OCD reported by Pauls et al. (1986), who suggested that the two illnesses may be a different manifestation of the same gene(s). In a recent NIMH study, 20% of personally interviewed first-degree relatives (i.e., parents and siblings) of the OCD probands met diagnostic criteria for OCD (Lenane et al. 1990). Interestingly, the primary OCD symptom in the affected family member was usually different from that of the proband, suggesting genetic transmission rather than modeling. Integrating these neuroanatomical and neurophysiologic hypotheses with those of genetic susceptibility and environmental stressors remains a challenge.

Treatment

Behavioral Treatment

Although behavioral treatment has been used clinically with much success, it has not been systematically studied in children and adolescents. Pediatric case reports suggest that the techniques employed with adults (Marks 1987) appear to be appropriate for children (for reviews, see Berg et al. 1989a; Wolff and Rapoport 1988).

Response prevention is the most frequently implemented treatment and is frequently used in addition to other specific behavioral treatment techniques. In the largest pediatric behavioral study reported, Bolton et al. (1983) used response prevention for 15 obsessive adolescents and achieved good treatment results in 11. The most successful behavioral approach used with adults is response prevention with in vivo exposure. This has been used in only two studies (Apter et al. 1984; Zikis 1983), both of which reported its usefulness in the younger group. Behavior modification therapy may be less successful for patients with obsessions only (as opposed to both obsessions and compulsions), for those who are very young, and for those who are uncooperative. In conclusion, it appears that behavioral treatment for children with OCD is appropriate and should be considered as one of the treatments of choice.

Pharmacologic Treatment

The serotonin reuptake blockers (clomipramine, fluoxetine, and fluvoxamine) have been reported to be effective for adults with OCD based on controlled trials (for a review, see Zohar et al. 1987). Flament et al. (1985) and Leonard et al. (1989b) have shown that children respond equally well compared with adults to one of these medications: clomipramine. In the first study, 23 pediatric patients participated in a 10-week double-blind, placebo-controlled crossover study (Flament et al. 1985, 1987). Clomipramine (in dosages of 3 mg/kg) was significantly better than placebo in decreasing OCD symptomatology at week 5, and an improvement in symptoms was usually seen by 3 weeks. Of the 19 children who completed the trial, 75% had a moderate to marked improvement, reporting a significant decrease in time spent in OCD activities as well as in distress experienced.

The second study was a double-blind, crossover comparison of clomipramine and desipramine (a selective noradrenergic reuptake blocker) in 48 children and adolescents with OCD (Leonard et al. 1989b). Clomipramine was significantly better than desipramine in ameliorating the OCD symptoms at week 5, and in some cases a significant improvement could be seen as early as the third week of treatment. Desipramine was no more effective in improving OCD symptoms than placebo had been in the earlier study (Flament et al. 1985). In fact, when desipramine was given as the second active medication, many of the patients relapsed. Both clomipramine and desipramine were well tolerated at 3 mg/kg/day, and the side effects profiles for the two drugs were very similar.

Fluoxetine, another selective serotonin reuptake blocker, has been reported to be effective for the treatment of OCD in adults in open studies (Fontaine and Chouinard 1986; Jenike et al. 1989) and in a single-blind trial (Turner et al. 1985). Fluoxetine is approved for use as an antidepressant in adults. Its safety and efficacy in the pediatric age group have not yet been established, although there are a few reports in this age group. Riddle et al. (1989) concluded that fluoxetine appeared to be safe and well tolerated in dosages of 10–40 mg/day in a group of 10 children and adolescents with either primary OCD or Tourette's syndrome and OCD. Additionally, 15 adolescents who completed the NIMH trial and did not respond to clomipramine, or who could not tolerate its side effects, have been tried on fluoxetine without any untoward side effects. Most showed a favorable clinical response. These reports suggest that fluoxetine may prove useful in younger patients with OCD; this deserves further study.

Psychodynamic and Psychosocial Treatment

Jenike (1986) reviewed the psychotherapeutic interventions that are available for the treatment of OCD and concluded that "traditional psychodynamic psychotherapy is not an effective treatment for patients with obsessive-compulsive disorder as defined in the DSM-III [American Psychiatric Association 1980]; there are no reports in the psychiatric literature of patients who stopped ritualizing when treated with this method alone" (p. 113). Psychodynamic psychotherapy can play an important role by addressing both general and specific issues in the patient's life, such as the way OCD impacts on the individual's self-esteem, personal relationships, and outlook, and by encouraging compliance with the behavioral or psychopharmacologic therapies that are dealing more directly with the OCD symptomatology. Clearly, an individual with OCD cannot be understood out of context of his or her feelings, relationships, and past and present experiences. Character styles consistent with "obsessional defenses" and obsessive-compulsive personality are amenable to psychotherapy (for reviews, see Jenike 1986; Salzman 1983, 1986).

Family therapy is an important treatment for pediatric OCD patients because family discord, marital difficulties, problems of a specific family member, or inappropriate roles or boundaries will interfere with the family's and each individual's successful functioning and therefore ultimately with the long-term outcome of the identified patient (Hafner et al. 1981; Hoover et al. 1984; Lenane 1991). A complete family assessment is necessary as part of the initial diagnostic evaluation of every OCD child. Lenane (1989) described the family therapy treatment goal as involving the whole family in treatment, getting all behaviors out in the open, obtaining full and accurate understanding of how everyone participates in the OCD behavior, and reframing of less-than-positive behavior. By dealing with the specific family dynamic issues, the family is available to participate in the OCD treatment plan of the identified patient in constructive and positive ways.

Prognosis

In the only follow-up study of an epidemiologic sample, Berg et al. (1989b) reported that of the 16 adolescents who initially were diagnosed with OCD, 5 (31%) still met criteria at 2-year follow-up, and 4 (25%) had "subclinical" OCD. Interestingly, 2 (12%) of the original OCD cases no longer met criteria for OCD but did so for obsessive-compulsive personality. The authors speculated that some children and adolescents with early onset OCD might develop obsessive-compulsive personalities as means of coping with the disorder.

Follow-up studies of pediatric OCD patients indicate that at least half of the patients are still symptomatic as adults (Berman 1942; Hollingsworth et al. 1980; Warren 1965). Flament et al. (1990) found that of 25 patients seen 2–7 years after initial presentation, 17 (68%) still met diagnostic criteria for OCD, and 12 (48%) had an additional diagnosis (most often depression or anxiety); only 7 (28%) no longer met diagnostic criteria for any DSM-III disorder. Surprisingly, neither baseline measures nor a positive response to clomipramine treatment was able to predict long-term outcome. These poor results might be explained, among other things, by the fact that this group had not been actively treated during the 2- to 5-year interim period, and only 12 subjects had been on clomipramine for more than a few months.

The 48 children and adolescents from the subsequent clomipramine-desipramine study have been followed more intensively, with ongoing recommendations for appropriate treatments. In the initial 2-year assessment of 40 of these patients, 10 (25%) had no OCD symptoms, 22 (55%) had only mild symptoms, and 8 (20%) had moderate to severe symptomatology (Leonard et al. 1989a). No conclusions can be drawn about the underlying severity of the OCD illness because two-thirds of the patients in each of these three groups (no, mild, and moderate to severe symptoms) were on maintenance medication for their OCD at the time of follow-up (Leonard et al. 1989a). One hopes that with new treatments available, closer monitoring, and active encouragement to follow through on treatment recommendations, a better long-term outcome could be obtained for this group than that previously reported in the literature.

Research Issues

There are a number of important research issues for childhood onset OCD. It is not known which children respond better to behavioral treatment and which to drug treatment. It is presumed, but not yet demonstrated, that the availability of these two treatment modalities alters the long-term prognosis. A long-term comparison of the two approaches is indicated.

Identifying children at risk for OCD, through genetic or biological studies, is also a research priority. Leonard et al. (1990) found that the parents of children with OCD reported significantly more "marked" patterns of early ritualistic behavior in the children than did parents of normal control subjects. Prospective studies are needed to determine whether these findings represent "preclinical OCD" or are an artifact of biased recall. If an at-risk group is identified, what would be the result of prophylactic behavioral treatment or pharmacotherapy? Such interventions, if successful, would be important contributions to the clinical management and perhaps the long-term prognosis of this troubling disorder.

References

Adams PL: Obsessive Children. New York, Penguin Books, 1973

American Psychiatric Association: Diagnostic and Statistical Manual of Mental Disorders, 3rd Edition. Washington, DC, American Psychiatric Association, 1980

American Psychiatric Association: Diagnostic and Statistical Manual of Mental Disorders, 3rd Edition, Revised. Washington, DC, American Psychiatric Association, 1987

Apter A, Bernhout E, Tyano S: Severe obsessive compulsive disorder in adolescence: a report of eight cases. J Adolesc 7:349–358, 1984

Berg CZ, Rapoport JL, Wolff RP: Behavioral treatment for obsessive-compulsive disorder in childhood, in Obsessive-Compulsive Disorder in Children and Adolescents. Edited by Rapoport JL. Washington, DC, American Psychiatric Press, 1989a, pp 169–188

Berg CZ, Rapoport JL, Whitaker A, et al: Childhood obsessive compulsive disorder: a two-year prospective follow-up of a community sample. Journal of Child and Adolescent Psychiatry 28:528–533, 1989b

Berman L: Obsessive-compulsive neurosis in children. J Nerv Ment Dis 95:26–39, 1942

Black A: The natural history of obsessional neurosis, in Obsessional States. Edited by Beech HR. London, Methuen, 1978

Bolton D, Collins S, Steinberg D: The treatment of obsessive-compulsive disorder in adolescence: a report of fifteen cases. Br J Psychiatry 142:456–464, 1983

Cox CS, Fedio P, Rapoport JL: Neuropsychological testing of obsessive-compulsive adolescents, in Obsessive-Compulsive Disorder in Children and Adolescents. Edited by Rapoport JL. Washington, DC, American Psychiatric Press, 1989, pp 73–85

Despert L: Differential diagnosis between obsessive-compulsive neurosis and schizophrenia in children, in Psychopathology of Childhood. Edited by Hoch PH, Zubin J. New York, Grune & Stratton, 1955, pp 240–253

Flament MF, Rapoport JL, Berg CJ, et al: Clomipramine treatment of childhood compulsive disorder. Arch Gen Psychiatry 42:977–983, 1985

Flament MF, Rapoport JL, Murphy DL: Biochemical changes during clomipramine treatment of childhood obsessive-compulsive disorder. Arch Gen Psychiatry 44:219–225, 1987

Flament MF, Whitaker A, Rapoport JL: Obsessive compulsive disorder in adolescence: an epidemiological study. J Am Acad Child Adolesc Psychiatry 27:764–771, 1988

Flament MF, Koby E, Rapoport JL, et al: Childhood obsessive compulsive disorder: a prospective follow-up study. J Child Psychol Psychiatry 31:363–380, 1990

Fontaine R, Chouinard G: An open clinical trial of fluoxetine in the treatment of obsessive compulsive disorder. J Clin Psychopharmacol 6:98–101, 1986

Frankel M, Cummings JL, Robertson MM, et al: Obsessions and compulsions in Gilles de la Tourette's syndrome. Neurology 36:378–382, 1986

Hafner RJ, Gilchrist P, Bowling J, et al: The treatment of obsessional neurosis in a family setting. Aust N Z J Psychiatry 15:145–151, 1981

Hollingsworth C, Tanguey P, Grossman L, et al: Longterm outcome of obsessive compulsive disorder in children. Journal of the American Academy of Child Psychiatry 9:134–144, 1980

Hoover CF, Insel TR: Families of origin in obsessive compulsive disorder. J Nerv Ment Dis 172:207–215, 1984

Janet P: Les Obsessions et la Psychiatrie, Vol 1. Paris, Felix Alan, 1903

Jenike MA: Psychotherapy of the obsessional patient, in Ob-

obsessive compulsive disorder in five U.S. communities. Arch Gen Psychiatry 45:1094–1099, 1988

LaPlane D, Baulac M, Widlocher D, et al: Pure psychic akinesia with bilateral lesions of basal ganglia. J Neurol Neurosurg Psychiatry 47:377–385, 1984

Lenane M: Families and obsessive-compulsive disorder, in Obsessive-Compulsive Disorder in Children and Adolescents. Edited by Rapoport JL. Washington, DC, American Psychiatric Press, 1989, pp 237–249

Lenane MC: Family therapy for children with obsessive-compulsive disorder, in Current Treatments of Obsessive-Compulsive Disorder. Edited by Pato MT, Zohar J. Washington, DC, American Psychiatric Press, 1991, pp 103–113

Lenane MC, Swedo S, Leonard H, et al: Psychiatric disorders in first degree relatives of children and adolescents with obsessive compulsive disorder. J Am Acad Child Adolesc Psychiatry 29:407–412, 1990

Leonard HL, Swedo SE, Lenane ML, et al: A prospective 2-year preliminary follow-up of 48 children and adolescents with severe primary obsessive compulsive disorder. Paper presented at the annual meeting of the American Academy of Child and Adolescent Psychiatry, New York, October 1989a

Leonard HL, Swedo S, Rapoport JL: Treatment of obsessive compulsive disorder with clomipramine and desipramine in children and adolescents: a double-blind crossover comparison. Arch Gen Psychiatry 46:1088–1092, 1989b

Leonard HL, Goldberger EL, Rapoport JL, et al: Childhood rituals: normal development or obsessive compulsive symptoms? J Am Acad Child Adolesc Psychiatry 29:17–23, 1990

Luxenberg JS, Swedo SE, Flament MF, et al: Neuroanatomical abnormalities in obsessive-compulsive disorder detected with quantitative X-ray computed tomography. Am J Psychiatry 145:1089–1093, 1988

Marks IM: Fears, Phobias and Rituals: Panic Anxiety and Their Disorders. Oxford, UK, Oxford University Press, 1987

Pauls DL, Towbin K, Leckman J, et al: Gilles de la Tourette syndrome and obsessive compulsive disorder: evidence supporting a genetic relationship. Arch Gen Psychiatry 43:1180–1182, 1986

Rapoport JL: Annotation, child obsessive-compulsive disorder. J Child Psychol Psychiatry 27:285–289, 1986

Riddle M, Hardin M, King R, et al: Fluoxetine treatment of children and adolescents with Tourette's and obsessive compulsive disorders. Paper presented at the annual meeting of the American Academy of Child and Adolescent Psychiatry, New York, October 1989

Rutter M, Tizard J, Whitmore K: Education, Health and Behavior. London, Longmans, 1970

Salzman L: Psychoanalytic therapy of the obsessional patient. Current Psychiatric Therapy 9:53–59, 1983

Salzman L: Psychotherapy of the obsessional patient, in Obsessive Compulsive Disorders: Theory and Management. Edited by Jenike MA, Baer L, Minichiello WE. Littleton, MA, PSG Publishing, 1986, pp 113–123

Swedo SE, Shapiro MB, Grady CL, et al: Cerebral glucose metabolism in childhood onset obsessive-compulsive disorder. Arch Gen Psychiatry 46:518–523, 1989a

Swedo SE, Rapoport JL, Cheslow DL, et al: High prevalence of obsessive compulsive symptoms in patients with Sydenham's chorea. Am J Psychiatry 146:246–249, 1989b

Swedo SE, Rapoport JL, Leonard HL, et al: Obsessive compulsive disorder in children and adolescents: clinical phenomenology of 70 consecutive cases. Arch Gen Psychiatry 46:335–341, 1989c

Turner SM, Jacob RG, Beidel DC, et al: Fluoxetine treatment of obsessive compulsive disorder. J Clin Psychopharmacol 5:207–212, 1985

Von Economo C: Encephalitis Lethargica: Its Sequelae and Treatment. Translated by Newman KO. New York, Oxford University Press, 1931

Warren W: A study of adolescent psychiatric inpatients and the outcome six or more years later. J Child Psychol Psychiatry 6:141–160, 1965

Wise SP, Rapoport JL: Obsessive-compulsive disorder: is it basal ganglia dysfunction? in Obsessive-Compulsive Disorder in Children and Adolescents. Edited by Rapoport JL. Washington, DC, American Psychiatric Press, 1989, pp 327–344

Wolff R, Rapoport JL: Behavioral treatment of childhood obsessive compulsive disorder. Behav Modif 12:252–266, 1988

Zikis P: Treatment of an 11-year-old obsessive compulsive ritualizer and Tiqueur girl with in vivo exposure and response prevention. Behavior Psychotherapy 11:75–81, 1983

Zohar J, Insel TR: Obsessive compulsive disorder: psychobiological approaches to diagnosis, treatment and pathophysiology. Biol Psychiatry 22:667–687, 1987

Zohar J, Mueller EA, Insel TR, et al: Serotonergic responsivity in obsessive-compulsive disorder. Arch Gen Psychiatry 44:946–951, 1987

Chapter 30

Simple Phobia, Social Phobia, and Panic Disorders

Henrietta L. Leonard, M.D.
Judith L. Rapoport, M.D.

Definition

According to DSM-III-R (American Psychiatric Association 1987), simple phobias are persistent fears of specific stimuli, such as animals, insects, blood, heights, closed spaces, or airplanes. When faced with that object or situation, the individual experiences significant anxiety, although he or she may recognize that the fear is unreasonable.

Social phobia is a persistent fear of a social situation in which a person might be scrutinized or might do something that would be embarrassing or humiliating. Examples include being unable to speak in public, to eat in front of others, to urinate in a public bathroom, or to answer questions in social settings. The social setting provokes great anxiety, and the individual recognizes this fear as unreasonable or excessive (American Psychiatric Association 1987).

Panic disorder is characterized by recurrent panic attacks, which are discrete periods of "intense fear or discomfort" accompanied by specific somatic symptoms. In panic disorder, there is great anticipatory anxiety because of the uncertainty as to when an attack will reoccur (American Psychiatric Association 1987).

Diagnostic Criteria

Simple phobia "is a persistent fear of a circumscribed stimulus" (American Psychiatric Associa-

tion 1987, p. 243) that provokes immediate anxiety. To meet DSM-III-R criteria (Table 30-1), the avoidant behavior must interfere in a person's normal routine or social relationships, or there must be marked distress about having the fear. The stimulus is either avoided or endured with intense anx-

Table 30-1. DSM-III-R diagnostic criteria for simple phobia

A. A persistent fear of a circumscribed stimulus (object or situation) other than fear of having a panic attack (as in panic disorder) or of humiliation or embarrassment in certain social situations (as in social phobia).
   Note: Do not include fears that are part of panic disorder with agoraphobia or agoraphobia without history of panic disorder.
B. During some phase of the disturbance, exposure to the specific phobic stimulus (or stimuli) almost invariably provokes an immediate anxiety response.
C. The object or situation is avoided, or endured with intense anxiety.
D. The fear or the avoidant behavior significantly interferes with the person's normal routine or with usual social activities or relationships with others, or there is marked distress about having the fear.
E. The person recognizes that his or her fear is excessive or unreasonable.
F. The phobic stimulus is unrelated to the content of the obsessions of obsessive-compulsive disorder or the trauma of posttraumatic stress disorder.

Source. Reprinted with permission from American Psychiatric Association 1987.

Table 30-2. DSM-III-R diagnostic criteria for social phobia

A. A persistent fear of one or more situations (the social phobic situations) in which the person is exposed to possible scrutiny by others and fears that he or she may do something or act in a way that will be humiliating or embarrassing. Examples include: being unable to continue talking while speaking in public, choking on food when eating in front of others, being unable to urinate in a public lavatory, hand trembling when writing in the presence of others, and saying foolish things or not being able to answer questions in social situations.

B. If an Axis III or another Axis I disorder is present, the fear in A is unrelated to it, e.g., the fear is not of having a panic attack (panic disorder), stuttering (stuttering), trembling (Parkinson's disease), or exhibiting abnormal eating behavior (anorexia nervosa or bulimia nervosa).

C. During some phase of the disturbance, exposure to the specific phobic stimulus (or stimuli) almost invariably provokes an immediate anxiety response.

D. The phobic situation(s) is avoided, or is endured with intense anxiety.

E. The avoidant behavior interferes with occupational functioning or with usual social activities or relationships with others, or there is marked distress about having the fear.

F. The person recognizes that his or her fear is excessive or unreasonable.

G. If the person is under 18, the disturbance does not meet the criteria for avoidant disorder of childhood or adolescence.

Specify generalized type if the phobic situation includes most social situations, and also consider the additional diagnosis of avoidant personality disorder.

Source. Reprinted with permission from American Psychiatric Association 1987.

Table 30-3. DSM-III-R diagnostic criteria for panic disorder

A. At some time during the disturbance, one or more panic attacks (discrete periods of intense fear or discomfort) have occurred that were 1) unexpected, i.e., did not occur immediately before or on exposure to a situation that almost always caused anxiety, and 2) not triggered by situations in which the person was the focus of others' attention.

B. Either four attacks, as defined in criterion A, have occurred within a four-week period, or one or more attacks have been followed by a period of at least a month of persistent fear of having another attack.

C. At least four of the following symptoms developed during at least one of the attacks:
1. Shortness of breath (dyspnea) or smothering sensations
2. Dizziness, unsteady feelings, or faintness
3. Palpitations or accelerated heart rate (tachycardia)
4. Trembling or shaking
5. Sweating
6. Choking
7. Nausea or abdominal distress
8. Depersonalization or derealization
9. Numbness or tingling sensations (paresthesias)
10. Flushes (hot flashes) or chills
11. Chest pain or discomfort
12. Fear of dying
13. Fear of going crazy or of doing something uncontrolled

Note: Attacks involving four or more symptoms are panic attacks; attacks involving fewer than four symptoms are limited symptom attacks (see agoraphobia without history of panic disorder).

D. During at least some of the attacks, at least four of the C symptoms developed suddenly and increased in intensity within 10 minutes of the beginning of the first C symptom noticed in the attack.

E. It cannot be established that an organic factor initiated and maintained the disturbance, e.g., amphetamine or caffeine intoxication, hyperthyroidism.

Note: Mitral valve prolapse may be an associated condition, but does not preclude a diagnosis of panic disorder.

Source. Reprinted with permission from American Psychiatric Association 1987.

iety, and the individual sees his or her fear as unreasonable or excessive.

To meet DSM-III-R diagnostic criteria for social phobia (Table 30-2), the social situation must elicit tremendous anxiety, resulting in interference in functioning or marked distress about experiencing the fear. Understanding that the fear is excessive does not relieve the anxiety. The diagnosis of social phobia is precluded for those under 18 years of age who meet criteria for avoidant disorder of childhood or adolescence.

To meet the DSM-III-R criteria for panic disorder (Table 30-3), an individual must have had at least four panic attacks within a 4-week period, or one of the attacks must have been followed by at least

a month of persistent fear of having an attack. Four of the following specific symptoms must have occurred during the panic attack: shortness of breath, dizziness, palpitations, trembling, sweating, choking, nausea, a feeling of depersonalization, numbness, flushes or chills, chest pain, or a fear of dying or of going crazy.

Table 30-4. DSM-III-R diagnostic criteria for panic disorder with agoraphobia

A. Meets the criteria for panic disorder.

B. Agoraphobia: Fear of being in places or situations from which escape might be difficult (or embarrassing) or in which help might not be available in the event of a panic attack. (Include cases in which persistent avoidance behavior originated during an active phase of panic disorder, even if the person does not attribute the avoidance behavior to fear of having a panic attack.) As a result of this fear, the person either restricts travel or needs a companion when away from home, or else endures agoraphobic situations despite intense anxiety. Common agoraphobic situations include being outside the home alone, being in a crowd or standing in a line, being on a bridge, and traveling in a bus, train, or car.

Specify current severity of agoraphobic avoidance:

Mild: Some avoidance (or endurance with distress), but relatively normal life-style, e.g., travels unaccompanied when necessary, such as to work or to shop; otherwise avoids traveling alone.

Moderate: Avoidance results in constricted life-style, e.g., the person is able to leave the house alone, but not to go more than a few miles unaccompanied.

Severe: Avoidance results in being nearly or completely housebound or unable to leave the house unaccompanied.

In Partial Remission: No current agoraphobic avoidance, but some agoraphobic avoidance during the past six months.

In Full Remission: No current agoraphobic avoidance and none during the past six months.

Specify current severity of panic attacks:

Mild: During the past month, either all attacks have been limited symptom attacks (i.e., fewer than four symptoms), or there has been no more than one panic attack.

Moderate: During the past month attacks have been intermediate between "mild" and "severe."

Severe: During the past month, there have been at least eight panic attacks.

In Partial Remission: The condition has been intermediate between "In Full Remission" and "Mild."

In Full Remission: During the past six months, there have been no panic or limited symptom attacks.

Source. Reprinted with permission from American Psychiatric Association 1987.

Panic disorder can exist either with or without agoraphobia (Tables 30-4 and 30-5). Little is known, however, about agoraphobia in the pediatric age group.

Clinical Findings

Simple Phobia

Many normal children experience fears and anxieties; at what point the anxiety becomes "clinical" can be a fine distinction. Lapouse and Monk (1959) reported that 43% of interviewed mothers acknowledged that their children had seven or more fears, and 15% stated that their children exhibited anxious behaviors (thumb sucking, teeth grinding, nail biting). Ollendick (1983) reported that of 217 children from 3 to 11 years of age, the average number of extreme fears ranged from 9 to 13. The numerous general fears and anxieties of children decrease with age, and the specific focus of the fear changes (Graziano et al. 1979).

In assessing the fears of children and adolescents, it is most important to maintain a developmental perspective, as some fears are common and appropriate at young ages. (An excellent review of the development of fears in children and adolescents is available elsewhere [Marks 1987].) However, the distinction is primarily made by severity of anxiety and impairment in functioning. Infants' fears diminish during the preschool years, although the fear of strangers may persist as "shyness." Preschool children are typically afraid of strangers, the dark, animals, or imaginary creatures. Elementary-school-aged children are more apt to be afraid of animals, darkness, their own safety, or thunder and lightening. Older children are more concerned with health, social, and school fears (Maurer 1965). Adolescent fears may focus more on failure, sex, or agoraphobia (Marks 1987). If the fears persist into older ages or if there is interference or distress associated with them, then

Table 30-5. DSM-III-R diagnostic criteria for panic disorder without agoraphobia

A. Meets the criteria for panic disorder.
B. Absence of agoraphobia, as defined above.

Specify current severity of panic attacks, as defined above.

Source. Reprinted with permission from American Psychiatric Association 1987.

these fears need to be evaluated as to their clinical importance.

Phobias based on fears of animals, darkness, water, snakes, or insects usually begin in childhood. The fear of blood or injury and of animals typically begins before the age of 7. These phobias are not usually linked to a specific traumatic event, and they usually occur for no specific reasons (Marks and Gelder 1966). Normal developmental fears of animals usually decrease around the age of 9 or 11 (Angelino et al. 1956). It would be unusual for a phobia of animals or dogs to begin in adolescence or adulthood, unless there was a specific traumatic event. The most common adult forms of phobias (e.g., heights, closed spaces, plane trips) do begin in the adult years.

A very interesting and common phobia with childhood onset is that of blood injury (Marks 1988). Having a medical procedure such as venipuncture, dental work, or blood donation, or even hearing the word *blood*, descriptions of surgery, or news reports of accidents, can precipitate a dramatic reaction of tachycardia, vasovagal bradycardia, and syncope. Mild fear of blood is certainly common in children, estimated to be 44% of 6- to 8-year-olds and 27% of 9- to 12-year-olds (Lapouse and Monk 1959). A true blood phobia has been estimated to occur in 2%–4.5% of children and adults (Marks 1988). Marks also commented on the female preponderance of the illness and the history of a family member with the identical phobia. Marks reported successful treatment with behavioral techniques using exposure therapy.

A true phobia for school ("school phobia") must be distinguished from separation anxiety disorder, overanxious disorder, depression, or conduct disorder (truancy). School phobia is discussed in greater detail by Leonard and Rapoport (Chapter 28, this volume). Briefly, in school phobia, the refusal to attend school is based on fearing something specific about the school situation, such as fearing a specific teacher or peer, taking a shower after gym, or something on the way to school. In most cases, there is a gradual onset, with increasing resistance to attending school. Somatic symptoms are frequent, and the child's stated reasons for avoiding school can be varied and unrelated to the underlying fear (Marks 1987).

In conclusion, phobias do start in childhood and need to be differentiated from normal developmental fears. The importance of identifying a clinical phobia lies in treating the resulting anxieties and disruptions in one's life.

Social Phobia

Those who have social phobia have a fear of performing (speaking, writing, eating, using public bathrooms) in the presence of others. Little is known about social phobia in childhood. It can be difficult to distinguish social phobia from overanxious or avoidant disorder.

Most of the research data differentiating these conditions come from studies of social phobic adults who retrospectively recall the onset of their symptoms in childhood or adolescence. Solyom et al. (1986) compared 47 social phobic adults, 80 agoraphobic adults, and 72 simple phobic adults. The social phobic adults experienced their first phobic symptoms earlier than the agoraphobic adults but later than the simple phobic adults. The simple phobic patients retrospectively recalled the age of onset of their first symptoms to be 12.8 years, with onset of illness at 16.0 years; the social phobic patients reported their age of onset at 16.6 years for symptoms and 23.5 years for illness. Agoraphobic patients had the latest onset age, with 24.5 and 26.0 years for symptoms and illness, respectively. These data from adult social phobic patients support the distinction between agoraphobia and simple phobia. Others have also reported clinical and demographic data showing social phobia to be distinct from the other phobias and anxiety disorders (Liebowitz et al. 1985). The disorder is more common in males (Solyom et al. 1986). Social phobia seems to begin between 15 and 20 years of age and to have a chronic, unremitting course (Marks et al. 1987; Solyom et al. 1986).

In conclusion, although social phobia is reported to begin in early to middle adolescence, it clinically is not entirely clear how social phobia is distinguished from overanxious or avoidant disorders. Research is needed to study children and adolescents with this disorder.

Panic Disorder

Until recently, it was not believed that panic disorder could be diagnosed in children (Gittelman-Klein and Klein 1988). As a result, little is known about agoraphobia in children. Agoraphobia almost inevitably follows panic disorder. Studies of adults with panic disorder have reported that many patients retrospectively recalled the onset to be in childhood or adolescence (Sheehan et al. 1981a). The first report to describe panic attacks in a child, however, was in 1984.

Van Winter and Stickler (1984) reported on a 12-year-old boy with a 4-year history of panic attacks who was of the fourth generation in his family to suffer from this condition. The authors described six additional patients (five girls and one boy, ages 9–17 years) who had panic attacks, with ages of onset ranging from 9 to 16. All but one had relatives with panic attacks. Herskowitz (1986) reported on four children and adolescents, ages 9–16, who presented with symptoms of "dizzy spells, tiredness, blackout spells, and rapid breathing" who were subsequently diagnosed as having panic disorder. Vitiello et al. (1987) was the first to report two cases of panic disorder in prepubertal children using structured psychiatric interviews. Two boys, ages 8 and 10, who were referred for separation anxiety with school phobia symptomatology met diagnostic criteria for panic disorder. Both boys had had the onset of their symptoms prior to age 5. One boy had mitral valve prolapse documented on echocardiogram. Panic disorder was present in both patients' families for three generations.

In 136 consecutively hospitalized children, Alessi and Magen (1988) reported on 7 (5.15%) cases of panic disorder. These four boys and three girls were all prepubertal (age range, 7–12 years) and reported their mean age of onset of panic symptoms to be at 8.3 ± 3.6 years (range, 3–12). Comorbidity was significant; six had separation anxiety disorder and four had depression (either major depressive disorder or dysthymic disorder). The authors cautioned against misdiagnosing true panic disorder as school phobia, separation anxiety, conduct disorder, or depression, although they acknowledged the comorbidity of these disorders.

Moreau et al. (1989) studied 220 children, ages 6–23, who were offspring of depressed parents. The authors also found that panic disorder can have its onset in prepubertal years. On structured interviews, 7 children had panic symptoms, with 6 actually meeting DSM-III (American Psychiatric Association 1980) criteria for panic disorder. The age of onset ranged from 5 to 18 years (4 prepubertal). Two subjects still met diagnostic criteria at 2-year follow-up. The clinical picture was identical to that seen in adults, and the mean number of symptoms was 6.1. All the cases of panic disorder were in the children of depressed parents, and none were found in the children of nondepressed control parents. Of the 6 cases, 4 met criteria for separation anxiety disorder and 4 for major depression, with the onset of the panic disorder being either concurrent with or subsequent to the depressive or separation anxiety disorder diagnosis. Not surprisingly, parents were better than the children in recalling past episodes of the child's panic attacks.

Panic disorder with or without agoraphobia typically has its onset in adult life, although there may be an association with childhood anxiety, specifically separation anxiety disorder or excessive fearfulness (Gittelman and Klein 1984). Klein (1964) noted that half of a sample of female adult panic patients with agoraphobia had a history of separation anxiety or school phobia. Interestingly, the agoraphobic adults with a history of school phobia had an earlier age of onset for the agoraphobia than did those without this history. The exact explanation for this relationship is not clear. Perhaps the childhood anxiety and avoidance symptoms might represent early manifestations of the same disorder, might predispose the adult to develop agoraphobia, or might reflect some more common anxiety symptomatology (Klein 1964).

Kagan et al. (1984, 1987) and Reznick et al. (1986) reported on "behavioral inhibition to the unfamiliar," which is a description of a group of children who are irritable as infants, shy and fearful as toddlers, and cautious, quiet, and introverted when school age. Rosenbaum et al. (1988) hypothesized that behavioral inhibition to the unfamiliar may be a predisposing characteristic in children at risk for panic disorder and agoraphobia later in life. Rosenbaum et al. compared children of parents having panic disorder with agoraphobia with those from psychiatric comparison groups. The children of probands with panic disorder with agoraphobia, either with or without comorbid major depressive disorder, had a significantly higher rate of behavioral inhibition. This high prevalence of behavioral inhibition in the offspring of adults with panic disorder with agoraphobia suggests that these children may be at risk for anxiety in childhood and later in adult life. The authors hypothesized that behavioral inhibition may be a precursor of or marker for a later affective or anxiety disorder or perhaps a nonspecific early precursor of later psychopathology. However, it is clear that not all children with behavioral inhibition go on to develop an anxiety disorder. Behavior inhibition is prevalent in the offspring of adults in treatment for panic disorder with agoraphobia, but it is not clear what is attributable to biology and what to environment, nor whether this inhibition leads to anxiety disorders later in life.

The relationship between parental psychiatric diagnoses and anxiety diagnoses in the offspring has been reviewed elsewhere (Leonard and Rapoport 1989). Weissman et al. (1984) studied children of adult probands with anxiety disorder, major depression, and matched normal control subjects. Of the children of the parents with both depression and panic attacks, 42% had an anxiety diagnosis. Children of the parents with depression *and* panic and/or agoraphobia had a higher rate of phobias. Depression plus agoraphobia or panic disorder increased a child's risk for an anxiety disorder. In summary, panic disorder can start in childhood; however, the childhood antecedents of adult panic disorder are unclear and deserve prospective study.

Differential Diagnosis

In simple phobia, there is a *specific* stimulus that produces the anxiety; in panic disorder, the fear of "having the panic attack" predominates. By definition, panic attacks cannot be triggered by a social situation in which the person was the focus of attention, such as in social phobia. Typically, in simple phobia, the very specific nature of the stimulus (e.g., animals, heights, subways) distinguishes it from social phobia, in which the fear is about embarrassment in social settings. Simple phobia is differentiated from posttraumatic stress disorder because the avoidance in posttraumatic stress disorder is directly related to the traumatic event. The avoidance in obsessive-compulsive disorder is related to the content of an obsession, as exemplified by, for example, avoiding dirt or germs. Anxiety that is related primarily to separation from mother and/or father should be classified under separation anxiety disorder.

The distinction between social phobia and avoidant disorder of childhood can be more problematic. Technically, social phobia is for a specific social situation, whereas in avoidant disorder the shrinking from contact with unfamiliar people would be more general and diffuse. This needs clarifying in the final version of DSM-IV.

Epidemiology

There are few pediatric psychiatric epidemiologic studies, and no large study could be found specifically for anxiety disorders in this child and adolescent population. A thorough review of the epidemiologic studies that have been done on a pediatric population is available elsewhere (Orvaschel and Weissman 1986).

Anderson et al. (1987) used the DSM-III standardized Diagnostic Interview Schedule for Children in a comprehensive study of 792 11-year-old New Zealand children. The 1-year prevalence was 2.4% (19 cases) for simple phobia and 0.9% (7 cases) for social phobia. No cases of panic disorder were reported.

Rutter et al. (1970) screened the total population of 10- and 11-year-olds on the Isle of Wight. They reported a prevalence rate for "serious fears" of 0.7%, with animals, darkness, school, and disease phobias the most common. Of 2,199 children, 30 (1.4%) had "anxiety disorder" (which did not include the 7 cases of obsessional anxiety).

Kashani and Orvaschel (1988) reported a 6-month prevalence rate of anxiety disorders in 150 community-based 14- to 16-year-olds on the basis of structured psychiatric interviews using DSM-III criteria. In this study, 26 (17.3%) adolescents met diagnostic criteria for at least one anxiety diagnosis; and 13 (8.7%) were severe enough that they had functional impairment. Unfortunately, the prevalence of the specific anxiety diagnoses is not given except for the fact that 7 (4.6%) of the 13 severe cases had a phobic disorder. There is no reference to cases of panic disorder.

Epidemiologic studies with adults frequently report (by retrospective recall) a childhood onset to their symptoms. Three sites of the National Institute of Mental Health Epidemiologic Catchment Area Program of about 3,000 *adults* found the prevalence rate of panic disorder to be 0.6%–1.0%. These adults retrospectively recalled the onset of their symptoms to peak at 15–19 years of age, with some individuals reporting childhood onset (Von Korff et al. 1985). The prevalence rates cannot be verified until adolescent epidemiologic studies are done.

Etiology

The etiology of panic disorder and social phobia is unknown. Fears can manifest themselves from no previous experience (innate) or after a small stimulus (prepotent); others are more learned (Marks 1987). Typically, simple phobias have been understood as stemming from a fright from the first encounter with the phobic stimulus, which results in a classical conditioning paradigm.

However, agoraphobia and social phobia do not fit the classical conditioning paradigm well because of the lack of correspondence with a precipitating factor and the more generally high level of anxiety

(Solyom et al. 1986). Perhaps, in those two disorders, the normal developmental stage of fear of strangers, which usually disappears by age 4, may for whatever reason continue (i.e., not be completely unlearned or mastered).

Liebowitz et al. (1985) speculated that social phobic persons who exhibit heightened autonomic arousal during the stressful situations might have greater or more sustained increases in catecholamine release or might be more sensitive to normal stress-mediated catecholamine elevations. No family studies of social phobic patients have been done, although Torgersen (1979) noted that monozygotic twins were more concordant than dizygotic twins for social phobic features. Liebowitz (1987) speculated that cognitive factors and biological hyperreactivity combined with developmental, biological, and psychological influences may be involved in social phobia.

Crowe et al. (1983) reported an increased rate of panic disorder in 278 first-degree relatives of 41 probands with panic disorder compared with relatives of normal control subjects (17.3% versus 1.8%). No family studies for social or simple phobias could be located.

Treatment

Simple Phobia

Currently, there are no indications for psychopharmacologic interventions for childhood phobias. Phobic adults have not been responsive to tricyclic agents (Klein 1964) and barely if at all responsive to beta-blockers (Bernadt et al. 1980; Gaind et al. 1975). A review of the pharmacologic treatment of phobic disorders is available elsewhere (Noyes et al. 1986).

Childhood phobias have traditionally been treated with insight-oriented psychodynamic therapy. However, the most successful treatments appear to be the desensitization behavioral techniques based on a learning theory model. Systematic desensitization involves teaching a child relaxation techniques and then exposing the child to progressively more distressful stimuli. When the child feels anxious after exposure to the feared object, the relaxation technique is invoked. This technique can be done in vitro; however, in vivo is generally more successful (Ultee et al. 1982). A variety of other behavioral approaches have been reported. Mod-

eling behavioral techniques involves having the child watch another person performing the anxiety-provoking situation. Flooding involves directly exposing the individual to the stimulus until the severe anxiety subsides. Excellent reviews of the behavior treatments of phobias are available elsewhere (Barrios and Hartmann 1981; Marks 1987; Ollendick and Francis 1988).

Social Phobia

No systematic treatment studies could be found for children or adolescents with social phobia. In adult-controlled studies, pharmacotherapy and behavioral therapy have shown efficacy. Two controlled studies have shown phenelzine (a monoamine oxidase inhibitor) to be superior to placebo for social phobic patients (Liewbowitz et al. 1988; Shea-Gelernter et al. 1988). Four controlled studies suggest that monoamine oxidase inhibitors are superior to placebo for mixed diagnostic groups of agoraphobic patients with social phobia (for reviews, see Liebowitz 1987; Liebowitz et al. 1985). Although open trials of beta-blockers suggested their efficacy, they did not prove to be superior to placebo in the two small controlled studies (Falloon et al. 1981; Shea-Gelernter et al. 1988). The results of behavioral therapy using desensitization or exposure, social skills training, and cognitive restructuring suggest that those approaches are very effective. (For reviews, see Liebowitz 1987; Mattick et al. 1989; Ost et al. 1980.)

With so little information available about the phenomenology of social phobia in childhood, and even less available information on its treatment, it is speculative to suggest any specific regimen. It goes without saying that a complete diagnostic evaluation should include an assessment of the anxieties and stresses that an individual and family face. At this point, a combination of psychodynamic therapy with behavioral therapy should be considered in the treatment of social phobia.

Panic Disorder

Adult studies have reported the efficacy of tricyclic antidepressants, monoamine oxidase inhibitors, and benzodiazepines (Sheehan et al. 1981b; Spier et al. 1986) for panic disorder. There are no controlled studies for the psychopharmacologic treatment of panic disorder in children. Case reports have described the efficacy of imipramine (Herskowitz 1986; Sverd 1988; Van Winter and Stickler 1984). Others have reported cases of children in whom alprazolam (Herskowitz 1986; Van Winter and Stickler 1984) either alone or in combination with imipramine was found to be helpful. Pfefferbaum et al. (1987) found alprazolam (0.375–3.0 mg/day) to be useful for 13 children with cancer to treat the anticipatory and acute situational anxiety prior to painful procedures. (In these children, "panic" was used descriptively rather than as meeting DSM-III-R criteria.) Biederman (1987) reported on the success of clonazepam (0.5–3.0 mg) for three prepubertal children with "panic symptoms" with a coexisting diagnosis of either separation anxiety disorder or overanxious disorder. Biederman acknowledged the diagnostic shortcoming of the "panic-like symptoms" and warned that a positive pharmacologic response should not be equated with validating a diagnosis. Kutcher and MacKenzie (1988) extended this finding to four adolescents meeting DSM-III criteria for panic disorder. An open trial of clonazepam (fixed dose of 0.5 mg twice daily) significantly decreased panic attack frequency and severity as reported at day 7 and day 14. The authors concluded that clonazepam may be an effective treatment for panic attacks and baseline anxiety in adolescents and at a dose lower than that reported for adults. All four patients continued their medication for a mean of 4 months (range, 3–6 months).

These studies suggest that childhood onset panic disorder may be similar in its pharmacologic response to that seen in adults. More systematic studies are necessary.

Prognosis

Little is known about how children with simple phobia do later in life. In a 5-year follow-up study of an epidemiologic sample, Agras et al. (1972) found that of the 10 children diagnosed with phobias, all had either improved or recovered. Hampe et al. (1973) saw phobic children at 2-year follow-up and found that 80% were symptom free but that 7% had "serious fear reactions." Since simple phobias are amenable to behavioral treatment, one might hypothesize that treated patients would have a better long-term outcome.

Because these diagnoses have only recently received attention in children, the long-term outcome of children with social phobia and panic disorder is presently unknown. Whether children and adoles-

cents with social phobia or panic disorder develop anxiety or affective disorders as adults, therefore, is also unknown.

Research Issues

No specific studies exist in the literature describing either the phenomenology of social phobia in children and adolescents or its treatment. Research is clearly needed. Little more is known about panic disorder in childhood, since it was first described only in 1984. Both treatment and longitudinal studies are needed for this disorder. Simple phobias remain the best described of these diagnoses, but few studies distinguish between exaggerated fears and the clinical cases. Whether other treatments besides behavioral techniques are useful also deserves further attention.

References

Agras WS, Chapin HN, Oliveau DC: The natural history of phobia. Arch Gen Psychiatry 26:315–317, 1972

Alessi NE, Magen J: Panic disorder in psychiatrically hospitalized children. Am J Psychiatry 145:1450–1452, 1988

American Psychiatric Association: Diagnostic and Statistical Manual of Mental Disorders, 3rd Edition. Washington, DC, American Psychiatric Association, 1980

American Psychiatric Association: Diagnostic and Statistical Manual of Mental Disorders, 3rd Edition, Revised. Washington, DC, American Psychiatric Association, 1987

Anderson JC, Williams S, McGee R, et al: DSM-III disorders in preadolescent children. Arch Gen Psychiatry 44:69–76, 1987

Angelino H, Dollins J, Mech EV: Trends in the "fears and worries" of school children. J Genet Psychol 89:263–267, 1956

Barrios BA, Hartmann DP: Fears and anxieties in children, in Behavioral Assessment of Childhood Disorders. Edited by Mash EJ, Terdal LG. New York, Guilford, 1981, pp 196–262

Bernadt MW, Silverstone T, Singleton W: Beta-adrenergic blockade in phobic subjects. Br J Psychiatry 137:452–457, 1980

Biederman J: Clonazepam in the treatment of prepubertal children with panic-like symptoms. J Clin Psychiatry 48:38–41, 1987

Crowe RR, Noyes R, Pauls DL, et al: A family study of panic disorder. Arch Gen Psychiatry 40:1065–1069, 1983

Falloon I, Lloyd G, Harpin R: Real-life rehearsal with nonprofessional therapists. J Nerv Ment Dis 169:180–184, 1981

Gaind R, Suri AK, Thompson J: Use of beta blockers as an adjunct in behavioral techniques. Scott Med J 20:284–286, 1975

Gittelman R, Klein DF: Relationship between separation anxiety and panic and agoraphobic disorders. Psychopathology 17(suppl 1):56–65, 1984

Gittelman-Klein R, Klein DF: Adult anxiety disorders and childhood separation anxiety, in Handbook of Anxiety, Vol 1: Biological and Cultural Perspectives. Edited by Roth M, Noyes R Jr. New York, Elsevier, 1988, pp 213–229

Graziano AM, DeGiovanni IS, Garcia K: Behavioral treatment of children's fears: a review. Psychol Bull 86:804–830, 1979

Hampe E, Noble H, Miller LC, et al: Phobic children one and two years posttreatment. J Abnorm Psychol 82:446–453, 1973

Herskowitz J: Neurologic presentations of panic disorder in childhood and adolescence. Dev Med Child Neurol 28:617–623, 1986

Kagan J, Reznick JS, Clarke C, et al: Behavioral inhibition to the unfamiliar. Child Dev 55:2212–2225, 1984

Kagan J, Reznick JS, Snidman N: The physiology and psychology of behavioral inhibition in young children. Child Dev 58:1459–1473, 1987

Kashani JH, Orvaschel H: Anxiety disorders in mid-adolescence: a community sample. Am J Psychiatry 145:960–964, 1988

Klein DL: Delineation of two drug-responsive anxiety syndromes. Psychopharmacologia 5:397–408, 1964

Kutcher SP, MacKenzie S: Successful clonazepam treatment of adolescents with panic disorder. J Clin Psychopharmacol 8:299–300, 1988

Lapouse R, Monk MA: Fears and worries in a representative sample of children. Am J Orthopsychiatry 29:223–248, 1959

Leonard HL, Rapoport JL: Anxiety disorders in childhood and adolescence, in American Psychiatric Press Review of Psychiatry, Vol 8. Edited by Tasman A, Hales RE, Frances AJ. Washington, DC, American Psychiatric Press, 1989, pp 162–179

Liebowitz MR: Social phobia. Mod Probl Pharmacopsychiatry 22:141–173, 1987

Liebowitz MR, Gorman JM, Fyer A, et al: Social phobia: review of a neglected anxiety disorder. Arch Gen Psychiatry 42:729–736, 1985

Liebowitz MR, Gorman JM, Fyer AJ, et al: Pharmacotherapy of social phobia: an interim report of a placebo control comparison of phenelzine and atenolol. J Clin Psychiatry 49:252–257, 1988

Marks IM: Fears, Phobias, and Rituals. New York, Oxford University Press, 1987

Marks I: Blood injury phobia: a review. Am J Psychiatry 145:1207–1213, 1988

Marks IM, Gelder MG: Different ages of onset in varieties of phobia. Am J Psychiatry 123:218–221, 1966

Mattick RP, Peters L, Clarke JC: Exposure and cognitive restructuring for social phobia: a controlled study. Behavior Therapy 20:3–23, 1989

Maurer AL: What children fear. J Genet Psychol 106:265–277, 1965

Moreau D, Weissman M, Warner V: Panic disorder in children at high risk for depression. Am J Psychiatry 146:1059–1060, 1989

Noyes R, Chaudry DR, Domingo DV: Pharmacologic treatment of phobic disorders. J Clin Psychiatry 47:445–452, 1986

Ollendick TH: Reliability and validity of the revised fear survey schedule for children (FSSC-R). Behav Res Ther 21:685–692, 1983

Ollendick TH, Francis G: Behavioral Assessment and Treatment of Childhood Phobias. Behav Modif 12:165–204, 1988

Orvaschel H, Weissman MM: The epidemiology of anxiety disorders in children, in Childhood Anxiety Disorders. Edited by Gittelman R. New York, Guilford, 1986, pp 58–72

Ost JG, Jerremalm A, Johansson J: Individual response patterns and the effects of different behavioral methods in the treatment of social phobia. Behav Res Ther 19:1–16, 1980

Pfefferbaum B, Overall JE, Boren HA, et al: Alprazolam in the treatment of anticipatory and acute anxiety in children with cancer. J Am Acad Child Adolesc Psychiatry 26:532–535, 1987

Reznick JS, Kagan J, Snidman N: The physiology and psychology of behavioral inhibition in young children. Child Dev 51:660–680, 1986

Rosenbaum JF, Biederman J, Gersten M, et al: Behavioral inhibition in children of parents with panic disorder and agoraphobia. Arch Gen Psychiatry 45:463–470, 1988

Rutter M, Tizard J, Whitmore K: Education, Health and Behavior. New York, John Wiley, 1970

Shea-Gelernter C, Cimbolic P, Tancer ME, et al: Cognitive behavioral and pharmacological treatments for social phobia: a preliminary controlled study. Paper presented at the 141st annual meeting of the American Psychiatric Association, Montreal, Canada, May 1988

Sheehan DV, Sheehan KE, Minichiello WE: Age of onset of phobic disorders: a re-evaluation. Compr Psychiatry 22:544–553 1981a

Sheehan DV, Ballenger J, Jacobson G: Relative efficacy of monoamine oxidase inhibitors and tricyclic antidepressants in the treatment of endogenous anxiety, in Anxiety: New Research and Changing Concepts. Edited by Klein DF, Rabkin J. New York, Raven, 1981b, pp 47–67

Solyom L, Ledwidge B, Solyom C: Delineating social phobia. Br J Psychiatry 149:464–470, 1986

Spier SA, Tesar GE, Rosenbaum JF, et al: Treatment of panic disorder and agoraphobia with clonazepam. J Clin Psychiatry 47:238–242, 1986

Sverd J: Imipramine treatment of panic disorder in a boy with Tourette's syndrome. J Clin Psychiatry 49:31–32, 1988

Torgersen S: The nature and origin of common phobic fears. Br J Psychiatry 134:343–351, 1979

Ultee CA, Griffioen D, Schellekens J: Reduction of anxiety in children: a comparison of the effects of systematic desensitization in vitro and systematic desensitization in vivo. Behav Res Ther 20:61–67, 1982

Van Winter JT, Stickler GB: Panic attack syndrome. J Pediatr 105:661–665, 1984

Vitiello B, Behar D, Wolfson S, et al: Panic disorder in prepubertal children (letter). Am J Psychiatry 144:525–526, 1987

Von Korff MR, Eaton WW, Keyl PM: Epidemiology of panic attacks and panic disorder. Am J Epidemiol 122:970–981, 1985

Weissman MM, Leckman JE, Merikangas KR, et al: Depression and anxiety disorders in parents and children. Arch Gen Psychiatry 41:845–852, 1984

Chapter 31

Posttraumatic Stress Disorder

Robert S. Pynoos, M.D., M.P.H.
Kathi Nader, D.S.W.
John S. March, M.D., M.P.H.

The clinical symptoms of posttraumatic stress disorder (PTSD)—reexperiencing, avoidance, and emotional constriction—were alluded to as early as 1666 by Samuel Pepys, a victim of the Great London Fire (Daly 1983). While the symptom profile can be traced to Sigmund Freud's (1939/1964) construct of positive and negative symptoms associated with "psychic trauma" in early childhood, PTSD first appeared in DSM-III (American Psychiatric Association 1980) as an adult disorder, and only with DSM-III-R (American Psychiatric Association 1987) was specific reference to the symptom presentation in children made. There has been a tendency among adults, including child psychiatrists, to expect children to have less serious, more transient reactions than adults (Benedek 1985). Clinical descriptive studies of children exposed to disaster (Newman 1976), kidnapping (Terr 1979), and violence (Pynoos and Eth 1985) have revised current psychiatric opinion.

Over the past decade, the study of PTSD in children and adolescents has become progressively more systematic and rigorous. Comparable findings suggest that, while the childhood presentation is influenced by constitution, age, developmental phase, prior life experience, and family or cultural milieu, the disorder in children and adolescents is similar to that found in adults (Nader et al. 1990; Pynoos et al. 1987; Yule and Williams 1990). There are also important influences on the intrapsychic, interpersonal, emotional, cognitive, and neurobiological development of children.

Diagnostic Criteria and Clinical Findings

To establish the diagnosis of PTSD, four criteria must be satisfied: 1) exposure to a traumatic stressor (see Table 31-1), 2) reexperiencing, 3) avoidance or numbing of general responsiveness, and 4) persistent increased arousal. The criteria point to important clinical parameters in the phenomenology of the disorder. DSM-III-R criteria are given in Table 31-2.

The Stressors

The most recent empirical literature confirms the primacy of exposure; that is, that the objective magnitude of the stressor is directly proportional to the risk of developing the disorder (March 1990). At the same time, PTSD is shaped by the singular impact the trauma holds for each child.

Children are as susceptible as adults to the typical traumatic stressors. Some stressors are more common to children (e.g., kidnapping, serious animal bites, or severe injury due to burns, accidental shootings, or hit-and-run accidents). Criminal victimization is more commonly due to sexual molestation (Goodwin 1988) or physical abuse (Green 1983) than, for example, armed assault. Children are also at special risk of witnessing violence to a family member (e.g., rape or murder, suicide behavior, or spousal or sibling abuse).

Societal conditions influence the type of trau-

Table 31-1. The stressor criteria for a diagnosis of PTSD

Objective features
  Serious threat to life or physical integrity
  Witnessing serious threat, harm, or grotesque death
  In some cases, learning about violent threat/harm to close friend or relative
  Sudden destruction of home or community
Salient subjective responses
  Intense fear, terror; horror; coercion; helplessness
Magnitude
  Intensity; duration; suddenness; personal impact
  Sufficient to be markedly distressing to almost anyone
Range of stressors reported in children
  Kidnapping and hostage situations
  Exposure to violence, including terrorism, gang violence, sniper attacks, war atrocities
  Witnessing rape, murder, and suicide behavior
  Sexual or physical abuse
  Severe accidental injury, including burns, hit-and-run accidents
  Life-threatening illness; life-endangering medical procedures
  Train, airplane, ship, severe automobile accidents
  Major disasters

matic events to which children are likely to be exposed. Changing family patterns contribute to rates of intrafamilial sexual molestation. Occurrences around the world lead to significant exposures of children and adolescents to extrafamilial violence (e.g., inner-city violence, civil war atrocities, torture, or state terrorism). The impact of disasters varies, not only by the severity of, for example, an earthquake or hurricane, but by building standards, advanced communication and evacuation, or disaster recovery efforts.

Reexperiencing Phenomena

Traumatic experiences involve intense perceptual experiences and internal moment-to-moment appraisals of the threat and of possible intervention. The event may remain in prolonged active memory storage, constantly threatening to intrude and disrupt normal information processing (Horowitz 1976). Recurrent intrusive and distressing images, sounds, smells, or impressions often point to moments of extreme horror or helplessness during the event (e.g., the impact from a flying object; the sight of the stabbing; the murderous eyes of the rapist; or the sight of the motionless, blood-covered body). Additionally, children mentally return to their ex-

perience, searching for ways to offset traumatic helplessness or to alter the outcome in thought and fantasy. Intrusive images may incorporate mental modifications that minimize or protect the children from the full horror of the experience, for example, by altering their proximity to the immediate danger or freezing the action before irreversible injury.

Children's traumatic dreams include repetitions of aspects of the experience, depictions of other life-threatening dangers, or, over time, more general fearful dreams (e.g., in young children, of being pursued by monsters). These dreams depict direct personal threat, even death, or threat of harm to others, especially family members, and they renew emotions associated with the experience. A boy wounded after a massacre dreamed of his family dying in earthquakes. Recall of the dreams 2 years later produced persistent distress.

Traumatic play refers to the repetitive dramatization in play of elements or themes of the event (e.g., scenes of violence, or "tornado" or "earthquake" games). Children may involve siblings or peers in their traumatic play (Terr 1985). As with traumatic images, this play may recur because the child alters the action, for example, by compulsively catching the bullet before it strikes. With time, the incorporation of traumatic elements may impede play's normative uses. The degree to which children's traumatic play either provokes anxiety or provides temporary relief is related to a number of factors (Nader and Pynoos 1991). This play may go unnoticed by parents unless it is overtly distressing, dangerous, violent, suicidal, or sexually precocious.

Reenactment behavior refers to unconscious replication of some aspect of the experience. In younger children, the behavior may be an "action memory" (Furman 1973; Terr 1988). For example, a preschool child who was trapped in a well began to squeeze herself into small spaces. Adolescents, especially, may seek out opportunities to engage in reenactment behavior or thrill seeking and thus attempt to take command of the situation. The reenactment behavior of adolescents can be dangerous because of their access to guns, automobiles, and drugs. Traumatic reminders may elicit the behavior. Whenever one adolescent felt helpless to meet a personal demand or confrontation, he would lie down on the floor in the way he had during a hostage taking.

Traumatic reminders include the external circumstances of the event and the internal emotional and physical reactions of the child. Their role in

Table 31-2. DSM-III-R diagnostic criteria for posttraumatic stress disorder

A. The person has experienced an event that is outside the range of usual human experience and that would be markedly distressing to almost anyone, e.g., serious threat to one's life or physical integrity; serious threat or harm to one's children, spouse, or other close relatives and friends; sudden destruction of one's home or community; or seeing another person who has recently been, or is being, seriously injured or killed as the result of an accident or physical violence.

B. The traumatic event is persistently reexperienced in at least one of the following ways:
   1. Recurrent and intrusive distressing recollections of the event (in young children, repetitive play in which themes or aspects of the trauma are expressed)
   2. Recurrent distressing dreams of the event
   3. Sudden acting or feeling as if the traumatic event were recurring (includes a sense of reliving the experience, illusions, hallucinations, and dissociative [flashback] episodes, even those that occur upon awakening or when intoxicated)
   4. Intense psychological distress at exposure to events that symbolize or resemble an aspect of the traumatic event, including anniversaries of the trauma

C. Persistent avoidance of stimuli associated with the trauma or numbing of general responsiveness (not present before the trauma), as indicated by at least three of the following:
   1. Efforts to avoid thoughts or feelings associated with the trauma
   2. Efforts to avoid activities or situations that arouse recollections of the trauma
   3. Inability to recall an important aspect of the trauma (psychogenic amnesia)
   4. Markedly diminished interest in significant activities (in young children, loss of recently acquired developmental skills such as toilet training or language skills)
   5. Feeling of detachment or estrangement from others
   6. Restricted range of affect, e.g., unable to have loving feelings
   7. Sense of a foreshortened future, e.g., does not expect to have a career, marriage or children, or a long life

D. Persistent symptoms of increased arousal (not present before the trauma), as indicated by at least two of the following:
   1. Difficulty falling or staying asleep
   2. Irritability or outbursts of anger
   3. Difficulty concentrating
   4. Hypervigilance
   5. Exaggerated startle response
   6. Physiologic reactivity upon exposure to events that symbolize or resemble an aspect of the traumatic event (e.g., a woman who was raped in an elevator breaks out in a sweat when entering any elevator)

E. Duration of the disturbance (symptoms in B, C, and D) of at least one month.

Specify delayed onset if the onset of symptoms was at least six months after the trauma.

Source. Reprinted with permission from American Psychiatric Association 1987.

renewing physiologic and psychological reactivity accounts for some of the phasic nature of the disorder. The unexpected nature of reminders may re-evoke a sense of unpreparedness and lack of control. Common reminders include the following: circumstances (e.g., location, time, preceding activity, clothes worn); precipitating conditions (e.g., high winds after a tornado, arguing); other signs of danger (e.g., staring eyes); unwanted results (e.g., fixed and dilated eyes; blood); endangering objects (e.g., trees, broken glass, weapons); and a sense of helplessness (e.g., cries for help, crying, fast heartbeat, a sinking feeling, ineffectualness, or moments of aloneness). Normal school procedures and academic exercises may serve as reminders. For

example, a fire drill may re-evoke a sense of prior emergency, or a civics class discussion of judicial proceedings may kindle fear and rage over the trial of a father's assassin.

Avoidance or Numbing of General Responsiveness

The intensity of traumatic emotions (Janet's "vehement emotions" [see Van der Kolk and Van der Hart 1989]) or immediate "affective blocking" (Krystal 1978) may result in a "contraction of the ego" (Kardiner 1941) to protect against overwhelming emotions. Of the symptom criterion, emotional constriction is the most difficult to measure. The report of emotional numbing appears to be a developmentally acquired self-perception, perhaps beginning in early adolescence. Rather than reporting feeling "numb," younger children report not wanting to know how they feel, tell of feeling alone with their subjective experience, or describe efforts to keep an emotion from emerging (e.g., by going to sit alone). Parents are not always aware of this sense of aloneness or isolation because the child may continue to cling or to seek comfort.

Children may become avoidant of specific thoughts, locations, concrete items, themes in their play, and human behaviors that remind them of the incident. They may discontinue pleasurable activities to avoid excitement or fear. Traumatic avoidance may selectively restrict daily activity or may generalize to more phobic behavior. Diminished activity may represent a preoccupation with intrusive phenomena, a depressive reaction, an avoidance of affect-laden states or of traumatic reminders, or an effort to reduce the risk of further trauma. Active behaviors, such as disruptions in the classroom, may be attempts to distract from intrusive thoughts or anxieties (e.g., yelling out bad words when there are high winds after a tornado).

Although initial clinical attention suggested a relative absence of major amnesia in children, recent studies have demonstrated a variety of memory disturbances (Pynoos and Nader 1989a). These disturbances may be introduced during recall rather than perception or storage. Children may omit moments of extreme life threat (at times, screened by detailed recounting of other fearful moments); may distort proximity, duration or sequencing; may introduce premonitions; and may in other ways minimize their life threat. In fact, dissociative memory disturbances may also occur, especially in response to physical coercion, molestation, or abuse.

Loss of acquired skills presents differently at varying ages. Younger children may become less verbal, even mute, and enuretic; thumb sucking may appear or increase. School-age children may show more inconsistency in behavior and mood, report forgetting recently acquired knowledge, and perform household chores as they did when younger. Adolescents may report becoming confused like a younger child at being asked too many questions at once, and then cry or appear to have a tantrum. Posttrauma decisions by adolescents may express feelings of increased dependence or rejection of traumatic helplessness by deciding against

leaving home or pursuing college, or by premature efforts to enter adulthood.

Increased States of Arousal

Symptoms of increased arousal reflect both tonic and phasic physiologic activity, and they tend to reinforce the disorder. The child is "on alert," ready to respond to any environmental threat (Kardiner 1941). Especially in school-age children, physiologic reactivity may include somatic symptoms as a form of reexperiencing.

The sleep disturbance of PTSD refers to a serious disturbance in sleep physiology that may persist for months, even years. It may reflect relative changes in sleep stages and mark the onset of parasomnia. Environmental noises may easily arouse the child. Sleep may be fitful and not restful. Lack of sleep and intrusive phenomena can lead to problems in concentration that acutely disrupt school performance.

Hypervigilance and exaggerated startle may alter a child's usual behavior by leading to chronic efforts to ensure personal security or the safety of others. These recurrent "bouts" of fear may seriously change a child's emerging self-concept. Despite their absence from DSM-III-R criteria, incident-specific fears commonly occur in children. Fears are particularly evident during times of vulnerability (e.g., in the bathroom, at bedtime) or in response to specific reminders. Lastly, temporary or chronic difficulty in modulating aggression can make children act more irritable and easy to anger, resulting in a reduced tolerance of the normal behaviors, demands, and slights of peers and family members, and possibly in unusual acts of aggression or social withdrawal.

Differential Diagnosis

After a catastrophic event, treatment planning may entail multiple diagnoses. Attunement to the traumatic experience when considering the overall symptom picture may help to alleviate a misdiagnosis. Anxiety and depression are common adjuncts to PTSD, and the associated disorders may appear in conjunction with posttraumatic stress reactions. As secondary adversities accumulate or when an associated bereavement is accompanied by self-punitive thoughts and a pervasive anhedonia, major depression, a common cause of secondary comorbidity in PTSD, should be independently assessed and treated.

A wide range of anxiety symptoms commonly occur following traumatic experiences. During a traumatic event, children may experience increased attachment behaviors, such as worries about the safety of family members or friends. Specific symptoms of separation anxiety may be present (e.g., clinging in response to a traumatic reminder; morbid fears of catastrophe befalling family members; nightly checking on the safety of a family member; continued apprehension about a sibling being out of sight) and, at times, warrant a diagnosis of separation anxiety disorder. Prior threats to important attachment bonds (e.g., parental illness, separation, or divorce) or constitutional proneness may contribute to posttrauma anxiety reactions. Simple phobias, which result from frightening or injurious encounters, can be distinguished from PTSD by the absence of reexperiencing phenomena or tonic changes in arousal behavior.

Primary obsessive-compulsive disorder is easily distinguished from PTSD by the absence of an antecedent qualifying stressor. After violence, rituals such as checking door locks occur in response to obsessional concerns about safety. Obsessional thoughts of contamination or washing rituals may occur after sexual assault. Rarely, obsessive-compulsive disorder develops in the context of PTSD by secondary generalization. Schizophrenia, the delusional disorders, and brief reactive psychoses are readily distinguished from PTSD on the basis of minimal criteria overlap, dissimilarities between psychotic intrusive thoughts and PTSD reexperiencing, and the presence of otherwise intact reality testing in PTSD.

PTSD can exacerbate or even mimic the "externalizing" disorders. Before diagnosing oppositional-defiant disorder, conduct disorder, or attention-deficit disorder, it is important to rule out PTSD as the cause of the child's deteriorating school performance, alteration in attentional ability, new-onset irritability, or aggression. Traumatic events can also exaggerate preexisting conduct or learning disorders, which in turn can hamper the ability of the child to process traumatic experiences. Such reciprocal exacerbation may be especially characteristic of substance-abusing children, who may come to rely on drugs as a maladaptive coping strategy.

A history of recurrent or repeated trauma may serve as one of several complex antecedents to borderline personality disorder (Herman et al. 1989). Therefore, symptoms of self-mutilation, sexual or aggressive play, and suicidal behaviors in children with incipient borderline personality disorder or narcissistic or antisocial disorders should always raise the question of reenactment behavior and prompt a search for traumatic antecedents. Repeated victimization may result in demonstrable contradictory behaviors across different contexts— in their extreme, multiple personality or other dissociative disorders (Putnam 1985).

Children with other major Axis I diagnoses (e.g., major affective disorder or schizophrenia) may be at added risk of exposure to specific traumatic stressors because of psychotic, violent, or suicidal parental behavior or assortative mating with a violent or abusive partner. On the inpatient child psychiatry unit, care must be taken to identify previous traumatic experiences and yet to avoid overreading PTSD as responsible for the entire clinical picture. On the other hand, adolescents severely traumatized, for example, by a violent massacre, may demonstrate subsequent dangerous, volatile, and substance-abusing behavior that prompts a host of diagnoses without consideration of PTSD as a primary diagnosis. Severe trauma-avoidant behavior may lead the clinician away from exploring traumatic antecedents.

Finally, it is important to recognize the normative nature of many reactions, especially during the initial weeks following a traumatic event. The diagnosis of an adjustment disorder is appropriate when the stressor is less extreme than in PTSD, when the full criteria for PTSD are not met, and when there is less interference with personality functioning.

Course

The clinical course of PTSD is highly variable and depends on circumstantial factors (the stressor), child-intrinsic factors, coping and resiliency, and extrinsic influences that govern the recovery environment. In general, the more severe the stressor (i.e., intensity, duration, suddenness, personal impact), the more prolonged the course (Pynoos and Nader 1989b). For those stressors with mild exposure and minimum personal impact, the symptoms usually diminish within days or weeks of the event. For adults, acute PTSD tends either to resolve within 3–4 months or to follow a chronic course (Rothman and Foa 1989). A chronic course can be expected when the child has been exposed to multiple injury and mutilation, numerous losses of life, or massive destruction. Exposure to cries of distress or witnessing mutilation, associated feelings of guilt, and issues of human accountability intensify and complicate reprocessing. Involvement in civil or criminal proceedings, as an unavoidable reminder and an adjudicator of blame, necessarily influences trauma resolution. Multiple adversities significantly add to the risk of comorbidity and, therefore, to the seriousness of the clinical condition.

Chronic or repetitive trauma is associated with profound restrictions in emotional responsiveness, pervasive interpersonal avoidant behavior, atypical modulation of aggression, and increased frequency of dissociative responses. The cumulative effects may deeply affect character formation, including severe disturbances in object relations, affect tolerance, and impulse control. By the time children reach adulthood, there may be a multiplicity of clinical presentations.

The symptom complex, its duration, and resolution are affected by a number of adversities that commonly follow tragedies, including relocation, attendance at a new school, separation from siblings, involuntary unemployment of a parent, and increased financial difficulties. In addition, there may be continued medical procedures and rehabilitation for physical injuries and disability and a difficult reintegration back into school. Children exposed to war atrocities may also suffer malnutrition, deprivation, family disruption, loss, immigration, and resettlement.

When the violence or disaster results in the death of a family member or friend, there is an important interplay between traumatic and grief reactions. First, continued preoccupations with the circumstances of the death lead to alterations in the bereavement course. Second, psychological "dissynchrony" occurs among family members with different degrees of exposure (Pynoos and Nader 1990).

Developmental issues influence children's appraisals of threat, attribution of meaning, emotional and cognitive means of coping, toleration of their reactions, expectations about recovery, and effectiveness in addressing secondary life changes. Perhaps because of constitution, temperament, or experiential factors, children differ in the degree of general or specific avoidant behavior or cognitive discrimination between reminders and the original traumatic stimulus. Shy or anxious children may be inclined to overgeneralize or display more social reticence. Depressed children may suffer undue guilt. Impulsive children may increase their problematic behaviors. Children may experience a renewal of symptoms or concerns because of prior stressful events, and, in the case of prior trauma, these reactions may significantly prolong recovery.

The family environment has a major influence on a child's symptoms and course. The younger the child, the more appraisal of threat and subsequent symptoms reflects parental reactions. As in other child psychiatric disorders, parental psychopathology can adversely affect children's resiliency and adaptation. In addition, traumatized parents may excessively depend on their children for support, become overprotective, and prohibit temporary regressions or open communication.

Etiology

Social learning theory, psychoanalytic theory, and neurobiological hypotheses provide three interrelated etiologic views on the causal role of a traumatic stressor, the relative importance of personal impact, and the tenacity of the arousal disturbance. In the two-factor conditioning model derived from social learning theory, PTSD is conceptualized as a stimulus-driven anxiety disorder in which both classical (factor one) and instrumental (factor two) conditioning play important roles (Kirkpatrick et al. 1985).

In classical conditioning, the stressor or traumatic event, acting as an unconditioned stimulus, elicits an unconditioned (reflexive) response in the child characterized by extreme fear and the cognitive perception of helplessness. Associated cognitive, affective, physiologic, and environmental cues comprise conditioned stimuli, which in turn become capable of eliciting a conditioned response in the form of PTSD symptoms. Subsequently, via instrumental conditioning, affected children quickly learn by trial and error that avoidance behaviors and other rituals reduce arousal. These behaviors preclude the extinction of trauma-based anxiety and foster stimulus generalization (Fairbank and Nicholson 1987). Although the prominent place given cognitive cuing separates this model from more historical Pavlovian or stimulus-response models, the crucial point is that the stressor shapes the disorder, especially those aspects involving fear conditioning.

Psychoanalytic theory also provides a two-factor model based on Sigmund Freud's (1926/1959) definition of traumatic helplessness as arising out of a situation where "external and internal, real and instinctual dangers converge" (p. 168). The nature, content, and intensity of these two sets of dangers are influenced by type of exposure, developmental maturity, auxiliary parental ego functions (including as a protective shield), experiential growth, and intrafamilial context. Elements of the traumatic experience may be singled out for special meaning because of prior experience or current importance (A. Freud 1937/1965), and a special "traumatic configuration" (Lindy 1985) may result.

In this model, mentation about the traumatic experience is never merely replication but always includes modification. For example, "denial in fantasy," "identification with the aggressor," and "reparative fantasies" were proposed as special mental operations used by children to address external threat and damage (A. Freud 1937/1965). Current studies suggest that the mental reworkings are more complex than implied by traditional usage of these terms (Pynoos and Nader, in press). Furthermore, ongoing maturity and experiential growth may initiate a reprocessing, which, through new understandings and added symbolic attributions, alleviates or exacerbates prior traumatic reactions. Finally, by focusing on disruption of the synthetic functions of the ego, this model emphasizes the role trauma plays in shaping character (S. Freud 1939/1964) and in corresponding defects in the sense of self, which may leave children more vulnerable to future life stresses (Greenacre 1952).

Neurobiological hypotheses about PTSD emerge from complementary studies of neurophysiology and neurochemistry. Animal experimentation has elucidated the neurophysiology of the fear-enhanced startle pathway, its adrenergic neurochemistry, and the pharmacologic effects of various agents (Davis 1986). Because inhibitory modulation of the startle reaction does not mature until approximately 8 years of age, it may be most vulnerable to compromise by traumatic stress, as demonstrated in a preliminary study of children exposed to violent trauma (Ornitz and Pynoos 1989).

Both trauma-induced noradrenergic dysregulation and phasic autonomic hyperresponsivity to trauma-related cues may occur. Evidence includes a heightened sympathetic response to trauma-specific stimuli, increased levels of urinary catecholamines, reduced alpha$_2$- and beta$_2$-adrenergic platelet binding, and subtle dysregulation in hypothalamic-pituitary-adrenal axis function (Krystal et al. 1989). There appear to be more similarities between the biological profiles of PTSD and panic disorder, as distinct from that of depression (Friedman 1988). In addition, there is recent experimental support for a phasic opioid-mediated stress-induced analgesia that is reversible by naloxone (Pittman et al. 1990). Finally, central serotonergic metabolism is associated with the control of threat-mediated impulsivity in primates (Soubrie 1986) and perhaps with PTSD as well, thereby accounting for some of the similarities between PTSD and obsessive-compulsive disorder, a putative serotonergic disorder (March et al. 1989). Future investigations of traumatized children need to be rooted in a sound understanding of developmental neurobiology.

Treatment

Although there is a lack of comparative treatment studies, a sufficient body of clinical knowledge has emerged to suggest a number of therapeutic guidelines (Pynoos and Nader 1990; Terr 1989). Type and duration of interventions often hinge on the amount of therapeutic attention needed to address trauma-associated external and internal dangers, and the related child-intrinsic and child-extrinsic factors. Despite advances in treatment, the primary public health concern should remain preventing the precipitating events.

Psychological First Aid

The goal of psychological first aid is to provide important initial emotional relief through immediate psychological services and age-appropriate interventions. After disasters or community violence, the school classroom is an optimum setting to identify children at risk for posttrauma stress reactions, to minimize the fear of recurrence and its continued interference with everyday activities or tasks, and to normalize the recovery process. The classroom is also an excellent site for addressing issues of dying and loss (Pynoos and Nader 1988).

The Initial Consultation

Therapeutic approaches to PTSD nearly all incorporate cognitive and emotional reprocessing of traumatic memories. The traumatic cues, the emotional meaning, and the personal impact are embedded in the details of the experience, and the clinician must be prepared to hear everything, however horrifying or sad.

Special interview techniques may be necessary to assist children to explore their subjective experiences thoroughly, and to help them understand the meaning of their responses (Nader and Pynoos 1991; Pynoos and Eth 1986). The consultant can help legitimize children's feelings and reactions and assist them in maintaining self-esteem. Children are assisted in identifying traumatic reminders that elicit intrusive imagery, intense affective responses, and psychophysiologic reactions. At the end of the interview, these reminders can be shared with parents to enhance their support and understanding.

Brief Therapy

Although trauma debriefing and consultation will prove adequate for some children, many severely exposed and other at-risk children will require extended therapeutic interventions. Traumatic experiences may involve many complex traumatic moments, even within a short period of time. Therefore, brief therapy may be needed to permit adequate reworking, including reactions to the first anniversary. There is often a progression toward the most terrifying and irreversibly damaging moments. To avoid incomplete emotional processing (Rachman 1980), special attention is paid to omissions, spatial misrepresentations, and altered focus, which indicate a suppression of normal fears. Implosive therapy (flooding), in contrast to desensitization, was found to be effective treatment for fear-related memories in one child with PTSD (Saigh 1986).

Brief therapy also permits contextual understanding of the trauma within the life situation and culture of the child and family. In monitoring acute disturbances in the child's normal development, the clinician can attend to the impact on phase-specific narcissistic vulnerabilities, psychosexual conflicts, and cognitive confusions. By remaining attentive to secondary changes in the child's life, the clinician can assist the child and family so that they may improvise in their practical responses.

Psychopharmacology and Arousal Behavior

In the future, the select use of medications to reduce arousal behavior will likely become more central to the care of childhood PTSD. A trial of medication is indicated when there is a marked and persistent sleep disturbance; continued and disruptive hypervigilance or exaggerated startle; or chronic, distressing physiologic reactivity to trauma-related cues. The goal is to reduce chronicity, functional impairment, and alterations in identity.

As we enter a new era of psychopharmacology, the pharmacologic agent, dosage, and method of monitoring efficacy will be directed at select neurophysiologic effects. Each of the reportedly useful agents to attenuate PTSD symptoms (e.g., tricyclic antidepressants, propranolol, and clonidine) has a different effect on brain-stem mechanisms (Krystal et al. 1989). For example, antidepressants do not reduce fear-enhanced startle, whereas the other agents do. Clonidine both reduces baseline startle and is most potent at eliminating fear-enhanced exaggerated startle. Preliminary evidence suggests that clonidine can help normalize sleep physiology secondary to PTSD-induced parasomnia, leading to immediate behavioral improvement at home and in school. A report by Famularo et al. (1988) described the use of propranolol in treating the arousal symptoms in children exposed to sexual assault. Serotonin-uptake–inhibiting agents such as clomipramine and fluoxetine, which seem to enhance impulse control across a wide range of psychiatric disturbances, may also prove useful in the treatment of PTSD.

Family Intervention

The family provides the key site for reinstating a sense of safety and security. The supportive behaviors of family and friends have been found to contribute to children's recovery (Lystad 1984). Family members may require their own therapeutic intervention before they can adequately attend to their children's reactions. A primary goal of family therapy is to help family members validate and legitimize each other's psychological course, thereby facilitating continued mutual support. Otherwise, there can be estrangement or impatience among family members.

Parenting skills can be enhanced through education regarding posttraumatic stress reactions, realistic expectations about the course of recovery, differing psychological agendas, the management of temporary regressions, and the importance of encouraging open communication between the family and their children.

Group Interventions

The small group (Yule and Williams 1990) offers the opportunity to reinforce the normative nature of reactions and recovery (including grief), to share mutual concerns and traumatic reminders, to address common fears and avoidant behavior, to increase tolerance for disturbing affects, to provide early attention to depressive reactions, and to aid recovery through age-appropriate and situation-specific problem solving. Especially for adolescents, groups can be a valuable tool to address temporary disturbances in peer relationships.

Long-Term Treatment

Many of the techniques and goals of long-term treatment are common to child psychotherapy or psychoanalysis (Ruben 1974). However, recognition that emotional meaning remains embedded in the traumatic experience is a constant feature of therapeutic work. Attention is given to revised intrapsychic conflicts and narcissistic accommodations and to traumatic influences on character formation. As has been proposed for children of divorce (Wallerstein 1990), a pulsed intervention model may be appropriate, in which an acute phase of treatment is followed by planned periods of consultation. After the initial treatment, the clinician would see a child at certain critical junctures, determined by anticipated or reported reminders and by the child's developmental challenges.

Long-term treatment permits ongoing exploration of the meanings of overly concretized mental representations and gives the opportunity to expand a child's symbolic usage. With assistance, prior action memories can become part of the "verbal self" (Stern 1985). Previous trauma, including chronic or repetitive trauma, may lead to oscillations between past and present experiences. Intrafamilial violence requires attention to the preexisting relationship with the perpetrator, the deceased, or the injured; to issues of identification and conflict of loyalty; to bereavement; to vulnerabilities secondary to a chronic impulse-ridden environment; and to the stigma and legacy.

When the trauma is violent and massive, a critical goal is to return a child to a normal developmental path with a maturing conscience and, as a result, to help alleviate dangerous unconscious reenactment behavior, especially during adolescence. Intervention fantasies, especially unresolved revenge fantasies, and preoccupation with rescue or reparative roles need to be worked through. Resolution of associated psychosexual disturbances may further extend the treatment.

Children face a unique challenge in integrating their traumatic experience(s) into a developmentally changing inner model of the world (Horowitz and Zilberg 1983). The clinician who joins them in this demanding task faces his or her own unique challenge and reward.

References

American Psychiatric Association: Diagnostic and Statistical Manual of Mental Disorders, 3rd Edition. Washington, DC, American Psychiatric Association, 1980

American Psychiatric Association: Diagnostic and Statistical Manual of Mental Disorders, 3rd Edition, Revised. Washington, DC, American Psychiatric Association, 1987

Benedek EP: Children and psychic trauma: a brief review of contemporary thinking, in Post-traumatic Stress Disorder in Children. Edited by Eth S, Pynoos RS. Washington, DC, American Psychiatric Press, 1985, pp 1–16

Daly RR: Samuel Pepys and posttraumatic stress disorder. Br J Psychiatry 143:64–68, 1983

Davis M: Pharmacological and anatomical analysis of fear conditioning using the fear-potentiated startle paradigm. Behav Neurosci 100:814–824, 1986

Fairbank J, Nicholson R: Theoretical and empirical issues in the treatment of posttraumatic stress disorder in Vietnam veterans. J Clin Psychol 43:44–55, 1987

Famularo R, Kinscherff R, Fenton T: Propranolol treatment for children with acute post-traumatic stress disorder. Am J Dis Child 142:1244–1247, 1988

Freud A: Normality and pathology in childhood (1937). London, Hogarth Press, 1965

Freud S: Inhibitions, symptoms and anxiety (1926), in The Standard Edition of the Complete Psychological Works of Sigmund Freud, Vol 20. Translated and edited by Strachey J. London, Hogarth Press, 1959, pp 75–175

Freud S: Moses and monotheism (1939), in The Standard Edition of the Complete Psychological Works of Sigmund Freud, Vol 23. Translated and edited by Strachey J. London, Hogarth Press, 1964, pp 1–137

Friedman M: Toward a rational pharmacotherapy for post-traumatic stress disorder. Am J Psychiatry 145:281–285, 1988

Furman RA: A child's capacity for mourning, in The Child in His Family: The Impact of Disease and Death. New York, John Wiley, 1973, pp 225–231

Goodwin J: Posttraumatic symptoms in abused children. Journal of Traumatic Stress 1:4, 1988

Green A: Dimensions of psychological trauma in abused children. Journal of the American Academy of Child Psychiatry 22:231–237, 1983

Greenacre P: Trauma, Growth and Personality. New York, International Universities Press, 1952

Herman JL, Perry JC, van der Kolk BA: Childhood trauma in borderline personality disorder. Am J Psychiatry 146:490–495, 1989

Horowitz M: Stress Response Syndromes. Northvale, NJ, Jason Aronson, 1976

Horowitz M, Zilberg N: Regressive alterations of the self concept. Am J Psychiatry 140:283–284, 1983

Kardiner A: The Traumatic Neuroses of War. New York, Hoeber, 1941

Kirkpatrick D, Veronen L, Best C: Factors predicting psychological distress among rape victims, in Trauma and Its Wake. Edited by Figley C. New York, Brunner/Mazel, 1985

Krystal H: Trauma and affects. Psychoanal Study Child 33:81–116, 1978

Krystal J, Kosten T, Perry B, et al: Neurobiological aspects of PTSD: review of clinical and preclinical studies. Behavior Therapy 20:177–193, 1989

Lindy JD: The trauma membrane and other clinical concepts derived from psychotherapeutic work with survivors of natural disasters. Psychiatric Annals 15:153–160, 1985

Lystad M: Children's response to disaster: family implications. International Journal of Family Psychiatry 5:41–60, 1984

March J: The nosology of post-traumatic stress disorder. Journal of Anxiety Disorders 4:61–82, 1990

March J, Gutzman L, Jefferson J, et al: Serotonin and treatment in obsessive compulsive disorder. Psychiatr Dev 7:1–18, 1989

Nader K, Pynoos RS: Play and drawing techniques as tools for interviewing traumatized children, in Play, Diagnosis and Assessment. Edited by Schaeffer C, Gitlan K, Sandrgun A. New York, John Wiley, 1991, pp 375–389

Nader K, Pynoos RS, Fairbanks L, et al: Childhood PTSD reactions one year after a sniper attack. Am J Psychiatry 147:1526–1530, 1990

Newman CJ: Children of disaster: clinical observations at Buffalo Creek. Am J Psychiatry 133:306–312, 1976

Ornitz EM, Pynoos RS: Startle modulation in children with posttraumatic stress disorder. Am J Psychiatry 146:7, 1989

Pittman RK, van der Kolk BA, Orr SP, et al: Naloxone-reversible analgesic response to combat-related stimuli in posttraumatic stress disorder: a pilot study. Arch Gen Psychiatry 47:541–544, 1990

Putnam FW: Dissociation as a response to extreme trauma, in The Childhood Antecedents of Multiple Personality. Edited by Kluft RP. Washington, DC, American Psychiatric Press, 1985, pp 66–97

Pynoos RS, Eth S: Children traumatized by witnessing acts of personal violence: homicide, rape, or suicide behavior, in Post-traumatic Stress Disorder in Children. Edited by Eth S, Pynoos RS. Washington, DC, American Psychiatric Press, 1985, pp 17–43

Pynoos RS, Eth S: Witness to violence: the child interview. Journal of the American Academy of Child Psychiatry 25:306–319, 1986

Pynoos RS, Nader K: Psychological first aid and treatment approach to children exposed to community violence: research implications. Journal of Traumatic Stress 1:445–473, 1988

Pynoos RS, Nader K: Children's memory and proximity to violence. J Am Acad Child Adolesc Psychiatry 28:236–241, 1989a

Pynoos RS, Nader K: Prevention of psychiatric morbidity in children after disaster, in OSAP Prevention of Mental Disorders, Alcohol and Other Drug Use in Children and Adolescents (DHHS Publ No ADM-89-1646). Edited by Shaffer D, Philips I, Enzer NB. Washington, DC, U.S. Government Printing Office, 1989b, pp 225–271

Pynoos RS, Nader K: Children's exposure to violence and traumatic death. Psychiatric Annals 20:334–344, 1990

Pynoos RS, Nader K: Issues in the treatment of posttraumatic stress in children and adolescents, in The International Handbook of Traumatic Stress Syndromes. Edited by Wilson JP, Raphael B. New York, Plenum (in press)

Pynoos RS, Frederick C, Nader K, et al: Life threat and posttraumatic stress in school-age children. Arch Gen Psychiatry 44:1057–1063, 1987

Rachman S: Emotional processing. Behav Res Ther 18:51–60, 1980

Rothman B, Foa E: Subtypes of PTSD and duration of symptoms. Position paper prepared for DSM-IV Anxiety Disorders Work Groups, PTSD Subgroup, 1989

Ruben M: Trauma in the light of clinical experience. Psychoanal Study Child 29:369–387, 1974

Saigh PA: In vitro flooding in the treatment of a 6-year-old boy's post-traumatic stress disorder. Behav Res Ther 24:685–688, 1986

Soubrie P: Reconciling the role of central serotonin neurons in human and animal behavior. Behavioral and Brain Sciences 9:319–364, 1986

Stern D: The Interpersonal World of the Infant. New York, Basic Books, 1985

Terr L: Children of Chowchilla: study of psychic trauma. Psychoanal Study Child 34:547–623, 1979

Terr LC: Children traumatized in small groups, in Post-traumatic Stress Disorder in Children. Edited by Eth S, Pynoos R. Washington, DC, American Psychiatric Press, 1985, pp 45–70

Terr L: What happens to early memories of trauma?: a study of twenty children under age five at the time of documented traumatic events. J Am Acad Child Adolesc Psychiatry 27:96–104, 1988

Terr L: Treating psychic trauma in children. Journal of Traumatic Stress 2:3–20, 1989

van der Kolk BA, van der Hart O: Pierre Janet and the breakdown of adaptation in psychological trauma. Am J Psychiatry 146:1530–1540, 1989

Wallerstein JS: Preventive interventions with divorcing families: a reconceptualization, in Preventing Mental Health Disturbances in Childhood. Edited by Goldston SE, Yager J, Heinicke CM, et al. Washington, DC, American Psychiatric Press, 1990, pp 167–185

Yule W, Williams RM: Post-traumatic stress reactions in children. Journal of Traumatic Stress 3:279–295, 1990

Section VII

Eating and Nutritional Disorders

Chapter 32

Eating and Nutritional Disorders of Infancy and Early Childhood

Irene Chatoor, M.D.

eeding is an early and significant form of interaction between mothers and infants. The investigation of feeding and eating behaviors of parents and infants has been viewed as a way to understand the emotional development of infants in general and the syndrome of failure to thrive in particular. Feeding is a powerful criterion by which mothers validate their competence as a parent. Infants who gag every time food is placed in their mouth or who outright refuse to open their mouth are a challenge to any parent and professional.

In this chapter, I describe various disturbances in eating and growth in infants and young children and attempt to address the diagnostic, etiologic, and therapeutic issues involved.

Failure to Thrive

Failure to thrive is a common problem in pediatrics. The term describes infants and young children who demonstrate failure in physical growth, often with delay of social and motor development. The diagnosis is made when the child's decelerated or arrested growth results in weight and height measurements that fall below the third percentiles on the Boston Growth Standards or demonstrate a persistent deviation below the established growth curve across two major percentiles over time (Woolston 1985).

Since 1908, when Chapin alerted pediatricians to the failure of growth and development associated with poverty and institutional care of infants and young children, research has revealed an awkward and, in many cases, not useful dichotomy, namely the differentiation of organic from nonorganic failure to thrive. Spitz (1945) gave new importance to Chapin's observations of nonorganic failure to thrive, demonstrating severe retardation of growth and development in infants raised in institutions. He called this syndrome "hospitalism." Spitz (1946) also demonstrated that infants suffered from failure to thrive and "anaclitic depression" if their mothers were abruptly withdrawn when the infant was between 6 and 12 months of age. Goldfarb's (1945) classic studies of the serious developmental disturbances of adolescents raised in institutions added weight to the argument that relative maternal deprivation was also a cause of failure to thrive. Over the years, there have been a variety of studies exploring the social factors contributing to failure to thrive, and a number of labels have been used to describe the etiology of nonorganic failure to thrive: 1) environmental failure to thrive (Barbero and Shaheen 1967); 2) psychosocial deprivation (Caldwell 1971); 3) maternal deprivation (Patton and Gardner 1962); 4) deprivation dwarfism (Silver and Finkelstein 1967); and 5) psychosocial dwarfism (Reinhart 1979). Commonly, nonorganic failure to thrive is thought to reflect a failure or relative absence of adequate maternal care and warmth.

While these studies explored the etiology of nonorganic failure to thrive, there has been a gradual appreciation of the many organic diseases that can lead to failure to thrive. These two perspectives led to a diagnostic division of the disorder into organic failure to thrive and non-organic failure to thrive. More recently, several authors have suggested that there is a third category of failure-to-thrive patients who present a combination of organic and nonorganic factors in the etiology of their growth disturbance (Casey et al. 1984; Homer and Ludwig 1981).

In 1983, Chatoor and Egan reported nine cases of failure to thrive and dwarfism due to food refusal, suggesting that this condition should be considered a separation disorder. Later, because of its similarities with anorexia nervosa, the authors renamed the syndrome infantile anorexia nervosa (Chatoor 1989; Chatoor et al. 1988b). Because of the diversity in etiology of failure to thrive and the awareness of various types of nonorganic, organic, and mixed types of failure to thrive, a developmental classification of feeding disorders associated with failure to thrive was suggested by Chatoor et al. (1984a, 1985). This classification incorporates a multifactorial etiology of the failure-to-thrive syndrome, including various organic and inorganic factors that can create, exacerbate, or be a sequela of the infant's growth problem. The developmental classification of feeding disorders draws from Greenspan and Lourie's (1981) stages of early infant development and from Mahler et al.'s (1975) concept of separation and individuation. Chatoor et al. (1984a, 1985) has classified three stages of feeding development in which adaptive and maladaptive behaviors in both the infant and the mother can be identified: 1) homeostasis, 2) attachment, and 3) separation.

Disorder of Homeostasis

In the first few months of life, the infant's task is to achieve regulation of state. The infant must form basic cycles and rhythms of sleep and wakefulness, feeding, and elimination. The infant must progress from a state of nutritional equilibrium in utero and reflex sucking in the first few days of life to one in which the infant controls the onset and termination of feedings by signals of hunger and satiation. To feed successfully, the infant must achieve a state of calm alertness. This requires a sensitive caregiver who can interpret the infant's cues and facilitate the infant's regulation of sleep and feedings. Brody and Axelrod (1970), who studied the feeding interactions of 122 mother-infant pairs, described three

parental variables (i.e., high empathy, moderate control, and high efficiency) that seemed to characterize successful feeding.

Feeding problems at this stage of development can stem from constitutional characteristics or medical difficulties of the infant. For example, infants with a labile autonomic nervous system have more difficulty in self-regulation. They are easily overstimulated and are commonly referred to as "colicky." It takes a sensitive and patient caregiver to regulate the stimulation for these infants in a way that allows them to settle down to be able to eat or sleep. On the other hand, some infants are so passive or tire out so quickly during feedings that the caregiver needs to wake them up or stimulate them to feed adequately. Particularly infants with cardiac or respiratory disease who are compromised in their breathing and infants with immature oral motor development tire out easily during feedings. These feeding difficulties frequently generate anxiety in the mother or lead to maternal depression. The mother experiences a sense of inadequacy because mothers tend to measure their competence as mother by their ability to feed their infant. Anxiety and depression, in turn, make it more difficult for these mothers to read their infants' cues and to optimize their feedings. Mother and infant become caught in a vicious cycle that frequently leads to failure to thrive of the infant and frustration, anxiety, and depression on the part of the mother.

The importance of these early months for the infant's development of self-regulation was highlighted by Dowling (1977), who studied seven infants born with esophageal atresia. Dowling followed the first group of infants, who had only gastrostomy feedings for the first months of life, until they were big enough for corrective surgery. However, after surgery, with a functional esophagus in place, these infants had severe difficulties learning to suck, chew, and swallow; they seemed to have no awareness of hunger and lacked motivation to eat or to play. They demonstrated marked delays in motor and language development. Dowling found that all these sequelae could be prevented by offering simultaneous sham feedings to infants who were receiving gastrostomy feedings only.

As demonstrated in this study by Dowling (1977), early regulation of feeding has a significant impact on the overall motivation and drive of the infant. Successful self-regulation of the infant lays the foundation for the next stage of development, whereas feeding difficulties early in life frequently leave infant and mother vulnerable for problems during the following stages of development.

Disorder of Attachment

Having achieved some capacity for self-regulation, the adaptive infant is able to mobilize and engage caregivers in increasingly complex interactions. Around 6 weeks of age, the infant begins to smile in a social way in response to the adult's face. This is usually seen by the caregiver as a sign that the infant is evolving into a real person.

Attachment develops within a reciprocal relationship. Either partner can facilitate or impede the process. Evidence of good attachment behavior includes mutual eye contact, smiling, reciprocal vocalizations, and mutual physical closeness expressed through cuddling and molding. Because at this point of development many of the infant's interactions with the caregiver occur around feedings, regulation of food intake is closely linked to the infant's affective engagement with the caregiver. Consequently, if the infant is not engaged in a meaningful relationship with a primary caregiver, this lack of attachment is usually marked by lack of physical, cognitive, and emotional growth and development. As Spitz pointed out in his early studies on "hospitalism" (1945) and "anaclitic depression" (1946), the lack of a primary caregiver, as well as the sudden withdrawal of the mother in the first year of life, leads to loss of appetite, depressed affect, drop in developmental quotient, and failure to thrive. The literature on nonorganic failure to thrive has primarily concerned itself with the exploration of this particular type of failure to thrive. Much has been written about the mothers whose infants suffer from this type of growth disorder. Fishhoff et al. (1971) found that 10 of the 12 mothers with failure-to-thrive infants demonstrated character disorders, whereas only 2 were considered psychoneurotic. Evans et al. (1972) distinguished three groups of parents with failure-to-thrive infants and classified them along a continuous spectrum of psychopathology. In the first group, the mothers had experienced the loss of an important person and suffered from acute depression. The second group of mothers had experienced repeated losses, were living in deprived conditions, showed severe depression, and appeared helpless and overwhelmed. The third group showed the most severe psychopathology. In this group, the moth-

ers were openly hostile and very angry in their interactions with the infants.

Fraiberg et al. (1975) pointed to the lack of nurturing in the mother's own infancy and childhood and the lack of a satisfying relationship with another emotionally supportive person, leading to the mother's inability to nurture her infant. A more recent study by Main and Goldwyn (1984) systematically explored the mother's attachment behaviors from her childhood into adult life and revealed that the mother's experience of her own mother as rejecting was related to specific distortions in her cognitive processes, to rejection of her infant, and to the infant's avoidant insecure attachment as observed in the laboratory. Gordon and Jamieson (1979) studied attachment in 12 19-month-old infants who had been hospitalized during the first year of life with a diagnosis of nonorganic failure to thrive and compared them with matched control subjects. Six of the 12 nonorganic failure-to-thrive infants and 2 of the 12 control infants were classified as insecurely attached. In addition, nonorganic failure-to-thrive infants showed marked inhibition of affect during separation from the mother. In an unpublished study by Chatoor et al., 20 infants with failure to thrive classified as attachment disorders and 20 infants matched by age, sex, and race, who were feeding and thriving well, were observed with their mothers during 20 minutes of feeding and 10 minutes of play. In both situations, the clinical group showed less mother-infant reciprocity as evidenced in less visual and vocal engagement, less physical closeness, and lack of pleasure in their interactions. During the feeding, the mothers of the failure-to-thrive infants were less contingent to the infant's cues; during the play, they were more oblivious to the infant's activities.

As described in DSM-III-R (American Psychiatric Association 1987) under reactive attachment disorder of infancy, infants with this condition frequently do not receive well-baby care and may be seen by the pediatrician only when they present with a complicating physical illness, usually infections, or "vomiting," which frequently turns out to be rumination. Rumination is a symptom characterized by the regurgitation of food that may then be partially or completely rechewed, reswallowed, or expelled. Because rumination frequently occurs when the infant is alone, it is not easily diagnosed. The symptom appears to serve the infant both for self-stimulation and tension relief (Chatoor et al. 1984b). It is a rare but severe and often life-threatening disorder in this young age group.

These infants with attachment problems demonstrate poorly developed social responsiveness. They frequently avoid gaze and appear listless and apathetic. Some infants seem to be hypervigilant when scanning the environment but look away when approached closely. When these infants are picked up, they are unable to cuddle and mold to the caregiver's body. They usually show disturbance in body tone, being floppy or rigid. Many are developmentally delayed.

Treatment. Treatment for these infants needs to be individualized and should address the physical and developmental needs these infants present. Because of the complexity of the issues involved, a multidisciplinary team comprised of a pediatrician, nutritionist, physical or occupational therapist, social worker, and child psychiatrist is generally required. Because of the large number of personnel involved, the seriousness of the disorder, and the degree of malnutrition, hospitalization is frequently necessary for a thorough assessment and initiation of nutritional rehabilitation.

During the hospitalization, a number of specialized infant-directed interventions can be carried out. They include nutritional rehabilitation, developmental stimulation, and emotional nurturance. It is important to assign a primary-care nurse and to limit the number of alternate caregivers as much as possible to facilitate a special relationship between the primary caregivers and the infant. Improvement in the infant's health and affective availability can then be used to activate the mother and engage her in the treatment process to form an alliance for treatment after discharge. As Harris (1982) pointed out, ''[C]hanges in growth and cognition are frequently rapid; changes in personality and behavior are much slower. Recovery from growth failure does not indicate that the parent child relationship is adequate; it is only a first step'' (pp. 240–241).

Because the mothers frequently present with a variety of social and psychological disturbances, their problems need to be explored while work goes on with the infant. As pointed out above, many of the mothers have experienced deprivation or losses during their own childhood and avoid engaging in any therapeutic relationship. It is important to look for and identify whatever positive behavior a mother demonstrates toward her infant to use it as a building block to bolster her competence as a mother. Nurturance of the mother is a first and critical step in the treatment to facilitate her potential to nurture the infant. However, some mothers are too impaired to move beyond their distrust and avoidance of those who want to help. The hospitalization of the infant provides a critical time to assess whether the mother can be engaged in a therapeutic relationship or whether the infant needs to be placed in alternate care.

A critical period follows the hospitalization of the infant. Fraiberg et al. (1975) pointed to the importance of the parent-infant work to facilitate attachment. They emphasized the need to address the mother's painful experiences of the past—the ''ghosts'' from the mother's childhood—to free her from repetition of those same experiences and allow her to become a different mother to her infant. Not only the mother but also the family in its relationship to the mother-infant pair needs to be considered in the treatment process. Drotar et al. (1979) pointed to the role of the family as a stress-buffering or stress-producing system. These authors suggested a family-centered outreach program in the home. The approaches by both Fraiberg et al. and Drotar et al. are home-based because the social impoverishment and severe avoidance behavior of these mothers frequently make office-based interventions impossible. On the other hand, home-based treatment teams are not always available, and sometimes the pathology of the mother and the disruptions in the family are so severe that the infant needs to be placed in alternate care.

Disorder of Separation (Infantile Anorexia Nervosa)

Between 6 months and 3 years, both motoric and cognitive maturation propel the infant into the next stage of development, the period of separation and individuation, as defined by Mahler et al. (1975). As the infant begins to crawl away from the mother, he becomes increasingly aware of his separateness and must confront the developmental issues of autonomy versus dependency. His new cognitive capacities allow him to understand the relationship between cause and effect and he learns that his actions elicit certain reactions from his caregivers. This awareness becomes evident in the increasing intentionality and willfulness observed during this period of development. Part of this learning process involves somatopsychological differentiation (Greenspan and Lieberman 1980). The infant begins to understand and differentiate a variety of somatic sensations, such as hunger, satiety, or tiredness, from emotional feelings, such as anger, frustration, or need for affection. As with the earlier developmental stages, both partners of the dyad contribute to the successful resolution of this process: the infant, by clearly signaling his somatic versus his emotional needs; the caregiver, by reading the infant's signals correctly and by responding in a contingent manner. For example, when the infant cries, the mother then must determine whether the infant is hungry or tired or in need of comfort and affection. Her response needs to address the infant's expression of his specific need. When the infant stops eating, the mother must determine whether the infant is feeling sated, seeking attention, or expressing anger and refusing her food in protest.

A clinical report by Chatoor and Egan (1983) described the diagnosis and treatment of an eating disorder that starts during the developmental period of separation and individuation and is characterized by food refusal or extreme food selectivity and undereating. The authors called it a separation disorder and later, because of its similarities to anorexia nervosa, infantile anorexia nervosa (Chatoor 1989; Chatoor et al. 1988b). The onset of this disorder is usually between 6 months and 3 years, with a peak onset around 9 months of age. The parents report a history of the infant's food refusal or extreme food selectivity and undereating despite all efforts to increase food intake. The feeding difficulties stem from the infant's thrust for autonomy. Mother and infant become embroiled in conflicts over autonomy and control, which primarily manifest during the feeding situation. This leads to a battle of wills over the infant's food intake. Characteristically, parents mention that they have tried "everything" to get the infant to eat. This usually means coaxing, cajoling, bargaining, distracting, or forcing food into the infant's mouth. This separation-related conflict interferes with the infant's development of somatopsychological differentiation. The process of learning to distinguish somatic sensations, such as hunger and satiety, from emotional feelings, such as affection, anger, or frustration, is clouded by noncontingent responses by the parent to cues coming from the infant. As a result of this confusion of somatic and psychological feeling states, the infant's eating is controlled by his emotional experiences instead of by his physiologic needs.

A study of 42 infants with infantile anorexia nervosa and 30 control subjects, matched by age, sex, and race, revealed significant differences in mother-infant interactions between the two groups (Chatoor et al. 1988b). The feeding-disordered group demonstrated less dyadic reciprocity, less maternal contingency, more dyadic conflict, and a struggle for control. This group's play was also characterized by less dyadic reciprocity, more dyadic conflict, less maternal responsiveness to the infant's needs, and more maternal intrusiveness.

These results are striking in that the mothers and infants of the feeding-disordered group clearly lacked the reciprocal exchange observed in the control group. The mothers of the infants with infantile anorexia nervosa were more self-directed and controlling, as evidenced by their missing and overriding the infants' signals. These mothers and infants seemed out of step with each other during their interactions. However, the mother's negative affects of anger, frustration, and sadness were mirrored by her infant's affect.

Bruch (1973) and Selvini (1981) have postulated that such dysfunctioning in the mother-infant relationship underlies the development of anorexia nervosa during adolescence. From detailed reconstruction of the developmental histories of her patients, Bruch concluded that "there was a paucity of appropriate and confirming responses by the parent to signals indicating the child's needs and other forms of self expression" (p. 55). Bruch postulated that appropriate responses to cues coming from the infant, in the biological as well as in the intellectual, social, and emotional fields, are necessary for the child to organize the significant building blocks for development of self-awareness and self-effectiveness. If a mother's reactions are continuously inappropriate, neglectful, or oversolicitous, the child will experience confusion. Rizzuto et al. (1981) proposed that the abnormal development of the anorectic adolescent is caused by the mother's inability to reflect back to the baby the baby's own self—her inability to fulfill the mirror role of the mother as proposed by Winnicott (1971).

The clinical assessment revealed two major groups of mothers who seemed unable to negotiate successfully issues of autonomy versus dependency with their infants during this developmental phase of separation and individuation. One group of mothers seemed to be more comfortable with the infant's autonomy during play, but had developed a "blind spot" when dealing with the infant during feeding. These dyads had usually experienced some transient feeding difficulties when the infant was ill, which seemed to have "sensitized" the mother to worry excessively about the infant's growth. These mothers seemed to feel insecure in their roles as mothers and measured their competence by how well their infant ate. Because of high anxiety during feeding, these mothers were unable to read the infant's cues correctly. Feeding became an increasingly frustrating task as the toddler refused to eat in an effort to assert more autonomy and control.

Another group of mothers reported intense conflicts with their own mothers during their growing years, which had continued into the adult years. They had been informed of poor childhood eating behaviors by their mothers or remembered their own battles over food during childhood. While these young mothers appeared to make conscious efforts to be loving and caring toward their infants, they had trouble tolerating their own negative or angry feelings toward them because those feelings represented "being like my mother." They did not want to be harsh and punitive like their own mothers, but they lacked the emotional experience of alternative role models. To be the caring and understanding mother they had yearned for during their childhood, these mothers exerted great effort to feed their infants, unable to recognize the infant's grabbing for the spoon or holding on to the dish as a sign of an attempt at autonomy and self-feeding. They appeared overdetermined to feed the infant and to control the feeding, believing they were more effective than the infant in getting food into the infant's mouth. When the infants refused to open their mouths, cried, or arched their backs in protest, these mothers were unable to interpret these behaviors correctly; instead, they felt frustrated and rejected by the infants. They then exerted greater effort, bargaining, begging, and distracting the infants. However, the more effort that was expended, the more resistant the infants became to eating mother's way, and the more skillful they grew in eliciting mother's attention by refusing to eat. Although most mother-infant dynamics are described by these two groups, other mother-infant interactions indicated variations in conflict over issues of autonomy versus dependency.

The fathers of infants with separation disorders presented a varied picture. In some cases they were intimately involved in the care of the infants and were as much drawn into the infant's battle over food as were the mothers. In other cases, the fathers were physically or emotionally removed from the family and left the care of the infant almost completely in the hands of the mother. Some fathers were emotionally removed from the child as a result of marital conflict.

The infants were observed to have certain temperamental characteristics. They were persistent and frequently forceful or provocative in the expression of their wants. They seemed to observe their mothers carefully and displayed an "I dare you mother" attitude. Some showed mild delays in gross motor development but seemed cognitively age-appropriate.

Treatment. The focus of treatment is on improving communication between parents and infant to facilitate the development of somatopsychological differentiation as part of the separation and individuation process of the infant, using a two-step therapeutic approach. The first step involves a cognitive-behavioral intervention aimed at helping the parents understand and promote the development of their infant's somatopsychological differentiation. The therapist begins the intervention by meeting with both parents and explaining the developmental conflict of their infant around autonomy and dependency and the expression of this conflict through food refusal.

Following this explanation of the infant's developmental conflicts, the parents are provided with behavioral techniques aimed at allowing the infant more autonomy during feeding, while setting limits on inappropriate, maladaptive behaviors. They are given some general "food rules": 1) facilitate self-feeding by offering finger food, a second spoon, or a little dish with food while feeding the infant; 2) feed the infant at regular times and don't offer milk and snacks between these regular meal and snack times to allow the infant to experience hunger; and 3) limit mealtimes to 30 minutes and terminate the meal earlier if the infant refuses to eat, throws food or eating utensils in anger or to provoke the parents, or plays with the food without eating. To facilitate somatopsychological differentiation, to help the infant distinguish physiologic hunger for food from emotional hunger for attention, the parents are encouraged to separate mealtimes from playtimes. They are asked to deal with the infant's food intake in a neutral manner, neither playing games to distract the infant to sneak a bite into the infant's mouth nor exaggerating their approval for every mouthful the infant swallows. Parents also are requested to withhold expressions of disapproval and frustration if the infant eats little or nothing. They are reassured that experiencing hunger is the only means of inducing the infant to eat. In this way, the infant's attention can be focused on his inner state of hunger or satiety rather than on his interactions with the parents. Parents are encouraged to introduce a playtime after the meal to provide appropriately the attention they previously showered on the infant when trying to induce the infant to eat.

Parents who are able to support one another can apply this approach. Usually, within a few days or weeks, they succeed in changing the infant's eating pattern. However, parents who are in conflict with one another, or mothers who struggle with unresolved issues of control stemming from their own childhood, cannot follow through with these behavioral instructions. In these cases, the second phase of treatment can involve couples therapy to address these unresolved marital conflicts, or individual psychotherapy for the mother to deal with her struggle over control by bringing out the "ghosts" from her childhood, as Fraiberg et al. (1975) described so pointedly. Some parents are resistant to therapy and change. Long-term follow-up studies of these infants are not available.

Food Refusal

Food refusal is one of the most frequently listed feeding problems. However, the literature offers very little classification and understanding of this symptom. Palmer et al. (1975) proposed a descriptive classification of various feeding behaviors in young infants, ranging from mealtime tantrums to delay in self-feeding. Jenkins et al. (1980) examined the symptomatology of all 359 infants aged 6–36 months in a London borough and reported that 6% of the mothers complained of significant feeding problems in their infants in the first year of life. The rate climbed to 24% at 18 months of age, and 34% ate poorly at 36 months of age. Chatoor et al. (unpublished manuscript) studied the interactions of 140 healthy and well-thriving infants, ranging in age from 1 month to 3 years, and their mothers during feeding and during play. Between 12 and 18 months, these infants and mothers showed a striking increase in conflict and decrease in reciprocity during feeding. During this age period, most infants made the transition to self-feeding. Most of the conflict in these dyads centered around who was putting the food into the infant's mouth, the mother or the infant. Many infants protested through food refusal if not allowed enough autonomy dur-

ing the feeding. After 18 months, infants and mothers seemed to have resolved these conflicts, and mealtime again became a pleasurable time of being together, with the infants primarily feeding themselves. This time of transition to self-feeding is also most commonly the time of onset of the eating disorder described earlier in this chapter as infantile anorexia nervosa, which is characterized by food refusal. In addition, Chatoor et al. (1988a) observed another eating disorder characterized by partial or total food refusal that they described as a posttraumatic feeding disorder.

Posttraumatic Feeding Disorder

This feeding disorder is most commonly seen in infants who have been medically ill and undergone painful manipulation of the oral cavity by insertion of tubes or vigorous suctioning, infants who have experienced pain during feeding because of esophageal reflux, or infants who have had episodes of gagging and choking during feedings. Infants who have undergone these adverse experiences appear to associate anything related to feeding with pain, and they show fear in anticipation of feedings. Some show distress when approached with the bottle or become fearful when touched in the perioral area. In some infants, the anticipatory fear of being fed is so severe that they cry or vomit at the sight of the bottle or the high chair. On the other hand, parents report that when these infants are drowsy and unaware of what they are doing, they are able to drink from the bottle.

From a study of five latency-age children, Chatoor et al. (1988a) observed that one incident of choking was enough to lead to severe fear of eating and choking and resulted in food refusal. These children had many symptoms of a posttraumatic stress disorder. They were preoccupied with the fear of choking and dying; they dreamed of choking or dying, and they avoided any activity that could be associated with choking. One boy was afraid to play with his dog out of fear the dog's hair would get in his mouth and choke him. Some children were afraid to go to sleep out of fear of choking to death while asleep.

It is difficult to say what the inner experience of a young nonverbal infant may be. However, the affective expressions of infants provide a window to their inner life. The behavior of these infants clearly indicates that they are frightened and that the fear seems to be aroused by the anticipation of eating. Since this fearful refusal to eat frequently follows traumatic oral experiences, Chatoor et al. (1988a) called it a "posttraumatic feeding disorder." In severe cases, it is characterized by refusal to have anything put in the mouth, and in milder or in partially treated cases, by refusal to chew or swallow solid food. If the infant is forced to open his mouth and if he is fed forcefully, severe distress is triggered, and the infant becomes even more fearful the next time around. The infant seems to have no awareness of hunger or to be too frightened to respond to feelings of hunger. The infant will become dehydrated and would probably die unless fed via a nasogastric or gastrostomy tube.

In time, secondary complications of this feeding disorder develop. If the infant refuses to put anything in his mouth over weeks, months, or years, the infant does not get any practice in sucking, chewing, and swallowing. The infant does not learn how to move his tongue in the side of the mouth and move food effectively to the pharynx to be swallowed. When the infant finally relaxes enough and puts food in his mouth, the infant frequently chokes and gags. This evokes old fears, and again the infant refuses to accept food in his mouth.

In addition, as the infant matures cognitively, he becomes more aware of cause and effect in his interactions with his caregivers. The infant learns to anticipate certain emotional responses and behaviors in his caregivers, whether he refuses to eat or whether he puts some food in his mouth. The food refusal usually arouses such intense feelings of anxiety, anger, or frustration in the parents that they try anything to get the infant to eat. As mentioned earlier, this includes coaxing, cajoling, bargaining, pleading, distracting, or forcing food down the infant's throat. Since nothing seems to work, the parents become inconsistent, trying one method after another, and feeding time becomes a highly emotional experience for infant and parent. The infant learns to exercise control over the parents' emotions and behaviors by opening or closing his mouth. This severely interferes with the infant's development of somatopsychological differentiation—the ability to differentiate somatic sensations, such as hunger or satiety, from emotional feeling states, such as need for affection and feelings of anger and frustration (Chatoor et al. 1985). This process perpetuates the infant's inability to recognize feelings of hunger and to associate eating with the relief of hunger feelings. These secondary complications, the lack of development of oropharyngeal coordi-

nation and of somatopsychological differentiation, perpetuate the feeding disorder.

Treatment. All these factors must be considered if treatment is to be effective. As a first step, it is important to help the parents understand the dynamics of a posttraumatic feeding disorder to enable them to become active participants in the treatment. The treatment of the infant involves three steps.

The first step is desensitization. The infant needs to be desensitized to the fear of eating. This is best done after thorough exploration of what seems to trigger anticipatory anxiety about eating. Frequently, the sight of the bottle or placement in the high chair is enough to distress the infant. These objects should be presented without association of feeding until the infant is comfortable and can tolerate being exposed to them. If the infant is frightened to be touched around the mouth, the mother should engage in pleasurable touching until the infant is comfortable to open his mouth, mouth a toy, or take a spoon without fear. Since mothers are frequently so upset that it is hard for them to break out of the old patterns, it might be necessary to have a professional initiate the desensitization process and model for the mother. Once the infant is able to mouth toys without fear, food can be introduced.

The second step is introduction of food. It is important to begin with water to avoid the association of feeding with milk. Also, the infant might have difficulty with oropharyngeal coordination and gag or choke, and this is less likely and less harmful when drinking water. Once the infant is comfortable with drinking water, juices and then milk can be introduced. It is very important that a professional assess the infant's oromotor coordination and work with the infant directly on chewing and swallowing semisolids that dissolve in the mouth, before any type of food is introduced that can lead to choking. Again, a hierarchy of solid food should be followed. Meats should be kept until last to avoid frightening choking experiences. During this stage, the emphasis is on teaching the infant oromotor skills. Since many infants like to imitate, modeling the placing of food in the mouth and how to chew and swallow is very helpful. As long as the infant works on desensitization and oromotor coordination, there should be no emphasis on the amount of food taken in, and positive reinforcement should be liberally given to newly acquired skills (e.g.,

"You opened your mouth nicely, that was good chewing, good swallowing").

The third step is regulation of food intake. Once the infant has fairly good feeding skills, the experience of hunger becomes an important new goal. This is the time to work on the regulation of tube feedings. Continuous infusion at night and fewer bolus feedings during the day need to be considered to make the infant hungry at feeding time. It is important that the parents do not exert pressure on the infant to eat more and allow the infant to learn how to regulate his intake according to his physiologic needs. This usually requires time and patience.

In summary, the posttraumatic feeding disorder has become a new challenge in the treatment of severely ill infants. There are many intertwining factors that contribute to this severe feeding disorder, which requires an integrated multidisciplinary team approach for successful intervention.

Pica

Pica is defined as the persistent eating of a nonnutritive substance. Infants and toddlers with this disorder typically eat plaster, paint, paper, clothing, hair, animal droppings, sand, or pebbles. Lead poisoning is the most common complication associated with the eating of paint and plaster. Neurologic complications of chronic lead poisoning may present with hyperactivity, short attention span, mental retardation, and convulsive disorder. Another complication associated with pica is the development of a bezoar, a ball of hair, plant, or chemical substances undigestible in the intestinal tract. Tricho (hair) and phyto (plants) bezoars are reported to account for more than 90% of the reported clinical cases (DeBakey and Ochsner 1938). Millican et al. (1962), who surveyed the prevalence of pica in three groups of children aged 1–6 years, reported that pica occurred in 32% of a black low-income group, in 10% of a white middle- and upper-income population, and was the highest, 55%, in a group of children hospitalized for accidental poisoning. The prevalence of pica dropped sharply in both high- and low-income groups after the age of 3 years. Wortis et al. (1962) reported that of 272 premature infants they followed, at the age of 30–33 months, 22% had pica. Millican et al. (1968) postulated that the higher incidence of pica in the black low-income group was partially due to the cultural acceptance of pica. They observed that 63%

of mothers with children with pica had pica themselves. Gutelius et al. (1962) reported that 87% of children with pica had mothers and/or siblings with pica.

Various hypotheses have been proposed to explain the phenomenon of pica. Organic, psychodynamic, socioeconomic, and cultural factors have been implicated in the etiology of this disorder. There are reports of pica induced in rats by iron deficiency (Woods and Weisinger 1970) or by a low-calcium diet (Jacobson and Snowdon 1976). Some clinical studies confirm the association between iron deficiency and pica (Lanzkowsky 1959; Reynolds et al. 1968), whereas Gutelius et al. (1962) concluded that, in a double-blind study, intramuscular iron was no more effective than saline injection in reducing pica.

Millican et al. (1979) proposed a multifactorial etiology where constitutional, developmental, emotional, socioeconomic, and cultural factors interact with one another. They observed that young children with pica showed a high degree of other oral activities, such as thumb sucking and nail biting. Millican et al. interpreted the ingestion of inedible substances as a distorted form of instinctual seeking of gratification and as a defense against the loss of security caused by lack of parental availability and nurture. They reported that these children experienced frequent separations from one or both parents, followed by replacement by inadequate or rapidly changing caregivers. In addition, these authors observed that the mothers seemed to encourage oral gratification in response to the child's expression of anxiety or distress. They would offer the pacifier or the bottle with milk in response to the infant's distress as substitute for their personal involvement in helping the infant cope. Singhi et al. (1981) reported on the role of psychosocial stress in the families of children with pica and found a strong association with maternal deprivation, parental neglect and child beating, impoverished parent-child interactions, and disorganized family structure. Vermeer and Frate (1979) pointed to the cultural acceptance of pica, especially in rural families of African lineage.

Some studies stress the seriousness of this disorder. Millican et al. (1962) reported on the psychopathology associated with pica. As a group, the younger children were somewhat retarded in their use of speech and showed conflicts about their dependency needs and aggressive feelings. Half of the adolescents evidenced some degree of depression, and several had personality disorders, primarily passive-dependent type or borderline. Many continued to engage in other forms of oral activities (e.g., thumb sucking; nail biting; aberrant food habits; tobacco, alcohol, and drug abuse).

Treatment. Treatment must reflect the various factors that appear to contribute to this disorder. Lourie (1977) proposed a psychoeducational treatment approach. Mothers need to be taught the dangers of pica and helped to become more available to their children. This requires social support for the mothers who may be economically deprived and socially isolated. The mother's depression or other psychopathology needs to be addressed before the mother will be able to nurture and supervise her infant or toddler more adequately. The child's nutritional state needs to be monitored and iron deficiency and lead poisoning need to be treated if indicated.

References

American Psychiatric Association: Diagnostic and Statistical Manual of Mental Disorders, 3rd Edition, Revised. Washington, DC, American Psychiatric Association, 1987

Barbero GJ, Shaheen E: Environmental failure to thrive: a clinical review. J Pediatr 71:638–644, 1967

Brody S, Axelrod S: Anxiety and Ego Formation in Infancy. New York, International Universities Press, 1970

Bruch H: Eating Disorders, Obesity, Anorexia Nervosa, and the Person Within. New York, Basic Books, 1973

Caldwell BM: The effects of psychosocial deprivation on human development in infancy, in Annual Progress in Child Psychiatry and Child Development. New York, Brunner/Mazel, 1971, pp 3–22

Casey PH, Bradley R, Wortham B: Social and nonsocial home environments and infants with nonorganic failure to thrive. Pediatrics 73:348–353, 1984

Chapin HD: A plan of dealing with atrophic infants and children. Archives of Pediatrics 25:491–496, 1908

Chatoor I: Infantile anorexia nervosa: a developmental disorder of separation and individuation. J Am Acad Psychoanal 17:43–64, 1989

Chatoor I, Egan J: Nonorganic failure to thrive and dwarfism due to food refusal: a separation disorder. Journal of the American Academy of Child Psychiatry 33:294–301, 1983

Chatoor I, Schaefer S, Dickson L, et al: Nonorganic failure to thrive: a developmental perspective. Pediatr Ann 13:829–843, 1984a

Chatoor I, Dickson L, Einhorn A: Rumination: etiology and treatment. Pediatr Ann 13:924–929, 1984b

Chatoor I, Dickson L, Schaefer S, et al: A developmental classification of feeding disorders associated with failure to thrive: diagnosis and treatment, in New Directions in Failure to Thrive: Research and Clinical Practice. Edited by Drotar D. New York, Plenum, 1985, pp 235–258

Chatoor I, Conley C, Dickson L: Food refusal after an incident of choking: a posttraumatic eating disorder. J Am Acad Child Adolesc Psychiatry 27:105–110, 1988a

Chatoor I, Egan J, Getson P, et al: Mother-infant interactions in infantile anorexia nervosa. J Am Acad Child Adolesc Psychiatry 27:535–540, 1988b

DeBakey M, Ochsner A: Bezoars and concretions: comprehensive review of literature with analysis of 303 collected cases and presentation of 8 additional cases. Surgery 4:934–964, 1938

Dowling S: Seven infants with esophageal atresia: a developmental study. Psychoanal Study Child 32:215–256, 1977

Drotar D, Malone C, Negray J: Psychosocial intervention with families of children who fail to thrive. Child Abuse Negl 3:927–935, 1979

Evans SL, Reinhart JB, Succop RA: Failure to thrive: a study of 45 children and their families. Journal of the American Academy of Child Psychiatry 11:440–457, 1972

Fishhoff J, Whitten CF, Pettit MG: A psychiatric study of mothers of infants with growth failure secondary to maternal deprivation. J Pediatr 79:209–215, 1971

Fraiberg S, Anderson E, Shapiro V: Ghosts in the nursery. Journal of the American Academy of Child Psychiatry 14:387–421, 1975

Goldfarb W: Psychological privation in infancy and subsequent adjustment. Am J Orthopsychiatry 15:247–255, 1945

Gordon AH, Jamieson JC: Infant-mother attachment in patients with nonorganic failure to thrive syndrome. Journal of the American Academy of Child Psychiatry 18:251–259, 1979

Greenspan SI, Lieberman AF: Infants, mothers and their interaction: a quantitative clinical approach to developmental assessment, in The Course of Life, Vol 1: Infancy and Early Childhood. Edited by Greenspan SI, Pollock GH. Rockville, MD, National Institute of Mental Health, 1980, pp 271–312

Greenspan SI, Lourie RS: Developmental structuralist approach to classification of adaptive and pathologic personality organizations: infancy and early childhood. Am J Psychiatry 138:725–735, 1981

Gutelius MF, Millican FK, Layman EH, et al: Children with pica: treatment of pica with iron given intramuscularly. Pediatrics 29:1018–1023, 1962

Harris JC: Nonorganic failure to thrive syndromes, in Failure to Thrive in Infancy and Early Childhood. Edited by Accardo PY. Baltimore, MD, University Park Press, 1982

Homer C, Ludwig S: Categorization of etiology of failure to thrive. Am J Dis Child 135:848–851, 1981

Jacobson JL, Snowdon CT: Increased lead ingestion in calcium deficient monkeys. Nature 162:51–52, 1976

Jenkins S, Bax M, Hart H: Behavioral problems in preschool children. J Child Psychol Psychiatry 21:5–17, 1980

Lanzkowsky P: Investigation into the etiology and treatment of pica. Arch Dis Child 34:140–148, 1959

Lourie RS: Pica and lead poisoning. Am J Orthopsychiatry 41:697–699, 1977

Mahler MS, Pine F, Berman A: The Psychological Birth of the Human Infant. New York, Basic Books, 1975

Main M, Goldwyn R: Predicting rejection of her infant from mother's representation of her own experiences: implications for the abused abusing interactional cycle. Child Abuse Negl 8:203–217, 1984

Millican FK, Lourie RS, Layman EM, et al: The prevalence of ingestion and mouthing of nonedible substances by children. Clinical Proceedings of the Children's Hospital of the District of Columbia 18:207–214, 1962

Millican FK, Layman EM, Lourie RS, et al: Study of an oral

fixation: pica. Journal of the American Academy of Child Psychiatry 7:79–107, 1968

Millican FK, Dublin CC, Lourie RS: Pica, in Basic Handbook of Child Psychiatry, Vol 2: Disturbances in Development. Edited by Noshpitz JD. New York, Basic Books, 1979, pp 660–666

Palmer S, Thompson RJ Jr, Linscheid TR: Applied behavior analysis in the treatment of childhood feeding problems. Dev Med Child Neurol 17:333–339, 1975

Patton RG, Gardner LI: Influence of family environment on growth: the syndrome of "maternal deprivation." Pediatrics 30:957–962, 1962

Reinhart JB: Failure to thrive, in Basic Handbook of Child Psychiatry, Vol 2: Disturbances in Development. Edited by Noshpitz JD. New York, Basic Books, 1979, pp 593–599

Reynolds RD, Binder HJ, Miller MB, et al: Pagophagia and iron deficiency anemia. Ann Intern Med 69:435–440, 1968

Rizzuto AM, Peterson RK, Reed M: The pathological sense of self in anorexia nervosa. Psychiatr Clin North Am 4:471–487, 1981

Selvini PM: Self-Starvation. Northvale, NJ, Jason Aronson, 1981, pp 43–60

Silver H, Finkelstein M: Deprivation dwarfism. J Pediatr 70:317–324, 1967

Singhi S, Singhi P, Adwani GB: Role of psychosocial stress in the cause of pica. Clin Pediatr 20:783–785, 1981

Spitz R: Hospitalism: an inquiry into the psychiatric conditions of early childhood. Psychoanal Study Child 1:53–74, 1945

Spitz R: Anaclitic depression: an inquiry into the psychiatric conditions of early childhood. Psychoanal Study Child 2:313–342, 1946

Vermeer DE, Frate DA: Geophagia in rural Mississippi: environmental and cultural contexts and nutritional implications. Am J Clin Nutr 32:2129–2135, 1979

Winnicott DM: Playing and Reality. New York, Basic Books, 1971

Woods SC, Weisinger RS: Pagophagia in the albino rat. Science 169:1334–1336, 1970

Woolston J: Diagnostic classification: the current challenge in failure to thrive research, in New Directions in Failure to Thrive: Research and Clinical Practice. Edited by Drotar D. New York, Plenum, 1985, pp 225–233

Wortis H, Rue R, Heimer C, et al: Children who eat noxious substances. Journal of the American Academy of Child Psychiatry 1:537–547, 1962

Chapter 33

Anorexia Nervosa

David B. Herzog, M.D.
Eugene V. Beresin, M.D.

norexia nervosa is an elusive and note-worthy disorder among predominantly adolescent and adult females. It is characterized by extreme weight loss, body-image disturbance, and an intense fear of becoming obese. Preoccupation with food is a commonly associated feature.

As a diagnosis, anorexia nervosa has been recognized by the medical community since the turn of the century. Medical accounts of the physical manifestations of anorexia nervosa resemble Allbutt's (1910) highly detailed description:

> A young woman thus afflicted, her clothes scarcely hanging together on her anatomy, her pulse slow and slack, her temperature two degrees below the normal mean, her bowels closed, her hair like that of a corpse—dry and lustreless, her face and limbs ashy and cold, her hollow eyes the only vivid thing about her—this wan creature whose daily food intake might lie on a crown piece, will be busy with mother's meetings, with little sister's frocks, with university extension and with what you please else of unselfish effort, yet on what funds God only knows. (p. 398)

The anorexia nervosa of the 20th century has historical correlates in the religiously inspired cases of "anorexia mirabilis" of female saints such as Catherine of Siena (1347–1380), where fasting noted female holiness; in the "miraculous maids" of the Reformation period, such as Eva Fleigen in 1599, where fasting indicated humility and underscored purity; and in the cases of "fasting girls" such as Sarah Jacob, the "Welsh Fasting Girl," during the Victorian era (1870s), when the transition between fasting as a sign of divine intervention to fasting

as a medical and scientifically explainable state began (Brumberg 1988). The investigation of anorexia nervosa in the 20th century has focused on the psychological, physiologic, psychodynamic, psychosocial, and now the multidimensional factors and biological/genetic vulnerabilities of this population (Yates 1989).

In this chapter, we will focus on the diagnostic criteria, clinical findings, differential diagnoses, epidemiology, etiology, treatment, and prognosis of anorexia nervosa.

Diagnostic Criteria

Anorexia nervosa typically has its onset in an adolescent female who perceives herself to be overweight. Anorexic patients commonly lose weight by restricting their food intake and intensely exercising, by purging after meals by laxative or diuretic abuse and/or vomiting, or by use of diet pills. Anorexia nervosa occurs less frequently in males. While the course of anorexia in males does not differ from that of females, detection is often more difficult.

The DSM-III-R (American Psychiatric Association 1987) criteria for anorexia nervosa are given in Table 33-1.

Anorexia nervosa and bulimia nervosa may coexist. Anorexia nervosa can be referred to as "restrictive anorexia" when weight is lost secondary to restrictive dieting or as "bulimic anorexia" when weight is lost as a result of binging and purging behaviors. The etiologic relationship between bulimia nervosa and anorexia nervosa remains un-

Table 33-1. DSM-III-R diagnostic criteria for anorexia nervosa

A. Refusal to maintain body weight over a minimal normal weight for age and height, e.g., weight loss leading to maintenance of body weight 15% below that expected; or failure to make expected weight gain during period of growth, leading to body weight 15% below that expected.

B. Intense fear of gaining weight or becoming fat, even though underweight.

C. Disturbance in the way in which one's body weight, size, or shape is experienced, e.g., the person claims to "feel fat" even when emaciated, believes that one area of the body is "too fat" even when obviously underweight.

D. In females, absence of at least three consecutive menstrual cycles when otherwise expected to occur (primary or secondary amenorrhea). (A woman is considered to have amenorrhea if her periods occur only following hormone, e.g., estrogen, administration.)

Source. Reprinted with permission from American Psychiatric Association 1987.

clear at present. Approximately 30%–50% of patients with anorexia nervosa develop symptoms of bulimia during the course of the disorder (Russell 1979). However, Kassett et al. (1988) often observed that bulimia precedes the onset of anorexia nervosa. When contrasted with restrictive anorexic patients, bulimic anorexic patients tend to be more distressed, depressed, dramatic, impulse disordered, overwhelmed, and at risk of medical impairment (Edwin et al. 1988); their families differ as well (Humphrey 1989; Strober et al. 1982).

Clinical Findings

Physical Symptoms

Common physical complaints include cold intolerance, dizziness, constipation, abdominal discomfort, and bloating. Despite her malnutrition, the anorexic patient is often hyperactive; lethargy is worrisome as it may be an indication of cardiovascular compromise or severe depression.

Physical Examination

Anorexic patients often wear multiple layers of bulky oversized clothing and appear younger than their chronological age. Cachexia and breast atrophy are observable. The skin is often dry and may be yellow-tinged as a result of carotenemia. Bradycardia, hypotension, hypokalemia, growth of lanugo hair, alopecia, and edema of the lower extremities are common (Herzog and Copeland 1985). Dental enamel erosion and lesions on the dorsal surfaces of the hands, Russell's sign (Russell 1985), are noted in anorexic patients who vomit.

Medical Complications

Medical complications, which can be life threatening, are present in the cardiovascular, hematologic, gastrointestinal, renal, neurologic, endocrine, and skeletal systems of the body. Death is frequently ascribed to inanition, but the exact cause of death is often unclear.

Cardiovascular complications. Electrocardiographic abnormalities are common among anorexic patients and normalize on refeeding. Low voltage, bradycardia, T-wave inversions, and ST segment depression may be found separately or in conjunction with arrhythmias, such as supraventricular premature beats or ventricular tachycardia (with and without exercise). In a study of anorexic and bulimic adolescents, Palla and Litt (1988) found 95% of strict dieters and 92% of vomiting or purging anorexic patients to have heart rates of less than 60 beats per minute during their hospital stays. Prolonged QT intervals and emetine-induced myocardial damage may be life threatening (Gottdiener et al. 1978). However, anorexic patients may have a long-standing bradycardia because of regular exercise. It is not often possible to predict which of these patients will ultimately have life-threatening cardiac consequences.

Hematologic changes. Mild anemia may be expected in 30% of cases, and leukopenia may be present in up to 50% of cases (Myers et al. 1981; Warren and Van de Wiele 1973). Refeeding reverses these symptoms. Immune properties seem to remain intact despite nutritional deficiencies.

Gastrointestinal complications. Decreased gastric motility and delayed gastric emptying are often found in restrictive anorexic patients (Mitchell 1984). Metaclopramide has been used successfully to increase motility and to decrease dyspeptic flatulence. Although pancreatic disease is unusual, pancreatitis has been reported in some cases. Liver enzymes and amylase levels may be elevated, but will reverse with refeeding. Acute gastric dilatation and rupture, and acute vascular compression of the duodenum leading to intestinal obstruction, are rare but carry a high mortality rate (Saul et al. 1981).

Renal abnormalities. Dehydration results in increased levels of blood urea nitrogen. Polyuria is often experienced by this population and may be traced to the decrease in renal concentrating capacity and an abnormality in vasopressin secretion, which may produce a partial diabetes insipidus (Vigersky et al. 1975). Peripheral edema is present in 20% of cases, usually during refeeding and rehydration (Silverman 1983). Restoration of weight reverses these symptoms, although vasopressin abnormalities may persist for some time.

Neurologic abnormalities. Neurologic abnormalities are rarely found on physical examination. Crisp et al. (1968) noted electroencephalographic abnormalities in 10% of anorexic patients. Examination of the sella turcica by radiograph is normal in anorexic patients. In a small number of patients, computed tomography scans reveal cortical atrophy and ventricular dilatation, which may not be reversible on weight gain. Extensive neurologic assessment is usually unwarranted, except in atypical presentations such as in prepubertal females, male patients, and those patients who show no response to treatment.

Endocrine complications. A hallmark of anorexia nervosa is amenorrhea, which most often results from starvation-induced hypogonadism. However, in one-third of patients, amenorrhea predates weight loss and antedates weight recovery. Clinical signs of hypothyroidism may be present and are due to decreased levels of triiodothyronine. Primary hypothyroidism is rare, as serum thyroxine and thyroid-stimulating hormone levels are usually in the low normal to normal range. Patients diagnosed with diabetes mellitus may induce further complications by manipulating insulin intake to regulate their weight (Szmukler 1984; Szmukler and Russell 1983).

Skeletal complications. Clinical reports of skeletal fractures in anorexic patients have encouraged bone density studies of these patients. Rigotti et al. (1984) found that women with amenorrhea of at least 2 years' duration were at increased risk for osteopenia. Biller et al. (1989) found that those women whose onset of anorexia nervosa occurred prior to the attainment of peak bone formation (mid to late teens) and whose amenorrhea persisted into adulthood were at greater risk for osteopenia than women whose amenorrhea began in adulthood (even when the duration of amenorrhea was controlled). Hypercortisolism and hypoestrogenism are proposed causal mechanisms of the osteopenia and warrant further investigation.

Psychological Assessment

Anorexic patients constitute a heterogeneous psychiatric population. Psychopathology can range from mild to profound impairment within the confines of a single eating disorder to, in the more severe cases, comorbid characterological, mood, anxiety, or psychotic disorders (Hudson 1984). Some patients may appear high functioning at the first interview but demonstrate more impairment after a few sessions, or vice versa.

The prototypic anorexic patient manifests severe body-image distortion, interoreceptive disturbance, and a pervasive sense of ineffectiveness (Bruch 1973). Personality characteristics distinctive of anorexic adolescents include obsessional traits, interpersonal insecurity, minimization of emotional expression, perfectionism, excessive conformance, rigid control over impulses, heightened industriousness, competitiveness, envy, and responsibility (Crisp et al. 1979; Strober 1980). Ambivalence about sexual and emotional maturation, separation anxiety, and fears of being controlled are typical areas of conflict.

Comorbid depressive disorder is common in anorexic patients. In a study of 30 inpatient and 60 outpatient anorexic, bulimic, and mixed cases, 77% of patients received a lifetime diagnosis of major affective disorder, 13% displaying bipolar disorder and 63% displaying major depression (Hudson et al. 1983b). Similar results were found by Herzog (1984), in whose study 55% of anorexic patients met criteria for major depressive disorder. Onset of a major mood disorder and anorexia nervosa is variable: mood disorders can precede the onset, have simultaneous onset, or antedate the onset of anorexia nervosa (Hudson et al. 1983b; Piran et al. 1985). Anxiety disorders, kleptomania, substance abuse (among bulimic anorexic patients), obsessive-compulsive disorder, psychosis, and personality disorders are also prevalent comorbid disorders (Hudson et al. 1983b, 1984; Piran et al. 1985). In our experience, the most commonly associated personality disorders include avoidant, schizoid, borderline, and narcissistic disorders.

The affective range of expression for anorexic patients is highly variable. On a mental status examination, the anorexic patient may be cheerful and hyperactive; may be in a nearly hypomanic state; or may appear sad and hypoactive, seemingly depressed. Most often, the patient's affect is quite restricted, and depressive features, although not openly acknowledged, may be inferred from the patient's behavior (e.g., neurovegetive signs and symptoms, social isolation, or depressive thought content). Suicidal ideation may be present. There is usually a very limited capacity for self-observation, psychological mindedness, or personal insight. Cognitive impairments, such as diminished attention, concentration, and short-term memory, or obsessional thinking about food may be starvation induced.

Differential Diagnoses

Initial medical assessment must address the possibility that organic illness may mimic signs and symptoms of eating disorders (Palla and Litt 1988). Physical disorders that have clinical symptoms in common with anorexia nervosa include diabetes mellitus, Crohn's disease, colitis, thyroid disease, and brain tumors. Anorexia nervosa may occur concurrently with these disorders. Psychiatric disorders that may manifest weight loss and purging include conversion disorder, schizophrenia, and mood disorders (Garfinkel et al. 1983).

Epidemiology

Lifetime prevalence of anorexia nervosa, according to large-scale population and archival surveys, is in the range of 0.1%–0.7% (Cullberg and Engstrom-Lindberg 1988; Lucas et al. 1988). Student populations have also been researched extensively. Crisp et al. (1976) found a 1% incidence rate of current treated and untreated cases of anorexia in British private secondary school populations. Concern about weight and shape among young girls is widespread. Prevalence of dieting concern and weight preoccupation measured in children, grades 3–6, showed that 45% reported wanting to be thinner, 39% had tried to lose weight, and 6.9% scored within the high-risk of the Eating Attitudes Test (Maloney et al. 1989).

Approximately 90%–95% of anorexic patients are women. Age of onset ranges from 8 years to the mid-30s, with bimodal peaks at 13–14 and 17–18 years (Halmi et al. 1979). In the majority of studies, the socioeconomic/ethnic status of anorexic women is typically middle to upper-middle class, Caucasian families (Crisp et al. 1976; Jones et al. 1980; Mann et al. 1983; Szmukler 1983, 1985). However, a survey by Pope et al. (1987) indicated an equal presence of anorexia nervosa among lower socioeconomic status women in a nonstudent population. Prepubertal females are presenting with anorexia nervosa with increasing frequency.

Etiology

High-Risk Populations

Populations most likely to be at a greater risk for anorexia, because of occupational and recreational environments, include ballet dancers (Garner et al. 1985), male long-distance runners (Yates et al. 1983), and models (Garner et al. 1980). Each of these areas require highly focused attention on weight and appearance and on lean body mass. Other susceptible groups include chronically ill women with diseases such as cystic fibrosis (Pumariega et al. 1986); diabetic women (Rodin et al. 1986); women with mood disorders, particularly depression (Garfinkel et al. 1987); and those women in professions that require high standards of achievement and appearance (Herzog et al. 1985, 1987b). Although men comprise a smaller statistical group of anorexic patients, particular subgroups that are more susceptible to anorexia nervosa include athletes (e.g., runners, wrestlers) and male homosexuals (Andersen 1990).

Sexual abuse is commonly found among clinical populations of anorexic patients. Sloan and Leichner (1986) found 5 of 6 concurrent cases and 9 of 23 subsequent cases on an inpatient unit to have histories of incest and sexual assault. In a study of 158 patients admitted to an eating disorders unit, 60 reported a history of sexual abuse: 8 of the sexually abused patients were diagnosed with anorexia nervosa, and 24 of the sexually abused patients had a diagnosis of anorexia nervosa and bulimia nervosa (Hall et al. 1989).

Pathogenesis

Some theorize that anorexia nervosa results from an arrest at an early developmental stage (Bruch 1973). Others view anorexia nervosa as a family problem where the anorexic person is the identified patient. Still others view anorexia nervosa as a form of mood disorder.

Individual development. Anorexia nervosa can be understood psychodynamically as a compromise solution in the patient's attempt to solve intrapsychic conflicts. In this framework, eating symptoms are seen as a behavioral manifestation of emotional conflict. Purging behaviors such as exercising and vomiting help the anorexic patient achieve affective homeostasis by allowing the patient to rid herself of painful affect and retain a sense of accomplishment by furthering weight loss (Herzog et al. 1987a).

Early developmental theory hypothesizes that the infant's primary sense of trust in others, self-confidence, positive self-esteem, gratification of basic physical and emotional needs, and accurate awareness of her affective and interoceptive sensations are dependent on a caregiver, typically the mother, who responds appropriately to her child. The mother's empathic attunement to her child's experience and needs both confirms their validity and, hopefully, satisfies them, since the infant is virtually totally dependent on the mother. When a mother imposes her own needs on the child, there may be serious consequences in one or more areas noted above. This may be clearly demonstrated in the feeding situation. The mother who responds appropriately to her child's cues of hunger provides biological gratification and nurturance; demonstrates a validation of the child's interoceptive sensation of hunger; and instills a sense of confidence in the child that her needs can be recognized, understood, valued, and satisfied by another person. However, when feeding takes place out of the mother's need to quiet the child rather than in response to the child's hunger, the child develops uncertainty about her inner states and her ability to evoke care from her mother. The child feels drawn to comply with the needs of her mother to maintain the fragile connection between mother and child on which the child's survival depends (Bruch 1982). This very same compliance and primacy of the mother's needs over the child's can occur in many areas besides the feeding situation. When experiences of this kind occur repeatedly, the child feels increasingly controlled, exploited, and devalued,

although such feelings are often denied, repressed, or repudiated to protect the mother. The last thing the child wants to do is to alienate the mother on whom she depends. Moreover, anorexic mothers are generally caring, devoted women and are not easy targets for scorn or ingratitude.

From an object-relational viewpoint, the child's disturbed relationship with the mother affects the child's ability to integrate her own aggression and hostility. Typically, mothers of anorexic patients are self-sacrificing and almost saintly in their care of others and denial of their own impulses and appetites. However, the apparent selfless nurturance of others often derives from an inner sense of badness, unworthiness, and insecurity and, as such, is not really attuned to the particular needs of others as much as it is attuned to the needs of the self. Such mothers are always trying to make something right in the effort to elevate their own self-esteem, protect their inner fragility, and mitigate a pervasive fear of loss. They, like their daughters, are exquisitely sensitive to perceived rejection, hostility, and conflict. This particular mother-daughter relationship makes it exceedingly difficult for the child to own, experience, and express aggression directed toward the mother. The child must disavow or defend against her anger, since wielding it could result in loss of mother either by her destruction or by abandonment. Hostility is projected and relegated to the external world, which is then viewed as dangerous and untrustworthy.

Approval and affection are seen as volatile states that can quickly become negative and disapproving. Ambivalence is poorly tolerated. The anorexic patient protects herself from the hostile elements by using ritualistic algorithms of good and bad (Gordon et al. 1989; Kernberg 1975). Although the anorexic patient's aggression is fiercely denied and projected, unconsciously it is deeply recognized, further contributing to low self-esteem and profound guilt. Aggression serves the anorexic patient in a self-directed punitive attack combined with a passive-aggressive assault on the family. Concomitantly, the inner experience is not of aggression but rather of a noble, ascetic, powerful activity that makes her feel special and misunderstood by the world.

The self-psychological perspective views anorexia nervosa as a defensive structure mobilized to cope with a disruption in the parent-child relationship (Geist 1989). Maternal failures of empathy and admiration result in the daughter's overcompliance with maternal wishes. The anorexic patient turns to her father for her emotional needs of empathy and admiration. The closeness present between father and daughter prior to sexual maturity is threatened during adolescence (Geist 1984). The underdeveloped physical state of anorexic patients may be understood as an attempt to preserve this preadolescent relationship.

Parental roles. The family structure of many anorectic patients, with an overly giving mother who is unable to take for herself and a powerful father who demands deference and unquestioned loyalty, compounds the child's sense of ineffectiveness (Gordon et al. 1989). The daughter, faced with the prospect of a submissive and subordinate life in a world of powerful and demanding men, is bound by loyalty to mother and the father's expectations of outward harmony (Gordon et al. 1989). Sexual maturity represents separation from a dependent mother and attraction toward a man like her father. Anorexia nervosa, then, is a compromise between the Scylla of maternal loyalty and the Charybdis of male dominance.

Family perspectives. While anorexia nervosa has not been conclusively found to result from errant family dynamics, family theory and family therapy have been useful in providing support and a theoretical context for the anorexic family. Family theorists attempt to understand anorexia nervosa in the context of family interaction in which the family is the unit of dysfunction and treatment. The identified patient is viewed as the symptom-bearer of the larger family unit.

Anorexic families often present a happy, conflict-free exterior that serves to mask feelings of mistrust, lack of intimacy between parents, enmeshment, overprotection, rigidity, and lack of conflict resolution (Minuchin et al. 1978). The role of the anorexic daughter serves to divert attention from impending family conflict; her symptoms serve as a stabilizing force for the family. As the anorexic daughter becomes increasingly thin, she becomes increasingly dependent and inseparable from the family (Minuchin 1984).

Recent empirical work with anorexic and normal families focused on their dynamic-interactive characteristics has confirmed clinical findings relative to "normal" families. Humphrey (1989) found parents of anorexic patients to be both "too nurturant" and "too neglectful." Excessive nurturance seemed to undermine the daughter's efforts at separation;

her attempts at genuine self-expression were neglected.

Biological factors. Mood disorders are common among anorexic patients. Several studies have reported that 50%–60% of anorexic patients meet criteria for major depressive disorder and 35%–40% of anorexic patients meet criteria for moderate or endogenous depression (Cantwell et al. 1977; Hendren 1983; Herzog 1984; Piran et al. 1985). The relationship between eating disorders and mood disorders remains unclear. One hypothesis suggests that eating disorders are variants of mood disorders due to neurochemical similarities. Conversely, it has been hypothesized that mood disorders result from eating disorders as a consequence of starvation (Hatsukami et al. 1984; Swift et al. 1986). Controlled family studies of anorexic patients have suggested a familial risk of mood disorders among first- and second-degree relatives of anorexic patients (Biederman et al. 1985; Gershon et al. 1984; Hudson et al. 1983a; Rivinus et al. 1984; Strober et al. 1990; Winokur et al. 1980). Strober et al. (1990) and Biederman et al. (1985) observed that increased morbid risk for mood disorders in first- and second-degree relatives was associated with the depressed anorexic subpopulation.

The presence of comorbid mood disorders in anorexic patients and the presence of familial mood disorders have stimulated neurochemical research in this population. Starvation itself produces extensive changes in hypothalamic and metabolic functioning, although it has been difficult to elicit abnormalities specific to anorexia nervosa. Anorexia nervosa is associated with changes in the noradrenergic, serotonergic, dopaminergic, and opioid neurotransmitter systems and with alterations in neuromodulators such as corticotropin-releasing hormone (Fava et al. 1989). Abnormalities have been noted in the production of cerebrospinal fluid levels of 3-methoxy-4-hydroxyphenyglycol, 5-hydroxyindoleacetic acid, homovanillic acid, beta-lipotropin, adrenocorticotrophic hormone, beta-endorphin, *N*-terminal fragment of proopiomelanocortin in the cerebrospinal fluid, and cortisol. Differences in prolactin response to L-tryptophan in dieting states have suggested alterations in brain 5-hydroxytryptamine-mediated responses (Goodwin et al. 1987). Nearly all these levels normalize after weight gain. Anorectic patients also exhibit decreased levels of cerebrospinal fluid norepinephrine and an elevated ratio of cerebrospinal fluid to plasma arginine vasopressin for long periods after weight gain (Gold et al. 1983).

Genetic factors in the transmission of anorexia among family members are at the forefront of anorexia research. In a study of monozygotic and dizygotic female twins, Holland et al. (1984) found a concordance rate for anorexia nervosa of 55% in the monozygotic twins and 7% in dizygotic twins. Later, Holland et al. (1988) found a 56% concordance rate in monozygotic twins and a 5% rate in dizygotic twins. Studies of first- and second-degree relatives of anorexic patients have found a significantly greater rate of anorexia nervosa in relatives of anorexic patients as compared with relatives of control subjects (Strober et al. 1990). Theander (1970) reported a sibling risk rate of 6.6% for anorexia nervosa of 94 female anorexic patients. These studies provide a foundation for future genetic studies.

Biological research on mechanisms of perception and taste in anorexia nervosa have probed the relationship between eating behaviors and taste percepts. Hypotheses about this relationship have formulated that a possible abnormal sensory response to high-caloric foods may be responsible for binging behaviors. An alternate view, the set-point hypothesis, would expect emaciated anorexic patients to show initially elevated taste preferences for caloric-dense foods followed by decreased levels after nutritional therapy. Drewnowski et al. (1987) found elevated optimal sugar-to-fat ratios among both restrictive and bulimic anorexic patients compared with those of control subjects. Such differences seem to be consistent despite weight gain. Abnormal taste profiles may be an enduring characteristic in the eating-disordered patient.

Treatment

Treatment of anorexia nervosa presents unique difficulties to the clinician. Anorexia nervosa is largely an ego-syntonic disorder. Since anorexic patients, unlike bulimic patients, do not feel there is a problem, anorexic patients do not commonly present themselves for treatment except at the insistence of a pediatrician, parents, friends, or an athletic coach. Patients may not come for medical attention until they have lost considerable weight (Maloney and Klykylo 1983). Anorexic patients often present themselves to clinicians to elicit help in "getting their family off their back" or to assuage family member wishes. Frequently, there is a great deal of resistance or ambivalence toward treatment. In the face of divisive family issues, family members may attempt to split treating clinicians on the basis of differing opinions. Patients and their families may evoke reactions of anger, stress, and helplessness in medical personnel (Brotman et al. 1984).

Evaluation of the anorexic patient should incorporate a team approach and include medical, psychiatric, family, and nutritional assessments. The first decision in the evaluation of the anorexic patient is often to determine whether inpatient treatment is indicated.

The clinician should be observant of ways of connecting with the reluctant or openly resistant patient. Usually an initial alliance will draw on some area of acknowledged difficulty, including symptoms such as restlessness, irritability, insomnia, hyperactivity, cold intolerance, poor concentration, family problems, or social isolation. In the absence of an identified problem, the clinician may develop an alliance by empathetically understanding the patient's perspective, such as her irritation and indignation that others around her will not leave her alone. Her condition forces others to pay attention and take control when, paradoxically, this is precisely what she fears. This pattern of a literal starvation for attention and caregiving, coupled with stoic isolation and passive, fearful, or (rarely) overtly hostile resistance, is played out in dyadic control struggles, both within the family and with the clinician. Hence it takes an interplay of sensitivity, empathy, and respect for the anorexic patient, with steadfast adherence to basic "bottom lines" of physical safety, for an adequate psychological assessment or treatment plan to proceed.

Inpatient Treatment

Inpatient treatment of anorexia nervosa is mandated by the severity of the patient's physical and psychological status. Although hospitalization is frequent, it must be viewed as one phase in long-term treatment that will also include outpatient care.

Suggested criteria for hospitalization of child and adolescent anorexic patients by the American Academy of Child and Adolescent Psychiatry are listed in Table 33-2. Inpatient treatment should incorporate a comprehensive psychiatric evaluation, psychological testing, a thorough medical examination, appropriate laboratory studies to determine the patient's physiological status, and close observation (Andersen et al. 1985). During the course of hospitalization, it is necessary to utilize a team ap-

Table 33-2. Guidelines for hospitalization of anorexic patients

Justification for admission

A. Presence of severe or persistent medical complications that threaten life or health to the point of producing impairment that renders outpatient treatment management ineffective.

Complications include one major and three minor or six minor:

Major complications

Weight <25%, either emaciated or cathexic
Hypoglycemic syncope or "gray outs"
Severe fluid and electrolyte imbalance
Cardiac arrhythmia
Severe dehydration

Minor complications

Moderate malnutrition, weight <15%
Recalcitrant vomiting
Bradycardia
Hypotension
Hypothermia
Lanugo
Amenorrhea for three consecutive cycles
Acute starvation
Vasomotor instability
Minor electrolyte imbalance or hypoglycemia
Hypothyroidism
Nutritional anemia
Exercise-induced injury
Impaired renal functioning
Intestinal atony

B. Patient who has stabilized on medical or pediatric inpatient service and then transferred to child and adolescent psychiatric/eating disorder treatment.

C. Failure of 2 months of weekly outpatient medical psychotherapy to produce expected weight and appropriate eating patterns.

Source. Adapted from the American Academy of Child and Adolescent Psychiatry (Stevenson 1989).

proach that includes a psychiatrist, nutritionist, family therapist, recreational therapist, educator, and a nursing staff trained in eating disorders.

Hospitalization may take place on either a pediatric or a psychiatric ward. Patients with severe depression in the midst of a family crisis or in severe denial can be managed more effectively on a psychiatric ward; those primarily needing nutritional repletion can often be managed adequately on a medical ward. The decision of where to hospitalize must take into consideration the staff's ex-

perience and comfort in dealing with an anorexic patient.

One innovative treatment design is the pediatric day-care unit (Danziger et al. 1988), where parents are incorporated as part of the day-to-day interventions of patient care. This approach seeks to eliminate the punitive aspects of patient separation from parents. Parental supervision of patient behavior and meals aids in the restoration of positive patient and parental interaction as well as the natural hierarchy of the family.

The inpatient treatment program must have a nutritional rehabilitation protocol to which all treating clinicians can agree. The physician must explain the treatment regimen in detail to the patient prior to hospitalization. It is essential that the staff, the patient, and the family are aware that the administration of a feeding regimen is a life-saving act rather than a punishment. At the time of admission, a target weight for discharge should be established. The patient need not actually reach ideal body weight during the hospital stay; the target weight, however, must be sufficiently high to protect her from bordering on a medically precarious state. This target weight should be maintained for a period of time prior to discharge. Once the patient has reached the target weight, a reasonable range should be established to allow for day-to-day fluctuations. The success of the protocol depends on the ability of the staff to be open, honest, empathic, and firm (but not inflexible) in its implementation. Once weight is increased to a medically stable level, the patient will be more psychologically amenable to other treatment modalities.

Outpatient Treatment

The core outpatient treatment for anorexic patients should include ongoing medical management as well as individual and family psychotherapy. Additional treatment options include nutritional counseling, group therapy, and pharmacotherapy. The treatment program should be tailored to the needs of the individual.

Psychotherapy. The goal of psychotherapy is to help the patient achieve capacities for self-regulation that are more adaptive than her current eating behaviors. Patient and/or family denial of the existence of a "problem" poses a difficult barrier to the formation of a therapeutic alliance. Denial of the illness by the patient or her family is an attempt to maintain a solution, albeit costly, to deeply rooted feelings of despair and inadequacy. Initially, the therapist must establish trust by acknowledging the patient's ongoing pain and recognizing the multiple determinants of the disorder (social, psychopathologic, genetic, biological, behavioral, and familial). The patient is often reassured by the therapist's knowledge about eating disorders and relieved to find the therapist neither minimizing nor repulsed by her symptoms. The patient's physical condition may dictate close attention to medical status. Clinicians should create a "therapeutic envelope" designed to provide a safety net for the patient should weight or vital sign indications fall below agreed-on minimums (Hamburg et al. 1989). The continuation of outpatient therapy may be contingent on the patient's maintenance of a minimum weight requirement (Bruch 1988). The establishment of clear guidelines regarding weight, vital signs, and hospitalization should be established early in treatment and can be formalized as a contract. It is only in the context of medical safety that the work of therapy can proceed. Over the course of treatment, the therapist may be challenged to respect the psychological needs of the patient to be very thin while holding steadfastly to protecting the patient's life.

A wide range of psychotherapeutic theoretical orientations and techniques have been advocated in the treatment of anorexic patients, including supportive, psychoeducational, cognitive behavioral, and insight-oriented therapies. Within the latter category, considerable variations are demonstrated in object-relations, ego psychological, self psychological, or traditional psychoanalytic approaches. Bruch (1973) cautioned that some features of the latter method may be harmful to anorexic patients. The silence of traditional psychoanalytic therapy is often understood by the anorexic patient as rejection and interpretations as demands for compliance, thus perpetuating the destructive cycle of constant concessions to the needs of others. Although specific techniques may differ among the schools of psychotherapy, these approaches share common elements that are therapeutic for the anorexic patient.

Since a fundamental problem for the anorexic patient is thought to lie in the earliest dyadic relationship, the therapist must be aware of the patient's deep distrust of relationships and the motives of others. The therapist, above all, should be empathic and accurately mirror the perceived wants, needs, and feelings of the patient. The therapist

should be patient, undemanding, reliable, consistent, and flexible. The therapist should be able to bear the patient's affect and demonstrate that relationships can sustain anger, conflict, and misunderstanding (Beresin et al. 1989). Empathic failures should be seen as inevitable and be mended promptly. As in all psychotherapy, empathy and caring are perfectly consistent with limit setting. The therapist must make it abundantly clear that the success of psychotherapy depends on at least minimal nutritional and physical requirements.

Psychotherapy with the anorexic patient is a slow, difficult process. Transferential anger and evaluation, suspension of therapy, struggles with monetary and time boundaries, critical illness, and hospitalization may appear throughout the course of therapy. Erroneous assumptions are discussed, and conflicts that may be embodied in the eating symptom may be addressed. Over time, the experience of the therapist's consistency in care and boundary maintenance may also facilitate the patient's ability to make effective use of additional forms of treatment, such as group therapy or pharmacotherapy.

Group therapy. Group therapy for teenage anorexic patients is primarily an inpatient modality. Anorexic patients often express little interest in group treatment, because they are socially avoidant and mistrustful. Moreover, their competitiveness can result in substantial weight loss for group members unless there are at least a few members who are well on their way toward recovery. Group therapy has evolved from friendships formed by patients on inpatient units, the common feelings of being misunderstood, and the vulnerability of discharged patients in the 6- to 8-week postdischarge period (Rollins and Piazza 1981). The goal of an inpatient group is to decrease feelings of isolation in the patient by creating a nonthreatening environment in which patients may share thoughts and feelings (Piazza et al. 1983). Patients find it helpful to learn that their feelings and symptoms are also experienced by others.

Self-help groups provide information, support, and encouragement to patients with eating disorders and to their families. Often these groups provide an initial outreach to patients in the community. Outside contact is encouraged among members, and feelings of self-worth and hope are reinforced.

Family therapy. Family therapy may be introduced initially to the family as a means of support for coping with the adolescent's anorexia. It is not often clear that family problems have led to the onset or maintenance of the eating disorder. Yet families are uniformly affected by anorexia nervosa. Dealing with an eating-disordered family member is a severe challenge. Family therapies employ a variety of techniques with anorexic families.

One technique is the reformulation of the child's "disease" to the "symptom" of the family in distress. The identified patient is empowered to see herself as potentially well, while the communication and affective patterns of other family members are addressed and restructured to provide support and tolerable independence to the patient (Minuchin 1984; Minuchin et al. 1978).

Indirect interventions may be used as a means of modifying the family's rigid beliefs and behavioral patterns. Paradoxical interventions are used when an open approach to the problem is likely to provoke denial or resistance in the family. The patient may be urged not to give up her problems too quickly as the consequences of the behavioral change are outlined. The family's reaction may be to proceed in the opposite direction of the therapist's instruction in order to maintain control and integrity (Schwartz et al. 1985).

A similar strategy is to reframe the "problem" of the patient as the "solution" to the family's multiple dilemmas. The problem then becomes viewed as a larger familial process in which all members play a part rather than the individual's illness (Selvini-Palazzoli 1978).

Ultimately, family therapy seeks to provide a "safe" holding environment for the children and the parents of the nuclear family. One goal of therapy is to discuss openly and to resolve any issues of incomplete or nonexistent individuation and separation in the family. Issues from a parent's childhood family that are transferred onto the children may be addressed. The therapist may "parent" all members of the family so that greater self-understanding and individuation can be achieved (White 1983).

Pharmacotherapy. Psychotropic medication should be prescribed only in the context of psychotherapy. Drug therapy has been much more successful in the treatment of bulimia nervosa than anorexia nervosa (see Barber, Chapter 34, this volume). Cyproheptadine and amitriptyline have been found to be statistically superior to placebo in short-term inpatient trials, but clinical efficacy has yet to be demonstrated. Clomipramine, lithium, thiothixene, pimozide, sulpiride, and naloxone have yielded negative or equivocal results.

Pharmacotherapy, however, can be a useful adjunct to the treatment of these patients. All comorbid disorders (e.g., obsessive-compulsive disorder, depression, and anxiety disorder) should be treated with the appropriate medication. Sometimes the prescription of antianxiety agents prior to meals can be useful in helping the anorexic patient manage the anxiety she experiences when she consumes a modest amount of food. The use and effects of the medication should be explained carefully to the anorexic patient to avoid misconceptions by the patient and to encourage family support of the treatment. Medication should be monitored very closely. Initially, low dosages are necessary to reduce possible side effects in this exquisitely sensitive population.

The following principles are essential in prescribing psychotropic medication to malnourished, dehydrated, and physically compromised patients who are often resistant to such treatment:

1. Educate the patient and family about the use and effects of medication to avoid misconceptions by the patient and to encourage family support.
2. Select the specific target symptoms (e.g., obsessions, depression).
3. Start at a low dose and increase slowly.
4. Follow serum levels of the medication, vital signs, and electrocardiograms.

Additional treatment options. Anorexic patients often have difficulty negotiating the transition between inpatient and outpatient programs. Additional treatment options for this population include residential treatment programs, halfway houses, and day-hospital group treatment programs.

In some cases, it is unsafe or inappropriate for the anorexic patient to return to the parental home. Options for continued treatment in such circumstances may be residential treatment or, for older adolescents or young adults, a halfway house. In extreme cases in which parental contact repeatedly results in additional weight loss for the patient, it may be prudent to instruct or confront the parents, seek voluntary change of the patient's residence, pursue legal stabilization through parental retention of custody and appointment of a guardian, or facilitate voluntary or involuntary transfer of custody to the state (Harper 1983).

Piran and Kaplan (1989) developed a day-hospital group treatment program that incorporates the closely supervised and highly scheduled environment of an inpatient setting. This treatment program offers an alternative to hospitalization for those patients who require such a structured environment.

Prognosis

Outcome

Outcome for anorexia nervosa can be assessed in terms of mortality, weight, eating attitudes and behaviors, menstruation, and psychological functioning. In a 5-year posthospitalization follow-up, 70%–75% of anorexic patients were found to be better, 20%–30% of patients were chronically ill, and 5% had died (Herzog et al. 1988). At 10-year follow-up posthospitalization of 76 anorexic women, Eckert et al. (1990) found a mortality rate of 6%; none of the women died by suicide. Herzog et al. (1988) found 24% of deaths reported due to suicide in a survey of 13 outcome studies.

Eckert et al. (1990) found high percentages of psychological problems such as depression (80%), suicide attempts (21%), social and general anxiety (55%), obsessive thinking (66%), compulsive behaviors (70%), perfectionism (87%), and boredom (69%) at 10-year follow-up. Underweight women tended to reveal more psychological problems during the follow-up period ($r = .05$). Cantwell et al. (1977) found that 33% of the adolescent patients had an affective disorder at a mean follow-up of 4 years.

In a review of long-term outcome studies, Swift (1982) obtained conflicting results regarding the correlation between better prognosis and early onset (defined 11–15 years of age) of anorexia nervosa. At present, there are no clear predictors of outcome for the anorexic population.

Course

Approximately 50% of anorexic patients engage in binging and purging behaviors during the course of the disorder (Casper et al. 1980). Some restrictive anorexic patients will become bulimic during the process of recovery (Garfinkel and Garner 1982). As with normal-weight bulimic patients, bulimic anorexic patients commonly have comorbid substance abuse and kleptomania disorders (Bulik 1987).

Do anorexic patients ever get well? Beresin et al. (1989) reported on 13 severely ill anorexic patients who were assessed to be recovered on the basis of weight, menses, eating attitudes and behaviors, body image, and psychosocial and psychiatric adjustment. They found that among the factors most helpful in the process of recovery were "therapeutic" relationships with professionals, friends, and family members. The presence of another person who relates to the anorexic patient honestly, and who encourages expression of the patient's feelings, allows the anorexic patient to break out of her solitary existence, clarify distortions in perceptions and thought, develop trust in people, and, above all, consolidate a strong sense of self.

Research Issues

Research in anorexia nervosa is advancing. Investigating valid and reliable diagnostic criteria is a priority. Additional research is necessary to address the subdivision of anorexia nervosa in the upcoming DSM-IV into restrictive and bulimic subtypes 1) to explore the necessity of amenorrhea as a symptom for diagnosis and 2) to address the relationship between anorexia nervosa and bulimia nervosa.

Family studies of anorexia nervosa will increase our understanding of the role of genetics in the etiology of this disorder. Prospective longitudinal studies on the naturalistic course of anorexia nervosa will establish base rates of short-interval and long-term recovery, chronicity, and morbidity.

Further research on the neurochemistry (neurotransmitter systems and neuromodulators) of anorexia nervosa and on changes in the central nervous system that precede onset is necessary to increase our understanding of the pathophysiology and to develop more effective pharmacologic and cognitive-behavioral treatments (Fava et al. 1989).

Research on the pattern of sensory responsiveness to sweetness and fat during childhood or early adolescence may determine early psychobiological markers for eating disorders (Grill 1985). Investigations of osteoporosis, potentially a frequent and severe complication of anorexia nervosa, will elucidate mediating mechanisms and appropriate treatment.

The current financial climate in medical care mandates outcome research on the effects of 3- to 6-month hospitalization on weight maintenance, eating attitudes, and nutritional stabilization. Similarly, since psychotherapy is still the outpatient "treatment of choice" in anorexia nervosa, the exploration into how psychotherapy works (i.e., comparison of different psychotherapy techniques) is a high priority.

Conclusion

Anorexia nervosa is a life-threatening disorder that has come to the forefront of public attention over the course of the past 30 years. The successful collaboration of clinical researchers from all disciplines is necessary to further our understanding of the pathogenesis and treatment of this disorder.

References

Allbutt TC: Neuroses of the stomach and of other parts of the abdomen, in A System of Medicine, Vol 3. Edited by Allbutt TC, Rolleston HD. London, MacMillan, 1910, p 398

American Psychiatric Association: Diagnostic and Statistical Manual of Mental Disorders, 3rd Edition, Revised. Washington, DC, American Psychiatric Association, 1987

Andersen AE: Diagnosis and treatment of males with eating disorders, in Males with Eating Disorders. Edited by Andersen AE. New York, Brunner/Mazel, 1990, pp 133–162

Andersen AE, Morse CL, Santmyer KS: Inpatient treatment for anorexia nervosa, in Handbook of Psychotherapy for Anorexia Nervosa and Bulimia. Edited by Garner DM, Garfinkel PE. New York, Guilford, 1985, pp 311–343

Beresin EV, Gordon C, Herzog DB: The process of recovering from anorexia nervosa, in Psychoanalysis and Eating Disorders. Edited by Bemporad JR, Herzog DB. New York, Guilford, 1989, pp 103–130

Biederman J, Rivinus RM, Kemper K, et al: Depressive disorders in relatives of anorexia nervosa patients with and without a current episode of nonbipolar major depression. Am J Psychiatry 142:1495–1497, 1985

Biller BMK, Saxe V, Herzog DB, et al: Mechanisms of osteoporosis in adult and adolescent women with anorexia nervosa. J Clin Endocrinol Metab 68:548–554, 1989

Brotman AW, Stern TA, Herzog DB: Emotional reactions of house officers to patients with anorexia nervosa, diabetes, and obesity. International Journal of Eating Disorders 3:71–77, 1984

Bruch H: Eating Disorders. New York, Basic Books, 1973

Bruch H: Anorexia nervosa: therapy and theory. Am J Psychiatry 139:1531–1538, 1982

Bruch H: Conversations With Anorexics. Edited by Czyzewski D, Suhr MA. New York, Basic Books, 1988

Brumberg JJ: Fasting Girls: The Emergence of Anorexia Nervosa as a Modern Disease. Cambridge, MA, Harvard University Press, 1988

Bulik CM: Drug and alcohol abuse by bulimic women and their families. Am J Psychiatry 144:1604–1606, 1987

Cantwell DP, Sturzenberg S, Burroughs J, et al: Anorexia nervosa: an affective disorder? Arch Gen Psychiatry 33:1039–1044, 1977

Casper RC, Elke ED, Halmi KA, et al: Bulimia: its incidence and clinical importance in patients with anorexia nervosa. Arch Gen Psychiatry 37:1030–1040, 1980

Crisp AH, Fenton GW, Scotton L: A controlled study of the EEG of anorexia nervosa. Br J Psychiatry 114:1149–1160, 1968

Crisp AH, Palmer RL, Kalucy RS: How common is anorexia nervosa: a prevalence study. Br J Psychiatry 128:549–554, 1976

Crisp AH, Hsu RL, Stonehill L: Personality, body weight and ultimate outcome in anorexia nervosa. Br J Psychiatry 40:335–352, 1979

Cullberg J, Engstrom-Lindberg M: Prevalence and incidence of eating disorders in a suburban population. Acta Psychiatr Scand 78:314–319, 1988

Danziger Y, Carol CA, Varsano I, et al: Parental involvement in treatment of patients with anorexia nervosa in a pediatric day-care unit. Pediatrics 81:159–162, 1988

Drewnowski A, Halmi KA, Pierce B, et al: Taste and eating disorders. Am J Clin Nutr 46:442–450, 1987

Eckert ED, Halmi KA, et al: Outcome in anorexia nervosa. Paper presented at the International Conference on Eating Disorders, New York, April 1990

Edwin D, Andersen AE, Rosell F: Outcome prediction by MMPI in subtypes of anorexia nervosa. Psychosomatics 29:273–282, 1988

Fava M, Copeland PM, Schweiger U, et al: Neurochemical abnormalities of anorexia nervosa and bulimia nervosa. Am J Psychiatry 146:963–971, 1989

Garfinkel PE, Garner DM: Anorexia Nervosa: A Multidimensional Perspective. New York, Brunner/Mazel, 1982, pp 327–352

Garfinkel PE, Garner DM, Kaplan AS: Differential diagnosis of emotional disorders that cause weight loss. Can Med Assoc J 129:939–945, 1983

Garfinkel PE, Garner DM, Goldbloom DS: Eating disorders: implications for the 1990's. Can J Psychiatry 32:624–630, 1987

Garner DM, Garfinkel PE, Schwartz D: Cultural expectations of thinness in women. Psychol Rep 47:483–491, 1980

Garner DM, Garfinkel PE, Rockert W, et al: A prospective study of eating disturbances in the ballet. Psychother Psychosom 48:170–175, 1985

Geist RA: Psychotherapeutic dilemmas in the treatment of anorexia nervosa: a self-psychological perspective. Contemporary Psychotherapy Review 2:268–288, 1984

Geist RA: Self-psychological reflections on the origins of eating disorders, in Psychoanalysis and Eating Disorders. Edited by Bemporad JR, Herzog DB. New York, Guilford, 1989, pp 5–27

Gershon ES, Schreiber JL, Hamovit JR, et al: Clinical findings in patients with anorexia nervosa and affective illness in their relatives. Am J Psychiatry 141:1419–1422, 1984

Gold PW, Kaye W, Robertson GL, et al: Abnormalities in plasma and cerebro-spinal fluid arginine vasopressin in patients with anorexia nervosa. N Engl J Med 308:1117–1123, 1983

Goodwin GM, Fairburn CG, Cowen PJ: Dieting changes serotonergic function in women, not men: implications for the aetiology of anorexia nervosa? Psychol Med 17:839–842, 1987

Gordon C, Beresin E, Herzog DB: The parent's relationship and the child's illness in anorexia nervosa. J Am Acad Psychoanal 17:29–42, 1989

Gottdiener JS, Gross HA, Henry WL, et al: Effects of self-induced starvation on cardiac size and function in anorexia nervosa. Circulation 58:426–433, 1978

Grill HJ: Physiological mechanisms in conditioned taste aversions, in Experimental Assessments and Clinical Applications of Conditioned Food Aversions. Edited by Braveman NS, Bronstein P. Ann NY Acad Sci 443:67–88, 1985

Hall RC, Tice L, Beresford TP, et al: Sexual abuse in patients with anorexia nervosa and bulimia. Psychosomatics 30:73–79, 1989

Halmi KA, Casper RC, Eckert ED, et al: Unique features associated with the age of onset of anorexia nervosa. Psychiatry Res 1:209–215, 1979

Hamburg P, Herzog DB, Brotman AW, et al: The treatment resistant eating disordered patient. Psychiatric Annals 19:494–499, 1989

Harper G: Varieties of parenting failure in anorexia nervosa: protection and parentectomy, revisited. Journal of the American Academy of Child Psychiatry 22:134–139, 1983

Hatsukami DK, Mitchell JE, Eckert ED: Eating disorders: a variant of mood disorders? Psychiatr Clin North Am 7:349–365, 1984

Hendren R: Depression in anorexia nervosa. Journal of the American Academy of Child Psychiatry 22:59–62, 1983

Herzog DB: Are anorexic and bulimic patients depressed? Am J Psychiatry 141:1594–1597, 1984

Herzog DB, Copeland PM: Medical progress: eating disorders. N Engl J Med 313:295–303, 1985

Herzog DB, Pepose M, Norman DK, et al: Eating disorders and social maladjustment in female medical students. J Nerv Ment Dis 173:734–740, 1985

Herzog DB, Hamburg P, Brotman AW: Psychotherapy and eating disorders: an affirmative view. International Journal of Eating Disorders 6:545–550, 1987a

Herzog DB, Borus JF, Hamburg P, et al: Substance abuse, eating behaviors and social impairment of medical students. Journal of Medical Education 62:651–657, 1987b

Herzog DB, Keller MB, Lavori PW: Outcome in anorexia nervosa and bulimia nervosa: a review of the literature. J Nerv Ment Dis 176:131–143, 1988

Holland AJ, Hall A, Murray R, et al: Anorexia nervosa: a study of 34 twin pairs. Br J Psychiatry 145:414–419, 1984

Holland AJ, Sicotte N, Treasure J: Anorexia nervosa: evidence for a genetic basis. J Psychosom Res 32:561–571, 1988

Hudson JI, Pope HG, Jonas JM, et al: Family history study of anorexia nervosa and bulimia. Br J Psychiatry 142:428–429, 1983a

Hudson JI, Pope HG, Jonas JM, et al: Phenomenologic relationship of eating disorders to major affective disorder. Psychiatry Res 9:345–354, 1983b

Hudson JI, Pope HG, Jonas JM: Psychosis in anorexia nervosa and bulimia. Br J Psychiatry 145:420–423, 1984

Humphrey LL: Observed family interactions among subtypes of eating disorders using structural analysis of social behavior. J Consult Clin Psychol 57:206–214, 1989

Jones DJ, Fox MM, Babigian HM, et al: Epidemiology of anorexia nervosa in Monroe County, New York, 1960–1976. Psychosom Med 42:551–558, 1980

Kassett JA, Gwirtsman HE, Kaye WH, et al: Pattern of onset of bulimic symptoms in anorexia nervosa. Am J Psychiatry 145:1287–1288, 1988

Kernberg O: Borderline Conditions and Pathological Narcissism. Northvale, NJ, Jason Aronson, 1975

Lucas AR, Beard CM, O'Fallon WM, et al: Anorexia nervosa in Rochester, Minnesota: a 45-year study. Mayo Clin Proc 63:433–442, 1988

Maloney M, Klykylo WM: An overview of anorexia nervosa, bulimia, and obesity in children and adolescents. Journal of the American Academy of Child Psychiatry 22:99–107, 1983

Maloney M, McGuire J, Daniels SR, et al: Dieting behavior and eating attitudes in children. Pediatrics 84:482–489, 1989

Mann AH, Wakeling A, Wood K, et al: Screening for abnormal eating attitudes and psychiatric morbidity in an unselected population of 15-year-old schoolgirls. Psychol Med 13:573–580, 1983

Minuchin S: Family Kaleidoscope. Cambridge, MA, Harvard University Press, 1984

Minuchin S, Rosman BL, Baker L: Psychosomatic Families: Anorexia Nervosa in Context. Cambridge, MA, Harvard University Press, 1978

Mitchell JE: Medical complications of anorexia nervosa and bulimia. Psychiatr Med 1:229–255, 1984

Myers TJ, Parkerson MD, Witter BA, et al: Hematologic findings in anorexia nervosa. Conn Med 45:14–17, 1981

Palla B, Litt IF: Medical complications of eating disorders in adolescents. Pediatrics 81:613–623, 1988

Piazza E, Carni JD, Kelly J, et al: Group psychotherapy for anorexia nervosa. Journal of the American Academy of Child Psychiatry 22:276–278, 1983

Piran N, Kaplan AS (eds): A Day Hospital Group Treatment Program for Anorexia Nervosa and Bulimia Nervosa (Eating Disorders Monogr Ser No 3). New York, Brunner/Mazel, 1989

Piran N, Kennedy S, Garfinkel PE, et al: Affective disturbance in eating disorders. J Nerv Ment Dis 173:395–400, 1985

Pope HG, Champoux RF, Hudson JI: Eating disorder and socioeconomic class: anorexia nervosa and bulimia in nine communities. J Nerv Ment Dis 175:620–623, 1987

Pumariega AJ, Pursell J, Spock A, et al: Eating disorders in adolescents with cystic fibrosis. Journal of the American Academy of Child Psychiatry 25:269–275, 1986

Rigotti NA, Nussbaum SR, Herzog DB, et al: Osteoporosis in women with anorexia nervosa. N Engl J Med 311:1601–1606, 1984

Rivinus TM, Biederman J, Herzog DB: Anorexia nervosa and affective disorders: a controlled family history study. Am J Psychiatry 141:1414–1418, 1984

Rodin G, Daneman D, Johnston L, et al: Anorexia nervosa and bulimia in insulin-dependent diabetes mellitus. Int J Psychiatry Med 16:46–57, 1986

Rollins N, Piazza E: Anorexia nervosa: a quantitative approach to follow-up. Journal of the American Academy of Child Psychiatry 20:167–183, 1981

Russell GFM: Bulimia nervosa: an ominous variant of anorexia nervosa. Psychol Med 9:429–448, 1979

Russell GFM: Anorexia and bulimia nervosa, in Child and Adolescent Psychiatry: Modern Approaches. Edited by Rutter M, Hersov L. Oxford, UK, Blackwell Scientific, 1985, pp 625–637

Saul SH, Dekker A, Watson CG: Acute gastric dilatation with infarction and perforation. Gut 22:978–983, 1981

Schwartz R, Barrett MJ, Saba G: Family therapy for bulimia, in Handbook of Psychotherapy for Anorexia Nervosa and Bulimia. Edited by Garner DM, Garfinkel PE. New York, Guilford, 1985, pp 280–307

Selvini-Palazzoli M: Self-Starvation: From Individual to Family Therapy in the Treatment of Anorexia Nervosa. Northvale, NJ, Jason Aronson, 1978

Silverman JA: Clinical and metabolic aspects of anorexia nervosa. International Journal of Eating Disorders 2:159–166, 1983

Sloan G, Leichner P: Is there a relationship between sexual

abuse or incest and eating disorders? Can J Psychiatry 31:656–660, 1986

Stevenson K: Guidelines for peer review of child and adolescent psychiatric treatment including substance abuse disorders and eating disorders, in DuPrat MM, Stevenson K: Child and Adolescent Psychiatric Illness: Guidelines for Treatment Resources, Quality Assurance, Peer Review and Reimbursement. Washington, DC, American Academy of Child and Adolescent Psychiatry, March 1989

Strober M: Personality and symptomatological features in young, nonchronic anorexia nervosa patients. J Psychosom Res 24:353–359, 1980

Strober M, Salkin B, Burroughs J, et al: Validity of the bulimia-restrictor distinction in anorexia nervosa: parental personality characteristics and family psychiatric morbidity. J Nerv Ment Dis 170:345–351, 1982

Strober M, Lampert C, Morrell W, et al: A controlled family study of anorexia nervosa: evidence of familial aggregation and lack of shared transmission with affective disorders. International Journal of Eating Disorders 9:239–253, 1990

Swift WJ: The long-term outcome of early onset anorexia nervosa. J Am Acad Child Adolesc Psychiatry 21:38–46, 1982

Swift WJ, Andrews D, Barklage NE: The relationship between affective disorder and eating disorders: a review of the literature. Am J Psychiatry 143:290–299, 1986

Szmukler GI: Weight and food preoccupation in a population of English schoolgirls, in Understanding Anorexia Nervosa and Bulimia. Edited by Burgman GJ. Ross Laboratories, OH, Fourth Ross Conference on Medical Research, 1983, pp 21–27

Szmukler GI: Anorexia nervosa and bulimia in diabetics. J Psychosom Res 28:365–369, 1984

Szmukler GI: Implications of anorexia nervosa and bulimia. Br Psychiatry Res 19:143–153, 1985

Szmukler GI, Russell GFM: Diabetes mellitus, anorexia nervosa and bulimia. Br J Psychiatry 142:305–308, 1983

Theander S: Anorexia nervosa: a psychiatric investigation of 94 female patients. Acta Psychiatr Scand Suppl 214:1–194, 1970

Vigersky RA, Loriaux DL, Andersen AE, et al: Anorexia nervosa: behavioral and hypothalamic aspects. Clinical Endocrinology and Metabolism 5:517–535, 1975

Warren MP, Van de Wiele RL: Clinical and metabolic features of anorexia nervosa. Am J Obstet Gynecol 117:435–449, 1973

White M: Anorexia nervosa: a transgenerational system perspective. Fam Process 22:255–273, 1983

Winokur A, March V, Mendels J: Primary affective disorder in relatives of patients with anorexia nervosa. Am J Psychiatry 137:695–698, 1980

Yates A: Current perspectives on the eating disorders, I: historical, psychological and biological aspects. J Am Acad Child Adolesc Psychiatry 28:813–828, 1989

Yates A, Leehay K, Shisslak CM: Running: an analogue of anorexia? N Engl J Med 308:251–255, 1983

Chapter 34

Bulimia Nervosa

Joan K. Barber, M.D.

Definition

Bulimia[1] as a *symptom* has long been recognized as 1) an expected consequence of starvation; 2) a result of cultural attitudes toward food (e.g., the Roman vomitoriums); 3) a condition associated with brain disease; or even, 4) in rare instances, a symptom associated with a major psychiatric syndrome (e.g., schizophrenia).

Bulimia as a *syndrome* has been an "official" diagnosis only since DSM-III (American Psychiatric Association 1980). Sporadic outbreaks of bingeing and vomiting to control weight were anecdotally reported long before 1980. It is rare but still possible to find older women patients who report having binged and purged throughout most of their lifetime to control their weight. Bulimia, or bulimia nervosa, appears, in retrospect, to have been increasing since the late 1970s.

Diagnostic Criteria

DSM-III and DSM-III-R (American Psychiatric Association 1987) criteria for anorexia do not include bingeing or purging in the definition of the syndrome. Yet repeatedly one reads of patients still labeled anorexic despite extensive histories of bingeing and purging. The diagnosis of anorexia nervosa should be limited to individuals who practice food restriction only (with or without excessive exercise). Bulimia nervosa should be reserved for patients who binge and purge. Both groups of patients share intense obsessions and preoccupations with food, weight, and body contour. Specialists who work with patients with eating disorders increasingly recognize that eating disorders represent a continuum of symptoms, and that the division into anorexia nervosa, bulimia nervosa, and eating disorders not otherwise specified may be found to be more arbitrary than actual (Abraham and Beumont 1982; Casper et al. 1980). The DSM-III-R (American Psychiatric Association 1987) criteria for bulimia nervosa are given in Table 34-1.

Clinical Findings

Clinical History

Bingeing patients come in all sizes and ages. The majority of bulimia nervosa patients are postadolescent and older. Among the obese patients are individuals who binge without purging. This group is most frequently older individuals who repeatedly have used very low-caloric commercial diet plans.

Most studies report that bulimia nervosa occurs at a later age than anorexia nervosa. The history of an episode of anorexia nervosa, anorecticlike episodes, or a severely restrictive (less than 1,000 kcal/day) diet is found in most bulimic patients (J. K. Barber, unpublished data, 1990). Only rarely does the binge-purge syndrome begin de novo. The anorecticlike syndrome may last 6 months or less;

---

[1]Bulimia [Greek: *bous* (ox) plus *limos* (hunger)] is defined as an abnormal increase in the sense of hunger. It is of interest that *bulimia* has become the primary word used to describe this behavior. *Cynorexia* [Greek: *kyon* (dog) plus *orexis* (appetite)] would appear to be a better companion word to *anorexia*.

Table 34-1. DSM-III-R diagnostic criteria for bulimia nervosa

A. Recurrent episodes of binge eating (rapid consumption of a large amount of food in a discrete period of time).
B. A feeling of lack of control over eating behavior during the eating binges.
C. The person regularly engages in either self-induced vomiting, use of laxatives or diuretics, strict dieting or fasting, or vigorous exercise in order to prevent weight gain.
D. A minimum average of two binge eating episodes a week for at least three months.
E. Persistent overconcern with body shape and weight.

Source. Reprinted with permission from American Psychiatric Association 1987.

only rarely does it include the body distortion that was once believed to be an essential feature of anorexia nervosa.

Binging patients generally report a preoccupation with food, weight, and body contour that consumes more than 85% of their time during waking hours. They often underestimate their general ability and work well below their capacity (as suggested by their undergraduate and postgraduate scholastic achievement). Almost uniformly their self-esteem is reported as low; these patients are overly preoccupied with the opinion of others (resulting in excessive overpersonalization and misunderstanding of others' behavior or statements), and they have great difficulty expressing their negative emotions directly or in a timely way. Social isolation may become severe in patients after many years of symptoms. Other coping skills atrophy in the presence of the anxiety reduction so commonly experienced after bingeing and purging. Perfectionism is frequently seen in patients with eating disorders. Failure to adhere to their planned intake by consuming as little as 50–100 extra calories often becomes the justification for a "real" binge in order to have enough food in their stomach to make vomiting easier. College-age patients often have made few or no decisions about life goals. This is possibly the primary result of the all-consuming preoccupation with contour and food, but also becomes a powerful defense against having to make decisions of any kind.

Depression is frequently seen in all types of patients with eating disorders. Patients with anorexia nervosa are especially subject to depression (probably secondary to starvation). Among bulimic patients, lower-weight patients with depression outnumber normal or overweight depressed patients (Cooper and Fairburn 1986). The dysphoric mood in bulimic patients may be secondary to the disturbed eating pattern rather than to a primary depression (Johnson-Sabine et al. 1984). Recovery from the bulimic behavior does not appear to be related to the recovery per se of the depression (Herzog 1988).

Absence of menses or irregular periods often are seen even in normal-weight patients. Diminished sexual drive is reported in both male and female low-weight patients. Sexual behavior varies from extreme degrees of promiscuity to virginal avoidance of any sexual contact. Similarly, acting out or delinquent behavior, which was at one time believed to distinguish bulimic patients from anorexic patients, is characteristic of only a minority of bulimic patients.

The family history of bulimic patients often reveals that an excessive concern about weight and appearance existed in their mothers. It is not uncommon to find that the mothers' weights (women usually 40–60 years old) are remarkably low. Depression is often reported in family members, but rarely can one assess its severity in the description given by patients (Yates 1989).

Physical Findings

Bulimic and purging patients may reveal findings largely dependent on the degree of purging, starvation, dehydration, and/or electrolyte disturbance.

Vomiting alone is often accompanied by fluctuating degrees of salivary gland hypertrophy. An increase in dental caries, gum recession, and enamel erosion is frequently observed by dentists; this may progress to a need for extensive restorative dentistry. Streaking of blood in the vomitus is not unusual, but frank bleeding may herald the very rare and life-threatening gastric or esophageal tear.

Low-weight patients with bulimia nervosa may demonstrate all or most of the findings of a hypometabolic or hypothalamic syndrome. These findings would include hypotension, orthostatic hypotension, bradycardia, cold skin, low body temperature, and extremities often showing variable degrees of livedo reticularis or cyanotic discoloration of the nail beds. Purging patients may also show evidence of dehydration with poor skin turgor. Hair loss may be reported by the patient.

Patients frequently complain of fullness, and abdominal distention may be seen on physical examination. Neurologic examination is usually within normal limits, except for absent or sluggish deep tendon reflexes with a slow return.

The mental status examination is usually within normal limits. Very-low-weight patients may appear apathetic or at times irritable. Changes in the level of consciousness or in the ability to concentrate suggest a delirium. This is usually secondary to electrolyte changes or severe dehydration; such patients require emergency hospitalization.

Laboratory Studies

Purging patients have chronic losses of electrolytes, especially when multiple types of purging are employed. Those who abuse laxatives and diuretics are at risk for developing cardiac arrhythmias that is secondary to potassium depletion. Electrocardiography is helpful in identifying those at risk for arrhythmias when premature ventricular contractions or elongation of the Q-T interval are found.

Elevated serum renin and aldosterone levels accompanied by diminished excretion of sodium, potassium, and chloride in a 24-hour urine specimen are common in purging patients (Velhuis et al. 1979). This information is useful in predicting the severity of the sodium retention and water weight gain that occur frequently when purging activity stops (J. K. Barber, unpublished data).

Resting metabolic rates are very helpful in documenting the presence of a hypometabolic state (i.e., secondary to starvation). Many patients have values that are 40%–55% of normal. It is of interest that circulating thyroid hormones (i.e., thyroxine, triiodothyronine uptake, FT4 index, thyroid-stimulating hormone) are normal in virtually all patients (J. K. Barber, unpublished data). Radiologic studies, beyond a routine chest film, are usually not necessary. Heart size is known to parallel the changes in body weight in starving patients or in low-weight patients with bulimia nervosa or anorexia nervosa.

Certain laboratory studies should be obtained routinely in all patients. Anemia, usually iron deficiency type, is found occasionally. Serum cholesterol and lipoproteins should be drawn because, despite the presence of a starved state, the occasional patient is found to have marked elevations in both cholesterol and low-density lipoproteins.

Differential Diagnosis

The differentiation between anorexia nervosa and bulimia nervosa may be very difficult, especially if bingeing and purging are "allowed" in diagnosing anorexia. Because of the confusion, there is some consideration to limit the anorexia diagnosis to food restrictors only.

The other possible but rare causes of bulimia include schizophrenia, the Kleine-Levin syndrome, the Klüver-Bucy syndrome, Parkinson's disease, prolactin-secreting pituitary tumors, and tumors of the hypothalamus.

Epidemiology

Certain facts about the distribution of the bulimic syndrome are agreed on: 1) food must be abundant; 2) the syndrome is social-class related; 3) most patients are female; and 4) most patients are young (Hart and Ollendick 1985).

Estimates of prevalence range from 1.9% of a general population (Cooper and Fairburn 1986) to around 4% of a college population (Drewnowski et al. 1988). Anecdotal reports from girls' boarding schools suggest that these figures may underestimate actual incidence (e.g., "Every bathroom always smells of vomit"). Occasional bingeing and vomiting (but not meeting criteria for a DSM-III-R diagnosis) may be quite common among college women (Button and Whitehouse 1981). Among minority groups, patients with eating disorders are found to occur in upwardly mobile families where achievement, competition, and perfectionism are stressed along with acceptance of cultural attitudes about desirable body form (Silber 1986).

Etiology

The concept of biopsychosocial causation of disease is well documented for eating disorders. Social pressure for thinness has preoccupied women for at least 40 years. Media emphasis on diet and contour and a powerful diet-obesity industry feed on each other. Kindergarten teachers report that girls aged 4–6 years are worried about being too fat; chubby children suffer social disapproval and rejection. Thinness in women has become equated with higher educational and vocational status.

Psychological factors reported by bulimic patients include childhood maladjustment and increased psychiatric morbidity in the family. Personality features include difficulty in self-regulation, social discomfort, rejection dysphoria, and high achievement goals that are diverted to the pursuit of thinness (Johnson and Connors 1987). The bulimic patient views the environment as more stressful, less predictable, and less desirable than do control patients (Heilbrun and Bloomfield 1986; Cattenach and Rodin 1988). Bulimic patients may view minor stresses as near-catastrophic.

The heterogeneity of bulimic patients makes it difficult to derive a unified theory of atypical development that "explains" the syndrome. There is general agreement, however, on the role of bingeing and vomiting in reducing anxiety and stress. Regardless of how the binge behavior begins (e.g., as a result of starvation or de novo), it rapidly can become a powerful defensive tool that appears to overpower many other coping devices. Some bulimic patients with a long-standing illness have so atrophied their coping skills that their only significant psychological defense is to resort to another episode of bingeing and purging.

In addition to the physical effects of starvation[2] (reduced metabolic rate, weakness, orthostatic hypotension, bradycardia, polyuria, delayed gastric emptying time), Keyes et al. (1950) in their study documented typical psychological responses to semistarvation. These symptoms are also commonly seen in individuals with eating disorders—namely, inability to concentrate and sustain mental effort, "emotional instability," irritability, depression, and obsessive preoccupation with food (Keyes et al. 1950).

---

[2]Human semistarvation (or starvation) has different consequences if it occurs during wartime (e.g., World War II civilians, concentration camp victims, or prisoners of war) and famines. In these circumstances, the effects of disease, poor housing, specific dietary deficiencies, and chronic psychological stress intensify the consequences of the caloric restriction per se. The seminal study of human starvation was reported by Keyes et al. (1950). Although this study lacks today's sophisticated knowledge of neurophysiology and neuroendocrinology, it remains a landmark in the understanding of what happens to normal individuals who are malnourished. In this study of normal male volunteers, the effects of caloric restriction were not accompanied by inadequate housing, poor clothing, contaminated food, water supplies, and the fears and uncertainty of day-to-day living. As a consequence, despite the severe caloric restriction and weight loss, these volunteers were not as severely affected as World War II populations. The Minnesota volunteers in Keyes et al.'s study lived under conditions similar to those individuals who today reduce their caloric intake by food restriction and/or by purging techniques (e.g., individuals with a variety of diagnosable eating disorders).

Other biological factors favoring continuation of a binge-and-purge syndrome include mechanisms of increased endorphin production as a result of ingesting large quantities of food or through vomiting. The majority of patients who binge report some altered mental state (e.g., "not thinking about anything," not aware of the taste of food after the first bites, feeling drowsy, feeling "spacey" or even "high" during the binge). There is a small minority of patients who are primarily vomiters; they report similar mental states after vomiting. It has been speculated that in binge vomiting, the increases in beta-endorphins may actually create an auto-addiction (Fullerton et al. 1988). Yager (1984) reported that entertainers and public speakers may diminish stage fright by vomiting before going on stage.

Starvation (inadequate consumption of necessary calories) probably plays a key role in the development of bingeing behavior. The work by Keyes et al. (1950) on human starvation documents many behaviors that recently were believed to be an important part of a psychological syndrome—namely, the intense obsession and preoccupation with food, depression, and emotional instability. The psychological survival mechanisms (obsession about food) may be induced during so-called dieting (actually starvation). The insatiable appetite, which usually occurs after the diet (especially low-caloric diets, e.g., less than 1,000 kcal/day) has ended, produces the familiar situation of rapid regain of weight to above starting levels.

A syndrome of "restrained eating" (not yet diagnosable as an eating disorder) has been reported in many young girls who alternately diet and overeat. In a study done in San Francisco (Mellin et al. 1986), some 38% of 9-year-olds and 80% of 10-year-olds were reported to have had this eating pattern. One might suspect that eventually some of these younger individuals will begin to gain excessive weight, which may be the precursor for the initiation of vomiting to control weight gain.

Many reports document apparent changes in levels of neurotransmitters. Many of these changes probably reflect the degree of starvation, bingeing, dehydration, and purging activities. None is believed to have etiologic significance.

Treatment

Treatment of bulimia nervosa remains controversial, probably because of the complexity of the underlying psychopathology (Yates 1990). All methods of treatment (inpatient or outpatient, antidepressant or no drugs, psychoanalytic or behavioral or cognitive therapy, individual or family, group or individual plus group) are successful some of the time, but it is unlikely that any one method always succeeds. Age of patient, degree of starvation, degree and types of symptoms, overall adequacy of coping skills, and motivation to change are all of importance in making a treatment plan. Young adolescent patients, forced into treatment by concerned parents, rarely have sufficient motivation to change behaviors and thus make poor candidates for outpatient treatment. Recidivism, however, is high also in these patients after inpatient treatment.

Patients with evidence of starvation must be considered to have a physiologic survival drive to overeat. Restoration of a normal eating pattern is a first goal for most patients (Mitchell and Eckert 1987). Education about good nutrition (food selection and caloric content) is essential. Most patients fail to recognize that hypothalamic mechanisms are far more responsible for weight control than their own attempts to juggle weight by small increases or decreases in food intake.

It is important for therapists to be well informed about nutrition to be able to monitor a patient's effort to return to a normal eating pattern. Early in treatment, it is helpful for the patient to keep a log of food consumption and to attempt to make connections among emotional states, stress, and the impulse to binge or purge. Eating three meals a day (with the composition of diet repetitious and boring) is a useful structure for patients to change misconceptions about the weight-gaining potential of foods and to reduce the rumination about foods to be eaten at the next meal.

With purging patients who have elevations in renin and aldosterone and a low urinary excretion of sodium, potassium, and chloride, special attention must be given to prepare them for possible rapid weight gain when purging is stopped. Water retention in purging patients is similar to that found in patients with chronic diuretic use or abuse (Mitchell et al. 1988; Velhuis et al. 1979). Concepts such as "wet" weight and "dry" weight need to be reinforced. Patients benefit from being taught how to measure degrees of edema (using pretibial pressure); this may reassure them that weight gain is the result of water and not fat.

Patients with any evidence of severe electrolyte disturbance, especially those patients with electro-cardiographic evidence of premature ventricular contractions or a prolonged Q-T interval, require inpatient care with monitoring.

Many clinicians who work with eating-disordered patients recognize the importance of group therapy. Groups may be open or closed, homogeneous or heterogeneous (for types of eating disorder), or time limited or time unlimited. Open, time-unlimited, heterogeneous groups have some advantages. There are advantages to age segregation; the problems of teenagers are very different from those of college students or mature women. Group therapy is especially useful in dealing with low self-esteem, the fearfulness of others' opinions, and the inability to be direct in expression of emotion.

The issue of the use of antidepressant medication in the treatment of bulimia nervosa has not yet been resolved. The use of tricyclic or other antidepressant drugs should be reserved for patients with significant depression and not used routinely (Mitchell and Groat 1984). A strategy of waiting until eating behavior has become more or less normal before making a decision to use an antidepressant has resulted in some settings in virtually no tricyclic usage at all. Other medications (antipsychotics, lithium, antianxiety agents, and anticonvulsants) have been tried and have been helpful in the occasional patient, but they do not appear to have any general usefulness. Opiate blockers need study and may have a therapeutic role for some patients (Jonas and Gold 1986).

Most eating-disorder specialty clinics are aware that treatment for bulimia nervosa requires long-term intervention. Recidivism after hospitalization is believed to be high (although there are few reports of this in the literature) and suggests that hospitalization should be seen only as a beginning to far more lengthy treatment. Multidisciplinary approaches are probably essential to the success of any program; other professionals to be involved in treatment should include nutritionists, pediatricians, internists, and/or endocrinologists.

Individual treatment appears to be necessary for most patients. There is some agreement that psychodynamic therapy and especially psychoanalytic therapy are not successful as a beginning form of treatment, which is similar to results found in the psychoanalytic treatment of alcoholism or drug addiction. Individual treatment must focus on key issues; these are usually diminished self-worth, over-concern about the opinion of others, difficulty in the expression of negative emotions, poor coping skills in interpersonal stress, perfectionism, and inability to make decisions about the future. The cognitive therapy approach is very useful, especially in giving patients a structured way of dealing with their many distortions and misperceptions. Low-weight patients are often poor candidates for psychotherapy, and a useful approach may be to reserve psychotherapy until after weight recovery (Mitchell and Eckert 1987).

Therapists should be familiar with nutritional facts, and part of individual therapy must be educational in helping patients realize that their ideas about food, weight control, and essential caloric intake are mistaken.

References

Abraham SF, Beumont PJV: How patients describe bulimia or binge eating. Psychol Med 12:625–635, 1982

American Psychiatric Association: Diagnostic and Statistical Manual of Mental Disorders, 3rd Edition. Washington, DC, American Psychiatric Association, 1980

American Psychiatric Association: Diagnostic and Statistical Manual of Mental Disorders, 3rd Edition, Revised. Washington, DC, American Psychiatric Association, 1987

Button EJ, Whitehouse A: Subclinical anorexia nervosa. Psychol Med 11:509–516, 1981

Casper RC, Eckert ED, Halmi KA, et al: Bulimia: its incidence and clinical importance in patients with anorexia nervosa. Arch Gen Psychiatry 37:1030–1035, 1980

Cattenach L, Rodin J: Psychosocial components of the stress process in bulimia. International Journal of Eating Disorders 7:75–88, 1988

Cooper PJ, Fairburn CG: The depressive symptoms of bulimia nervosa. Br J Psychiatry 148:268–274, 1986

Drewnowski A, Yee DK, Krahn DD: Bulimia in college women: incidence and recovery rates. Am J Psychiatry 145:753–755, 1988

Fullerton DT, Swift WJ, Getto CJ, et al: Differences in the plasma beta-endorphin level of bulimics. International Journal of Eating Disorders 7:191–200, 1988

Hart KJ, Ollendick TH: Prevalence of bulimia in working and university women. Am J Psychiatry 142:851–854, 1985

Heilbrun AB, Bloomfield DL: Cognitive differences between bulimic and anorectic females. International Journal of Eating Disorders 5:209–222, 1986

Herzog DB: Eating disorders, in New Harvard Guide to Psychiatry. Edited by Nicholi AM Jr. Cambridge, MA, Harvard University Press, 1988, pp 434–445

Johnson C, Connors ME: The Etiology and Treatment of Bulimia Nervosa. New York, Basic Books, 1987

Johnson-Sabine EC, Wood KH, Wakeling A: Mood changes in bulimia nervosa. Br J Psychiatry 145:512–516, 1984

Jonas JM, Gold MS: Naltrexone reverses bulimic symptoms. Lancet 1:807, 1986

Keyes A, Brozek J, Henschel A, et al: The Biology of Human Starvation. Minneapolis, MN, University of Minnesota Press, 1950

Mellin LM, Scully S, Irwin CE: Disordered eating characteristics in preadolescent girls. Paper presented at the annual meeting of the American Dietetic Association, Las Vegas, NV, October 1986

Mitchell JE, Eckert ED: Scope and significance of eating disorders. J Consult Clin Psychol 55:628–634, 1987

Mitchell JE, Groat R: A placebo-controlled, double-blind trial of amitryptiline in bulimia. J Clin Psychopharmacol 4:186–193, 1984

Mitchell JM, Pomeroy C, Seppala M, et al: Pseudo-Bartter's syndrome, diuretic abuse, idiopathic edema, and eating disorders. International Journal of Eating Disorders 7:226–237, 1988

Silber TJ: Anorexia nervosa in blacks and Hispanics. International Journal of Eating Disorders 5:121–128, 1986

Strober M, Katz JL: Do eating disorders and affective disorders share a common etiology? A dissenting opinion. International Journal of Eating Disorders 6:171–189, 1987

Velhuis JB, Bardin CW, Demers LM: Metabolic mimicking of Bartter's syndrome by covert vomiting. Am J Med 66:361–363, 1979

Yager J: Bulimia. Resident & Staff Physician 30:44–58, 1984

Yates A: Current perspectives on the eating disorders, I: history, psychological and biological aspects. J Am Acad Child Adolesc Psychiatry 28:813–828, 1989

Yates A: Current perspectives on the eating disorders, II: treatment, outcome, and research directions. J Am Acad Child Adolesc Psychiatry 29:1–9, 1990

Chapter 35

Obesity of Infancy and Childhood

Joseph L. Woolston, M.D.

Considerable attention has been focused on the eating disorders of early childhood that result in growth failure, such as failure to thrive and rumination. In contrast, the eating disorders that result in excessive weight gain have been virtually ignored. DSM-III-R (American Psychiatric Association 1987) has reinforced this prejudice by refusing to classify any form of obesity as an eating disorder. Instead, it describes obesity as a physical disorder. As a result of this lack of interest in obesity of early childhood, there are many widely held misconceptions about its etiology, course, and even heterogeneity of subtypes. This state of clinical indifference about the fundamentals of infantile obesity makes a scientific strategy for intervention difficult.

The first step in the elucidation of any new field of study is a consensual operational definition that is phenomenologically accurate. In the study of obesity, there needs to be an easy, accurate, reliable method of defining the clinical condition. Since obesity denotes being excessively fat, the operational definition must differentiate the condition of having excessive adipose tissue for chronological age from simply being heavy for chronological age. Triceps skin-fold thickness (Garn and Clark 1976) and an obesity index using weight gain, suprailiac skin fold, and waist circumference (Crawford et al. 1974) are two well-standardized measurements that appear to satisfy the requirements for a useful, operational definition of obesity. A simpler, if slightly less valid, measure of obesity is defined by exceeding 120% of ideal body weight for height for a given age and sex. Specifically, ideal body weight for height is calculated by dividing actual weight by the expected weight for a given age and sex and height percentile.

The Natural History of Infantile and Childhood Onset Obesity

Developmental Evolution

The study of the natural history of obesity in infancy and early childhood is in its beginning stages. Data about the typical course of this disorder are contradictory. The most widely held belief is that obesity of early onset is a chronic and steadily progressive disorder with very few remissions. In a study by Charney et al. (1976), 36% of infants who exceeded the 90th percentile in weight were reported to be overweight as adults, as opposed to 14% of average or lightweight infants. Eid (1970) found that infants who were gaining weight rapidly were four times more likely to be obese by age 8 years than infants who were gaining weight at a normal rate. This grim prognosis has been buttressed by a network of theory and experimental data about fat-cell proliferation in early childhood and its deleterious impact on appetite and weight gain later in life.

However, more recent workers (Poskitt 1980; Shapiro et al. 1984) reported that obesity in infancy is a poorer predictor of childhood obesity later in childhood than was believed previously. Poskitt (1980) showed that the relative risk of an overfat infant becoming an overfat 5-year-old was about 2.5 times that for a normal infant. Of 203 children,

40% were overweight (>110% ideal body weight) or obese (>120% ideal body weight) as infants. By age 5 years, 13.5% were overweight, and 2.5% were obese. Most overweight infants did not become overweight children, but 60% of the 27 overweight 5-years-olds also were overweight in infancy. Poskitt's findings indicate that fatness in infancy leads to an increased chance of fatness in early childhood, but this risk is less than was thought previously. Shapiro et al. (1984) studied 450 6-month-old infants whom they followed for 8½ years. They found that of the 26 children (17 boys) who were obese at 6 months, fewer and fewer remained obese at subsequent annual measurements, until only 1 remained obese at 9 years. In contrast, infants who were not obese at 6 months but who later became obese at ages 4–8 years were much more likely to be obese at 9 years.

This rather poor correlation between obesity in infancy and obesity in later childhood calls into question the notion of relentlessly progressive obesity that is triggered by fat-cell proliferation in infancy or early childhood. Rather than there being a critical phase in infancy for fat-cell proliferation, it is more likely that the degree and duration of obesity are the major determinants of total adipose cell number in humans (Kirtland and Gurr 1979; Knittle et al. 1979). Poskitt (1980) reported that very little multiplication of adipose cells takes place in infancy. The natural increase in size of those adipose cells present at birth is sufficient to account for almost all of the increase in fat stored in the first year without any increase in cell number.

Epidemiology, Social Factors, and Eating Habits

The incidence and prevalence of obesity in early childhood are not nearly as well studied as in obesity in adulthood. The few studies indicate that the prevalence rate of obesity is 5%–10% of preschool-age children (Maloney and Klykylo 1983). Occasionally, "epidemics" of infantile obesity have been reported with prevalence rates of 16.7% of infants under 12 months of age (Shukla et al. 1972). These epidemics appear to be caused by culturally determined misinformation or fads about infant-feeding practices (Shukla et al. 1972; Taitz 1971). The well-publicized and best documented epidemic occurred in England between 1960 and 1975 (Taitz 1977). At that time, English parents were encouraged to follow the maxim that "one cannot overfeed a young baby." Parents commonly used full

cream milk powder with added sucrose as baby formula, and in many parts of England mothers were encouraged to introduce solids at a very early stage. By 1973, the dangers of infantile obesity and hypertonic dehydration were well publicized. Between 1971 and 1976, the rate of 6-week-old infants being fed unmodified milk powder went from 90% to 0%, and the rate of infants above the 50th percentile in weight went from 79% to 43% (Taitz 1977). In a closely analogous fashion, nonorganic failure to thrive has been reported to occur as a result of parental misconceptions about diet (Pugliese et al. 1987; Woolston 1983). In a more classic picture, obesity appears to be related to cultural practices, since it covaries with social class.

Obesity in females is nine times more common in social classes III and IV than in social classes I and II (Stunkard et al. 1972). The prevalence of obesity is linked to the socioeconomic status of the parents almost as strongly as it is to the subject's own social class (Goldblatt et al. 1965). This finding argues that socioeconomic status is linked to obesity in a causal, rather than a simple associative, manner, perhaps mediated through culturally determined eating habits and contemporary dietary misconceptions.

Genetic-Familial Factors

A family-line analysis of obesity indicates that there is a strong correlation between the fatness of parents and their children. For example, by age 17, the children of obese parents have three times the chance of being obese as the children of lean parents. If one sibling is fat, there is a 40% chance that a second sibling will be fat (Garn and Clark 1976). If two siblings are fat, there is an 80% chance that the third sibling will be fat. Although these data seem to support a genetic basis for obesity, one must keep other nongenetic, but family-related, factors in mind. The same study that reported the sibling data indicated that if one spouse is fat, there is a 30% chance that the other spouse also will be fat (Garn and Clark 1976). Obviously this finding cannot be explained by genetic factors.

The familial factors related to infantile obesity are less clear. Poskitt (1980) reported that there was no significant difference between the number of overweight and normal-weight infants with one or both parents overweight. By 5 years of age, however, 78% of the overweight and only 35% of the normal-weight children had at least one parent overweight. This was a significant difference and showed that the relative risk of a child's being overweight with at least one parent overweight was more than five times that of a child with two normal-weight parents.

Well-designed genetic studies involving monozygotic-dizygotic concordance and adoption samples (Stunkard et al. 1986) support a strong genetic contribution to all forms of body habitus ranging from fatness to thinness.

Temperament

Although temperament has become a focus of study in pediatrics and child psychiatry (Thomas and Chess 1977), it has been generally neglected in research about childhood onset obesity. This lack of investigation is surprising since temperament potentially could be associated with the development and course of obesity in three separate ways: 1) etiologic factors (e.g., low activity output); 2) correlates or consequences (e.g., social undesirability might result in negative peer interactions and social withdrawal); and 3) problems in management (low persistence would interfere with treatment compliance) (Carey et al. 1988). Since temperament has been demonstrated to have a major genetic determination (Wilson and Mathany 1986), it may be one mediating factor for the genetic contribution of obesity. To date, one study has demonstrated an association between eight difficult temperament characteristics and rapid weight gain and obesity in middle childhood (Carey et al. 1988).

Organic Factors

One of the primary foci by clinicians who are exploring the etiology of infantile obesity is the discovery of specific organic dysfunctions that produce endogenous obesity. This endogenous form of obesity is in contradistinction to exogenous obesity, in which there is no physical dysfunction other than consuming an excess caloric intake. Endogenous forms are caused by discrete genetic, endocrinologic, or neurologic syndromes, including Prader-Willi, Klinefelter's, Fröhlich's, Laurence-Moon-Biedl, Kleine-Levin, and Mauriac syndromes. Of special research interest is that Prader-Willi syndrome appears to be associated with a microdeletion of the proximal long arm of chromosome 15, band q 11.2. (Donlon 1988). In a sur-

prising and currently unexplainable turn of events, Angelman's syndrome, or the "happy puppet" syndrome, appears to be associated with the same microdeletion (Donlon 1988).

Although these organic causes of obesity frequently are searched for as an etiology for obesity in early childhood, they are quite rare. In addition, one easy rule of thumb can distinguish between exogenous and endogenous obesity. Children with endogenous obesity usually are below the 25th percentile in height and have delayed bone age, whereas children with exogenous obesity are above the 50th percentile in height and have an advanced bone age.

Psychogenic Factors

Studies of psychopathology in obese adults have been as contradictory as studies of other aspects of obesity. Although many authors have reported no objective data indicating an increased incidence of psychopathology in obese adolescents and adults (McCance 1961; Shipman and Plesset 1963), others have reported just the opposite (e.g., Bruch 1973; Stunkard 1975). Silverstone (1969) attempted to reconcile these discrepant reports by differentiating between late onset obesity secondary to a gradual accumulation of fat and early onset obesity characterized by a sudden increase in fatness that was the result of anxiety-driven overeating.

Very little is known about psychopathology in infantile obesity. In one of the few reports about this problem, Kahn (1973) described a sample of 73 obese children less than 3 years old. He found that 32% of these young children showed a sudden weight gain associated with a major and traumatic separation from their primary caregivers. This report is suggestive of a discrete syndrome related to traumatic separation that results in a sudden onset of obesity.

A second type of psychogenic obesity of infancy and early childhood occurs in the context of a disorganized family in which the child's needs are poorly perceived and even more poorly differentiated (Christoffel and Forsyth 1985). Typically, any sign of distress in the infant or toddler is responded to by feeding and/or neglect.

The observed psychosocial characteristics parallel features described in failure to thrive of psychosocial origin (Barbero and Shaheen 1967; Leonard et al. 1966). Children with this form of psychogenic obesity are from families in which there is severe disruption and disorganization. Factors that contribute to and are an expression of family dysfunction include separation of the parents, alcohol or drug abuse by the parents, and failure to maintain a stable and constant living environment. There often is denial about the severity—or even the existence—of the problem, and there often is poor medical care, failure to follow through with management plans, and, sometimes, hostility toward health professionals. The common behavioral outcome in all cases was the parents' inability to set limits, which also was evident in other parent-child interactions. Maternal depression clearly was evident in some cases. The severe family disorganization, in addition to being related to the etiology of obesity, presents a major obstacle to treatment. Case reports (Boxer and Miller 1987; Woolston and Forsyth 1989) describe a high level of parental noncompliance, direct undermining, and parents' lack of participation in the treatment of their child.

Classification Schema for Infantile Obesity

One of the most obvious explanations for the contradictory results of various studies is that obesity in this age group is an etiologically heterogeneous syndrome. Many authors (e.g., Maloney and Klykylo 1983; Stunkard 1975, 1980) have identified multiple factors that contribute to the development of obesity, including emotional, socioeconomic, genetic, developmental, energetic, and neurologic factors.

However, virtually no attempts have been made to subdivide forms of juvenile onset obesity into phenomenologically homogeneous groupings. Although such an attempt might be seen as reductionism, it seems to be warranted by the clear evidence of heterogeneity in this syndrome. The first point of differentiation in this subtyping schema should be between endogenous and exogenous obesity. Endogenous obesity should be classified according to specific organic etiology. Exogenous obesity should be subdivided into simple excessive caloric intake, genetic-familial, psychogenic, and mixed.

Obesity of Simple Excessive Caloric Intake

Obesity of simple excessive caloric intake results when a primary caregiver overfeeds the infant as a result of misinformation or cultural practice. There is no evidence of psychopathology in the infant or the caregiver, and there is a negative family history for obesity. This form of infantile obesity is relatively responsive to dietary intervention, assuming that the cultural attitudes that influence feeding can be modified. The age of onset can range from the neonatal period to early childhood, and the course may be rapid or gradual.

Genetic-Familial Obesity

In genetic-familial obesity, there is a presumption of an underlying genetic or familial vulnerability to obesity. There is no evidence of psychopathology or nutritional misinformation, but there is a positive family history for obesity. In addition, the child may have characteristics associated with a so-called difficult temperament (less rhythmical-predictable and persistence-attention). Although both the age of onset and course are variable, most commonly the obesity is gradual and progressive, starting by the fifth or sixth year of life. Intervention has rather poor results, especially if it is introduced after the obesity has been established for several years.

Psychogenic Obesity

In psychogenic obesity, there may be a negative family history for obesity and no evidence of nutritional misinformation, but there is strong evidence of psychopathology in the infant and/or the primary caregiver. Currently there is evidence to describe two specific types of psychogenic obesity: one related to a traumatic separation from the primary caregiver, and the other related to severe, chronic familial disorganization. This first form of obesity has a sudden onset (usually before age 3 years) and can progress rapidly. Intervention must address the psychological, as well as the nutritional, needs of the child and primary caregiver. Since the etiology is related more to psychological issues than genetics, the results of intervention will be more variable than the rather poor prognosis for familial obesity. The second type of psychogenic obesity is associated with severely disorganized families in which the child's developmental needs are either ignored or misperceived. In these families, infants and toddlers are fed at the slightest sign of distress.

Obesity of Mixed Etiology

In obesity of mixed etiology, more than one of the previously listed etiologies are found. Rather obviously, infants who are overfed and have a positive family history for obesity and who have significant psychological disturbances will have a very resistant form of obesity. Each factor will act synergistically to maintain the obesity despite vigorous intervention. A clustering of these three etiologic factors is not uncommon.

Treatment Implications

In the past, evaluation and treatment of infantile and childhood obesity have utilized a model of linear causality. Typically, there is a search for a specific cause, especially "organic" or endogenous. This search usually is a futile one since endogenous obesity is quite rare and virtually never occurs in children over the 25th percentile in height. The focus then is turned to a very narrow nutritional approach. Although this focus is closer to the biological underpinnings of the problem, notably a positive balance between caloric intake and expenditure, it frequently ignores the powerful psychosocial influences that are permitting or encouraging the child to overeat and underexercise. As is appropriate for any complex, multifactorial, chronic disorder, assessment and treatment must occur in the context of a multidisciplinary team approach (Boxer and Miller 1987; Woolston and Frosyth 1989). Ideally, this team consists of a pediatrician, developmental psychologist, child psychiatrist, social worker, nurse, and nutritionist. The team assesses the child's pediatric, developmental, psychiatric, familial, adaptive, functional, and maturational status. Because of the complexity and severity of this disorder, an inpatient evaluation may be required. Engagement of the family is the most important variable in successful treatment.

A full medical assessment of the child must be performed to evaluate the concomitants and the sequelae of obesity, as well as possible causes. Such disorders as slipped femoral epiphysis, diabetes mellitus, hypoxia, papilledema, sleep apnea, hypertension cardiomegaly, pneumonia, polycythemia, and Pickwickian syndrome may result from obesity and must be treated vigorously. The need for vigorous treatment in the Pickwickian syndrome is imperative, since the respiratory hypoventilation and daytime hypersomnolence as sequelae of severe obesity have a reported mortality rate of 40% in children (Boxer and Miller 1987). Because there appears to be a correlation between severe familial disorganization and some cases of infantile obesity, the pediatrician should evaluate the child for other medical problems associated with neglect, such as inadequate immunization, lead poisoning, iron deficiency, and tuberculosis.

A careful developmental, cognitive, and emotional assessment needs to be done to define various psychological and developmental strengths and weaknesses. If the child is older than 30 months, the developmental psychologist should contact the appropriate educators to assess and enroll the child in an early intervention school program. The child should be evaluated for specific psychiatric disorders, such as attention-deficit hyperactivity disorder, anxiety disorders, mood disorders, and oppositional disorder.

In addition to evaluating all aspects of family functioning, potential mental health and social resources for the family need to be assessed. The overall nutritional state of the child, the caloric intake for weight maintenance, and perhaps the nutritional status of other family members should be determined. The daily functioning of the child and family, including feeding and other mealtime behaviors, will be ascertained, and specific behaviors that need to be eliminated or strengthened will be determined. In this manner, the team must evaluate the overall strengths and weaknesses of the child and family to discover the multiple factors for the child's excessive caloric intake and inadequate caloric expenditure.

The various factors that contribute to the disorder must be addressed as appropriate by each member of the treatment team. As with other severe growth and eating disorders, removal of the child from the home sometimes is necessary. This most restrictive alternative must be reserved as a relatively undesirable intervention since the problem frequently reemerges when the child returns to the home.

References

American Psychiatric Association: Diagnostic and Statistical Manual of Mental Disorders, 3rd Edition, Revised. Washington, DC, American Psychiatric Association, 1987

Barbero G, Shaheen E: Environmental failure to thrive: a clinical interview. J Pediatr 73:690–698, 1967

Boxer GH, Miller BD: Treatment of a 7-year-old boy with obesity-hypoventilation (Pickwickian syndrome) on a psychosomatic inpatient unit. J Am Acad Child Adolesc Psychiatry 5:798–805, 1987

Bruch H: Eating Disorders: Obesity, Anorexia Nervosa and the Person Within. New York, Basic Books, 1973

Carey WB, Heguik RL, McDevitt SC: Temperamental factors associated with rapid weight gain and obesity in middle childhood. Developmental and Behavioral Pediatrics 9:194–198, 1988

Charney E, Chamblee H, McBride M, et al: The childhood antecedents of adult obesity: do chubby infants become obese adults? N Engl J Med 195:6–9, 1976

Christoffel KK, Forsyth BWC: The ineffective parent, childhood obesity syndrome. Paper presented at the 25th annual meeting of the Ambulatory Pediatric Association, 1985

Crawford PB, Keller CA, Hampton MC, et al: An obesity index for six-month-old children. Am J Clin Nutr 27:706–711, 1974

Donlon TA: Similar molecular deletions on chromosome 15 q 11.2 are encountered in both the Prader-Willi and Angelman syndrome. Hum Genet 80:322–328, 1988

Eid EE: Follow-up study of physical growth of children who had excessive weight gain in the first six months of life. Br Med J 2:72–76, 1970

Garn SM, Clark DC: Trends in fatness and the origins of obesity: Ad Hoc Committee to Review the Ten-State Nutrition Survey. Pediatrics 57:443–456, 1976

Goldblatt PB, Moore ME, Stunkard AJ: Social factors in obesity. JAMA 192:1039–1044, 1965

Kahn EJ: Obesity in children, in The Psychology of Obesity: Dynamics and Treatment. Edited by Kiell N. Springfield, IL, Charles C Thomas, 1973, pp 109–112

Kirtland J, Gurr MI: Adipose tissue hypercellularity: a review, 2: the relationship between cellulocity and obesity. Int J Obes 3:15–55, 1979

Knittle JC, Timmers K, Ginsberg-Fellner F, et al: The growth of adipose tissue in children and adolescents. J Clin Invest 63:239–246, 1979

Leonard M, Rhymes J, Solnit AJ: Failure to thrive in infants. Am J Dis Child 111:600–612, 1966

Maloney MJ, Klykylo WM: An overview of anorexia nervosa, bulimia and obesity in children and adolescents. Journal of the American Academy of Child Psychiatry 22:99–107, 1983

McCance C: Psychiatric factors in obesity. Unpublished dissertation for diploma in psychological medicine, University of London, London, 1961

Poskitt EME: Obese from infancy: a re-evaluation. Topics in Pediatrics 2:81–89, 1980

Pugliese MT, Weyman-Daum M, Moses N, et al: Parental health beliefs as a cause of nonorganic failure to thrive. Pediatrics 80:175–182, 1987

Shapiro LR, Crawford PB, Clark MJ: Obesity prognosis: a longitudinal study of children from age six months to nine years. Am J Public Health 74:968–972, 1984

Shipman MG, Plesset M: Anxiety and depression in obese dieters. Arch Gen Psychiatry 8:530–535, 1963

Shukla A, Forsyth AA, Anderson CM, et al: Infantile overnutrition in the first year of life: a field study in Dudley Worcestershire. Br Med J 4:507–515, 1972

Silverstone JT: Psychological factors in obesity, in Obesity: Medical and Scientific Aspects. Edited by Baird IM, Howard AN. London, E & S Livingstone, 1969, pp 45–55

Stunkard AJ: Obesity, in American Handbook of Psychiatry, 2nd Edition, Vol 4. Edited by Reiser MF (Arieti S, Editor-in-Chief). New York, Basic Books, 1975, pp 767–786

Stunkard AJ: Obesity, in Comprehensive Textbook of Psychiatry III. Edited by Kaplan HI, Freedman AM, Sadock BJ. Baltimore, MD, Williams & Wilkins, 1980, pp 1872–1882

Stunkard AJ, d'Aquill E, Fox S, et al: Influence of social class on obesity and thinness in children. JAMA 221:579–584, 1972

Stunkard AJ, Foch TT, Hrubec Z: A twin study of human obesity. JAMA 256:51–54, 1986

Taitz L: Infantile overnutrition among artificially fed infants in the Sheffield region. Br Med J 1:315–316, 1971

Taitz L: Obesity in pediatric practice: infantile obesity. Pediatr Clin North Am 24:107–122, 1977

Thomas A, Chess S: Temperament and Development. New York, Brunner/Mazel, 1977

Wilson RS, Mathany AP: Behavioral-genetics in infant temperament: the Louisville Twin Study, in The Study of Temperament: Changes, Continuities and Challenges. Edited by Plomin R, Dunn J. Hillsdale, NJ, Lawrence Erlbaum, 1986, pp 81–97

Woolston JL: Eating disorders in infancy and early childhood. Journal of the American Academy of Child Psychiatry 22:114–121, 1983

Woolston JL, Forsyth B: Obesity of infancy and early childhood: a diagnostic schema, in Advances in Clinical Child Psychology, Vol 12. Edited by Lahey BB, Kazdin AE. New York, Plenum, 1989, pp 179–192

Section VIII

Tic and Movement Disorders

Chapter 36

Tic, Stereotypy, and Habit Disorders

Robert A. King, M.D.
James F. Leckman, M.D.
Donald J. Cohen, M.D.

Definition

Tics are abrupt, purposeless, recurrent, stereotyped movements or sounds. They are frequently experienced as being involuntary or as occurring in response to an irresistible impulse. Classically, tics may be suppressed or deferred for brief periods of time. The frequency of tics can vary considerably over the course of a day in response to changing environmental circumstances; over the course of weeks to months, a pattern of "waxing and waning" of tic symptoms is common. Tics may mimic exactly voluntary movements or speech, or they may have even an exaggerated or more "forceful" character.

Sudden, brief, meaningless tics occurring singly are considered *simple tics*; in contrast, *complex tics* involve movements or vocalizations orchestrated into longer or more "purposeful"-appearing constellations. Common simple motor tics include grimaces, rapid head or limb jerks, shrugs, and abdominal tensing. Among the most common simple vocal tics are sniffs, barks, coughs, guttural throat clearing, and other expiratory vocalizations. Examples of complex motor tics are biting, throwing, hitting, skipping, touching objects or self, and gestures, which may be obscene (copropraxia) or compulsive imitations (echopraxia). Complex vocal tics can include dysfluencies and aberrations in prosody through formed syllables, words, or phrases; such phrases often take the form of stereotyped ejaculations (for example, "shut up!" "you

bet!"), obscenities (coprolalia), or echo phenomena (echolalia).

Among affected individuals, the intensity, frequency, and diversity of tics combine to create a wide gamut of severity. At one end of the spectrum stand transient, monosymptomatic tics that occur passingly in a large number of school-age children. At the other extreme stand the persistent, variegated multiple vocal and motor tics of Tourette's syndrome. In some individuals, tics appear as apparently isolated phenomena. In others, they may be associated with learning difficulties, impulsivity, inattentiveness, emotional lability, and obsessive-compulsive phenomena.

The diagnosis of a *tic disorder* implies distress or impairment in self-esteem, social functioning, or performance at school or work because of the presence of tics. The ubiquity and diversity of tics pose difficult classification problems that cannot be satisfactorily answered at present, given our ignorance of the clinical epidemiology, natural history, and underlying etiology of tics. For example, there are not yet reliable descriptive or threshold criteria (in terms of frequency, duration, or diversity) that can satisfactorily distinguish those tics that carry greater comorbidity or more ominous prognostic implications from those tics that are more benign.

The classification of tic disorders in DSM-III-R (American Psychiatric Association 1987) distinguishes three specific disorders: transient tic disorder, chronic motor or vocal tic disorder, and Tourette's disorder. The DSM-III-R schema distinguishes these disorders by means of precise criteria for frequency, persistence, and variety of tics. However, these criteria are more or less arbitrary; despite a spurious air of precision, it is unclear to what extent the frequency and duration criteria demarcate distinctive syndromes with differing etiologies, symptomatic concomitants, or clinical course.

The DSM-III-R criteria for tic disorders are given in Table 36-1.

Clinical Findings

Transient Tic Disorder

Transient tics are very common in prepubertal children, with boys more often affected than girls. The most common transient tics involve the face, head, neck, or arms. When the lower extremities are involved or multiple tics are present, the syndrome may be hard to differentiate from general fidgetiness. Transient vocal tics are much rarer. Transient tics are usually mild and run a waxing and waning course, which is often exacerbated by stress, excitement, or boredom. Children are often unaware of their tics or may try to rationalize them away (e.g., "I just sniffed because I had a cold"). Indeed, repetitive blinking, sniffing, or throat clearing often results in visits to the optometrist, allergist, or pediatrician, respectively. Transient tics in childhood are by definition time limited and, in most cases, benign. However, in the absence of a positive family tic history, there are no clear clinical guidelines to predict which mild motor tics of recent onset will remit and which will persist or effloresce.

Chronic Motor or Vocal Tic Disorder

By definition, this condition is more persistent than transient tic disorder. As with other tic disorders, chronic motor or vocal tic disorder runs a waxing and waning course, manifests a broad range of severity, and appears to be exacerbated by stress, arousal, or fatigue. The most common chronic tics are motor ones, especially those of the face, head, neck, and arms. In evaluating adults with chronic tics, a careful history often reveals that the tics have been present since childhood. Indeed, in retrospect, some such individuals may have met the criteria for Tourette's syndrome as children, but, following an amelioration of their symptoms in late adolescence, now manifest only chronic motor tics as a residual condition.

Table 36-1. DSM-III-R diagnostic criteria for tic disorders

Tourette's disorder (syndrome)

A. Both multiple motor and one or more vocal tics have been present at some time during the illness, although not necessarily concurrently.
B. The tics occur many times a day (usually in bouts), nearly every day or intermittently throughout a period of more than one year.
C. The anatomic location, number, frequency, complexity, and severity of the tics change over time.
D. Onset before age 21.
E. Occurrence not exclusively during psychoactive substance intoxication or known central nervous system disease, such as Huntington's chorea and postviral encephalitis.

Chronic motor or vocal tic disorder

A. Either motor or vocal tics, but not both, have been present at some time during the illness.
B. The tics occur many times a day, nearly every day, or intermittently throughout a period of more than one year.
C. Onset before age 21.
D. Occurrence not exclusively during psychoactive substance intoxication or known central nervous system disease, such as Huntington's chorea and postviral encephalitis.

Transient tic disorder

A. Single or multiple motor and/or vocal tics.
B. The tics occur many times a day, nearly every day for at least two weeks, but for no longer than twelve consecutive months.
C. No history of Tourette's or chronic motor or vocal tic disorder.
D. Onset before age 21.
E. Occurrence not exclusively during psychoactive substance intoxication or known central nervous system disease, such as Huntington's chorea and postviral encephalitis.

Tic disorder not otherwise specified

Tics that do not meet the criteria for a specific tic disorder. An example is a tic disorder with onset in adulthood.

Source. Reprinted with permission from American Psychiatric Association 1987.

Tourette's Syndrome (Chronic Motor and Phonic Tic Disorder)

This eponymic condition was first described in 1885 by Georges Gilles de la Tourette, who noted what he considered its cardinal features: convulsive muscular jerks, inarticulate cries, and coprolalia. He also noted that individual symptoms waxed and waned and that, although some patients' tic symptoms worsened over time, there was no general mental deterioration.

The initial symptoms of Tourette's syndrome most frequently appear in prepuberty from age 5 to 10 years. Initially, they may resemble the transient motor tics of childhood in that they are often mild, transient, and involve the face, head, or upper extremities. With time, however, the tics become persistent and increase in diversity and distribution, often progressing from the upper parts of the body to involve the trunk and legs (rostral-caudal progression). Most motor tics are initially simple ones (e.g., blinks, arm or head jerks, grimaces), but with time more complex motor tics such as biting, clapping, touching, or skipping may appear, as well as echopraxis.

The onset of motor tics usually precedes that of vocal tics by a year or two. However, in some cases, simple vocal tics such as sniffing or compulsive throat clearing may be the harbingers of the disorder. Initial vocal tics are most often simple and include clicks, chirps, throat clearing, grunts, and squeaks. Later, vocal tics may increase in complexity, with inappropriate blurting out of formed syllables, words, and phrases or compulsive repetition of either the patient's own utterances (palilalia) or those of others (echolalia). Speech fluency and prosody may be paroxysmally altered. Despite its traditional association with the syndrome, coprolalia usually does not appear until around puberty and occurs in only about one-third of cases.

The variety and patterning of tics are virtually inexhaustible. Individual tics may wax and wane over weeks or months or even disappear, only to be replaced in time by others. Tics may occur singly or as part of complex combinations of motor and vocal tics involving many parts of the body. Their frequency may range from isolated occurrences a few times per week to torrential bouts that last for hours and leave the patient and those around the patient frightened and exhausted. The intensity of tics may vary from those so minimal that only the patient is aware of them, to explosive outbursts that resound throughout the house or result in physical damage to the self or surroundings. In rare cases, disfigurement or even blindness may result from violent motor tics (e.g., self-hitting).

Children, especially young ones, may be unaware of, deny, or minimize their symptoms. Efforts may be made to camouflage the ticlike nature of a gesture (e.g., by disguising a head toss as a brushing back of the hair) or to substitute a less objectionable exclamation for an offensive one (e.g., "Sh-sh" or "Sugar!"). Patients may be able to suppress tics more or less successfully for a period of time (e.g., in church or while performing), but experience a paroxysm of tics once they relax their guard. As a result, teachers and parents may have divergent impressions of tic severity or be misled into thinking that the tics are voluntary and could be eliminated if only the child would exert more willpower. Tics markedly decrease during sleep and are exacerbated by stress, excitement, fatigue, and illness.

When tic symptoms are prominent, they frequently take a serious toll on children's self-esteem and social confidence. Beyond exposing the child to gibes and reproaches, the tics leave the child feeling out of control of his or her own body and mental processes. The very boundaries of the self and the distinction between what is actively willed versus what is involuntarily experienced are called into question (Cohen 1980).

Associated Conditions

Not all of the psychological difficulties of the child with Tourette's syndrome result from stigma or shame. Impulsivity, distractibility, emotional lability, and learning difficulties are often associated with the syndrome and may even antedate the onset of tics. Indeed, for many children, these associated symptoms are potentially greater sources of social and functional impairment than are the tics per se (Stokes et al. 1988).

By adolescence, compulsions and obsessions may make their appearance. Some compulsions, such as tapping, kissing, biting, and sexual touching, may be impossible to distinguish from complex motor tics. Other obsessions and compulsions may range from ordering behaviors (e.g., "evening up") or needing to get an action "just right" through full-blown ego-dystonic obsessions and compulsions (e.g., repetitive washing and checking) (Grad et al. 1987). Careful inquiry often reveals recurrent, intrusive, and unwanted thoughts or images (frequently concerning aggression, sex, or other emotionally charged issues), as well as a relentless preoccupation with resisting compulsive urges. By adulthood, as many as 55%–90% of patients with Tourette's syndrome also meet the criteria for an associated diagnosis of obsessive-compulsive disorder (Pauls et al. 1986).

Case Example

Andy first developed eye blinking and facial grimaces at age 9, about 6 months after the tragic death of a beloved older brother in an automobile accident. At first, his symptoms were attributed to a bad case of poison ivy, but they persisted after the rash cleared. Over the next several months, Andy developed additional motor tics, which included head jerks, shoulder shrugs, and hand and arm movements; in addition, he began to grunt and make throat-clearing sounds. About 2 years later, after his father saw a television program on the disorder, the diagnosis of Tourette's syndrome was finally made. Andy was begun on haloperidol, which markedly decreased his symptoms, but he felt sedated and complained of "feeling like a zombie." At school, Andy's performance was mediocre because of attentional difficulties, the disruption caused by his tics, and fights with peers who teased him. Over the next 7–8 years, Andy and his family maintained regular contact with the Tourette's syndrome clinic team, who came to be important sustaining figures for him. His vocal tics remained simple ones, but at times his motor tics included pounding and hitting objects. Over the years, Andy's motor tics waxed and waned, but were only partially controlled by trials of clonidine, clonazepam, and/or pimozide. In the face of an unsettled home situation and economic hardship, Andy finished high school, obtained a job as a maintenance worker, and moved into an apartment of his own. Despite his tics, Andy was popular with girls and maintained a close circle of friends. However, his ability to drive, on which his job depended, was periodically compromised by violent arm jerks.

One day, at age 19, while having lunch with an infirm elderly aunt, Andy was suddenly seized by an intrusive urge and mental image of smashing her in the face with his fist. Although no stranger to fistfights with peers, Andy was dismayed by what he felt to be a horrific, repugnant urge and quickly found a pretext to flee the room. Similar ego-alien thoughts and urges began to trouble Andy at work and at home, most often directed toward weak or infirm figures for whom he in fact had fond feelings. For example, Andy had to flee a family gathering when he found himself preoccupied with thoughts of kicking his pregnant cousin in the abdomen. These intrusive thoughts and urges became so upsetting that Andy feared he was going crazy and even contemplated killing himself or moving across country to protect his loved ones. Getting up his courage to confide these thoughts to the clinic's nurse specialist, Andy was greatly relieved to learn that such obsessions and compulsions represented a facet of Tourette's syndrome. However, despite the addition of fluoxetine to his regimen of pimozide, these thoughts remained both deeply upsetting and

distracting, and finally culminated in Andy quitting his job.

Differential Diagnosis

In its fully developed form, with both simple and complex motor and phonic tics present, Tourette's syndrome is easily distinguished from other neurologic conditions. However, when motor tics occur in isolation, as in the other tic disorders or prodromal phase of Tourette's syndrome, the differential diagnosis must include a variety of other dyskinesias: myoclonus, choreoathetosis, dystonia, akathisia, paroxysmal and tardive dyskinesias, and excessive startle syndromes (Fahn and Erenberg 1988). The presentation and natural history of the tic disorders are usually sufficiently distinctive to permit diagnosis on clinical grounds without extensive diagnostic tests. In few other situations besides the tic disorders does one find the confluence of childhood onset and abrupt but intermittent movements that are temporarily suppressible. The distribution, timing, and kinesthetics of tics usually distinguish them from the unilateral pattern of ballismus; the twisting, frequently sustained movements of dystonia; and the inability to sustain contractions that characterizes chorea. Clinical context is also a helpful guide. For example, acute and tardive akathisias and dyskinesias are usually associated with starting or stopping neuroleptic medication. Chorea often occurs in the context of a genetic or metabolic disorder (e.g., Wilson's disease or Huntington's chorea) or autoimmune reaction to streptococcal infection (as in Sydenham's chorea).

Epidemiology

Tics are common among children, with the highest apparent prevalence between 7 and 11 years of age. Community surveys find as many as 13% of boys and 11% of girls are reported by their parents to have "tics" (Zahner et al. 1988). However, community prevalence estimates vary widely with the survey method and question wording used. Most existing estimates are probably overly inclusive and do not indicate clinical significance.

In contrast to tic behaviors, there are few systematic data on the epidemiology of tic disorders as delineated by the DSM-III-R criteria of severity and persistence. At one time, Tourette's syndrome was considered extremely rare. With greater public and professional awareness, many more cases now come to clinical attention. At the same time, it has become clearer that there exist many mild, previously undiagnosed cases. Although surveys of cases coming to clinical attention provide a rough estimate, they underestimate the true prevalence of the disorder by omitting many undiagnosed or mild cases. Among children under 18 years of age, a statewide community survey of North Dakota health personnel found prevalence rates for Tourette's syndrome of 9.3 and 1.0 per 10,000 for boys and girls, respectively; among adults, however, the prevalence rates were much lower, 0.77 per 10,000 for men and 0.22 per 10,000 for women (Burd et al. 1986). Thus, as other studies confirm, children are more likely to be identified than adults, and males are more commonly affected than females.

Etiology

Recent advances in understanding the pathogenesis of Tourette's syndrome provide a working model that may serve as a paradigm for other childhood onset neuropsychiatric disorders: 1) an apparent genetically determined vulnerability, 2) age-dependent expression of symptoms reflecting maturational factors, 3) sexual dimorphism, 4) stress-dependent fluctuations in symptom severity, and 5) apparent environmental influences on the phenotypic expression of the underlying genotype (Leckman et al. 1988d).

Genetic Factors

Monozygotic twin pairs show a markedly higher concordance rate for Tourette's syndrome (53%) than do dyzygotic twins (only 8%); if concordance is measured by the broader criteria of the presence of *any* tics in the co-twin, the monozygotic concordance rate increases to 77% versus 23% for dizygotic twin pairs (Price et al. 1985). These figures suggest a strong genetic factor in Tourette's syndrome as well as a common genetic determinant for both Tourette's syndrome and milder tic symptoms. However, as discussed below, the finding that there exist monozygotic pairs discordant for tics also suggests that nongenetic factors play a role in determining the phenotypic expression of the presumed genetic vulnerability to Tourette's syndrome.

Family studies indicate that at least 65%–90% of cases of Tourette's syndrome are familial. However, these same studies suggest that what is transmitted in the families of probands with Tourette's syndrome is not simply vulnerability to Tourette's syndrome per se but rather vulnerability to a broad range of tic or obsessive-compulsive symptoms (Pauls and Leckman 1986, 1988; Pauls et al. 1986). Thus the phenotypic expression of the presumed Tourette's syndrome genotype is highly variable, with the inherited diathesis manifesting itself in the form of tics and/or obsessive-compulsive symptoms of varying severity. Gender-related, stress-related, and other as yet poorly understood factors appear to modify the form and severity of phenotypic expression.

Family studies that have examined the prevalence of either tic disorder or obsessive-compulsive disorder in first-degree relatives of probands with Tourette's syndrome suggest that the vulnerability to these disorders is best explained in such families by the model of an autosomal dominant trait with very high penetrance (close to 100%) for males and lower penetrance (about 70%) for females (Pauls and Leckman 1986). Furthermore, in females, as compared with males, the gene may be more likely to manifest itself as obsessive-compulsive disorder rather than a tic disorder. The range of tic disorder among affected individuals includes transient tic disorder, chronic tic disorder, and Tourette's syndrome. Thus, to a significant extent, the various tic disorders may not represent discrete entities but rather points on a spectrum of symptomatic severity in the expression of a common underlying genetic vulnerability.

One unanswered question concerns the extent to which genetic factors related to Tourette's syndrome play a predisposing role in the common transient tics of childhood. As noted earlier, as many as 13% of school-age boys are reported to have tics. Although stress and anxiety are often observed to exacerbate such tics, the role of constitutional factors in the genesis of transient tics is unknown. Analysis of one large kindred with a high density of individuals with Tourette's syndrome or chronic multiple tics revealed two family members with histories of nonrecurrent transient tics; the pedigree of at least one of these individuals indicated that he was an obligate carrier of the putative Tourette's syndrome gene (Kurlan et al. 1988). It thus appears that, in at least some individuals, transient tic disorder may represent a mild phenotypic expression of the Tourette's syndrome gene and a marker of genetic risk for that individual's offspring. Whether there exist other forms of transient tics that are not genetically determined (phenocopies) or have alternate genetic determinants (genocopies) remains to be determined.

The family data also point to common genetic factors at work in both tic disorders and in some cases of obsessive-compulsive disorder (Pauls and Leckman 1988; Pauls et al. 1986). As previously noted, obsessive-compulsive disorder is a common associated diagnosis in patients with Tourette's syndrome. Furthermore, first-degree relatives of Tourette's syndrome patients have an increased prevalence of obsessive-compulsive disorder, which may occur unaccompanied by any tic symptoms. This increased risk of obsessive-compulsive disorder among the first-degree relatives is unaffected by whether the probands have Tourette's syndrome plus obsessive-compulsive disorder or Tourette's syndrome alone. This suggests that the obsessive-compulsive disorder seen in such families represents an alternative phenotypic expression of the Tourette's syndrome gene. Although the Tourette's syndrome gene probably accounts for only a minority of cases of obsessive-compulsive disorder, the clinical manifestations of the obsessive-compulsive disorder associated with the Tourette's syndrome gene appear clinically indistinguishable from those in cases of obsessive-compulsive disorder occurring in the absence of a family history of tic disorder. Interestingly enough, tics or other abnormal movements are found in 20% of patients carrying a primary diagnosis of obsessive-compulsive disorder, especially those who are male or younger or whose obsessive-compulsive disorder is of recent onset (Swedo et al. 1989c).

Neuroanatomical Correlates

Speculations concerning the neuroanatomical substrate of Tourette's syndrome (as well as that of obsessive-compulsive disorder) have focused heavily on the basal ganglia and their cortical, thalamic, and midbrain connections (Chappel et al. 1990; Rapoport 1989). The basal ganglia are rich in dopamine and other neurotransmitters implicated in the pathogenesis of Tourette's syndrome by neuropharmacologic evidence. With their extensive connections to the sensorimotor and associational cortex, the basal ganglia appear to play a crucial role in integrating sensorimotor information and

motor control (Albin et al. 1989). Dysfunction of these structures and their associated neurotransmitter systems underlies other movement disorders, such as Parkinson's disease, Huntington's chorea, Sydenham's chorea, and encephalitis lethargica, conditions that, like Tourette's syndrome, involve abnormalities of both movement and emotive behavior. Postmortem studies of a small number of Tourette's syndrome patients' brains have suggested altered neurotransmitter levels in the basal ganglia (Anderson et al., unpublished data; Haber et al. 1986). Pilot positron-emission tomography studies of adult patients with Tourette's syndrome have found increased glucose metabolism in the basal ganglia (Chase et al. 1984), a finding paralleled by imaging studies that implicate the caudate in childhood onset obsessive-compulsive disorder (Swedo et al. 1989a).

Neurochemical Correlates

The most promising research into the pathogenesis of tic disorders concerns possible defects in neurotransmitter or neuromodulator regulation. The most intensively studied systems have been those mediated by various amino acid and monoamine neurotransmitters and the neuropeptides located in the basal ganglia and related brain structures (Chappel et al. 1990; Leckman et al. 1988c, 1988d).

Support for the role of altered dopaminergic functioning in Tourette's syndrome comes from the clinical observation that neuroleptics such as haloperidol and pimozide, which preferentially block central dopaminergic D_2 receptors, are clinically useful in partially suppressing tics in most patients with Tourette's syndrome. In contrast, dopaminergic agonists such as L-dopa, d-amphetamine, methylphenidate, and cocaine frequently exacerbate tics. Given the complex interaction of these drugs with the D_1 and D_2 receptor systems, located differentially in various cortical and subcortical structures, the relative roles of these two systems are unclear.

Dopaminergic fibers originating in the substantia nigra and the ventral tegmental area connect these nuclei and related portions of the basal ganglia to the associative cortex, the limbic system, and the locus coeruleus (the principal regulator of noradrenergic tone in the central nervous system). Additional evidence implicating altered dopamine regulation in Tourette's syndrome comes from the observation that abnormal movements and obsessive-compulsive behaviors may be seen in postencephalitic patients following viral infections that affect the dopaminergic neurons of the basal ganglia and in patients with Sydenham's chorea, a poststreptococcal autoimmune condition affecting these same structures (Swedo et al. 1989b). Cerebrospinal fluid levels of the dopamine metabolite homovanillic acid are apparently reduced in patients with Tourette's syndrome (Leckman et al. 1988d). However, preliminary positron-emission tomography imaging studies of central dopamine receptors have yet to find consistent changes in D_2 receptor density or distribution. Thus the nature of the altered dopaminergic functioning implicated in Tourette's syndrome remains unclear as well as the question of whether this abnormality is primary or secondary to defects in other neurotransmitter systems.

A possible role for the noradrenergic system in the pathogenesis of Tourette's syndrome is suggested by the observation that stress exacerbates many tics and that clonidine, an alpha$_2$-adrenergic receptor blocker, may ameliorate some tics. However, there are few other supporting data for the importance of noradrenergic mechanisms.

The endogenous opioid system, including dynorphin and Met-enkephalin, have also been implicated in the pathophysiology of Tourette's syndrome, as well as in other movement disorders involving the basal ganglia. These opiates are known to interact with central dopaminergic neurons and to have a broad range of motor and behavioral effects. Elevated levels of cerebrospinal fluid dynorphin A [1–8] have been found in patients with Tourette's syndrome (Leckman et al. 1988c). Furthermore, postmortem study of the brains of a small number of patients with Tourette's syndrome has found decreased levels of dynorphin A [1–17] in the substantia nigra (S. N. Haber, unpublished data, 1986).

The ambiguity of the evidence regarding specific neurotransmitters' role in the pathogenesis of Tourette's syndrome reflects the complexity of the pathophysiologic mechanisms involved and the relative crudeness of the investigational methods currently available. The interactions between the various neurotransmitter systems in the basal ganglia and associated structures are complex (Albin et al. 1989). For example, although D_2-receptor blockers diminish tics in many individuals, their ultimate therapeutic effect may be exerted many synapses removed from the dopaminergic neurons on which they have their immediate impact. Furthermore, it is also possible

that tic disorders may be biologically heterogeneous so that a given neurotransmitter mechanism might play a role in some, but not in other, forms of the disorder.

Nongenetic Factors

Although the vulnerability for Tourette's syndrome is apparently transmitted as an autosomal rather than sex-linked dominant trait, gender-specific factors may influence the expression of the gene. For example, the tic disorder phenotype may be more penetrant in males compared with females (Pauls and Leckman 1988). The nature of these gender-specific influences on the phenotypic expression of the gene is unclear. Because the tic symptoms of Tourette's syndrome usually begin well before puberty, it seems likely that the pubertal activation of the hypothalamic-pituitary-gonadal axis is not responsible for the sexual dimorphism found in the expression of the Tourette's syndrome gene. Prenatal androgen levels are known to have dramatic and permanent effects on the functional organization of the developing nervous system. It is thus possible that androgens or other gender-related factors favoring symptomatic expression of the Tourette's syndrome gene exert their effects prenatally on the developing male nervous system.

The lack of complete concordance for tics among monozygotic twins provides additional evidence that nongenetic factors influence the phenotypic expression of the Tourette's syndrome gene. Supporting the notion that these mediating factors may operate prenatally, Leckman et al. (1987) reported that in monozygotic pairs discordant for Tourette's syndrome, the twin who subsequently developed tics was uniformly the twin with the lower birth weight.

Although there have been contradictory reports regarding the association between perinatal difficulties and later tics (Pasamanick and Kawi 1956; Shapiro et al. 1988), stressful maternal life circumstances during pregnancy and the severity of first trimester nausea and/or vomiting appear to be risk factors for the later development of tic disorder (Leckman et al. 1990). Leckman et al. (1984) hypothesized that postnatal stresses may also sensitize genetically vulnerable individuals in such a way as to favor the later emergence of tics.

Treatment

Treatment must begin with a careful, comprehensive evaluation of the patient's psychological, social, and educational or vocational adjustment. The diagnosis of an identifiable tic disorder does not obviate the need for a thorough medical, developmental, family, and psychosocial history and assessment. The impact of the symptoms on the patient's self-concept, family and peer relations, and classroom participation must be assessed in the context of the patient and family's overall strengths and weaknesses.

Structured instruments are helpful adjuncts in collecting and summarizing symptom data and provide useful baseline information for any therapeutic intervention (Leckman et al. 1988a). The Yale Global Tic Severity Scale (Leckman et al. 1989) and the Shapiro Tourette Syndrome Severity Scale (Shapiro et al. 1988) are two reliable and valid clinical rating instruments used to inventory and quantify current tic symptoms. Although standardized videotaping may be useful in assessing and recording current tic behavior, fluctuations in patients' tic behavior in response to the clinical setting may make it difficult to obtain a representative sample of tic behavior (Goetz et al. 1987). The Yale-Brown Obsessive Compulsive Scale (Goodman et al. 1989) is a reliable instrument developed to assess and quantify obsessive-compulsive behavior in adults; as of this writing, a childhood version is under development.

The challenges facing patients with tic disorders (and their families) vary with both the changing manifestations of the disorder and the vicissitudes of normal development. Because chronic tic disorder and Tourette's syndrome represent chronic conditions, the ongoing availability of a supportive clinician is an invaluable asset for both patient and family in anticipating and dealing with difficulties.

Supportive, Educational, and Psychotherapeutic Interventions

By the time consultation is sought, the child's symptoms are often already caught up in a web of anxious apprehensions or blameful attributions. Education about the nature and course of tic disorders can ameliorate this burden, but it is essential to learn what shared and private meanings the symptoms and diagnosis carry for the patient and family. (These idiosyncratic meanings may become apparent only in the course of extended clinical contact.) For example, helping the child, parents, and school understand the child's symptoms as manifestations of a neuropsychiatric disorder can help "decriminalize" symptoms previously regarded as willful, provocative, or "crazy." Parents are usually relieved to learn that, in contrast to the extreme picture often presented in the lay press, most cases are not relentlessly progressive and improve by adulthood. When the condition is familial, its heritable aspects may be painful for families to contemplate. Parents often feel guiltily responsible for a condition that appears to come from their side of the family. When one of the parents also has symptoms of the disorder, his or her own experiences may provide either a valuable source of empathy or a burdensome impetus to repudiate or overidentify with the child's difficulties. Ongoing attention to such issues and support for the parents and child in coping with symptoms are essential elements of care.

Collaboration with the school can be very helpful in further destigmatizing the child's behavior, obtaining needed special educational services, and gaining the teachers' support in dealing with peer ostracism or teasing.

It is now generally accepted that chronic tic disorders are not *caused* by psychological factors. However, symptoms are often exacerbated by stress or emotional arousal, and, in turn, the tic disorders are themselves the source of considerable psychosocial difficulty. Thus although psychotherapy cannot be expected to eliminate chronic tics, it may nonetheless play an important role in reducing stress, addressing low self-esteem, and ameliorating family or internal conflicts that relate to the tics.

The local and national Tourette Syndrome Association can provide educational materials, advocacy resources, and valuable emotional support through contact with other children with Tourette's syndrome and their families.

Pharmacologic Treatment

As with other disorders, medication is indicated in tic disorder only when potential benefits appear to outweigh potential side effects. In children with Tourette's syndrome, the indications and choice of medication will differ, depending on whether the target symptoms are the tics themselves or the associated symptoms of inattention, impulsivity, or obsessive-compulsive disorder. There is no evidence that medication affects the prognosis or underlying course of the illness.

Physical discomfort, social stigmatization, and interference with classroom participation are all indications for a trial of medication for tics. The most potent medications for tics are haloperidol and pimozide, two neuroleptics that are relatively specific D_2-receptor antagonists. About 60%–90% of patients with Tourette's syndrome respond to these medications and experience a mean reduction in symptom severity of about 65% (Shapiro and Shapiro 1988; Shapiro et al. 1989). Medication is best started at a low dose (0.25 mg of haloperidol or 1 mg of pimozide), with gradual increments of the same amount every 1–2 weeks if the symptoms remain severe. Increases and decreases in dose should be made slowly, since the therapeutic response to medication is often gradual; in addition, rebounds in tic severity following abrupt withdrawal of medication can obscure the underlying course of the symptoms.

Despite the potency of the neuroleptic drugs, their side effects often limit their usefulness. Evidence of acute dystonias, akathisia, drowsiness, cognitive blunting, dysphoria, and separation anxiety often necessitates reducing or discontinuing these medications. The possibility of tardive dyskinesias also makes the chronic use of these agents problematic. Both pimozide and haloperidol have been reported to cause cardiac conduction abnormalities; hence, a baseline electrocardiogram is desirable before initiating medication. Because of haloperidol's marginally greater efficacy and pimozide's potentially greater cardiac effects, haloperidol may be the preferable agent with which to begin neuroleptic treatment.

Because of the neuroleptics' frequent side effects, it is wise to limit their use to the severer cases of Tourette's syndrome or to those unresponsive to other medication. An alternative first-choice medication for tics, especially in mild cases, is clonidine, an alpha-adrenergic antagonist that, while less potent and less consistently effective than the neuroleptics, is safer (Leckman et al. 1988b). Unlike the neuroleptics, which are usually given in a single bedtime dose to reduce sedation, clonidine must be given every 3–4 hours during the day to maintain tic control. Clonidine is best started with a single 0.05 mg dose each morning. If this is tolerated well, additional 0.05 mg doses are added at weekly intervals, first at noon and then after school. If tics are troublesome in the evening, an additional suppertime dose may be added. If necessary, the strength of each dose may be gradually increased in small increments up to a total daily of about 0.3 mg; beyond this level, side effects usually become problematic. The response to clonidine is most often gradual, often requiring 8–12 weeks to become apparent, and in some cases up to a year to develop fully. Beyond reducing tics, clonidine also frequently has a beneficial effect on the inattentiveness, distractibility, and emotional lability found in many children with Tourette's syndrome; indeed, clonidine has also been found useful in some children with attention-deficit hyperactivity disorder in the absence of Tourette's syndrome (Hunt et al. 1985).

The principal side effect of clonidine is sedation, which occurs in about 10%–20% of patients; this drowsiness is dose related and usually decreases over time. Other side effects include irritability, dry mouth, orthostatic hypotension, and, rarely, exacerbations of preexisting cardiac arrhythmias.

Over and above the tics per se, the inattention, distractibility, or obsessions and compulsions that accompany Tourette's syndrome may require pharmacologic intervention. Because stimulants frequently exacerbate tics, their use in children with Tourette's syndrome remains controversial (Golden 1988). For those children whose inattentiveness is not ameliorated by clonidine, a cautious trial of a tricyclic, such as desipramine, in low doses may be the best choice (Riddle et al. 1988).

Obsessive-compulsive symptoms may plague older patients with Tourette's syndrome, even when the tics have diminished spontaneously or in response to medication. Fluoxetine, a selective serotonin reuptake inhibitor, has proven useful in such cases (Riddle et al. 1990). Although other serotonergic agents, such as fluvoxamine and clomipramine, seem theoretically promising, there are few systematic data on their antiobsessional efficacy in Tourette's syndrome.

Patients with tic disorders and their families should be cautioned about all drug use, both licit and illicit. Sympathomimetics ranging from decongestants through amphetamine and cocaine markedly exacerbate tics. Older patients may experiment with alcohol, nicotine, or cannabinoids in an attempt to self-medicate their tics.

Research Issues

Research into the pathogenesis and treatment of tics is progressing on many fronts. Advances in imaging techniques such as magnetic resonance imaging and spectroscopy, positron-emission tomography, single photon emission tomography, and regional cerebral blood flow promise to shed light on the pathophysiology and neuroanatomy of Tourette's syndrome and related disorders. The development of brain banks and new immunohistochemical techniques will facilitate postmortem neuropathologic studies of Tourette's syndrome. Basic neurophysiologic research into the functioning of the basal ganglia and their neurotransmitter systems will be an important adjunct to understanding the pathophysiology of Tourette's syndrome.

Ongoing studies of high-risk families with high prevalences of tic disorder and/or obsessive-compulsive disorder pursue several goals. First, linkage studies of such families utilizing new recombinant techniques may permit locating and characterizing the putative Tourette's syndrome gene, as well as clarifying how it exerts its pathogenic effect; this in turn may facilitate the development of therapeutic agents. Second, identification of individuals in such families who are genetically at risk for Tourette's syndrome and related conditions will facilitate the study of how nongenetic factors influence the pathogenesis of these conditions. However, the development of markers that can prospectively identify as yet asymptomatic children carrying the Tourette's syndrome gene will pose the double challenge of how to avoid stigmatization and how to intervene preventively to minimize the development of symptomatic illness.

References

Albin RL, Young AB, Penney JB: The functional anatomy of basal ganglia disorders. Trends Neurosci 12:366–375, 1989

American Psychiatric Association: Diagnostic and Statistical Manual of Mental Disorders, 3rd Edition, Revised. Washington, DC, American Psychiatric Association, 1987

Burd L, Kerbeshian L, Wikenheiser M, et al: Prevalence of Gilles de la Tourette's syndrome in North Dakota adults. Am J Psychiatry 143:787–788, 1986

Chappel P, Leckman JF, Pauls D, et al: Biochemical and genetic studies of Tourette's syndrome: implications for treatment and future research, in Application of Basic Neuroscience to Child Psychiatry. Edited by Deutsch S, Weizman A, Weizman R. New York, Plenum, 1990, pp 241–260

Chase TN, Foster NL, Fedio P, et al: Gilles de la Tourette syndrome: studies with the fluorine-18-labeled fluorodeoxyglucose positron emission tomographic method. Ann Neurol (Suppl) 15:175, 1984

Cohen DJ: The pathology of the self in primary childhood au-

tism and Gilles de la Tourette syndrome. Psychiatr Clin North Am 3:383–402, 1980

Fahn S, Erenberg G: Differential diagnosis of tic phenomena: neurologic perspective, in Tourette's Syndrome and Tic Disorders. Edited by Cohen DJ, Bruun RD, Leckman JF. New York, John Wiley, 1988, pp 41–54

Gilles de la Tourette G: Study of a neurologic condition characterized by motor incoordination accompanied by echolalia and coprolalia (1885) (translated by Goetz CG, Klawans HL), in Gilles de la Tourette Syndrome. Edited by Friedhoff AJ, Chase TN. New York, Raven, 1982, pp 1–16

Goetz CG, Tanner CM, Wilson RS, et al: Clonidine and Gilles de la Tourette syndrome: double-blind study using objective rating methods. Ann Neurol 21:307–310, 1987

Golden GS: The use of stimulants in the treatment of Tourette's syndrome, in Tourette's Syndrome and Tic Disorders: Clinical Understanding and Treatment. Edited by Cohen DJ, Bruun RD, Leckman JF. New York, John Wiley, 1988, pp 317–325

Goodman WK, Price LH, Rasmussen SA, et al: The Yale-Brown Obsessive Compulsive Scale. Arch Gen Psychiatry 46:1006–1011, 1989

Grad LR, Pelcovitz D, Olson M, et al: Obsessive-compulsive symptomatology in children with Tourette's syndrome. J Am Acad Child Adolesc Psychiatry 26:69–73, 1987

Haber SN, Kowall NW, Vonsattel JP, et al: Gilles de la Tourette's syndrome: a postmortem neuropathological and immunohistochemical study. J Neurol Sci 75:225–241, 1986

Hunt RD, Minderaa R, Cohen DJ: Clonidine benefits children with attention-deficit disorder and hyperactivity: report of a double-blind, placebo crossover therapeutic trial. Journal of the American Academy of Child Psychiatry 24:617–629, 1985

Kurlan R, Behr J, Medved L, et al: Transient tic disorder and the spectrum of Tourette's syndrome. Arch Neurol 45:1200–1201, 1988

Leckman JF, Cohen DJ, Price RA, et al: The pathogenesis of Gilles de la Tourette's syndrome: a review of data and hypothesis, in Movement Disorders. Edited by Shah AB, Shah NS, Donald AG. New York, Plenum, 1984, pp 257–272

Leckman JF, Price RA, Walkup JT, et al: Nongenetic factors in Gilles de la Tourette's syndrome (letter). Arch Gen Psychiatry 44:100, 1987

Leckman JF, Towbin KE, Ort SI, et al: Clinical assessment of tic disorder severity, in Tourette's Syndrome and Tic Disorders: Clinical Understanding and Treatment. Edited by Cohen DJ, Bruun RD, Leckman JF. New York, John Wiley, 1988a, pp 55–78

Leckman JF, Walkup JT, Cohen DJ: Clonidine treatment of Tourette's syndrome, in Tourette's Syndrome and Tic Disorders: Clinical Understanding and Treatment. Edited by Cohen DJ, Bruun RD, Leckman JF. New York, John Wiley, 1988b, pp 103–116

Leckman JF, Riddle MA, Berrettini WH, et al: Elevated CSF dynorphin A [1–8] in Tourette's syndrome. Life Sci 43:2015–2033, 1988c

Leckman JF, Riddle MA, Cohen DJ: Pathobiology of Tourette's syndrome, in Tourette's Syndrome and Tic Disorders: Clinical Understanding and Treatment. Edited by Cohen DJ, Bruun RD, Leckman JF. New York, John Wiley, 1988d, pp 103–116

Leckman JF, Riddle MA, Hardin MT, et al: The Yale Global Tic Severity Scale: initial testing of a clinician-rated scale of tic severity. J Am Acad Child Adolesc Psychiatry 28:566–573, 1989

Leckman JF, Dolnansky ES, Hardin MT, et al: Perinatal factors in the expression of Tourette's syndrome: an exploratory study. J Am Acad Child Adolesc Psychiatry 29:220–226, 1990

Pasamanick B, Kawi A: A study of the association of prenatal and perinatal factors in the development of tics in children. J Pediatr 48:596–601, 1956

Pauls DL, Leckman JF: The inheritance of Gilles de la Tourette syndrome and associated behaviors: evidence for autosomal dominant transmission. N Engl J Med 315:993–997, 1986

Pauls DL, Leckman JF: The genetics of Tourette's syndrome, in Tourette's Syndrome and Tic Disorders: Clinical Understanding and Treatment. Edited by Cohen DJ, Bruun RD, Leckman JF. New York, John Wiley, 1988, pp 91–101

Pauls DL, Towbin KE, Leckman JF, et al: Gilles de la Tourette's syndrome and obsessive-compulsive disorder. Arch Gen Psychiatry 43:1180–1182, 1986

Price RA, Kidd KK, Cohen DJ, et al: A twin study of Tourette syndrome. Arch Gen Psychiatry 42:815–820, 1985

Rapoport JL (ed): Obsessive-Compulsive Disorder in Children and Adolescents. Washington, DC, American Psychiatric Press, 1989

Riddle MA, Hardin MT, Cho SC, et al: Desipramine treatment of boys with attention-deficit hyperactivity disorder and tics: preliminary clinical experience. J Am Acad Child Adolesc Psychiatry 27:811–814, 1988

Riddle MA, Hardin MT, King R, et al: Fluoxetine treatment of children and adolescents with Tourette's syndrome and obsessive-compulsive disorders: preliminary clinical experience. J Am Acad Child Adolesc Psychiatry 29:45–48, 1990

Shapiro AK, Shapiro ES: Treatment of tic disorders with haloperidol, in Tourette's Syndrome and Tic Disorders: Clinical Understanding and Treatment. Edited by Cohen DJ, Bruun RD, Leckman JF. New York, John Wiley, 1988, pp 267–280

Shapiro AK, Shapiro ES, Young JG, et al (eds): Gilles de la Tourette Syndrome, 2nd Edition. New York, Raven, 1988

Shapiro ES, Shapiro AK, Fulop G, et al: Controlled study of haloperidol, pimozide, and placebo for the treatment of Gilles de la Tourette's syndrome. Arch Gen Psychiatry 46:722–730, 1989

Stokes A, Bawden H, Camfield P, et al: Factors associated with the adjustment of children with Tourette's syndrome. Paper presented at the annual meeting of the American Academy of Child and Adolescent Psychiatry, Seattle, WA, October 1988

Swedo SE, Schapiro MB, Grady CL, et al: Cerebral glucose metabolism in childhood-onset obsessive compulsive disorder. Arch Gen Psychiatry 46:518–523, 1989a

Swedo SE, Rapoport JL, Cheslow DL, et al: High prevalence of obsessive-compulsive symptoms in patients with Sydenham's chorea. Am J Psychiatry 146:246–249, 1989b

Swedo SE, Rapoport JL, Leonard H, et al: Obsessive-compulsive disorder in children and adolescents: clinical phenomenology of 70 consecutive cases. Arch Gen Psychiatry 46:335–341, 1989c

Zahner GEP, Clubb MM, Leckman JF, et al: The epidemiology of Tourette's syndrome, in Tourette's Syndrome and Tic Disorders: Clinical Understanding and Treatment. Edited by Cohen DJ, Bruun RD, Leckman JF. New York, John Wiley, 1988, pp 79–80

Section IX

Disorders in Somatic Function

Chapter 37

Sleep Disorders: Infancy Through Adolescence

Thomas F. Anders, M.D.

Polysomnographic (PSG) recording of sleep during the past 30 years has expanded our knowledge about the organization and regulation of sleep and waking. Sleep-wake evaluations in a sleep laboratory have become a helpful clinical diagnostic tool. At the same time, professionalization has occurred. The American Sleep Disorders Association certifies clinical laboratories and the technicians who record sleep. The American Board of Sleep Disorders Medicine and Clinical Polysomnography certifies clinicians. This new specialty comprises an interdisciplinary group of professionals. However, just as sleep-wake assessments in child and adolescent psychiatry remain uncommon, child and adolescent psychiatrists are underrepresented in this group.

A number of psychophysiologic systems are routinely recorded by polysomnography in a sleep laboratory. Typically, subjects are instrumented for all-night recording of peripheral muscle tone, eye movements, and cardiac and respiratory activity, and electroencephalograms (EEGs) are obtained. Eye movement patterns, muscle tone, and the EEG are the primary parameters used to score rapid eye movement (REM) and non-rapid eye movement (NREM) sleep. Patterns of obstructed breathing, heart rate irregularity, and episodic behavior during sleep are associated features useful in diagnosing specific sleep disorders.

Until recently, recordings have been largely confined to nighttime in a laboratory. Sleeping in an unfamiliar sleep laboratory is disruptive of normal sleep and requires adaptation by recording over several nights. These constraints have made sleep research with young subjects especially difficult. Both subjects and their parents are reluctant to sleep away from home, especially if they do not have a sleep problem and are being asked to serve as normal control subjects. Ambulatory polysomnography monitoring has greatly expanded the scope of sleep research by providing opportunities for home recording and for 24-hour recording.

The Physiology of Sleep States

Aserinsky and Kleitman (1955) are credited with the first modern descriptions of the two states of sleep, now widely known as REM and NREM sleep. REM sleep has been called active or paradoxical sleep because, in contrast to patterns of slowed neurophysiologic and neurochemical activity expected in sleep, metabolic processes are, paradoxically, active (Kales 1969). The brain's electrical activity recorded on the EEG during REM sleep resembles wakefulness. Neuronal firing, neurotransmitter turnover, and metabolic activity also resemble patterns of waking. Mental activity during REM sleep is vigorous and is reported as dreams. Thus, during REM sleep, an individual appears asleep, but for the most part the central nervous system is highly activated.

We know from the sleep laboratory why individuals appear so peaceful during REM sleep when their brains are so active (Berger 1969). The limbs of sleepers in REM sleep are "paralyzed" by the active inhibition of peripheral muscle tone. We also know from animal studies that when the brain centers responsible for this inhibition of peripheral muscle tone are transected, the animals exhibit motor disinhibition. They are behaviorally active during REM sleep, seeming to "act out" the content of their visual imagery. Transected cats will exhibit hissing and defensive posturing, as if attacking a predator or defending themselves (Jouvet and DeLorme 1965). A recently described REM parasomnia in humans (described below) seems to represent a clinical analogy of this experimental transection.

In contrast to the psychophysiologic activation of REM sleep, NREM sleep is characterized by the more expected, basal, organized patterns of physiologic inhibition. The muscle tone inhibition of REM sleep ceases, as do the REM bursts. Both respiration and heart rate are slowed in rate and more regular in rhythm. The EEG is synchronized with specific slower frequency wave forms, such as sleep spindles, K-complexes, and delta waves that define four NREM sleep stages.

In newborns, only two sleep states, REM sleep and NREM sleep, can be distinguished. After the first 6 months of life, during NREM sleep, the specific EEG wave forms that are used to subclassify NREM sleep emerge. The EEG of stage 1 NREM sleep resembles the tracing of REM sleep; however, respiratory and heart rate patterns, muscle tone, and eye movement patterns are inhibited. The EEG of stage 2 NREM sleep contains K-complexes and sleep spindles. Stages 3 and 4 NREM sleep have varying amounts of slow, high-voltage synchronized delta waves.

Development of Sleep-Wake State Organization

The maturation reflected in the EEG is only one of the developmental changes that occurs during infancy. The proportional relationships to each other of REM and NREM sleep, the REM-NREM sleep cycle length, the sleep onset state, and diurnal influences on sleep-wake organization are four other areas that mature during childhood (Anders and Keener 1983).

Proportionately, REM sleep occupies approximately 20% and NREM sleep about 80% of total sleep time in adults. Stages 3 and 4 NREM sleep account for approximately 20% of all NREM sleep.

In neonates, REM sleep occupies 50% of total sleep time, and stage 4 sleep does not occur. REM and NREM sleep states alternate with each other in sleep cycles that recur periodically. In the adult, sleep cycles recur every 90 minutes on average, while in the infant, the cycle length is approximately 50 minutes.

In the adult, sleep typically begins with NREM stage 4 sleep, and the first third of the sleep period has most of the total night's stage 4 NREM sleep. That is, although REM-NREM cycles recur throughout the night, the percentage of NREM stage 4 sleep in a single cycle is greater during the early part of the night than later in the night. The proportion of REM sleep in a single sleep cycle is greater during the latter part of the night. In infants, sleep begins with an initial REM period, and sleep cycles throughout the night have as much REM sleep as NREM sleep. There are no early- and late-night differences in REM-NREM proportions. These shifts in the temporal organization of states during the course of a night's sleep reflect the maturation of internal central nervous system mechanisms that regulate the individual's biological clock.

Taken together, these developmental shifts represent a functional diminution in the prominence of REM sleep as maturation proceeds, suggesting that REM sleep plays an early ontogenetic role in the maturation of specific central nervous system pathways, especially the visual tracts (Roffwarg et al. 1966). An understanding of these changes in the organization and regulation of REM and NREM sleep is essential for understanding the specific sleep disorders that affect infants, children, and adolescents.

Sleep Disorders of Infants, Children, and Adolescents

The American Sleep Disorders Association revised the Diagnostic Classification of Sleep Disorders (Association of Sleep Disorders Centers 1979). Essentially, there are four major categories of sleep disorder: 1) disorders of initiating and maintaining sleep (the insomnias); 2) disorders of excessive somnolence; 3) parasomnias (unusual sleep-related behaviors and events); and 4) sleep cycle disorders (biorhythmic or chronobiological disorders). Like the maturation of sleep-wake state organization, sleep disorders in infants, children, and adolescents can be viewed from a developmental perspective. Although age distinctions are not ironclad, a developmentally oriented evaluation is useful in differential diagnosis, any treatment planning, and prognostic forecasting. In general, an age-appropriate, short-lived disturbance is less serious and requires less intervention than a disorder that appears earlier or persists beyond the usual age limits. The former most often reflects environmental disruptions or perturbations; the latter may reflect more significant organic or psychopathologic dysfunction.

Just as it is important to obtain a careful sleep history when evaluating children who present with sleep problems, so too is it important to inquire about sleep habits in all children who present with behavior problems. As described in more detail below, some attention-deficit and hyperactivity syndromes may represent disordered sleep. Growth retardation may also be associated with sleep pathology.

A sleep history requires a detailed description of all sleep-related symptoms in the child, and a thorough history of sleep problems and patterns in other family members. What is the age of onset of the problem? What is the frequency of the symptom in terms of events per week or per night, and what has been its course (stable, worsening, improving)? What time during the night or day does the symptom occur, in terms of both clock time and the time since falling asleep? For example, parasomnias are related to sleep onset and not to clock time. They generally occur 90–120 minutes after falling asleep. Phase delay syndromes are related to clock time. Bedtimes usually occur at times that are later than usual. Night terrors can be distinguished from nightmares in that the former occur during the first third of the sleep period in NREM stage 4 sleep, and the latter occur later in the night when REM sleep predominates.

The child's customary sleep habits are important to establish. What is the usual bedtime and rise time? How regular are sleep habits? What are the sleeping arrangements? With whom does the child share a room or bed? Do the child's symptoms disturb others? Are bedtime rituals present? How common are dreams and nightmares? How common are night waking, bet wetting, and snoring?

Finally, it is important to assess the effects of a nighttime sleep problem on daytime functioning. Is the child sleepy during the day or is the child alert and active? Does the child nap regu-larly? Do the nighttime symptoms encroach on normal social functions? For example, is the child embarassed to sleep at a friend's house or sleep away at camp?

Sleep Disorders in Infants and Toddlers (Birth–Age 3)

Sleeping through the night is the most common concern of parents during infancy. Night waking may be viewed as a precursor of difficulty in initiating and maintaining sleep. Parents of infants tend to expect continuous sleep periods of 3–4 hours punctuated by awakenings for feedings for the first 2–3 months of life, with longer periods at night and shorter periods (naps) during the day by 4 months of age. Some parents expect that their infants should sleep through the night shortly after birth. Sometimes health professionals prescribe hypnotics or antihistamines. More often, they counsel parents to let their baby cry.

Using maternal questionnaires, Moore and Ucko (1957) reported that 71% of infants begin to sleep through the night ("settle") by 3 months and 84% by 6 months of age. Settling is defined as sleeping from 12 midnight through 5 A.M. By 10 months of age, 90% of the infants in Moore and Ucko's study had settled. During the second half of the first year, however, and during the second year of life, 50% of the babies who had settled developed night-waking problems.

Research suggests that settling needs to be more carefully defined (Anders 1979). Using all-night, time-lapse video recording in the infant's home, in contrast to obtaining maternal questionnaire data, it was found that babies stay asleep for less time than their parents report. Since parents are usually asleep during the night and report only on infants who awaken and cry, infants who awaken and return to sleep on their own are reported as having slept through the night. Video studies demonstrate that most infants by 6 months of age awaken one or two times during the night after 5–6 hours, but one-third to one-half of awake infants are able to fall back asleep without calling for parental help.

This has led to the designation of infants as signalers (those who call for help when they awaken) and self-soothers (those who return to sleep on their own). There were no discernable differences in REM-NREM sleep state organization that distinguished the signalers from self-soothers. There were significant differences, however, in the way parents of signalers handled their infants at bedtime. Parents of signalers placed their infants into the crib already asleep. Self-soothers were much more likely to be put into their crib awake at sleep onset and allowed to fall asleep on their own. Self-soothers were more likely to use a sleep aid, such as a pacifier, to help them fall asleep on their own. Signalers, in contrast, were already asleep at sleep onset and did not use a sleep aid. In the middle of the night, after an awakening, the process was repeated. Self-soothers awakened for 3–5 minutes, but were able to fall asleep on their own. They frequently used their sleep aid to help them. Signalers awakened, became fussy, and began to cry. They seemed to use their parents as their sleep aid (J. Anders and L. Halpern, personal communication, June 1990).

During the second year of life, it is common for infants to resist bedtime and separation from their parents and to develop bedtime routines that make the transition easier. Infants with significant problems present with severe and intractable battles at bedtime associated with frequent and prolonged bouts of night waking that begin shortly after sleep onset and persist to rise time in the morning. Frequently, these more serious disorders are a source of family tension associated with significant conflict about managing the infant's sleep.

A number of strategies to assist families have been attempted. These range from advice that urges the parents to "let the infant cry" for 5–7 nights, to graduated withdrawal of parental presence by waiting for progressively longer periods of time before intervening (Ferber 1985), to a focus on the behaviors around going to bed and falling asleep. Since night waking may be associated with whether an infant is put into the crib awake or asleep at sleep onset, and whether a child struggles significantly at bedtime, the night-waking problem can be better understood as a problem of separation. Parents may benefit by "teaching" their children to separate and fall asleep on their own.

Sleep Problems in the Preschooler (Age 3–6)

The common problems of this age period are struggles around going to bed and nightmares. Preschoolers, especially if there are older siblings in the family, enjoy participating in the family's evening activities. Although separation anxiety per se does not play a major role at bedtime after the age of 3 years, frequently fears of the dark or fears of being alone take its place. Because daytime experiences for preschoolers are frequently exciting and overstimulating, calming down at bedtime may be difficult. More and more families have irregular schedules. Two working parents, or one working single parent, out of the home frequently, are common occurrences. Time with a parent may be a precious commodity that the toddler wishes to prolong. Day-care settings may be associated with overstimulation, leading to troubled sleep. The role of television in overstimulation and fear arousal remains unknown.

Whatever the causes, the preschool child may protest vigorously at bedtime in an attempt to lengthen the time to final lights out. Prolonged rituals that include repeated stories, returns for more hugs and kisses, another glass of water or snack, and pleas for "5 more minutes" are examples of such protestations. Insistence on falling asleep in the parent's bed or while lying next to and holding the parent is also an expression of this problem.

Dreams are usually reported by children after age 3 years (Foulkes 1982). Nightmares follow shortly thereafter. Dream content before age 8 is usually short and concrete. Dream symbolization and elaboration are uncommon. Nightmares are anxiety dreams that awaken the sleeping child. Nightmares occur during REM sleep and result in a fully awake and oriented child who remembers and recounts the content of the dream. Since REM sleep occurs most commonly in the latter third of the night, nightmares generally are noted in the early morning hours, after 2 A.M. Nightmares need to be distinguished from night terrors (to be described in more detail below).

A nightmare is frightening. Its content often deals with themes of being injured, lost, or abandoned. If nightmares become frequent, they can be another source of reluctance to go to bed at night. In the younger toddler, the action of nightmares is often represented by images of monsters and frightening animals. In older children, the content of nightmares typically contains more comprehensible human imagery.

Most commonly, nightmares and bedtime protestations are transient and "normal" occurrences that do not seriously disrupt family functioning. In the treatment of frequent and recurrent nightmares, and nightly, prolonged struggles at bedtime, the sources of anxiety need to be explored and interventions designed that can, as well as possible, address the child's needs for comfort, security, regularity of sleep habits, and protection from overstimulation.

A rare sleep disorder in the toddler can be classified as a disorder of excessive somnolence. Typically, the obstructive sleep apnea syndrome (Guilleminault and Stoohs 1990) has been observed in older adults. Daytime sleepiness is usually the presenting complaint and is the result of the accumulated sleep loss that is secondary to the repeated brief awakenings that follow each apneic episode. In some adults, there may be 250–300 sleep apnea arousals each night.

The toddler version of sleep apnea may present as failure to thrive. The multiple arousals at night seem to interfere with the secretion of growth hormone. Whereas the cause of the obstruction associated with sleep apnea in adults is frequently unknown, in toddlers it appears that obstruction is associated with hypertrophied tonsils and adenoids. When tonsillectomies were routinely performed in all children, a generation ago, the obstructive sleep apnea syndrome in preschoolers was unknown. Today, however, there are greater numbers of children who, after repeated ear, nose, and throat infections, develop hypertrophied tonsils and adenoids. Some of these youngsters experience obstructive sleep apnea during sleep and fail to grow properly. All evaluations for failure to thrive in children should inquire about sleep habits.

A presumptive diagnosis of obstructive sleep apnea can be entertained if the child snores. A characteristic high-pitched expiratory snore is associated with the sleeper's vigorous attempts to move air through an obstructed glottis. A cassette recorder at the bedside to record snoring can be used as an aid to diagnosis. A definitive diagnosis requires an evaluation in a sleep laboratory with polysomnography monitoring that includes respiration. A tonsillectomy and adenoidectomy should restore normal sleep and growth.

The School-Age Child (Age 5–13)

During latency, most infancy and toddler sleep problems subside. Some of the former bedtime rituals continue as habits that the child carries out. Need for a night-light might persist, or a child may read before falling asleep. A familiar stuffed animal may continue to serve as a companion in the night. A relatively uncommon but dramatic group of disorders, the parasomnias, appear during this age period. Parasomnias are sleep disorders in which episodes of nonwaking activity interrupt sleep suddenly and intermittently without disturbing sleep. The four most common parasomnias are night terrors (pavor nocturnus), sleepwalking (somnambulism), sleeptalking (somniloquy), and sleep-related enuresis. Night terrors often begin during the toddler and preschool period, but may persist into the school years. They are often misdiagnosed as nightmares.

Until recently, all of the parasomnias were considered to share a set of common physiologic properties unique to NREM stage 4 sleep (Anders and Keener 1983). In an expanded classification, however, both REM and NREM parasomnias have been defined (Mahowald and Rosen 1990). The NREM parasomnias generally occur at a particular point in the sleep cycle, at the end of an NREM stage 4 sleep period, just prior to a transition to REM sleep. Physiologically, NREM stage 4 sleep is the "deepest" stage of sleep. Sensory thresholds are highest, and it is difficult to arouse individuals. When aroused, subjects are generally disoriented, and their thinking is confused. There is no verbal recounting of mental activity. This contrasts with awakenings from REM sleep that are characterized by alertness, rapid orientation, and articulate recall of dream experiences. Awakenings from NREM stages 1 and 2 sleep are more like awakenings from REM sleep.

Broughton (1968) suggested that REM sleep that follows NREM stage 4 sleep may serve to "arouse" the subject from deep sleep. He speculated that in children who present with NREM stage 4 parasomnias, the central nervous system mechanisms that trigger the transition from stage 4 NREM sleep to REM sleep are immature or dysfunctional. The failure to enter REM sleep leads to a parasomnia arousal, which substitutes for the more normal activating effects of REM sleep. Thus NREM stage 4 parasomnias have also been called disorders of arousal (Broughton 1968).

In addition to the unique timing of NREM stage 4 parasomnias, just prior to an expected REM period, other common features of NREM parasomnias are 1) a predominance of males to females (6–8:1); 2) a strongly positive family history, along male lines; and, 3) retrograde amnesia for the event on the following morning. Children who present with parasomnias distress their families, but are themselves most often not aware of the episode. They usually do not awaken; if they do, they are disoriented and confused and fall rapidly back to sleep. In the morning, they have no recall of the event.

In general, NREM stage 4 parasomnias are easy to diagnose. The time of the episode after sleep onset is a key differential diagnostic feature, since, most often, NREM stage 4 sleep is limited to the first 3 hours of sleep. A night terror attack or sleepwalking episode, therefore, usually occurs approximately 90–120 minutes after sleep onset. Second, NREM stage 4 sleep is characteristically "deep," and individuals are difficult to awaken. Mental activity is not present during NREM stage 4 sleep. When individuals awaken, there is disorientation and confusion; there are no reports of dreaming.

Night terrors are characterized by a child's sudden arousal, accompanied by screaming and thrashing uncontrollably in bed. The child may appear glassy-eyed and stare without seeing; he or she does not respond to visual or verbal cues. In the laboratory, such an episode is characterized by continuous high-voltage delta waves on the EEG, characteristic of NREM stage 4 sleep. During a night terror attack, the child is not awake, but may appear to be highly agitated. Autonomic arousal, characterized by tachypnea, tachycardia, and diaphoresis, is obvious. Parental attempts at consolation are not effective. The attack terminates spontaneously after approximately 3–5 minutes, and the child transitions to REM sleep. Occasionally an attack may last 30 minutes. If parental intervention is sustained and vigorous, the child may awaken, but then is confused, disoriented, and unable to relate dream material. The child quickly returns to sleep and does not remember the episode on the following morning.

The clinical presentation of night terrors is distinct from that of nightmares. Nightmares are associated with vivid dream imagery; a fully alert, frightened, and oriented youngster; and recollection of the episode in the morning. As described previously, nightmares are also more likely to occur during the latter third of the night when REM sleep predominates.

Sleepwalking, like night terrors, also occurs approximately 90–120 minutes after sleep onset. The child sits up in bed and may fidget for a period of time, or may leave the bed and "walk" to another location. There is generally no screaming, so that the child may be found in a new location in the morning. If sitting up or moving around the bed is the only manifestation of the parasomnia, then no one may be aware of the episode in the morning. The child does not recall the episode.

A popular misconception is that sleepwalking is purposeful. In general, sleepwalkers are poorly co-ordinated and are unable to carry out complex behaviors. In fact, sleepwalkers are in danger of injuring themselves, and parents need to be advised to "accident-proof" their child's sleeping environment to protect their child from harm. It is highly unlikely that a child or adolescent who leaves the house and takes a drive in the family car or who wanders to the kitchen to consume a midnight snack is sleepwalking. Sleepwalkers are unable to perform such complex behaviors.

Sleep talking, like sleepwalking and night terror attacks, generally is confined to NREM stage 4 sleep. Short cries or garbled utterances can be heard. Usually the content of the sleep utterance is unintelligible. The episode is short and not remembered in the morning.

NREM stage 4 parasomnias are considered to be familial, developmental immaturities of sleep state transition mechanisms. The most parsimonious treatment is reassurance of the child and family that the problem is transient, not serious, and requires no specific pharmacologic or psychotherapeutic intervention. Most often the child "outgrows" the parasomnia by the onset of adolescence. Protection of the sleeping subject from self-injury is critical. Since both sleep loss and excessive fatigue are associated with an increased need for NREM stage 4 sleep, and a heightened need for stage 4 sleep may be related to an increase in the frequency and intensity of parasomnias, additional advice to parents should include the importance of regular sleep habits with sufficient amounts of nighttime sleep. An after-school nap may also reduce any NREM stage 4 sleep deficit.

In extreme cases in which the parasomnia is so frequent that the child becomes too embarrassed to sleep over at a friend's house, or becomes inhibited in other usual daytime social activities, a benzodiazepine may be tried at bedtime. These drugs are usually effective, but termination of pharmacotherapy often results in a recurrence of the parasomnia. When parasomnias persist into adolescence, or present initially in adolescence, neurologic consultation and further medical evaluation are warranted to rule out a seizure disorder. Parasomnias frequently resemble seizures, and an EEG with nasopharyngeal electrodes may be warranted for persistent, intractable cases prior to prescribing benzodiazepines.

Sleep-related enuresis, by far the most common parasomnia, is discussed by Walsh and Menville (Chapter 38, this volume). It is generally not limited to NREM stage 4 sleep. A second clinical disorder that has expanded the definition of parasomnias to sleep interruptions beyond NREM stage 4 sleep is the REM sleep behavior disorder (Mahowald and Rosen 1990). Normally, tonic inhibition of peripheral muscle tone in REM sleep results in sleep paralysis. However, in affected children, this atonia is absent during REM sleep, resulting in vigorous and sometimes violent self-directed or other-directed motor attacks. REM sleep behavior disorder is a very rare disorder reported most commonly in older adult males; two cases in childhood have been reported, one in a child with associated brain-stem pathology (Schenck et al. 1986). The pathophysiology seems related to tumors or vascular malformations in brain-stem areas associated with REM muscle tone inhibition. Treatment remains symptomatic and supportive.

Sleep Disorders in Adolescence

Two classes of sleep disorders most commonly affect adolescents: disorders of excessive somnolence and phase delay syndromes. The disorder of excessive somnolence that begins in adolescence is narcolepsy, and the most common initial complaint is excessive sleepiness.

To assess quantitatively the amount of excessive daytime sleepiness that subjects with disorders of excessive somnolence experience, the Multiple Sleep Latency Test should be performed (Carskadon and Dement 1987). The test, carried out in a sleep laboratory, uses polysomnography to assess the amount of sleep that is obtained during five 20-minute trials, from mid-morning to early evening. At each time period, the subject is requested to try to fall asleep. The latency to sleep onset for each attempted "nap" represents how sleepy the individual is. The test, standardized for use with adults and for adolescents at different Tanner stages of puberty (Tanner 1962), has been shown to be a sensitive indicator of sleepiness and is significantly correlated with the amount of performance decrement associated with sleepiness.

Narcolepsy, a disorder of REM sleep, is characterized by episodic bouts of excessive daytime sleepiness leading to irresistible sleep attacks that intrude on waking (Guilleminault 1987). In the full-blown clinical syndrome, individuals suffer from four symptoms, referred to as the narcoleptic tetrad: 1) REM sleep attacks during wakefulness, 2) cataplexy, 3) hypnagogic hallucinations, and 4) sleep paralysis. This tetrad of symptoms represents REM activation at the wrong point in the temporal sequence of sleep-wake organization. Transitions from wakefulness to REM sleep are physiologic only during early infancy. After this period, REM sleep almost always follows NREM sleep. In narcolepsy, however, the REM nuclei in the brain are not inhibited by the waking state, but instead fire periodically, leading to REM sleep attacks that interrupt the waking state.

Cataplexy results from the sudden inhibition of peripheral muscle tone triggered by REM activation during wakefulness. The cataplectic subject suddenly becomes atonic and falls to the ground "paralyzed" until muscle tone is restored. The individual usually maintains consciousness and is aware of feeling paralyzed. Cataplectic attacks are often preceded by intense emotional outbursts, such as laughing, crying, or feelings of rage. These affective antecedents suggest pathways between the limbic system and the pontine nuclei that are activated in REM sleep.

Hypnagogic hallucinations refer to vivid, often frightening visual imagery that is experienced by narcoleptic patients while falling asleep. Again, these visual images represent the dreamlike mental activity of REM sleep occurring at sleep onset instead of later in the night. Similarly, sleep paralysis refers to muscle tone inhibition, as in cataplexy, that occurs at sleep onset.

It is unusual to have all four of the features of the tetrad when the disorder first manifests itself. Short REM latencies (the time to the initial REM period) and frank sleep onset REM periods are the first symptoms to appear at the time of puberty. Excessive daytime sleepiness with brief REM micro-sleep attacks follows. Cataplexy becomes problematic at a later age. The diagnosis requires a comprehensive evaluation. A positive family history is suggestive. Any combination of symptoms of the narcoleptic tetrad further substantiates the diagnosis. The youngster with narcolepsy characteristically feels refreshed on awakening from a sleep attack. This contrasts to the disorientation and feelings of persistent fatigue that accompany brief naps associated with disorders of excessive somnolence secondary to other causes. The definitive diagnosis of narcolepsy requires polysomnographic evaluation in a sleep laboratory. Sleep onset REM periods are pathognomonic.

The treatment of narcolepsy is largely symptomatic. The psychoactive class of pharmacologic agents, methylphenidate and dextroamphetamine, are palliative in warding off sleepiness and suppressing

REM activity. However, tolerance is likely to develop. Supportive counseling with encouragement not to resist sleep attacks is often helpful. Work and school schedules that provide opportunities for brief naps are also useful.

In one study of young adults with narcolepsy who were asked to reconstruct the onset of their illness retrospectively, the most common misdiagnosis made by professionals who evaluated them as adolescents was hyperactivity disorder (now classified as attention-deficit hyperactivity disorder) (Navalet et al. 1976). These adults remembered that they were constantly fidgeting to ward off feelings of sleepiness. Both teachers and practitioners labeled these behaviors as hyperactive. Although narcolepsy is a rare disorder, occurring in only approximately 4 in 10,000 individuals, and hyperactivity is a much more common disorder, estimated to occur in 7%–10% of school-age children, all children who present with attention-deficit hyperactivity disorder or other hyperactivity syndromes should be given the benefit of a careful sleep history. Specific questions that focus on symptoms of the narcoleptic tetrad and on a family history of sleep disorders should be asked.

A second, more common sleep disorder that occurs in adolescents meets the criteria of phase delay syndrome (Thorpy et al. 1988). Both academic and social pressures mount sharply during adolescence. Typically, adolescents begin to complain of feeling tired, an unusual complaint for preadolescent youngsters, and frequently sleep longer hours on weekends than on school days. Adolescents are often ready to go to bed at any time, and sleep late in the morning whenever possible. These behaviors contrast sharply with the tireless, high-energy preadolescent child who never wants to go to bed.

Careful studies of the sleep needs of adolescents have demonstrated repeatedly that adolescents after puberty need more sleep, particularly NREM stage 4 sleep, than younger children. The increased physiologic sleep need seems related to the endocrinologic changes of pubertal development, as determined by Tanner staging (Carskadon et al. 1980; Tanner 1962). This endocrine-associated sleep need is coupled with heightened social pressures, including staying up late studying or socializing. The combination amounts to a significant sleep deficit that many adolescents experience. It is the size of the sleep deficit that largely accounts for the increased daytime sleepiness.

The phase delay, however, results from the fact that as adolescents stay up later and later at night-time, and wake up later and later in the morning, the circadian regulation of sleep, including the many physiologic functions that are triggered by sleep onset, becomes progressively delayed. As the body's timing mechanisms get shifted, it becomes more difficult physiologically to fall asleep and wake up at the usual hours. Adolescents thus find themselves in a perpetual condition of jet lag. That is, their biological clock becomes reset at a time different from the demands of their social and academic life.

Sufficient sleep, at least 8 hours a night, at regular, socially acceptable times is of particular importance during adolescence. When sleep debts accumulate by force of circumstances, napping should be encouraged. Once a phase delay syndrome is chronic and persistent, phase advance methods of resetting the biological clock may be necessary (Ferber 1987). The diagnosis of this condition can usually be made from the history alone. Occasionally, however, adolescents are poor reporters and misrepresent both the degree of their sleepiness and the phase disturbances of their sleep. Multiple Sleep Latency Test evaluations and a night in the sleep laboratory may clarify confusing pictures.

Disordered Sleep in Medical and Psychiatric Conditions

There is less information about sleep-wake state disorganization in children and adolescents who suffer from medical and psychiatric conditions than for adults (Kales and Tan 1969). Even the disruptions of sleep presumably associated with the common childhood illnesses are, by and large, anecdotal reports not supported by systematic research. Since several laboratory conditions, such as ambient temperature and unfamiliar surroundings, have been shown to affect sleep, it is likely that children with fevers or obstructed breathing or who are sleeping in new settings will experience fragmented sleep.

Children who live in institutions are reported to have sleep characterized by short sleep periods, repeated nighttime awakenings, and phase delay disorders. Children with mental retardation and autistic-like syndromes also suffer from frequent night awakenings and phase shifts (Okawa and Sasaki 1987). In general, disorganization of REM and NREM sleep parameters per se is associated only with profound syndromes of brain damage (Feinberg 1969). All of these studies, however, focus on small samples of referred populations and rely on parental or custodial reports of sleep behavior. Few polysomnographic studies of randomly selected members of these populations have been attempted. Such sampling bias promotes overreporting of sleep pathology.

Similarly, sleep disruption in children with psychiatric disorders remains controversial. Although it has been clearly demonstrated that adults with major depressive disorder suffer from a characteristic array of indicators of disturbed sleep, including disruptions of sleep-related endocrine regulation, these indicators are not regularly present in the sleep of children and adolescents who exhibit major depressive disorder (Dahl and Puig-Antich 1990). The sleep of depressed adults is characterized by a short initial REM latency and fragmented ultradian regulation with multiple arousals and early morning awakening. The circadian peak of early morning cortisol excretion is blunted. Although a few reports have suggested changes comparable to those noted in adult depression, these studies are characterized by small sample sizes, a failure to provide for laboratory adaptation, and the use of inadequately diagnosed subjects. More carefully controlled, larger studies have failed to replicate the disrupted patterns of sleep-wake disorganization noted in depressed adults, although the endocrine changes have been noted in children (Dahl and Puig-Antich 1990).

Similarly, in the few studies of children with attention-deficit disorder (or hyperactivity), despite parental complaints of disturbed sleep, the sleep-wake state organization in a sleep laboratory was unaffected (Greenhill et al. 1983; Kaplan et al. 1987; Small et al. 1971). Again, a paucity of studies, characterized by small samples and heterogeneous diagnostic groupings, contributes to inadequate definitive conclusions. The waking behavioral hyperactivity associated with excessive somnolence, both from narcolepsy and from the obstructive sleep apnea syndrome, has already been described.

Finally, studies that examine the effects of alcohol and other chemicals on sleep generally report two patterns of sleep-wake state disorganization (Lumley et al. 1987). There is reduction in REM sleep and fragmentation of sleep by multiple arousals during agitated states of hallucinosis and withdrawal, and there are periods of prolonged atypical "drugged" sleep during states of intoxication. These results are difficult to interpret, however. The pharmacologic effects of chemicals, both prescription and nonprescription, vary by dose, chronicity of use, and chemical structure of the compound. Initially, use of most sedative drugs leads to increased sleep, then habituation and tolerance develop, leading to chronic sleep deprivation, particularly REM deprivation.

Both hypnotics and alcohol are frequently misused for insomnia that masks underlying disorders of anxiety and depression. After periods of such misuse, it is often not clear whether inappropriate drug use led to disordered sleep, or whether disordered sleep-wake organization precipitated the course of self-medication. Careful studies of the effects of substance abuse on sleep-wake state organization in children and adolescents have not been done.

Research Issues

It is clear that we have learned a great deal about sleep-wake state maturation, regulation, and organization during early childhood and adolescence. Our research has allowed us to be more informed clinicians. Many disorders, such as the parasomnias and the disorders of excessive somnolence, were previously missed entirely or misdiagnosed. Often symptoms of these disorders were labeled as psychogenic and treated predominantly by psychotherapy. Although we are still not certain of the pathogenesis of some of the syndromes, our ability to diagnose them better and, on occasion, to prescribe more specific, palliative treatments provides reassurance to children and their families and avoids the stigma of inappropriate or inaccurate diagnoses.

Yet, other than physical restitution, primarily associated with NREM stage 4 sleep, we are still uncertain about the functions of sleep in general and of REM sleep in particular. Why is there more REM sleep in immature individuals, and why is NREM stage 4 sleep seemingly so important in early childhood and adolescence? It has been speculated that information processing occurs during REM sleep so that daytime experiences, especially novel experiences, are converted from short-term to long-term memories during REM sleep. Since young infants and children presumably experience many more new and novel bits of information each day, perhaps they require more time in REM sleep for this information-processing function.

Similarly, it is known that growth hormone is secreted primarily during NREM stage 4 sleep. Since early childhood and adolescence are periods of rapid growth, it is possible that the increased need for this state during these developmental periods provides the substrate for increased growth hormone secretion.

The relationships between sleep-state organization and physical and mental health in children and adolescents are only beginning to be explored. The informed clinician must be concerned about sleep-wake state organization in all children who present with physical and psychological disorders. A careful sleep history that examines the regularity of sleep habits, appropriate amounts of sleep, disruptions of sleep, and the behaviors associated with going to bed each night should be obtained in every evaluation. When disruptions of sleep are reported, the careful timing of the event in relation to going to bed and falling asleep is critical in making a diagnosis. Recognizing the associated characteristics of specific parasomnias, in terms of alertness and orientation surrounding the event, also helps to substantiate a clinical impression. Occasionally, a bedside cassette tape recorder, activated at bedtime by a parent, helps capture sleep disruptions for clinical review.

When symptoms are frequent and cause significant distress for families, a specialist evaluation in a sleep disorders center is indicated. Most often, however, the sleep disorders of children and adolescents are transitory and can easily be diagnosed by a careful history. Rarely are medications indicated. Sound, informed advice and reassurance are usually sufficient.

It is necessary to understand nighttime sleep-wake state organization in the broader context of daytime activity and circadian regulation. The emerging field that investigates these disorders from the 24-hour perspective is known as chronobiology. As polysomnographic recording equipment becomes ever more miniaturized and automated for long-term recording, it will soon be possible to study larger groups of children over longer periods of time in their home environments. Only then will it be possible to make more definitive statements about etiology of, natural history of, and treatment efficacy for childhood sleep disorders.

References

Anders T: Night waking in infants during the first year of life. Pediatrics 63:860–864, 1979

Anders T, Keener M: Sleep-wake state development and disorders of sleep in infants, children and adolescents, in Developmental-Behavioral Pediatrics. Edited by Levine M, Carey W, Crocker A, et al. Philadelphia, PA, WB Saunders, 1983, pp 596–606

Aserinsky E, Kleitman N: A motility cycle in sleeping infants as manifested by ocular and gross bodily activity. J Appl Physiol 8:11–13, 1955

Association of Sleep Disorders Centers: Diagnostic Classification of Sleep and Arousal Disorders, ed 1 (Prepared by the Sleep Disorders Classification Committee, HP Roffwarg, Chairman). Sleep 2:99–121, 1979

Berger R: Physiological characteristics of sleep, in Sleep: Physiology and Pathology. Edited by Kales A. Philadelphia, PA, JB Lippincott, 1969, pp 66–79

Broughton R: Sleep disorders: disorders of arousal? Science 159:1070–1078, 1968

Carskadon M, Dement W: Sleepiness in normal adolescents, in Sleep and Its Disorders in Children. Edited by Guilleminault C. New York, Raven, 1987, pp 53–66

Carskadon M, Harvey K, Duke P, et al: Pubertal changes in daytime sleepiness. Sleep 2:453–460, 1980

Dahl R, Puig-Antich J: Sleep disturbances in child and adolescent psychiatric disorders. Pediatrician 17:32–37, 1990

Feinberg I: Sleep in organic brain conditions, in Sleep: Physiology and Pathology. Edited by Kales A. Philadelphia, PA, JB Lippincott, 1969, pp 131–147

Ferber R: Solve Your Child's Sleep Problem. New York, Simon & Schuster, 1985

Ferber R: Circadian and schedule disturbances, in Sleep and Its Disorders in Children. Edited by Guilleminault C. New York, Raven, 1987, pp 165–180

Foulkes D: Children's Dreams: Longitudinal Studies. New York, John Wiley, 1982

Greenhill L, Puig-Antich J, Goetz R, et al: Sleep architecture and real sleep measures in prepubertal children with attention-deficit disorder with hyperactivity. Sleep 6:91–101, 1983

Guilleminault C: Narcolepsy and its differential diagnosis, in Sleep and Its Disorders in Children. Edited by Guilleminault C. New York, Raven, 1987, pp 181–194

Guilleminault C, Stoohs R: Obstructive sleep apnea syndrome in children. Pediatrician 17:46–51, 1990

Jouvet M, DeLorme F: Locus coeruleus et Sommeil paradoxical. C R Soc Biol (Paris) 159:895–899, 1965

Kales A: Sleep: Physiology and Pathology. Philadelphia, PA, JB Lippincott, 1969

Kales A, Tan T: Sleep alterations associated with medical illnesses, in Sleep: Physiology and Pathology. Edited by Kales A. Philadelphia, PA, JB Lippincott, 1969, pp 148–157

Kaplan B, McNicol J, Conte R, et al: Sleep disturbances in preschool-aged hyperactive and nonhyperactive children. Pediatrics 6:839–844, 1987

Lumley M, Roehrs T, Askel D, et al: Ethanol and caffeine effects on daytime sleepiness/alertness. Sleep 10:306–312, 1987

Mahowald M, Rosen G: Parasomnias in children. Pediatrician 17:21–31, 1990

Moore T, Ucko L: Night waking in early infancy, Part I. Arch Dis Child 32:333–342, 1957

Navalet Y, Anders T, Guilleminault C: Narcolepsy in children, in Narcolepsy: Advances in Sleep Research, Vol 3. Edited by Guilleminault C, Dement W, Passouant P. Holliswood, NY, Spectrum, 1976, pp 171–177

Okawa M, Sasaki H: Sleep disorders in mentally retarded and brain impaired children, in Sleep and Its Disorders in Children. Edited by Guilleminault C. New York, Raven, 1987, pp 171–177

Roffwarg H, Muzio J, Dement W: Ontogenetic development of the human sleep-dream cycle. Science 152:576–582, 1966

Schenck C, Bundlie S, Patterson A, et al: Chronic behavior disorders in a 10-year-old girl and episodic REM and NREM sleep movements in an 8-year-old brother. Sleep Research 15:162, 1986

Small A, Hibi S, Feinberg I: Effects of dextroamphetamine sulfate on EEG sleep patterns of hyperactive children. Arch Gen Psychiatry 25:369–380, 1971

Tanner J: Growth at Adolescence, 2nd Edition. Oxford, UK, Blackwell Scientific, 1962

Thorpy M, Korman E, Spielman A, et al: Delayed sleep-phase syndrome in adolescents. J Adolesc Health Care 9:22–27, 1988

Chapter 38

Disorders of Elimination

Thomas Walsh, M.D.
Edgardo Menvielle, M.D.

The disorders of elimination, enuresis and encopresis, represent a failure to achieve or maintain control of bodily functions. These disorders are not uncommon and have the potential to cause significant distress for both the child and family. They present to a variety of health professionals, on occasion as a symptom of other disorders. In this chapter, the causes, sequelae, and treatment of each of these disorders are reviewed.

Functional Enuresis

Functional enuresis is the repeated involuntary or intentional discharge of urine beyond the expected age of control (in the absence of a definable physical abnormality). According to DSM-III-R (American Psychiatric Association 1987), the disorder is present when there are at least two episodes per month for children up to age 6 and one episode per month for older children (Table 38-1). Primary enuresis occurs in children who have never been dry for an extended period; secondary enuresis is the reemergence of wetting after a continuous period of control of 6 months or longer. Enuresis may be characterized as nocturnal (the most common), diurnal (more frequent in children under 5), and mixed.

Clinical Features

Primary enuresis accounts for about 80% of patients. Left untreated, the remission rate is 10%–

20% per year, which gradually increases with age; it can therefore be viewed as a self-limiting disorder, with 1% continuing into adulthood (Forsythe and Redmond 1974).

Although most children with enuresis do not have a coexisting psychiatric disorder, the prevalence of emotional-behavioral disorders is greater than in the general population (Essen and Peckham 1976; Rutter et al. 1973). Coexisting disorders include encopresis, developmental delays, and sleep disorders. No association has been demonstrated between enuresis and tics, nail biting, temper tantrums, fire setting, or cruelty to animals (Felthous and Bernhard 1978; Oppel et al. 1968).

Psychosocial impairment in children with enuresis can be a function of the effect of enuresis on the child's self-esteem, the degree to which the disorder causes social isolation and ostracism by peers, and the negative response of caregivers (e.g., anger, punishment, and rejection). Impairment may be a result of coexisting disorders. While the number of enuretic children with coexisting emotional-behavioral problems is small, children for whom help is sought may have more behavioral symptoms (Couchells et al. 1981).

Differential Diagnosis

A diagnosis of functional enuresis assumes the absence of identifiable physical causes. Any condition causing increased urine output can cause enuresis; thus diabetes mellitus and diabetes insipidus must be considered, as well as increased fluid intake with psychogenic causes. Urinary tract infection, espe-

Table 38-1.   DSM-III-R diagnostic criteria for functional enuresis

A. Repeated voiding of urine during the day or night into bed or clothes, whether involuntary or intentional.
B. At least two such events per month for children between the ages of five and six, and at least one event per month for older children.
C. Chronologic age at least five, and mental age at least four.
D. Not due to a physical disorder, such as diabetes, urinary tract infection, or a seizure disorder.

Specify primary or secondary type.
   Primary type: the disturbance was not preceded by a period of urinary continence lasting at least one year.
   Secondary type: the disturbance was preceded by a period of urinary continence lasting at least one year.

Specify nocturnal only, diurnal only, or **nocturnal and diurnal.**

Source. Reprinted with permission from American Psychiatric Association 1987.

cially in girls, must be ruled out, as must seizure disorders, renal insufficiency, neurologic disorders that affect bladder innervation, neuroleptic-induced enuresis, and urinary tract anatomical abnormalities. All of these can be readily ruled out by careful clinical assessment based on history, physical examination, urinalysis, and urine culture when necessary, with further assessment only as clinically indicated.

Epidemiology

Bed-wetting is as common in girls as in boys between 4 and 6 years old, with the ratio increasing steadily after that, so that by age 11, boys are twice as likely to be bed-wetters. Nocturnal enuresis occurs in 15% of 5-year-olds, with a decrease of about 15% per year thereafter. At age 7, 15% of boys wet less often than once per week, and 7% wet at least once per week, with those with enuresis referred for treatment most commonly coming from the latter group (Shaffer 1985).

Approximately 75% of enuretic children have a first-degree relative with a history of enuresis. When both parents have a positive history, 77% of the children are enuretic; when one parent is affected, 44% of the children are enuretic (Bakwin 1973). The relationship of enuresis to a range of psychosocial factors, including family, social, and economic background, once was thought to be significant but has since been questioned (Fergusson et al. 1986).

Etiology

No single cause of enuresis has been identified. Primary enuresis has been viewed as representing a maturational delay, with multiple factors contributing to this theory. Genetic studies have found a high incidence of enuresis in parents and siblings of bed-wetters (Bakwin 1973). There is an association of developmental delay with enuresis that may partially account for the high rate of coincident psychiatric disorders (Shaffer 1985). In addition, it has been suggested that some enuretic children do not have the normal decreased urine output at night based on the failure to develop a circadian variation in vasopressin (antidiuretic hormone) release (Norgaard et al. 1989); however, the clinical significance of this suggestion remains subject to further investigation.

The concept of enuresis as a disorder of sleep has been investigated, with the conclusion that there is no association of enuresis with any particular stage of sleep (Mikkelson et al. 1980). Enuresis has been related to abnormalities in bladder size, function, or anatomy, but these anatomical factors appeared to account for only a small minority of patients.

Secondary enuresis can be a manifestation of stress in children, especially between the ages of 4 and 6. Environmental stressors, such as a move to a new home, birth of a sibling, hospitalization, or child abuse, may cause a transient regression in bladder control. There have been psychodynamic explanations proposed for enuresis, viewing the symptom as a manifestation of castration anxiety, repressed sexual or aggressive drive, a masturbatory equivalent, or an immature form of gratification (Katan 1926; Sperling 1965). Although there is no evidence to support that enuresis has a symbolic meaning, there is a relationship between psychiatric disorder and enuresis, with cause and effect being different in individual cases (Rutter et al. 1973).

Treatment

Multiple treatment modalities exist for functional enuresis. However, one point is central to the application of them all: that enuresis is for the most part a benign disorder that is self-limited. Reassurance and support are necessary to avoid secondary emotional effects on self-esteem and family relationships, and the development of shame and guilt from the symptoms. Excessive investigation and overaggressive treatment of all types should be avoided.

Any treatment course should be preceded by a period of observation during which there is open discussion of the problem, tracking of symptoms by use of a chart, and positive reinforcement of dry periods. Simple interventions such as late fluid restrictions and encouraging nighttime urination may be tried at this point. This pretreatment period sometimes produces remission of symptoms.

The most effective treatment for primary enuresis is the use of the enuresis alarm, a conditioning device employing an alarm that is triggered by the child's voiding. Various designs of this apparatus are available, from the traditional "bell and pad" to more compact and sensitive systems. Explanations for the success of this treatment are based on behavioral theories, including classical conditioning, avoidance learning, and social learning. The success rate for the enuresis alarm is good, with reports of initial response of 60%–80% with some relapse. Because of the relapse rate, a second course of treatment is often necessary (Forsythe and Butler 1989). Dry bed training (including positive reinforcement for inhibiting urination, retention control training, positive practice nighttime awakening, cleanliness training, and aversive consequences) has been used, but does not appear to be effective when used in the absence of an enuresis alarm. For maximum effect, compliance must be addressed in the use of the enuresis alarm. With the significant potential for failure of the family to continue use of the enuresis alarm, there must be a sensitivity to a family's difficulties in sustaining treatment with guidance and support. Despite the fact that the enuresis alarm is the most effective treatment, only 5% of surveyed physicians recommended its use, with the majority using less effective or ineffective methods (Shevlov et al. 1981).

A number of pharmacologic agents have been used with some success to treat enuresis. Tricyclic antidepressants and desmopressin have proved beneficial. Stimulants, sedatives, and anticholinergic agents have not.

Tricyclic antidepressants, especially imipramine, have been widely studied and used in the treatment of enuresis (Bindelglas and Dee 1978). The mechanism of action of imipramine is uncertain.

Three possible theories—antidepressant action, alteration in sleep, and anticholinergic action—have not been substantiated (Rapoport et al. 1980). Effective doses are in the 25–75 mg range, with a decrease in frequency of wetting in most cases, but total remission in only about 30%; significant relapse occurs after discontinuation of imipramine. The potential cardiac side effects and the risk of fatal toxicity on overdose need to be considered in the use of imipramine.

Desmopressin, an analog of the antidiuretic hormone vasopressin, has been found to be effective in patients with nocturnal enuresis who do not have normal diurnal variation of antidiuretic hormone secretion (Klauber 1989). The postulated mechanism is a decrease in nighttime urine output to a point that does not exceed bladder capacity, thus eliminating nighttime wetting.

In general, pharmacologic interventions are useful in situations in which it is important to achieve rapid short-term relief from symptoms, when symptoms become the source of conflict in relationships within a family, or when the symptoms create or exacerbate maladaptive behavior in the child and other methods have failed.

The decision to treat is an important one for an individual child; the benefits of treatment need to justify an often prolonged and complex process. Although most enuretic children are not psychiatrically disturbed, those who seek help are under more stress and are more symptomatic. Since it appears that children can have improved self-concept following successful treatment and that treatment failure does not have adverse emotional effects, treatment is justified when help is sought (Moffatt 1989).

Prognosis

Since enuresis is for the most part self-limiting and effective treatment is available, prognosis is good. In children in whom there are coexisting disorders or significant secondary emotional complications, appropriate intervention is necessary for successful outcome.

Functional Encopresis

According to DSM-III-R (American Psychiatry Association 1987), functional encopresis is the repeated voluntary or involuntary passage of feces

Table 38-2. DSM-III-R diagnostic criteria for functional encopresis

A. Repeated passage of feces into places not appropriate for that purpose (e.g., clothing, floor), whether involuntary or intentional. (The disorder may be overflow incontinence secondary to functional fecal retention.)
B. At least one such event a month for at least six months.
C. Chronologic and mental age, at least four years.
D. Not due to a physical disorder, such as aganglionic megacolon.

Specify primary or secondary type.
  Primary type: the disturbance was not preceded by a period of fecal continence lasting at least one year.
  Secondary type: the disturbance was preceded by a period of fecal continence lasting at least one year.

Source. Reprinted with permission from American Psychiatric Association 1987.

into places not appropriate for that purpose in children at least 4 years old and with a mental age of at least 4, and not due to a physical disorder (Table 38-2). The frequency required is at least one such event a month for at least 6 months.

Clinical Features

In primary encopresis, the disturbance is not preceded by a period of fecal continence; secondary encopresis is preceded by a period of fecal continence lasting at least 1 year. The secondary type may account for as many as 50%–60% of all the cases (Walker et al. 1988). Different types of encopresis can be described based on the outcome of bowel training, awareness of defecation, presence of chronic constipation, and psychological precipitants of soiling episodes. In children who achieve adequate bowel control but who deposit feces in inappropriate places in response to family stress or as a purposeful act, the soiling episode may represent a reversible behavioral disorganization or regression under stress or an act of angry defiance or reprisal toward the caregivers. Children who have never achieved appropriate bowel control and who may have a history of inadequate, unsuccessful toilet training may be unaware of the soiling or may be aware but unable to control it. Retentive encopresis is the most common variety (85%–95%). These children have either never achieved bowel control or achieved control but proper functioning is not maintained because of retention of feces leading to fecal impaction and overflow. This group

has infrequent bowel movements and frequent accidents (often more than two a day) in the form of small stains of liquid stool (Doleys 1983; Levine 1982).

Deliberate smearing of feces as a covert expression of anger should be differentiated from smearing that takes place accidentally in the child's attempt to clean or hide feces passed involuntarily. Children may wish to avoid situations that may lead to embarrassment, and some children may attempt to hide soiled clothes and deny the soiling, appearing mortified when the problem is discussed. Others appear either unconcerned or unaware. The majority of children with functional encopresis do not appear to have significant behavioral problems (Gabel et al. 1986). However, children referred to a psychiatrist may represent a more severely affected group with more coexisting behavioral or family problems (Friman et al. 1988).

Epidemiology

Functional encopresis is a problem estimated to affect between 1.5% and 7.5% of elementary-school-aged children (Walker et al. 1988). This wide range of reported incidence is due to variation in the diagnostic criteria used in the various studies. Secondary encopresis rarely starts after the age of 8. Primary encopresis apparently is more common in lower socioeconomic classes and is three to four times more common in males than in females. It is generally believed that encopresis is frequently underreported (Doleys 1983; Hersov 1985).

Etiology

No single pathophysiologic or psychodynamic explanation accounts for encopresis. The most persuasive arguments point to a combination of maturational factors interacting with social factors.

Children with retentive encopresis are chronically constipated. Constipation may be the result of a combination of various factors. The retention of feces may start as a result of painful defecation because of an anal fissure, a struggle between the parent and the child over bowel training, or a phobic avoidance of the toilet based on a real or imaginary negative experience. When constipation is set, it leads to fecal impaction, and liquid feces tend to leak around the impaction. The child's attempts to prevent involuntary passage of feces by anal contraction may increase the amount of retained feces. With rectal distention, the internal anal sphincter becomes weak and underresponsive and there is a decreased sensation of passage of feces through the rectum. The child may lose awareness of the passage of stools. In primary encopresis, constipation is often established before the child has mastered bowel control skills.

Psychodynamic factors generally focus on the mother-child relationship. Proposed causes are rigid perfectionistic parents, coercive training, and the mother's ambivalence toward the child's need for autonomy (Anthony 1957; Easson 1960; Pinkerton 1958). Family constellation factors, such as the uninvolved-passive father and the domineering, overinvolved or depressed mother, have been implicated as well (Bemporad et al. 1971).

Differential Diagnosis

Functional encopresis must be distinguished from structural organic causes of encopresis, such as aganglionic megacolon (Hirschsprung's disease). Although severe cases of aganglionic megacolon are detected soon after birth, mild cases may go undetected until later in life. Functional encopresis should also be distinguished from chronic or intermittent diarrhea due to organic disorders such as Crohn's disease or irritable bowel syndrome.

Treatment

The goal of treatment for encopresis is the regular independent use of the toilet and the resolution of coexisting problems. The therapeutic approach should be based on the type of encopresis, with the simultaneous use of medical, behavioral, and psychotherapeutic interventions as indicated. Careful evaluation, including both medical and psychosocial assessment, and a period of observation with recording of soiling accompanied by open discussion of the symptoms should precede any intervention. Medical and behavioral interventions vary according to the characteristics of each child's soiling. The treatment principles for children who retain feces include education of the child and the parents about the problem, disimpaction, and bowel control training. Education about the symptom, the mechanism of retention, and the rationale for the intervention is used as the initial strategy to recruit both parent and child as active participants collaborating to solve the problem (Landman and Rappaport 1985).

A necessary medical intervention is to remove the blockage of feces in the bowel. This is usually done with the use of enemas. After the bowel is clean, a combination of several management measures is used to prevent reimpaction and to gain continence control. Diet modification with an increase of the child's intake of dietary fiber and water is useful to facilitate bowel function and to prevent impaction. To increase the chance of bowel movements in the toilet utilizing the gastroileal reflex, 10-minute sittings 20 minutes after meals are prescribed. Appropriate bowel movements and accident-free days are reinforced through praise or tangible rewards. Aversive consequences for soiling accidents, such as showering and washing the soiled clothes, are useful (Doleys 1983; Gerber and Meyer 1965; Houts and Peterson 1986; Young 1973).

When psychopathology is present in the individual and family, appropriate psychotherapeutic intervention is indicated. Associated psychopathology may be a factor in the etiology of encopresis, especially in children who have demonstrated adequate bowel control. In other cases, it may be a result of the encopresis and may impede the effectiveness of the bowel control training. While psychiatric intervention is necessary to treat coexisting primary psychiatric disorders, psychotherapy may also be needed to treat secondary maladaptive patterns even though self-esteem may improve with relief of the symptoms. Family therapy is necessary to disengage the child and family from interactions that perpetuate the problem (Margolies and Gilstein 1983–1984).

Prognosis

There is a gradual decline in incidence of functional encopresis from a peak age of 6 years in boys and 8 years in girls, to almost complete disappearance by age 16. Soiling at night has a poorer prognosis than soiling during the day. Other indicators of poor prognosis are a nonchalant attitude, associated conduct problems, and soiling as an expression of aggression (Landman and Rappaport 1985; Levine 1982).

Research Issues

With maturational factors being so important in both enuresis and encopresis, further research is needed to explore the relationship between the two, to attempt to define the pathophysiology of each, and to explore common links to other developmental disorders. In addition, the relationship between maturational and emotional factors needs further investigation.

References

American Psychiatric Association: Diagnostic and Statistical Manual of Mental Disorders, 3rd Edition, Revised. Washington, DC, American Psychiatric Association, 1987

Anthony EJ: An experimental approach to the psychology of childhood: encopresis. Br J Med Psychol 30:146–175, 1957

Bakwin H: The genetics of enuresis, in Bladder Control and Enuresis. Edited by Kolvin I, MacKeith RC, Meadow SR. London, Heinemann Medical, 1973, pp 73–77

Bemporad JR, Pfeifer CM, Gibbs L, et al: Characteristics of encopretic patients and their families. Journal of the American Academy of Child Psychiatry 10:272–292, 1971

Bindelglas PM, Dee G: Enuresis treatment with imipramine hydrochloride: a 10-year follow-up study. Am J Psychiatry 135:1549–1552, 1978

Couchells SM, Johnson SB, Carter R, et al: Behavioral and environmental characteristics of treated and untreated enuretic children and matched nonenuretic controls. J Pediatr 99:812–816, 1981

Doleys DM: Enuresis and encopresis, in Handbook of Child Psychopathology. Edited by Ollendick TH, Hersen M. New York, Plenum, 1983, pp 201–226

Easson RI: Encopresis-psychogenic soiling. Can Med Assoc J 82:624–628, 1960

Essen J, Peckham C: Nocturnal enuresis in childhood. Dev Med Child Neurol 18:577–589, 1976

Felthous AR, Bernhard H: Enuresis, firesetting, and cruelty to animals: the significance of two thirds of this triad. J Forensic Sci 45:240–246, 1978

Fergusson DM, Horwood LJ, Shannon FT: Factors related to the age of attainment of nocturnal bladder control: an 8-year longitudinal study. Pediatrics 78:884, 1986

Forsythe WI, Butler RJ: Fifty years of enuretic alarms. Arch Dis Child 64:879–885, 1989

Forsythe WI, Redmond A: Enuresis and spontaneous cure rate of 1,129 enuretics. Arch Dis Child 49:259, 1974

Friman PC, Matthews JR, Finney JW, et al: Do encopretic children have significant behavioral problems? J Pediatr Psychol 11:375–383, 1988

Gabel S, Hegeders AM, Wald A, et al: Prevalence of behavior problems and mental health utilization among encopretic children: implications for behavioral pediatrics. J Dev Behav Pediatr 7:293–297, 1986

Gerber H, Meyer V: Behavior therapy and encopresis: the complexities involved in treatment. Behav Res Ther 2:227–231, 1965

Hersov L: Faecal soiling, in Child and Adolescent Psychiatry: Modern Approaches, 2nd Edition. Edited by Rutter M, Hersov L. St. Louis, MO, CV Mosby, 1985, pp 482–489

Houts AC, Peterson JK: Treatment of a retentive encopretic child using contingency management and diet modification with stimulus control. J Pediatr Psychol 11:375–383, 1986

Katan A: Experiences with enuretics. Psychoanal Study Child 2:24–55, 1926

Klauber GT: Clinical efficacy and safety of desmopressin in the treatment of nocturnal enuresis. J Pediatr 114 (suppl):719, 1989

Landman GB, Rappaport L: Pediatric management of severe treatment-resistant encopresis. J Dev Behav Pediatr 6:349–351, 1985

Levine MD: Encopresis: its potentiation, evaluation and alleviation. Pediatr Clin North Am 29:315–330, 1982

Margolies R, Gilstein K: A systems approach to the treatment of chronic encopresis. Int J Psychiatry Med 13:141–151, 1983–1984

Mikkelson EJ, Rapoport JL, Nee L, et al: Childhood enuresis, I: sleep patterns and psychopathology. Arch Gen Psychiatry 37:1139–1145, 1980

Moffatt MEK: Nocturnal enuresis: psychologic implications of treatment and nontreatment. J Pediatr 114 (suppl):697, 1989

Norgaard JP, Rittig S, Djurhuus JC: Nocturnal enuresis: an approach to treatment based on pathogenesis. J Pediatr 114 (suppl):705, 1989

Oppel WC, Harper PA, Rider RV: Social, psychological and neurological factors associated with enuresis. Pediatrics 42:627–641, 1968

Pinkerton P: Psychogenic megacolon in children: the implications of bowel negativism. Arch Dis Child 33:371–398, 1958

Rapoport JL, Mikkelson EJ, Zavardil A, et al: Childhood enuresis, II: psychopathology, tricylic concentration in plasma, and antienuretic effect. Arch Gen Psychiatry 37:1146–1152, 1980

Rutter M, Yule W, Graham P: Enuresis and behavioral deviance, in Bladder Control and Enuresis. Edited by Kolvin I, MacKeith RC, Meadow SR. Philadelphia, PA, JB Lippincott, 1973, pp 137–147

Shaffer D: Enuresis, in Child Psychiatry: Modern Approaches, 2nd Edition. Edited by Rutter M, Hersov L. Oxford, UK, Blackwell Scientific, 1985, pp 465–481

Shevlov SP, Gundy J, Weiss JC, et al: Enuresis: a contrast of attitudes of parents and physicians. Pediatrics 67:707, 1981

Sperling M: Dynamic considerations and treatment of enuresis. Journal of the American Academy of Child Psychiatry 4:19–31, 1965

Walker CE, Milling L, Bonner B: Incontinence disorders: enuresis and encopresis, in Handbook of Pediatric Psychology. Edited by Routh D. New York, Guilford, 1988, pp 263–298

Young GC: The treatment of childhood encopresis by conditioned gastro-ileal reflex training. Behav Res Ther 11:499–503, 1973

Chapter 39

Concept and Classification of Psychosomatic Disorders

Gregory K. Fritz, M.D.
Larry K. Brown, M.D.

Since Socrates and Hippocrates, physicians have concerned themselves with psychosomatic relationships. Lipowski (1977, p. 234) noted that Gaub, a professor of medicine in Leyden in the mid-1700s, wrote, "The reason why a sound body becomes ill or an ailing body recovers very often lies in the mind. Contrariwise, the body can frequently both beget mental illness and heal its offspring." Heinroth coined the term *psychosomatic* in 1818 and was a strong, if little noted, advocate of the importance of considering the impact of mental life on the physical health of an individual (Whittkower 1974). Psychiatry and the psychosomatic approach became increasingly isolated in the 19th century at the same time as the science of medicine—anatomy, microbiology, and biochemistry—made great progress while embracing Virchow's principle of cellular pathology (Whittkower 1974).

The psychosomatic movement began in Germany and Austria in the 1920s and 1930s in response to the increasing mechanization of medicine. Franz Alexander brought the psychosomatic movement to the United States from Germany, and focused his psychoanalytic research energies on psychosomatic problems. Alexander's group studied patients with seven disorders (asthma, peptic ulcer, rheumatoid arthritis, ulcerative colitis, neurodermatitis, thyrotoxicosis, and essential hypertension), which have been identified in the past as *the* psychosomatic diseases. Each of the seven was postulated to have a specific psychodynamic conflict as its etiologic base. In asthma, for example, strong, unconscious dependency wishes and a concomitant fear of separation were thought to constitute its psychological roots; the wheezing was seen as a suppressed cry for the mother. Alexander's "specificity theories" have received little empirical validation over the years, but the creativity of his concepts make his book *Psychosomatic Medicine: Its Principles and Applications* an enduring contribution to the field (Alexander 1950). At about the same time, Flanders Dunbar (1954) pursued her own specificity theory, in which she proposed that particular personality types characterized patients with a specific psychosomatic disease. Her description of the "ulcer personality," the "arthritic personality," and so on, predated the currently postulated Type A personality. Recent studies have shown that the presence of a chronic illness in general, rather than characteristics of a specific disorder, accounts for much of the significant psychological variation between chronically ill and healthy children (Hilliard et al. 1985).

Currently, psychosomatic theories of disease emphasize the complexity and nonlinearity of mind-body relationships. Each chronic disease is seen as a heterogeneous entity comprised of subforms, each with a different clinical picture. Individuals with the same disorder may vary genetically, physiologically, and psychologically. Their own reactions to the illness, their personal habits and behavior, and those of individuals in their social setting contribute to the predisposition, presentation, and course of the disease.

Biopsychosocial Model

The development of the biopsychosocial model (Engel 1980) focused attention on the interactions among all of the contextual levels in an illness, from the organ to the societal. As vividly described by Engel, even something as apparently physical as a venipuncture interacts with the patient's psychological state (e.g., frustration, self-blame) and caregiver's attitudes, and, in a spiral of interactions, ultimately affects further physical states, hospital course, and friendships. An understanding of these transactional effects requires that we thus view every illness as psychosomatic in nature. The complex interplay between mind and body is further reinforced by research in oncology, immunology, and wellness behavior that challenges our conventional views of cause and effect.

Psychological forces are speculated to play an important role in a diverse range of major somatic illnesses, from cancer progression to immune functioning. For example, in a well-controlled follow-up study of women with metastatic breast cancer, Spiegel et al. (1989) found that psychotherapy could improve the quality and length of life for patients. In a random sample of 86 cancer victims, researchers were surprised to find that, at the 10-year follow-up, the therapy group lived an average of 37 months, compared with 19 months for the control group.

Ader (1974) first presented data showing that immunological reactivity could be classically conditioned. Rats prone to develop autoimmune disease were given cyclophosphamide to suppress the immune system. The cyclophosphamide was paired with a saccharin-flavored solution in a conditioning paradigm. The saccharin solution was repeated every 3 days, and the subsequent mortality rate was found to correlate with the amount of solution given in the conditioning trial. The saccharin that had been conditionally paired with cyclophosphamide then subsequently functioned as an immune suppressant. This general phenomenon has been replicated and extended to show that cell-mediated immunity can also be conditioned (Cohen and Ader 1988). Preliminary data (Smith and McDaniel 1983) indicate that immune conditioning can also occur in humans. In this research, psychological factors have been implicated in modifying the delayed hypersensitivity or tuberculin reaction. Volunteers were injected several times with tuberculin and saline in different arms. When tuberculin was substituted for saline in the "saline bottle" and injected in the arm that had previously received saline, the resulting hypersensitivity response was markedly diminished. It appears likely that the immune system is integrated with psychological processes and that this regulatory balance helps explain the effect of psychological factors in disease progression (Rogers 1989). The converse, the extent to which immune functioning influences behavior, remains to be explored.

A human example of immune-psychological relationships is provided by research on the health implications of psychotherapy. In 42 patients undergoing radiotherapy for cancer, weekly psychotherapy was associated with reduced emotional and physical signs of distress, as compared with a control group of patients (Forester et al. 1985). Pennebaker et al. (1988) asked healthy college students to write about either traumatic or trivial events for 4 days. Writing about a traumatic experience was associated with a decrease in health center use and an improvement in blastogenic response of T-lymphocytes to two mitogens. These examples and more detailed recent writing (Rogers 1989; Weiner 1989) illustrate the complex relationships between mind, brain, and body. Such research suggests that not only do these relationships exist, but psychotherapy could be cost effective in improving health care.

Stages of Psychosomatic Involvement

The biopsychosocial model emphasizes interactions at any level and in any direction among components. Linear, cause-and-effect models are not adequate to explain the diversity of findings described above. For the purpose of clinical practice, it is useful to delineate phases of the illness process as 1) vulnerability to disease, 2) symptom onset, 3) recurrence, 4) maintenance of the disease state, and 5) living with or reacting to the illness. The extent to which psychological factors exert a significant influence on a particular illness phase will vary from case to case. Together, these influential factors constitute the psychosomatic component for an individual patient.

There is abundant evidence that certain behaviors increase one's vulnerability to future disease. The adverse health consequences of smoking, overeating, and drug abuse are generally recognized. The three leading causes of death in teenagers, in fact, are the results of "behavioral misadventures": accident, homicide, and suicide (Paulson 1988). The clear relationship between behavioral risks (needle sharing, unprotected intercourse) and human immunodeficiency virus (HIV) infection is a current, poignant, and lethal example of an important instance in which behavior determines vulnerability to disease. A change in psychological state, even without altering observable behavior, may also influence health. Individuals who have experienced a major stress are then more susceptible to illness. This relationship is clear with adults, in whom a change in immune functioning has been documented following death of a spouse (Rogers 1989). Similar immune changes in children can be presumed to occur after parental death or divorce or even after less significant, but additive, life upsets.

Psychological factors may precipitate the onset of a disorder or may influence the timing of symptom presentation. Failure to thrive in infancy secondary to maternal and child attachment dysfunction is perhaps the clearest example (Benoit et al. 1989; Chatoor and Egan 1983). The types of attachment dysfunctions are varied and largely nonspecific. In adolescents, the onset of eating disorders is undoubtedly a result of psychological, sociocultural, and biological forces (Yates 1989). The importance of psychological factors is highlighted by the fact that one-third to one-half of young women who develop anorexia cease to menstruate *before* significant weight loss occurs (Halmi 1974). It has been suggested that psychological stress could trigger the onset of diabetes mellitus, given the ability of stress in normal control subjects to stimulate hormones that oppose insulin's action, but this relationship remains uncertain (Barglow et al. 1986; Hauser and Pollets 1979; Leaverton et al. 1980).

The role of psychological dysfunction in affecting the reoccurrence of acute diabetic episodes is better defined. In teenagers with diabetes mellitus, stress experiences have been associated with poor short-term (fasting blood sugar) and long-term (glycosylated hemoglobin) measures of glucose control (Hanson and Pichert 1986; Schwartz et al. 1986). In children with asthma, psychological stress will sometimes precipitate attacks, and case reports of fatal childhood attacks reveal the frequent emotional triggers of attacks in those patients (Fritz et al. 1987). Similarly, some skin disorders, particularly atopic dermatitis, are thought to be multiply

determined by genetic factors, elevated IgE antibodies, and emotional precipitants. Flares in the dermatitis often occur in conjunction with emotionally stressful periods, perhaps mediated by the immune system (Engels 1982). In hemophilia, high emotional arousal can increase bleeding tendency, apparently without trauma. Whether this tendency is due to changes in the vascular bed caused by neuroendocrine changes or due to inadvertent, unrecognized self-injury is unclear (Mattson and Kim 1982).

Psychological factors can serve a maintenance function for chronic illnesses by a diverse set of mechanisms. When there is a common underlying biological dysfunction, psychological factors may act synergistically with the physical. Alternatively, psychological factors may influence patient or family noncompliance with the medical regimen and subsequent increased morbidity. Asthma and depression, for example, have both been associated with relatively increased cholinergic activity (Nadi et al. 1984). In severe depression, the increased activity has been reported in metabolites of central cholinergic neurotransmitters; in asthma, peripheral increased parasympathetic tone results in bronchoconstriction. A similar imbalance in both conditions could account for the worsening of both states concurrently and additively. Some research on asthma (Kinsman et al. 1982) indicates that a particular pattern of psychological response to the illness defines a patient at risk for psychologically maintained morbidity. An increased rate of rehospitalization was found in patients with high levels of nonspecific anxiety and in those with great disregard of symptoms. Middle levels of anxiety and responsiveness to symptoms are probably associated with the most adaptive coping and disease monitoring (Fritz 1987). In cystic fibrosis, substantial attention to diet must be paid by the family and health care staff (Roy et al. 1984). For a small group of teenage girls with cystic fibrosis, the disease interacts with their developing self-image and eating behavior to produce an atypical eating disorder, further complicating treatment of the original medical disorder (Pumariega et al. 1986).

Illness at Developmental Levels

The child's level of psychosocial development will influence reactions to a new illness or the progression of a chronic disorder. More detailed reviews exist elsewhere of the relationship between developmental stage and chronic illness (McCollum 1981) and acute hospitalization (Mrazek 1986). The general impact of an illness on children at differing ages will be summarized in the following paragraphs. The nature and extent of reaction are impossible to predict. No single factor causes poor adjustment, and in fact most children and families continue to be functional (Pless and Pinkerton 1975; Stabler 1988).

Infancy

In infancy, severe illnesses may produce intense emotional reactions in new parents at the very time they are trying to become a family, rather than a marital couple. Parents with little child-rearing experience have great difficulty separating problems with their baby into illness-related and normal disturbances. In some cases, the predictable guilt, horror, and disbelief associated with illness or handicap in an infant can damage parental-child attachment, leading to chronic dysfunction. Generally, ultimate adaptation is good, and some follow-up studies of oncology survivors have found that the earlier the illness, the better the long-term functioning (Koocher et al. 1980).

Preschool

Preschoolers are verbal and increasingly motoric. Chronic illness and repeated hospitalization cause restriction of activities and may impair early, needed socialization experiences. Because of the preschoolers' egocentrism, illnesses may be psychologically associated with a sense of wrongdoing or punishment. Parents, at the same time, may become confused as to the degree of strictness that is required. Misbehavior, which normally emerges in this stage, may become extreme, or the wish to be "naughty" may be overly controlled in the "perfect" child. In both cases, the normal, balanced internalization of family rules has been interrupted.

Latency Age

Latency-age children can employ causal thinking and are more observant of their own bodily reactions. Consequently, they can understand their illness in some logical detail. Dramatic misconceptions can still exist if professionals are not careful to use developmentally appropriate words, as in the case of the frightened boy in the X-ray department who thought the "CAT" scanner contained a ferocious feline. At this age, children's reports of symptomatology are increasingly used to make treatment decisions. Research with asthmatic children has shown a high degree of variation among individuals in their ability to perceive accurately changes in peak flow rate (Fritz et al. 1990). The accuracy of these children may be influenced by their cognitive level and by emotional factors. A sense of mastery and achievement, especially in school, is normally acquired by children at this age. Illness that interferes with school performance or is disruptive of normal peer activities can damage self-esteem. Efforts to improve academics (e.g., tutoring, teacher conferences, or neuropsychiatric assessment) or enhance allowed physical activities (e.g., noncontact sports for hemophilia patients) can pay large dividends.

Teens

In teenagers, illnesses can impact on their struggle for autonomy, their physical-sexuality development, and their peer relationships. Illness can force dependence on parents and physicians to a degree not found in healthy teenagers. The perception of immaturity by adults, due to delayed growth in secondary sexual characteristics, can reinforce this dependence. Compliance problems often result when the illness and its treatment become involved in a teenager's conflictual struggle for independence. Fully developed autonomy actually enhances the teenager's adoption of reasonable therapeutic goals. Likewise, compliance with salicylate therapy in teenagers with rheumatoid arthritis increases with better developed autonomy (Litt et al. 1982). Physical and sexual maturation may be delayed by chronic illness. Boys who are late in developing are rated as less mature, popular, or confident than their peers. For girls, maturing at the same rate as their peers is associated with greatest confidence (Gross and Duke 1980). Many reports document the tendency of healthy people to ignore the emerging sexuality of those with physical disabilities. Being treated as asexual can greatly inhibit normal sexual exploration. The importance of adequate, timely, medical care on sexuality development is highlighted by the recent follow-up report of 80 women with congenital adrenal hyperplasia (Mulaikal et al. 1987). Of those patients whose vaginal reconstruction had resulted in an inadequate introitus, 64% had not had any sexual experiences, compared with 23% in those with an adequate repair.

Family reactions to an ill child are equally complex and dependent on prior family patterns, coping styles, and experiences with illness. Reactions of fear, anger, loneliness, and guilt seem universal (Featherstone 1980). Marital strain seems inevitable, and some research (Breslau and Davis 1986) has found a greater rate of divorce and depressive symptoms in mothers of children with chronic illness. For many illnesses, such as cancer and AIDS, the ambiguity and social anxiety are unsettling (Comaroff and Maguire 1981; Krener and Miller 1989). In the face of acute illness, siblings can be relatively neglected by parents and health care workers. Reactions of jealousy, overprotectiveness, and survival guilt are common. Some programs for the chronically ill have specific components for siblings to address these issues.

Assessment

A comprehensive medical evaluation assesses the role of psychological factors in the course of a chronic illness or the occurrence of a physical symptom. The psychological component of the diagnostic process should get "equal billing" with physical and laboratory components. It should be introduced directly as a relatively routine part of the process, and it should take place concurrently with other diagnostic studies, rather than be withheld as a last resort. The nature of psychosomatic interactions dictates that physicians involved in the comprehensive evaluation communicate effectively with one another before, during, and after the diagnostic process. This fact seems too obvious to need emphasis, but adequate communication is far from the rule in most settings.

The child psychiatrist assessing psychosocial factors in a pediatric patient needs to approach the case with several principles in mind. First, a significant psychosomatic element is possible with every disorder; there are no diagnostic categories that, when discovered, rule out an associated, major psychological component. Second, even in diseases in which psychosocial factors have been widely recognized, such as asthma, diabetes, and ulcerative colitis, it is possible for the psychological components to be of minimal importance for a particular child's illness. Individuals, not disorders, have

psychosomatic relationships. Third, a lack of satisfying findings on physical or laboratory examination is not adequate evidence for ascribing a psychological explanation to a specific case. Psychiatric evaluation should reveal a combination of intrapsychic and environmental factors of sufficient magnitude and likelihood to impact the course of the disorder before psychosocial intervention is undertaken. Finally, a lack of typical, major psychopathology diagnosable in either the child or the family does not preclude the possibility that psychological factors are influencing the illness to a significant degree.

Psychological evaluation of a child with a physical illness entails essentially the same thorough approach described previously in this volume (see Section II on assessment and diagnosis), with some additions and areas of emphasis. Especially important in the history is a chronology of the relationship between physical symptoms and emotional or stressful periods. With ongoing involvement, having the child and/or parents keep a journal in which important variables are tracked with daily entries can be an important asset in understanding a complicated picture. Standard assessment instruments, which are becoming increasingly common in psychiatric practice, may be of limited use with children who are physically ill, because disease-related symptoms (e.g., fatigue, somatic concerns, sleep disturbances, medication side effects) complicate efforts to quantify such psychological phenomena as depression and anxiety. However, several questionnaires have been developed specifically for assessing children and families with medical problems, and they may be useful in the evaluation process. Examples include the following:

- The Eating Attitudes Test (Garner and Garfinkel 1979) is a 40-item measure of the symptoms of eating disorders that is readily applicable in a clinical setting.
- The High Sensitivity Cognitive Screen (Faust and Fogel 1989) is a 20-minute interview-based test designed to detect subtle or delineated cognitive deficits in an assessment short of formal neuropsychological evaluation, useful for patients aged 13 and older.
- The Coping Health Inventory for Parents (McCubbin et al. 1983) is an 80-item checklist in which parents report their response to the management of family life with a chronically ill child. Different coping patterns are quantified.

The Varni/Thompson Pediatric Pain Questionnaire (Thompson and Varni 1986) is an instrument developed to quantify pain in children. Easy to administer at the bedside, the questionnaire is an adjunct to clinical assessment.

In addition to these and other standardized questionnaires, physiologic measures can be helpful in the psychosomatic assessment of specific children. Examples include pulmonary function testing (especially the use of a peak flow meter at home), ambulatory electroencephalogram monitoring (useful in distinguishing various types of seizure disorders and pseudoseizures), and parental use of a videocamera at home to record unusual episodes or symptoms.

Treatment

The early specificity theorists were motivated by the hope that if they could identify a psychological etiology for a psychosomatic disease, then a psychological therapy could treat or cure it. Psychoanalysis and dynamic psychotherapy proved not to be as effective as expected. It remains true that the multifactorial etiology of chronic illness means that even intensive psychological intervention will not "cure" the disorder. However, there are a number of approaches available to the child psychiatrist that, singly or in combination, can be of major benefit to patients with a particular illness. These interventions will be described below in order of increasing intensity and investment.

Education

The most straightforward psychologically based intervention to impact the psychosomatic component of an illness is education. Misunderstanding, nonadherence to the regimen, poor judgment about symptom management, and faulty communication with medical professionals frequently contribute to much of the morbidity associated with chronic pediatric illnesses. Thus effective education is increasingly seen as worthwhile and cost effective for patients and their families. Formal educational programs; educational books, tapes, and coloring books; computer programs; and videotapes have been developed for many chronic illnesses, although their availability is uneven. Child psychiatrists consult-

ing on pediatric units frequently encounter patients whose understanding of their illness and its treatment is inadequate. Arranging for the appropriate education is a critical step toward improving the child's situation.

A review by Fritz (1987) described the characteristics and success of educational interventions in the promotion of self-management in childhood asthma; the findings pertain in principle to many other chronic illnesses as well. Educational programs for chronically ill children and their parents should strive to make them experts on their illness (consistent with levels of development) to help them become sophisticated partners with the physician in managing the illness, minimizing morbidity, and maximizing normal functioning. The bywords of such expertise are "active," responsible," and "knowledgeable." Such educational programs typically utilize a group format. In the group meetings, information is presented about the physiology of the illness and about the appropriate use and effects of medications. Often provided is guidance on stress management, environmental manipulation, and communication with physicians. Peer contact and support are usually encouraged; behavioral management and relaxation training may also be included. Educational programs should not ignore or minimize parental involvement in the treatment of the illness, no matter what the age of the affected child. Finally, an effective program recognizes the variable needs of each group of individuals and is sufficiently flexible to allow some modifications when needed.

Consultation

Consultation-liaison psychiatry represents a major clinical application of psychosomatic principles. Frequently, the child psychiatrist's first involvement with a child with a chronic illness comes when the pediatrician requests consultation. The effectiveness of the psychiatric input in the case depends to a large degree on the manner in which the plan for psychiatric consultation is presented to the patient and the family. Psychiatric consultation is described as one of a number of components of comprehensive care; the patient and family are assured of the pediatrician's continuing role in providing primary care. When the consultation is presented in this light, the pediatrician's firm belief in the desirability of the psychiatric involvement is communicated, and the patient and parents usually find the psychological evaluation acceptable.

The child psychiatrist can usefully suggest indicators for psychiatric referral (Fritz 1983). Such indicators include 1) the association of environmental stress with exacerbation or flares of the illness; 2) unusual preoccupation or indifference to the illness on the part of the child or the parents; 3) poorly controlled symptoms despite an adequate medical regimen; 4) parents' or patient's difficulty recognizing improvement and seeming to need the illness; and 5) significant countertransference reactions evoked in the primary physician. Nonpsychiatrists rarely use their own feelings of anger, rejection, or protectiveness, evoked by the patient, as useful data, but an effective liaison relationship can help them do so.

Outpatient Psychiatric Intervention

Outpatient psychiatric intervention will be recommended for a substantial group of the patients seen in consultation. The mode of treatment is determined on an individual basis; there is no particular disorder that implies or rules out a given intervention.

Individual and family therapy are commonly utilized in psychosomatic problems as they are with other psychiatric disorders. However, several caveats must be borne in mind when undertaking such therapy with a child or family in which there is a chronic pediatric illness. First, the therapist must respect the reality of the medical situation. While intrapsychic factors are always relevant, the stressors associated with a chronic or potentially fatal illness should not be underestimated or minimized. Second, the therapist must respect the need for somatic language and symptoms. When outpatient therapy does not "take" with psychosomatic cases, the problem is often a matter of the language differences between the therapist, who uses psychological language, and the patient and family, who think and speak in terms of physical illness, medical problems, and somatic dysfunction. Confronting this somatic disposition early in therapy and attempting to deal with the "real" or "underlying" issues often lead to the patient's sense of being misunderstood or out of place. Finally, the therapist must respect the patient's creativity in discovering coping solutions. The same standards for judging mental health, utilization of defenses,

and developmental progression that have evolved for physically healthy children often do not apply or are only partially relevant to children with chronic illness.

Behavioral techniques have been increasingly employed with children with chronic illnesses. Relaxation training is the most common of these, and it has been applied in treatment of a number of chronic disorders, including asthma, pain syndromes, cystic fibrosis, and cancer. The usefulness of relaxation training is disputed, since outcome studies vary in the results they report (Erskine and Schonell 1979; Richter and Dahme 1982). The major question frequently concerns the clinical relevance of small but statistically significant changes in a given physiologic parameter. When biofeedback is added to the relaxation training—typically, information on frontalis muscle tension is provided—the result may be improved. Behavioral therapy with contingent reinforcement is also used to enhance compliance and to reduce the illness behavior that impairs functioning. The behavioral approaches have been so generally effective that most large pediatric centers utilize health care psychologists working in conjunction with psychiatrists (Fritz 1990).

The patient's school life may be compromised by a variety of factors operative in chronic illness: frequent school absence, cognitive impairment, disfigurement, or delay in physical maturation. The psychiatrist's contact with school personnel needs to be active and can range from phone contact to teacher conferences, to planning an educational program on chronic illness for classmates of the patient (Henning and Fritz 1983). A current example of community alarm and classroom anxiety associated with pediatric illness is the reentry of children with HIV infection. Physician involvement can decrease fear regarding the initial case and can extend, in a primary prevention fashion, to helping schools plan for longer-range issues and even consultation regarding appropriate curriculum development (Brown and Fritz 1988).

Psychosomatic Inpatient Treatment

Hospitalization on a pediatric psychosomatic unit is the most intensive psychological intervention. Such a unit has been described in detail by Steiner et al. (1982). The service is designed for patients with symptoms that disrupt development and have been refractory to outpatient medical and psychological interventions. The staff on an acute pediatric ward usually has neither the time nor the training to deal with the psychological complexities these cases present. In contrast, most psychiatric wards lack the capacity to provide the acute medical care needed to manage the medical crises or provide the medical treatment that various chronic illnesses require. The psychosomatic unit provides daily group and individual therapy; a highly structured milieu that incorporates behavioral modification approaches, such as contracting and a token economy; and frequent family sessions. The specific goals and therapeutic strategies are individually tailored, and close communication between pediatricians and psychiatrists is assiduously maintained. Such units are now common in many medical centers, and they have made an important contribution to the care of children with psychosomatic disorders.

References

Ader R: Letter to the editor. Psychosom Med 36:183–184, 1974

Alexander F: Psychosomatic Medicine: Its Principles and Application. New York, WW Norton, 1950

Barglow P, Berndt D, Burns W, et al: Neuroendocrine and psychological factors in childhood diabetes mellitus. Journal of the American Academy of Child Psychiatry 25:785–793, 1986

Benoit D, Zeanah C, Barton M: Maternal attachment disturbances in failure to thrive. Infant Mental Health Journal 10:185–202, 1989

Breslau N, Davis G: Chronic stress and major depression. Arch Gen Psychiatry 43:309–314, 1986

Brown L, Fritz G: AIDS education in the schools: literature review as a guide for curriculum planning. Clin Pediatr (Phila) 27:311–316, 1988

Chatoor I, Egan J: Nonorganic failure to thrive and dwarfism due to food refusal: a separation disorder. Journal of the American Academy of Child Psychiatry 22:294–301, 1983

Cohen N, Ader R: Immunomodulation by classical conditioning, in Psychological, Neuropsychiatric, and Substance Abuse Aspects of AIDS. Edited by Bridge TP, Mirsky AF, Goodwin FK. New York, Raven, 1988, pp 199–202

Comaroff J, Maguire P: Ambiguity and the search for meaning: childhood leukemia in the modern clinical context. Soc Sci Med 15B:115–123, 1981

Dunbar F: Emotions and Bodily Changes. New York, Columbia University Press, 1954

Engel G: The clinical application of the biopsychosocial model. Am J Psychiatry 137:535–544, 1980

Engels W: Dermatologic disorders. Psychosomatics 23:1209–1219, 1982

Erskine J, Schonell M: Relaxation therapy in bronchial asthma. J Psychosom Res 23:131–137, 1979

Faust D, Fogel B: The development and initial validation of a sensitive bedside cognitive screening test. J Nerv Ment Dis 177:25–30, 1989

Featherstone H: A Difference in the Family: Living With a Disabled Child. New York, Basic Books, 1980

Forester B, Kornfeld D, Fleiss J: Psychotherapy during radiotherapy: effects on emotional and physical distress. Am J Psychiatry 142:22–27, 1985

Fritz G: Childhood asthma: a psychosomatic review. Psychosomatics 24:959–967, 1983

Fritz G: Psychological issues in assessing and managing asthma in children. Clin Rev Allergy 5:259–271, 1987

Fritz GK: Consultation-liaison in child psychiatry and evolution of pediatric psychiatry. Psychosomatics 31:85–90, 1990

Fritz G, Rubinstein S, Lewiston N: Psychological factors in fatal childhood asthma. Am J Orthopsychiatry 57:253–257, 1987

Fritz GK, Klein RB, Overholser JC: Accuracy of symptom perception in childhood asthma. J Dev Behav Pediatr 11:69–73, 1990

Garner D, Garfinkel P: The Eating Attitudes Test: an index of the symptoms of anorexia nervosa. Psychol Med 9:273–279, 1979

Gross R, Duke P: The effect of early versus late physical maturation on adolescent behavior. Pediatr Clin North Am 27:71–77, 1980

Halmi K: Anorexia nervosa: demographic and clinical features in 94 cases. Psychosom Med 36:18–26, 1974

Hanson S, Pichert J: Perceived stress and diabetes control in adolescents. Health Psychol 5:439–452, 1986

Hauser S, Pollets D: Psychological aspects of diabetes mellitus: a critical review. Diabetes Care 2:227–232, 1979

Henning J, Fritz GK: School reentry in childhood cancer. Psychosomatics 24:959–967, 1983

Hilliard JP, Fritz GK, Laviston NJ: Levels of aspiration of parents for their asthmatic, diabetic and healthy children. J Clin Psychol 41:587–597, 1985

Kinsman R, Dirks J, Jones N: Psychomaintenance of chronic physical illness, in Handbook of Clinical Health Psychology. Edited by Millon T, Green C. New York, Plenum, 1982, pp 435–465

Koocher G, O'Malley J, Gogan J, et al: Psychological adjustment among pediatric cancer survivors. J Child Psychol Psychiatry 21:163–173, 1980

Krener P, Miller F: Psychiatric response to HIV spectrum disease in children and adolescents. J Am Acad Child Adolesc Psychiatry 28:596–605, 1989

Leaverton R, White C, McCormick C, et al: Parental loss antecedent to childhood diabetes mellitus. Journal of the American Academy of Child Psychiatry 19:678–689, 1980

Lipowski Z: Psychosomatic medicine in the seventies: an overview. Am J Psychiatry 134:233–244, 1977

Litt I, Cuskey W, Rosenberg A: Role of self-esteem and autonomy in determining medication compliance among adolescents with juvenile rheumatoid arthritis. Pediatrics 69:15–17, 1982

Mattson A, Kim S: Blood disorders. Psychiatr Clin North Am 5:345–356, 1982

McCollum A: The Chronically Ill Child: A Guide for Parents and Professionals. New Haven, CT, Yale University Press, 1981

McCubbin MA, Patterson JM, et al: CHIP—Coping Health Inventory for Parents: an assessment of parental coping patterns in the care of the chronically ill child. Journal of Marriage and the Family 45:359–370, 1983

Mrazek D: Pediatric hospitalization: understanding the stress from a developmental perspective, in The Psychosomatic Approach: Contemporary Practice of Whole-Person Care. Edited by Christie M, Mellett P. New York, John Wiley, 1986, pp 164–196

Mulaikal R, Migeon C, Rock J: Fertility rates in female patients with congenital adrenal hyperplasia due to 21-hydroxylase deficiency. N Engl J Med 316:178–182, 1987

Nadi N, Nurnberger J, Gershon E: Muscarinic cholinergic receptors on skin fibroblasts in familial affective disorder. N Engl J Med 311:225–230, 1984

Paulson JA: The epidemiology of injuries in adolescents. Pediatr Ann 17:84–96, 1988

Pennebaker J, Kiecolt-Glaser J, Glaser R: Disclosure of traumas and immune function: health implications for psychotherapy. J Consult Clin Psychol 56:239–245, 1988

Pless I, Pinkerton P: Chronic Childhood Disorder: Promoting Patterns of Adjustment. Chicago, IL, Year Book Medical, 1975

Pumariega A, Pursell J, Spock A, et al: Eating disorders in adolescents with cystic fibrosis. Journal of the American Academy of Child Psychiatry 25:269–275, 1986

Richter R, Dahme B: Bronchial asthma in adults: there is little evidence for the effectiveness of behavioral therapy and relaxation. J Psychosom Res 26:533–540, 1982

Rogers M: The interaction between brain behavior and immunity, in Psychosomatic Medicine: Theory, Physiology and Practice, Vol 1. Edited by Cheren S. Madison, WI, International Universities Press, 1989, pp 279–330

Roy C, Darling P, Weber A: A rational approach to meeting macro- and micronutrient needs in cystic fibrosis. J Pediatr Gastroenterol Nutr 3(suppl 1):154–162, 1984

Schwartz L, Springer J, Flaherty J, et al: The role of recent life events and social support in the control of diabetes mellitus. Gen Hosp Psychiatry 8:212–216, 1986

Smith G, McDaniel S: Psychologically mediated effect on the delayed hypersensitivity reaction to tuberculin in humans. Psychosom Med 45:65–70, 1983

Spiegel D, Bloom J, Kraemer H, et al: Effect of psychosocial treatment on survival of patients with metastatic breast cancer. Lancet 2:888–891, 1989

Stabler B: Perspectives on chronic health problems, in Child Health Psychology. Edited by Melamed B, Matthews K, Routh D, et al. Hillsdale, NJ, Lawrence Erlbaum, 1988, pp 251–263

Steiner H, Fritz G, Hilliard D, et al: A psychosomatic approach to childhood asthma. J Asthma 19:111–121, 1982

Thompson K, Varni J: A developmental cognitive-behavioral approach to pediatric pain assessment. Pain 25:283–296, 1986

Weiner H: Dynamics of the organism: implications of recent biological thought for psychosomatic theory and research. Psychosom Med 51:608–635, 1989

Wittkower E: Historical perspective of contemporary psychosomatic medicine. Int J Psychiatry Med 5:309–319, 1974

Yates A: Current perspectives on the eating disorders, I: history, psychological and biological aspects. J Am Acad Child Adolesc Psychiatry 28:813–828, 1989

Chapter 40

The Somatoform Disorders

Michael Jellinek, M.D.
David B. Herzog, M.D.

The interaction between psyche and soma remains an enigma. Although illnesses fit on various points of an "organic" to "functional" continuum, every disorder has physiologic and psychological features. The term *psychosomatic* has been used to categorize a number of disorders in which there appears to be a loss or alteration of physical function secondary to psychological factors (Graham 1985).

Traditionally, a psychosomatic disorder was understood through hysterical conversion models, with the child's physical symptoms providing "a solution" to an emotional conflict. In this model, there is minimal evidence for organic disease, and the child is not as worried as one might expect because the illness is supported and reinforced by emotional needs.

Historically, chronic diseases were also felt to be associated with characterological traits (Reiser 1985), rather than those traits being highlighted by the demands of the disorder (Burke et al. 1989; Mrazek et al. 1987). When the boundaries between the psychological and physiologic are less clear, however, this model fails. Is a child at greater risk for asthmatic progression or repeated viral infection if depressed or living in a home stressed by parental discord? How is the stress mediated? What are the interactive changes in neurotransmitters, neuroendocrine pathways, or immunologically related susceptibility? How do these factors interact with a child's genetic vulnerability to a chronic disease such as asthma (Mrazek 1986) or diabetes mellitus (Brand et al. 1986; Johnson 1988)? Confusing the issue further is the fact that many children with organic disease suffer secondary emotional consequences that often lead to further physical consequences, for example, diabetic ketoacidosis resulting from poor compliance, "volitional" or "manipulative" asthma attacks (Matus 1981), or pseudoseizures.

In addition, many children presenting with psychiatric disorders also have multiple physical complaints. Livingston et al. (1988) found that between 25% and 39% of children admitted to a psychiatric hospital had physical symptoms, including headache, food intolerance, abdominal pain, nausea, and dizziness.

For many aspects of the interaction between psyche and soma, we do not yet know what questions to ask and have no valid and reliable biochemical, behavioral, or psychological measures. Studies tend to be retrospective and focus on numbers too small for multifactorial analysis. Thus we are left with our clinical judgment (Esman et al. 1985) to differentiate whether we are dealing with a largely 1) psychological disorder; 2) physiologic disease; 3) psychological aspects of a chronic disease; 4) physical-psychological manifestations of a disease that is emerging (e.g., abdominal pain in someone who will later develop inflammatory bowel disease); or 5) complex diagnoses, such as behaviorally involved seizure disorders (e.g., complex partial seizures) or pain syndromes (e.g., reflex sympathetic dystrophy). For the purposes of this chapter, we will highlight the psychological aspects of disorders that are medical or chronic.

Children routinely communicate through their physical complaints, such as being tired or having a stomachache. In a large study of more than 47,000 children in pediatric primary care, Starfield et al. (1980) found that between 5.7% and 10.8% of these children could be categorized as having psychosomatic symptoms. Abdominal pain and asthma led the list, followed by headache, constipation, and dysmenorrhea. For most psychosomatic complaints, reassurance and time seemed effective. In terms of more serious disorders, such as failure to thrive, severe asthma, diabetes, and epilepsy, there remains an ongoing debate as to the extent psychological issues directly cause acute or chronic disease. In a critical review, Graham (1985) stated that there is insufficient evidence to conclude that life stresses or personality style result in or cause chronic disease. He favored research on a complex, multifactorial model. In discussing the psychosomatic features of serious adolescent disorders (anorexia nervosa, asthma, inflammatory bowel disease, and diabetes), Schowalter (1983) supported Minuchin et al.'s (1975) conceptualization of three major contributing factors: 1) a family organization that encourages somatization, 2) a child involved in parental conflict, and 3) physiologic vulnerability. As research into genetics, neuroscience, and epidemiology proceeds, the clinician faced with psychosomatic illness must gather information from pediatric and psychiatric perspectives and must develop a comprehensive treatment plan, relying on clinical judgment.

Psychological Aspects of Chronic Disease

For the child and family, chronic disease is experienced as a major loss that has a substantial impact on day-to-day life. Every chronic disease has a profile of psychological costs at different ages (Perrin 1990). The impact of the disease varies by the child's age, the nature of the illness, and the secondary effects on family life (Geist 1979; Taylor 1985).

The toddler with a serious *seizure disorder* will face daily medication, restrictions on activities, the possible stigma of a helmet, and interference with learning either from the seizures or as a side effect of the medication. As a young child, the seizures may limit activities and peer interactions. Instead of having school as a place to build self-esteem and social skills, every day may be a struggle to save face and not feel inferior or rejected. As an adolescent, the years of being supported and sheltered by the family give way to the desperate need for autonomy and acceptance by peers. Seizures in adolescents are frightening to the individual trying to achieve a sense of autonomy and control and to peers who feel their friend may suddenly die in front of their eyes. Seizure disorders interrupt such common but critical activities as driving a car. The medications will seem a burden, a daily symbol of inferiority and of being different.

The child with *diabetes* faces the preoccupation of daily injections, diet, and blood testing (Feinkelstein 1986). The very young diabetic will have to gain the earliest sense of autonomy in the midst of "good control." Parents are forced by the illness to be more involved than development otherwise would dictate at every stage of childhood. Parents must cope with their own feelings about "control" and the feelings of guilt for passing on the genetic vulnerability. How should they instill the discipline needed? How much is needed? How responsible will they feel when their child becomes ketotic or hypoglycemic? How can they help their adolescent face the limits of diabetes amid the developmental need for power and limitlessness? How can they best prevent, delay, and then help their child and themselves adjust to the beginnings of "complications" and permanent limitations?

Cystic fibrosis (Drotar et al. 1981) presents a different set of challenges. For all but the most severely affected children, the diagnosis is made early, followed by a long period of good health. Nevertheless, this long grace period is dependent on frequent physical therapy, an exercise program, and multiple medications. Sustained parental involvement is required in the roles of a physical therapist several times a day, a cheerleader for exercise that by adolescence is a burdensome reminder of respiratory limitations, and a pharmacist for the 15 and more pills needed every day. Although antibiotic therapy and emphasis on nutrition are increasing the life expectancy of children with cystic fibrosis so that many will live into their 20s and 30s, older adolescents face the noisy breathing, shortness of breath, repeated hospitalizations, hemoptysis, and deaths of clinic friends.

For children with *cancer* (Selter 1990), there is the overall life-and-death struggle, the intense sense of feeling sick with repeated chemotherapy, and the dread of recurrence.

For those with *inflammatory bowel disease*, there is the fear of embarrassment, the need to be near a bathroom, extended bouts of pain, and the likely prospect of major surgery. For many families, the stresses of illness are sadly compounded by the burdens associated with high quality care and multiple medications.

Remarkably, most children, if given information, empathic care, and parental support, adapt very well to the burdens of their illness. Although at times of stress there may be regression, depression, poor compliance, and anger or frustration, children with chronic disease can continue their emotional development with remarkably little dysfunction. Orr et al. (1984) found that most children with chronic disease did well psychosocially, but those with ongoing impairment were at higher risk for dysfunction. Studies of specific disorders, such as diabetes (Frisch and Bode 1990) and cystic fibrosis (Khaw 1990), show only a mildly increased risk of psychosocial dysfunction. Psychosocial follow-up studies, however, suffer from difficulties in measurement of intrapsychic distress, self-esteem, and social functioning. Days absent from school or grades are convenient but superficial measures. Assessing peer relationships, self-esteem, or the deeper emotional impact of the disease on the child and family is methodologically much harder.

"Functional" Disorders

Disorders such as recurrent abdominal pain pose different problems (Ernst et al. 1984; Hodges et al. 1984; McGrath et al. 1983). The pediatric evaluation reveals no organic etiology, and yet the child continues to complain. There may be a number of diagnostic procedures available, but they may be too invasive given the child's overall good health. Still other disorders have some initial physical finding, such as the neurologic and vascular findings in reflex sympathetic dystrophy, but the pain dysfunction continues long after the resolution of overt organic signs. Rather than focusing on inappropriately aggressive efforts to define the specific etiologic basis for the child's complaint, it is useful to consider the extent of dysfunction. How much does the symptom interfere with psychosocial development? Most mild dysfunction resolves with time, reassurance, warm soaks, analgesics, and so on. Moderate and severe dysfunction becomes labeled as psychosomatic.

A minor foot bruise may evolve into a painful limp. The child will continue to limp and then may be unable to walk. Abdominal pain, often present only during the daytime, may prevent the child from going to school and may secondarily affect peer relationships. Parents will become increasingly concerned. If the illness is serving to resolve an intrapsychic conflict, the child will seem too ready to accept the consequences of the illness. If there is an unconscious dyadic purpose, then the illness will lead to increased, often regressive, enmeshment between a parent, often the mother, and child. If the symptoms are based in family tensions, then the parents will unite by focusing too narrowly on the child's medical needs. All of these solutions to intrapsychic and interpersonal conflicts avoid anger, sadness, and disclosure of secrets, but at the price of normal development and the risk of medical intervention. If the underlying stresses are severe, or if the dynamics of the family are highly resistant to psychological perspectives, then the medical risks can become substantial. The vague nature of the physical complaints and parental determination to find an organic cause will result in eventually finding some physician who will be more aggressive or invasive than is often times necessary.

Evaluation

Evaluating the child to assess the psychological consequence of chronic disease requires the usual comprehensive perspective and knowledge of the particular features of the disorder. Evaluating a child with psychosomatic complaints requires special skills. The atmosphere is typically pressured, as the family considers the psychiatric assessment as an indicator that their primary care physician or even subspecialist has "missed the boat" in finding an etiology. Psychosomatic diagnoses are made by exclusion. Since certainty is impossible, parents will use the inevitable doubt to press for further medical diagnostic procedures. Every test cannot be done, and thus the broader pediatric or psychiatric evaluation will be conducted amid nagging doubts. The child and family will be reluctant to talk about psychological issues, since they have had to express emotional conflicts in actions, symptoms, and dysfunction rather than words. "Doctor shopping" is common and often neglects the needs of the child.

The child psychiatrist's approach must be gentle, patient, and nonconfrontational. The consequences of the disorder, the dysfunction, should be the focus, rather than etiology. The pediatric follow-up and diagnostic workup should be continued at an appropriate level of intensity and invasiveness. Ancillary medical services, such as dietitians or physical therapists, should be used to treat the symptom. At a minimum, such medical treatment gives the child respect, understanding, and a gradual "way out" without acknowledging an exclusively psychological explanation.

Psychiatric Treatment

In addition to medical interventions, the child psychiatrist must make a clear decision to accept a psychosomatic child and family into treatment. Such a decision requires gaining the trust of the family, a trust based on an empathic approach and investment of time. Toward the end of the evaluation, patterns will emerge as to the specific nature of the conflict. Unresolved anger and losses, secrets, and unmet needs will be identified as relevant for treatment independent of a psychosomatic symptom. As treatment progresses, the physical complaint loses its priority and energy; rather than disappearing, the symptom no longer interferes with functioning. The child may well need individual therapy to deal with the internal defenses that are too dependent on displacement, depression, and regression. Family therapy may be needed to help the members function more autonomously and be open and direct in their communications. If marital issues have made the child the "identified" but inappropriate patient, then couples sessions will be required to focus on the sources of marital discord.

Working With Pediatricians

Added to the complexity of the evaluation and treatment plan is the child psychiatrist's relationship with the referring pediatrician. The families of these children have often intimidated one or more pediatricians and have refused previous efforts at child psychiatric referral. The pediatrician's first call will often be marked by frustration and requests for help in how to get such a family to agree to a referral. Several suggestions may be useful:

1. Avoid coming to a final etiologic diagnosis. The pediatrician should suggest that both the physical and the psychological avenues require further exploration.
2. Focus on the psychosocial history, common sources of stress, family psychiatric history, and emotional consequences of the

dysfunction. By gathering sufficient detailed information, the pediatrician may be able to identify clear psychological needs that are quite distinct from the symptoms.
3. Suggest focusing on dysfunction rather than diagnosis. Thus the child psychiatric evaluation is justified clearly by the dysfunction rather than a pursuit of the etiology.
4. Suggest patience, with the hope that time will foster a sufficient relationship.
5. Suggest an "if . . . , then" approach. Let the pediatrician note concern and doubt about future diagnostic procedures, but willingness to pursue additional noninvasive efforts. If this last round of diagnostic tests is negative, then the family should agree in advance to accept a referral.
6. Initiate the child psychiatric consultation on day 1 if pediatric hospitalization is necessary. Delaying a child psychiatric evaluation until after the other workups have been completed will communicate to the family that the child psychiatric evaluation is a last resort, not as important as the other referrals, and, given the short length of stay, not a priority.
7. Some families, despite the best efforts of both the pediatrician and the child psychiatrist, will refuse the referral. Acknowledge to the pediatrician that this is part of the family problem and not a question of the pediatrician's competency.
8. Suggest to the pediatrician that the child may be at risk for abuse if the family continues to pursue high-risk, invasive evaluations. Rarely, referral to the state department of social service is the only approach that will protect the child from needless surgery.

If the pediatrician is able to make a successful referral, then prompt action and careful attention to communication are essential. In outpatient settings, the child psychiatrist should call the pediatrician back and discuss the key stages of the assessment process. On inpatient consultations, the child psychiatrist should suggest a "team meeting" involving the primary care nurse, pediatrician, any ancillary medical services such as physical therapy, house staff, and the child psychiatrist. Bringing the team together and developing a comprehensive, unified treatment plan will provide a structure that is helpful to the child and family in following through on the treatment efforts. Any indication of a breakdown in communication or the family's poor compliance with a treatment plan is an indication of serious concern and should be addressed at an early point. Ignoring such signals will lead to discharges against medical advice, time-consuming arguments among the team, and ultimately the poor care of the child.

Conclusion

Psychosomatic illnesses require a multidisciplinary approach to both diagnosis and treatment. In an evaluation of these disorders, Schowalter (1983) recommended 1) establishing clear clinical collaboration between pediatricians and child psychiatrists; 2) coordinating medical and psychiatric treatment (neither continuing without the other); 3) developing a patient-pediatrician partnership; 4) focusing therapy on encouraging adolescent separation from parents; 5) viewing the symptom as a carrier for family issues; and 6) supporting behavioral gains with efforts that will change feelings and attitudes. Implementing these guidelines given the inherent psychological stubbornness of psychosomatic disorders will continue to be a challenge for both pediatricians and child psychiatrists.

Research Issues

The future holds the promise of both more understanding and greater complexity. In addition to what is already known concerning psychodynamics and family systems, there will be major contributions from the fields of genetics, endocrinology, and immunology. The findings of strong genetic factors in depression, alcoholism, and attention-deficit hyperactivity disorder certainly suggest that, beyond psychological identification, the transmission of somatic vulnerabilities includes a major genetic component. The research concerning the interaction of endocrinologic and immunological humoral factors makes it quite likely that we will have to redefine our views for most of the disorders thought to be psychosomatic and for some that even now are considered purely organic (Olweus et al. 1988). The hint of what is to come may be evident in the research concerning suppression of immunological function during depression in adults (O'Donnell et al. 1988). Obviously much work needs to be done to confirm and expand these findings and then assess if they are applicable to children. Integrating future research with the contributions of environmental factors, including stress, parent behavior, the child's personality, and development, will continue to provide challenges to the child psychiatrist functioning as researcher, consultant, or clinician.

References

Brand AH, Johnson JH, Johnson SB: Life stress and diabetic control in children and adolescents with insulin-dependent diabetes. J Pediatr Psychol 11:481–495, 1986

Burke P, Meyer V, Kochshis S, et al: Obsessive-compulsive symptoms in childhood: inflammatory bowel disease and cystic fibrosis. J Am Acad Child Adolesc Psychiatry 28:525–527, 1989

Drotar D, Doershuk CF, Stern RC, et al: Psychosocial functioning of children with cystic fibrosis. Pediatrics 67:338–343, 1981

Ernst AR, Routh DK, Harper DC: Abdominal pain in children and symptoms of somatization disorder. J Pediatr Psychol 9:77–86, 1984

Esman A, Hertzig ME, Lewis NB, et al: Grand rounds in child psychiatry: a case of psychogenic pain. Journal of the American Academy of Child Psychiatry 24:781–787, 1985

Feinkelstein R: Living with insulin-dependent diabetes mellitus, in Clinical Diabetes Mellitus: A Problem Oriented Approach. Edited by Davidson JK. New York, Thieme-Stratton, 1986, pp 544–550

Frisch L, Bode H: Diabetes mellitus, in Massachusetts General Hospital Handbook of Psychiatric Aspects of General Hospital Pediatrics. Edited by Jellinek MS, Herzog DB. Chicago, IL, Year Book Medical, 1990, pp 124–131

Geist RA: Onset of chronic illness in children and adolescents: psychotherapeutic and consultative intervention. Am J Orthopsychiatry 49:4–23, 1979

Graham PF: Psychosomatic relationships, in Child Psychiatry: Modern Approaches, 2nd Edition. Edited by Rutter M, Hersov L. St. Louis, MO, Blackwell Scientific, 1985, pp 599–613

Hodges K, Kline JJ, Barbero G, et al: Life events occurring in families of children with recurrent abdominal pain. J Psychosom Res 28:185–186, 1984

Johnson SB: Psychological aspects of childhood diabetes. J Child Psychol Psychiatry 29:729–738, 1988

Khaw KT: Cystic fibrosis, in Massachusetts General Hospital Handbook of Psychiatric Aspects of General Hospital Pediatrics. Edited by Jellinek MS, Herzog DB. Chicago, IL, Year Book Medical, 1990, pp 132–137

Livingston R, Taylor JL, Crawford SL: A study of somatic complaints and psychiatric diagnosis in children. J Am Acad Child Adolesc Psychiatry 27:185–187, 1988

Matus I: Assessing the nature and clinical significance of psychological contributions to childhood asthma. Am J Orthopsychiatry 51:327–341, 1981

McGrath PJ, Goodman JT, Firestone P, et al: Recurrent abdominal pain: a psychogenic disorder? Arch Dis Child 58:888–890, 1983

Minuchin S, Baker L, Rosman BL, et al: A conceptual model of psychosomatic illness in children. Arch Gen Psychiatry 32:1031–1032, 1975

Mrazek DA: Childhood asthma: two central questions for child psychiatry. J Child Psychol Psychiatry 27:1–5, 1986

Mrazek DA, Casey B, Anderson I: Insecure attachment in severely asthmatic preschool children: is it a risk factor? J Am Acad Child Adolesc Psychiatry 26:516–520, 1987

O'Donnell M, Silove D, Wakefield D: Current perspectives on immunology and psychiatry. Aust N Z J Psychiatry 22:366–382, 1988

Olweus D, Mattsson A, Schalling D, et al: Circulating testosterone levels and aggression in adolescent males: a causal analysis. Psychosom Med 50:261–272, 1988

Orr DP, Weller SC, Satterwhite B, et al: Psychosocial implications of chronic illness in adolescence. J Pediatr 104:152–157, 1984

Perrin J: Chronic illness, in Massachusetts General Hospital Handbook of Psychiatric Aspects of General Hospital Pediatrics. Edited by Jellinek MS, Herzog DB. Chicago, IL, Year Book Medical, 1990, pp 90–97

Reiser MF: Changing theoretical concepts in psychosomatic medicine, in Child and Adolescent Psychiatry: Modern Approaches, 2nd Edition. Edited by Rutter M, Herzov L. St. Louis, MO, Blackwell Scientific, 1985, pp 477–500

Schowalter JE: Psyche and soma of physical illness during adolescence. Psychosomatics 24:453–461, 1983

Selter L: Oncology, in Massachusetts General Hospital Handbook of Psychiatric Aspects of General Hospital Pediatrics. Edited by Jellinek MS, Herzog DB. Chicago, IL, Year Book Medical, 1990, pp 142–149

Starfield B, Gross E, Wood M, et al: Psychosocial and psychosomatic diagnoses in primary care of children. Pediatrics 66:159–167, 1980

Taylor DC: Psychological aspects of chronic sickness, in Child and Adolescent Psychiatry: Modern Approaches, 2nd Edition. Edited by Rutter M, Herzov L. St. Louis, MO, Blackwell Scientific, 1985, pp 614–619

Section X

Special Issues in Childhood and Adolescence

Chapter 41

Substance Use and Abuse

George W. Bailey, M.D.

Few problems affect the physical, emotional, and social well-being of American youth and their families as pervasively and as profoundly as substance abuse. Although youthful substance abuse is not new, the current problem is qualitatively and quantitatively different from previous times.

What used to be considered deviant behavior practiced by a small group of fringe youth has become the "statistical norm." Despite this, substance use and abuse is not normative behavior in children and adolescents (American Academy of Child and Adolescent Psychiatry 1987b).

Despite recently declining trends in youthful substance use (Johnston et al. 1989), the numbers of children and adolescents continuing to use drugs and the types of drugs they are using are alarming. Also, the age of first use is lower, and the types of drugs used are more serious and their use frequently entails stiffer legal penalties than ever before (Johnston et al. 1989).

Definition

The literature on substance abuse is large, diverse, and scattered throughout many different disciplines. Most current knowledge is based on studies using adult male alcoholics as the model. Data from these studies are extrapolated to other substances of abuse and then applied to children and adolescents.

Chemical dependency is the generic term used to describe the final stage of serious substance abuse, although there is question regarding applying its definition to children and adolescents (Bukstein et al. 1989). It is generally accepted to mean the com-

pulsive use of chemicals and the inability to resist the impulse to use them despite negative consequences in major areas of one's life.

Epidemiology

It is important to know who is using psychoactive substances, what and how they are using them, and to what extent.

Psychoactive substance use and abuse affects three groups of children and adolescents: children of substance abusing parents, those youth who actively take drugs: and those involved in trafficking drugs (Bailey 1989a). Within each group, there is a broad spectrum of substance use and abuse, and any individual youth may experience this in a variety of different ways.

A high index of suspicion is important for all adolescents; however, some youths are more at risk than others for development of substance abuse. These high-risk groups include children of substance abusers; victims of physical, sexual, or psychological abuse; school dropouts; pregnant teenagers; economically disadvantaged youth; antisocial and delinquent youth; youth with mental health problems, especially depressed and suicidal youth; and physically disabled youth (Kumpfer 1987).

Legal Drugs of Abuse

Alcohol is the leading legal drug of abuse despite its illegal use in underage children and adolescents. Beer and wine (especially wine coolers) (Johnson 1988) are the preferred alcoholic beverages, with hard liquor a less popular choice.

The most commonly used tobacco products are cigarettes; cigars; pipe tobacco; and, more recently, smokeless tobacco, such as "snuff" and chewing tobacco (Connolly et al. 1986).

Nonprescription medications are an important source of legal substances of abuse (Johnston et al. 1987; Roush et al. 1980). These over-the-counter medications are easily attainable at pharmacies and grocery and convenience stores and provide ready access to psychoactive substances. They are common sources of antihistamines, atropine, bromides, caffeine, ephedrine, pseudoephedrine, phenylpropanolamine, and amphetamine-like substitutes (Pentel 1984).

Psychiatrists and other physicians are often sources for prescription psychoactive medications. These include stimulants, benzodiazepines, barbiturates and other sedative-hypnotics, tricyclic medications, narcotic and nonnarcotic analgesics, and antimuscarinics (Dilsaver 1986).

Anabolic steroids are a new source of abusable drugs (Johnson et al. 1989; Krowchuk et al. 1989). Typically used to enhance body build and athletic ability, these drugs also have some important psychoactive properties (Pope and Katz 1988).

Volatile inhalants are important and potentially dangerous legal substances of abuse (Ron 1986; Skuse and Burrell 1982; Westermeyer 1987). They are often the drug of choice for younger and economically disadvantaged children because they are cheap, easily accessible, and present in most every household. Most young inhalant abusers abandon them after a few years of use and advance to other mind-altering drugs (McHugh 1987). Typical inhalants include volatile gases (gasoline and butane) (Evans and Raistrick 1987a, 1987b); toluene products (glues, acrylic paints, paint thinners, automotive products); halogenated hydrocarbons (freon, degreasers, solvents, spot removers, typewriter correction fluid); and nitrous oxide (dental anesthetics, whipped cream propellants, automotive power boosters) (McHugh 1987). "Poppers" or "snappers" (amyl, *n*-butyl, isobutyl nitrites) are popular volatile inhalants. These alkyl nitrites are often sold as "room deodorants" and "liquid incense," with a reputation for enhancing sexual excitement (McHugh 1987).

Illegal Drugs of Abuse

Cannabinoids are the most commonly abused illegal substances. No longer considered to be benign substances, they produce significant biological, cognitive, psychological, and interpersonal impairments (Haas 1987; Janowsky et al. 1979; Schwartz 1987; Schwartz et al. 1987, 1989; Tunving 1987).

Cocaine, in the form of powder, free base, and the highly addictive "crack," has created more profound changes in human behavior than any other illegal drug in history (Kirsch 1986). Hepatitis, bacterial endocarditis, sepsis, and human immunodeficiency virus (HIV) are not infrequent consequences of intravenous cocaine use. Many youth attempt to avoid these and the fear of needles by turning to smokable crack. Also, some use crack in combination with drugs generally not associated with youthful substance use, such as heroin and opioids. Other combinations include crack with phencyclidine, methamphetamine, and synthetic compounds.

Synthetic analogs are biochemical variations of federally controlled drugs that mimic the effects of narcotics, stimulants, and hallucinogens (Kirsch 1986). They are difficult to control legally and typically are undetectable by usual toxicologic means. These highly dangerous drugs do not warrant the glamorized label of "designer drugs" since they produce significant morbidity and mortality.

Clinicians have many available sources regarding the extent of legal and illegal substances use. The National Institute on Drug Abuse sponsors four major surveys: Monitoring the Future Study (National High School Senior Survey); the National Household Survey on Drug Abuse; National Adolescent School Health Survey; and the Drug Abuse Warning Network. These are available free of charge through the National Clearinghouse for Alcohol and Drug Information.[1]

The stage concept (DuPont 1984; Kandel 1975, 1982; Kandel and Logan 1984; Kandel et al. 1978a, 1978b; Macdonald 1984) is very useful in understanding the progressive development of substance use and abuse in youth. In Kandel's concept, youths begin their use of substances with legal and relatively "less serious" drugs (alcohol and tobacco) and progress through a series of stages to illegal, "more serious" drugs. These stages are 1) use of beer or wine, 2) use of cigarettes or hard liquor, 3) use of marijuana (Kandel's primary "gateway" drug) and 4) use of illicit drugs other than marijuana. Donovan and Jessor (1983) suggested that "problem drinking" occurs as a stage after marijuana and before heroin and cocaine. Kandel also posited that youths do not typically abandon drugs

---

[1]PO Box 2345, Rockville, MD 20852.

used at earlier stages, but tend to carry them over into other stages. This leads to a very common and important aspect of youthful substance abuse: multiple drug use.

Diagnostic Considerations

Both DSM-III (American Psychiatric Association 1980) and DSM-III-R (American Psychiatric Association 1987) are of limited value in making the diagnosis of psychoactive substance use and abuse in youth. Both fail to distinguish between preadolescent, adolescent, and adult substance use and abuse (Bailey 1989b), and both lack valid and reliable age-appropriate diagnostic criteria (Bukstein et al. 1989).

Diagnosing youthful psychoactive substance use and abuse requires a comprehensive and multifaceted assessment process. Clinicians must rely on a variety of methods to do so. Diagnostic information may be obtained from the following sources.

History

Most children and adolescents deny substance use and abuse as a problem. Nevertheless, the history is a very important source of information. Knowing what, when, and how to ask appropriate historical questions is critical. There are several helpful reviews on interviewing techniques (e.g., Anglin 1987; Farrow and Deisher 1988; Felice and Vargish 1984). Listening to what a patient has to say and what is left unsaid is most telling. Information obtained in this manner needs verification by parents, teachers, referral sources, and others involved. Family history is very important in assessing for substance use and abuse. A thorough, careful three-generational genogram, using as many family members as possible, will significantly increase the yield of important information (Baker et al. 1987).

Examinations

The physical and neurologic examinations are integral parts of any substance abuse evaluation. Clinicians choosing not to perform their own examinations should refer to colleagues for this critical aspect of the comprehensive assessment. In addition, any youth suspected of substance use and abuse warrants a formal mental status examination. It is important to look for evidence of both acute and chronic impairments.

Laboratory

Definitive routine screening tests for substance use and abuse in pediatric or adolescent populations are currently lacking (Farrow et al. 1987). Abramovitz (1985) hypothesized that this may be true because youthful substance abusers may exhibit acute, usually time-limited, complications, yet appear well in intervening periods despite their continued substance use.

Screening for sexually transmitted diseases, including HIV, is warranted in many substance-abusing youth. If indicated, this process should be done following careful informed discussion.

Toxicology screens are widely used, yet remain controversial. Several excellent reviews are available regarding general information (MacKenzie et al. 1987; Schwartz and Hawks 1985; Stewart 1982); moral, ethical, philosophical, and legal considerations (Goldsmith 1988; King 1987; Silber 1987); and the concordance of toxicology screens with historical and clinical data (Silber et al. 1987).

Clinical indicators for using toxicology screens include the following: 1) all adolescents with psychiatric symptoms; 2) high-risk adolescents (e.g., children of substance abusers, runaways, delinquents); 3) adolescents with changes in mental status or performance; 4) adolescents with acute behavior changes; 5) adolescents with recurrent respiratory ailments; 6) adolescents with recurrent accidents or unexplained somatic symptoms; and 7) adolescents for whom abstinence is to be monitored (Gold and Dackis 1986).

Clinicians have several major responsibilities regarding toxicologic screening: 1) to know when, where, and how to order it; 2) to have a general knowledge of common laboratory methods of toxicologic analysis, including the advantages and disadvantages of each; and 3) to understand and interpret these findings to patients, families, and consultees (Bailey 1989b).

Drug interference by other pharmacologically active agents may complicate drug screening. This is particularly important with multiple drug users (Stewart 1982) and those individuals who deliberately use adulterants to confound results. In addition, clinicians should be familiar with conditions that produce false-negative and false-positive results (MacKenzie et al. 1987).

A negative screen does not necessarily mean that drug use is absent; nor does a positive screen necessarily mean that drugs are causing the immediate symptoms or that the youth is under the influence at the time of the test (Stewart 1982). Any presumptive positive screen requires confirmation by a well-documented reference procedure, such as gas chromatography–mass spectrometry (Stewart 1982).

A confirmed positive drug screen is only one step in an otherwise critical process. Appropriate utilization of these clinical data must be integrated into a comprehensive clinical assessment and cogent presentation to the child and his or her family (Bailey 1989b). The interpretation of positive drug screens requires that physicians be knowledgeable about medicine, pharmacology, drug kinetics, and drug effects (Goldsmith 1988).

Assessment Instruments

Assessment tools are available as screening instruments, semistructured and structured diagnostic interviews, and self-report scales. Examples of screening instruments include the CAGE Test (Ewing 1984; Ewing and Rouse 1970) and the Children of Alcoholics Screening Test (Jones 1983). Both can be valuable tools for clinicians (Bailey 1989b).

The Minnesota Chemical Dependency Adolescent Assessment Package is an example of a semistructured and structured diagnostic instrument. This is a multidimensional assessment package consisting of a self-report chemical abuse problem severity inventory; a self-report inventory of personal, family, and social factors that predispose, perpetuate, or accompany adolescent chemical involvement; and a structured interview organized around DSM-III-R diagnostic criteria for psychoactive substance use disorders (Winters and Henley 1988).

Another example is the Teen-Addiction Severity Index (Kaminer et al., in press), which is a semistructured instrument based on McLellan et al.'s (1980) adult Addiction Severity Index. It assesses chemical usage, school status, employment-support status, family relationships, peer-social relationships, legal status, and psychiatric status.

Surveys on drug use and individual diagnostic assessments rely heavily on self-report despite the possibility of under- and overreporting. Barnea et al.'s (1987) review of the literature, and their own longitudinal adolescent study using self-report techniques, showed a high rate of cross-sectional and longitudinal reliability. Silber et al. (1987) also showed good concordance between self-report and urine toxicology screens in adolescent patients.

Clinical Findings

Youthful substance abuse is probably the most commonly missed pediatric diagnosis (Macdonald 1984). This is due in part to nonspecific and variable clinical presentations and delays between the onset of substance use and clinical detection (Williams et al. 1989).

Clinical findings depend on the type, amount, frequency, and time of last use of psychoactive substances. They also may be complicated and confounded by multiple drug use.

The most common findings on physical examination are alterations in vital signs; weight loss; chronic fatigue; chronic cough, respiratory congestion, and red eyes; poor attention to personal hygiene; constipation; and general apathy and malaise. Accidents and injuries are also important clinical markers. They may imply incidents that occur while under the influence, manifestations of physical or sexual abuse, or suicidal behavior.

The neurologic examination may reveal soft neurologic signs, gait or coordination disturbances, paresthesias, nystagmus, and seizure activity.

On the formal mental status examination, there may be acute and chronic changes, such as alterations in level of consciousness; deterioration in memory; impaired attention, concentration, and other cognitive abilities; disorientation and dissociative states; illusions and hallucinations; and disordered thought. Low self-esteem, guilt, worthlessness, and suicidal ideations are also common. For stimulants (particularly cocaine), mood changes may be manifested by intense euphoria and stimulation followed by restlessness, fatigue, somnolence, irritability, aggression, depression, and suicidal ideations.

Children of substance abusers represent a particularly vulnerable group. Most is known about children of alcoholics (El-Guebaly and Offord 1977; Russell et al. 1985), yet literature is increasing on children of other substance abusers (e.g., Deren 1986). Children of substance abusers are susceptible on a variety of fronts. Prenatal exposure to alcohol (e.g., Little et al. 1982; Macdonald and Blume 1986; Rosett et al. 1983; Streissguth et al. 1980), cocaine (Chasnoff et al. 1986, 1987), marijuana (Petersen 1987), and other substances (Sonderegger 1986) is associated with biological and psychological disturbances. Children of substance abusers also may be at risk for AIDS and other sexually transmitted diseases because of their parent's sexual and drug-abusing behaviors.

Children of alcoholic parents often have associated psychiatric disturbances, such as attention-deficit hyperactivity disorder; conduct disorder; learning and language disorders; anxiety disorders; affective disorders; eating disorders; personality disorders; ingrained personality traits, including compulsive overachieving, low self-esteem, denial of feelings, and difficulty with interpersonal relations (Bennett et al. 1988; Russell et al. 1985); and posttraumatic stress disorder (Cermack 1988). They also are significantly more likely to become alcoholics (Goodwin 1985; Schuckit 1985b) and to marry substance abusers (Woititz 1983).

Differential Diagnosis

Poor school performance; oppositional, noncompliant, and aggressive behaviors; and changes in mood, sleep appetite, attitude, attire, music, and social relationships are all nonspecific signs and symptoms of substance abuse in children and adolescents. Many disturbances may cause these ubiquitous findings. It is important that clinicians carefully and appropriately assess these myriad clinical presentations to determine the exact etiology. This is a matter of differential diagnosis.

The use and abuse of alcohol and other drugs may present in combination with psychosocial disorders. This is a matter of dual diagnosis (i.e., substance abuse and psychiatric illness). The association between substance abuse and psychiatric illness has been clearly documented (e.g., Bukstein et al. 1989; Demilio 1989; Groves et al. 1986; Lavik and Onstad 1986). Such associations include anxiety and eating disorders (Bukstein et al. 1989), unipolar depression (Deykin et al. 1987; Kashani et al. 1985), bipolar illness (Famularo et al. 1985), antisocial behavior (Cantwell 1978; Clayton 1986; Robins 1978), attention-deficit hyperactivity disorder (Gittelman et al. 1985), borderline personality disorder (Loranger and Tullis 1985), physical and sexual abuse (Behling 1979; Schiff and Cavaiola 1988), and suicide (Fowler et al. 1986; Rich et al. 1988).

The issue of triple diagnosis (i.e., substance abuse, psychiatric illness, and physical illness) is insufficiently explored. One condition encompassing these issues is the association between psychoactive substance use and abuse and AIDS. AIDS, AIDS-related complex, and seropositivity with HIV are major public health issues, and their association with substance use and abuse is well established (e.g., Petersen 1987). There is growing evidence that this problem is spreading down the age spectrum to infants, children, and adolescents (Drucker 1986).

Although the primary spread of HIV in substance abusers is by intravenous drug taking and needle sharing, one cannot discount the importance of adolescent heterosexual and homosexual activity. More HIV-infected persons are entering substance abuse treatment programs, and many learn of their HIV status as part of a substance abuse assessment (Drucker 1986).

The AIDS–substance abuse association creates a unique set of circumstances with extensive ramifications for clinicians and the public. This association significantly affects prevention, diagnosis, and treatment (Batki et al. 1988) and has a major impact on medical-legal issues, such as disclosure and confidentiality (Pascal 1987).

Etiology

Psychoactive substance use, abuse, and dependency are excellent examples of conditions reflecting a biopsychosocial determination. These conditions are determined by multiple factors, including genetic vulnerability, environmental stressors, social pressures, psychiatric problems, and individual personality characteristics (Newcomb et al. 1986).

Biological Factors

Most efforts to link psychoactive substance abuse and biology deal with the transmission of alcoholism. Twin (see Cloninger et al. 1989), family (Cotton 1979), and adoption studies (Cadoret et al. 1980, 1986; Cloninger et al. 1981) document a strong genetic component to the predisposition to develop alcoholism. Several behavioral (Schuckit 1984, 1985a), biochemical (Schuckit et al. 1987a, 1987b), and electrophysiologic studies (Begleiter et al. 1984, 1987) in high-risk youth support the role of biological influences. Data examining the biological underpinnings of drugs of abuse other than alcohol are also emerging (e.g., Cadoret et al. 1986).

Psychological Factors

Psychological factors are important determinants of youthful substance use and abuse. However, determining which factors are primary and which are secondary may be difficult. Often, behavioral traits, such as rebelliousness, poor school performance, delinquency, and criminal behavior (Kandel 1982), and personality traits, such as low self-esteem, anxiety, depression, and lack of self-control, predate the onset of substance abuse (Carroll 1981; Kandel 1981).

To understand adolescent problem drinking, Jessor and Jessor (1977) developed a conceptual framework called the problem-behavior theory. Three major indices of psychosocial variation are involved: the personality system, the perceived environmental system, and the behavioral system. Within each system, there are variables that predict the likelihood of problem drinking. In the personality system, variables include lowered value on and expectation of personal achievement and greater desire for independence, decreased religiosity, and a heightened sense of alienation. Variables in the perceived environmental system are reduced parental behavior control and only minimal disapproval of drinking, greater influence by friends, and available models for drinking. Finally, those in the behavioral system include deviant acts such as lying, stealing, aggression, performing poorly academically, and tolerating these behaviors in others. Some believe this problem-behavior model also applies to other substances of abuse (Williams et al. 1989).

Social Factors

The important social antecedents of substance use and abuse include parental and peer substance use and their approval of such use; the adolescent's own beliefs and norms about substance use and its harmfulness; a predisposition toward nonconformity; rebellion and independence; low academic performance and motivation; and engaging in "problem behaviors" reflecting deviance from appropriate adolescent behavior (Semlitz and Gold 1986).

Maternal drug use, low self-esteem, depression, psychological distress, poor relationships with parents, low sense of social responsibility, and lack of religious commitment are other important social determinants (Newcomb et al. 1986).

Environmental substance use patterns are pow-erful predictors of problems in children and adolescents. For example, parents of adolescents who use illicit drugs are more likely to be illicit drug users themselves (Harford and Grant 1987). Social contexts outside the home are also important variables. Where and with whom young people use substances and the meaning and structure of drinking situations play critical roles in the initiation and maintenance of substance abuse (Harford and Grant 1987).

Treatment

There are multiple treatment philosophies and modalities for youthful substance abuse. Most treatment programs share general features, such as abstinence from substances of abuse; group therapy with other substance abusers; adjunctive use of self-help groups, such as Alcoholics Anonymous (AA), Narcotics Anonymous (NA), and Cocaine Anonymous (CA); and the philosophy that the problem is "arrested" rather than cured (Hoffman et al. 1987b). Most treatment programs also use the 12-step principles based on the AA model (Ehrlich 1987).

Treatment settings include outpatient treatment, inpatient treatment followed by aftercare, and residential or therapeutic communities. The latter may include day treatment or initial out-of-the-home placement.

Outpatient

This is the most common, yet often most difficult, form of treatment. Several reasons account for this: denial of the problem by the youth or family, mistrust of adult intrusiveness, unwillingness to abstain, refusal to relinquish substance-using peers, and lack of motivation (Wheeler and Malmquist 1987).

Semlitz and Gold (1986) outlined the following as indicators for outpatient treatment: absence of acute medical or psychiatric problems; absence of chronic medical problems precluding outpatient treatment; willingness to abstain from psychoactive substances; cooperation with random urine screening; previously successful outpatient treatment; family interest and involvement in the treatment process; and self-motivation for treatment.

Outpatient treatment uses community resources, such as hotlines; alcohol and drug counseling services; information centers; specialized emergency room staffs or crisis teams; halfway houses; educational, occupational, and vocational services; social and legal services; self-help groups; and community mental health centers.

More structured types of outpatient services include substance abuse counseling (intended to limit progression of use), aftercare (see below), day treatment as an alternative to inpatient or residential treatment, and various family educational and assistance programs (Wheeler and Malmquist 1987).

Inpatient

There are myriad inpatient substance abuse treatment programs. Many use the Minnesota Model, which provides a structured, time-limited inpatient stay of generally less than 2 months. The treatment philosophy, which is based on the disease concept of chemical dependency, uses an AA-like 12-step recovery program.

Some inpatient facilities are "28-day" programs that emphasize detoxification from chemicals and narrowly focused treatment of the substance abuse only. This highly controversial type of treatment program is problematic since, using strict diagnostic criteria, less than 5% of those entering an inpatient treatment program require specific medical detoxification, and most have additional psychosocial problems (CATOR 1986).

Many inpatient treatment programs are for dually diagnosed youths. These programs assess and treat the substance abuse problem and underlying psychiatric disorders.

The better inpatient treatment programs use a comprehensive, multidisciplinary biopsychosocial assessment and require active family involvement in the process. Education of the chemically dependent youth and the family is a major focus. Other psychotherapeutic interventions include individual (especially in those with concomitant psychiatric problems), group (social skills, assertiveness training, leisure activity and planning), and family therapy. Academic and vocational interventions are also important, and attendance at AA, NA, and CA meetings is required.

Staff in such inpatient programs are multidisciplinary. They ideally consist of child and adolescent psychiatrists, pediatricians or adolescent specialists, psychologists, chemical dependency counselors, nurses, teachers, and occupational and/

or recreational therapists. Legal consultation is often available also.

Specific guidelines for determining the need for child and adolescent inpatient hospitalization (including treatment for substance abuse) have been established (American Academy of Child and Adolescent Psychiatry 1987a), and the integral role of the child and adolescent psychiatrist in such treatment has been delineated (American Academy of Child and Adolescent Psychiatry 1989).

Aftercare

Adolescents face the greatest temptation and difficulty maintaining abstinence immediately following discharge from inpatient treatment. Aftercare is designed to continue their specific substance abuse treatment on an outpatient basis. Aftercare activities involve intensive, partial-day-treatment programs, weekly aftercare meetings, or both.

Self-help groups (e.g., AA, NA, CA) are an integral aspect of aftercare. "Working the 12 Steps" and "ninety meetings in ninety days" are common expectations of this phase of treatment.

Residential-Therapeutic Community

Youth in need of this type of treatment typically have serious additional psychiatric, behavioral (generally antisocial), and other social and family problems and unsuccessful inpatient stays (Wheeler and Malmquist 1987).

Therapeutic communities are highly structured, drug-free, nonpermissive residential settings staffed primarily by paraprofessional program graduates in their own recovery. Treatment involves intensive daily routines involving group therapy (typically highly confrontational), individual counseling, tutorial learning sessions, remedial and formal education, and daily "community" work chores and responsibilities. Accepting one's role and responsibilities within the community are major focuses in this form of treatment, with lengths of stay varying from 6 months up to 2 years.

Finding the most appropriate treatment for a specific child or adolescent is often a difficult task, limited in large part by available options. The optimum arrangement would provide a broad continuum of treatment services, with each child or adolescent entering at the most appropriate level of care based on a careful, comprehensive individualized diagnostic assessment. Within such a system, there is the option of transition from higher to lower levels of care and vice versa, as clinically indicated.

An example of a comprehensive, well-designed approach to such a treatment continuum is the Cleveland Admission, Discharge and Transfer Criteria for adolescent chemical dependency (Hoffman et al. 1987a). These criteria encompass the important variables that make substance abuse treatment of youths different from that of adults: the importance of developmental level; the need for extended treatment periods due to the complexity of issues in youth and comorbidity with psychiatric and medical conditions; and family psychopathology and family involvement in the treatment process.

There are six levels of care based on the following variables: potential for withdrawal problems, comorbid physical and psychiatric complications, impairment in life function, attitude toward treatment, relapse potential, and nature of the environment necessary for recovery. The six levels of care are: 1) adolescent mutual/self-help; 2) adolescent low-intensity outpatient treatment; 3) adolescent intensive after-school treatment; 4) adolescent structured all-day treatment; 5) adolescent medically supervised intensive inpatient treatment; and 6) adolescent medically managed, intensive inpatient evaluation unit. Criteria and indications for treatment of dually diagnosed youths and of those needing extended care or transitional living programs are included.

Prevention

There are three major approaches to prevention of psychoactive substance use and abuse: school-based, community-based, and family-focused prevention programs (Ezekoye et al. 1986). Two promising additional approaches are also under study: multicomponent prevention programs and environmental public policy approaches (Kumpfer 1989).

School-based Programs

The school-based programs include cognitive, affective-interpersonal, alternative, behavioral skills training, and comprehensive school climate approaches. Cognitive programs tend to increase alcohol and drug knowledge without definitively decreasing or delaying the onset of use (Moskowitz 1983).

The affective-interpersonal programs, directed at increasing self-concept, understanding of feelings and interpersonal relationships, and awareness of the communication and decision-making processes, show little effectiveness in decreasing use, changing attitudes, or delaying the onset of use (Moskowitz et al. 1984).

Alternative programs are based on the theoretical assumption that providing youth with skills and competency building "alternative highs" reduces substance use and abuse. The effectiveness of such programs is equivocal (Schaps et al. 1981). Some youths actually increase use when the program is associated with entertainment, sports, social, extracurricular, and vocational activities, whereas those youths associated in programs with academic and religious activities and hobbies tend to decrease use (Swisher and Hu 1983).

The school-based behavioral prevention programs consist of two general approaches: the social influences approach and the personal-social skills training. The social influences approach (Evans et al. 1978) focuses on influences that promote substance use (e.g., parental, peer, media pressures) and promotes coping skills to resist these influences. The personal-social skills training approach builds on the principles of the social influence model in addition to acquiring additional generic personal and social skills (Botvin and Wills 1985). While both approaches are effective, particularly when combined (Botvin 1986), several researchers suggest that the peer pressure notion as a primary determinant is too simplistic (e.g., Moskowitz 1983; Sheppard et al. 1985).

Community-based Programs

Community-based programs are aimed at the media and at parent and community groups (e.g., Blum et al. 1976). All have equivocal results (Kumpfer 1989).

Family-focused Prevention Strategies

Family-focused prevention strategies involve parent training and family skills training (e.g., Forehand and McMahon 1982; Patterson 1982), various forms of family therapy (e.g., Klein et al. 1977), and family self-help groups.

In a three-pronged Strengthening Families Program, Kumpfer and DeMarsh (1986) found parent training, childrens' social skills training, and family skills training successful in reducing the children's risk factors. In combination, these three components decreased the use of alcohol and drugs in older children, and, despite varying degrees of dysfunction, most parents developed more effective parenting skills that favorably affected risk factors for their children.

Multicomponent Approaches

Multicomponent approaches are more recent strategies that incorporate school, family, community, and mass media components. Data to date suggest this combined approach has a synergistic effect that may increase the effectiveness of all components (Kumpfer 1989).

Environmental and Regulatory Changes

Another approach involves environmental and regulatory changes to prevent alcohol and drug abuse. Such changes include increasing excise tax and price (Grossman et al., unpublished manuscript); decreasing availability by increasing the minimum purchase age (e.g., Williams and Lillis 1985); reducing the number of outlets selling alcohol for off-premise consumption (MacDonald and Whitehead 1983); restricting sales at public events (Whittman 1985); regulating the content of advertising for alcoholic beverages (Mosher and Wallack 1981); and increasing counteradvertising (Wallack 1984).

Prognosis

The untreated use of psychoactive substances by children and adolescents has several possible outcomes. Some youth experiment and stop; others continue to use casually without significant consequences. Some use regularly, with varying degrees of difficulty in the major areas of their lives. Some progress to chemical dependency. Some die.

Fortunately, data suggest that most youth "mature out" of substance abuse (Jessor 1985; Kandel and Logan 1984). Unfortunately, it is impossible to predict definitively the course any individual youth will take.

Determining treatment outcome involves several factors, including an understanding of the principles that affect prognosis (e.g., Friedman and Glickman 1987; Holmberg 1985; Kandel et al. 1986); agreement on what constitutes successful treatment outcome (e.g., abstinence versus controlled use versus successful life function); a determination of how to measure treatment outcome (e.g., treatment effect versus "maturing out" effects); factors relating to relapse (Saunders and Allsop 1987); and correlation between short-term and long-term treatment outcome.

Hoffman et al. (1987b) identified six difficulties that need addressing before adequate assessment of treatment efficacy can be accomplished. These are 1) differences in perspectives and definitions of substance-related problems by referral sources; 2) differential characteristics of patient populations; 3) differential characteristics of treatment programs; 4) lack of categorization of patient-treatment match; 5) lack of measurement of an adolescent's individual treatment response; and 6) failure to identify and use appropriate outcome variables.

Research Issues

The foremost task for future direction in this area is development of appropriate research designs and studies specifically addressing the special developmental and biopsychosocial needs of children and adolescents. Following this process, basic psychiatric research is needed in all aspects of the problem: pathogenesis, prevention, diagnosis, and treatment.

Attention should be focused on high-risk youth, in particular, children of substance abusers. Clarification and delineation of standardized terminology and appropriate diagnostic criteria as they apply to children and adolescents are particularly important. Research in individualized assessment techniques and treatment plans, treatment efficacy, relapse prevention, and evaluation of treatment outcome are also critical.

References

Abramovitz M (ed): Acute drug abuse reactions. Medical Letter 27:77–80, 1985

American Academy of Child and Adolescent Psychiatry: Guidelines for treatment resources, quality assurance, peer review and reimbursement. Washington, DC, American Academy of Child and Adolescent Psychiatry, 1987a

American Academy of Child and Adolescent Psychiatry: Position statement on substance abuse, part I: the nature and extent of the problem. Washington, DC, American Academy of Child and Adolescent Psychiatry, 1987b

American Academy of Child and Adolescent Psychiatry: Position statement: inpatient hospital treatment of children and adolescents. Washington, DC, American Academy of Child and Adolescent Psychiatry, 1989

American Psychiatric Association: Diagnostic and Statistical Manual of Mental Disorders, 3rd Edition. Washington, DC, American Psychiatric Association, 1980

American Psychiatric Association: Diagnostic and Statistical Manual of Mental Disorders, 3rd Edition, Revised. Washington, DC, American Psychiatric Association, 1987

Anglin TA: Interviewing guidelines for the clinical evaluation of adolescent substance abuse. Pediatr Clin North Am 34:381–398, 1987

Bailey GW: Children, adolescents and substance abuse: an overview. Paper presented at the annual meeting of the American Academy of Child and Adolescent Psychiatry, October 1989a

Bailey GW: Current perspectives on substance abuse in youth. J Am Acad Child Adolesc Psychiatry 28:151–162, 1989b

Baker NJ, Berry S, Adler L: Family diagnoses missed on a clinical inpatient service. Am J Psychiatry 144:630–632, 1987

Barnea Z, Rahau G, Teichman M: The reliability and consistency of self-reports on substance use in a longitudinal study. Br J Addict 82:891–898, 1987

Batki SL, Sorenson JL, Faltz B, et al: Psychiatric aspects of treatment of IV drug abusers with AIDS. Hosp Community Psychiatry 39:439–441, 1988

Begleiter H, Poresz B, Bihari B, et al: Event-related brain potentials in boys at high risk for alcoholism. Science 225:1493–1496, 1984

Begleiter H, Poresz B, Rawlings R, et al: Auditory recovery function and P3 in boys at high risk for alcoholism. Alcohol 4:315–321, 1987

Behling DW: Alcohol abuse as encountered in 51 incidences of reported child abuse. Clin Pediatr (Phila) 18:87–91, 1979

Bennett LA, Wolin SJ, Reiss D: Cognitive, behavioral, and emotional problems among school-age children of alcoholic parents. Am J Psychiatry 145:185–190, 1988

Blum R, Blum E, Garfield E: Drug Education: Results and Recommendations. Lexington, MA, Lexington Books, 1976

Botvin GJ: Substance abuse prevention research: recent developments and future directions. J Sch Health 56:369–374, 1986

Botvin GJ, Wills TA: Personal and social skills training: cognitive-behavioral approaches to substance abuse prevention, in Prevention Research: Deterring Drug Abuse in Children and Adolescents. Edited by Bell C, Battles C. Rockville, MD, National Institute on Drug Abuse, 1985, pp 8–49

Bukstein OG, Brent DA, Kaminer Y: Comorbidity of substance abuse and other psychiatric disorders in adolescents. Am J Psychiatry 146:1131–1141, 1989

Cadoret RJ, Cain CA, Grove WM: Development of alcoholism in adoptees raised apart from alcoholic biological relatives. Arch Gen Psychiatry 37:561–563, 1980

Cadoret RJ, Troughton E, O'Gorman TW, et al: An adoption study of genetic and environmental factors in drug abuse. Arch Gen Psychiatry 43:1131–1136, 1986

Cantwell DP: Hyperactivity and antisocial behavior. Journal of the American Academy of Child Psychiatry 17:252–262, 1978

Carroll JK: Perspectives on marijuana use and abuse and rec-

ommendations for preventing abuse. Am J Drug Alcohol Abuse 8:259–282, 1981

CATOR: Chemical Abuse/Addiction Treatment Outcome Registry. St. Paul, MN, CATOR, 1986

Cermack T: A Time to Heal. New York, St Martins Press, 1988

Chasnoff IJ, Burns WJ, Schnoll SH, et al: Effects of cocaine on pregnancy outcome. NIDA Res Monogr 67:335–341, 1986

Chasnoff IJ, Burns KA, Burns WJ: Cocaine use during pregnancy: perinatal morbidity and mortality. Neurotoxicol Teratol 157:686–690, 1987

Clayton RR: Multiple drug use: epidemiology, correlates and consequences. Recent Dev Alcohol 4:7–38, 1986

Cloninger CR, Bohman M, Sigvardsson S: Inheritance of alcohol abuse: cross-fostering analysis of adopted men. Arch Gen Psychiatry 38:861–868, 1981

Cloninger CR, Dinwiddie SH, Reich T: Epidemiology and genetics of alcoholism, in American Psychiatric Press Review of Psychiatry, Vol 8. Edited by Tasman A, Hales RE, Frances AJ. Washington, DC, American Psychiatric Press, 1989, pp 293–308

Connolly GN, Winn DM, Hecht SS, et al: The re-emergence of smokeless tobacco. N Engl J Med 314:1020–1027, 1986

Cotton NS: The familial incidence of alcoholism: a review. J Stud Alcohol 40:89–116, 1979

Demilio L: Psychiatric syndromes in adolescent substance abusers. Am J Psychiatry 146:1212–1214, 1989

Deren S: Children of substance abusers: a review of the literature. J Subst Abuse Treat 3:77–94, 1986

Deykin EY, Levy JC, Wells V: Adolescent depression, alcohol, and drug abuse. Am J Public Health 77:178–182, 1987

Dilsaver SC: Antimuscarinic agents as substances of abuse: a review. J Clin Psychopharmacol 8:14–22, 1986

Donovan JE, Jessor R: Problem drinking and the dimension of involvement with drugs: a Guttman scalogram analysis. Am J Public Health 73:468–472, 1983

Drucker E: AIDS and addiction in New York City. Am J Drug Alcohol Abuse 12:165–181, 1986

DuPont RL: Getting Tough on Gateway Drugs: A Guide for the Family. Washington, DC, American Psychiatric Press, 1984

Ehrlich P: 12-Step principles and adolescent chemical dependence treatment. J Psychoactive Drugs 19:311–317, 1987

El-Guebaly N, Offord DR: The offspring of alcoholics: a critical review. Am J Psychiatry 134:357–365, 1977

Evans AC, Raistrick D: Patterns of use and related harm with toluene-based adhesives and butane gas. Br J Psychiatry 150:773–776, 1987a

Evans AC, Raistrick D: Phenomenology of intoxication with toluene-based adhesives and butane gas. Br J Psychiatry 150:769–773, 1987b

Evans RI, Rozelle RM, Mittlemark MB et al: Deterring the onset of smoking in children. Journal of Applied Social Psychology 8:125–135, 1978

Ewing JA: Detecting alcoholism: the CAGE questionnaire. JAMA 252:1905–1907, 1984

Ewing JA, Rouse BA: Identifying the hidden alcoholic. Paper presented at the 29th International Congress on Alcohol and Drug Dependence. Sydney, Australia, 1970

Ezekoye S, Kumpfer KL, Bubowski W: Childhood and Chemical Abuse: Prevention and Intervention. New York, Haworth Press, 1986

Famularo R, Stone K, Popper C: Preadolescent alcohol abuse and dependence. Am J Psychiatry 140:1187–1189, 1985

Farrow JA, Deisher R: A practical guide to the office assessment of adolescent substance abuse. Pediatr Ann 15:675–684, 1988

Farrow JA, Rees JM, Worthington-Robert BS: Health, developmental, and nutritional status of adolescent alcohol and marijuana abusers. Pediatrics 79:218–223, 1987

Felice ME, Vargish W: Interviewing and evaluation of the adolescent, in Practice of Pediatrics. Edited by Kelly VE. Hagerstown, MD, Harper & Row, 1984, pp 7–14

Forehand RL, McMahon RJ: Helping the Non-Compliant Child: A Clinician's Guide to Parent Training. New York, Guilford, 1982

Fowler RC, Rich CL, Young D: San Diego suicide study, II: substance abuse in young cases. Arch Gen Psychiatry 43:962–965, 1986

Friedman AS, Glickman NW: Effects of psychiatric symptomatology on treatment outcome for adolescent male drug abusers. J Nerv Ment Dis 175:425–430, 1987

Gittelman R, Mannuzza S, Shenker R, et al: Hyperactive boys almost grown up, I: psychiatric status. Arch Gen Psychiatry 42:937–947, 1985

Gold MS, Dackis GA: Role of the laboratory in the evaluation of suspected drug abuse. J Clin Psychiatry 47:17–23, 1986

Goldsmith MF: Drug testing upheld, decried: physicians asked to decide. JAMA 259:2341–2342, 1988

Goodwin DW: Alcoholism and genetics: the sins of the fathers. Arch Gen Psychiatry 42:171–174, 1985

Groves JB, Batey SR, Wright HH: Psychoactive drug use among adolescents with psychiatric disorders. Am J Hosp Pharm 43:1714–1718, 1986

Haas AP: Long-term outcome of heavy marijuana use among adolescents. Pediatrician 14:77–82, 1987

Harford TC, Grant BF: Psychosocial factors in adolescent drinking contexts. J Stud Alcohol 48:551–557, 1987

Hoffman NG, Halikas JA, Mee-Lee D: The Cleveland Admission, Discharge and Transfer Criteria: Model for Chemical Dependency Treatment Programs. Cleveland, OH, The Greater Cleveland Hospital Association, 1987a

Hoffman NG, Sonis WA, Halika JA: Issues in the evaluation of chemical dependency treatment programs for adolescents. Pediatr Clin North Am 34:449–459, 1987b

Holmberg MB: Longitudinal studies of drug abuse in a fifteen-year-old population, 2: antecedents and consequences. Acta Psychiatr Scand 71:80–91, 1985

Janowsky DS, Clopton PL, Leichner PP, et al: Interpersonal effects of marijuana. Arch Gen Psychiatry 36:781–785, 1979

Jessor R: Adolescent problem drinking: psychosocial aspects and developmental outcomes, in Proceedings: NIAAA-WHO Collaborating Center Designation Meeting and Alcohol Research Seminar. Washington, DC, U.S. Government Printing Office, 1985

Jessor R, Jessor SL: Problem Behavior and Psychological Development: A Longitudinal Study of Youth. New York, Academic, 1977

Johnson EM: Wine coolers: they're not a "soft" drink, in Schools Without Drugs: The Challenge. Washington, DC, U.S. Department of Education, 1988

Johnson MD, Jay S, Shoup B, et al: Anabolic steroid use by male adolescents. Pediatrics 83:921–924, 1989

Johnston LD, O'Malley PM, Bachman JG: Psychotherapeutic, licit, and illicit use of drugs among adolescents. J Adolesc Health Care 8:36–51, 1987

Johnston LD, O'Malley PM, Bachman JG: Illicit drug use, smoking, and drinking by America's high school students, college students, and young adults, 1975–1987. Rockville, MD, National Institute on Drug Abuse, 1988

Johnston LD, Bachman JG, O'Malley PM: High school senior survey; monitoring the future study. Rockville, MD, National Institute on Drug Abuse, 1989

Jones JW: The Children of Alcoholics Screening Test. Chicago, IL, Camelot Unlimited, 1983

Kaminer Y, Bukstein O, Tarter RE: The Teen Addiction Severity Index (T-ASI): rationale and reliability. Int J Addict (in press)

Kandel DB: Stages in adolescent involvement in drug use. Science 190:912–914, 1975

Kandel DB: Frequent marijuana use: correlates, possible effects, and reasons for using and quitting. Paper presented at the American Counsel on Marijuana Conference: Treating the Marijuana Dependent Person, Bethesda, MD, 1981

Kandel DB: Epidemiological and psychosocial perspectives on adolescent drug use. Journal of the American Academy of Child Psychiatry 21:328–347, 1982

Kandel DB, Logan JA: Patterns of drug use from adolescence to young adulthood, I: periods of risk for initiation, continued use, and discontinuation. Am J Public Health 74:660–666, 1984

Kandel DB, Kessler R, Margulies R: Adolescent initiation into stages of drug use: a developmental analysis, in Longitudinal Research on Drug Use: Empirical Findings and Methodological Issues. Edited by Kandel DB. Washington, DC, Hemisphere-Wiley, 1978a, pp 75–100

Kandel DB, Kessler R, Margulies R: Antecedents of adolescent initiation into stages of drug abuse: a developmental analysis. Journal of Youth and Adolescence 7:13–40, 1978b

Kandel DB, Davies MA, Karus D, et al: The consequences in young adulthood of adolescent drug involvement. Arch Gen Psychiatry 43:746–754, 1986

Kashani JH, Keller MB, Solomon N, et al: Double depression in adolescent substance abusers. J Affective Disord 8:153–157, 1985

King NMP: Moral and legal issues in screening for drug use in adolescents. J Pediatr 111:249–250, 1987

Kirsch MM: Designer Drugs. Minneapolis, MN, Compcare Publishers, 1986

Klein NC, Alexander JF, Parson BV: Impact of family systems intervention on recidivism and sibling delinquency: a model of primary prevention and program evaluation. J Consult Clin Psychol 45:469–474, 1977

Krowchuk DP, Anglin TM, Goodfellow DB, et al: High school athletes and the use of ergogenic aids. Am J Dis Child 143:486–489, 1989

Kumpfer KL: Prevention of drug abuse: a critical review of risk factors and prevention strategies. Paper prepared for the American Academy of Child and Adolescent Psychiatry's Project Prevention: An Intervention Initiative, October 1987

Kumpfer KL: Children, adolescents and substance abuse: a review of prevention strategies. Paper presented at the annual meeting of the American Academy of Child and Adolescent Psychiatry, New York, October 1989

Kumpfer KL, DeMarsh J: Family oriented interventions for prevention of chemical dependency in children and adolescents, in Children and Chemical Abuse: Prevention and Early Intervention. Edited by Ezekoye S, Kumpfer KL, Bukowski W. New York, Haworth, 1986, pp 100–126

Lavik NJ, Onstad S: Drug use and psychiatric symptoms. Acta Psychiatr Scand 73:437–440, 1986

Little RE, Graham JM, Samson HH: Fetal alcohol effects in humans and animals. Adv Alcohol Subst Abuse 1:103–125, 1982

Loranger AW, Tullis EH: Family history of alcoholism in borderline personality disorders. Arch Gen Psychiatry 42:153–157, 1985

Macdonald DI: Drugs, drinking and adolescents. Am J Dis Child 138:117–125, 1984

Macdonald DI, Blume SB: Children of alcoholics. Am J Dis Child 140:750–754, 1986

MacDonald S, Whitehead P: Availability of outlets and consumption of alcoholic beverages. Journal of Drug Issues, Fall 1983, pp 477–486

MacKenzie RG, Cheng M, Haftel AJ: The clinical utility and evaluation of drug screening techniques. Pediatr Clin North Am 34:423–438, 1987

McHugh MJ: The abuse of volatile substances. Pediatr Clin North Am 34:333–340, 1987

McLellan TA, Luborsky L, Woody GE, et al: An improved diagnostic evaluation instrument for substance abuse patients: the Addiction Severity Index. J Nerv Ment Dis 168:26–33, 1980

Mosher JF, Wallack LM: Government regulation of alcohol advertising: protecting industry profits versus promoting the public health. J Public Health Policy 2:333–353, 1981

Moskowitz JM: Preventing adolescent substance abuse through drug education. NIDA Res Monogr 47:233–249, 1983

Moskowitz JM, Malvin J, Schaeffer G: The effects of drug education at follow-up. Journal of Alcohol and Drug Education 30:45–49, 1984

Newcomb MD, Maddahian E, Bentler PM: Risk factors for drug use among adolescents: concurrent and longitudinal analysis. Am J Public Health 76:525–531, 1986

Pascal CB: Selected legal issues about AIDS for drug abuse treatment programs. J Psychoactive Drugs 19:1–12, 1987

Patterson GR: Coercive Family Process. Eugene, OR, Castalia, 1982

Pentel P: Toxicity of over-the-counter stimulants. JAMA 252:1898–1903, 1984

Petersen RC (ed): Drug abuse and drug abuse research: the second triennial report to Congress. Rockville, MD, National Institute on Drug Abuse, 1987

Pope HG, Katz DL: Affective and psychiatric symptoms associated with anabolic steroid use. Am J Psychiatry 145:490–497, 1988

Rich CL, Fowler RC, Fogarty LA, et al: San Diego suicide study, III: relationships between diagnosis and stressors. Arch Gen Psychiatry 45:589–592, 1988

Robins LN: Sturdy childhood predictors of adult antisocial behavior: replications from longitudinal studies. Psychol Med 8:611–622, 1978

Ron M: Volatile substance abuse: a review of possible long-term neurological, intellectual and psychiatric sequelae. Br J Psychiatry 148:235–246, 1986

Rosett HL, Weiner L, Lee A, et al: Patterns of alcohol consumption and fetal development. Obstet Gynecol 61:539–546, 1983

Roush GC, Thompson WD, Berberian RM: Psychoactive medicinal and non-medicinal drug use among high school students. Pediatrics 66:709–715, 1980

Russell M, Henderson C, Blume SB: Children of alcoholics: a review of the literature. New York, Children of Alcoholics Foundation, 1985

Saunders B, Allsop S: Relapse: a psychological perspective. Br J Addict 82:417–429, 1987

Schaps E, DiBartolo R, Moskowitz J, et al: Primary prevention evaluation research: a review of 127 impact studies. Journal of Drug Issues 11:17–43, 1981

Schiff M, Cavaiola A: The presentation of dual diagnosis in an adolescent chemical dependence unit. Alcoholism Treatment Quarterly 5:261–271, 1988

Schuckit MA: Subjective responses to alcohol in sons of alcoholics and control subjects. Arch Gen Psychiatry 41:879–884, 1984

Schuckit MA: Ethanol-induced changes in body sway in men at high alcoholism risk. Arch Gen Psychiatry 42:375–379, 1985a

Schuckit MA: Genetics and the risk for alcoholism. JAMA 254:2614–2617, 1985b

Schuckit MA, Gold E, Rich C: Plasma cortisol levels following ethanol in sons of alcoholic and control subjects. Am J Psychiatry 144:942–945, 1987a

Schuckit MA, Gold E, Rich C: Serum prolactin levels in sons of alcoholics and control subjects. Am J Psychiatry 144:854–859, 1987b

Schwartz RH: Marijuana: an overview. Pediatr Clin North Am 34:305–317, 1987

Schwartz RH, Hawks RL: Laboratory detection of marijuana use. JAMA 254:788–792, 1985

Schwartz RH, Hoffman NG, Jones R: Behavioral, psychosocial, and academic correlates of marijuana usage in adolescents. Clin Pediatr 26:264–270, 1987

Schwartz RH, Gruenwald PJ, Klitzner M, et al: Short-term memory impairments in cannabis-dependent adolescents. Am J Dis Child 143:1214–1219, 1989

Semlitz L, Gold MS: Adolescent drug abuse: diagnosis, treatment and prevention. Psychiatr Clin North Am 9:455–473, 1986

Sheppard M, Wright D, Goodstadt M: Peer pressure and drug use: exploding the myth. Adolescence 20:949–958, 1985

Silber TJ: Adolescent marijuana use: screening and ethics. Adolescence 22:363–370, 1987

Silber TJ, Getson P, Ridley S, et al: Adolescent marijuana use: concordance between questionnaire and immunoassay for cannabinoid metabolites. J Pediatr 111:299–302, 1987

Skuse D, Burrell S: A review of solvent abusers and their management by a child psychiatric out-patient service. Hum Toxicol 1:321–329, 1982

Sonderegger TB: Overview of perinatal substance abuse: research and clinical perspectives. Neurobehavioral Toxicology and Teratology 8:325–327, 1986

Stewart DC: The use of the clinical laboratory in the diagnosis and treatment of substance abuse. Pediatr Ann 11:669–682, 1982

Streissguth AP, Landesman-Dwyer S, Martin JC, et al: Teratogenic effects of alcohol in humans and laboratory animals. Science 209:353–361, 1980

Swisher JD, Hu TW: Alternatives to drug abuse. NIDA Res Monogr 47:9–15, 1983

Tunving K: Psychiatric aspects of cannabis use in adolescents and young adults. Pediatrician 14:83–91, 1987

Wallack L: The prevention of alcohol-related problems: recommendations for public policy initiatives. Berkeley, CA, Prevention Research Center, 1984

Westermeyer J: The psychiatrist and solvent-inhalant abuse: recognition, assessment, and treatment. Am J Psychiatry 144:903–907, 1987

Wheeler K, Malmquist J: Treatment approaches in adolescent

chemical dependency. Pediatr Clin North Am 34:437–447, 1987

Whittman FD: Reducing environmental risk of alcohol problems. Berkeley, CA, Prevention Research Center, 1985

Williams RA, Feibelman ND, Moulder C: Events precipitating hospital treatment of adolescent drug abusers. J Am Acad Child Adolesc Psychiatry 28:70–73, 1989

Williams TP, Lillis RP: Changes in alcohol consumption by eigh-teen-year-olds following an increase in New York's purchase age to nineteen. Paper presented at the National Council on Alcoholism, National Alcoholism Forum, Washington, DC, 1985

Winters K, Henley G: The Personal Experience Inventory. Los Angeles, CA, Western Psychological Services, 1988

Woititz JG: Adult Children of Alcoholics. Pampano Beach, FL, Health Communications, 1983

Chapter 42

Gender Identity and Psychosexual Disorders

Kenneth J. Zucker, Ph.D.
Richard Green, M.D., J.D.

Definition

In this chapter, we provide an overview of gender identity and psychosexual problems in children and adolescents. Three terms—gender identity, gender role, and sexual orientation—are useful in organizing one's thinking about gender identity and psychosexual problems.

Gender identity refers to a person's basic sense of self as a male or a female. It includes both the awareness that one *is* a male or a female and an affective appraisal of such knowledge. Based on work with intersex children, Money et al. (1957) concluded that gender identity typically appears in its nascent form between the ages of 2 and 3 years. More recent empirical studies have demonstrated that children in this age range, typically by about 30 to 36 months, are able to categorize other people by gender (Etaugh et al. 1989; Leinbach and Fagot 1986; Paluszny et al. 1973; Thompson 1975) and, presumably, themselves.

Gender role refers to a person's adoption of cultural markers of masculinity and femininity. In children, gender role preference can be indexed in a variety of ways, including toy interests, role and fantasy play, and personality attributes. Conceptually, one can consider a child to be primarily masculine or feminine, based on the child's pattern of gender role behavior. Alternatively, one can view a child as both masculine and feminine (androgynous), masculine, feminine, or neither masculine nor feminine (undifferentiated). Over the past 30 years, dozens of studies have been conducted on gender role behavior in children (see Huston 1983).

Almost without exception, these studies have shown that the sexes differ significantly with regard to several sex-typed attributes, including toy and fantasy play (e.g., Fagot 1977), peer affiliation preference (e.g., Maccoby and Jacklin 1987), aggression (e.g., Maccoby and Jacklin 1974, 1980), activity level (e.g., Eaton and Enns 1986), and rough-and-tumble play (e.g., DiPietro 1981).

Lastly, sexual orientation refers to the pattern of a person's erotic responsiveness. Heterosexual, bisexual, and homosexual are the three sexual orientations most commonly described by contemporary nosologists in sexology, although age of the sexual partner (either in fantasy or behavior) is also an important factor to consider. Gender identity and gender role are typically viewed as developmentally prior to the emergence of sexual orientation, although this view is not held universally. More detailed consideration of these three terms can be found elsewhere (e.g., Green 1974; Money 1973, 1985, 1988; Stoller 1968a).

Diagnostic Criteria

In DSM-III-R (American Psychiatric Association 1987), six diagnoses are of relevance with regard to gender identity and psychosexual problems during childhood and adolescence:

1. Gender identity disorder of childhood (GIDC) (Table 42-1)
2. Gender identity disorder not otherwise specified
3. Transsexualism (Table 42-2)

Table 42-1.   DSM-III-R diagnostic criteria for gender identity disorder of childhood

For Females

A. Persistent and intense distress about being a girl, and a stated desire to be a boy (not merely a desire for any perceived cultural advantages from being a boy), or insistence that she is a boy.

B. Either (1) or (2):
  1. Persistent marked aversion to normative feminine clothing and insistence on wearing stereotypical masculine clothing, e.g., boys' underwear and other accessories
  2. Persistent repudiation of female anatomic structures, as evidenced by at least one of the following:
      a) An assertion that she has, or will grow, a penis
      b) Rejection of urinating in a sitting position
      c) Assertion that she does not want to grow breasts or menstruate

C. The girl has not yet reached puberty.

For Males

A. Persistent and intense distress about being a boy and an intense desire to be a girl or, more rarely, insistence that he is a girl.

B. Either (1) or (2):
  1. Preoccupation with female stereotypical activities, as shown by a preference for either cross-dressing or simulating female attire, or by an intense desire to participate in the games and pastimes of girls and rejection of male stereotypical toys, games, and activities
  2. Persistent repudiation of male anatomic structures, as indicated by at least one of the following repeated assertions:
      a) That he will grow up to become a woman (not merely in role)
      b) That his penis or testes are disgusting or will disappear
      c) That it would be better not to have a penis or testes

C. The boy has not yet reached puberty.

Source. Reprinted with permission from American Psychiatric Association 1987.

4. Gender identity disorder of adolescence or adulthood, nontranssexual type (Table 42-3)
5. Transvestic fetishism (Table 42-4)
6. Sexual disorder not otherwise specified

During childhood, only the first two of these six diagnoses are of relevance. In adolescence, however, all but the first diagnosis may be used as gender identity and psychosexual concerns become more differentiated, in part, because of the increased salience of erotic behavior. Thus, in addition to concerns around gender identity proper, which can be diagnosed as transsexualism; gender identity disorder of adolescence or adulthood, nontranssexual type; or gender identity disorder not otherwise specified, the clinician must also be attentive to paraphiliac behavior (transvestic fetishism) or distress regarding one's sexual orientation, most typically in homosexuality (sexual disorder not otherwise specified).

The reliability and validity of the GIDC diagnosis have received attention. Based on chart data from 36 consecutive referrals to a child and adolescent gender identity clinic, Zucker et al. (1984) found very high agreement on whether the child met DSM-III (American Psychiatric Association 1980) criteria for GIDC. It also was found that the children who met the complete diagnostic criteria were, on average, more cross-gendered in their behavior than were the children who did not meet the complete diagnostic criteria.

Among demographic variables, age of the child at assessment has been most consistently associated with the GIDC diagnosis. Based on 108 consecutive referrals, Zucker (1991) found that the children who received the GIDC diagnosis were significantly younger than were the children who did not (6.4 years versus 9.0 years, respectively). In part, this finding appears related to older children's tendency not to verbalize the wish to be of the opposite sex, which is a distinct criterion for GIDC (see Table 42-1). Clinical evidence may suggest continued discomfort with gender identity concerns, but the older child may be more aware of social convention and thus not verbalize concerns, at least during an initial assessment.

These findings have led to the question of whether it is appropriate to retain in DSM-IV the wish to be of the opposite sex as a distinct criterion (Zucker 1991). It has been suggested that the criteria be

Table 42-2.   DSM-III-R diagnostic criteria for transsexualism

A. Persistent discomfort and sense of inappropriateness about one's assigned sex.
B. Persistent preoccupation for at least two years with getting rid of one's primary and secondary sex characteristics and acquiring the sex characteristics of the other sex.
C. The person has reached puberty.

Specify history of sexual orientation: **asexual, homosexual, heterosexual,** or **unspecified.**

Source. Reprinted with permission from American Psychiatric Association 1987.

Table 42-4.   DSM-III-R diagnostic criteria for transvestic fetishism

A. Over a period of at least six months, in a heterosexual male, recurrent intense sexual urges and sexually arousing fantasies involving cross-dressing.
B. The person has acted on these urges, or is markedly distressed by them.
C. Does not meet the criteria for gender identity disorder of adolescence or adulthood, nontranssexual type, or transsexualism.

Source. Reprinted with permission from American Psychiatric Association 1987.

collapsed across points A and B (see Table 42-1), with four or five characteristics required for a GIDC diagnosis. Table 42-5 shows the proposed changes in the DSM-III-R diagnostic criteria prepared by the DSM-IV Subcommittee on Gender Identity Disorders and Transsexualism, under the auspices of the working group on child and adolescent psychiatric disorders. These new criteria would probably lead to fewer false negative diagnoses.

Although the validity of the diagnosis of transsexualism is beyond dispute, the DSM-III-R criteria pose some practical problems, particularly the criterion regarding duration of the condition: "Persistent preoccupation for at least two years with getting rid of one's primary and secondary sex characteristics" (American Psychiatric Association 1987, p. 76). Because irreversible physical interventions in minors are risky (cf. Dulcan and Lee 1984), the practical dilemma for adolescents re-

Table 42-3.   DSM-III-R diagnostic criteria for gender identity disorder of adolescence or adulthood, nontranssexual type

A. Persistent or recurrent discomfort and sense of inappropriateness about one's assigned sex.
B. Persistent or recurrent cross-dressing in the role of the other sex, either in fantasy or actuality, but not for the purpose of sexual excitement (as in transvestic fetishism).
C. No persistent preoccupation (for at least two years) with getting rid of one's primary and secondary sex characteristics and acquiring the sex characteristics of the other sex (as in transsexualism).
D. The person has reached puberty.

Specify history of sexual orientation: **asexual, homosexual, heterosexual,** or **unspecified.**

Source. Reprinted with permission from American Psychiatric Association 1987.

volves around treatment (e.g., institution of hormonal therapies or surgical procedures). Moreover, there is disagreement among clinicians regarding the extent to which transsexualism can be truly consolidated in the adolescent years. Thus the 2-year criterion, which is obviously arbitrary although of some practical utility (see Money and Ambinder 1978), may be too short in some cases. On the other hand, clinical experience suggests that in some cases transsexualism can be quite consolidated by the age of 15 or 16 (see Newman 1970), but the appropriate treatment path for minors is mined by a host of often times complex legal and practical issues.

There have been no formal empirical studies examining the diagnosis of transvestic fetishism in adolescents. The diagnostic criteria for transvestic fetishism (see Table 42-4) are sufficiently "loose" to make their use with adolescents not particularly difficult. Clinically, one encounters adolescents who display a range of fetishistic cross-dressing (e.g., wearing women's underwear while masturbating versus complete cross-dressing accompanied by erotic arousal). Conceptually, one should be interested in whether such behavior represents a preference (cf. Freund 1974). With adolescents, this is not always clear, since many youngsters display considerable heterosexual arousal and interaction without the use of feminine apparel. The DSM-III-R criteria for transvestic fetishism do not, however, address the issue of erotic preference.

Clinical Findings

Phenomenology

Because the majority of empirical research has focused on children with GIDC, the clinical findings

Table 42-5. DSM-IV draft diagnostic criteria for gender identity disorder (children)

A. A profound and persistent cross-gender identification manifested in children by at least four of the following:
  1. Repeatedly stated desire to be, or insistence that he or she is, the opposite sex
  2. In girls, insistence on wearing stereotypical masculine clothing; in boys, preference for cross-dressing or simulating female attire
  3. Strong preference for cross-sex roles in fantasy play or persistent fantasies of being the opposite sex
  4. Intense desire to participate in the games and pastimes of the opposite sex
  5. Strong preference for playmates of the opposite sex
  In adolescents and adults, by symptoms such as a stated desire to be the opposite sex, frequent passing as the opposite sex, desire to live as or be treated as the opposite sex or the sense that one has the typical feelings and reactions of the opposite sex
B. Persistent discomfort with one's assigned sex or sense of inappropriateness in that gender role manifested in children by any of the following:

  In boys, assertion that his penis or testes are disgusting or will disappear, or assertion that it would be better not to have a penis, or aversion towards rough-and-tumble play and rejection of male stereotypical toys, games, and activities.

  In girls, rejection of urinating in a sitting position or an assertion that she does not want to grow breasts or menstruate, assertion that she has or will grow a penis, or persistent marked aversion toward normative feminine clothing.

  In adolescents and adults, by symptoms such as preoccupation with getting rid of one's primary and secondary sex characteristics (e.g., request for hormones, surgery, or other procedures to physically alter sexual characteristics to simulate the opposite sex) or statements that one was born into the wrong sex.

For sexually mature individuals, specify history of sexual attraction: toward males, females, both, neither, unspecified.

---

reported in this section focus primarily on this diagnosis. Children with GIDC present with a rather coherent set of behavioral signs. In a boy, this would include the following: making verbal statements that he is, or would like to be, a girl; cross-dressing in girls' or women's clothing; having a preference for culturally stereotypic feminine toys and activities; emulating females in fantasy play; having a preference for girls as playmates; displaying feminine or effeminate motoric movements; having a high-pitched or effeminate voice; expressing dislike of his sexual anatomy (e.g., concealing his penis; sitting to urinate to embellish the fantasy of having female genitalia); and being averse to rough-and-tumble play and group sports. In a girl, the inverse is observed. Of particular note is the intense aversion to culturally stereotypic girls' clothing and the desire to have her hairstyle look like that of a boy, such that a naive observer would perceive her as a male. Taken together, these characteristics point to the child's very strong cross-gender identification, and several research studies have established their discriminant validity, or relative uniqueness (Green 1987; Zucker 1985, 1991).

The study of the child's actual sense of gender identity has been somewhat more complicated. Most children with GIDC "know" that they are male or

female; that is, if they are asked the question "Are you a boy or a girl?" they answer correctly (Zucker et al. 1988). Some of these youngsters, however, do not seem to know the answer or else are "confused" about their gender status (i.e., whether they are male or female). In part, this may be a developmental phenomenon, but it also may be a sign of the severity of the overall condition (cf. Stoller 1968b). The child's internal representation of gender has been harder to study, although clinical experience suggests that the stability of the gender sense can be quite labile in some children. Zucker (unpublished data) has been working on a semistructured interview schedule designed to assess the degree of gender identity conflict and dysphoria in individual children. The following vignette is with a nearly 7-year-old girl (IQ = 123) who, by parent report, meets the DSM-III-R criteria for GIDC:

Interviewer (I): Are you a girl or a boy?
Child (C): For real life or pretend?
I: Real.
C: Girl.
I: Are you a boy?
C: Yeah, pretend.
I: When you grow up, will you be a Daddy or a Mommy?

C: If I get a sex change, a Daddy.
I: Could you ever grow up to be a Mommy?
C: If I don't get a sex change.
I: Are there any good things about being a girl?
C: No.
I: Are there any things that you don't like about being a girl?
C: . . . wearing dresses, playing with girls' stuff, playing with girls . . .
I: Do you think it is better to be a girl or a boy?
C: Boy.
I: Can you tell me why?
C: Get to do different things and I prefer these . . . wear different things, imagine a boy wearing a dress and wearing pink, that's "grossitating." I break all my pink crayons.
I: In your mind, do you ever think that you would like to be a boy?
C: Yes.
I: Can you tell me why?
C: More fun . . .
I: In your mind, do you ever get mixed up and you're not really sure if you are a girl or a boy?
C: No.
I: Do you ever feel more like a boy than like a girl?
C: Yes.
I: Tell me more about that.
C: I play with lots of boys . . .
I: . . . In your dreams, are you a girl, a boy, or sometimes a girl and sometimes a boy?
C: Boy.
I: Tell me about the dreams . . .
C: Robbers stealing jewelry for our wives . . .
I: Do you ever think that you really are a boy?
C: Yes.
I: Tell me more about that.
C: Just get to point "na-ha," I can't make up my mind.

Age of Onset

Green (1976) reported that the age of onset of cross-gender behaviors is typically during the preschool years. In his sample of boys, for example, 55% were cross-dressing by their third birthday, 80% were cross-dressing by their fourth birthday, and 90% were cross-dressing by their fifth birthday. Many experienced clinicians have observed repetitive, intense cross-gender behaviors to appear even before a child's second birthday. Clinical data on girls (Zucker 1989) reveal a similar age of onset. It is important to note that among more typical children a display of various gender role behaviors also can be observed during this period in the life cycle. This similarity suggests that the underlying mechanisms for both patterns may be the same, albeit mirror images.

Associated Psychopathology

In DSM-III-R, it is stated that "some of these children, particularly girls, show no other signs of psychopathology. Others may display serious signs of disturbance, such as social withdrawal, separation anxiety, or depression" (p. 72). What are the data regarding the presence of other types of psychopathology in children with GIDC? If other forms of psychopathology are present, how is the association with GIDC to be understood?

Unfortunately, omnibus-structured interview schedules that cover the gamut of childhood psychopathology have not been conducted on this clinical population. Several smaller-scale empirical studies, almost exclusively with boys with GIDC, have, however, reported on the presence of general psychopathology (Bates et al. 1973, 1979; Coates and Person 1985; Lowry and Zucker 1990; Rekers and Morey 1989; Tuber and Coates 1989; Zucker 1985, 1990a). These studies suggest that boys with gender identity problems display levels of general psychopathology similar to those of matched psychiatric control children and greater than those of normal control children. For example, on the Child Behavior Checklist (Achenbach and Edelbrock 1981), a parent-report instrument of behavior problems, boys with GIDC have been shown to display behavior problems at a level comparable to that of the clinic-referred standardization sample (Coates and Person 1985; Zucker 1990a). On this particular instrument, "internalizing" problems were somewhat more common than "externalizing" problems (Zucker 1990a), which is consistent with clinical observations that many of these boys experience anxiety, depression, and social withdrawal. More generally, it should be noted that the overall functioning of children with GIDC varies considerably. Some of these youngsters show major personality dysfunction and often require intensive intervention for these problems in their own right. On the other hand, some youngsters show minimal behavioral psychopathology and function quite well in the different environments of daily life.

Biophysical Markers

By observation, it is apparent that the vast majority of children with GIDC do not suffer from biological abnormalities in sexual differentiation, such as the different intersex conditions, that might, on theoretical grounds, explain the condition. Because sex hormone levels are so low during childhood (Si-zonenko 1978), it is unlikely that a standard endocrine assessment would detect abnormalities. Green (1976) and Rekers et al. (1979) reported normal XY karyotypes. Green also found that the feminine boys he studied did not differ in height and weight from control boys (Roberts et al. 1987), although they were hospitalized more often before their participation in the study.

Differential Diagnosis

Diagnostic Issues in Children

There are several diagnostic issues that require consideration in relation to GIDC. In boys, there is a type of cross-dressing that appears to be quite different from the type of cross-dressing that is part of the clinical picture in GIDC. In the latter, cross-dressing encompasses a range of behaviors, including the wearing of dresses, women's shoes, and jewelry, all of which enhance the fantasy or desire to be like the opposite sex. In the former, cross-dressing is limited to the use of undergarments such as panties and nylons. As with boys with GIDC, the cross-dressing has a compulsive and self-soothing flavor to it. However, it is not accompanied by other signs of cross-gender identification; in fact, apart from the cross-dressing, these boys are conventionally masculine. Many male adolescents and adults who carry the diagnosis of transvestic fetishism recall such cross-dressing during childhood; however, there have been no prospective studies of prepubertal boys engaging in this form of cross-dressing to see what proportion, if any, develop transvestic fetishism.

When all of the clinical signs of GIDC are present, there is little difficulty in making the diagnosis. If one accepts the idea of a spectrum of cross-gender identification, then there is more room for ambiguity, and one must be prepared to identify what Meyer-Bahlburg (1985) referred to as the "zone of transition between clinically significant cross-gender behavior and mere statistical deviation from the gender norm" (p. 682).

Friedman (1988), for example, suggested that there is a subgroup of boys who are "unmasculine," but not feminine. Based on clinical experience, Friedman argued that these boys suffer from a "persistent, profound feeling of masculine inadequacy which leads to a negative valuing of the self" (p. 199). Although not described in the formal clinical literature, there is probably a subgroup of girls as well who are "unfeminine," but not masculine, and who may suffer from similar feelings. Although these youngsters would not meet DSM-III-R criteria for GIDC, the residual diagnosis of gender identity disorder not otherwise specified could be employed in such cases.

For girls, the main differential diagnostic issue concerns the distinction between GIDC and what is known in popular culture as "tomboyism." According to *Webster's* (1990), a tomboy is "a girl of boyish behavior." Green et al. (1982) studied a community sample of "tomboys" and found that, compared with a control group of "non-tomboys," they displayed a greater number of masculine traits, such as a preference for boys as playmates, interest in rough-and-tumble play, and play with guns and trucks. In many respects, the cross-gender behavior of such tomboys is similar to the masculine gender role preferences of girls referred clinically for gender identity concerns (Zucker 1989). Based on critiques of the DSM-III criteria for GIDC in girls (e.g., Zucker 1982), the DSM-III-R criteria for GIDC in girls were modified in the hope of better differentiating these two groups of girls. Clinical experience suggests that at least three characteristics are useful in making a differential diagnosis. First, girls with GIDC express a profound unhappiness with their female gender status; in contrast, Green (1980) noted that the girls in his sample of tomboys were "generally *content being female*" (p. 262, emphasis in original). Second, girls with GIDC display a marked aversion to culturally defined feminine clothing and will do their utmost to avoid having to wear it. Their refusal to wear "girl's clothes" under any circumstance often precipitates clinical referral. Although tomboys prefer functional and casual clothing (Green et al. 1982), they do not display the same type of rigid rejection of feminine clothing. Third, girls with GIDC, unlike tomboys, often verbalize or act out their discomfort with their sexual anatomy.

Diagnostic Issues in Adolescence

There are at least four types of psychosexual problems that the clinician will encounter among adolescents (Bradley and Zucker 1990). Clinical experience suggests that persistent cross-gender identification throughout childhood is a risk factor for transsexualism. As noted earlier, DSM-III-R specifies a 2-year period in which there is a "persistent preoccupation" with ridding oneself of the primary and secondary sex characteristics. It is important to evaluate the fixedness of the desire to change sex, since therapeutic decisions will be influenced by the adolescent's openness to consider alternatives to sex reassignment (Newman 1970). From a differential diagnostic standpoint, the diagnosis of gender identity disorder of adolescence or adulthood, nontranssexual type can be used for individuals whose desire to change sex does not quite fit the criteria for transsexualism. Whether gender identity disorder of adolescence or adulthood, nontranssexual type is actually a distinct clinical syndrome is, however, far from clear.

The second psychosexual problem that can be observed in adolescents involves individuals who have a history of GIDC or a subclinical variant. These adolescents show various signs of cross-gender identification, yet do not voice a desire to change sex. They are circumspect about their sexual orientation, so it is not possible to classify them as homosexuals. These youngsters often are referred because of continued social ostracism. Many of these adolescents are able to acknowledge distress about not fitting in because of their cross-gender behavior. In these cases, the residual diagnosis of gender identity disorder not otherwise specified could be used to indicate that the adolescent continues to struggle with gender identity concerns.

A third type of psychosexual problem involves adolescents who have been referred because of homosexual behavior or orientation. Many of these adolescents have a history of GIDC or a variation of it, perhaps akin to the unmasculinity described by Friedman (1988; see also Friedman and Stern 1980). Although the reason for referral varies, it is important to rule out continuing concerns about gender identity. For adolescents distressed about their sexual orientation, the diagnosis of sexual disorder not otherwise specified can be given.

The last type of psychosexual problem is, as far as we know, the exclusive province of adolescent males. It concerns cross-dressing associated with sexual arousal. As noted earlier, the extent of the cross-dressing varies, and there is no problem, in principle, in employing the diagnosis of transvestic fetishism. As noted with adult transvestites, a heterosexual orientation predominates. A history of GIDC is not part of the clinical picture, although some of these boys think about sex-reassignment surgery and are at risk for transsexualism. Because the clinical course of heterosexual transsexualism

seems to develop more slowly than that of homosexual transsexualism (Blanchard et al. 1987), this may account for why it is relatively uncommon to encounter an adolescent transvestite who is also strongly gender dysphoric. It should be noted that the diagnosis of transsexualism is an exclusionary criterion for transvestic fetishism in DSM-III-R, but this seems to be clinically inaccurate since the two disorders may well co-occur (Blanchard and Clemmensen 1988).

Epidemiology

Prevalence

There have been no studies designed to assess specifically the prevalence of gender identity disorders in children. If one accepts the assumption that GIDC is associated with later transsexualism, then conservative estimates of prevalence might be inferred from epidemiologic data on this condition. According to one citation (Meyer-Bahlburg 1985), the number of adult transsexuals is small: 1 in 24,000–37,000 men and 1 in 103,000–150,000 women. This may be a mild underestimate, since the data are derived, in part, on the number of persons attending specialty clinics that evaluate adults for hormonal and surgical sex reassignment, and not all gender-dysphoric adults make themselves known. On the other hand, it should be recognized that GIDC is associated with homosexual transsexualism, but not heterosexual (or nonhomosexual) transsexualism (Blanchard et al. 1987). Since in men homosexual transsexualism accounts for only about half of the male patients seen (Blanchard et al. 1987), one has to consider this in drawing conclusions about the prevalence of GIDC.

The literature on the epidemiology of homosexuality might also help gauge the prevalence of GIDC. Unfortunately, the true prevalence of exclusive, or nearly exclusive, homosexuality remains a source of contention (Fay et al. 1989). According to Whitam and Mathy (1986), the better designed studies regarding prevalence suggest a rate of 2%–6%, at least for men. Another problem is that the retrospective literature on childhood cross-gender behavior in homosexual men and women often does not indicate how to classify cases as cross-gendered versus not cross-gendered. Moreover, cases classified as cross-gendered would not necessarily meet the complete diagnostic criteria for GIDC in DSM-

III-R. Despite these problems, it should be noted that all major retrospective studies show that homosexual adults recall substantially more childhood cross-gender behaviors than do heterosexual adults (e.g., Bell et al. 1981; Harry 1982; Saghir and Robins 1973; Whitam and Mathy 1986).

Liberal estimates of prevalence can be derived from studies on children in whom individual cross-gender behaviors have been assessed. For example, on the Child Behavior Checklist (Achenbach and Edelbrock 1981), the percentage of mothers of nonreferred boys aged 4–13 years (and grouped at 2-year intervals) who endorsed the item "behaves like opposite sex" ranged from 0.7% in boys aged 12–13 to 6.0% in boys aged 4–5. Among nonreferred girls, maternal endorsement of this item was higher, ranging from 9.6% to 12.9%. For the item "wishes to be of the opposite sex," the endorsement was lower for both sexes, ranging from 0% to 5.0% in specific sex by age groupings. These kinds of data no doubt overestimate "caseness," although this method of data collection might be a reasonable screening device for more intensive evaluation (cf. Pleak et al. 1989).

Incidence

There are no adequate epidemiologic data that can address the question of whether there has been a change in the incidence of GIDC over the years.

Referral Rates

Prevalence and incidence issues aside, there has been a consistent observation that boys are more often referred than girls for gender identity concerns. The most systematic data on this point come from the first author's (K.J.Z.) clinic in Toronto, Canada, with a referral ratio of about 6:1 of boys to girls.

There are at least two explanations for this strong sex difference in referral rates. First, it may well be that boys are more vulnerable to gender identity disorder than are girls, much as they are to a variety of other child psychiatric conditions (Eme 1979). Second, cultural factors appear more related to differential tolerance of cross-gender behavior in boys than in girls. In childhood, cross-gender behavior in girls is subject to less negative sanctions than it is in boys by both peers and parents (Fagot 1985; Green 1976; Green et al. 1982; Langlois and Downs

1980; Zucker et al. 1985). Moreover, adults are more likely to link cross-gender behavior in boys to atypical outcomes, such as homosexuality, than they are in girls (Antill 1987; Martin 1990). Zucker (1989) provided some data to suggest that girls with GIDC need to display more extreme behaviors than boys to elicit a referral. Thus it is possible that cases of girls with GIDC are under-referred because of the greater acceptance of girlhood masculinity.

Etiology

Biological Mechanisms

The search for biological determinants of human psychosexual development—gender identity, gender role, and sexual orientation—is still in a rudimentary state, despite a great deal of effort on the part of many researchers. There is disagreement on several issues. Do biological factors exert fixed versus predisposing influences on the components of psychosexual development? Can animal models be useful in understanding human phenomena? Are there unwanted "political" implications of advancing a biological explanation for human psychosexual development? These questions and others have been subject to intense debate within the field over the years.

At present, researchers have failed to identify a biological anomaly or variant associated specifically with GIDC. There is evidence, however, that certain behavioral traits linked to biological processes may characterize children with GIDC. The relation of GIDC to biological variables relies on data from "allied" populations, from which generalizations might be made.

Prenatal sex hormones. Although circulating sex hormones probably have little causal effect on gender identity, gender role, and sexual orientation, considerable attention has been accorded to the influential role of the prenatal hormonal environment and its effect on psychosexual differentiation. Experimental studies—from mice to monkeys—have shown quite clearly how manipulation of the prenatal hormonal milieu can affect postnatal sex-dimorphic behavior.

Is there evidence that prenatal hormonal variations in humans, due to either endogenous anomalies or exogenous manipulation, exert effects that are consistent with those that have been observed in lower animals? Reviews of this complex literature (e.g., Ehrhardt and Meyer-Bahlburg 1981) suggest that there is enough consistency to pursue the lead.

Consider, for example, studies of girls and women with congenital adrenal hyperplasia, a particularly illuminating form of pseudohermaphroditism. This autosomal recessive disorder is associated with enzyme defects that result in abnormal adrenal steroid biosynthesis. Because of the high level of androgen production during fetal development, masculinization of the external genitalia is common. Based on data from lower animals and from theory, it has been presumed that some "masculinization" of the organ of behavior, the brain, may also have occurred.

As reviewed elsewhere (Berenbaum 1990; Dittmann 1989; Ehrhardt and Meyer-Bahlburg 1981), there is evidence that the gender role behavior of girls with congenital adrenal hyperplasia is more masculine and/or less feminine than that of unaffected control subjects. The impact of congenital adrenal hyperplasia on gender identity is less clear, although the percentage who express some ambivalence about being female or who have been reared as boys (in part because the condition was untreated) is probably higher than among girls in the general population. Recent adult follow-up studies of girls with congenital adrenal hyperplasia suggest that there are higher rates of bisexuality and homosexuality and lower rates of marriage and sociosexual experiences than would be expected otherwise (Dittmann et al. 1990; Money et al. 1984; Mulaikal et al. 1987).

Despite the rather obvious role of the hormonal anomaly in explaining the overall pattern, it is important to note that individual differences in "outcome" occur, and the determinants of such variation remain open to debate to date (see, e.g., Berenbaum 1990; Dittmann et al. 1990; Ehrhardt and Baker 1974). It is not clear, for instance, to what extent differences result from the severity of the disorder, from biomedical sequelae of the condition, or from social factors, such as how parental understanding of the condition might affect their socialization techniques vis-à-vis gender.

Can this body of data help explain the genesis of GIDC? As noted earlier, no identifiable hormonal anomaly seems to characterize children with this disorder. Perhaps, however, less pronounced variations in the prenatal hormonal milieu that do not affect genital differentiation, but do account,

in part, for intrasex differences in the expression of sex-dimorphic behavior, play a role. For example, an avoidance of rough-and-tumble play and a low activity level are part of the clinical picture in boys with GIDC. Both of these behaviors show a strong sex dimorphism (Eaton and Enns 1986) and are probably partly determined by biological factors. Such behavioral traits, coupled with the anxiety often observed clinically in such boys (Bradley 1985; Coates 1990), may set in motion a complex chain of psychosocial sequelae that predispose to cross-gender identification (see, e.g., Green 1987).

Physical appearance. In Stoller's (1968a, 1975) study of extremely feminine boys, he noted that their mothers commented on their physical beauty as infants, particularly the face. Although Stoller (1975) suggested that this may have been a bit of an exaggeration, he appears to have been impressed by these boys' physical appearance: "We have noticed that they often have pretty faces, with fine hair, lovely complexions, graceful movements, and—especially—big, piercing, liquid eyes" (p. 43). In Stoller's view, the boy's physical beauty fueled the mother's conscious and unconscious desires to feminize her son.

Green (1987; Green et al. 1985; Roberts et al. 1987) systematically studied physical attractiveness in a large sample of feminine and control boys. Blind ratings of audiotaped interviews showed that the parents of the feminine boys were more likely than the parents of the control boys to describe their sons during infancy as "beautiful" and "feminine." Interestingly, Green (1987) found that degree of recalled beauty correlated with ratings of maternal encouragement of feminine behavior. Green's data suggest that these boys may well have objective physical properties that distinguish them from control subjects. On the other hand, it is easy to see how "retrospective distortion" can be implicated in explaining these data.

More recently, Zucker et al. (in press) reported physical attractiveness data on a group of boys with GIDC and clinical control boys. Colored photographs of both groups of boys were taken at the time of assessment (mean age, 8.1 years). College students then made ratings of these pictures for five adjectives: attractive, beautiful, cute, handsome, and pretty. The raters were blind to group status, being informed only that they would be viewing pictures of boys. The boys with GIDC were rated as significantly more attractive than the clinical control boys on all five traits. Thus these data nicely complement and extend the previous findings of Stoller (1968a) and Green (1987). Nevertheless, interpretation of the data remains complex. On the one hand, these data may reflect objective, biophysical differences in the appearance of feminine versus control boys. On the other hand, they may reflect the effects of social shaping of physical appearance. In other words, physical appearance may be a predisposing factor in the development of GIDC or it may serve to perpetuate the disorder, as a result of social shaping.

Psychosocial Mechanisms

Several psychosocial factors have been thought to play a role in either the genesis or the perpetuation of GIDC. Most of these factors have been better studied in boys than in girls, and some of them have been held to be sex specific. A few of the more prominent hypotheses are discussed here.

Social reinforcement. Do parents shape or influence sex-dimorphic behavior in their children? As it turns out, this very simple question has proven to be exceedingly difficult to answer. If one turns to the normative literature, it becomes apparent how complicated the matter actually is (see, e.g., Fagot 1985; Fagot and Leinbach 1989; Lytton and Romney 1991). Perhaps a general conclusion is that parents do play a role in influencing patterns of sex-dimorphic behavior, but not in the simplistic way that social learning theorists, from their academic armchairs, so readily expected the situation to be.

When one asks the parents of children with GIDC to recall their initial responses to cross-gender behaviors, such as cross-dressing and cross-sex toy play, there is reasonable evidence to suggest that tolerance, or nonresponsiveness, was very common (Green 1987). Actual encouragement of these behaviors appears to be more common than negative or discouraging reactions.

Initial parental tolerance or encouragement of cross-gender behavior may therefore be of some etiologic significance. The reasons for such tolerance appear to be quite variable, including parental values and goals regarding psychosexual development; feedback from a professional that the behavior is within normal limits and "only a phase"; parental conflicts around issues of masculinity and

femininity; and parental psychopathology and discord, which leave the parents relatively preoccupied and thus unresponsive to their child's behavior.

Mother-child and father-child relationships. In Stoller's (1968a, 1975, 1979) clinical studies, he described an overly close relationship between mother and son and a distant, peripheral father-son relationship. Stoller (1985) has held that such qualities are of etiologic relevance: "The more mother and the less father, the more femininity" (p. 25). Stoller (1985) argued that GIDC in boys is a "developmental arrest . . . in which an excessively close and gratifying mother-infant symbiosis, undisturbed by father's presence, prevents a boy from adequately separating himself from his mother's female body and feminine behavior" (p. 25).

Green (1987) assessed the amount of shared time between parents of feminine boys and parents of control subjects during the first 5 years of life. The fathers of feminine boys reported spending less time with their sons from the second to fifth year than did the fathers of controls. In contradiction to the overcloseness hypothesis, the mothers of feminine boys also reported spending less time with their sons than did the mothers of controls.

The data on father-son shared time are quite consistent with a large body of clinical literature, whereas the mother-son data are not. Negative findings are difficult to interpret, particularly when they have not been consistently replicated. In this instance, they are difficult to reconcile with data showing that feminine boys feel closer to their mothers than to their fathers (Green 1987). Perhaps qualitative features of the mother-son relationship, such as attunement to each other's feelings, would have been a more sensitive index of the dyad's nature. It is also possible that relative time spent with mother versus father would have yielded differences between Green's feminine boys and control boys.

As of yet, systematic studies on parent-child relationships have not been conducted for girls with GIDC. Preliminary clinical observations (Bradley 1980; Green 1974; Stoller 1975; Zucker 1989) suggest that the mother-daughter relationship is often conflictual and not close, leading to what might be described as a "disidentification" from the mother (cf. Greenson 1968). In some instances, there is a devaluing of femininity and an overvaluing of masculinity, which seem to be encouraged by the parents. Many of these girls tend to admire what their fathers do. In other cases, they appear to be quite frightened of their fathers and seem to develop the belief that they need to be quite strong and powerful to be safe. These preliminary clinical studies suggest that there may well be marked differences in the qualitative aspects of the parent-child relationship in gender-disturbed boy and girls.

Maternal psychosexual development. Based on clinical data, Stoller (1968a) reported that mothers of very feminine boys had childhood psychosexual conflicts. Although initially feminine, he argued that "a degree of masculinity beyond what usually [would] be called tomboyishness" (p. 298) developed following a breach in the father-daughter relationship. A desire to be a male was relinquished at puberty, yet sociosexual experience was minimal, and, as adults, these women married distant men with whom sexual relations were poor. These women appeared to be uncomfortable with their femininity: "While these women have a feminine quality, inextricably woven in is this other, difficult to describe but easy to observe use of certain boyish or 'neuter' external features" (p. 298).

Green's (1987) effort to verify Stoller's (1968a) observations yielded mixed results. Mothers of feminine boys were more likely than the mothers of the control boys to describe themselves as tomboys (Green et al. 1985), but they did not differ with regard to their recall of specific sex-typed behaviors (Green 1987). The two groups of mothers also did not differ with regard to the extent of adolescent sociosexual experience. Finally, Green's (1987) trait assessment of childhood masculinity-femininity did not provide strong support for the possibility that less severe signs of cross-gender behavior were present. From these data, it would appear that mothers of very feminine boys, on average, do not have grossly atypical psychosexual histories. Perhaps other aspects of psychosexuality need to be studied, such as the mother's current attitude toward men and her concurrent views regarding masculinity and femininity.

General psychopathology. Little systematic study has been given to the presence of general dysfunction, such as psychiatric disorder and marital discord, in the parents of children with GIDC. The evidence is certainly suggestive that these parents display pathologic traits greater than would be expected in the general population (Marantz and Coates 1991; Wolfe 1990). Assuming these preliminary data hold up, there are two main questions to pursue. First, will there be any specificity to the parental difficulties or will they simply be typical of what is observed in the parents of other children with psychiatric difficulties? Second, how, if at all, do these difficulties play a direct role in the development of the child's gender identity disorder? A rather simple hypothesis might be that the degree of parental dysfunction and marital discord is associated with tolerance of cross-gender behavior, perhaps because the parents are not functioning optimally and thus are less sensitive about developments in the child. If large enough samples could be generated, causal-modeling techniques could be used to test different hypothesized pathways leading to the development of gender identity disorder in the child.

Treatment

The treatment of children with GIDC has utilized behavior therapy, psychodynamic psychotherapy, family therapy, and eclectic combinations of these approaches. Detailed reviews of the treatment literature can be found elsewhere (Zucker 1985, 1990b; Zucker and Green 1989).

It goes without saying that the theoretical lens through which one views psychopathology influences how treatment issues will be conceptualized. For example, proponents of behavior therapy (e.g., Rekers 1977) have focused largely on the development of techniques to modify specific sex-typed behaviors such as cross-dressing and exclusive play with opposite-sex toys, whereas psychodynamically oriented clinicians view gender identity disorder in the context of family pathology and associated personality psychopathology in the child (Coates and Person 1985; Meyer and Dupkin 1985) and place as much emphasis on treating these problems as the gender identity symptomatology itself. Thus what (or whom) should be treated is determined by how the clinician attempts to understand the psychopathology.

Unfortunately, the empirical basis of treatment efficacy for children with GIDC is weak, much like the treatment efficacy for many types of childhood psychopathologies (Kazdin 1990). Comparative studies of different types of treatment approaches are simply not available; thus any claim of superiority, particularly with regard to long-term effects, is unwarranted (cf. Meyer and Sohmer 1983; Rekers 1986). Again, it should be noted that this is a problem that cuts across many areas of childhood psychopathology (Shaffer 1984). These caveats aside, several of the more salient treatment approaches will be discussed.

Behavior Therapy

Rekers (1977, 1985) and his colleagues have provided the most systematic information regarding behavioral approaches. Using different types of behavioral techniques, such as differential social attention or reinforcement, the token economy, and self-regulation, there is evidence that specific sex-typed behaviors can be either reduced or increased in their frequency. The techniques have been subject to two main limitations: stimulus specificity and response specificity. The first term refers to the phenomenon of a behavior reappearing (e.g., cross-dressing) in the absence of the stimulus condition under which it was modified (e.g., parental negative sanctions, new environment). The second term means that the treatment does not generalize or influence untreated behaviors, although they appear to be of the same type as the treated behavior. Thus a procedure might modify cross-dressing, but not generalize to play with dolls, if that behavior was not specifically subject to formal treatment techniques.

Despite these limitations, an overall analysis of the behavior therapy case report literature suggests some impact on the presenting problem and apparently an impact on the child's overall sense of gender identity (Zucker 1985). There are, however, no published long-term follow-ups of children treated by behavior therapy techniques. Green (1987) reported that two boys who were treated by Rekers followed-up in his own prospective study were bisexual. Thus Rekers' (1986) recent claim—that from "the result of my research studies, it now appears that a preventive treatment for transvestism, transsexualism, and some forms of homosexuality has indeed been isolated" (p. 28)—has not yet been demonstrated with empirical data.

Psychotherapy

The psychotherapy literature consists of a couple dozen case reports (see Zucker 1985, 1990b). Unlike the use of quantitative data in the behavior therapy case report literature, the psychotherapy literature is much more descriptive and qualitative in nature. Comparative trials of psychotherapy versus other forms of treatment, or even no treatment, have not

been carried out. Although difficult to quantify, the impression one gets from studying this literature is that many of the children had made gains by the end of their therapy. Because many of the parents of these children were in therapy and because in some instances the child received additional, concurrent treatments (e.g., as an inpatient), the precise mechanisms of change are often difficult to disentangle.

Elsewhere we have identified discernible themes in the psychotherapy case report literature (Zucker 1985, 1990b; Zucker and Green 1989). These include an emphasis on the significance of the emergence of cross-gender behavior during the preoedipal years, with concomitant attention to early object relations and general ego functioning. Attention is given to understanding the impact of the mother-child and father-child relationships on the formation of the gender symptomatology and the parental psychodynamics that putatively underlie the parents' tolerance for the cross-gender behavior. Some authors conceptualize the gender behavior as representing symptoms of underlying pathologic phenomena in the child. In a sense, then, this literature takes a more contextual approach in understanding the gender identity disorder than does the behavior therapy literature.

Prognosis

Green (1987) provided the most detailed information regarding long-term follow-up of boys with GIDC. Green originally assessed 66 extremely feminine boys and 56 control boys at a mean age of 7.1 years (range, 4–12). About two-thirds of the boys in each of these groups were reevaluated at a follow-up mean age of 18.9 years (range, 14–24). Sexual orientation in fantasy and behavior was assessed by means of a semistructured interview schedule. Using Kinsey scale criteria, all 35 control boys were heterosexual in fantasy at follow-up. Of the 25 control boys who had experienced sexual relations, one was classified as bisexual, and the remainder were classified as heterosexual. In contrast, of the 44 feminine boys, 33 (75%) were classified as either bisexual or homosexual; of the 30 feminine boys who had experienced sexual relations, 24 (80%) were classified as either bisexual or homosexual. Only one of the feminine boys, who was sexually attracted to males, was seriously entertaining the notion of sex reassignment surgery. Thus homosexuality rather than (homosexual) transsexualism appears to be the most common long-term outcome associated with GIDC.

Why was transsexualism not a common outcome in Green's (1987) study? There are two main explanations. First, as noted by Weinrich (1985), the low base rate of transsexualism would require large sample sizes, even within the population of gender-disturbed children. Second, it is possible that the assessment process and, when it occurs, treatment alter the natural history of gender identity disorder. Clinical experience and observation suggest that it is only those children who have not moved away from extreme cross-gender identification that remain at risk for transsexualism (McCauley and Ehrhardt 1984). Zucker et al. (1986) found that the persistence of gender dysphoria, including the wish for sex reassignment, was considerably higher among patients first assessed in adolescence and followed up later compared with patients who were first assessed in childhood and followed up in adolescence (Zucker and Bradley 1989). It may be then that developments at or near the transition from childhood to adolescence may be important in differentiating a transsexual outcome from other outcomes.

Research Issues

The phenomenology of GIDC has now been well described. There are excellent assessment tools now available for diagnostic workups (see Green 1987; Zucker 1991). Perhaps what needs to be better understood is the concept of "gender dysphoria" as it applies to young children, since it is in fact this feeling state that is the sine qua non of the parent disorder, transsexualism.

The psychobiology of gender identity, gender role, and sexual orientation remains an area of intense study. So far, it appears that gross biological abnormalities will not prove to be of importance (see, e.g., Gladue 1988; Gooren 1988, 1990; Meyer-Bahlburg 1984). The exact effects of prenatal sex hormones on postnatal sex-dimorphic behavior continue to be an area of great interest; however, other areas of biological sex research also may yield new insights. Recent studies regarding genetic (Buhrich et al. 1991; Eckert et al. 1986; Mitchell et al. 1989), familial (Bailey et al. 1991; Blanchard and Sheridan, in press; Pillard and Weinrich 1986), and neuropsychological (e.g., Gladue et al. 1990; McCormick et al. 1990; Sanders and Ross-Field 1987) correlates of psychosexual be-

havior may provide other ways of studying the role of biological phenomena.

Psychosocial research also has yielded important leads. It is now clear how complex early social interaction is vis-à-vis gender (e.g., Fagot and Leinbach 1989). Microsocial observations of the behavior of children with gender identity disorder may help to clarify the complexities in early interactions with significant others. There also needs to be greater attention to the assessment of general psychopathology, both in the child and in the parents. Elucidating how general psychopathology serves as a risk factor for this disorder will be of great importance. Finally, the interconnection between gender identity disorder and later sexual orientation suggests that a better understanding of the development of eroticism is required in its own right (Zucker 1990a). To date, the processes underlying erotic development have not been well described. Hopefully, advances on all of these fronts will sharpen our understanding of psychosexual development in the years to come.

References

Achenbach TM, Edelbrock CS: Behavioral problems and competencies reported by parents of normal and disturbed children aged four through sixteen. Monogr Soc Res Child Dev 46 (1, Serial No 188), 1981

American Psychiatric Association: Diagnostic and Statistical Manual of Mental Disorders, 3rd Edition. Washington, DC, American Psychiatric Association, 1980

American Psychiatric Association: Diagnostic and Statistical Manual of Mental Disorders, 3rd Edition, Revised. Washington, DC, American Psychiatric Association, 1987

Antill JK: Parents' beliefs and values about sex roles, sex differences, and sexuality: their sources and implications, in Sex and Gender. Edited by Shaver P, Hendrick C. Newbury Park, CA, Sage, 1987, pp 294–328

Bailey JM, Willerman L, Parks C: A test of the maternal stress theory of human male homosexuality. Arch Sex Behav 20:277–293, 1991

Bates JE, Bentler PM, Thompson SK: Measurement of gender deviant development in boys. Child Dev 44:591–598, 1973

Bates JE, Bentler PM, Thompson SK: Gender-deviant boys compared with normal and clinical control boys. J Abnorm Child Psychol 7:243–259, 1979

Bell AP, Weinberg MS, Hammersmith SK: Sexual Preference: Its Development in Men and Women. Bloomington, IN, Indiana University Press, 1981

Berenbaum SA: Congenital adrenal hyperplasia: intellectual and psychosexual functioning, in Psychoneuroendocrinology: Brain, Behavior, and Hormonal Interactions. Edited by Holmes CS. New York, Springer-Verlag, 1990, pp 227–260

Blanchard R, Clemmensen LH: A test of the DSM-III-R's implicit assumption that fetishistic arousal and gender dysphoria are mutually exclusive. Journal of Sex Research 25:426–432, 1988

Blanchard R, Sheridan PM: Sibship size, sibling sex ratio, birth order, and parental age in homosexual and nonhomosexual gender dysphorics. J Nerv Ment Dis (in press)

Blanchard R, Clemmensen LH, Steiner BW: Heterosexual and homosexual gender dysphoria. Arch Sex Behav 16:139–152, 1987

Bradley SJ: Female transsexualism: a child and adolescent perspective. Child Psychiatry Hum Dev 11:12–18, 1980

Bradley SJ: Gender dysphorias in childhood: a formulation, in Gender Dysphoria: Development, Research, Management. Edited by Steiner BW. New York, Plenum, 1985, pp 175–198

Bradley SJ, Zucker KJ: Gender identity disorder and psychosexual problems in children and adolescents. Can J Psychiatry 35:477–486, 1990

Buhrich N, Bailey JM, Martin NG: Sexual orientation, sexual identity and sex-dimorphic behaviors in male twins. Behav Genet 21:75–96, 1991

Coates S: Ontogenesis of boyhood gender identity disorder. J Am Acad Psychoanal 18:414–438, 1990

Coates S, Person ES: Extreme boyhood femininity: isolated behavior or pervasive disorder? Journal of the American Academy of Child Psychiatry 24:702–709, 1985

DiPietro JA: Rough-and-tumble play: a function of gender. Dev Psychol 17:50–58, 1981

Dittmann RW: Pranatal Wirksame Hormone und Verhaltensmerkmale von Patientinnen mit den Beiden Klassichen Varianten des 21-Hydroxylase-Defektes. New York, Peter Lang, 1989

Dittmann RW, Kappes ME, Kappes MH: Sexual behavior in adolescent and adult females with congenital adrenal hyperplasia. Neuroendocrinology Letters 12:283, 1990

Dittmann RW, Kappes MH, Kappes ME, et al: Congenital adrenal hyperplasia, II: gender-related behavior and attitudes in female salt-wasting and simple-virilizing patients. Psychoneuroendocrinology 15:421–434, 1990

Dulcan MK, Lee PA: Transsexualism in the adolescent girl. Journal of the American Academy of Child Psychiatry 23:354–361, 1984

Eaton WO, Enns LR: Sex differences in human motor activity level. Psychol Bull 100:19–28, 1986

Eckert ED, Bouchard TJ, Bohlen J, et al: Homosexuality in monozygotic twins reared apart. Br J Psychiatry 148:421–426, 1986

Ehrhardt AA, Baker SW: Fetal androgens, human central nervous system differentiation, and behavior sex differences, in Sex Differences in Behavior. Edited by Friedman RC, Richart RM, Vande Wiele RL. New York, John Wiley, 1974, pp 33–51

Ehrhardt AA, Meyer-Bahlburg HFL: Effects of prenatal hormones on gender-related behavior. Science 211:1312–1318, 1981

Eme RF: Sex differences in childhood psychopathology: a review. Psychol Bull 86:574–595, 1979

Etaugh C, Grinnell K, Etaugh A: Development of gender labeling: effect of age of pictured children. Sex Roles 21:769–773, 1989

Fagot BI: Consequences of moderate cross-gender behavior in preschool children. Child Dev 48:902–907, 1977

Fagot BI: Beyond the reinforcement principle: another step toward understanding sex-role development. Developmental Psychology 21:1097–1104, 1985

Fagot BI, Leinbach MD: The young child's gender schema: environmental input, internal organization. Child Dev 60:663–672, 1989

Fay RE, Turner CF, Klassen AD, et al: Prevalence and patterns of same-gender sexual contact among men. Science 243:338–348, 1989

Freund K: Male homosexuality: an analysis of the pattern, in Understanding Homosexuality: Its Biological and Psychological Bases. Edited by Loraine JA. Lancaster, UK, Medical and Technical Publishing, 1974, pp 25–81

Friedman RC: Male Homosexuality: A Contemporary Psychoanalytic Perspective. New Haven, CT, Yale University Press, 1988

Friedman RC, Stern LO: Juvenile aggressivity and sissiness in homosexual and heterosexual males. J Am Acad Psychoanal 8:427–440, 1980

Gladue BA: Hormones in relationship to homosexual/bisexual/heterosexual gender orientation, in Handbook of Sexology, Vol 6: The Pharmacology and Endocrinology of Sexual Function. Edited by Sitsen JMA. Amsterdam, Elsevier, 1988, pp 388–409

Gladue BA, Beatty WW, Larson J, et al: Sexual orientation and spatial ability in men and women. Psychobiology 18:101–108, 1990

Gooren LJG: An appraisal of endocrine theories of homosexuality and gender dysphoria, in Handbook of Sexology, Vol 6: The Pharmacology and Endocrinology of Sexual Function. Edited by Sitsen JMA. Amsterdam, Elsevier, 1988, pp 410–424

Gooren LJG: The endocrinology of transsexualism: a review and commentary. Psychoneuroendocrinology 15:3–14, 1990

Green R: Sexual Identity Conflict in Children and Adults. New York, Basic Books, 1974

Green R: One-hundred ten feminine and masculine boys: behavioral contrasts and demographic similarities. Arch Sex Behav 5:425–446, 1976

Green R: Patterns of sexual identity development in childhood: relationship to subsequent sexual partner preference, in Homosexual Behavior: A Modern Reappraisal. Edited by Marmor J. New York, Basic Books, 1980, pp 255–266

Green R: The "Sissy Boy Syndrome" and the Development of Homosexuality. New Haven, CT, Yale University Press, 1987

Green R, Williams K, Goodman M: Ninety-nine "tomboys" and "non-tomboys": behavioral contrasts and demographic similarities. Arch Sex Behav 11:247–266, 1982

Green R, Williams K, Goodman M: Masculine or feminine gender identity in boys: developmental differences between two diverse family groups. Sex Roles 12:1155–1162, 1985

Greenson RR: Dis-identifying from mother. Int J Psychoanal 49:370–374, 1968

Harry J: Gay Children Grown Up: Gender Culture and Gender Deviance. New York, Praeger, 1982

Huston AC: Sex-typing, in Handbook of Child Psychology, 4th Edition, Vol 4: Socialization, Personality, and Social Development. Edited by Hetherington EM. New York, John Wiley, 1983, pp 387–467

Kazdin AE: Psychotherapy for children and adolescents. Annu Rev Psychol 41:21–54, 1990

Langlois JH, Downs AC: Mothers, fathers, and peers as socialization agents of sex-typed play behaviors in young children. Child Dev 51:1237–1247, 1980

Leinbach MD, Fagot BI: Acquisition of gender labels: a test for toddlers. Sex Roles 15:655–666, 1986

Lowry CB, Zucker KJ: Is there an association between separation anxiety disorder and gender identity disorder in boys? Paper presented at the meeting of the International Academy of Sex Research, Sigtuna, Sweden, August 1990

Lytton H, Romney DM: Parents' differential socialization of boys and girls: a meta-analysis. Psychol Bull 109:267–296, 1991

Maccoby EE, Jacklin CN: The Psychology of Sex Differences. Stanford, CA, Stanford University Press, 1974

Maccoby EE, Jacklin CN: Sex differences in aggression: a rejoinder and reprise. Child Dev 51:964–980, 1980

Maccoby EE, Jacklin CN: Gender segregation in childhood. Advances in Child Development and Behavior 20:239–287, 1987

Marantz S, Coates S: Mothers of boys with gender identity disorder: a comparison of matched controls. J Am Acad Child Adolesc Psychiatry 30:310–315, 1991

Martin CL: Attitudes and expectations about children with nontraditional and traditional gender roles. Sex Roles (in press)

McCauley E, Ehrhardt AA: Follow-up of females with gender identity disorders. J Nerv Ment Dis 172:353–358, 1984

McCormick CM, Witelson SF, Kingstone E: Left-handedness in homosexual men and women: neuroendocrine implications. Psychoneuroendocrinology 15:69–76, 1990

Meyer JK, Dupkin C: Gender disturbance in children: an interim clinical report. Bull Menninger Clin 49:236–269, 1985

Meyer JK, Sohmer BH: Gender problems in children. Drug Therapy 13:43–56, 1983

Meyer-Bahlburg HFL: Psychoendocrine research on sexual orientation: current status and future options. Prog Brain Res 61:375–398, 1984

Meyer-Bahlburg HFL: Gender identity disorder of childhood: introduction. Journal of the American Academy of Child Psychiatry 24:681–683, 1985

Mitchell JE, Baker LA, Jacklin CN: Masculinity and femininity in twin children: genetic and environmental factors. Child Dev 60:1475–1485, 1989

Money J: Gender role, gender identity, core gender identity: usage and definition of terms. J Am Acad Psychoanal 1:397–403, 1973

Money J: The conceptual neutering of gender and the criminalization of sex. Arch Sex Behav 14:279–290, 1985

Money J: Gay, Straight, and In-Between: The Sexology of Erotic Orientation. New York, Oxford University Press, 1988

Money J, Ambinder R: Two-year, real-life diagnostic test: rehabilitation versus cure, in Controversy in Psychiatry. Edited by Brady JP, Brodie HKH. Philadelphia, PA, WB Saunders, 1978, pp 833–845

Money J, Hampson JG, Hampson JL: Imprinting and the establishment of gender role. Archives of Neurology and Psychiatry 77:333–336, 1957

Money J, Schwartz M, Lewis VG: Adult erotosexual status and fetal hormonal masculinization and demasculinization: 46,XX congenital virilizing adrenal hyperplasia and 46,XY androgen-insensitivity syndrome compared. Psychoneuroendocrinology 9:405–414, 1984

Mulaikal RM, Migeon CJ, Rock JA: Fertility rates in female patients with congenital adrenal hyperplasia due to 21-hydroxylase deficiency. N Engl J Med 316:178–182, 1987

Newman LE: Transsexualism in adolescence: problems in evaluation and treatment. Arch Gen Psychiatry 23:112–121, 1970

Paluszny M, Beit-Hallahmi B, Catford JC, et al: Gender identity and its measurement in children. Compr Psychiatry 14:281–290, 1973

Pillard RC, Weinrich JD: Evidence of familial nature of male homosexuality. Arch Gen Psychiatry 43:808–812, 1986

Pleak RR, Meyer-Bahlburg HFL, O'Brien JD, et al: Cross-gender behavior and psychopathology in boy psychiatric outpatients. J Am Acad Child Adolesc Psychiatry 28:385–393, 1989

Rekers GA: Assessment and treatment of childhood gender problems, in Advances in Clinical Child Psychology, Vol 1. Edited by Lahey BB, Kazdin AE. New York, Plenum, 1977, pp 267–306

Rekers GA: Gender identity problems, in Handbook of Clinical Behavior Therapy With Children. Edited by Bornstein PA, Kazdin AE. Homewood, IL, Dorsey, 1985, pp 658–699

Rekers GA: Inadequate sex role differentiation in childhood: the family and gender identity disorders. Journal of Family and Culture 2:8–37, 1986

Rekers GA, Morey SM: Personality problems associated with childhood gender disturbance. Italian Journal of Clinical and Cultural Psychology 1:85–90, 1989

Rekers GA, Crandall BF, Rosen AC, et al: Genetic and physical studies of male children with psychological gender disturbances. Psychol Med 9:373–375, 1979

Roberts CW, Green R, Williams K, et al: Boyhood gender identity development: a statistical contrast of two family groups. Developmental Psychology 23:544–557, 1987

Saghir MT, Robins E: Male and Female Homosexuality: A Comprehensive Investigation. Baltimore, MD, Williams & Wilkins, 1973

Sanders G, Ross-Field L: Neuropsychological development of cognitive abilities: a new research strategy and some preliminary evidence for a sexual orientation model. Int J Neurosci 36:1–16, 1987

Shaffer D: Notes on psychotherapy research among children and adolescents. Journal of the American Academy of Child Psychiatry 23:552–561, 1984

Sizonenko PC: Endocrinology in preadolescents and adolescents, I: hormonal changes during normal puberty. Am J Dis Child 132:704–712, 1978

Stoller RJ: Sex and Gender, Vol 1: The Development of Masculinity and Femininity. New York, Science House, 1968a

Stoller RJ: Male childhood transsexualism. Journal of the American Academy of Child Psychiatry 7:193–209, 1968b

Stoller RJ: Sex and Gender, Vol 2: The Transsexual Experiment. London, Hogarth Press, 1975

Stoller RJ: Fathers of transsexual children. J Am Psychoanal Assoc 27:837–866, 1979

Stoller RJ: Presentations of Gender. New Haven, CT, Yale University Press, 1985

Thompson SK: Gender labels and early sex role development. Child Dev 46:339–347, 1975

Tuber S, Coates S: Indices of psychopathology in the Rorschachs of boys with severe gender identity disorder: a comparison with normal control subjects. J Pers Assess 53:100–112, 1989

Webster's Ninth New Collegiate Dictionary. Springfield, MA, Merriam-Webster, 1990, p 1241

Weinrich JD: Transsexuals, homosexuals, and sissy boys: on the mathematics of follow-up studies. Journal of Sex Research 21:322–328, 1985

Whitam FL, Mathy RM: Male Homosexuality in Four Societies: Brazil, Guatemala, the Philippines, and the United States. New York, Praeger, 1986

Wolfe SM: Psychopathology and psychodynamics of parents of boys with a gender identity disorder of childhood. Unpublished doctoral dissertation, The City University of New York, 1990

Zucker KJ: Childhood gender disturbance: diagnostic issues.

Journal of the American Academy of Child Psychiatry 21:274–280, 1982

Zucker KJ: Cross-gender-identified children, in Gender Dysphoria: Development, Research, Management. Edited by Steiner BW. New York, Plenum, 1985, pp 75–174

Zucker KJ: Girls with the gender identity disorder of childhood. Paper presented at the meeting of the Society for Sex Therapy and Research, Tucson, AZ, 1989

Zucker KJ: Psychosocial and erotic development in cross-gender- identified children. Can J Psychiatry 35:487–496, 1990a

Zucker KJ: Treatment of gender identity disorders in children, in Clinical Management of Gender Identity Disorders in Children and Adults. Edited by Blanchard R, Steiner BW. Washington, DC, American Psychiatric Press, 1990b, pp 25–47

Zucker KJ: Gender identity disorder, in Child Psychopathology: Diagnostic Criteria and Clinical Assessment. Edited by Hooper SR, Hynd GW, Mattison RE. Hillsdale, NJ, Lawrence Erlbaum, 1991, pp 305–342

Zucker KJ, Bradley SJ: Gender identity and sexual orientation in cross-gender-identified children: a follow-up in adolescence. Paper presented at the meeting of the Society for Research in Child and Adolescent Psychopathology, Miami, FL, February 1989

Zucker KJ, Green R: Gender identity disorder of childhood, in Treatments of Psychiatric Disorders: A Task Force Report of the American Psychiatric Association, Vol 1. Washington, DC, American Psychiatric Association, 1989, pp 661–670

Zucker KJ, Finegan JK, Doering RW, et al: Two subgroups of gender-problem children. Arch Sex Behav 13:27–39, 1984

Zucker KJ, Wilson DN, Stern A: Children's appraisals of sex-typed behavior in their peers. Paper presented at the meeting of the Society for Research in Child Development, Toronto, 1985

Zucker KJ, Bradley SJ, Gladding JA: A follow-up study of transsexual, transvestitic, homosexual, and "undifferentiated" adolescents. Paper presented at the meeting of the International Academy of Sex Research, Amsterdam, September 1986

Zucker KJ, Kuksis M, Bradley SJ: Gender constancy judgments in cross-gender-identified children. Paper presented at the meeting of the International Academy of Sex Research, Minneapolis, MN, August 1988

Zucker KJ, Wild J, Bradley SJ, et al: Physical attractiveness in boys with gender identity disorder. Arch Sex Behav (in press)

Chapter 43

Adjustment and Reactive Disorders

Norbert B. Enzer, M.D.
Susan Delavan Cunningham, M.D.

Adjustment disorder has been a very frequently used diagnosis in child and adolescent psychiatry. A survey of 441,429 children and adolescents admitted to selected private psychiatric hospitals, public mental hospitals, general hospitals, and psychiatric clinics in 1975 showed that adjustment reaction was the most common diagnosis for those admitted to inpatient and outpatient services—30% and 45%, respectively (Sowder et al. 1975).

Despite the number of children and adolescents who have been diagnosed as having an adjustment disorder, there is relatively little research regarding these disorders, and the definition and criteria for diagnosis continue to be controversial. Treatment outcomes and prognosis are also unclear, although by definition these disorders are transient.

Definition

The definition of adjustment disorder has undergone modification with every change in the diagnostic scheme. Reactive disorder is a term suggested by the Group for the Advancement of Psychiatry (GAP) Committee on Child Psychiatry in 1966. It describes a condition similar to the condition described as adjustment disorder in DSM-II (American Psychiatric Association 1968), but it emphasizes different aspects of the disorder (i.e., the state of the child rather than the stressor or the reaction itself). All the DSM definitions and the GAP report concur that the disorder involves a stressor and a person reacting to that stressor in a way considered

maladaptive or somehow not with an expected "healthy" response.

Whatever the name and whatever the criteria, the diagnosis is frequently used, and the criteria often are not strictly applied. Various reasons for this are given. Kranzler (1988) noted that there is "diagnostic hedging [or a] fear of stigmatizing patients with a more 'serious' diagnosis" (p. 814). It may be that the characteristics of these disorders make it difficult to apply criteria in the same way they can be applied to other disorders. Furthermore, children and adolescents may be brought for evaluation at a time in their development or during a period in the genesis of psychopathology prior to the presentation of a history and symptom pattern that is consistent with another more specific disorder.

DSM-III-R (American Psychiatric Association 1987) describes adjustment disorder as "a reaction to an identifiable psychosocial stressor (or multiple stressors) that occurs within three months of onset of the stressor(s)" (p. 330). The characteristics of the "maladaptive" reaction are described, and it is specified that the disturbance cannot have lasted more than 6 months. If symptoms have been present more than 6 months, it is necessary to use another diagnosis. This makes it difficult to apply the diagnostic criteria to very real conditions often seen in clinical practice of child and adolescent psychiatry. Children react to stressors such as divorce, illness or death in the family, natural disasters, violent experiences, or abuse for varying periods of time and often for more than 6 months. Yet they may not have symptoms that fulfill the criteria for other more specific diagnoses. The child may react emotionally with fearfulness, sadness, irritability, or lability; with specific symptoms such as nightmares or phobialike avoidance; or with behavior pattern changes, such as declining school performance, withdrawal, or aggression. Yet the clinical situation may not meet the criteria for a specific mood, anxiety, or conduct disorder.

It has been difficult to define this disorder precisely in the various diagnostic schema. Perhaps that is because of the nature of the disorder itself. Fabrega et al. (1987) made this point in their study of patients with adjustment disorder. They noted:

> The clinician will naturally find recognized illness conditions showing clearly delineated symptom profiles. However, the clinician must also be prepared to find conditions that do not show such properties, but, that, nonetheless, require intervention and/or disposition. The latter may include marginal and/or transitional categories of illness as well as conditions that do not meet criteria of illness. (p. 567)

Fabrega et al. studied patients, age 19 and older, at a 24-hour walk-in psychiatric clinic. All were considered somewhat stressed, since they had presented themselves to the clinic for services. The subjects were evaluated using a semistructured format, and a diagnosis was given. The diagnostic formulation used the multiple axes of DSM-III (American Psychiatric Association 1980). The study showed adjustment disorder to be a condition that could be differentiated from "not ill" or a specific disorder using a multiaxial approach. Fabrega et al. felt that their study validated the utility of the designation of adjustment disorder, as a transitional or marginal disorder; subjects with adjustment disorder differed from those "not ill" and from those with specific disorders.

This study did not follow the course of patients with adjustment disorder; however, given the nature of the disorder, it may be less definite than the DSM criteria specify. Since none of the subjects were less than 19 years of age, the results cannot be directly applied to children or even to younger adolescents.

Diagnostic Criteria

DSM-III-R describes specific criteria for adjustment disorder as shown in Table 43-1. Severity of the stressor(s) and the stressor itself are to be indicated on Axis IV. Table 43-2 illustrates the differences

Table 43-1. DSM-III-R diagnostic criteria for adjustment disorder

A. A reaction to an identifiable psychosocial stressor (or multiple stressors) that occurs within three months of onset of the stressor(s).
B. The maladaptive nature of the reaction is indicated by either of the following:
   1. Impairment in occupational (including school) functioning or in usual social activities or relationships with others
   2. Symptoms that are in excess of a normal and expectable reaction to the stressor(s)
C. The disturbance is not merely one instance of a pattern of overreaction to stress or an exacerbation of one of the mental disorders previously described.
D. The maladaptive reaction has persisted for no longer than six months.
E. The disturbance does not meet the criteria for any specific mental disorder and does not represent uncomplicated bereavement.

Source. Reprinted with permission from American Psychiatric Association 1987.

among three of the DSM schemes and the GAP classification.

There have been numerous complaints regarding the lack of strictness in application of the diagnostic criteria. There are, however, difficulties in applying them to real clinical situations and especially so for children or adolescents who are in the process of developing. DSM-III-R requires that the reaction to the stressor occur within 3 months. However, some reactions are delayed, and some stressors continue and change. Also, DSM-III-R does not take into account the interaction of stressors with developmental changes in children or adolescents. The significance of important life events, the capacity of a child to adapt, and the potential reactions vary enormously with the child's developmental stage. For example, Hetherington (1979), stated that "the experience of divorce will differ qualitatively for children of varying ages rather than the trauma being more or less intense" (pp. 852–853). There are developmental differences in cognitive abilities, coping strategies, and available support systems. The recency of the divorce is only one factor. Strictly applied, if the child or adolescent is still experiencing difficulty after 6 months, another diagnosis must be used. Adjustment to parental divorce may take much longer than 6 months, and yet the child may not fit the category of a specific disorder.

Although never an official diagnostic classifica-

Table 43-2. Comparison of diagnostic criteria for adjustment and reactive disorders

	DSM-II (1968) (Transient situational disturbance)	DSM-III (1980) (Adjustment disorder)	DSM-III-R (1987) (Adjustment disorder)	GAP (1966) (Reactive disorder)
Nature of stressor	"Overwhelming[ly]" environmental	Variable; specified and coded Axis IV	Same as DSM-III	Variable; common and unusual—"emotionally traumatic"
Duration of stress	Acute	Acute, chronic, or periodic	Same as DSM-III	Acute, chronic, or periodic
Course	Symptoms diminish after removal of the stress. If they continue, a new diagnosis is necessary.	Disorder occurs within 3 months of onset of stressor. Disorder resolves when stressor disappears or when new level of adaptation occurs.	Disorder occurs within 3 months of onset of stressor. If symptoms continue for more than 6 months, a new diagnosis is necessary.	"Transient" or "temporary," but may become chronic
Age	Subtyped according to developmental stage	Developmental stage not specified. May begin at any age.	Same as DSM-III	Developmental stage specified
Symptoms	Variable, including psychoses	Maladaptive reaction with impaired social or occupational functioning or excessive reaction. Psychoses excluded. Disorder is subtyped according to symptoms.	Same as DSM-III	Variable, including psychoses
Other psychiatric disorders	No apparent "underlying mental disorders" present	Other disorders may be present.	Other disorders may be present.	Other disorders may be present.
Dynamic factors, previous level of functioning, endowment of child or adolescent	Not emphasized	Axis V codes adaptive functioning in the past year. Endowment, dynamic factors not considered.	Same as DSM-III	Dynamic state and meaning to child and parents emphasized. "Past experiences," "endowment," "level of development," and "adaptive resources" are considered.

tion, the GAP report is important historically and appears to avoid some of these difficulties. There is no time specified between the stress and the onset of symptoms, although there must be a (presumed) causal relationship. There is a greater emphasis on the child's developmental stage and the significance of the stressor to that child. The GAP classification assumes a remission of symptoms with alleviation of the stressor, but makes the point that

the reaction can become chronic. If it does not interfere with development, it continues to be called a reactive disorder.

Clinical Findings

The clinical characteristics vary considerably from child to child and may vary from time to time in the same child. In some cases, symptoms may be present only in a particular setting (e.g., the school or at home). In others, the reaction may be apparent in most areas of the child's life. The severity of the symptoms is not necessarily related to the severity of the stressor. "The pretraumatic state may be more important in predicting the type and severity of the person's reaction than the trauma itself. Variables such as the person's sex, age, temperament, and previous traumatic experiences are all crucial" (Woolston 1988, p. 281). Particularly in children, what may appear to be a "minor" stress may produce rather intense reactions.

DSM-III-R subtypes adjustment disorder according to the primary symptoms. Several of the subtypes are "partial syndromes of specific disorders" (American Psychiatric Association 1987, p. 329). If the full syndrome is present, the specific disorder should be diagnosed; for example, if a child is reacting to a loss with a full depressive syndrome, depending on the symptoms, major depressive disorder or dysthymic disorder would be diagnosed. Despite there being a reaction to a loss, adjustment disorder with depressed mood is not the diagnosis. Table 43-3 lists the nine subtypes of adjustment disorders in DSM-III-R.

The GAP report describes a variable picture under reactive disorder; there can be behavioral, psychological and/or physical symptoms. "Part of the reaction may represent adaptive attempts, as in regression or withdrawal, while part may be a sign of adaptive failure" (Group for the Advancement of Psychiatry 1966, p. 223). Woolston (1988) proposed five conceptual models of adjustment disorders, four of which describe mechanisms by which an environmental stressor may stimulate a series of responses that can lead to perpetuation of symptoms after the stressor has been reduced or eliminated.

Certainly it is evident that some events, such as divorce, lead to additional changes for the child or adolescent. There may be economic hardship, geographic moves, changes in relationships with each parent, and so on, which require adaptation. Although a child may adjust to the divorce itself, these other changes may lead to difficulties and the development of symptoms.

Differential Diagnosis

DSM-III-R lists three conditions, and we've added two more, to consider in the differential diagnosis.

Conditions Not Attributable to a Mental Disorder That Are a Focus of Attention or Treatment (V Codes)

This would be similar to Fabrega et al.'s (1987) "not ill" category. There has been a stressor and a reaction, but the symptoms are not excessive or maladaptive. The so-called healthy response of the GAP system might be included here. As noted in DSM-III-R, clinical judgment is important in making the differentiation.

Personality Disorders

Reactions to stress are often problematic for the patient with a personality disorder. However, the symptoms of a personality disorder are not temporary, and the problematic style continues. Exacerbations in behavioral patterns associated with a personality disorder are not usually diagnosed as an adjustment disorder. New symptoms, not previously present, however, may warrant such a diagnosis.

This distinction may be particularly important to consider for children and adolescents for whom early intervention could be of great benefit. It was once thought that difficulties in adolescence and "turmoil" were normal (Freud 1958). As Masterson (1968) and Offer et al. (1981) pointed out, however, it is not normal. Troubled adolescents can benefit from intensive treatment.

Psychological Factors Affecting Physical Condition

This diagnosis requires the presence of a physical disorder in which "psychological factors contribute to the initiation or exacerbation of a physical condition. . . . [At times, there] may be only a single symptom, such as vomiting" (American Psychiatric Association 1987, p. 333). Children and adolescents with physical disorders (e.g., migraine headaches, diabetes, asthma, arthritis, acne) may react to environment stress, which may be related to their disorders, such as limitations imposed by the disorder or the treatment, requiring the reactions of peers or family members; or problems with self-esteem, body image, or their own attitudes about the illness. There may be an exacerbation of symptoms in reaction to unrelated environmental stressors. Properly, these children should be separated

Table 43-3. Types of adjustment disorder in DSM-III-R

Code the type according to the predominant symptoms. Specify the stressor(s) and its (their) severity on Axis IV.

Adjustment disorder with anxious mood
This category should be used when the predominant manifestation is symptoms such as nervousness, worry, and jitteriness.

Adjustment disorder with depressed mood
This category should be used when the predominant manifestation is symptoms such as depressed mood, tearfulness, and feelings of hopelessness.

Adjustment disorder with disturbance of conduct
This category should be used when the predominant manifestation is conduct in which there is violation of the rights of others or of major age-appropriate societal norms and rules. *Examples:* truancy, vandalism, reckless driving, fighting, defaulting on legal responsibilities.

Adjustment disorder with mixed disturbance of emotions and conduct
This category should be used when the predominant manifestations are both emotional symptoms (e.g., depression, anxiety) and a disturbance of conduct (see above).

Adjustment disorder with mixed emotional features
This category should be used when the predominant manifestation is a combination of depression and anxiety or other emotions. The major differential is with depressive and anxiety disorders. *Example:* an adolescent who, after moving away from home and parental supervision, reacts with ambivalence, depression, anger, and signs of increased dependence.

Adjustment disorder with physical complaints
This category should be used when the predominant manifestation is physical symptoms, e.g., fatigue, headache, backache, or other aches and pains, that are not diagnosable as a specific Axis III physical disorder or condition.

Adjustment disorder with withdrawal
This category should be used when the predominant manifestation is social withdrawal without significantly depressed or anxious mood.

Adjustment disorder with work (or academic) inhibition
This category should be used when the predominant manifestation is an inhibition in work or academic functioning occurring in a person whose previous work or academic performance has been adequate. Frequently there is also a mixture of anxiety and depression. *Example:* inability to study or to write papers or reports.

Adjustment disorder not otherwise specified
Disorders involving maladaptive reaction to psychosocial stressors that are not classifiable as specific types of adjustment disorder. *Example:* an immediate reaction to a diagnosis of physical illness, e.g., massive denial and noncompliance, that is too maladaptive to be categorized as the V Code V15.81, Noncompliance with Medical Treatment.

Source. Adapted with permission from American Psychiatric Association 1987.

diagnostically from those children who may react to stress with physical complaints such as fatigue, headaches, abdominal pain, changes in sleep or eating patterns, or with regressions in toileting or language development.

The birth of a sibling, a change of school, a geographic move, a financial crisis, or family conflict may evoke a variety of symptoms related to physical or physiologic functions in children and in some adolescents. Young children, particularly those who have been recently toilet trained, may revert to wetting or soiling when reacting to a stressor. Some may show infantile patterns of eating and sleep

difficulties where these did not exist before. Lethargy, complaints of fatigue, or pains of one sort or another may occur at almost any age.

Posttraumatic Stress Disorder

The stressor is considered "outside the range of usual human experience" (American Psychiatric Association 1987, p. 250), and nearly everyone would find it distressing. The symptoms, specified in DSM-III-R, include reexperiencing the trauma in some way (e.g., flashbacks or dreams). There is an avoidance of reminders of the event or "numbing of general responsiveness" (p. 250). There are also symptoms of intensified arousal (e.g., sleep problems or other somatic symptoms). In children, this can be an important consideration. Although the response may be delayed and memory of the event repressed, a variety of psychological and physical symptoms may be present.

Specific Disorders (e.g., Anxiety Disorder/Mood Disorder)

If the full symptom picture is present, the diagnosis of the specific disorder should be given.

Epidemiology

Although there are few epidemiologic studies of adjustment disorder, it is probably quite common. In describing the results of their longitudinal study, Chess and Thomas (1984) noted that "the great majority of the clinical cases in childhood (40 out of 45) . . . were adjustment disorders with mild cases predominant" (p. 54). In speaking of reactive disorders, Kessler (1979) stated, "The incidence of reactive disorders is universal; it is difficult to conceive of a human being progressing from infancy through adolescence without trauma sufficient to interfere, at least temporarily, with psychosocial development" (p. 177).

Adjustment disorders and reactive disorders occur at all ages. DSM-III-R does not subtype adjustment disorder according to age or developmental level; however, it does acknowledge that some individuals may be more vulnerable than others. The GAP report does make a differentiation according to developmental stages. It appears that there may be a difference in the disorder at various ages in vulnerability, severity, and outcome.

The early years of childhood may represent a phase of particular vulnerability. Kessler (1979, p. 177) noted, "Although reactive disorders occur at all ages, the infant and preschool child are more vulnerable to a wider range of environmental assaults or lack of support." Similarly, Chess and Thomas (1984) indicated that most of the adjustment disorder cases seen in their study presented in the preschool years, followed by those cases in the 6- to 8-year-old group.

A study by Andreasen and Wasek (1980) and a follow-up of that study by Andreasen and Hoenk

(1982) addressed the differences between adolescents and adults diagnosed with adjustment disorder. Differences appeared in severity, symptoms, duration, and outcome. Adolescents often had a more severe illness than adults that lasted longer. More adolescents were hospitalized for a longer time, and more had been distressed for a longer time before being seen. Nearly half of the adolescents had experienced symptoms for more than a year; only a quarter of the adults had been symptomatic that long.

The clinical picture differed, with more behavioral and acting-out symptoms among the adolescents and more depressive symptoms for the adults (although more than half of the adolescents also demonstrated depressive symptoms). Stressors varied and, as Andreasen and Wasek (1980) noted, often did not meet the DSM-II criteria for being "overwhelming." School problems were clearly the most common stressors in adolescents (60.3%), followed by parental rejection (27.1%), alcohol and drug problems (26.1%), and parents separated or divorced (25.1%).

Andreasen and Hoenk (1982) found that "the adolescents had a considerably poorer outcome in terms of both number and type of diagnoses" (p. 585). Only 44% of the adolescents were "completely well" with "no significant problems during the follow-up period," whereas 71% of the adults had "no significant problems." It also seemed that the diagnoses were more severe than for the adults: "Substantially more adolescents developed Major Depressive Disorder, Antisocial Personality, and Alcohol/Drug Use Disorder" (p. 585). Several adolescents also had become schizophrenic.

These studies used DSM-II and DSM-III criteria. Some of those adolescents might not fit the present criteria for adjustment disorder. For example, if there were psychotic symptoms, adjustment disorder could not be a primary diagnosis. Hospitalization would also be more difficult. The study does, however, make an important point for the careful evaluation of adolescents in distress. Some may be in the beginning stages of a serious disorder. As Fabrega et al. (1987) termed it, adjustment disorder may be a "transitional disorder" on the way to a specific disorder for some patients.

Etiology

Adjustment disorders are multiply determined, and often there is not a simple one-to-one correlation between an event and the outcome. In general, adjustment disorders are considered to be the result of a child or adolescent reacting to a stress. There are a number of factors about the child or adolescent to be taken into account, as well as a number of aspects of the stressor and the environment to consider.

Children and adolescents vary in vulnerability; there are differences in past experiences, endowment, temperament, and coping mechanisms. Developmental stage and capacity of the support system are other variables. A child who has had some experience with mastering difficulties, has good health, has good cognitive capacities, has an easy temperament (i.e., adaptable), and has a supportive environment will fare better than children who do not have those advantages. A child who has had no experience in mastering difficulties, has been overwhelmed, has poor health, has problems with learning, has a difficult temperament, and has an inconsistent, poor quality support network will be more vulnerable.

Developmental level probably also contributes to vulnerability. Kranzler (1988) stated that "there are certain points in a child's development, particularly at transitional phases, at which he may be more vulnerable to a pathological rather than a growth response to stress" (p. 822).

Stressors vary in duration, intensity, and their nature. Some stressors would be considered stressful for anyone; others would be stressful only for some. The GAP report emphasizes individual variability, stating:

> In making the diagnosis of reactive disorder the dynamic state and reaction of the child should be emphasized rather than the degree of stress . . .
> relatively mild stimuli may produce a reactive disorder in a particular child depending on its meaning to the child, his parents. (Group for the Advancement of Psychiatry 1966, p. 223)

DSM-III-R indicates that severity of the stressor is important and that it should be coded on Axis IV, along with the specific stressor. However, it also notes:

> The severity of the reaction is not completely predictable from the intensity of the stressor. People who are particularly vulnerable may have a more severe form of the disorder following only a mild or moderate stressor, whereas others may have only a mild form of the disorder in response to a marked and continuing stressor. (American Psychiatric Association 1987, p. 329)

It would seem important to consider all of these aspects of the stressor as significant. There are individual meanings attached to events, but the intensity and duration of the stressor also contribute to difficulty. A divorce might be a welcome relief, but if there are continuing intense visitation and financial battles in which the child is caught, the stress is different than it is for a child whose parents are able to resolve conflicts or at least not put the child in the middle of their battles with each other.

The environment must also be considered. The child's reaction to a stressor often influences a change in the environment, which may yield a new stress. Changes may interact with each other and compound the symptoms.

Sameroff and Fiese (1989) posited a "transactional model" of interaction between the environment and the developing child that takes into account the complex relationships and reactions. This model permits a level of understanding that can lead to specific interventions.

Treatment

Immediate treatment works to relieve stress and symptoms as well as serving a preventive purpose:

> Not uncommonly, children and adolescents who experience reactive disorders and are not treated, later succumb to adult life stress-producing situations in a similar fashion. Earlier life failure at coping with stressors may be a culmination of repeated disproportionately intense life responses and vulnerability. (Mishne 1986, p. 220)

Appropriate intervention can assist in the development of improved coping abilities and a sense of mastery, in addition to symptom relief.

Treatment should be preceded by an evaluation of the child or adolescent and his or her environment. Detailed information about the duration, intensity, and nature of the stressor and its meaning to the child or adolescent should be obtained. The child's developmental level, past history, ego strengths, and coping abilities are important factors to consider. The pertinent family, school, and community systems should be assessed for contribution to the difficulty and interaction with the child's responses, as well as the ability to be supportive.

Medications are not used in children as frequently as they are in adults, and their effects are often less certain. However, sedatives, antianxiety agents, and other medications with sedative side effects have all been used on a short-term basis, with anecdotal reports of good results. Sometimes symptom relief is needed before other issues can be addressed.

The stressor and its meaning can be addressed in individual therapy (or sometimes in a group setting). One of the brief therapy formats that includes a specific focus and time limit, as described by Dulcan (1984), might be a useful approach.

The child or adolescent can gain insight into the nature of the stressor; misinterpretations can be clarified and a sense of mastery can be encouraged by helping the child develop adaptive coping skills as well as supporting those adaptive skills already present.

It is essential to understand the context of the stressor in the child's environment. In some cases, it may be possible to eliminate, reduce the impact of, or avoid a stressor. Anxiety about going to school may reflect real or perceived threats at school or on the way to school, whether riding a bus or walking. Children may report the "threats" or actual events. Sometimes they may not, because of real or imagined threats of retaliation or because the child believes his or her feelings are unacceptable. Some situations may require protection and active direct intervention by adults. Physical and sexual abuse are extreme examples of such situations. There are, however, some situations in which the particular stress cannot be avoided or eliminated (e.g., death of a family member, divorce, or geographic family moves).

In other situations, it might be possible to eliminate a particular stressor, but it may not be in the best interest of the child to do so. When interpersonal conflicts with a teacher or peers and disappointments in achievement in school, on the playground, in sports, or outside school activities precipitate symptoms, it may be more productive in the long run for a child to learn to cope with and adapt to such situations than to avoid or eliminate them. It is a matter of clinical judgment to determine what level of environmental intervention is needed and appropriate.

Interventions with the parents and family, school, and community can be made, again, based on an assessment. Sometimes, especially with young children, interventions with parents are all that is needed to resolve stress and to relieve symptoms.

Helping parents to understand the limits of the young child's capacities, the meaning of the stressful situation to the child, their own reaction to the situation, and their child's reactions, and offering them specific direction in their own behavior, not only can help to relieve the current problem, but also can build skills and perspectives useful in the future.

With older children and adolescents, parent or family work is often only part of the treatment plan. Individual work is usually necessary because of the varied meanings attached to stressors and the greater complexity of environmental influences. In some cases, work with the entire family will be beneficial.

Prognosis

DSM-III-R assumes that the prognosis for adjustment disorder is good. After the stress is eliminated or there is a "new level of adaptation," the disorder is expected to end. The GAP report makes a different prediction for reactive disorder, saying the outcome can be determined only at follow-up. The GAP report noted that "although the majority of these disorders may be transient or temporary, a variety of forces can lead to more chronically incapacitating pictures" (Group for the Advancement of Psychiatry 1966, p. 224).

There have been few outcome studies of adjustment disorder. As noted above, Andreasen and Hoenk's (1982) follow-up study indicated that the outcome for adolescents was not as favorable as the authors had expected. Andreasen and Hoenk also found that there were no predictors of diagnosis from the symptoms present at the initial evaluation. Those who later developed an antisocial personality tended to have more behavioral symptoms; however, this was not a statistically significant difference.

The Chess and Thomas (1984) longitudinal study showed that those who were diagnosed with adjustment disorder in their early years were more likely to have symptoms continuing into adolescence than were those with an onset later in childhood. If symptoms had disappeared by adolescence, the adolescent tended to continue to do well through early adulthood. However, if symptoms did continue into adolescence, the adolescent tended to get worse, and that course continued through early adulthood.

There are a number of factors that are probably important prognostically, including vulnerability of the child, the developmental level of the child at the time of the original problem, the nature and duration of the stressor, the nature and time of treatment, support systems, environmental interventions, and successive life circumstances.

Research Issues

More studies on adjustment disorder in children and adolescents are clearly needed. It would be beneficial to explore differences in clinical findings, course, and prognosis according to age and developmental level. Studies on individual vulnerability (and resilience), interventions, and outcome are needed. A likely problem area will be in the definition of adjustment disorder. The DSM-III-R restriction of duration to 6 months leaves a number of people who cannot be categorized, if their symptoms do not fit the criteria for other disorders. Virtually all the questions regarding epidemiology, treatment, and prognosis remain to be addressed by future research.

References

American Psychiatric Association: Diagnostic and Statistical Manual of Mental Disorders, 2nd Edition. Washington, DC, American Psychiatric Association, 1968

American Psychiatric Association: Diagnostic and Statistical Manual of Mental Disorders, 3rd Edition. Washington, DC, American Psychiatric Association, 1980

American Psychiatric Association: Diagnostic and Statistical Manual of Mental Disorders, 3rd Edition, Revised. Washington, DC, American Psychiatric Association, 1987

Andreasen NC, Hoenk PR: The predictive value of adjustment disorders: a follow-up study. Am J Psychiatry 139:584–590, 1982

Andreasen NC, Wasek P: Adjustment disorders in adolescents and adults. Arch Gen Psychiatry 37:1166–1170, 1980

Chess S, Thomas A: Origins and Evolution of Behavior Disorders From Infancy to Early Adult Life. New York, Brunner/Mazel, 1984

Dulcan MH: Brief psychotherapy with children and their families: the state of the art. Journal of the American Academy of Child Psychiatry 23:544–551, 1984

Fabrega H, Mezzich H, Mezzich AC: Adjustment disorder as a marginal or transitional illness category in DSM-III. Arch Gen Psychiatry 44:567–572, 1987

Freud A: Adolescence. Psychoanal Study Child 13:255–278, 1958

Group for the Advancement of Psychiatry: Psychopathological Disorders in Childhood: Theoretical Considerations and a Proposed Classification (Vol 6, Rep No 62). New York, Group for the Advancement of Psychiatry, 1966

Hetherington EM: Divorce: a child's perspective. Am Psychol 34:852–853, 1979

Kessler ES: Reactive disorders, in Basic Handbook of Child Psychiatry, Vol 2: Disturbances in Development. Edited by Noshpitz JD. New York, Basic Books, 1979, pp 173–184

Kranzler EM: Adjustment disorders, in Handbook of Clinical Assessment of Children and Adolescents, Vol 2. Edited by Kestenbaum CJ, Williams DT. New York, New York University Press, 1988, pp 812–828

Masterson JF: The psychiatric significance of adolescent turmoil. Am J Psychiatry 124:1549–1554, 1968

Mishne JM: Clinical Work With Adolescents. New York, Free Press, 1986

Offer D, Ostrov E, Howard XI: The mental health professional's concept of the normal adolescent. Arch Gen Psychiatry 38:149–152, 1981

Sameroff AJ, Fiese BH: Conceptual issues in prevention, in Prevention of Mental Disorders, Alcohol and Other Drug Use in Children and Adolescents (DHHS Publ No ADM-89-1646). Edited by Shaffer D, Philips I, Enzer NB. Rockville, MD, U.S. Department of Health and Human Services, 1989, pp 23–53

Sowder B, Burt M, Rosenstein M, et al: Use of psychiatric facilities by children and youth. Washington, DC, U.S. Department of Health and Human Services, 1975

Woolston JL: Theoretical considerations of the adjustment disorders. J Am Acad Child Adolesc Psychiatry 27:280–287, 1988

Chapter 44

Child Physical Abuse

Arthur H. Green, M.D.

Definition

Child physical abuse refers to a nonaccidental physical injury inflicted on a child by a parent or guardian and encompasses the total range of physical injury. Child abuse is differentiated from child neglect, which refers to the failure of the parent or guardian to provide the child with adequate physical care and supervision. The legal definitions of child abuse stated in the New York State Child Protective Services Act of 1973 are as follows:

Definition of Child Abuse: An "abused child" is a child less than 16 years of age whose parent or other person legally responsible for his care:

1. Inflicts or allows to be inflicted upon the child serious physical injury, or
2. Creates or allows to be created a substantial risk of serious injury, or
3. Commits or allows to be committed against the child an act of sexual abuse as defined in the penal law.

Diagnostic Criteria

The possibility of physical abuse must be considered in every child who presents with an injury. A careful history and physical examination should be performed if one suspects an inflicted injury. The examination should include a routine X-ray survey of all children under 5 years of age and laboratory tests to rule out the possibility of an abnormal bleeding tendency.

While there is no single physical finding or diagnostic procedure that can confirm the diagnosis of child abuse with absolute certainty, the presence of the following signs and symptoms obtained from the history, physical examination, and observation of the child and the child's parent(s) is suggestive of an inflicted injury.

History

1. Unexplained delay in bringing the child for treatment following the injury.
2. History is implausible or contradictory.
3. History is incompatible with the physical findings.
4. There is a history of repeated suspicious injuries.
5. The parent blames the injury on a sibling or a third party.
6. The parent claims that the injury was self-inflicted.
7. The child had been previously taken to numerous hospitals for the treatment of injuries.
8. The child accuses the parent or caregiver of injuring him or her.
9. The parent has a prior history of abuse as a child.
10. The parent has unrealistic and premature expectations of the child.
11. The parent demonstrates a lack of concern about the injury.

Physical Findings

1. Pathognomonic "typical" injuries commonly associated with physical punishment, such as bruises on the buttocks and lower back and bruises in the genital area or inner thigh, may be inflicted after the child wets or soils or is resistant to toilet training. Bruises and soft tissue injuries at different stages of healing are signs of repeated physical abuse. Bruises of a special configuration, such as hand marks, grab marks, strap marks, and pinch marks, usually indicate abuse.
2. Certain types of burns are typically inflicted, such as multiple cigarette burns, scalding of hands or feet, burns of the perineum and buttocks.
3. Abdominal trauma leading to a ruptured liver or spleen.
4. Subdural hematoma with or without skull fracture.
5. Radiologic signs, such as subperiosteal hemorrhages, epiphyseal separations, metaphyseal fragmentation, periosteal shearing, and periosteal calcifications.
6. Eye injuries, including retinal hemorrhage, dislocated lens, and detached retina.
7. Cephalhematoma caused by hair pulling.
8. Multiple rib fractures caused by blows to the chest or back.
9. Ear injuries, including twisting injuries of the lobe, bruises of the pinna, and ruptured tympanic membrane with hemorrhage and hematoma formation.
10. Spiral fractures caused by a forcible twisting of an arm or leg.

Differential Diagnosis

Several bone diseases, such as osteogenesis imperfecta, congenital syphilis, osteomyelitis, infantile cortical hyperostosis, and spina bifida, may result in fractures and pathologic alterations in the bones, which may resemble lesions caused by physical abuse. These diseases may be identified by characteristic radiologic findings.

Bleeding disorders, such as purpura or hemophilia, might simulate inflicted soft tissue injuries resulting in bleeding. The bleeding disorders may be detected by coagulation studies, including a platelet count, bleeding time, prothrombin time, and thrombin time.

Inflicted injuries are often claimed to be "accidents" by the parents, and true accidental injuries are fairly common in young children. However, these may be distinguished from inflicted injuries by the absence of the "typical" abusive history and physical findings outlined previously.

Infants and toddlers may occasionally be injured by older siblings. These attacks may be motivated by rivalry and jealousy of the "baby," who is perceived as the favorite of the parents. The abusive sibling often has a history of prior abuse or scapegoating.

Clinical Findings

Physically abused children and their parents are frequently identified by typical constellations of pathologic personality traits and psychological symptoms and by their deviant patterns of family interaction.

The first descriptions of physically abusing parents in the 1960s and 1970s consisted of clinical observations of relatively small numbers of parents who battered their children. These early investigations often attributed the propensity for abuse to discrete personality traits or psychological disorders. However, many of these traits were present in large numbers of nonabusing parents as well. The failure of the early studies to use control groups led to faulty generalizations and conclusions. More recent research in this field has been based on theories of multiple causality, in which parental factors are believed to interact with environmental and sociocultural variables and the characteristics of the child, with physical abuse as a final outcome.

Recent observations of physically abusing parents suggest that the following characteristics might predispose them to be assaultive to their children.

Background of Deprivation and Abuse

The ability to care for a child is greatly influenced by the parent's own childhood experiences with caregivers. Steele (1976) and Green (1980) stressed the importance of deprivation, neglect, and physical abuse in the backgrounds of abusing parents. Negative interactions with their own parents (Kadushin and Martin 1981), including child abuse (Court 1975), and negative feelings toward fathers in abusing mothers (Oates 1986) were all characteristics of abusing parents.

Low Self-Esteem

Controlled studies of abusing mothers by Rosen and Stein (1980), Evans (1980), and Anderson and Lauderdale (1982) revealed that these mothers scored significantly lower than normal control mothers on standardized scales measuring self-esteem. This finding may reflect chronic rejection and criticism and other negative childhood experiences of these women.

Psychopathology and Psychiatric Impairment

There is evidence that the rather high prevalence of psychiatric disorders in abusing parents is related to their potential for abuse. Psychopathy was reported in abusing fathers by Smith et al. (1973) and in abusing parents by Paulson (1976). Baldwin and Oliver (1975) found that 34% of parents of severely abused children had been psychiatric inpatients. Kaplan et al. (1983) found that abusing fathers were frequently diagnosed as alcoholic, antisocial personality, and labile personality, while their nonabusing spouses often suffered from major depressive disorder.

Green (1979) described a typical pattern in child abusing fathers characterized by extreme jealousy of their spouse's attention toward the target child based upon maternal deprivation and unresolved sibling rivalry.

Cognitive Impairment

Smith et al. (1973) reported that almost half of their sample of abusing mothers were of borderline or subnormal intelligence when tested with the short form of the Wechsler Adult Intelligence Scale (Wechsler 1955). Baldwin and Oliver (1975) reported that 30% of the 65 abusing mothers they studied were of borderline or moderately retarded intelligence. Starr et al. (1978) observed that abusing mothers had significantly lower IQ scores than did mothers of children hospitalized for medical emergencies.

Environmental Stress

The importance of environmental stress as an etiologic factor in child abuse has been in part predicated on the high percentage of low socioeconomic status multiproblem families involved in official reports of child abuse. The 1977 national survey by the American Humane Association (1979) of reported cases of maltreatment indicated that the median family income of abusing and neglecting families was $5,361, or 36% of the United States median income of $16,009. Strauss (1980), Starr et al. (1978), and Chapa (1978) demonstrated a correlation between stressful events experienced by parents and the incidence of child abuse. The abusing parents experienced more stressful situations than did nonabusing controls.

Social Isolation

Starr et al. (1978) and Wolock and Horowitz (1977) described their samples of abusing mothers as more socially isolated than nonabusing control mothers. Salzinger et al. (1983) explored the social networks of abusing mothers and found that they had smaller peer networks and spent less time with their networks than did a control group of nonabusing mothers.

In summary, abusing parents may exhibit a wide variety of characteristics, such as childhood exposure to inadequate and often times abusive caregivers, low self-esteem, psychiatric disorders, cognitive impairment, and increased environmental stress and social isolation, which are likely to exert a cumulative negative impact on their parenting ability and contribute to their "abuse proneness." Their social isolation and paucity of peer contacts reduce their exposure to potentially normal and corrective parenting models.

Characteristics of Abused Children

The abused child is traumatized not only by the repeated physical assault by the parent, but also by the long-term pathologic climate of child-rearing on which the abuse is superimposed. This includes harsh or punitive disciplinary methods, scapegoating, gross under- or overstimulation, and insensitivity to the child's needs, all of which have an adverse long-term cumulative impact on the child. The following signs and symptoms are frequently present in physically abused children.

Anxiety Disorders

Green (1985) described anxiety states, sleep disturbances, nightmares, and psychosomatic complaints in abused children as immediate sequelae of the physical assault. Some of these anxiety-ridden children satisfied DSM-III-R (American Psychiatric Association 1987) criteria for posttraumatic stress disorder by exhibiting repetitive, traumatic play expressing themes of the abuse, flashbacks, constriction of affect and avoidance of events associated with the abuse, and symptoms of increased arousal such as excessive irritability, hypervigilance, and startle reactions. Kempe (1976) observed that abused children were hypervigilant, anxious, and fearful in relating to adults and expected punishment and criticism.

Paranoid Reactions and Mistrust

Green (1978a) described how the abused child's early and pervasive exposure to parental rejection, assault, and deprivation undermines the ability to achieve basic trust because of the expectation of similar maltreatment from other adults and parental figures. Ounstead (1972) described the syndrome of "frozen watchfulness," referring to the expression of hypervigilance and fearfulness in the abused infant or young child as the environment is scanned for potentially abusive individuals. This hypervigilant reaction in early childhood might act as a precursor to subsequent paranoid behavior.

Poor Self-Image

Green (1978a) described the impaired self-concept in physically abused children as an end result of chronic physical and emotional scarring, humiliation, and scapegoating, reinforced by each new episode of abuse. Children who are repeatedly threatened with beatings and abandonment eventually believe that this comes as a result of their own misbehavior, regardless of their actual innocence. A study by Oates (1986) demonstrated that physically abused children scored significantly lower on the Piers-Harris Self-Concept Scale than did normal children.

Depression and Suicidal Behavior

Gaensbauer and Sands (1979) described social and affective withdrawal, diminished capacity for plea-

sure, and a proneness toward negative affects such as distress, sadness, and anger in a group of abused infants. Green (1978a) reported sadness, depression, and self-deprecatory ideation in physically abused children. Green (1981) also described a "core affective disorder" in abused children as a consequence of their early exposure to assault, scapegoating, and unpredictable and unempathic parenting. Green (1978b) also documented evidence of self-destructive behavior in 40% of a sample of latency-aged abused children. This behavior, which consisted of self-mutilation, suicide attempts, or suicidal ideation, was frequently precipitated by parental beatings or threatened abandonment by parental figures. Allen and Tarnowski (1989) reported a higher incidence of depression and hopelessness in a group of physically abused children than in nonabused control children. The abused children also exhibited a more external locus of control, indicating that they do not feel that their actions have an impact on environmental events.

One might regard the self-destructive behavior as a means of submitting to the murderous wishes of the abusing parent, yet some adaptive and defensive motives might be present. For example, the child's self-injury or provocation of abuse from the environment might represent a sensation of mastery and control over the more terrifying parental beatings that occur spontaneously and without warning. Many abused children ultimately adopt a pain-dependent life-style of repetitive "victimlike" relationships with sadistic love objects modeled after the abusing parent, which may represent the child's attempt to repeat and master the traumatic impact of the original abuse.

Impaired Impulse Control

Aggressive and assaultive behavior has been described in abused toddlers by George and Main (1979) and in abused school-age children by Livingston (1987) and Green (1978a). According to Green (1978a), these problems with impulse control are determined by the child's use of "identification with the aggressor" as a major defense mechanism, based on their identification with their own violent parents. Loss of impulse control is further enhanced by the presence of central nervous system dysfunction. Victims of physical abuse often engage in disruptive behavior in school and delinquent and antisocial behavior during adolescence and are at risk for battering their future offspring.

Cognitive and Developmental Impairment

Abused children frequently display cognitive and intellectual impairment and delayed development on standardized IQ and developmental tests (Elmer and Gregg 1967; Martin 1972; Morse et al. 1970; Smith 1975). In controlled studies, Oates (1986) and Sandgrund et al. (1974) reported depressed IQ scores compared with nonabused control subjects. In some cases, the cognitive impairment might have preceded the maltreatment and even provoked it. Speech and language impairments in abused children might be caused by an inhibition of these functions if a child is frequently beaten while crying or vocalizing.

Central Nervous System Impairment

Neurologic impairment has been documented in several retrospective studies of abused children (Baron et al. 1970; Smith and Hanson 1974), but the etiology of this impairment is unclear. Martin et al. (1974) reported that numerous abused children with skull fractures and subdural hematomas were neurologically intact, while many abused children without head injury exhibited neurologic deficits. Green et al. (1981b) reported that 52% of abused children without head injury demonstrated neurologic impairment compared with 14% of the nonabused control subjects. However, the abused sample was not significantly more damaged than a neglected, nonabused comparison group, suggesting that the adverse physical and psychological environment associated with maltreatment, such as perinatal trauma, poor infant care, nutritional deficiency, and abnormal sensory stimulation, may be more damaging to the central nervous system than the physical assault.

Parent-Child Interaction in Physically Abusing Families

As might be expected, observations of parent-child interaction in abusing families reveal substantial deviations from the norm. Burgess and Conger (1977) reported lower rates of overall interaction, with less positive forms of contact and higher rates of negative behavior in abusing and neglecting families compared with normal control families. Gaensbauer and Sands (1979) observed impaired reciprocity in mother-infant interactions in cases of child abuse. The infants often failed to respond to their mothers' attempts to initiate interaction, often resulting in parallel play. Wasserman et al.'s (1983) study of abusing and nonabusing mother-infant dyads revealed that the abusing mothers interacted less with their infants and often ignored them. These mothers were less verbal and were often unsuccessful in engaging their infants in play. The nonabusing mothers were more verbal, demonstrated more positive affect, and were more successful in engaging their babies in games and other interactions.

These observations suggest that the abusing dyad might be locked into a mutually reinforcing negative spiral, in which the mother lacks the positive affective behavior required to engage her infant, who, in turn, is less likely to respond to the mother's attempts at initiating play. A vicious cycle may ensue, consisting of ineffective maternal responsiveness, withdrawal and discomfort in the infant, and further frustration in the mother, leading to asynchrony and a lack of reciprocity in the mother-infant relationship.

Epidemiology

Kempe et al.'s (1962) classic description of the "battered child syndrome" stimulated nationwide interest in child abuse, which soon became recognized as a major pediatric and social problem. Between 1963 and 1965, all 50 states passed laws requiring medical reporting of child abuse and neglect, and child protective services were established throughout the country. Improved reporting procedures have recently demonstrated the true magnitude of the problem. According to the findings of the national incidence study of child abuse and neglect carried out in 1986 (Department of Health and Human Services 1988), almost two million children were found to be maltreated. Some 5.7 of 1,000 children, or 358,300, were estimated to be physically abused, and 2.8 of 1,000 children, or 211,100, were emotionally abused; 2.5 of 1,000 children, or 155,900, were sexually abused. About one million children were identified as neglected; the major categories of neglect were subdivided into educational, physical, and emotional neglect. Of the physically abused children, 2.8 of 1,000, or 173,700, were described as injured or impaired. There were significant increases in the incidence of both physical abuse and neglect compared with the findings from the prior study period of 1981. These estimates of the incidence of maltreatment are consistent with the findings of the National Committee for the Prevention of Child Abuse (Cohn 1983), which estimated that more than one million children are severely abused annually, with 2,000–5,000 deaths occurring from physical abuse.

Etiology

The search for a simple explanation or cause of physical abuse has been elusive and unproductive. Most experts in the field believe that multiple etiologic factors operating in the parents, children, and the environment interact to produce an abusive outcome. For example, an abuse-prone parent (determined by impulsivity and childhood exposure to maltreatment), caring for a vulnerable, at-risk child, who might be unresponsive or hyperactive, might proceed to abuse the child in the presence of adverse environmental conditions, such as social isolation or the lack of a supportive spouse or substitute caregiver.

Belsky (1980) proposed a similar multifactorial model for child abuse. He conceptualized child maltreatment as a social and psychological phenomenon that is multiply determined by forces at work in the individual (ontogenetic development) and in the family (microsystem) and the culture (macrosystem) in which the individual and family are embedded. The contributions of the child to maltreatment would occur in the microsystem, and environmental stresses would operate in the exosystem. Societal attitudes toward violence and corporal punishment would represent the influence of the macrosystem.

Green (1980) sought to explain the high incidence of abuse among multiproblem families of lower socioeconomic status by the impact of poverty on each of the major variables associated with physical abuse. Lower socioeconomic status contributes to an increase in environmental stress through family disorganization, unemployment, inadequate income, poor housing, and excessively large numbers of children. Poor inner-city families provide a background conducive to the development of abuse-prone personality traits, such as the traditional use of physical punishment and authoritarian forms of child-rearing, which may be transmitted from generation to generation. The higher incidence of perinatal trauma and inadequate infant care in these families contributes to the physical and psychological deviancy that makes children vulnerable to abuse and scapegoating. Green (1980) considered the variables of environmental stress, parental personality traits, and characteristics of the child as a complementary series of factors leading to physical abuse and neglect, which changes as one ascends the socioeconomic ladder. For example, middle-class abusers would be likely to demonstrate more abuse-prone personality traits that might be more easily provoked by milder stressful conditions than would poverty-ridden abusing parents. Middle-class parents are less likely to be cited for neglect, as they possess the material resources to provide for the basic physical needs of their children and the ability to employ substitute caregivers. The compromised child-rearing of middle- and upper-class parents on the basis of abuse-prone personality traits may be compensated for by delegating parenting responsibility to nursemaids and boarding schools. The stressful conditions of poverty faced by lower-class parents, on the other hand, may trigger maltreatment in the relative absence of abuse-prone personality traits.

Treatment

The major goal of treatment is to protect the child from further injury and strengthen the family and its child-rearing capacity. Intervention should attempt to modify the pathologic personality traits of the abusing parent in a supportive setting, reduce the environmental stress, and reverse the symptoms and sequelae of abuse in the children. If possible, the children should remain at home. If the risk for further injury is too great, the children should be temporarily placed outside of the home.

The first objective with the abusing parents is to provide immediate crisis intervention to alleviate family conflict and environmental stressors. Once the family is stabilized, individual therapy may be employed to establish a trusting, supportive relationship with the parent. This therapy is designed to improve the parent's devalued self-image, to reverse the misperceptions of the child that lead to scapegoating, to interpret the link between current abusive practices and the parent's own childhood experiences of maltreatment, and to provide the parents with a positive child-rearing model for identification and information about parenting and child development. Parenting education will also be designed to help parents develop nonabusive disciplinary and child-rearing techniques. Successful intervention should enable parents to derive pleasure from the child.

The traditional outpatient psychiatric intervention must be greatly modified if these objectives are to be attained. A crisis-oriented multidisciplinary treatment program with a strong outreach component is the most appropriate type of intervention for these families. The facility may be hospital or community based, and it should provide the following comprehensive services: counseling and psychotherapy, parenting education, group and family therapy, outreach services, and crisis intervention.

Therapeutic intervention with the children must deal with each of the major psychopathologic sequelae of physical abuse previously outlined. The acute traumatic reactions and anxiety disorders may be relieved by allowing the child to master the trauma through a controlled repetition of the event using symbolic reenactments with dolls, puppets, drawings, and so on. Strengthening of impulse control is enhanced by imposing limits on the direct expression of aggression, such as hitting or destroying play materials and encouraging the verbalization of anger. Improvement of self-esteem gradually takes place during the child's exposure to the climate of warmth and acceptance generated by the therapist, which also gradually neutralizes the child's mistrust and hypervigilance. The child needs to be told that the beatings resulted from parental problems rather than as a consequence of the child's "badness." The presence of specific learning disabilities or behavior problems might require remedial intervention or placement in a special class.

Abused infants and preschool children may be treated in a therapeutic nursery designed to assess and improve the pathologic parent-child interaction. Therapeutic involvement with the parent-child dyad is geared to eliminate distortions in the parent's perceptions of the child, to help the parent understand the cues and signals of the child, and to identify and change mutually frustrating aspects of the parent-child interaction.

Prognosis

The prognosis in child abuse depends on the capacity of the parent to modify his or her abusive

caregiving practices and to improve parenting skill. The prognosis for the child is related to the ability to reverse his or her psychopathology and cognitive impairment. The overall prognosis for abuser and victim will therefore be related to the availability and efficacy of intervention.

The results of a nationwide evaluation of federally funded demonstration programs providing treatment services to abusing and neglecting families have been disappointing (Cohn and Daro 1987). In this evaluation 30% of this population reabused or reneglected their children during their involvement with the program. Only 42% of the parents were judged by their therapists as having a reduced potential for maltreatment at the termination of treatment. However, the children exhibited higher rates of improvement, in the range of 70%. Green et al. (1981a) reported a more successful treatment outcome in a multidisciplinary hospital-based program, with two-thirds of the abusing parents demonstrating some improvement, with a recidivism rate of 16%. Parents who sought help voluntarily and who were able to acknowledge abuse and other problems had a greater potential for improvement than parents who entered the program involuntarily and never admitted the abuse or a need for treatment. The better treatment results in this study were thought to be a result of the availability of outreach services, such as home visiting and service-oriented telephone advocacy.

There have been no other follow-up studies dealing with the effectiveness of intervention with abused children. However, clinical observations (Green 1980; Kempe and Kempe 1978) suggest that intervention with the children is usually successful, providing the abuse is eliminated from the environment. Successfully treated children not only demonstrate a reduction in their abuse-related symptomatology, but also are less likely to repeat the violent behavior with their offspring or others in the next generation. Although the capacity for change in abusing parents is less likely than in their child victims, the slight-to-moderate probability for improvement in these parents warrants referral in most cases to a specialized treatment program, considering the alternatives of no treatment or placement of the children in foster care.

Research Issues

Promising areas of research with abusing parents include the assessment of psychiatric impairment by the use of standardized psychiatric interviews and exploration of the coping styles and psychophysiologic responsiveness of the parents to child-related stressors, which would permit the deployment of more individually tailored and biologically oriented treatment strategies. The effectiveness of a wide variety of treatment modalities should be determined, such as individual versus group or family interventions and behavioral versus psychodynamically oriented techniques. Research is needed on the relative effectiveness of various outreach modalities, such as home visiting, assignment of homemakers or foster-grandparents in the home, and the use of crisis hot lines. Further exploration of the deviant aspects of mother-infant interaction in abusive and high-risk dyads would be helpful in developing more specific intervention strategies in a therapeutic nursery setting. It would also be valuable to conduct prospective, longitudinal studies dealing with the impact of preventive intervention with mother-infant dyads deemed to be at risk for abuse.

Areas for research with physically abused children might include long-term follow-up studies of treated and nontreated victims of abuse, which would yield information regarding the effectiveness of treatment and the natural development of long-term sequelae in the untreated children. It would also be useful to carry out a long-term prospective follow-up study of abused children in the foster care system, contrasting their developmental, educational, and psychiatric status with that of comparable abuse victims who remain with their natural families.

References

Allen DM, Tarnowski KJ: Depressive characteristics of physically abused children. J Abnorm Child Psychol 17:1–11, 1989

American Humane Association: National Study on Child Neglect and Abuse Reporting. Denver, CO, AHA, 1979

American Psychiatric Association: Diagnostic and Statistical Manual of Mental Disorders, 3rd Edition, Revised. Washington, DC, American Psychiatric Association, 1987

Anderson S, Lauderdale M: Characteristics of abusive parents: a look at self-esteem. Child Abuse Negl 6:285–293, 1982

Baldwin J, Oliver J: Epidemiology and family characteristics of severely abused children. British Journal of Preventative Social Medicine 29:205–221, 1975

Baron M, Bejar R, Sheaff P: Neurological manifestations of the battered child syndrome. Pediatrics 45:1003–1007, 1970

Belsky J: Child maltreatment: an ecological integration. Am Psychol 35:320–335, 1980

Burgess RL, Conger RD: Family interaction patterns related to child abuse and neglect: some preliminary findings. Child Abuse Negl 1:269–277, 1977

Chapa D: The relationship between child abuse/neglect and substance abuse contrasting Mexican-American and Anglo families: interim report. San Antonio, TX, San Antonio Child Abuse Project Civic Organization, February 1978

Cohn AH: An Approach to Preventing Child Abuse. Chicago, IL, National Committee for the Prevention of Child Abuse, 1983

Cohn AH, Daro D: Is treatment too late?: what ten years of evaluative research tells us. Child Abuse Negl 11:433–442, 1987

Court J: Nurture and nature: the nurturing problem, in Concerning Child Abuse. Edited by Franklin AW. New York, Churchhill Livingstone, 1975, pp 106–112

Department of Health and Human Services: Study findings: study of national incidence and prevalence of child abuse and neglect. Washington, DC, Department of Health and Human Services, 1988

Elmer E, Gregg CS: Developmental characteristics of abused children. Pediatrics 40:596–602, 1967

Evans A: Personality characteristics and disciplinary attitudes of child-abusing mothers. Child Abuse Negl 4:179–187, 1980

Gaensbauer T, Sands K: Distorted communication in abused/neglected infants and their potential impact on caretakers. Journal of the American Academy of Child Psychiatry 18:236–250, 1979

George C, Main M: Social interactions of young abused children: approach, avoidance and aggression. Child Dev 50:306–318, 1979

Green AH: Psychopathology of abused children. Journal of the American Academy of Child Psychiatry 17:92–103, 1978a

Green AH: Self-destructive behavior in battered children. Am J Psychiatry 135:579–586, 1978b

Green AH: Child abusing fathers. Journal of the American Academy of Child Psychiatry 18:270–282, 1979

Green AH: Child Maltreatment: A Handbook for Mental Health and Child Care Professionals. New York, Jason Aronson, 1980

Green AH: Core affective disturbance in abused children. J Am Acad Psychoanal 9:435–446, 1981

Green AH: Children traumatized by physical abuse, in Post-Traumatic Stress Disorder in Children. Edited by Eth S, Pynoos RS. Washington DC, American Psychiatric Press, 1985, pp 133–154

Green AH, Power E, Steinbook B, et al: Factors associated with successful and unsuccessful intervention with child abusing families. Child Abuse Negl 5:45–52, 1981a

Green AH, Voeller K, Gaines R, et al: Neurological impairment in battered children. Child Abuse Negl 5:129–134, 1981b

Helfer RE, McKinney J, Kempe R: Arresting or freezing the developmental process, in Child Abuse and Neglect: The Family and Community. Edited by Helfer R, Kempe C. Cambridge, MA, Ballinger, 1976, pp 55–73

Kadushin A, Martin J: Child Abuse: An Interactional Event. New York, Columbia University Press, 1981

Kaplan S, Pelcovitz D, Salzinger S, et al: Psychopathology of parents of abused and neglected children and adolescents. Journal of the American Academy of Child Psychiatry 22:238–244, 1983

Kempe CH, Silverman F, Steele B, et al: The battered child syndrome. JAMA 181:17–24, 1962

Kempe R, Kempe C: Child Abuse. Cambridge, MA, Harvard University Press, 1978

Livingston R: Sexually and physically abused children. J Am Acad Child Adolesc Psychiatry 26:413–415, 1987

Martin H: The child and his development, in Helping the Battered Child and His Family. Edited by Kempe C, Helfer R. Philadelphia, PA, JB Lippincott, 1972

Martin H, Beezely P, Conway E, et al: The development of abused children. Adv Pediatr 21:25–73, 1974

Morse W, Sahler O, Friedman S: A 3-year follow-up study of abused and neglected children. Am J Dis Child 120:439–446, 1970

Oates K: Child Abuse and Neglect: What Happens Eventually? New York, Brunner/Mazel, 1986

Ounstead C: Essay on developmental medicine, in Psychiatric Aspects of Medical Practice. Edited by Mandelbrote B, Gelder MG. London, Staples Press, 1972

Paulson M, Schwener G, Bendel R: Clinical applications of the Pd, Ma and (OH) experimental MMPI scales to further understanding of abusive parents. J Clin Psychol 32:558–564, 1976

Rosen B, Stein M: Women who abuse their children. Am J Dis Child 134:947–950, 1980

Salzinger S, Kaplan S, Artemyeff C: Mothers' personal social networks and child maltreatment. J Abnorm Psychol 92:68–76, 1983

Sandgrund A, Gaines R, Green A: Child abuse and mental retardation: a problem of cause and effect. American Journal of Mental Deficiency 79:327–330, 1974

Smith SM: The Battered Child Syndrome. London, Butterworths, 1975

Smith SM, Hanson R: 134 battered children: a medical and psychological study. Br Med J 3:666–670, 1974

Smith SM, Hanson R, Noble S: Parents of battered babies: a controlled study. Br Med J 4:388–391, 1973

Starr R, Seresnie S, Steinlaus J: Social and psychological characteristics of abusive mothers. Paper presented at the annual meeting of the Eastern Psychological Association, Washington, DC, May 1978

Steele B: Violence within the family, in Child Abuse and Neglect: The Family and Community. Edited by Helfer R, Kempe C. Cambridge, MA, Ballinger, 1976, pp 3–23

Strauss M: Social stress and marital violence in a national sample of American families. Ann NY Acad Sci 347:229–250, 1980

Wasserman G, Green A, Allen R: Going beyond abuse: maladaptive patterns of interaction in abusing mother-infant pairs. Journal of the American Academy of Child Psychiatry 22:245–252, 1983

Wechsler D: Wechsler Adult Intelligence Scale. New York, Psychological Corporation, 1955

Wolock I, Horowitz B: Factors relating to levels of child care among families receiving public assistance in New Jersey: first report (DHEW Grant No 90-C-418). Washington, DC, National Center on Child Abuse and Neglect, Office of Child Development, 1977

Chapter 45

Child Sexual Abuse

Alayne Yates, M.D.

Sexual abuse is a common occurrence. It is usually not reported. Sexual abuse often continues for years and can produce long-term emotional damage. Although there are many programs designed to detect, counteract, and prevent sexual abuse, the services that exist tend to be underfunded and overwhelmed by a deluge of case referrals. Treatment helps many, but not all, abused children. Although every state has some sort of mandated reporting of sexual abuse, the extent to which individual states detect abuse and fund service programs varies enormously.

The concern about sexual abuse first arose as part of society's larger concern about violent abuse and the emotional damage that abused children suffer. However, sexual abuse seems to be only distantly related to violent abuse in that both forms of abuse may be found more frequently in dysfunctional families. However, sexually abused girls do not report higher levels of family violence than do girls who have not been abused (Finkelhor 1984).

Sexual abuse could be construed as a social rather than a psychiatric problem because of its association with low-income families, limited parental education, and a higher rate of social disruption (Finkelhor 1984). However, sexual abuse is a psychiatric problem because it can lead to immediate and long-term emotional sequelae in children. Abused youngsters may suffer from problems such as anxiety, depression, somatization, or posttraumatic stress disorder. They may be left with a sense of guilt or badness (Sgroi 1982) and a distorted perception of the body and sexuality. When children experience pleasure from the sexual encoun-

ters, the sense of badness may be intensified. After intrafamilial abuse is discovered, children may be rejected by the parents or removed from the home. Because of this, the children may become anxious, depressed, or guilty. The children may care for the abuser and may be upset at the punishment. They may also feel responsible for the family disruption.

Child and adolescent psychiatrists may need to address the possibility of sexual abuse in even the most routine child and family evaluations. Psychiatrists must be alert to the possibility of abuse when a child displays heightened eroticization. They need to be able to take a sexual history directly from the child—a history that includes expectable as well as abnormal sexual experiences. They need to be aware of the indicators of possible abuse in the family: a rigid, patriarchal structure; poor marital relationship; role confusion; vague boundaries; and social isolation. They may need to coordinate services and plan treatment, and they should know what services are available. They may be asked to organize a multidisciplinary approach for sexually abused children in foster care. These children often need individual, group, and family therapy as well as a tight behavioral program, coordination with the school, and support for the foster parents (Yates 1987).

Status of Research

Although we have learned a great deal about sexually abused children, their families, and those who perpetrate abuse, it is important to recognize the limits of our knowledge. Professionals report only about one-third of the cases of which they are aware (National Center for Child Abuse and Neglect 1981), and 90% of all cases are likely not to be reported (Franklin 1974). The reported cases may differ from those that are never reported in factors such as social class, degree of coercion, and family disruption. We are unable to determine if this is the case because all children who are suspected of being abused must be reported and are therefore subject to intervention and treatment. The children who are available for study may have been interviewed on multiple occasions, been separated from family members, been through the courts, received therapy, and so on. Because of this, the effect of the abuse can be confused with the effect of intervention, family disruption, therapy, etc. Because of these and other problems, we are unable to make categorical statements about the effects of sexual abuse (Widom 1988). However, we can in fact make meaningful comparisons between subgroups of abused children, such as girls versus boys, maternal versus paternal versus stranger, and younger versus older children.

The study of sexual abuse suffers from several methodological problems in that sexual abuse has never been adequately or reliably defined (Fromuth and Burkhart 1987). In some studies, sexual abuse includes a chance encounter with an exhibitionist, voyeurism, fondling, and sex play between children. If abuse is defined as a deleterious influence or trauma, these events would not necessarily qualify. Other studies are underinclusive, narrowly defining sexual abuse as a long-term sexual relationship with a much older individual. Most studies do not control for contextual variables, such as coercion or whether the child is nurtured by the abuser. A molestation by an older peer may be lumped with abuse by relatives, baby-sitters, and teachers, without regard for the context in which the events occurred. There is usually no effort to control for the duration or intensity of the abuse, or the child's perception of the event(s).

It is the child's perception of the abuse that is the critical determinant of emotional damage. Yet in most research studies, the child's perception is not taken into account; many investigators continue to assume that all molestation must be traumatic. If the sexual abuse consists of fondling, a chance encounter with an exhibitionist, or a game of "doctor" with other children, the child may perceive these events as normal, nonabusive, and nonharassing (Vander Mey

1988). Of the sexual encounters in childhood, described by adults, 20% do not involve any physical contact, and 53% involve only some sort of sexual fondling (Finkelhor 1984).

Despite the inherent limitations in the study of sexual abuse, significant progress has been made in gaining a more objective understanding of the phenomenon. There appears to be a trend toward greater depth and increasing ideological restraint in the study of sexual abuse. In the last several years, there have been works published that attempt to establish an objective view of that which is known and that which is not known. Certain issues become increasingly apparent: 1) sexual abuse is a frequent event; 2) it can be associated with severe and persistent emotional damage; 3) many individuals who have been abused continue to function well; 4) false accusations sometimes do occur; 5) in certain instances, there has been more harm than good done through intervention; 6) the services available are often woefully inadequate; 7) children can be abused by the system in the investigative process and through court proceedings; and 8) we know very little about normal sexual development or how it is affected by molestation.

History

In the 16th and 17th centuries, families did not enjoy privacy as we know it now (Jackson 1990). Family members, employees, and servants would work, eat, and sleep under one roof and usually in the same room. There was no special provision made for children, who were viewed as inferior adults. Sexual matters were not concealed from children, and adults freely discussed sexual topics in front of them. Masturbation was tolerated, and sex play among children and between children and adults was expected. Children's sexual development was not regarded as troublesome, and, although sexual abuse undoubtedly existed, it was not identified as a problem.

In the early 19th century, literary romanticism began to influence affluent, well-educated parents. These parents began to view children as intrinsically innocent and asexual. This idea slowly became widespread, although it did not completely replace the earlier concepts. The function of the family was redefined as that of protecting the innocent child from the corrupting influences of the world. Parents concealed their own sexual interests and shielded children against sexual knowledge to preserve the children's "natural" state of innocence. Talk about sex in the schools and community was closely regulated.

The 20th century has been marked by a growing concern for the well-being of children. With the advent of effective birth control, families have become smaller, and each child is viewed as a special person. Children are no longer the property of the parents, and they are no longer expected to contribute to the family economy. They have the right to be protected and nourished. The concept that children have rights is the basis for the child advocacy movement and our effort to protect children from being sexually abused.

Although children may be better protected today, they tend to be confused and anxious about sexuality. They are told about the dangers of sexual abuse in dramatized prevention programs, but they are shielded from information about normal sexuality at school (Gebhard 1977; Thornberg 1972) and at home (Gagnon and Simon 1973). They may be scolded or cautioned about their sexual interests, but they are exposed to explicit sexual material through the media. They are warned about the dangers of AIDS, but they are led to expect that they should enjoy sexual experiences in adult life. How well children are able to sort out these ambiguities and contradictions is not known. Children's average, expectable attitudes about sexuality are difficult to assess, since there is a strong sanction about asking children questions about their sexual thoughts or experiences apart from the investigation of sexual abuse.

Prevalence

Kinsey et al. (1953) established that a great many women and quite a few men have experienced a sexual encounter at some time during their development. Today one-fifth to one-third of college women are thought to have experienced some form of sexual contact with an adult male during their development (Finkelhor 1979; Gagnon 1965; Landis 1956). The events range from seeing an exhibitionist in an alley or being fondled by a neighbor to long-term molestation. For about 15% of the women, the sexual experience is long term, and it most often involves a person within the family. The experience usually does not include intercourse.

There are two recent large-scale, random samplings of the prevalence of abuse in the general population. The National Center for Child Abuse and Neglect (1981) survey suggested that 5% of children are sexually abused by familiar adults. A national sampling by Finkelhor et al. (1990) indicated that 27% of women and 16% of men have a history of sexual abuse (broadly defined). Most of the sexual experiences are one-time events. The rates are higher for individuals who are raised in the West and who are reared in unhappy families. Abuse by fathers and stepfathers seems not to be as common as has usually been thought; it comprises only 6% of the total. Relatively few children are molested by strangers, but boys are more likely to be abused by strangers, whereas girls are more likely to be abused by family members.

A great deal more is known about the abuse of girls than the abuse of boys (Vander Mey 1988). Most estimates of the prevalence of abuse in males are thought to be low because boys are reluctant to talk about being molested, perhaps because they do not wish to admit vulnerability or to seem to be weak (Knopp 1986; Nasjleti 1980; Porter 1986). When boys are abused by males, they may be embarrassed by the implication that they might be homosexual. Yet the estimates of the number of males who have been abused run as high as 31% (Finkelhor 1987). Compared with abused girls, abused boys are more likely to be middle class, to be abused by women (Faller 1989; Vander Mey 1988), to be threatened, and to be forced to perform sexual acts (Pierce and Pierce 1985). Boys present a variety of reactions to having been abused, ranging from no loss of esteem (Rush 1980) to profound shame and a sense of powerlessness (Freeman-Longo 1986). Several samples of college men (Fritz et al. 1981; Fromuth and Burkhart 1989; Landis 1956) indicate that most sexually abused men do not experience serious long-term effects, although they may be more likely to express a homosexual preference than boys who have not been abused (Finkelhor 1981).

Men who have been sexually abused in childhood have been said to be very likely to become sexual abusers or rapists in adolescence or adulthood. It is true that a majority of adult male sex offenders report sexual abuse or trauma in childhood—most often by more than one person over an extended period (Groth and Freeman-Longo 1979), and it is true that older children who abuse younger children have often been molested by an adult (Johnson 1989). However, a great many individuals who have been abused do not become abusers. Although having been abused may serve as a risk factor for becoming an abuser, there must be many other factors involved.

There is a dramatic increase in the number of sexual abuse cases reported. However, the increase may be due to the greater awareness of sexual abuse, the advent of preventative programs, mandated reporting, or the availability of treatment, rather than an actual increase in numbers. Sexual abuse could be expected to decrease because of the preventative programs, the higher rate of detection, and longer incarceration for offenders. There may be less abuse because the husbands and wives in today's families achieve a more even balance of power. More traditional, less democratic family structures are associated with an increased risk of sexual abuse (Herman 1981; Swanson and Biaggio 1985). Lastly, the increased involvement of fathers in raising children may diminish the risk of sexual abuse. Fathers who care for the bodies of their infant sons and daughters seem to be at less risk of abusing the children later on (Parker and Parker 1986).

Theory

Finkelhor and Browne (1986) suggested that the extent to which the child is traumatized by sexual abuse is determined by four factors: traumatic sexualization, powerlessness, stigmatization, and betrayal. The sexualization stems from the premature stimulation; it leads to inappropriate, early sexual behavior in the service of nonsexual as well as sexual needs. The powerlessness is caused by the circumstances over which the child has no control; it leads to feelings of fear, anxiety, and helplessness. The stigmatization is secondary to the child's sense of being bad or damaged and the reactions of others after the abuse is discovered; it leads to feelings of shame and guilt. The betrayal stems from misuse at the hands of a person who is trusted; this leads to disillusionment and anger.

Schetky and Green (1988) cited a somewhat different list of factors that influence the sexually abused child's symptomatology and outcome. These are the age and developmental level of the child; the onset, duration, and frequency of the abuse; the degree of coercion and physical trauma; the relationship between the child and the perpetrator; the child's preexisting personality; and the interaction between acute and long-term variables. The man-

ner in which the system handles the case and the family's reaction after disclosure are important determinants of outcome also.

Incestuous Families

Because of their training in child development and psychopathology, child psychiatrists may be asked to assess and treat children who are alleged to be sexually abused. Most of these cases are of in-home molestation that involves a relative or relatives.

Fathers Who Abuse

High-achieving, apparently responsible, upper socioeconomic strata fathers may sexually abuse their children, but they are less likely to be detected and less likely to be convicted than lower socioeconomic class fathers. Studies of sexually abusive fathers describe these men as often controlling and intimidating (Herman 1981), as abusing alcohol, and as having unstable employment (Meiselman 1978). They are said to be socially inhibited and unable to develop relationships outside of the family; some are described as devoutly religious and adverse to forming an extramarital relationship when they are turned away by the spouse (Gebhard et al. 1965; Weinberg 1955).

Mothers Who Abuse

Self-report surveys indicate that a significant number of women are molesting children. Most of these cases are not reported, and we know little about these women. Although they were pictured in earlier case studies as psychotic or severely disordered and promiscuous, more recent investigations tend to depict them as lonely and emotionally deprived (Renshaw 1982).

Wives and Mothers

The spouses of sexually abusing fathers have been described as emotionally deprived, depressed, sexually unresponsive, and infantile (Lustig et al. 1966; Weiner 1962). These women may be dependent on the spouse and be unwilling to recognize the abuse because of the fear of marital disruption (Herman

1981; Meiselman 1978). They may reject the maternal role or transfer it to the daughter, who then becomes incestuously involved with the father. In this manner, they may be unconsciously recreating the abusive circumstances they experienced in childhood.

Once the incestuous relationship is established, it may continue for years. The mother may be working outside of the home so that she is unaware of the incestuous relationship. Her unavailability as a wife and mother may be part of the circumstance that fosters the sexual abuse. The mother may become aware of the abuse but refuse to intervene because she is dependent on her husband and afraid to be without his support. She may deny the possibility of abuse and reject the daughter when the daughter complains of being molested.

Daughters

Incestuously involved girls are described as physically and sexually attractive. They are likely to be the oldest or only daughter in the family, although other children may become involved as time goes by. The children who are selected by the abusive parents may be more likely to display physical problems or to be cognitively compromised. They may be alienated from or angry at the mother (Browning and Boatman 1977; Davies 1979; Gebhard et al. 1965; Goodwin et al. 1982).

The Abusive Format

The prototypic family at high risk for incest is marked by poor limit setting and little concern for the individual's privacy, belongings, or rights. The father assumes a dominant role, and the mother retreats to a position of passivity and dependency. The marital relationship deteriorates, and the mother may refuse intercourse. The father takes over many of the caregiving responsibilities toward the daughter, and the daughter, who receives little support from the mother, attempts to please the father by shouldering some of the maternal responsibilities (Herman 1981; Meiselman 1978; Mrazek et al. 1981; Schetky and Green 1988).

Emotional Consequences

Studies of women who identify themselves as abused indicate a higher rate of depression, psy-choneurosis, drug and alcohol abuse, and somatic anxiety (Bagley and Ramsey 1986; Peters 1976). Symptoms that have been associated with abuse (but that are also associated with a number of other circumstances) include mistrust, low self-esteem, anger, depression, school underachievement, hysterical traits, various somatic complaints, social withdrawal, impairment of body image, phobic behavior, behavioral disorders, accident proneness, and borderline personality disorder (Everstine and Everstine 1989; Schetky and Green 1988; Sgroi 1982). Of children who have been identified as abused, 21% present none of these symptoms (Conte and Schuerman 1987).

There are two symptom clusters that appear to be the direct result of sexual abuse: posttraumatic stress disorder and eroticized behavior. Posttraumatic stress disorder appears to be a frequent sequela of traumatic sexual abuse if the child has been raped, abducted, or forced into a position of profound helplessness. It is less frequently present when the child is older and is not threatened or forced. Although the criteria for posttraumatic stress disorder in childhood have not been defined (Benedek 1985), the symptoms may include fear and anxiety, various startle reactions, reenactment, sleep disturbance, flashbacks, constriction, regression, anger, and depression (Goodwin 1985). Symptoms may be severe and persistent, perhaps evolving into a chronic traumatic neurosis (Gelinas 1983).

Young children who have been molested over time often behave in a sexual manner with play materials or with other persons (Kolko et al. 1988; Yates 1982). The eroticized behavior seems either to be directly related to the length and intensity of the sexual contact (i.e., learned sexual responsiveness) or to be a defensive reenactment of the trauma in which the child assumes the role of the sexual aggressor (Schetky and Green 1988). Eroticized children are more likely than other children to draw genitals (Hibbard et al. 1987), and they may solicit sex from children and adults. They may be described as seductive, and they are at risk for further sexual abuse. They need protection, specialized foster placements, and treatment by well-trained therapists (Yates 1987).

Normal children become somewhat eroticized in the course of development. They may observe the parents' making love, sleep in crowded quarters, have oedipal fantasies, engage in sex play, observe animals mating, look at adult magazines, turn on the Playboy channel, and so on. Observing sexual activity seems to increase children's fantasy rather than their sexual activity, but when children observe the sexual activity of humans and animals with whom they can identify or when they are involved in frequent sex play, this can produce eroticized behavior that is similar to that of sexually abused children (Yates 1987). Eroticized behavior such as this can be confused with behavior secondary to a long-term molestation. Eroticized behavior warrants a sophisticated evaluation.

Civil Litigation

The court may ask a child psychiatrist to evaluate a child who is alleged to be damaged by witnessing or participating in a sexual act. This is a legitimate request. These are complex cases that require an understanding of child development, child psychopathology, child interviewing technique, and normal erotic development. Although children may be devastated by sexual molestation, this does not necessarily occur. Children may not be traumatized when they are fondled or when they view the genitals of a familiar adult, especially if they are accustomed to nudity and physical affection in the home. In other cases, children may perceive a sexual event as unpleasant or "yukky," but not as very disturbing or frightening.

The diagnosis of posttraumatic stress disorder can be misused, especially when civil litigation is involved. Posttraumatic stress disorder may be alleged solely on the history that the parents provide. Young children may not recall or be able to describe sleep disturbance, constriction of interests, or recurrent and intrusive recollections. The children may agree with whatever symptoms the parents describe. They may have been evaluated by inexperienced or unsophisticated examiners who are prejudiced toward the "discovery" of posttraumatic stress disorder by the history that the parents provide. A complete evaluation will require an assessment of the circumstances of the alleged molestation, of the child's perception of the events, and of the child's status and changes in status since the molestation. This may require a review of school records and interviews with individuals who know the child but who do not have a vested interest in the case.

False and Mistaken Allegations

Peters (1976), Goodwin et al. (1979), and Faller (1988) indicated a 3%–8% rate of unfounded or false ac-

cusations among children who are referred to an agency, program, or emergency room because of suspected abuse. The percentage of unfounded or false accusations seems to be much higher when the allegations occur in the course of custody and visitation disputes. The accusations in these disputes are often advanced by one parent against the other without the involvement of the child. If the parent alone advances the accusations, these accusations tend to be incorrect, but if the child initiates the accusations, they usually are correct (Yates and Musty 1988). In a rare instance, a preschool child may come to believe erroneously that a sexual event has transpired when it has not. The child may be manipulated by the parent or may strongly wish to believe that the parent is correct. The child may misinterpret affectionate caregiving behavior because of highly erotic, oedipal fantasies about the parent.

Children who make false or mistaken allegations may employ adult terminology such as "intercourse," or they may parrot the same story again and again. They may enjoy talking about the abuse and be eager to expand on the topic. They are less likely than truly abused children to provide realistic details or a logical sequence of events. They may become vague or evasive when they are questioned about the details, or they may look to the parent for help. Abused children are usually reluctant to speak of the sexual events; they are embarrassed, and the story may be painful for them to relate. Yet they may describe a logical series of events that are rich in detail and clearly beyond what a child of that age could be expected to know (Benedek and Schetky 1987; Schetky and Green 1988; Terr 1986).

A poor interviewing technique can lead to false accusations. Well-intended but naive workers may unconsciously encourage false accusations when they center all of their interest on sexual issues and uncritically accept whatever story the child produces as long as it is of a sexual or aggressive nature. Other examiners employ leading questions and may threaten the child with not going to the bathroom, eating, or going home until the child reveals what *really* happened (Benedek and Schetky 1987). A skilled examiner will allow the child to describe spontaneously what happened before asking for further information. If the child has been interviewed or interrogated before, the child may need several sessions before feeling comfortable with the examiner. Before the end of the assessment, the examiner needs to ask the child to reflect on the statements made (Nurcombe 1986; Yates 1990). "Did that really take place or is that something that you think might have happened?" or "Are you sure that is what really happened?" are ways in which the examiner can let the child know that accuracy is important. On the other hand, the examiner must be careful not to seem critical, judgmental, or confrontative; this could distort or impede the flow of information. The evaluation sessions should be taped whenever possible. The taping may obviate the need for additional assessments, and it may be used as evidence in court.

Considerable controversy has arisen over the use of the anatomically correct dolls. Untrained but enthusiastic workers have used the dolls to "grill" the children. The dolls need to be employed like other dolls and puppets in the playroom: to help children express themselves. They should be placed with the other toys, fully clothed, and the child should be allowed to explore the playroom and to choose freely among the play materials. Objective evaluations are obtained when the child spontaneously plays out or talks about sexual happenings. The examiner may then use the dolls to clarify or to help the child expand on the material (Yates 1988).

Following the individual interviews, the examiner may wish to observe the child with each of the parents. This is especially important if one of the parents has been accused of sexually abusing the child by the other parent in the context of a custody dispute. If the accusation is accurate, the child is likely to abreact or become silent when in the company of the abusive parent. If the accusation is inaccurate, the child is more likely to relate positively to the parent.

Intervention

When a parent is accused of sexually abusing a child, the first consideration is to protect the child. It is less harmful to the child if the parent who is suspected of the abuse leaves the home and the rest of the family remains intact. Unfortunately, there are many instances in which the child or children are removed from the home, abruptly and without any clear indication of when they will be returned. The identified child may be pressured by family members to recant, may be interrogated and evaluated many times, and may eventually be called to testify in court. These experiences have various consequences: some children are relieved and feel protected, whereas others are more devastated by the intervention than they were by the abuse. Some children are torn between their anger at, and love for, the abusive parent.

Therapy

Family, group, and individual therapies may be used singly or in combination to treat sexually abused children. The family approach described by Giarretto (1982) is especially useful when reunification is the goal. Groups for sexually abused children or adolescents are especially useful for support and redefinition in the immediate postdiscovery period. Individual therapy may be necessary if the child is severely disturbed or dysfunctional. Reconstructive individual therapy may be necessary to enable children who have been involved in long-term intrafamilial abuse to form relationships that are not based on (or in reaction to) the abusive relationship. In this case, the therapist's sex should be the same as that of the perpetrator.

Questions to Be Addressed

There are many more questions about sexual abuse than there are answers. The influence of family disruption, dysfunction, and rejection on outcome needs to be assessed. The role of the child's perception of the molestation, the child's ego functions, and the child's sense of mastery in preventing or ameliorating damage need to be determined. The effect of the family's expectation that the child will be damaged needs to be investigated. The effect of the prevention programs on normal sexual development also needs to be considered.

References

Bagley C, Ramsey R: Sexual abuse in childhood: psychosocial outcomes and implications for social work. Social Work in Human Sexuality 4:33–48, 1986

Benedek E: Children and psychic trauma: a brief review of contemporary thinking, in Post-Traumatic Stress Disorder in Children. Edited by Eth S, Pynoos RS. Washington, DC, American Psychiatric Press, 1985, pp 1–16

Benedek EP, Schetky DH: Problems in validating allegations of sexual abuse, II: clinical evaluation. J Am Acad Child Adolesc Psychiatry 26:916–921, 1987

Browning D, Boatman B: Incest: children at risk. Am J Psychiatry 134:69–72, 1977

Conte JR, Schuerman JR: Factors associated with an increased impact of child sexual abuse. Child Abuse Negl 11:201–211, 1987

Davies R: Some neuropsychiatric findings. Int J Psychiatry Med 9:115–121, 1979

Everstine DS, Everstine LE: Sexual Trauma in Children and Adolescents. New York, Brunner/Mazel, 1989

Faller KC: Child Sexual Abuse: An Interdisciplinary Manual for Diagnosis, Case Management and Treatment. New York, Columbia University Press, 1988

Faller KC: Characteristics of a clinical sample of sexually abused children: how boy and girl victims differ. Child Abuse Negl 13:281–291, 1989

Finkelhor DH: Sexually Victimized Children. New York, Free Press, 1979

Finkelhor D: The sexual abuse of boys. Victimology 6:76–84, 1981

Finkelhor D: Child Sexual Abuse: New Theory and Research. New York, Free Press, 1984

Finkelhor D: The sexual abuse of children: current research reviewed. Psychiatric Annals 17:233–241, 1987

Finkelhor D, Browne A: Initial and long-term effects: conceptual framework, in Sourcebook on Child Sexual Abuse. Edited by Finkelhor D. Beverly Hills, CA, Sage, 1986, pp 180–198

Finkelhor D, Hotaling G, Lewis IA, et al: Sexual abuse in a national survey of adult men and women: prevalence, characteristics, and risk factors. Child Abuse Negl 14:19–28, 1990

Franklin R: Incest in the middle class differs from that processed by the police. Clinical Psychiatry News, March 1974

Freeman-Longo RE: The impact of sexual victimization on males. Child Abuse Negl 10:411–414, 1986

Fritz GS, Stoll K, Wagner NN: A comparison of males and females who were sexually molested as children. J Sex Marital Ther 7:54–59, 1981

Fromuth ME, Burkhart BR: Childhood sexual victimization among college men: definitional and methodological issues. Violence and Victims 2:241–253, 1987

Fromuth ME, Burkhart BR: Long-term psychological correlates of childhood sexual abuse in two samples of college men. Child Abuse Negl 13:533–542, 1989

Gagnon JH: Female child victims of sex offenses. Social Problems 13:176, 1965

Gagnon JH, Simon W: Sexual Conduct. Chicago, IL, Aldine Publishing, 1973

Gebhard P: The acquisition of basic sex information. Journal of Sex Research 13:148–169, 1977

Gebhard P, Gagnon J, Pomeroy W, et al: Sex Offenders: An Analysis of Types. New York, Harper & Row, 1965

Gelinas D: The persisting negative effects of incest. Psychiatry 46:312–332, 1983

Giarretto H: A comprehensive child abuse sexual treatment program. Child Abuse Negl 6:263–278, 1982

Goodwin J: Post-traumatic symptoms in incest victims, in Post-Traumatic Stress Disorder in Children. Edited by Eth S, Pynoos RS. Washington, DC, American Psychiatric Press, 1985, pp 155–168

Goodwin J, Sahd D, Rada R: Incest hoax: false accusations, false denials. Bull Am Acad Psychiatry Law 6:269–276, 1979

Goodwin J, McCarty T, DiVasto P: Physical and sexual abuse of the children of adult incest victims, in Sexual Abuse: Incest Victims and Their Families. Edited by Goodwin J. Boston, MA, John Wright-PSC, 1982, pp 139–154

Groth AN, Freeman-Longo R: Men Who Rape: The Psychology of the Offender. New York, Plenum, 1979

Herman J: Father-Daughter Incest. Cambridge, MA, Harvard University Press, 1981

Hibbard RA, Roghmann K, Hoekelman RA: Genitalia in children's drawings: an association with sexual abuse. Pediatrics 79:129–137, 1987

Jackson S: Demons and innocents: Western ideas on children's sexuality in historical perspective, in Handbook of Sexology, Vol 7: Childhood and Adolescent Sexology. Edited by Perry ME. Amsterdam, Elsevier, 1990, pp 23–49

Johnson TC: Female child perpetrators: children who molest other children. Child Abuse Negl 13:571–585, 1989

Kinsey A, Pomeroy W, Martin C, et al: Sexual Behavior in the Human Female. Philadelphia, PA, WB Saunders, 1953

Knopp FH: Introduction, in Treating the Young Male Victim of Sexual Assault: Issues and Intervention Strategies. Edited by Porter E. Syracuse, NY, Safer Society Press, 1986

Kolko DJ, Moser JT, Weldy SR: Behavioral/emotional indicators of sexual abuse in child psychiatric inpatients: a controlled comparison with physical abuse. Child Abuse Negl 12:529–541, 1988

Landis JT: Experiences of 500 children with adult sexual deviation. Psychiatr Q Suppl 30:91–109, 1956

Lustig N, Dresser J, Spellman S, et al: Incest. Arch Gen Psychiatry 14:31–40, 1966

Meiselman K: Incest: A Psychological Study of Causes and Effects With Treatment Recommendations. San Francisco, CA, Jossey-Bass, 1978

Mrazek P, Lynch M, Bentovim A: Recognition of child sexual abuse in the United Kingdom, in Sexually Abused Children and Their Families. Edited by Mrazek P, Kempe H. New York, Pergamon, 1981, pp 134–171

Nasjleti M: Suffering in silence: the male incest victim. Child Welfare 59:269–275, 1980

National Center for Child Abuse and Neglect: Study Findings: National Study of Incidence and Severity of Child Abuse and Neglect. Washington, DC, National Center for Child Abuse and Neglect, 1981

Nurcombe B: The child as witness: competency and credibility. Journal of the American Academy of Child Psychiatry 25:473–480, 1986

Parker S, Parker H: Father-daughter sexual child abuse: an emerging perspective. Am J Orthopsychiatry 56:531–549, 1986

Peters JJ: Children who are victims of sexual assault and the psychology of offenders. Am J Psychother 30:398–421, 1976

Pierce R, Pierce LH: The sexually abused child: a comparison of male and female victims. Child Abuse Negl 9:191–199, 1985

Porter E (ed): Treating the Young Male Victim of Sexual Assault: Issues and Intervention Strategies. Syracuse, NY, The Safer Society Press, 1986

Renshaw D: Incest: Understanding and Treatment. Boston, MA, Little, Brown, 1982

Rush F: The Best Kept Secret: Sexual Abuse of Children. New York, McGraw-Hill, 1980

Schetky D, Green A: Child Sexual Abuse: A Handbook for Health Care and Legal Professionals. New York, Brunner/Mazel, 1988

Sgroi S: Handbook of Clinical Intervention in Child Sexual Abuse. Lexington, MA, Lexington Books, 1982

Swanson L, Biaggio M: Therapeutic perspectives on father-daughter incest. Am J Psychiatry 142:667–674, 1985

Terr LC: The child psychiatrist and the child witness: traveling companions of necessity, if not by design. Journal of the American Academy of Child Psychiatry 25:462–472, 1986

Thornberg H: A cooperative study of sex education sources. J Sch Health 62:88–91, 1972

Vander Mey BJ: The sexual victimization of male children: review of previous research. Child Abuse Negl 12:61–72, 1988

Weinberg K: Incest Behavior. New York, Citadel Press, 1955

Weiner I: Father-daughter incest. Psychiatr Q 36:607–632, 1962

Widom CS: Sampling biases and implications for child abuse research. Am J Orthopsychiatry 58:260–269, 1988

Yates A: Children eroticized by incest. Am J Psychiatry 139:482–485, 1982

Yates A: Psychological damage associated with extreme eroticism in young children. Psychiatric Annals 17:257–261, 1987

Yates A: Anatomically correct dolls: should they be used as the basis for expert testimony? J Am Acad Child Adolesc Psychiatry 27:387–388, 1988

Yates A: False and mistaken allegations of sexual abuse, in American Psychiatric Press Review of Psychiatry, Vol 10. Edited by Tasman A, Goldfinger SM. Washington, DC, American Psychiatric Press, 1991, pp 320–335

Yates A, Musty T: Erroneous allegations of molestation by preschool children. Am J Psychiatry 145:989–992, 1988

Chapter 46

Acquired Immunodeficiency Syndrome

Myron L. Belfer, M.D.
Kerim Munir, M.B.,B.S., M.P.H.

Acquired immunodeficiency syndrome (AIDS) is regarded by many as the most serious health threat confronting the United States (Fineberg 1988). Children (less than 13 years old) and adolescents (13–19 years old) have accounted for only 1%–2% of cases of AIDS reported to the Centers for Disease Control (CDC) (1990). The Public Health Service estimates suggest that by 1991 there will be more than 3,000 reported cases of children with AIDS and an estimated 10,000 children infected with the human immunodeficiency virus type 1 (HIV-1) (American Public Health Association 1989).

Pediatric AIDS (<13 years of age) occurs in three main groups: 1) behavior risk group—children born to mothers who are intravenous (IV) drug users and/or the sexual partners of HIV-infected males (81% of all pediatric cases); 2) transfusion or coagulation factor risk group—children infected pre-1985 by transfusions of contaminated blood, blood products, or clotting factors (16% of all pediatric cases); and 3) undetermined risk group (3% of all pediatric cases). Adolescent AIDS (13–19 years old) is categorized in three main groups: 1) behavior risk group—adolescents infected through high-risk sexual contact or IV drug use (75% of all adolescent cases); 2) transfusion or coagulation factor risk group—adolescents who have acquired AIDS

through transfusion of infected blood, blood products, or clotting factors (20% of all adolescent cases); and 3) undetermined risk group (5% of all adolescent cases).

As the number of AIDS cases increases and the illness becomes a more long-term medical care issue, child and adolescent mental health providers will need to be increasingly knowledgeable about HIV disease, to be trained to counsel individuals and families about possible exposure, and to provide the longer-term psychiatric care of the individuals living with a chronic illness as treatments prolong life.

AIDS in children and adolescents is preventable (Allen and Curran 1988). This provides a special challenge to child psychiatrists and others to be involved in prevention efforts aimed at high-risk parents, children, and adolescents. The key to interrupting HIV-1 transmission in young children and adolescents is the understanding and modification of the behaviors that put them at risk. The social conditions that sustain the epidemic of AIDS in children and adolescents include poor education, inadequate access to health and social services, homelessness, illicit drug use, poor attitudes about sexual responsibility, sexual abuse, and teenage prostitution (American Public Health Association 1989).

There now is a growing body of knowledge on the psychosocial and neuropsychological aspects of HIV-1 infection in children and adolescents. In this chapter, we review the relevant published reports on the clinical and the psychosocial epidemiology of HIV-1 disease in children and in

This work was presented, in part, at the 141st annual meeting of the American Psychiatric Association, Montreal, Canada, May 1988 and supported by National Institute of Mental Health Child and Adolescent Mental Health Academic Award MH-000826-01.

adolescents. The developmental and neuro-psychological aspects of HIV-1 disease in children are also reviewed since this is increasingly important for all professionals specializing in child and adolescent mental health. Finally, the prospects for and obstacles to AIDS education and prevention targeted for children and adolescents are discussed along with specialized care programs.

Definition

The CDC definition (Centers for Disease Control 1987) is based on three essential criteria: 1) history of a risk factor associated with AIDS, 2) laboratory evidence of immunodeficiency, and 3) evidence of HIV-1 infection. Multiple or recurrent bacterial infections and lymphoid interstitial pneumonia and pulmonary lymphoid hyperplasia are accepted as indicative of AIDS in children, but not among adults. For children less than 15–18 months of age whose mothers are thought to have had HIV-1 infection during the child's perinatal period, the laboratory criteria for HIV-1 infection are different, since the presence of HIV-1 antibodies in the child may represent the persistence of the passively acquired maternal antibodies (Ammann 1987; Rogers et al. 1989; Rubinstein 1986).

The incubation period, or the time from transmission to first detectable clinical disease, appears to be relatively shorter in children with intrauterine transmission than in adults (Auger et al. 1988). The data taken from the New York City and New York State case registries suggest that there may be two incubation period distributions: 1) short incubation period (median, 4.1 months) and 2) long incubation period (median, 6.1 years). The longer incubation period is comparable to that of 8.0 years previously reported for adolescents and adults. The long incubation periods also suggest that there is a large population of children who are maternally infected but who have not yet been diagnosed (Auger et al. 1988).

Pediatric AIDS

Incidence

As of February 1990, a cumulative total of 2,055 pediatric AIDS cases (less than 13 years old) has been reported in the United States in the following exposure categories: 1) 1,675 (82%) born to mothers who are with/at risk for AIDS/HIV infection; 2) 217 (11%) recipients of blood, blood components, or tissue; 3) 108 (5%) hemophilia/coagulation disorder; and 4) 55 (3%) undetermined. Of the total pediatric AIDS cases, 84% have been reported since 1985, 54% have died, and 82% were less than 5 years old. The incidence of pediatric AIDS has doubled annually since the beginning of the epidemic and shows no signs of slowing. In 1988, 1 of every 61 newborns in New York City was seropositive, with 1,000 such children born (*New York Times* 1989). Of all the pediatric AIDS cases at this writing, 50% have been reported from New York City; Newark, New Jersey; and Miami, Florida, and 84% have been reported from metropolitan areas (Des Jarlais and Friedland 1987; Friedland et al. 1985, 1987). The overall HIV-1 seroprevalence rate in New York State between November 30, 1987, and November 30, 1988, was 0.66% (1,816 newborns out of 276,609 births). The seroprevalence was 0.16% in upper New York State and 1.25% in New York City, the rates of seropositivity being highest in blacks (1.8%) and Hispanics (1.3%) compared with whites (0.13%) (Landesman and Willoughby 1989; Landesman et al. 1987; Novick et al. 1989).

Black and Hispanic children are more likely than white children to have IV drug-using mothers or mothers who were spouses or partners of IV drug users (Center for Disease Control 1989). The incidence rate in children of IV drug users is 12 times higher among black children and 9 times higher among Hispanic children than among white children (Centers for Disease Control 1986, 1989; Des Jarlais and Friedman 1987; Drucker 1986).

Transmission Categories

Parent with/at risk for HIV-1. The vertical transmission of HIV-1 to infants of seropositive women occurs by three possible routes: 1) in utero, through maternal-fetal circulation (Lapointe et al. 1985; Marion et al. 1986); 2) perinatal, during labor and delivery by exposure to mother's blood (Macchi et al. 1986; Pyun et al. 1987); and 3) postnatal, through infected breast milk, as suggested by case reports (Weinbreck et al. 1988; Ziegler et al. 1985) and by the high seroprevalence of HIV-1 in breast milk of seropositive mothers (Thiry et al. 1985). Many issues related to maternal-fetal transmission still remain poorly understood (Johnson et al. 1989; Ochs 1989). In utero transmission is the predominant route, and breast milk transmission is thought to be rare (Eichberg et al. 1988). The timing of infection has obvious relevance to interventions such as abortion, cesarean delivery, and withholding of breast milk.

Studies of HIV-1 seropositive pregnant women have reported perinatal transmission rates as high as 30%–50% (Blanche et al. 1989; European Collaborative Study 1988; Lallemant et al. 1989). It has been estimated that one-third of HIV-1 positive infants will have HIV-1 infection and/or AIDS by the age of 18 months and about one-fifth of this group will have died (Blanche et al. 1989; Pizzo et al. 1989). The longer incubation period of HIV-1 infection in some children may contribute to an underestimation of the mother-child transmission rate.

Blood transfusion. Screening of donated blood and plasma, heat treatment of clotting factor concentrates, and donor screening were begun in April 1985. These methods reduced the risk associated with transfused blood products from 1 in 100,000 to 1 in 1,000,000 transfused unit of blood (Centers for Disease Control 1985b). As of February 1990, the distribution of transfusion-acquired AIDS in children (less than 13 years old) was 56% white, 23% black, and 20% Hispanic (Centers for Disease Control 1990).

Hemophilia/coagulation disorder. The impact of AIDS in the hemophiliac population has been devastating (Hilgartner 1987; Roberts 1989). The seroprevalence of HIV-1 infection is high in patients with severe hemophilia. As of this writing, 58% of hemophiliac children have been infected. The seroprevalence of HIV-1 infection among the childbearing-age spouses or partners of hemophiliacs is also high, ranging from 15% to 18%. Despite the high HIV-1 seroprevalence, a smaller number of children with hemophilia than adults have progressed to AIDS (20% of HIV-1 adults versus 4% of HIV-1 children) (Hilgartner 1987). Child's age at the time of HIV infection is an important factor in identifying susceptibility and relatively long-term AIDS-free survival. The distribution of coagulation-factor–acquired AIDS cases in children (less than 13 years of age) is similar to that in transfusion-acquired cases: 72% white, 12% black, and 14% Hispanic (Centers for Disease Control 1990).

Clinical Classification of HIV-1 Infection in Children

Children can be clinically categorized using the following modification of the CDC's classification system for HIV-1 infection: 1) asymptomatic children with true infection status indeterminate; 2) moderate illness: symptomatic children except those with opportunistic infections (e.g., children with nonspecific disease manifestations, lymphoid interstitial pneumonitis, progressive neurologic disease, or recurrent bacterial infections); and 3) severe illness: children with opportunistic infections (e.g., *Pneumocystis carinii* pneumonia, disseminated cytomegalovirus, or pulmonary candidiasis).

Clinical Picture

The most common presentation of AIDS in young children is failure to thrive, with loss of developmental milestones. Fever, recurrent bacterial infections (pneumonia, septicemia, meningitis, or cellulitis), *Pneumocystis carinii* pneumonia or other opportunistic infections, chronic unexplained diarrhea, persistent oral candidiasis, and wasting also occur commonly (McLoughlin et al. 1987; Parks and Scott 1987). Other symptoms include lymphadenopathy (greater than 1 cm) at two or more noncontiguous sites, hepatomegaly, splenomegaly, recurrent otitis media, parotitis, or evidence of neuroencephalopathy (Pawha et al. 1986).

Compared with adults, children are much more commonly subject to recurrent and severe bacterial infections, with *Streptococcus* pneumonia, *Haemophilus* influenza, and salmonella reflecting a B-cell abnormality early in the course of HIV-1 infection (Andiman et al. 1985; Bernstein et al. 1985). Although T-cell abnormalities similar to those in adults also occur in children, lymphopenia tends to occur later in the course of infection. Lymphocytic interstitial pneumonitis, rare among adults, occurs in nearly half the cases in children (Joshi and Oleske 1986). *Pneumocystis carinii* pneumonia is one of the most common opportunistic infections in children, whereas Kaposi's sarcoma, a common malignancy in adults with AIDS, is exceedingly rare in children (Ammann 1987; Parks and Scott 1987).

HIV-1 can directly infect cells in the central nervous system (CNS) (Barnes 1986; Ho et al. 1985; Shaw et al. 1985). CNS manifestations of AIDS in children include motor dysfunction, encephalopathy, meningitis, seizures, and neoplastic involvement (Ammann 1987; Rogers et al. 1987). The latter includes primary CNS lymphomas, systemic lymphomas invading the meninges, and cerebral metastases secondary to Kaposi's sarcoma, otherwise very rare in children. An embryopathy attributed to in utero HIV-1 infection has been described consisting of microcephaly, prominent boxlike forehead, flattened nasal bridge, wide palpebral fissures, obliquity of the eyes, hypertelorism, blue sclerae, and patulous lips (Iosub et al. 1987; Marion et al. 1986). Others have not confirmed the presence of craniofacial dysmorphism in children exposed to intrauterine HIV-1 (Qazi et al. 1987), and the possibility of HIV-1-related dysmorphism is now abandoned by many clinicians. Neurologic symptoms or evidence of encephalopathy related to HIV-1 infection have consistently been noted in about 65% of children with HIV-1 (Ammann 1987; Pizzo et al. 1988). A devastating complication is neuropsychological deterioration characterized by progressive loss of developmental milestones and cognitive functioning (Belman et al. 1988). Apathy and psychomotor retardation may also be presentations of HIV-1 infection in young children.

Medical Assessment and Treatment

The enzyme-linked immunosorbent assay tests are run in duplicate on initially positive or borderline sera, with confirmation tests of positive results performed by Western blot test (Pizzo et al. 1988). Other tests include positive HIV-1 viral cultures or the polymerase chain reaction technique (Pezzela et al. 1989; Rogers et al. 1989). The laboratory findings include hypergammaglobinemia; decreased number of T lymphocytes or of CD4 helper cells, or both; reversed CD4/CD8 ratio; or cutaneous anergy. Nonfocal diffuse slowing on electroencephalogram, slight elevation of protein and cell count in cerebrospinal fluid, and cortical atrophy, ventricular dilation, or basal ganglia calcification in imaging studies may be associated findings.

To date, management of HIV-1 infection in children has been limited to supportive care (e.g., nutrition, passive immunization, and antibiotic therapy). As has been the case in adults with AIDS, there is evidence that treatment with the antiretroviral drug zidovudine (Retrovir or AZT) reduces morbidity in children under 13 years of age, especially in those with AIDS encephalopathy (Pizzo et al. 1988). The prognosis of intrauterine HIV-1

infected infants, especially those with clinical disease at age less than 6 months, is invariably poor (Novick and Rubinstein 1987).

Psychological Assessments

Comprehensive neuropsychological assessments appropriate to the child's age or stage of development are essential. These should include measures of general ability, adaptive behavior, language, attention, memory, and learning as well as visual and perceptual abilities and problem solving. HIV-related neuropsychological syndromes are difficult to recognize in the early stages of infection (Nurnberg et al. 1984; Perry and Jacobsen 1986). Infants and children born to IV drug-using mothers are likely to have developmental delays irrespective of HIV-1 infection; therefore, documentation of progressive loss of milestones (or a drop in psychometric scores) is important.

Psychiatric Aspects

The psychological reactions of young children with AIDS are comparable to those seen in children with catastrophic medical illness or cancer. Although features such as anxiety, sadness, nightmares, irritability, and "battle fatigue," depending on duration and severity of the disease and its treatment, are common, young children with AIDS face a unique set of adverse conditions. These include: 1) presence of physical illness in major attachment figure(s) (i.e., presence of AIDS in a parent); 2) current and past positive family history of psychiatric illness in parent(s) (e.g., substance abuse, depression, HIV-related organic brain disorders); 3) major life event(s) (e.g., death of a parent, foster care placement); and 4) poverty and social alienation.

Children who are old enough to attend school may experience estrangement, avoidance, and rejection by peers; disfiguring effects of wasting; ensuing lesions; and the complications of treatment. These burdens extend to their most intimate relationships at home, at school, and among peers and are exaggerated by the extreme uncertainty that characterizes the entire process.

In cases of perinatal AIDS, the emotions in the transmitting parent also have a significant impact on the child and range from his or her own fear of the disease, to guilt of passing on the virus to the child, and to the anger and shame of being a victim. These feelings are compounded by the uncertainty, until the age of 15 months, that an antibody-positive child may be truly infected. Quality of parental care and availability of substitute care by relatives or by friends are likely to be protective of the psychological well-being of children in such families.

Since early treatment, supportive care, and nutritional supplementation are considered essential in prolonging the quality and length of survival in perinatal AIDS, extraordinary efforts are necessary to avail and maintain them in treatment (Centers for Disease Control 1985a). It is important to encourage a therapeutic alliance with a key caregiver; to establish support teams, including counselors and social workers who will follow the family throughout the vicissitudes of illness; and to provide institutional care sensitive to the needs of these patients. Older siblings without HIV infection face the prospect of multiple losses of family members to AIDS and therefore need counseling as well as placement with other family members, friends, or foster parents. In some instances, the older siblings become the primary caregivers, with all the attendant problems faced by young parents and compounded by their own experience of loss.

Clinical Programs

There is a need to provide comprehensive and interdisciplinary care using case management to address medical and social needs and to ensure adequate health care financing and access to services and flexible responsiveness to needs of all children and families (Association for the Care of Children's Health 1989). Outside the hospital setting where multidisciplinary neonatal and infant nurseries are being established, a variety of foster care, day care, and home support programs for children with AIDS are being developed. The quality of parent involvement, parental health, and retention of staff in these intense settings are critical issues. The psychiatrists, along with other mental health professionals, have an important role to play in providing support, identifying depression, facilitating bonding, and treating the psychiatric sequelae in parents, children, and caregivers.

In areas where there has been effective preparation in the community and school by educators and mental health professionals, integration of children into schools has been possible. Where there has not been receptivity, children have been ex-

cluded and have become homebound. In these instances, limited tutoring and restricted activities have invariably isolated the children. Some unique activity-based programs sponsored by medical facilities treating children have helped to maintain a degree of socialization. Although special care centers are designed to meet the specific needs of HIV-1 infected children, they are not needed for reasons of infection control, nor should they become a means to segregate infected children.

Parents of children in day care centers or schools are not deemed to have the right to information regarding the HIV-1 status of other children. The decision to return to school should be based on the physical condition, development, and behavior of the child and the child's expected interaction with others as well as the overall risks and benefits to the child and others (American Academy of Pediatrics 1989).

Adolescent AIDS

Incidence

Adolescents at highest risk of HIV-1 infection are disenfranchised inner-city youths who use drugs and engage in unprotected sexual intercourse (heterosexual and homosexual) (Deisher et al. 1989; Eisenberg 1988; Hein 1989; Vermund et al. 1989). As of February 1990, a total of 504 adolescent AIDS cases (13–19 years old) have been reported to the CDC. If adolescents and young adults 13–21 years old are grouped together, they account for 1.2% of the total number of AIDS cases in the United States. Of the 380 male cases, 51% were white, 29% were black, and 18% were Hispanic. On the other hand, of the 124 female cases, 60% were black, 20% were white, and 18% were Hispanic. The statewide and CDC surveillance data invariably underreport cases, particularly from low HIV-1 seroprevalence regions. The incidence rate may be underestimated in view of the competing risks for mortality from accidents, homicide, and suicide, which although relatively rare may be proportionally high among those adolescents at most risk for HIV-1 infection.

The frequency of AIDS in the adolescent age group rises with increasing age. There are as many AIDS cases reported for young adults ages 20–21 as for adolescents ages 13–20. Given the long incubation period (greater than 8 years), it seems likely that many AIDS cases in the 20–29 years old age category acquired the infection during their adolescence.

Among adolescents with AIDS, there is a higher proportion of females than among adults with AIDS. The ratio of male-to-female adolescent cases is 3:1 in New York City and 7:1 in the United States (excluding New York City). The comparable adult male-to-female ratios are 7:1 in New York City and 15:1 in the United States (excluding New York City) (Vermund et al. 1989).

Transmission Categories

The data on adolescent AIDS cases reported to CDC by state health departments are grouped with adult AIDS cases into one of six transmission categories: 1) male homosexual or bisexual activity, 2) male homosexual or bisexual activity and IV drug use, 3) IV drug use, 4) heterosexual activity, 5) receipt of a transfusion of blood, blood products, or coagulation factors, and 6) other or unknown behavior (Vermund et al. 1989).

More than half of adolescent male AIDS cases reported homosexual contact, irrespective of whether they were from New York City or from the remainder of the United States; however, adolescents with AIDS are less likely than adults with AIDS to have acquired the infection by male homosexual activity. Heterosexual transmission accounts for 9% of all adolescent AIDS cases compared with 4% among all adult cases. About half of all adolescent female AIDS cases are reported to be from heterosexual transmission. The comparable figure for males is 2% for both adolescents and adults.

Adolescents are less likely than adults to have acquired AIDS by IV drug use. IV drug use is more frequently reported among adolescents with AIDS from New York City (23%) than adolescents outside New York City (14%). Among males, a history of IV drug use (with or without history of homosexual activity) is reported in 16% of adolescent AIDS cases in New York City, compared with 4% of adolescent AIDS cases for the remainder of the United States. The current cocaine epidemic among inner-city youth is occurring in the same urban centers with the highest seroprevalence of HIV infection. Cocaine may be used intravenously and is associated with disinhibition, unsafe sexual practices, and prostitution (Fullilove et al. 1990).

The transfusion group primarily includes adolescents who received transfusion of blood, blood products, or clotting factors prior to spring of 1985, when HIV-1 screening began in the United States (Centers for Disease Control 1985b). The incidence of AIDS in hemophiliac adolescents is nearly two times lower than in adults (Goedert et al. 1989).

Psychiatric Aspects

Preexisting or co-occurring high rates of mental disorders, high incidence of HIV-1-related neurologic and psychiatric syndromes, psychosocial stress, and negative societal reactions are common accompaniments of AIDS in adolescent populations. The neuropsychological effects of HIV-1 infection in adolescents have not been studied separately from those in adults. AIDS dementia complex associated with primary HIV-1 infection of the brain is likely to be a leading cause of cognitive, motor, and behavioral impairment (Grant et al. 1987; Navia et al. 1986). Initial complaints may include poor concentration and impairment of short-term memory and coordination. The psychological and behavioral symptoms may precede the sensory and motor neurologic deficits. As in adults, organic brain syndromes caused by HIV-1 infection (Beckett et al. 1987; Ostrow et al. 1988) may mimic functional psychiatric disorders, such as major depression (Faulstich 1987), paranoid or schizophreniform psychosis (Thomas and Szabaldi 1987), mania (Gabel et al. 1986), or obsessive-compulsive disorder (Fenton 1987; Nurnberg et al. 1984; Perry and Jacobsen 1986; Rundell et al. 1986).

The increased relative risk of suicide, either as an acute reaction to the distress of being informed about the infection or as a consequence of HIV-1-related psychiatric disorder (e.g., depression), has been documented in young males (ages 20–39 years) in New York City and California (Kizer 1988; Marzuk et al. 1988). Adolescents at risk for acquiring HIV-1 infection are also likely to be at high risk for suicide, stressing the need for vigilant psychiatric follow-up. This is particularly relevant among adolescent males, ages 15–19 years, since suicide represents the second most frequent cause of death in this age group (Brent et al. 1988; Shaffer 1988) and high rates of affective disorder, antisocial behavior, and substance abuse also co-occur.

The decision to admit HIV-1-infected children and adolescents to a psychiatric hospital rests with the child and adolescent psychiatrist and members of the treatment team, weighing the hospital's ability to manage the specific psychiatric condition and to ensure both the child's safety and that of other patients (American Academy of Child and Adolescent Psychiatry 1989). It is recommended that HIV-1 testing (with pre- and post-test counseling) should be reserved for those patients with risk factors for infection and done with written informed consent of the parent(s) or guardian(s).

Clinical Programs

Adolescents are particularly challenging to provide programming for because of limited information on HIV-1-infected gay youth, street youth, and youth in institutions (DiClemente et al. 1988; Goodman and Cohall 1989; Hein 1989). Unfortunately, much needs to be done because of the vulnerability of this group, the stigmatization, and often the lack of social, emotional, economic, and cognitive resources (Cates and Bowen 1989). HIV-1/AIDS identification and treatment efforts for adolescents will need to be closely linked to drug treatment programs, family planning, sexually transmitted diseases and perinatal clinics, programs for runaway and homeless youth, child protective services, and the juvenile courts.

Prevention

Risk Behaviors

Efforts to control HIV-1 infection in children and adolescents involve focusing on at-risk sexual behavior and needle sharing among IV drug users, as well as addressing a number of complex issues, including adolescent at-risk sexual behaviors, substance abuse, pregnancy, homelessness, prostitution, urban poverty, inadequate social services, poor education, and deficient health care services. As of this writing, there are no consistently effective means for altering the behaviors that relate to the most common modes of HIV-1 transmission: unprotected sexual intercourse (heterosexual and homosexual) and IV drug use (Eisenberg 1988).

There are parallels between the risk factors for teenage pregnancy and adolescent risk factors for transmission of HIV-1 infection: minority status, low socioeconomic status, low educational attainment, and history of poor family relationships (Maciak et al. 1987; Zuckerman et al. 1984). The United States leads the industrialized world in the rates of teenage pregnancy, abortion, and birth (Westoff et al. 1983). Continued efforts aimed both at delaying early sexual experiences among teens and encouraging the use of contraception are necessary to reduce the pregnancy rate and risk of HIV-1 seroconversion in teenagers.

Intensified efforts to identify infected infants as early as possible have two important implications: earlier treatment, which could improve the survival rates of infected infants, and earlier diagnosis of maternal infection, which could allow preventive intervention and reduce possible HIV transmission. Seropositive children are assumed to be infected unless they become seronegative; they require vigilant follow-up and need to have a low threshold for medical hospitalization.

Information about adolescent sexuality in general, and the extent of homosexual experiences in adolescence in particular, is derived from studies of adults retrospectively recalling their adolescent experiences (Remafedi 1987). Of adolescents ages 16–19, 17% of males report at least one homosexual experience (Sorensen 1973). Since the incidence of high-risk sexual experiences increases with age, it has been argued that outreach services for gay youth about AIDS should begin in early adolescence.

IV drug use (female and heterosexual male) represents 18% of all AIDS cases reported to the CDC (Centers for Disease Control 1989). Since IV drug-using adolescents are unlikely to respond to surveys or to attend school regularly, there are no reliable data to judge the extent of IV drug use among adolescents (McKirnan and Johnson 1986). Furthermore, crack cocaine use by adolescents is associated with impetuous sexual activity and bartering sexual services in exchange for the drug (Fullilove et al. 1990), and such adolescent risk-taking behaviors have consistently resisted preventive strategies (Robinson et al. 1986). Among high school students, cocaine abuse has slowly declined in 1989, but this trend is not representative of inner-city adolescents in high HIV-1 prevalence neighborhoods who do not attend school. Opiate use is on the increase (Johnston et al. 1987).

As of this writing, there are 900,000 homeless adolescents across the United States. This group of runaway or "throwaway" youth is characterized by multiple and often overlapping problems, including substance abuse, drug dealing, prostitution, and a history of legal and mental health interventions (Wolf 1990). High rates of other sexually transmitted diseases among them indicate their susceptibility to HIV-1 infection.

Children and adolescents who have been sexually abused or raped by HIV-1-infected individuals may themselves become infected (Gellert and Mascola 1989). Sexual abuse of children and adolescents is a serious and increasing public health problem. At least 250,000 cases of child sexual abuse are reported annually (Krugman 1986). Furthermore, a single molester or a rapist may commit an astonishingly high number of abusive acts (American Academy of Pediatrics 1988; Gellert and Mascola 1989).

Beliefs, Knowledge, and Attitudes

Children rank television, magazines, and radio as their best sources of information about AIDS (Brown and Fritz 1988). Some educational television programs are controversial in view of concerns raised by parents about possible adverse effects of such programs on young children (*Wall Street Journal* 1987). In an interview study of schoolchildren, 40% indicated that they would not touch someone with AIDS; in a telephone survey of children, 25% felt that children with AIDS should not attend school (Brown and Fritz 1988; Strunin and Hingson 1987).

Education and Prevention Programs

Efforts to intercept the AIDS epidemic rest on the development of effective health education to change the behavior that leads to disease transmission (Eisenberg 1989; Fineberg 1988; Sandberg et al. 1988). Yet educational efforts to date have been more successful in heightening awareness about AIDS than in producing sufficient changes in transmission behavior (Becker and Joseph 1988; Hingson et al. 1990).

Children are constantly evolving in their cognitive capacities, as well as their socialization and abstraction abilities. Thus any educational intervention aimed at imparting knowledge or promoting prevention must be repeated in a meaningful fashion at each evolving developmental stage. A one-time imparting of knowledge is virtually useless; sequential, reinforced teaching is needed. HIV transmission is a complex issue to communicate to young children, and very few age-appropriate materials currently exist (Foundation for Children With AIDS 1989; Fassler and McQueen 1990; Hausherr 1989; Quackenbush and Villarreal 1988, 1989). AIDS is identified as an illness and placed in the context of other known illnesses, and over time, issues of

transmission are introduced as are issues related to the transmission of other familiar illnesses. For a child with average intelligence, by age 10, educators can move beyond imparting knowledge about transmission to changing behavior. Ten-year-olds represent an important target group since, in many high-risk locales, sexual activity and substance abuse may be beginning or, more rarely, may have begun. Thus by this age, there is a small window of opportunity to address preventive education and behavior change. Soon thereafter, with the onset of adolescent risk-taking activity, emphasis must be placed on remediation rather than education or prevention.

In terms of psychological development, there needs to be a sense of self-esteem and a healthy sense of vulnerability. Unfortunately, for at-risk children and adolescents, development may already be compromised because of other realities of daily life. The conditions that place the adolescent at risk begin early and are affected by traumatic experiences. For adolescents with histories of sexual abuse or rape, information about AIDS is emotionally compounded (Gellert and Mascola 1989). Professionals who counsel sexual abuse victims remain concerned that the paucity of data on HIV-1 infection acquired through sexual abuse will delay preventive action. Historically, victims of sexual assault have been asked not to wash or douche prior to examination by a physician. A survey of Maryland hospitals has suggested that use of topical anti-HIV spermicidal agents such as nonoxynol-9 should be used as soon as possible after the assault, perhaps by the victim herself, or soon after arrival to the hospital (Foster and Bartlett 1989). The issue of HIV-1 testing should also be approached with caution in this risk group.

The knowledge of HIV-1 infection is likely to cause panic, acting-out, or suicidal behavior in some adolescents. In one study, 21% of the adolescents spontaneously reported that they would commit suicide if they had positive test results, highlighting the level of anxiety associated with the issue of testing in this age group (Goodman and Cohall 1989). Since teenagers usually have difficulty in perceiving probable future risks and think of the present in concrete terms, it may be difficult to help them understand such concepts as an incubation time that may take years before the development of AIDS (Haffner 1987).

An essential part of every preventive or educational program is to meet with a person with AIDS (Klitzner 1989). Studies have so far shown that while we can educate adolescents, we are not able to bring about comparable changes in behavior. Some of the failure results from the issue of poor self-esteem and sense of invulnerability—a "not me" attitude. Adolescents at most risk for HIV infection are those likely to see themselves as invulnerable to death or disease and those who tend to resist traditional preventive strategies.

Behavioral change in the potentially vulnerable heterosexual adolescent and young adult populations is uncommon, as is risk reduction in urban minorities (Becker and Joseph 1988). Only a few studies investigate the relationship of knowledge and attitudes to risk reduction (Fullilove et al. 1990; Hingson et al. 1990). As AIDS spreads beyond the initial risk groups, the ability to assess risk by sexual history becomes less meaningful. For adolescents and young adults, this has led some investigators to recommend use of condoms and spermicide containing nonoxynol-9 for all sexual encounters except long-standing monogamous relationships. Reduction in number and careful selection of partners are also recommended (Francis and Chin 1987; Hearst and Hulley 1988).

One encouraging finding that has emerged in some prevention programs is the increased level of worry about contracting AIDS reported by adolescents who engage in one or more high-risk behaviors. The prevention campaigns designed to reduce AIDS risk behavior need to be targeted to specific groups, coupled with widespread distribution of condoms (Fullilove et al. 1990; Hingson et al. 1990). Adolescents' sexual encounters are unplanned and often occur on the spot after drinking or drug use. Programs should help build the skills necessary for safer sex practices and should be targeted to specific, identifiable high-risk groups (Goodman and Cohall 1989; Kegeles et al. 1989; Sandberg et al. 1988). Newer programs are emphasizing peer education, peer-staffed hotlines, and other peer-related support activities accompanied by close supervision, reinforcement, and emotional support by responsible adults (Klitzner 1989).

So far, the lack of AIDS care training among psychiatrists has been of little consequence in some regions because of the low incidence of HIV infection in children and adolescents. This will change as child psychiatrists are increasingly called on in their roles as hospital, school, and day care consultants. As AIDS in children and adolescents becomes a chronic illness due to more effective, but noncurative interventions, psychiatrists as therapists are more likely to work directly with young

AIDS patients. The hospital staff caring for critically ill and/or bereaved children with AIDS are likely to feel unusually vulnerable to their own anxieties about death and failure. In the tradition of consultation services of general hospitals (Cassem 1987), psychiatrists can foster close working relationships with other hospital staff, becoming significant members of support teams in the comprehensive care of AIDS patients (Krener 1987; Krener and Miller 1989).

It is unlikely that by the time the adolescent storm of HIV infection is gathered, there will be a cure for AIDS. To date, development of a vaccine is a long-term prospect. Therefore, widespread educational and preventive programs remain the only hope of containing the epidemic. Child psychiatrists and other mental health professionals will need to be increasingly involved in this new frontier of the AIDS epidemic.

References

Allen JR, Curran JW: Prevention of AIDS and HIV infection: needs and priorities for epidemiologic research. Am J Public Health 78:381–386, 1988

American Academy of Child and Adolescent Psychiatry: Policy statement: AIDS and psychiatric hospitalization of children and adolescents. Washington, DC, American Academy of Child and Adolescent Psychiatry, June 1989

American Academy of Pediatrics: Pediatric guidelines for infection control of human immunodeficiency virus (acquired immunodeficiency virus) in hospitals, medical offices, schools, and other settings. Pediatrics 82:801–807, 1989

American Academy of Pediatrics: Rape and the adolescent. Pediatrics 81:595–597, 1988

American Public Health Association: Pediatric HIV infection: report of the special initiative on AIDS (APHA/SIA Report 6). Washington, DC, American Public Health Association, 1989

Ammann AJ: Pediatric acquired immunodeficiency syndrome. Information on AIDS for the Practicing Physician, AMA and National Council on Drugs 2:17–23, 1987

Andiman WA, Eastman R, Martin K, et al: Opportunistic lymphoproliferations associated with Epstein-Barr viral DNA in infants and children with AIDS. Lancet 2:8469–8470, 1985

Association for the Care of Children's Health: Building Systems of Care for Children with HIV Infection and Their Families. Washington, DC, Health Resources and Services Administration, Office of Maternal and Child Health, 1989

Auger I, Thomas P, De Grutolla V, et al: Incubation periods for paediatric AIDS patients. Nature 336:575–577, 1988

Barnes DM: Brain function decline in children with AIDS. Science 232:1196, 1986

Becker MH, Joseph JG: AIDS and behavioral change to reduce risk: a review. Am J Public Health 78:394–410, 1988

Beckett A, Summergrad P, Manscreck T, et al: Symptomatic HIV infection of the CNS in a patient without clinical evidence of immunodeficiency. Am J Psychiatry 144:1342–1344, 1987

Belman AL, Diamond G, Dickson D, et al: Pediatric acquired

immunodeficiency syndrome: neurologic syndromes. Am J Dis Child 149:29–35, 1988

Bernstein LJ, Krieger BZ, Novick B, et al: Bacterial infection in the acquired immunodeficiency syndrome in children. Pediatric Infectious Disease 4:472–475, 1985

Blanche S, Rouzioux C, Moscato MG, et al: A prospective study of infants born to women seropositive for human immunodeficiency virus type 1. N Engl J Med 320:1643–1648, 1989

Brent DA, Perper JA, Goldstein CE, et al: Risk factors for adolescent suicide: a comparison of adolescent suicide victims with suicidal inpatients. Arch Gen Psychiatry 45:581–588, 1988

Brown LK, Fritz GK: Children's knowledge and attitudes about AIDS. J Am Acad Child Adolesc Psychiatry 27:505–508, 1988

Cassem NH: The consultation service, in Psychiatry in a General Hospital: The First Fifty Years. Edited by Hackett TP, Weisman AD, Kucharski A. Littleton, MA, PSG Publishing Company, 1987, pp 33–39

Cates W, Bowen GS: Education for AIDS prevention: not our only voluntary weapon. Am J Public Health 79:871–874, 1989

Centers for Disease Control: Education and foster care of children infected with human T-lymphotropic virus type-III/lymphadenopathy-associated virus. MMWR 34:517–521, 1985a

Centers for Disease Control: Provisional Public Health Service inter-agency recommendations for screening donated blood and plasma for antibody to the virus causing acquired immunodeficiency syndrome. MMWR 34:5–7, 1985b

Centers for Disease Control: Acquired immunodeficiency syndrome among blacks and Hispanics: United States. MMWR 35:655–666, 1986

Centers for Disease Control: Classification system for human immunodeficiency virus (HIV) infection in children under 13 years of age. MMWR 36:225–230, 235, 1987

Centers for Disease Control: Update: acquired immunodeficiency syndrome associated with IVDU: U.S. 1988. MMWR 38:165–170, 233–235, 1989

Centers for Disease Control: HIV/AIDS Surveillance Reports, February 1990

Deisher RW, Farrow JA, Hope K, et al: The pregnant adolescent prostitute. Am J Dis Child 143:1162–1165, 1989

Des Jarlais DC, Friedman SR: HIV infection among intravenous drug users: epidemiology and risk reduction. AIDS 1:67–76, 1987

DiClement RJ, Boyer CB, Morales ES: Minorities and AIDS: knowledge, attitudes, and misconceptions among black and latino adolescents. Am J Public Health 78:55–57, 1988

Drucker E: AIDS and addiction in New York City. Am J Drug Alcohol Abuse 12:165–181, 1986

Eichberg JW, Allan JS, Cobb KE, et al: In utero transmission of an infant chimpanzee with HIV. N Engl J Med 319:722–723, 1988

Eisenberg L: Health education and the AIDS epidemic. Br J Psychiatry 154:754–767, 1989

European Collaborative Study: Mother-to-child transmission of HIV infection. Lancet 2:1039–1043, 1988

Fassler D, McQueen K: What's a Virus, Anyway? The Kids Book About AIDS. Burlington, VT, Waterfront Publications, 1990

Faulstich ME: Psychiatric aspects of AIDS. Am J Psychiatry 144:551–556, 1987

Fenton TW: AIDS-related psychiatric disorder. Br J Psychiatry 151:579–588, 1987

Fineberg HF: Education to prevent AIDS: prospects and obstacles. Science 239:592–596, 1988

Foster IM, Bartlett J: Anti-HIV substances to rape victims. JAMA 261:3407, 1989

Foundation for Children With AIDS: Children With AIDS Newsletter, Vol 1, November 1989, p 11

Francis DP, Chin J: The prevention of AIDS in the United States. JAMA 257:1357–1366, 1987

Friedland GH, Klein RS: Transmission of the human immunodeficiency virus. N Engl J Med 317:1125–1135, 1987

Friedland GH, Harris C, Butkus-Small C, et al: Intravenous drug abusers and the acquired immunodeficiency syndrome (AIDS): demographic, drug use and needle-sharing patterns. Ann Intern Med 145:1413–1417, 1985

Fullilove RE, Fullilove MT, Bowser BP, et al: Risk of sexually transmitted disease among black adolescent crack users in Oakland and San Francisco, Calif. JAMA 263:851–855, 1990

Gabel RH, Barnard N, Norko M, et al: AIDS presenting as mania. Compr Psychiatry 27:251–254, 1986

Gellert GA, Mascola L: Rape and AIDS. Pediatrics 83 (suppl):644, 1989

Goedert JJ, Kessler CM, Aledort LM, et al: A prospective study of human immunodeficiency virus type-1 infection and the development of AIDS in subjects with hemophilia. N Engl J Med 321:1141–1148, 1989

Goodman E, Cohall AT: Acquired immunodeficiency syndrome and adolescents: knowledge, attitudes, beliefs, and behaviors in a New York City adolescent minority population. Pediatrics 84:36–42, 1989

Grant I, Atkinson JH, Hesselink JR, et al: Evidence for early central nervous system involvement in the acquired immunodeficiency syndrome (AIDS) and other human immunodeficiency virus (HIV) infections: studies with neuropsychologic testing and magnetic resonance imaging. Ann Intern Med 107:828–836, 1987

Haffner DW: AIDS and adolescents: the time for prevention is now. Washington, DC, The Center for Population Options, November 1987

Hausherr R: Children and the AIDS Virus: A Book for Children, Parents & Teachers. New York, Clarion Books, 1989

Hearst N, Hulley SB: Preventing the heterosexual spread of AIDS: are we giving our patients the best advice? JAMA 259:2428–2432, 1988

Hein K: Commentary on adolescent acquired immunodeficiency syndrome: the next wave of the human immunodeficiency virus epidemic? J Pediatr 114:144–149, 1989

Hilgartner MW: AIDS and hemophilia. N Engl J Med 317:1125–1135, 1987

Hingson RW, Strunin L, Berlin B, et al: Beliefs about AIDS, use of alcohol and drugs, and unprotected sex among Massachusetts adolescents. Am J Public Health 80:295–299, 1990

Ho DD, Rota TR, Schooley RT, et al: Isolation of HTLV-III from cerebrospinal fluid and neural tissues of patients with neurological syndromes related to acquired immunodeficiency syndrome. N Engl J Med 313:1493–1497, 1985

Iosub S, Bamji M, Stone RK, et al: More on the immunodeficiency virus embryopathy. Pediatrics 80:512–516, 1987

Johnson JP, Nair P, Hines SE: Natural history and serologic diagnosis of infants born to human immunodeficiency virus infected women. Am J Dis Child 143:1147–1153, 1989

Johnston LD, O'Malley PM, Bachman JG: Drug use and related factors among American high school students and young adults: national trends, 1975–1986 (DHHS Publ No ADM-87-1535. Washington, DC, U.S. Government Printing Office, 1987)

Joshi VV, Oleske JM: Pulmonary lesions in children with the

acquired immunodeficiency syndrome: a reappraisal based on data in additional cases and follow-up study of previously reported cases. Hum Pathol 17:641–642, 1986

Kegeles SM, Adler NE, Irwin CE: Adolescents and condoms. Am J Dis Child 143:911–915, 1989

Kizer KW: AIDS and suicide in California. JAMA 260:1881, 1988

Klitzner M: AIDS prevention and education: recommendations of the work group. J Adolesc Health Care 10:45S–47S, 1989

Krener PK: Impact of the diagnosis of AIDS on hospital care of an infant. Clin Pediatr (Phila) 26:30–34, 1987

Krener P, Miller FB: Psychiatric response to HIV spectrum disease in children and adolescents. J Am Acad Child Adolesc Psychiatry 28:596–605, 1989

Krugman RD: Recognition of sexual abuse in children. Pediatr Rev 8:25–30, 1986

Lallemant M, Lallemant-Le-Coeur S, Cheynier D, et al: Mother-child transmission of HIV-1 and infant survival in Brazzaville, Congo. AIDS 3:643–646, 1989

Landesman SH, Willoughby A: HIV disease in reproductive age women: a problem of the present. JAMA 261:1326–1327, 1989

Landesman S, Minkoff H, Holman S, et al: Serosurvey of human immunodeficiency virus infection in parturients: implications for human immunodeficiency virus testing programs for pregnant women. JAMA 258:2701–2703, 1987

Lapointe N, Michand J, Pekovic D, et al: Transplacental transmission of HTLV-III virus. N Engl J Med 312:1325–1326, 1985

Macchi B, Verani P, Lazzarin A, et al: Evidence of HTLV-III/LAV intrauterine infection. Paper presented at the Second International Conference on AIDS, Paris, June 23–25, 1986

Maciak BJ, Spitz AM, Strauss LT, et al: Pregnancy and birth rates among sexually experienced U.S. teenagers—1974, 1980, 1983. JAMA 258:2069–2071, 1987

Marion RW, Wiznia AA, Hutcheon RG, et al: Human T-cell lymphotropic virus type-III (HTLV-III) embryopathy: a new dysmorphic syndrome associated with intrauterine HTLV-III infection. Am J Dis Child 140:638–640, 1986

Marzuk PM, Tierney H, Tardiff K, et al: Increased risk of suicide in persons with AIDS. JAMA 259:1333–1337, 1988

McKirnan DJ, Johnson T: Alcohol and drug use among "street" adolescents. Addict Behav 11:201–205, 1986

McLoughlin LC, Nord KS, Joshi VV, et al: Severe gastrointestinal involvement in children with the acquired immunodeficiency syndrome. J Pediatr Gastroenterol Nutr 6:517–524, 1987

Navia BA, Jordan B, Price RW: The AIDS dementia complex, I: clinical features of the AIDS dementia complex. Ann Neurol 19:525–535, 1986

New York Times: AIDS legacy: a growing generation of infants. New York Times, July 17, 1989, A1

Novick BE, Rubinstein A: AIDS: the paediatric perspective. AIDS 1:3–7, 1987

Novick LF, Berns D, Stricof R, et al: HIV seroprevalence in newborns in New York State. JAMA 261:1745–1750, 1989

Nurnberg HG, Prudic J, Fiori M, et al: Psychopathology complicating acquired immunodeficiency syndrome (AIDS). Am J Psychiatry 141:95–96, 1984

Ochs HD: The human immunodeficiency virus-infected infant (editorial). Am J Dis Child 143:1138–1139, 1989

Ostrow D, Grant I, Atkinson H: Assessment and management of the AIDS patient with neuropsychiatric disturbances. J Clin Psychiatry 49 (suppl):14–22, 1988

Parks WP, Scott CB: An overview of pediatric AIDS, in AIDS:

Modern Concepts and Therapeutic Challenges. Edited by Broder S. New York, Marcel Dekker, 1987, pp 245–262

Pawha S, Kaplan M, Fikrig S, et al: Spectrum of human T-cell lymphotropic virus type-III infection in children. JAMA 255:2299–2305, 1986

Perry S, Jacobsen P: Neuropsychiatric manifestations of AIDS-spectrum disorders. Hosp Community Psychiatry 37:135–142, 1986

Pezzela M, Rossi P, Lombardi V, et al: HIV viral sequences in seronegative people at risk detected by in situ hybridization and polymerase chain reaction. Br Med J 298:713–716, 1989

Pizzo PA, Eddy J, Falloon J, et al: Effect of continuous intravenous infusion of zidovudine (AZT) in children with symptomatic HIV infection. N Engl J Med 319:889–896, 1988

Pyun KH, Ochs HD, Dufford MTW, et al: Perinatal infection with human immunodeficiency virus: specific antibody responses by the neonate. N Engl J Med 317:611–614, 1987

Qazi QH, Sheikh TM, Fikrig S, et al: Lack of evidence for craniofacial dysmorphism in perinatal human immunodeficiency virus infection. J Pediatr 112:7–11, 1987

Quackenbush M, Villarreal S: Does AIDS Hurt? Educating Young Children About AIDS. Santa Cruz, CA, Network Publications, 1988

Quackenbush M, Villarreal S: Talking about AIDS with young children: focus, AIDS Health Project. San Francisco, CA, University of California, March 1989

Remafedi G: Homosexual youth: a challenge to contemporary society. JAMA 258:222–225, 1987

Roberts HR: The treatment of hemophilia: past tragedy and future promise. N Engl J Med 321:1188–1189, 1989

Robinson TN, Killen JD, Taylor B, et al: Perspectives on adolescent substance use: a defined population study. JAMA 258:2072–2076, 1986

Rogers MF, Thomas PA, Stracher ET, et al: Acquired immunodeficiency syndrome in children: report of the Centers for Disease Control national surveillance, 1982 to 1985. Pediatrics 79:1008–1014, 1987

Rogers MF, Ou CY, Rayfield M, et al: Use of polymerase chain reaction for early detection of the proviral sequences of human immunodeficiency virus in infants born to seropositive mothers. N Engl J Med 320:1649–1654, 1989

Rubinstein A: Pediatric AIDS. Curr Probl Pediatr 16:361–409, 1986

Rundell JR, Wise MG, Ursano RJ: Three cases of AIDS-related psychiatric disorders. Am J Psychiatry 143:777–778, 1986

Sandberg DE, Rotheram-Borus MJ, Bradley J, et al: Methodological problems in assessing AIDS prevention programs. Journal of Adolescent Research 3:413–418, 1988

Shaffer D: The epidemiology of teen suicide: an examination of risk factors. J Clin Psychiatry 49 (suppl):36–41, 1988

Shaw GM, Harper ME, Hahn BE, et al: HTLV-III infection in brains of children and adults with AIDS encephalopathy. Science 227:177–181, 1985

Sorensen RC: Adolescent Sexuality in Contemporary America. New York, Work Publishing, 1973

Strunin L, Hingson R: Acquired immunodeficiency syndrome and adolescents: knowledge, beliefs, attitudes and behaviors. Pediatrics 79:825–882, 1987

Thiry L, Sprecher-Goldberger S, Jonckheer T, et al: Isolation of AIDS virus from cell-free breast milk of three healthy virus careers. Lancet 2:891–892, 1985

Thomas CT, Szabaldi E: Paranoid psychosis as the first presentation of a fulminating lethal case of AIDS. Br J Psychiatry 151:693–695, 1987

Vermund SH, Hein K, Gayle HD, et al: Acquired immunodeficiency syndrome among adolescents: case surveillance profiles in New York City and the rest of the United States. Am J Dis Child 143:1220–1225, 1989

Weinbreck P, Loustaud V, Denis F, et al: Post-natal transmission of HIV-1 infection. Lancet 1:482, 1988

Westoff CF, Calot G, Foster AD: Teenage fertility in developed nations. Fam Plann Perspect 15:105–106, 1983

Wolf S: The health care needs of homeless and runaway youths. JAMA 263:811, 1990

Ziegler JB, Cooper DA, Johnson RO, et al: Postnatal transmission of AIDS-associated retrovirus from mother to infant. Lancet 1:896–898, 1985

Zuckerman BS, Walker DK, Frank DA, et al: Adolescent pregnancy: behavioral determinants of outcome. J Pediatr 105:857–863, 1984

Chapter 47

Suicide and Suicidality

Cynthia R. Pfeffer, M.D.

uicidality in children and adolescents had been an almost unheard of phenomenon before the mid-1970s. Clinicians expressed the belief that suicidal ideation or suicidal acts could not be defined before adolescence because of intrapsychic and developmental immaturity. In the 1970s and early 1980s, empirical studies began to report descriptions of suicidal children and adolescents (Cohen-Sandler et al. 1982; Pfeffer et al. 1979, 1980; Tishler and McKenry 1982). Shaffer (1982) acknowledged the existence of suicidal behavior in children and adolescents and posed an important question: "Is suicidal behavior a diagnosis or is it merely an epiphenomenon of a variety of different mental states each with its own and different determinants and prognoses?" (p. 414). Shaffer concluded that "existing studies do not provide evidence that suicidal children are a dis tinct diagnostic group in which one can expect to find characteristic dynamic or other antecedents" (p. 415).

In this chapter, I review recent research with the aim of highlighting whether there is evidence of diagnostic specificity for youth suicidality. The prevalence of suicide and nonfatal suicidal behavior in children and adolescents is outlined, and research on validating indicators or predictors of youth suicidality is presented. Such indicators encompass spheres of psychopathologic predictors, family factors, biological correlates, environmental stress, intrapsychic mechanisms related to imitation, outcome results, and intervention strategies.

Definition of Suicidal Behavior

Suicidal behavior in children and adolescents can be defined as a preoccupation or act that inten-

tionally aims to inflict injury or death to oneself. Suicidal behavior is episodic. The duration of an episode of suicidal ideation or action may be acute and brief or may last several hours or days. Repeated suicidal acts occur. Suicidal ideation or acts may occur in the preschool or preadolescent period or in adolescence. Although an intent to cause self-injury or to die is essential in the definition, it is not necessary that a youngster have a mature concept of the finality of death. The aim of the suicidal preoccupation or act is to die, regardless of what the concept of death means to a youngster (Pfeffer 1986).

Continuity of Suicidal Behavior

A much-debated issue is whether suicidal ideation, suicide attempts, and suicide are distinct, discontinuous phenomena. Pfeffer (1986) suggested that all these suicidal behaviors can be considered along a spectrum. Others (Carlson and Cantwell 1982) suggested that distinctions exist between youngsters with suicidal ideation and those who make suicide attempts. For example, Carlson and Cantwell reported that youngsters with suicidal ideation are more depressed than those who attempt suicide.

Research tends to support the notion of a continuity between youth suicidal ideation, suicide attempts, and suicide. Brent et al. (1986) studied 231 children and adolescents who were evaluated with the National Institute of Mental Health Diagnostic Interview Schedule for Children (Costello et al. 1982). The youngsters were evaluated for degree of suicidality, psychiatric symptoms, and psychiatric disorders. The results suggested a hierarchy of suicidal

507

behavior, ranging from no suicidal behavior to non-specific suicidal thoughts to specific suicidal ideation to suicidal acts. Another report (Brent et al. 1988) investigated the relation between suicide attempts and suicide; 27 adolescent suicide victims were compared with 56 suicidal psychiatric inpatients, among whom 18 had only suicidal ideation and 38 had attempted suicide. The results suggested a continuity in characteristics between adolescents who committed suicide and those who exhibited nonfatal suicidal behavior. Both groups of adolescents had high rates of affective disorders and family histories of affective disorders, antisocial disorders, and suicide. However, a firm conclusion about such a continuity in suicidal behavior could not be based on the findings of this study because differences between the suicidal groups were noted. For example, the adolescents who committed suicide had a higher prevalence of bipolar disorder and affective disorders with co-occurring diagnoses.

Another aspect of suicidal behavior involves the lethality of the method. A variety of factors are relevant in determining the degree of lethality of a suicidal act; these may include demographic characteristics and psychosocial factors. In one study (Brent 1987), charts of 131 adolescents consecutively psychiatrically hospitalized for suicide attempts were reviewed to identify factors associated with lethality. The results suggested that high medical lethality was most associated with being a male and having a diagnosis of an affective and/or substance abuse disorder and definite suicidal intent. Furthermore, these factors were similar to those in adolescents who committed suicide. The study also found that the lethality of an impulsive suicide attempt was most associated with the availability of a lethal suicide method (e.g., firearms). However, suicide intent and the severity of psychopathology were most associated with the lethality of non-impulsive suicide attempts.

Prevalence of Suicidal Behavior

With the recognition of exceedingly high suicide rates among 15–24-year-olds, which peaked at a rate of 13.6 per 100,000 in 1977 (Pfeffer 1986), research began to evaluate longitudinal trends in suicide rates among youth. Several issues became apparent. These were age or cohort effects, which encompass changes in suicide rates over the lives of individuals. A variety of studies (Goldney and

Table 47-1. Suicide rates in 1988 by age groups

Age group (years)	Suicide rate
1–14	0.6
15–24	12.8
25–34	15.5
35–44	14.3
45–54	14.8
55–64	15.7
65–74	16.8
75–84	28.9
85 and older	19.7

Note. Per 100,000 population.

Katsikitis 1983; Hellon and Solomon 1980; Murphy and Wetzel 1980; Solomon and Hellon 1980) found that as individuals age, suicide rates increase. This is especially true for white males. However, this relationship is not strictly progressive but bimodal, with a peak in suicide rates in the 25–34-year-old group and a slight decrease thereafter with a subsequent increase with age. This is illustrated in Table 47-1 for the suicide rates for different age groups per 100,000 population in 1988 (National Center for Health Statistics 1989).

Another trend in suicide rates is period effects, which indicate changes in suicide rates during particular historical periods (Holinger 1989). These trends are impossible to identify in 10–14-year-olds because the suicide rates for this age group have been consistently low. For the 15–24-year-olds, period effects are indicated by high rates in the 1930s, decreases in the 1940s to mid-1950s, and increases during the mid-1950s to 1980s.

The mechanisms underlying age or period effects for suicide rates require further study, but some explanations can be offered. One explanation is that the recent increase in youth suicide rates may be part of a general increase in problems such as depression, substance abuse, and divorce.

Holinger and Offer (1982) found that changes in the number of youths in the population are directly associated with changes in suicide rates among youth: a higher number of youths in the population is associated with higher suicide rates. One explanation for this relationship is more intense competition (e.g., for jobs, school openings) when there is a larger youth population. This intense competition produces stress and feelings of anxiety, despair, hopelessness, and worthlessness among those who are less successful.

Youth suicide rates also have increased because

Table 47-2. Comparison of suicide rates among age groups, 1985–1988

Year	All ages	5–14-year-olds	15–24-year-olds
1985	12.3	0.8	12.9
1986	12.8	0.8	13.1
1987	12.7	0.7	12.9
1988	12.3	0.6	12.8

Note. Per 100,000 population.

of an increased use of firearms, the most lethal method of suicide (Boyd and Moscicki 1986). Specifically, suicide by firearms for 10–24-year-olds has increased from 2.3 per 100,000 population in 1933 to 5.5 per 100,000 population in 1982. The rate for other suicide methods during this time went from 2.5 to 3.3 per 100,000 population. The most dramatic increase in firearm use occurred in the 1970s and 1980s. It also has been reported (Brent et al. 1987) that adolescent suicide victims who use firearms as a suicide method were 4.9 times more likely to have been drinking than were those adolescents who used other suicide methods. These researchers concluded that the greater availability of firearms and increased use of alcohol among teenagers were significant factors in the increased rates for youth suicide.

Table 47-2 compares rates of suicide from 1985 to 1988 in different age groups (National Center for Health Statistics 1989; Pfeffer 1986). These data reflect that suicide rates among 5–14-year-olds are quite low and that there has been a slight decrease in suicide rates in the last few years. Suicide was the third leading cause of death in 1987 for 15–24-year-olds, following accidents and homicide. It is highest in white males.

There are no central registries for nonfatal suicidal behavior. The lack of such data makes it difficult to have reliable rates on suicide attempts. Some reports on prevalence of suicide attempts (Harkavy-Friedman et al. 1987; Smith and Crawford 1986) have estimated that 9% of adolescents in the general population have attempted a suicide. Approximately 1% of preadolescents report a recent suicide attempt (Pfeffer et al. 1984).

Joffe et al. (1988) reported data on 3,294 youngsters in the Ontario Child Health Study. Among 14–16-year-olds in this large epidemiologic study, suicide attempts and suicidal ideation were more prevalent among girls than boys. The prevalences were 7.1% and 14.5%, respectively, for girls and 2.4% and 3.3%, respectively, for boys.

Rates of suicide and suicide attempts are higher among psychiatric patients than in the general population. Kuperman et al. (1988) reported that in a 4- to 15-year follow-up of 1,331 formerly hospitalized child psychiatric patients, suicide was nine times more frequent than expected in the general population. Pfeffer et al. (1988) reported that 34% of adolescent psychiatric inpatients were hospitalized because of a recent suicide attempt.

Predictors of Youth Suicidal Behavior

Predictors or risk factors for suicidal behavior encompass such domains as psychopathologic factors, family and environmental variables, and biological correlates.

Psychopathologic Factors

Three types of disorders are consistently associated with youth suicidal behavior. Symptoms of mood disorders, conduct disorder, and borderline personality disorder have been noted in studies of youth suicide and nonfatal suicidal behavior.

Among the psychological autopsy studies of youth suicide, a mixture of antisocial and affective symptoms are common. In a record review of 31 young adolescents who committed suicide, Shaffer (1974) found that 57% had mixed antisocial and affective symptoms, 17% had only antisocial symptoms, 13% had affective symptoms, and 15% did not have symptoms of these disorders. In this sample of youth suicide victims, four personality types were evident: impulsive, paranoid, withdrawn-uncommunicative, and perfectionistic. Furthermore, 46% had a prior history of suicidal ideation or acts. This study was limited by the absence of a comparison group.

Distinctions were noted between 20 adolescent suicide victims and 17 nonsuicidal adolescents matched to the suicide victims on demographic features (Shafii et al. 1985). Evidence of such antisocial behaviors as involvement with legal authorities, physical fights, stealing, and school suspension was shown by 70% of the suicide victims as compared with 24% of the nonsuicidal adolescents; 70% of the suicide victims, in contrast to 29% of the nonsuicidal adolescents, abused drugs or alcohol. There was a significantly higher prevalence of suicidal behavior among the suicide victims. This report did not describe symptoms of mood disorders.

Strong evidence for the relation of antisocial disorder and substance abuse was offered by the San Diego Suicide Study (Rich et al. 1986), which compared 150 suicide victims less than 30 years old with suicide victims older than 30 years. This study provided a developmental perspective by demonstrating that symptoms of affective disorders were more common in the older suicide victims but symptoms of antisocial problems and substance abuse were more prevalent in the younger individuals. For example, 78% of the older individuals had an affective disorder compared with 47% of the younger suicide victims. Specifically, major depressive disorder was more prevalent among the older individuals. Of the younger individuals, 12% compared with 2% of the older suicide victims had an antisocial personality; 88% of the younger suicide victims, in contrast to 39% of the older suicide victims, abused drugs. Overall, 90% of the total sample of suicide victims had a psychiatric disorder, suggesting that suicide is associated with defined psychopathology.

National vital statistics indicate that males commit suicide more than females. Shaffer (1988) compared 97 male and 17 female adolescent suicide victims with 65 males and 20 females who were considered nonsuicidal control subjects. Risk to commit suicide was increased by the presence of a history of a suicide attempt, major depression, substance abuse, and antisocial behavior. For males, risk was increased with the presence of history of a suicide attempt (risk increased 22.5 times), major depression (8.6 times), substance abuse (7.1 times), and antisocial behavior (4.4 times). For females, there was an increased risk by the presence of major depression (49.0 times), history of a suicide attempt (8.6 times), antisocial behavior (3.2 times), and substance abuse (0.8 times). Thus although the types of risk factors were similar for males and females, the degree of risk incurred by each factor differed for males and females. This study, like other psychological autopsy studies of youth suicide, highlights the important associations of affective and antisocial problems with adolescent suicide.

Significant associations have been found between nonfatal suicidal behavior and affective disorders, antisocial symptoms, and personality types. Apter et al. (1988) reported that, among 140 consecutive adolescent psychiatric inpatient admissions evaluated with the Schedule for Affective Disorders and Schizophrenia for School-Age Children (Kiddie-SADS) (Chambers et al. 1985), ratings

of suicidal behavior were higher among those diagnosed with a conduct disorder than those with a major depressive disorder. However, among the inpatients with conduct disorder, affective disorder, and schizophrenia, ratings for depression were significantly associated with ratings of suicidal behavior. This study suggests that symptoms of depression in adolescents with various psychiatric disorders are significant correlates of suicidal behavior. Robbins and Alessi (1985) described the types of symptoms of depression that are most associated with suicidal behavior in adolescent psychiatric inpatients. They studied 64 adolescent psychiatric inpatients and interviewed them with the Schedule for Affective Disorders and Schizophrenia; 33 adolescents had made at least one suicide attempt. Ratings of suicidal tendencies were significantly associated with such symptoms of depression as the following: depressed mood, negative self-evaluation, hopelessness, insomnia, poor concentration, anhedonia, guilt, worrying, low energy, poor appetite, indecisiveness, social withdrawal, and alcohol abuse. Among these variables, the best predictors of suicidal tendencies were depressed mood, anhedonia, and alcohol abuse.

The interactive effects between major depressive disorder and substance abuse were evaluated among 424 college students, 16–19 years old (Levy and Deykin 1989). Fifteen students (3.5%) reported having attempted suicide at some time in their lives. Furthermore, 1.9% had diagnoses of both major depression and substance abuse, 6.6% had only major depression, and 7.5% had only substance abuse. There was a significant association of major depression with suicidal ideation or attempts. Furthermore, substance abuse was an independent risk factor for suicidal behavior. For example, students with a substance abuse disorder had a 2.1- to 3.7-times higher risk of suicidal ideation or behavior. The presence of major depression was associated with equal rates of suicidal behavior for men and women. However, substance abuse was associated with higher suicidal behavior among men than among women. The significance of this study is that it evaluated suicidal risk in a nonclinical sample of adolescents.

Other studies (Delga et al. 1989; Inamdar et al. 1982) reported conflicting results on the prevalence of suicidal tendencies among psychotic and nonpsychotic adolescent inpatients. In a sample of adolescents admitted to a large urban municipal hospital (Inamdar et al. 1982), high rates of suicidal behavior were noted among psychotic adolescents.

However, in a voluntary psychiatric hospital, no differences were found in prevalence of suicidal behavior between psychotic and nonpsychotic adolescent inpatients. The variability in results of these studies may be reflective of the demographic and sociocultural backgrounds of the patients.

Evaluations in adolescent delinquent populations (Alessi et al. 1984; Miller et al. 1982) suggest that affective disorders, borderline personality disorder, and hyperactivity or impulsivity are significant correlates of suicidal behavior. These studies also lend support to the importance of affective disorder symptomatology and nonfatal suicidal behavior. Further evidence has been presented that among adolescent psychiatric inpatients with major depressive disorder, suicide attempts are more prevalent among those adolescents who have a borderline personality disorder (Friedman et al. 1983). Proneness to impulsivity, a specific characteristic of borderline personality disorder, may augment the likelihood of a suicide attempt in a depressed adolescent.

Prospective research in adult suicide victims (Beck et al. 1985) and research on adults who attempted suicide (Dyer and Kreitman 1984) suggest that hopelessness is a strong predictor of suicidal behavior. Hopelessness appears to be a stronger correlate of suicidal behavior than depression. A similar observation has been reported for preadolescent psychiatric inpatients (Kazdin et al. 1983), but not for minority female adolescents who attempt suicide (Rotheram-Borus and Trautman 1988). Additional research is warranted to determine the relations between youth suicidal behavior, depression, and hopelessness.

Family and Environmental Factors

Suicidal ideation and acts are inherently based on the interactions between intrapsychic functioning and external circumstances. This was specifically highlighted by the results of the psychological autopsy investigation of the San Diego Suicide Study (Rich et al. 1988), in which a relationship was found between specific psychiatric disorders and environmental stressors in suicide victims. The most common stressors of suicide victims were interpersonal loss or conflicts, economic problems, and illness. Interpersonal loss or conflict and economic problems were equally prevalent in those below and above age 30, but illness was more prevalent in the older group. Furthermore, more stresses of all types occurred in the suicide victims with substance abuse disorder than in suicide victims with only an affective disorder.

Other psychological autopsy studies of youth suicide victims identified such environmental stressors as disciplinary crises (Shaffer 1974) and mental illness in the family (Shaffer 1974, 1988; Shafii et al. 1985). Specific aspects of family emotional disturbance were suicidal behavior and emotional or physical abuse. For example, one study (Shafii et al. 1985) of 20 adolescent suicide victims and 17 nonsuicidal adolescents indicated that 60% of the adolescent suicide victims, compared with 24% of the nonsuicidal adolescents, had parents with emotional disorders. Shaffer (1988) reported that 41% of 97 male adolescent suicide victims, compared with 17% of 65 nonsuicidal male adolescents, had a family history of suicide. Among females, 33% of 17 suicide victims, compared with 13% of 20 nonsuicidal adolescents, had a family history of suicide. Associations between family psychopathology and nonfatal youth suicidal behavior have been documented in numerous studies (Pfeffer 1989). Furthermore, family interpersonal conflict, lack of cohesion, and low levels of impulse control have been observed in families of suicidal youngsters (Asarnow et al. 1987). Of particular note is the association between family violence (Pfeffer 1989), such as physical abuse (Deykin et al. 1985; Pfeffer et al. 1988), and youth suicidal behavior. For example, youngsters who had a history of physical abuse were four times more likely to attempt suicide than youngsters who did not have a history of physical abuse (Deykin et al. 1985).

Biological Correlates

Notwithstanding the recent avid interest in studying biological correlates of suicidal behavior, there is almost no research on this issue in children and adolescents. Despite the demonstrated associations of suicidal behavior in adults with amine metabolites (Mann and Stanley 1986), such data have not been published about youth populations. This kind of data can broaden our understanding of mechanisms leading to suicide or nonfatal suicidal acts in children and adolescents.

Outcome of Suicidal Youth

There are relatively few outcome studies of suicidal youth. Those studies undertaken have been limited by the lack of standardized measurements at initial and outcome times. In addition, the most consistently studied outcome has been suicide. Little data exist on other factors such as the relations between psychopathology and social function and suicidal behavior.

Follow-up studies range from short-term periods of 6 months to 5 years and long-term periods involving 7–15 years (Pfeffer 1988). Essentially, these studies document a low rate of suicide. A maximum of 4%–9% of youngsters who were studied had committed suicide at the time of follow-up.

Treatment and Prevention

Treatment of a suicidal child or adolescent encompasses a multifocal approach that aims primarily at altering a suicidal episode and reducing suicidal risk factors (Pfeffer 1986). Therefore, interventions are geared to decreasing accessibility to suicidal methods, delaying the possibility for suicidal action, and diminishing symptoms of psychiatric disorders. These aims can be accomplished by utilizing combinations of psychosocial and psychopharmacologic interventions. Enhancing environmental supports by alleviating family strife, decreasing symptoms of parental psychopathology, and fostering beneficial involvements with peers and nonfamilial adults are essential elements in the treatment of suicidal youngsters. Furthermore, intervention should be immediate whenever any suicidal potential is evident. Treatment should be maintained as long as acute suicidal risk prevails. Follow-up assessments are advisable to evaluate the youngster's stability in psychosocial functioning.

In recent years, suicide prevention programs have been developed as part of high school curricula. These programs aim to foster awareness of warning signs of suicidal behavior and skills in how to respond to suicidal tendencies recognized in one's peers. Most of these programs have not been evaluated with regard to their efficacy in decreasing suicidal acts. Spirito et al. (1988) reported on a school suicide prevention program for ninth-grade students in which the students' knowledge, attitudes, coping styles, sense of hopelessness, and helping behaviors were evaluated 10 weeks after completing the program. The results suggested that knowledge about suicide increased slightly. There was some impact on enhancing coping behaviors and decreasing hopelessness. However, attitudes about suicide were not changed significantly. In another

report, Shaffer et al. (1988) noted that results of their evaluation of such programs suggest a lack of effectiveness of school-based suicide prevention programs because such programs all aimed at a low-risk group of youngsters. Shaffer et al. reported that students have sound knowledge about suicidal behavior before being exposed to the suicide prevention curriculum, and prevention programs actually have little impact on changing students' misperceptions about suicidal behavior. Further study is warranted, especially to identify characteristics of school-based suicide prevention programs.

Other suicide prevention programs have been developed as a means of responding to the suicide of a student within a community. The aim of such programs is to contain the potential for suicidal behavior in peers. Efforts are specifically geared to minimizing a contagion effect or imitation of suicide. Advocates of youth suicide prevention favor a reduction in media coverage of youth suicide. These efforts are outgrowths of research describing an increased rate of youth suicide subsequent to nonfictional and fictional media presentations of youth suicide (Häfner and Schmidtke 1989; Phillips et al. 1989).

Summary

Suicide and nonfatal suicidal behavior in children and adolescents is an important mental health problem that requires extensive efforts for early identification and intervention. There is increasing evidence that specific risk factors are associated with youth suicidal behavior. The risk factors include such psychiatric disorders as affective, conduct, and substance abuse disorders. Environmental stresses include family discord and family psychopathology. A history of suicidal behavior predicts suicidal acts. Imitation of suicidal behavior is another risk factor.

Additional research is needed to delineate effective intervention and prevention strategies. Public health policies need to be developed, especially with regard to suicide prevention.

References

Alessi NE, McManus M, Brickman A, et al: Suicidal behavior among serious juvenile offenders. Am J Psychiatry 141:286–287, 1984

Apter A, Bleich A, Plutchik R, et al: Suicidal behavior, depression, and conduct disorder in hospitalized adolescents. J Am Acad Child Adolesc Psychiatry 27:696–699, 1988

Asarnow JR, Carlson G, Guthrie D: Coping strategies, self-perceptions, hopelessness, and perceived family environments in depressed and suicidal children. J Consult Clin Psychol 55:361–366, 1987

Beck AT, Steer RA, Kovacs M, et al: Hopelessness and eventual suicide: a 10-year prospective study of patients hospitalized with suicidal ideation. Am J Psychiatry 142:559–563, 1985

Boyd JH, Moscicki EK: Firearms and youth suicide. Am J Public Health 76:1240–1242, 1986

Brent DA: Correlates of the medical lethality of suicide attempts in children and adolescents. J Am Acad Child Adolesc Psychiatry 26:87–89, 1987

Brent DA, Kalas R, Edelbrock C, et al: Psychopathology and its relationship to suicidal ideation in childhood and adolescence. Journal of the American Academy of Child Psychiatry 25:666–673, 1986

Brent DA, Perper JA, Allman CJ: Alcohol, firearms, and suicide among youth: temporal trends in Allegheny County, Pennsylvania, 1960 to 1983. JAMA 257:3369–3372, 1987

Brent DA, Perper JA, Goldstein CE, et al: Risk factors for adolescent suicide: a comparison of adolescent suicide victims with suicidal inpatients. Arch Gen Psychiatry 45:581–588, 1988

Carlson GA, Cantwell DP: Suicidal behavior and depression in children and adolescents. Journal of the American Academy of Child Psychiatry 21:361–368, 1982

Chambers WJ, Puig-Antich J, Hirsch M, et al: The assessment of affective disorders in children and adolescents by semi-structured interview. Arch Gen Psychiatry 42:696–702, 1985

Cohen-Sandler R, Berman AL, King RA: Life stress and symptomatology: determinants of suicidal behavior in children. Journal of the American Academy of Child Psychiatry 21:178–186, 1982

Costello AJ, Edelbrock C, Kalas R, et al: The NIMH Diagnostic Interview Schedule for Children (DISC). Pittsburgh, PA, Department of Psychiatry, University of Pittsburgh, 1982

Delga I, Heinssen RK, Fritsch RC, et al: Psychosis, aggression, and self-destructive behavior in hospitalized adolescents. Am J Psychiatry 146:521–525, 1989

Deykin EY, Alpert JJ, McNamarra JJ: A pilot study of the effect of exposure to child abuse or neglect on adolescent suicidal behavior. Am J Psychiatry 142:1299–1303, 1985

Dyer JAT, Kreitman N: Hopelessness, depression, and suicidal intent in parasuicide. Br J Psychiatry 144:127–133, 1984

Friedman RC, Aronoff MS, Clarkin JF, et al: History of suicidal behavior in depressed borderline inpatients. Am J Psychiatry 140:1023–1026, 1983

Goldney RD, Katsikitis J: Cohort analysis of suicide rates in Australia. Arch Gen Psychiatry 40:71–74, 1983

Häfner H, Schmidtke A: Do televised fictional suicide models produce suicides? In Suicide Among Youth: Perspectives on Risk and Prevention. Edited by Pfeffer CR. Washington, DC, American Psychiatric Press, 1989, pp 117–141

Harkavy-Friedman JM, Asnis GM, Boeck M, et al: Prevalence of specific suicidal behaviors in a high school sample. Am J Psychiatry 144:1203–1206, 1987

Hellon CP, Solomon MI: Suicide and age in Alberta, Canada, 1951 to 1977: the changing profile. Arch Gen Psychiatry 37:505–510, 1980

Holinger PC: Epidemiologic issues in youth suicide, in Suicide Among Youth: Perspectives on Risk and Prevention. Edited

by Pfeffer CR. Washington, DC, American Psychiatric Press, 1989, pp 41–62

Holinger PC, Offer D: Prediction of adolescent suicide: a population model. Am J Psychiatry 139:302–307, 1982

Inamdar SC, Lewis DO, Siomopoulos G, et al: Violent and suicidal behavior in psychotic adolescents. Am J Psychiatry 139:932–935, 1982

Joffe RT, Offord DR, Boyle MH: Ontario Child Health Study: suicidal behavior in youth 12–16 years. Am J Psychiatry 145:1420–1423, 1988

Kazdin AE, French NH, Unis AS, et al: Hopelessness, depression, and suicidal intent among psychiatrically disturbed inpatient children. J Consult Clin Psychol 51:504–510, 1983

Kuperman S, Black DW, Burns TL: Excess suicide among formerly hospitalized child psychiatry patients. J Clin Psychiatry 49:88–93, 1988

Levy JC, Deykin EY: Suicidality, depression, and substance abuse in adolescence. Am J Psychiatry 146:1462–1467, 1989

Mann JJ, Stanley M: Psychobiology of Suicidal Behavior. New York, New York Academy of Sciences, 1986

Miller ML, Chiles JA, Barnes VE: Suicide attempters within a delinquent population. J Consult Clin Psychol 50:491–498, 1982

Murphy GE, Wetzel RD: Suicide risk by birth cohort in the United States, 1949 to 1974. Arch Gen Psychiatry 37:519–523, 1980

National Center for Health Statistics: Advance report of final statistics, 1988. Monthly Vital Statistics Report, Vol 39, no 7 (suppl). Hyattsville, MD, Public Health Service, 1989

Pfeffer CR: The Suicidal Child. New York, Guilford, 1986

Pfeffer CR: Suicidal behavior among children and adolescents: risk identification and intervention, in American Psychiatric Press Review of Psychiatry, Vol. 7. Edited by Frances AJ, Hales RE. Washington, DC, American Psychiatric Press, 1988, pp 386–402

Pfeffer CR: Family characteristics and support systems as risk factors for youth suicidal behavior, in Alcohol, Drug Abuse, and Mental Health Administration, Report of the Secretary's Task Force on Youth Suicide, Vol 2. Washington, DC, Alcohol, Drug Abuse, and Mental Health Administration, 1989, pp 71–87

Pfeffer CR, Conte HR, Plutchik R, et al: Suicidal behavior in latency-age children. Journal of the American Academy of Child Psychiatry 18:679–692, 1979

Pfeffer CR, Conte HR, Plutchik R, et al: Suicidal behavior in latency-age children: an outpatient population. Journal of the American Academy of Child Psychiatry 19:703–710, 1980

Pfeffer CR, Zuckerman S, Plutchik R, et al: Suicidal behavior in normal children: a comparison with child psychiatric inpatients. Journal of the American Academy of Child Psychiatry 23:416–423, 1984

Pfeffer CR, Newcorn J, Kaplan G, et al: Suicidal behavior in adolescent psychiatric inpatients. J Am Acad Child Adolesc Psychiatry 27:357–361, 1988

Phillips DP, Carstensen LL, Paight DJ: Effects of mass media news stories on suicide, with new evidence on the role of story content, in Suicide Among Youth: Perspectives on Risk and Prevention. Edited by Pfeffer CR. Washington, DC, American Psychiatric Press, 1989, pp 101–116

Rich CL, Young D, Fowler RC: San Diego suicide study, I: young versus old subjects. Arch Gen Psychiatry 43:577–582, 1986

Rich CL, Fowler RC, Fogarty LA, et al: San Diego suicide study,

III: relationships between diagnoses and stressors. Arch Gen Psychiatry 45:589–592, 1988

Robbins DR, Alessi NE. Depressive symptoms and suicidal behavior in adolescents. Am J Psychiatry 142:588–592, 1985

Rotheram-Borus MJ, Trautman PD: Hopelessness, depression, and suicidal intent among adolescent suicide attempters. J Am Acad Child Adolesc Psychiatry 27:700–704, 1988

Shaffer D: Suicide in childhood and early adolescence. J Child Psychol Psychiatry 15:275–291, 1974

Shaffer D: Editorial: diagnostic considerations in suicidal behavior in children and adolescents. Journal of the American Academy of Child Psychiatry 21:414–415, 1982

Shaffer D: The epidemiology of teen suicide: an examination of risk factors. J Clin Psychiatry 49:36–41, 1988

Shaffer D, Garland A, Gould M, et al: Preventing teenage suicide: a critical review. J Am Acad Child Adolesc Psychiatry 27:675–687, 1988

Shafii M, Carrigan S, Whittinghill JR, et al: Psychological autopsy of completed suicide in children and adolescents. Am J Psychiatry 142:1061–1064, 1985

Smith K, Crawford S: Suicidal behavior among "normal" high school students. Suicide Life Threat Behav 16:313–325, 1986

Solomon MI, Hellon CP: Suicide and age in Alberta, Canada, 1951 to 1977: a cohort analysis. Arch Gen Psychiatry 37:511–513, 1980

Spirito A, Overholser J, Ashworth S, et al: Evaluation of a suicide awareness curriculum for high school students. J Am Acad Child Adolesc Psychiatry 27:705–711, 1988

Tishler CL, McKenry PC: Parental negative self and adolescent suicidal attempts. Journal of the American Academy of Child Psychiatry 21:404–408, 1982

Chapter 48

Personality Disorders

Paulina F. Kernberg, M.D.

The existence of personality disorders in childhood and adolescence is controversial. Most textbooks on child psychiatry do not include personality disorder, regardless of the author's theoretical orientation, although there are a few that have addressed this issue (Adams and Fras 1988; Finch and Green 1979; Josephson and Porter 1979; P. Kernberg 1988; Lewis 1986).

As Lewis (1986) asserted, although the rate of change of personality in childhood and adolescence appears to be faster than in subsequent stages of the life cycle, this does not mean that personality does not exist. Instead, it means that personality disorders may be more difficult to diagnose. If one finds numerous personality traits in a child or adolescent that are maladaptive, inflexible, or rigid with continuity in time and across situations, one might consider the possibility of a specific personality disorder.

Frequently the thrust of development is not enough to counterbalance chronic deformations or distortions of the child's personality. Development proceeds, but along pathologic lines. All too often, only a DSM-III/DSM-III-R (American Psychiatric Association 1980, 1987) Axis I diagnosis is addressed in a child's diagnostic evaluation, overlooking an underlying Axis II personality disorder or developmental disorder, which will significantly affect the child's ultimate prognosis (Plakun 1989; Weissman et al. 1978). The current diagnostic nomenclature in DSM-III-R contributes to the controversy. Because children are not considered to have personality disorders, their chronic maladaptive ways of dealing with themselves and their environment are not specifically addressed in Axis II. The equivalent categories—avoidant disorder, oppositional defiant disorder, and severe conduct disorders—are placed in Axis I.

A Definition of Personality in Children and Adolescents

The concept of personality needs to be defined to consider the existence of personality disorders in children. DSM-III-R stated: "Personality traits are enduring patterns of perceiving, relating to, and thinking about the environment and oneself, and are exhibited in a wide range of important social and personality contexts" (American Psychiatric Association 1987, p. 335). Another useful definition comes from Fenichel (1945), who referred to personality as the ego's habitual modes of adjustment to the external world, the id, and the superego, and the characteristic ways of combining these modes with one another. Using the DSM-III-R definition, we can identify in children such personality traits as egocentricity, inhibition, cautiousness, self-confidence, sociability, activity, resentfulness, and oppositionalism in various combinations. If such traits become inflexible, maladaptive, and chronic across time and situations, causing significant impairment in the child's functioning and adaptiveness, then we are dealing with a personality disorder, regardless of age. Indeed, DSM-III-R indicates that manifestations of personality disorders may be recognizable by adolescence or earlier. Moreover, a requirement for the diagnosis of antisocial disorder is a severe, chronic conduct disorder and a pattern

515

of irresponsible and antisocial behavior since the age of 15.

As Rutter (1981) indicated, some concept of personality is needed to go beyond the notion that child psychopathology is simply a persistence of habits or behaviors. The concept of personality in children serves as the anchoring point for the organization of constitutional factors, experiences, traumas, and symptoms. Thus Rutter (1984) considered various kinds of continuity in his study of personality. Most relevant for personality development is the continuity of structural process or mechanism, which refers not to the form or quality of the personality, but to the psychological process in the underlying structure. This continuity may link patterns of behavior related to early experiences with some psychological outcome at a later date, such as a relationship between sexual abuse and borderline personality disorders.

Certainly personality traits and their expression are affected by the situational or interpersonal context, such as the presence or absence of the father in the attachment phase; the arrival of a new sibling; or whether the child is observed at home, at school, or with peers. Trait theories, however, recognize situational variability (Epstein 1979). Here it is important to consider the *effective environment*. Rutter and Garmezy (1983), for example, have demonstrated that institutionally reared children experience lasting effects through their late 20s, even though they are by then in entirely different environments. The concept of cumulative trauma, such as repeated separations or long-term sexual abuse, implies a consideration of personality development. Also, the concept of personality is required to understand how a child may actively induce, as it were, negative or positive environments, according to early experiences. For example, Pedersen et al. (1978) discussed the effect that a particular teacher may have on children. The effect of positive attitudes and work habits and the promotion of self-esteem increase the capacity of these children to profit from later education. Negative experiences in childhood, when not counteracted by positive supports later on, expose a lack of resilience and resourcefulness if circumstances again become unfavorable.

Personality Development

There is evidence of significant genetic contributions to such personality disorders as obsessive-compulsive personality disorder (Flament et al. 1988)

and antisocial personality disorder (Shields 1975; Shulsinger 1972). Biologically determined disorders, such as attention-deficit disorder or cognitive deficits due to perinatal factors, also contribute to the development of personality disorders (Andrulonis et al. 1981). Attention, memory, affect modulation, and spatial orientation are all cognitive functions that contribute to the formation of the child's representational world (Sandler and Rosenblatt 1962) and thus to personality. Attachment seems to have been confirmed as a determinant of personality development (Rutter 1985). Neglect, sexual abuse, physical violence, multiple separations, and psychiatric illness in the parents frequently contribute to the genesis of personality disorders, especially the impulsive character disorders (histrionic, borderline, narcissistic, and antisocial personality disorders). Indeed, one could start from the premise that any factor—genetic, constitutional, or environmental—that interferes with the normal integration and differentiation of the child's representational world (i.e., the self-representations and representations of others in interaction with the self, including affect links) will place the child at risk for a personality disorder. Traumatic experiences, as well as developmental disorders, also affect the formation of the representational world and, in turn, distort ego functions, superego functions, and the adaptive expression of affects, impulses, and wishes (Fenichel 1945).

Beres (1969) referred to character or personality development as a consistent pattern of adaptation to reality, whether normal or pathologic. He postulated that an early fixity of response in the child may presage serious psychopathology and that one can recognize in such a child an increasing reliance on certain defenses, pointing to the development of later character or personality structure. Consider, for example, the excessive use of projection in the paranoid character, action-proneness in the acting-out character, reaction formations in the obsessive character, and repression in the hysterical character. What is important is the precocious fixity of these defense patterns.

Hartmann (1958) linked individual differences in the early emerging ego functions to later choice of defense and, by implication, to choice of illness. He also introduced the hypothesis of individual differences at birth with regard to the infant's state of adaptiveness. Years later, Brazelton (1973) illustrated the extent of individual differences in processing internal and external stimuli. Although it is difficult to bridge neonatal and adult behavior, research findings point out that it is possible to observe continuities in some personality traits (Bronson 1967; Kagan 1984; Korner 1964; Looney et al. 1981; Rutter 1984). In this regard, Korner proposed that we study the style of development, instead of particular developmental processes—an approach that might contribute to the understanding of personality development in children.

Gardner and Moriarity (1968) observed that school-age youngsters could be grouped into "levelers" (global perceivers) or "sharpeners" (discriminate perceivers). The former showed greater difficulty in distinguishing similar stimuli in various sensory modalities—an incapacity that had a negative effect on learning tasks and recall. Gardner et al. noted that children between the ages of 9 and 13 had a perceptual style that was not only constant over time but also showed sex differences. Girls tended to be levelers, whereas boys were characteristically sharpeners. They found a definite correlation between these cognitive controls and defensive style, a correlation that continued over time. Their findings suggest that, even in normal children, there are characteristic ways of dealing with outside and inside stimuli that show stability across time.

Longitudinal Studies

Moss and Susman (1980) presented a summary of longitudinal studies of personality that—despite methodological differences—all indicated that infants have a personality profile. The New York longitudinal study found that the greatest stabilities in the period from age 3 months to at least 2 years were found in mood, adaptability, approach behavior, and intensity, and the least stable were in activity level and distractibility. The National Institute of Mental Health longitudinal study (Halverson and Waldrop 1976; Yang and Moss 1978) examined the role of environment and biological factors. For males, biological and temperamental influences were most important, whereas for females, environmental stimuli, such as the mother's interest in social behavior, seemed to account for behaviors like social responsiveness. Escalona and Heider (1959) predicted personality styles in preschool children from observations conducted between 4 and 32 weeks of age; sex role, interest patterns, activity patterns, and expressive behavior were successfully predicted. The Purdue longitudinal study (Martin 1964), which followed four preschool cohorts from 2 to 5 years of age, showed a high degree of stability in the relative amount of aggression and control dominance, as well as stability in dependency, autonomous achievement, and friendship-affiliation behavior.

Of children showing aggressivity at age 3 years, 68% showed this trait 5 years later (Richman et al. 1982). In another longitudinal study of personality development, children were seen between 2½ to 6 years of age, and then followed up each year from 6 to 12 years, during adolescence, and as young adults (Kagan and Moss 1962). Passivity was highly stable for boys and girls over the first 10 years of life. Independent orientation showed a moderate degree of stability over the first 10 years of life. Independence was stable for females over the 11-year span from 3 to 14; it was stable for males only from middle childhood to adolescence. Girls who were dependent on female adults during middle childhood established a dependent and passive relation with males during adulthood.

The same study found that aggression to peers but not to mother was highly stable over the first 10 years of life. Indirect aggression to peers, such as verbal attacks, was stable from the preschool years through adolescence. Over the span from childhood to adulthood, aggression was more stable for males than for females.

Nearly three-quarters of the severe conduct disturbances persisted between 10 and 15 years in the Isle of Wight study (Rutter and Graham 1973). It is worth noting that while passivity (an acceptable behavior for females but not for males) was stable from childhood to adulthood only for females, achievement (an acceptable behavior for both males and females) was stable for both sexes.

There was also a high degree of continuity between preschool sex-role behavior and adolescent behavior. Fixed sex interests were stable from childhood to adulthood for both sexes, especially for males. Social interaction traits were also predictive. Lack of spontaneity and social withdrawal during middle childhood and adolescence were predictive of adult social anxiety. Lastly, introspectiveness was predictive of a similar tendency during adulthood.

Diagnosis of Personality Disorder in Childhood

DSM-III-R will be used as a framework for organizing observations on child personality disorders. Children under age 18 who have the essential features of any of the conditions described for adults as personality disorders can be so diagnosed (taking modifications from developmental considerations into account). Cohen et al. (1983) reported that children may manifest persistent, unstable patterns of developmental deviations by the fourth year of life. From another perspective, Rapoport and Ismond (1990) indicated that equivalent "symptoms" diagnosed in childhood and persisting after age 18 are then classified under the corresponding adult personality disorder.

As further clinical research evidence accumulates and the concept of personality disorders in childhood becomes more familiar, the nomenclature in DSM-III-R for certain diagnoses in childhood or adolescence might be replaced with the corresponding personality disorder. For example, if all criteria are met, including those of severity and chronicity, avoidant disorder of childhood or adolescence corresponds to avoidant personality disorder (Rapoport and Ismond 1990), oppositional-defiant disorder corresponds to passive aggressive personality disorder, and pervasive developmental disorder corresponds to schizotypal personality disorder. All of the conduct disorders (solitary aggressive type and undifferentiated) can be subsumed in the Cluster B personality disorders (i.e., borderline, narcissistic, and antisocial personality disorders). At present, antisocial personality disorder requires that the conduct disorder start before age 15, and there is an injunction that the diagnosis of antisocial personality disorder should not be given under age 18. In my opinion, if a patient fulfills the criteria of antisocial personality disorder for 3 years or more, that diagnosis should be given, regardless of whether or not the patient is 18.

It is also important to emphasize that children and adolescents can be diagnosed as having borderline personality disorder rather than identity disorder—the corresponding adolescent category, which will be deleted in the upcoming DSM-IV.

In sum, if the personality disorder criteria are met and if the disturbance is pervasive and persistent, it is unlikely that the disorder will be limited to a developmental stage. In particular, the differences between a 15-, 16-, and 17-year-old from a developmental perspective are not sufficient to warrant avoiding a diagnosis of antisocial personality disorder, after several interviews with the patient and careful consideration of behavior, especially a lack of guilt and remorse and at least four of the following: inability to sustain consistent work behavior or equivalent behavior in an academic setting if the person is a student, failure to conform to social norms of lawful behavior, irritability and aggressiveness as indicated by repeated physical fights or assaults, failure to honor financial obligations, failure to plan ahead or impulsivity, lack of regard for the truth, recklessness with regard to personal safety or the safety of others, or lack of remorse (feels justified in having hurt, mistreated, or stolen from another).

Spectrum of Childhood Personality Disorders

As has been described for adults, personality disorders can be viewed along a spectrum from neurotic to borderline to psychotic.

Within the neurotic level of personality disorders, we find the passive-aggressive, dependent, avoidant, obsessive-compulsive, self-defeating, and sadistic personality disorders. To receive any of these diagnoses, children should meet the corresponding DSM-III-R criteria for adults in a descriptive sense, but they should also be looked at from a functional perspective. Do they have a sense of age-appropriate identity and cope with internal and external stresses by using more advanced mechanisms of defense such as repression, rationalization, or isolation? Most important, do they have a sense of and relationship to reality with intact reality testing?

Comparatively more severe disorders include the schizoid, paranoid, borderline, narcissistic, antisocial, and histrionic personality disorders, which all have a borderline personality organization (O. Kernberg 1976). There is a lack of integration of identity: of the self-concept and the concept of others.

The Sense of Identity

The sense of identity—the child's self-concept and representation or working schema of others—must be considered here as an important anchor or organizer of personality traits. Although identity consolidation is a predominant developmental task of adolescence, the school-age child already has an age-appropriate sense of identity. Between the ages of 6 and 12 years, children have a sense of "me-ness." They have a sense of who they are and of their own continuity throughout various activities (e.g., school, home, camp), through time (past, present, future), and with different persons.

Lower-level defense mechanisms predominate,

such as splitting, denial, projection, primitive idealization, devaluation, and omnipotent control. Moreover, the relationship to reality may be lost, but the capacity to test reality is preserved, and the child can regain reality contact with the clinician's support.

At the most severe end is the psychotic personality organization, which includes the schizotypal personality disorder. Here there is a fragmented and bizarre sense of identity with psychotic defense mechanisms, such as severe constriction, deanimation of animate objects (e.g., considering other people to be machines), and animation of inanimate objects (e.g., assuming that stuffed animals have a life of their own). These defenses are an attempt to keep massive anxiety and depression under control. In addition, there is a loss of the capacity to test reality and a loss of a relationship to reality.

In general, treatment recommendations follow this spectrum of personality disorders. For the "neurotic" personality disorders, clinicians tend to use predominantly psychosocial interventions, with the exception of obsessive-compulsive personality disorder, for which Rapoport and Ismond (1990) described the beneficial effects of clomipramine. For the borderline personality organization, individual supportive-expressive psychotherapy (P. Kernberg 1983b), group therapy (Scheidlinger 1982), or family therapy (Shapiro et al. 1975) is indicated, while medication may be used for specific target symptoms (Cantwell and Carlson 1978; O. Kernberg 1976; Petti 1981; Rockland 1989; Wiener 1985).

Finally, in the psychotic personality organization, treatment combines neuroleptics in low dosages with psychosocial interventions of a supportive nature, including environmental changes.

The application of adult criteria for personality disorders to children and adolescents has not yet been explored systematically in all categories. It is possible, for example, that Cluster A diagnoses, which include paranoid personality disorder, can be seen in adolescence as part of a mixed personality disorder with schizoid, schizotypal, or borderline personality disorder. Such is the case of Maria, a 15-year-old hospitalized for trying to kill her parents by cooking stews and muffins with rat poison and setting fires outside their bedroom door. Her parents, who came from Latin America, were deprecated by Maria as "minority WASPs." Except for one girlfriend, Maria felt there was nobody she could count on. Her own parents, she explained,

Table 48-1. DSM-III-R diagnostic criteria for histrionic personality disorder

A pervasive pattern of excessive emotionality and attention-seeking, beginning by early adulthood and present in a variety of contexts, as indicated by at least *four* of the following:

1. Constantly seeks or demands reassurance, approval, or praise.
2. Is inappropriately sexually seductive in appearance or behavior.
3. Is overly concerned with physical attractiveness.
4. Expresses emotion with inappropriate exaggeration, e.g., embraces casual acquaintances with excessive ardor, uncontrollable sobbing on minor sentimental occasions, has temper tantrums.
5. Is uncomfortable in situations in which he or she is not the center of attention.
6. Displays rapidly shifting and shallow expression of emotions.
7. Is self-centered, actions being directed toward obtaining immediate satisfaction; has no tolerance for the frustration of delayed gratification.
8. Has a style of speech that is excessively impressionistic and lacking in detail, e.g., when asked to describe mother, can be no more specific than, "She was a beautiful person."

Source. Reprinted with permission from American Psychiatric Association 1987.

deliberately annoyed her by ignoring her sensitivity to their "disgusting" eating habits and the way they talked. Moreover, she felt she could never forgive her parents for not controlling her older brother, who had physically abused her. She did not care what others thought of her; even when praised, she was convinced this was done solely for exploitation.

The diagnostic impression here was of a personality disorder not otherwise specified with paranoid, schizoid, and sadistic features. The recommended treatment in such cases is individual and family psychotherapy. Neuroleptics in minimal dosages may be tried to modulate the paranoid and more bizarre thinking.

Histrionic Personality Disorder

These cases refer to the milder form of the disorder, namely, hysterical personality disorder. The DSM-III-R criteria (Table 48-1) are a compromise between the classic hysterical personality and the histrionic personality disorder of DSM-III, which overlapped with borderline personality disorder. These children tend to appear outgoing, engaging, and charming, but are soon perceived as irritating and intrusive, impulsive, and more selfish than is normal for their age (P. Kernberg 1981). They crave attention, stimulation, and excitement. Hyperemotional, but in a superficial way, these children have a fickle and capricious quality. They lose friends as fast as they gain them. Their emotions are labile, erupting in theatrical outbursts or undergoing equally abrupt withdrawal.

The sexuality of the hysterical personality in childhood is deceptive. The provocative seductiveness is only superficially sexual; it really expresses identifications with seductive parents as a means of retrieving or maintaining love, or as an acting out of hostile manipulations. The hysterical child or adolescent seldom seeks a sexual partner in the adult sense, but absorbs instead an eroticized positive or negative attention from the parents or others. If the mother herself is hysterical or infantilizing or encourages competitiveness in her child, the child will identify with her. A hysterical personality can also result if the little girl manages to turn her father into a substitute mother by developing abnormally close ties with him because she is, or feels, deprived of adequate mothering. If this relationship becomes sexualized (because of her father's conflict), the child may later use this technique to get dependent gratification from other father figures at the cost of submission and passivity.

Most of these patients suffer from some deficit in their cognitive development, with inevitable limitations in learning tasks. They are so busy both acting on and repressing their sexual and aggressive impulses that they have little attention left for sublimated interest or learning. In addition, they are what Gardner and Moriarity (1968) described as "levelers"; that is, their cognitive style is characterized by lack of discrimination and a global approach to learning.

The main mechanisms of defense in the patient with histrionic personality disorder are repression of the awareness of sexual elements in their own behavior, reaction formation, and intellectualization to handle the anger and frustration. In more severe forms of histrionic personality disorder, defenses are more primitive, including projection and somatization.

Case Example 1

Jeannie, a 14½-year-old, was described as an expressive, easily excitable baby, pointing to some temperamental givens in her personality. Later, although she seemed generally able to control her affects, she had intense temper tantrums if something did not go her way. As a teenager, she was provocative but prudish,

exhibiting herself in a bikini, but expressing outrage if boys commented on her looks. Despite her attractive appearance, she behaved as a sexless, frozen person. She complained, as is frequent in personality disorders, of feelings of depression. During treatment, Jeannie demonstrated a global cognitive style. "I never seem to grasp the idea of a conversation," she complained. "I want to make sure that people will like me. . . . Usually, this results in my feeling forced. . . . What else can I say? I can never tell what is fair and what is unfair. It is a defense against really knowing." "Almost everything I do, I drop out of," she continued. "My older brother has kept his interest throughout the years, and by now he is a good piano player. I have it all there, but I can't seem to do anything with it. . . . I haven't done anything with my talents. It is almost as if you didn't have them."

In sum, Jeannie fit several criteria for the histrionic personality disorder, including overstatement and hyperbole in her speech, her constant search for praise and approval, inappropriate sexual seductiveness, exaggerated emotional expression (her temper outbursts and changing moods), a feeling of lack of genuineness, and self-centeredness.

Case Example 2

Tina, a 6-year-old, showed some characteristics of the hysterical personality disorder despite her much younger age. Tina's parents consulted me because of her extremely negative reactions to her brother, 3 years her junior. Since his birth, she had become very demanding, and no matter how much her parents did, she always felt that it was not enough. She also antagonized her peers. In school, nobody wanted to sit next to her. She could read very well, but her desk was a mess, and she was forever losing her pencils, as well as her library books, milk money, and notebook. During the diagnostic evaluation, Tina drew herself quite large, almost 20 inches tall, while she made her brother a fragment of a stick figure only 2 inches tall. There was a theatrical quality about her. Often she came in dragging a long scarf as if she were a grande dame. Overall, Tina showed constant need for praise and approval, problems in her relationships with others, exaggerated emotional expression, overconcern with physical appearance, and intense penis envy, as reflected in her intense negative reaction to her brother's genitals. Her seductive relationship to her father was evident in her kissing him on the mouth to say goodnight; with her mother, she complained of aches and pains, to obtain nurturing reactions.

Treatment

For the histrionic (or hysterical) personality disorder, child analysis or psychoanalytic psychotherapy, two to three times a week, is the treatment of choice, aimed at the maladaptive defenses, oral demandingness, envy of boys, and guilt about sexual feelings (P. Kernberg 1981). Specifically, the child's guilt about masturbatory fantasies, oedipal rivalry, and penis envy (expressed in a self-devaluatory body image), as well as the misuse of sexualized interactions to fulfill dependency needs, should be addressed. As the treatment progresses, character traits may be slowly transformed into symptoms of depression, anxiety, or even dissociation, which can be resolved through interpretive work in a therapeutic atmosphere of supportiveness and understanding.

Parental counseling also is advisable. Although cultural and individual differences play a role in hysterical pathology, the main contributing factor seems to be the parent-child relationship (Metcalf 1977). The hysterical patient's insatiable attention seeking may originate in part in partially frustrated attachment behaviors in infancy. In the two cases described, the mothers were uncomfortable and uncertain about their maternal role and were emotionally unavailable.

Parental counseling is particularly important given the variety of pathogenic interactions. Often, for example, the mother shows hysterical traits herself. Moreover, the parents may seem overtly to encourage the child to expect help or guidance from others, yet covertly to signal that obtaining this is beyond the child's competence, and it can be supplied only by the parents, encouraging in this way the child's demandingness. They may discourage the expression of anger, assertiveness, or anxiety, and encourage dependency and passivity instead. Further problems arise when parents are physically overstimulating, especially when they infantilize the child. As a result, the child may show an early and intense sexuality or eroticization and, in later life, may need to maintain a high level of egocentric and sexually oriented interactions to satisfy dependency needs.

There are somewhat different recommendations for treatment of cases at the more severe range of the spectrum, where histrionic personality overlaps with borderline personality disorder. Here the treatment should follow supportive-expressive approaches with psychotherapy twice a week for 1–3 years. Structured limits should be established. Parental counseling should include clarification of primitive defense mechanisms operating within the family.

Borderline Personality Disorder

Borderline personality in childhood has been described by various authors (Aarkrog 1977; Ekstein and Wallerstein 1954; Frijling-Schreuder 1969; Geleerd 1958; P. Kernberg 1983a; Kestenbaum 1983;

Table 48-2. DSM-III-R diagnostic criteria for borderline personality disorder

A pervasive pattern of instability of mood, interpersonal relationships, and self-image, beginning by early adulthood and present in a variety of contexts, as indicated by at least *five* of the following:

1. A pattern of unstable and intense interpersonal relationships characterized by alternating between extremes of overidealization and devaluation.
2. Impulsiveness in at least two areas that are potentially self-damaging, e.g., spending, sex, substance use, shoplifting, reckless driving, binge eating. (Do no include suicidal or self-multilating behavior covered in [5].)
3. Affective instability: marked shifts from baseline mood to depression, irritability, or anxiety, usually lasting a few hours and only rarely more than a few days.
4. Inappropriate, intense anger or lack of control of anger, e.g., frequent displays of temper, constant anger, recurrent physical fights.
5. Recurrent suicidal threats, gestures, or behavior, or self-multilating behavior.
6. Marked and persistent identity disturbance manifested by uncertainty about at least two of the following: self-image, sexual orientation, long-term goals or career choice, type of friends desired, preferred values.
7. Chronic feelings of emptiness or boredom.
8. Frantic efforts to avoid real or imagined abandonment. (Do not include suicidal or self-multilating behavior covered in [5].)

Source. Reprinted with permission from American Psychiatric Association 1987.

Mahler and Kaplan 1977; Masterson 1980; Pine 1974, 1983; Rosenfeld and Sprince 1963; Weil 1953). The descriptive symptomatology bears a resemblance to the diagnostic category for adult borderline personality disorder (Table 48-2), namely: 1) a pattern of unstable and intense interpersonal relationships, alternating between idealization and devaluation; 2) impulsiveness; 3) affective instability, or marked shifts in mood, usually lasting a few hours and only rarely lasting more than a few days; 4) inappropriate intense anger or lack of control of anger, frequent displays of temper, and recurring physical fights; 5) recurring suicidal threats, gestures, or behavior, or self-mutilating behavior; 6) marked and persistent identity disturbance, manifested by uncertainty about self-image, sexual orientation, type of friends, long-term goals, and/or preferred values; 7) chronic feelings of emptiness or boredom; and 8) frantic efforts to avoid real or imagined abandonment.

Petti and Law (1982), Dr. Jerome Liebowitz (personal communication 1981), and Bemporad et al. (1982) have demonstrated the applicability of DSM-III-R criteria to children in inpatient and outpatient settings. Similarly, Rapoport and Ismond (1990) recommended that borderline personality disorder "be diagnosed in children and adolescents, rather than the corresponding childhood category of identity disorder, provided that the personality disorder criteria are met and the nature of the disturbance is pervasive, persistent, and not limited to a developmental stage" (p. 61).

From a developmental perspective, borderline children have not accomplished tasks that normal preschool children have achieved; namely, they cannot tolerate separation from mother, lack established standards of bad and good, have an inability to express a wide variety of modulated feelings, and are uncertain about sexual distinctions (P. Kernberg 1979). Compared with their school-age peers, borderline children are not able to maintain a sense of sex and role identity through play, fantasy, and learning tasks. Impulse control remains poor, with unpredictable states. They do not show enjoyment of peer interactions and increased independence from parents. The Oedipus complex is not yet resolved through sublimatory channels and repression, as would be expected by 5 years of age.

The borderline adolescent, in turn, has not acquired a sense of identity or developed age-appropriate abstract thinking. There is little indication of emancipation and autonomy from the family, and the perceptions of the family tend to be unrealistic. Gender identity with the capacity for intimacy and heterosexual adjustment is not established, and masturbatory fantasies are primarily connected with various pregenital themes, such as sadistic or excretory activities.

Borderline children, in contrast to borderline adults, may report visual and auditory hallucinations, but kinesthetic and tactile hallucinations are rare. Visual and auditory hallucinations may be fostered if children are unable to express their aggression because their parents cannot contain or handle it. If these children have poor models for reality testing (Pine 1974), they may lose contact with reality (Geleerd 1958) while preserving the capacity for reality testing.

Play should be considered as an additional diagnostic descriptor in borderline children. These children do not play age appropriately. The play is compulsive (Weil 1953), with little evidence of enjoyment or of the capacity to resolve conflict through elaborations of fantasies. Games may be endlessly repeated, and the child may enter into elementary fantasy play more typical of much younger children (e.g., playing at eating or flying and falling). The incidence of play disruption is higher than in neurotic children; aggressive and sexual impulses infiltrate the play, so that intense anxiety follows, and the child is unable to continue playing unless aided by the therapist. In their fantasies, these children see themselves as omnipotent, and oral and anal sadistic themes predominate.

Relationships with peers are characterized by a sense of coercion and possessiveness, with idealization or abrupt devaluations and, occasionally, a phenomenon called "shadowing" (echoing and borrowing from a peer's identity). There is no empathy for others, as these youngsters relate to others as "props" or projections of part of themselves.

In my experience, the most important diagnostic criteria include an identity disorder; shifting levels of ego organization involving motor, cognitive, and affect modulation; and an inability to assume responsibility for one's own actions. There is a lack of a sense of "me-ness" and of gender identity, as well as an incapacity to be alone or a longing and fear of being left. Shifting levels of ego function account for the abrupt regressions, sudden lack of judgment, and impulsivity, as well as the disturbed relationship to reality (although the capacity to test reality is preserved). The use of primitive defenses, particularly splitting, projection, and denial, explains these children's difficulties in assuming responsibility for their actions; formation of an integrated conscience or superego is impaired. In addition, borderline children tend to show extreme ambivalence toward their siblings; sibling rivalry can become outright hatred, with sibling abuse. The splitting mechanism affects the relationship to the parents, not only in terms of bad and good, but also in establishing a relationship to the parents on a one-to-one basis. The child relates to the mother to the exclusion of the father, or to the father to the exclusion of the mother. A normal transitional object, in terms of timing and the kind of object, tends to be absent.

An unstable sense of identity is reflected in a sense of dependence on the "other" for survival, illustrating the personality disorder problem underlying severe separation anxiety problems. An alternative is to resort to narcissistic defenses, indicating a lack of need for anybody and denial of danger. These patients try at times to control others totally or to submit entirely to another's control to gain some sense of identity (P. Kernberg 1983a). Another attempt to gain identity can frequently be seen during treatment when they attribute the role of patient to the therapist while assuming the role of therapist. This can be done so vividly that the therapist literally feels as the patient does.

Depression frequently accompanies a borderline personality disorder (Gorton and Akhtar 1990). These children perceive themselves as without continuity, so they fail to anticipate gratification or even show it. They lack an age-appropriate capacity for realistic self-esteem or mastery. Their chronic feeling tone is one of apathy and anhedonia or worthlessness. They do not derive gratification because of lack of reciprocity in maternal/paternal or peer relationships. To the contrary, they are rejected and disliked for their primitive ways of relating to others. These children are unable to derive pleasure from play or to use play to discharge their frustrations and aggressions, which adds to their helplessness and hopelessness.

Lastly, the frequent coexistence of organicity (Andrulonis et al. 1981) makes for difficulties in learning and social interaction, which compound the child's depression. This multidetermined depression, coexisting with impulsivity and other characteristics, may account for the fact that suicide attempts are a frequent cause for hospitalization (Pfeffer 1983).

Family Assessment

The families of borderline adolescents (Shapiro et al. 1975) and children tend to foster and maintain borderline functioning. Parents tend to use the child narcissistically, for their own purposes. There is anxiety about supporting the child's autonomy and a denial of his or her independence. The defense mechanisms of splitting, devaluation, idealization, denial, and primitive forms of projection seen in the individual also operate in the family group.

Psychological Testing

In both structured and unstructured tests, borderline children show fluidity of associations, peculiar logic, and flights into fantasy, although not formal thought disorder. Even if their perceptual, motor, and intellectual capacities are intact, these children do not use them creatively or effectively. Overall, there is a deficit in adaptation (Leichtman and Nathan 1983). Object representations seem to be unrealistic and unidimensional. Human precepts tend to split into all-bad or all-good figures. Partial merger, in the sense of one person being attached to another, seems rather typical: for example, a patient may describe two-headed people or two elephants joined together at the tail. Themes of loss, separation, and abandonment, with helplessness and primitive aggression, appear. The tenuous sense of identity is illustrated by body-image distortions, anxiety about disappearance, strong identification with extraterrestrial beings, and visions of people about to explode.

Differential Diagnosis

Borderline personality disorder should be considered in such Axis I syndromes as severe conduct disorders, separation anxiety disorder, anorexia nervosa, bulimia nervosa, gender identity disorder, and elective mutism. In adolescents, as with adults, major affective disorder is frequently associated with borderline personality disorder. The specific developmental disorders have all been found in a significant percentage of borderline adolescents and young adults (Andrulonis et al. 1981).

Borderline children may have brief psychotic episodes related to stress, with paranoid symptoms, depersonalization, derealization, dissociation, and suicide attempts. However, these are different from psychosis (P. Kernberg 1983a). Typical psychotic processes include fragmentation, extreme hypochondriasis, animation of inanimate objects, deanimation of animate objects, formation of bizarre objects, and persistent delusions and hallucinations. The anxieties go beyond the ones of annihilation, but are characterized by fears of falling, losing oneself through dissolving, or disappearing. Lack of capacity to test reality, given the supports of clarification and confrontation, further delineates psychosis from borderline conditions. Psychotic patients' regressions to a symbolic state, with no boundaries between self and object, are to be contrasted with the borderline patients' fusion fantasies (P. Kernberg 1983a). Borderline children illustrate failures in the separation-individuation process, but not regression to an undifferentiated self. This formulation has practical implications in clarifying and understanding the reactions of the patient to the therapist.

Additional Considerations

The continuity of childhood borderline conditions into adulthood has been addressed, although as yet not in a conclusive manner (Blum 1974; O. Kernberg 1978; Mahler and Kaplan 1977; Pine 1974). Mahler and Kaplan described a boy who, during the separation-individuation phase, showed severe splitting and insecure, avoidant attachment and later developed a typical borderline personality. Dr. John Clarkin (personal communication, 1989), in an ongoing study of borderline personality disorders in adults, found that borderline patients typically reported that their symptoms started in childhood, a finding supported by Dr. Martha Linnehan (personal communication, 1988).

Case Example 1

Velia, cited by Kestenbaum (1983), already had no friends at 5 years old and by age 7 was prone to severe and uncontrollable rages, did not get along with other children, and abused younger children if she did not get her way. She had begun lying to her parents, stealing from her mother's purse, and tearing up her own clothes and hiding them. Despite high intelligence, Velia lacked the concentration to complete homework. She seemed constantly nervous, but denied that she had any problems. At times, she betrayed her anger and hostility in comments such as, "How would you like it if I put a live rattlesnake on your plate?" This 7-year-old often became violently upset with her therapist, exclaiming "You are dead; I killed you!" or "You are a mind reader and a witch; you made me think of awful things!" In this way, she showed her shifting levels of functioning, her tendency to projections, and her paranoid ideation. Abrupt regressions in ego states also existed, as when she soiled herself during sessions. Yet, in other sessions, Velia displayed positive emotions, telling the therapist that she wished to adopt her because she loved her as much as her grandmother. When followed up in adult life (Kestenbaum 1983), Velia demonstrated low achievement not commensurate with her intelligence, drug abuse, promiscuity, manipulative suicidal threats, and disturbances in close relationships. Beneath her seemingly good socialization lay a disturbed identity, shifting identifications with others, and a predominance of rageful affect rather than emotional warmth. There were also brief micropsychotic episodes under stress. In all, she fulfilled the criteria of adult borderline personality disorder, as outlined by Gunderson and Kolb (1978).

Case Example 2

Another case in point is that of Nick, a 7½-year-old who suffered from severe separation anxiety marked by an inability to sleep in his own room or to be left alone, day or night. Nick had no friends. Although he did well academically, he was shunned by everybody in his school. Indeed, a school transfer was necessary because he was continually scapegoated. He refused to bathe, put on his clothes backwards, chewed his shirts, swallowed his nasal mucus, and occasionally soiled his pants. Depressed and moody, he frequently talked about suicide. (At the time, the parents were talking about divorce, although this was kept from the child.) At 2 years old, Nick had been evaluated by a developmental specialist. He showed accelerated development in certain areas and retardation in others. Although his intellectual ability placed him in the superior range, he differed from most 2-year-olds in the way he used his abilities, illustrating the deficit in adaptive capacity described by Leichtman and Nathan (1983). For example, he conceptualized his environment to such a degree that his response to blocks did not reflect their potential use in building houses. His capacity for imaginative play was already lagging. At age 2, he was considered to be at risk.

Treatment

The treatment of the borderline patient should be multimodal, with the therapist giving attention to both the child and the environment. Family work should address the correction of intrafamilial interactions, especially splitting, projection, and denial among different family members, and the child's acceptance of the parents' relationship as a couple. Day hospitals, inpatient settings, and special school programs are only for the more severe forms of this disorder.

Psychoanalytically oriented psychotherapy should be conducted two to three times a week, for a minimum of 1–2 years. Play materials should be simple and lend themselves to gross motor activities (e.g., sponge balls, dart games, bowling equipment). Interventions should emphasize the "here-and-now" as a way of enhancing the child's reality-testing capacity. The child's perception of the therapist's actions and verbal interventions should also be clarified on an ongoing basis. Fantasy distortions need to be verbalized and shared to allow for secondary verbalization and clarification. The possibility of sharing primitive fantasies with the therapist will lower the child's anxiety and permit fantasies to be channeled through play, dreams, or even daydreams, rather than in impulse-ridden, self-destructive behaviors.

Working with the lack of ego and superego integration requires discussion of attempts at splitting, denial, omnipotent control, primitive projection, idealization, and devaluation. Often the child's body language evidences the splitting defense, and this should be clarified. Integration of the split sense of self is another important goal. Facilitating a sense of continuity across time and situations helps correct the unstable sense. The therapist serves as the container of different states, different frames of mind, that belong to one person, the child.

A focus on superego functions can help to neutralize aggressive impulses toward self and others and omnipotent traits that prompt the child to antisocial behaviors. The child's ability to empathize with others can be improved by providing feedback on the effect of the child's shifting functioning on the therapist.

The child also needs help in seeing the parents objectively in both their positive and their negative aspects, as well as support in grieving for what the parents are not. In this way, the child becomes able to see that parents have their own separate limitations, which are not caused by the child.

The various vicissitudes of differentiation, rapprochement, and pathologic symbiosis should be dealt with in the relationship between therapist and child. The so-called preoedipal conflicts around issues of trust or distrust—remaining the same or daring to become different, following or running away, being controlled or being in control, remaining dependent or becoming autonomous, being a boy or a girl or an undifferentiated neuter—all are aspects that can be discussed to enable the child to proceed with development into later stages.

Borderline children also may need help with their sense of body ego, especially given the frequent association with attention-deficit disorders and associated cognitive disorders, which can enhance their sense of instability. The child needs to be able to talk realistically about such deficits.

Finally, treatment should account for ego weakness and lack of impulse control. The ego defect or arrest is seen as resulting from such defenses as splitting, denial, projection, and regression; these can be interpreted in terms of their meanings and functions during the therapeutic work. In contrast, if the ego weakness is seen as irreversible, rather than as a form of defense, the possibility of change will not be considered, thus contributing to a self-fulfilling prophecy.

Additional Treatments

Through interactions with another child, in a group of two or with a small therapy group, the child learns how to listen, respond, maintain contact, negotiate, and conclude interactions in a step-by-step manner.

Medication can also be an important adjunct for the child with a borderline personality disorder. The choice depends on the target symptoms. Low-dosage neuroleptics may be helpful in reducing the child's disorganization and facilitating the internalization of therapeutic intervention. If the target symptom is depression, antidepressants such as imipramine and fluoxetine may be indicated. In general, the effects of medication should be reassessed from time to time as the child's psychological reorganization becomes stabilized.

Prognosis

The prognosis with borderline children is from guarded to good, depending on environmental factors and the possibility of access to effective treatment. Without treatment, however, the general consensus is that these children are at severe risk for the continuation of their borderline personality disorder, antisocial personality disorder, substance abuse, or other forms of more serious pathology in the schizophrenic and manic-depressive range (Kestenbaum 1983).

Narcissistic Personality Disorder

McGlashan and Heinssen (1989) described an overlap between narcissistic, antisocial, and borderline disorders; all share certain borderline features and a relative absence of schizophrenic and manic symptoms. They differ, however, in terms of narcissistic and antisocial traits. The three basic criteria for narcissistic personality disorder are a pervasive pattern of grandiosity, lack of empathy, and a hypersensitivity to the evaluation of others.

In more detail, the criteria (Table 48-3) are that the patient 1) reacts to criticism with feelings of rage, shame, or humiliation; 2) is interpersonally exploitative, taking advantage of others to achieve his or her own needs; 3) has a grandiose sense of self-importance, expects to be noticed as "special," and exaggerates achievements and talents; 4) believes that his or her problems are unique and can be understood only by other "special" people; 5) is preoccupied with fantasies of unlimited success, power, brilliance, beauty, or ideal love; 6) has a sense of entitlement; 7) requires constant atten-

Table 48-3. DSM-III-R diagnostic criteria for narcissistic personality disorder

A pervasive pattern of grandiosity (in fantasy or behavior), lack of empathy, and hypersensitivity to the evaluation of others, beginning by early adulthood and present in a variety of contexts, as indicted by at least *five* of the following:

1. Reacts to criticism with feelings of rage, shame, or humiliation (even if not expressed).
2. Is interpersonally exploitative: takes advantage of others to achieve his or her own ends.
3. Has a grandiose sense of self-importance, e.g., exaggerates achievements and talents, expects to be noticed as "special" without appropriate achievement.
4. Believes that his or her problems are unique and can be understood only by other special people.
5. Is preoccupied with fantasies of unlimited success, power, brillance, beauty, or ideal love.
6. Has a sense of entitlement: unreasonable expectation of especially favorable treatment, e.g., assumes that he or she does not have to wait in line when others must do so.
7. Requires constant attention and admiration, e.g., keeps fishing for compliments.
8. Lack of empathy: inability to recognize and experience how others feel, e.g., annoyance and surprise when a friend who is seriously ill cancels a date.
9. Is preoccupied with feelings of envy.

Source. Reprinted with permission from American Psychiatric Association 1987.

tion and admiration; 8) lacks empathy, being unable to recognize and experience how others feel; and 9) is preoccupied with feelings of envy.

Frequently, many of the features of histrionic, borderline, and antisocial personality disorders are also present in the narcissistic personality disorder (McGlashan and Heinssen 1989). Depressed mood is extremely common. Personal defeats or irresponsible behavior may be justified by rationalization or lying. There is no gratification in achievement. The superego is not well integrated and tends to be projected either to the outside, with paranoid anxieties, or to the body, with somatic and hypochondriacal symptoms. Typically, exploitativeness is also projected to the outside, so that there is extreme distrust of others.

Developmental Manifestations

There are some additional developmental manifestations characteristic of narcissistic children (P.

Kernberg 1989). First, there may be severe learning problems. Despite superior intelligence, these children can fail. Teachers report that these youngsters can be arrogant and haughty, feeling that nobody is entitled to tell them what to do. They either get the best grades or the worst, for they find it difficult to apply themselves to any study they feel is beneath their dignity. They do not enjoy their learning experience. All their activities have a "driven" quality, without interest in the activity for its intrinsic value. Activities and achievements are only means to satisfy the ongoing need for attention and admiration.

Problems with peers are codetermined by an inability to empathize with others and by intense feelings of envy. Any acknowledgment of difference is haughtily denied. Friends can only be friends when they are clones. Peers are related to with a feeling of entitlement that justifies exploitativeness. Friends can be overidealized or devalued if they become a source of envy, so that the whole relationship is disavowed. These youngsters tend to choose either a popular, pretty or handsome partner to reflect on their grandiosity or someone who is considered extremely ugly or "a freak," in that way enhancing their sense of worth by contrast with the devalued partner, who is under their control.

Narcissistic children may show gaze aversion—a sign that is rare in the general population, but typical of autistic children and sometimes found in youngsters with antisocial traits. For children with narcissistic personality disorder, avoiding eye contact helps to avoid the traumatic experience of not being acknowledged. In addition, it helps to avoid confrontation between their own grandiosity and the reflection from adults, who see them as vulnerable and self-deceiving.

The play of narcissistic children is disturbed. Between the ages of 3½ and 11 years, they quickly become bored with new toys and are inhibited in their play, particularly their fantasy play. Even in structured games, however, these children react to any defeat with rule changes, temper tantrums, and regressive reactions. As treatment proceeds and the narcissistic child engages in fantasy, the play is characterized by raw aggression: toys and dolls are dismembered and bleed to death, or the whole earth is massacred by a gun-wielding murderer without mercy. Initially, the play is pleasureless, but later sadistic enjoyment may occur. There is a proclivity to cheat and to change rules if the game does not go in their direction.

The need for constant attention and admiration

can disguise an inability to be alone. Separation anxiety may be "covered up" by haughtiness and devaluation. One 4-year-old patient dragged his mother into the playroom, only to have her sit there while he conducted himself in an aloof manner, as if he couldn't care less about her existence. However, if the mother attempted to leave the room or refused to accompany him into the playroom, he had a temper outburst. In adolescence, these patients may refuse to participate in sleep-overs or to go away to camp, claiming a lack of interest in these activities.

A preoccupation with self-image can be seen at times in a compulsive need to look in the mirror. There is an acute sense of vulnerability in self-regard, both psychological and physical.

Additional Developmental Considerations

In the diagnosis of narcissistic personality disorder in childhood, it is important to differentiate infantile narcissism from pathologic narcissism. Young children, for instance, normally have grandiose fantasies and make angry efforts to control mother and to keep themselves at the center of her attention. Fantasies of great power, wealth, and beauty are common in the preschool years. However, the normal child does not need to be universally admired as the sole owner of everything that is enviable and valuable. The demands are related to realistic needs and incapacities. When these needs are gratified, the child is satisfied. In contrast, in pathologic narcissism, the demands are excessive and can never be fulfilled.

Normal children are capable of warm gratitude when their demands are met, but narcissistic children tend to be cold and aloof, "entitled" at best. In the normal child, achievements enhance self-esteem and self-regard, are enjoyed, and enable the child to set new realistic goals. In contrast, in narcissistic children, successes or achievements offer fleeting satisfaction, as long as attention from others is obtained. Normal young children show genuine attachment and interest in others, at least when they are not frustrated, and they have the capacity to trust or depend on significant objects. The narcissistic child is unable to depend on other people and does not show genuine attachment and interest in others; on the contrary, these feelings are pretended to obtain gratification and to exploit others.

At least from school age on, normal children accept their positive and negative aspects and begin

striving toward ideals provided by parents or friends. In narcissistic children, the accepted aspects of the self are coalesced with the ideals, leading to the formation of a grandiose self, with projection of the negative aspects of the self onto the external world.

Rinsley (1989) postulated that although narcissistic personality disorder overlaps with borderline characteristics, it is developmentally different in the relationship to the mother. In the borderline child, there is an arrest of both separation and individuation processes. In contrast, in narcissistic personality disorder, there is a dissociation of these two processes, so a significant degree of individuation may be achieved in the face of separation failure. This leads to a pseudomature child and explains the separation anxiety.

Various developmental influences may present a risk for the formation of narcissistic personality disorder, such as having narcissistic parents, being adopted, being abused, being overindulged, losing a parent through death, or having a divorced parent who attempts to erase any traces of the child's identification with the other parent.

Treatment

The choice of treatment for narcissistic personality disorder is either psychoanalysis or intensive expressive-supportive psychotherapy two to three times a week. The goals are to uncover the primitive fantasies connected with the grandiose self and replace this pathologic self with normal infantile narcissism or, in adolescence, with normal narcissism. This requires the systematic clarification, confrontation, and interpretation of the narcissistic defenses, including omnipotent control, devaluation, idealization, and denial, in their expression in the relationship between the patient and the therapist (Egan and Kernberg 1984). Empathy with both the patient's libidinal, dependent wishes and his or her envious destructiveness is necessary. The therapist must be extremely cautious given the vulnerability of these patients—as one of them explained, "I feel like a turtle without a shell."

Concomitant parental counseling or family therapy is strongly recommended to work on maladaptive narcissistic defenses operating at the family level, which help to maintain the disorder. Often the child is seen as an extension of the parents and not as a separate and different person in his or her own right. On the other hand, at times these children may exert such control on family members with such effectiveness that the family submits to them; the child then becomes the "monster who needs to be appeased," fueling the sense of grandiosity. Counseling with the parents includes enabling them to empathize with the child's contradictory, subjective experience of grandiosity and vulnerability, including the child's intense envy of those who can enjoy things.

Case Example 1

Cathy was 9 years old when I first saw her. She was described by her parents as being overcontrolling, prone to temper outbursts, derogatory toward adults, calling her father and mother "dumb" and "stupid" in no uncertain terms. Because of her haughty and controlling manner, she did not have any friends. She was seen for 7 months, and most of these traits appeared to recede, but 3 years later, her parents consulted me again. Although Cathy was now doing very well at school, she did not have close friends. Her mother commented on her self-centeredness and indicated that Cathy did not know the subtleties of discretion or "loyalty." There was intense rivalry with her sister, 3 years her junior, and Cathy constantly disrupted family life. She was prone to temper tantrums and made her parents feel incompetent. She also devalued her mother's relationship with her father, saying she coudn't understand why her mother had married her father. Cathy had a poor body image and liked to cover herself with oversized sweatshirts. She had problems going away from home and felt chronically homesick at camp. Described as arrogant by her teachers, she avoided eye contact with adults. She did only things she could do easily and well. Left to her own devices, she was easily bored. Indeed, there was a constant sense of dissatisfaction and dysphoria, which she verbally denied.

Case Example 2

Adams and Fras (1988) described Lester, a 9-year-old with an expressive writing disorder who reacted to this deficit with personality characteristics that fit the criteria for narcissistic personality disorder. Any mention of his writing deficit precipitated a rage attack and reminders that he was "the smartest kid in his class." He bragged of his ability to dominate and exploit his age-mates, whom he called "dumb clods." He also talked grandiosely about his superior knowledge in physics and astronomy, and even challenged his therapist, asking whether he was famous for anything. He tried to control his parents' sex life, throwing screaming tantrums outside their bedroom door. He was bratty and obnoxious, and his parents felt powerless to help him.

Antisocial Personality Disorder

This diagnosis requires evidence of a full-fledged conduct disorder with the onset before age 15 and a pattern of irresponsible and antisocial behavior since the age of 15 (Table 48-4).

Case Example 1

Adams and Fras (1988) described the case of Sharwell, an 11-year-old boy who met the criteria for borderline personality disorder and, it could be added, for antisocial personality disorder (except for age). This child had been seen by psychiatrists since age 5, pointing to the chronicity and severity of his problems. He was expelled for assaultiveness, and already at age 11 had beaten and raped a 6-year-old girl. His anger was uncontrollable, and he had bizarre fantasies about violence, death, and destructiveness. Shifting ego states were indicated by his occasional lapses into baby talk. On admission to the inpatient unit, Sharwell was ingratiating and overly complimentary to the therapist, whom he considered the only good person; in contrast, he was abusive to the rest of the staff, threatening to kill them. He had no ability to control his cravings: he overate and had the table manners of a 2-year-old. He conned other children out of their belongings, their turns at bike riding, or their desserts at mealtimes. Similarly, he begged or borrowed from any gullible adult. Yet, despite his show of bravado, he described himself as "bad, dumb, fat, weird-looking, weak, and ugly."

Although Adams and Fras (1988) presented this case as a borderline personality, as I mentioned, it also fulfills the criteria for antisocial personality disorder. The child had a severe conduct disorder with highly aggressive behavior and assaultiveness (the rape). Uncontrollable anger and a pattern of irresponsible and antisocial behavior were evidenced in his outbursts of rage, in addition to failure to follow social norms, stealing, lying, and conning others for personal profit or pleasure.

Case Example 2

At 10 years of age, Tom was unable to accept criticism; he had little respect for authority, and his work patterns at school were careless and disorganized. In his peer relationships, he had to be "in charge"; if not, he would physically or verbally attack his peers. He showed a lack of regard for other people's property and on occasion stole. He didn't seem to feel guilty after misbehaving. Although at times he could appear as a likeable, successful student, in general he was a discipline problem at school, demanding constant attention.

On the Wechsler Intelligence Scale for Children, his verbal score was 97 and performance score 104. Picture arrangement was in the 91st percentile, pointing to his social smartness, but on similarities he scored in the 16th percentile. He demonstrated a good understanding of social causality and good

Table 48-4.   DSM-III-R diagnostic criteria for antisocial personality disorder

A. Current age at least 18.

B. Evidence of conduct disorder with onset before age 15, as indicated by a history of *three* or more of the following:
   1. Was often truant.
   2. Ran away from home overnight at least twice while living in parental or parental surrogate home (or once without returning).
   3. Often initiated physical fights.
   4. Used a weapon in more than one fight.
   5. Forced someone into sexual activity with him or her.
   6. Was physically cruel to animals.
   7. Was physically cruel to other people.
   8. Deliberately destroyed others' property (other than by fire setting).
   9. Deliberately engaged in fire setting.
   10. Often lied (other than to avoid physical or sexual abuse).
   11. Has stolen without confrontation of a victim on more than one occasion (including forgery).
   12. Has stolen with confrontation of a victim (e.g., mugging, purse-snatching, extortion, armed robbery).

C. A pattern of irresponsible and antisocial behavior since the age of 15, as indicated by at least *four* of the following:
   1. Is unable to sustain consistent work behavior, as indicated by any of the following (including similar behavior in academic settings if the person is a student):
      a) Significant unemployment for six months or more within five years when expected to work and work was available
      b) Repeated absences from work unexplained by illness in self or family
      c) Abandonment of several jobs without realistic plans for others
   2. Fails to conform to social norms with respect to lawful behavior, as indicated by repeatedly performing antisocial acts that are grounds for arrest (whether arrested or not), e.g., destroying property, harassing others, stealing, pursuing an illegal occupation.
   3. Is irritable and aggressive, as indicated by repeated physical fights or assaults (not required by one's job or to defend someone or oneself), including spouse- or child-beating.
   4. Repeatedly fails to honor financial obligations, as indicated by defaulting on debts or failing to provide child support or support for other dependents on a regular basis.
   5. Fails to plan ahead, or is impulsive, as indicated by one or both of the following:
      a) Traveling from place to place without a prearranged job or clear goal for the period of travel or clear idea about when the travel will terminate
      b) Lack of a fixed address for a month or more
   6. Has no regard for the truth, as indicated by repeated lying, use of aliases, or "conning" others for personal profit or pleasure.
   7. Is reckless regarding his or her own or others' personal safety, as indicated by driving while intoxicated, or recurrent speeding.
   8. If a parent or guardian, lacks ability to function as a responsible parent, as indicated by one or more of the following:
      a) Malnutrition of child
      b) Child's illness resulting from lack of minimal hygiene
      c) Failure to obtain medical care for a seriously ill child
      d) Child's dependence on neighbors or nonresident relatives for food or shelter
      e) Failure to arrange for a caretaker for young child when parent is away from home
      f) Repeated squandering, on personal items, of money required for household necessities
   9. Has never sustained a totally monogamous relationship for more than one year.
   10. Lacks remorse (feels justified in having hurt, mistreated, or stolen from another).

D. Occurrence of antisocial behavior not exclusively during the course of schizophrenia or manic episodes.

reality testing. On the other hand, despite his bravado, he evidenced low self-esteem.

In groups, Tom often showed off by doing breakdancing and was not particularly interested in playing with other kids, introducing unusual rules into a checkers game, for example, so that he could win.

He learned to behave well enough to be discharged, yet a few months later he reverted to severe temper tantrums, lied, stole small items, and had difficulty sitting still. At the time his parents were going through a divorce, with the father being verbally and physically abusive to the mother.

Tom was the product of an unplanned pregnancy of an unmarried woman. His father had displayed criminal behavior and had allegedly committed a murder; his mother was a drug addict. As a young child, Tom was accident prone. Later, he was truant from school and lied about doing his homework.

When interviewed at age 14, what was striking was his withholding of information, his secretiveness. He denied using drugs and complained that the physician was a "spy." He also indicated that his teachers disliked him and did not call on him although he knew the answers.

This boy was eventually killed in an automobile accident while playing "chicken" by lying in front of cars. His pet rabbit had been found dead earlier that day.

Case Example 3

Because he was 16 years old at the time of his evaluation, Sam was diagnosed as having severe conduct disorder, solitary type, instead of antisocial personality disorder. He had been stealing and lying since grammar school. Sam was the biological son of a man who had beaten and raped his mother. His mother was a substance abuser. In kindergarten, Sam was evaluated professionally when he poked a schoolmate with scissors. Although he was never officially charged with a crime, he was arrested by the police because of vandalism. He had day and night dreams of shooting and stabbing people. He also cut himself, stating "I feel relieved. . . . I had a weight on my shoulders and [now] I don't feel it anymore."

In his mental status examination, Sam did not show any formal thought disorder. Cognitive function was intact clinically, as was his reality testing, although he had heard voices inside his head: "They tell me I am bad." Despite his fantasies of suicide and homicide, he denied he would act on these. He was aware of his lack of remorse when he did hurt someone: "I am so cold. Things don't affect me. I have no conscience." He had some insight into the nature of his difficulties, commenting that if he had a lot of feelings, he just could not hold everything in: "It builds up and I explode."

During the psychiatric assessment, this boy murdered a neighbor. He did not complete the evaluation, because he was sent to a reform school.

Treatment

Psychotherapy is contraindicated for the child with antisocial personality disorder, because psychotherapy depends on the capacities for relationship and honesty, which are impaired in these patients. Behavior modification has had some positive responses in attempts to control aggression with token economy and time-out procedures, or contingency programs in which cessation of the behavior (e.g., stealing) leads to home visits. Par-

ent training has also been relatively successful based on parent report. Pharmacotherapy has been used for target symptoms, but the findings from these trials are inconclusive.

Berlin (unpublished manuscript) reported on a noncontingency milieu approach in which all contingencies are unpredictable and inconsistent in terms of punishment and rewards. The youngster is thrown into acute anxiety or depression, or even acute disorganization, which in turn makes the child more dependent on the staff and more treatable. The treatment lasts from a few weeks to 2 months.

Concluding Remarks

A study of personality development is closely linked with the issues of continuities and discontinuities in development, as summarized by Emde and Harmon (1984). Although discontinuities often concern specific times of developmental transformation or change, there are also times of qualitative shifts with new patternings in behavior. From a genetic point of view, there are processes that switch on and switch off in development, so that genetic mechanisms not only form the basis for stabilities, but can also account for discontinuities. Discontinuity, however, does not imply a lack of connectedness between early developments and later ones, as described by Rutter (1984). From a different perspective, Korner (1964) has described continuities in style that are related to temperament and dyadic relationships and continuities concerning competencies or skill, such as cognition.

Even biological models have to address these new perspectives on continuities. Despite the notion of critical periods, it has been found that adults can undergo structural alterations as a result of experience. Critical periods may relate more to the rate of connections and primacy of early patterns than to unique mechanisms in the immature brain. The plasticity of the brain is greater than anticipated.

Longitudinal studies may be able to clarify issues of continuity and discontinuity. For example, when the representational self emerges, an internalized set of intentions and role structures also begins to appear, so that it should then be more possible than before to identify continuities and behavioral connectedness. Another approach looks in more detail at heterotypic continuities, which relate to a given behavior that appears different at a later age because of developmental transformations.

Which aspects of personality are chosen for study certainly will affect the outcome. Personality traits organize themselves, and it is this organization that shows continuity, not the isolated traits. It is also important to appreciate the mutual influences of the observation of behavioral traits, and the environment, taking into account, for example, role expectations for the different sexes at school or at home. To talk about continuities requires that these continuities be related to the context in which they are studied.

Assessing Normality and Abnormality

Discussions of personality and personality disorders in the adult psychiatric literature (Frances 1986; Gorton and Akhtar 1990) indicate the controversy between categorical and dimensional taxonomy. Categorical taxonomy draws sharp boundaries between normality (no disorder present) and abnormality (disorder present). In contrast, dimensional taxonomy requires a quantitative assessment across a number of continuous dimensions, such as self-concept, interpersonal relations, and cognitive styles. Indeed, personality disorders viewed from a categorical perspective do not include patients who may have significant pathology, such as those who overlap Axis I and Axis II categories or have mixed atypical disorders. Moreover, more than one personality diagnosis may be present.

The same considerations can be applied to childhood psychopathology with certain modifications. For one, any boundary between normality and abnormality needs to be related to the developmental stage. State versus trait confusion can be significantly reduced if clinicians base their interview on collateral historical information and repeated interviews and observations, rather than on a single interview. Any diagnosis of personality disorder should fulfill these criteria: that there are inflexible and maladaptive behaviors causing significant impairment in social or occupational functioning, as well as subjective distress, and that these behaviors have been characteristic of the child's or adolescent's functioning for a period of 2 years or more, and have been exhibited in a wide range of important social and personal contexts. This proviso should reassure those clinicians who rightfully are concerned about overdiagnosis in childhood and adolescence.

Research Issues

The systematic exploration of personality disorders in childhood and adolescence remains to be done. Gutterman et al. (1987) reviewed five structured diagnostic interviews keyed to DSM-III criteria for psychiatric disorders in childhood and adolescence. Only one of the five interviews scheduled for children included the assessment of borderline, compulsive, histrionic, or schizotypal personality disorders. Yet treatment outcome may depend on the diagnosis of personality disorder.

It is important to clarify the Axis II category and the relationship between Axis II and Axis I diagnoses. To compound the problem, there is overlap within Axis II (Gorton and Akhtar 1990; McGlashan and Heinssen 1989). Looking at the Axis I and Axis II overlap, we find coexistence of affective disorders with a spectrum of personality disorders, including borderline, antisocial, dependent, hypomanic, narcissistic, histrionic, and self-defeating personality disorders. Schizophrenic disorders and even paranoid disorders may exist on a spectrum with Cluster A (or psychotic) personality disorders, while the anxiety disorders and social phobias coexist on a continuum with Cluster C (or neurotic) personality disorders. Organic brain disorders such as attention-deficit hyperactivity disorder seem frequently to be associated with the spectrum of borderline personality disorders. What is most interesting is that Axis II diagnoses may indicate a vulnerability to certain psychiatric illnesses, but they also may be the expression of chronic subsyndromal forms of specific psychiatric illnesses. Both could be attributed to a specific or particular developmental experience or genetic predisposition. What is most important is that personality comorbidity often predicts the disease course and treatment outcome in a variety of patients (Weissman et al. 1978).

In sum, the consideration of personality disorders in children and adolescents provides the clinician with a potentially useful tool for treatment planning, as well as for coordinating research efforts with the adult psychiatry field.

References

Aarkrog T: Borderline and psychotic adolescent: borderline symptomatology from childhood—actual therapeutic approach. Journal of Youth and Adolescence 6:187–197, 1977

Adams PL, Fras I: Beginning Child Psychiatry. New York, Brunner/Mazel, 1988

American Psychiatric Association: Diagnostic and Statistical Manual of Mental Disorders, 3rd Edition. Washington, DC, American Psychiatric Association, 1980

American Psychiatric Association: Diagnostic and Statistical Manual of Mental Disorders, 3rd Edition, Revised. Washington, DC, American Psychiatric Association, 1987

Andrulonis PA, Glueck BC, Stroebel CF, et al: Organic brain dysfunction and the borderline syndrome. Psychiatr Clin North Am 4:47–66, 1981

Bemporad JR, Smith HE, Hanson G, et al: Borderline syndromes in childhood: criteria for diagnosis. Am J Psychiatry 139:596–602, 1982

Beres D: Character formation in adolescence, in Psychoanalytic Approach to Problems and Therapy. Edited by Lorand S, Schneer H. New York, Delta Books, 1969, pp 1–9

Blum HF: The borderline childhood of the wolfman. J Am Psychoanal Assoc 22:721–742, 1974

Brazelton B: Neonatal behavior assessment scale, in Clinics in Developmental Medicine, No 50. Philadelphia, PA, JB Lippincott, 1973

Bronson WC: Adult derivatives of emotional expressiveness and reactivity control: developmental continuities from childhood to adulthood. Child Dev 38:801–817, 1967

Cantwell DP, Carlson GA: Stimulants, in Pediatric Psychopharmacology. Edited by Werry JS. New York, Brunner/Mazel, 1978, pp 171–207

Cohen DJ, Slaywitz SE, Young G, et al: Borderline syndromes and attention-deficit disorders of childhood, in The Borderline Child. Edited by Robson KS. New York, McGraw-Hill, 1983, pp 197–222

Egan J, Kernberg PF: Pathologic narcissism in childhood. J Am Psychoanal Assoc 32:39–62, 1984

Ekstein R, Wallerstein J: Observations on the psychology of borderline and psychotic children. Psychoanal Study Child 11:303–311, 1954

Emde RN, Harmon RJ: Entering a new era in the search for developmental continuities, in Continuities and Discontinuities in Development. Edited by Emde RN, Harmon RJ. New York, Plenum, 1984, pp 1–14

Epstein S: The stability of behavior: on predicting most of the people much of the time. J Pers Soc Psychol 37:1097–1126, 1979

Escalona SK, Heider GM: Prediction and Outcome. New York, Basic Books, 1959

Fenichel O: The Psychoanalytic Theory of the Neuroses. New York, WW Norton, 1945

Finch SM, Green JM: Personality disorders, in Basic Handbook of Child Psychiatry, Vol 2. Edited by Noshpitz J. New York, Basic Books, 1979, pp 235–248

Flament M, Whitaker A, Rapoport JL, et al: Obsessive compulsive disorder in adolescence: an epidemiological study. J Am Acad Child Adolesc Psychiatry 27:764–771, 1988

Frances AJ: Introduction to personality disorders, in Psychiatry, Vol 1. Edited by Michels R, Cavenar JO Jr, Brodie HKH, et al. New York, Basic Books, 1986, pp 1–6

Frijling-Schreuder E: Borderline states in children. Psychoanal Study Child 24:307–327, 1969

Gardner R, Moriarity A: Personality Development at Preadolescence: Exploration of Structure Formation. Seattle, WA, University of Washington Press, 1968

Geleerd E: Borderline states in childhood and adolescence. Psychoanal Study Child 13:279–295, 1958

Gorton G, Akhtar S: The literature on personality disorders, 1985–1988: trends, issues and controversies. Hosp Community Psychiatry 41:39–51, 1990

Gunderson J, Kolb J: Discriminating features of borderline patients. Am J Psychiatry 135:792–796, 1978

Gutterman EM, O'Brien JD, Young JG: Structured diagnostic interview for children and adolescents: current status and future directions. J Am Acad Child Adolesc Psychiatry 25:621–630, 1987

Halverson CF, Waldrop MF: Relations between preschool activity and aspects of intellectual and social behavior at age 7½. Developmental Psychology 12:107–112, 1976

Hartmann H: Ego Psychology and the Problem of Adaptation. New York, International Universities Press, 1958

Josephson MM, Porter RT (eds): Clinicians Handbook of Childhood Psychopathology. Northvale, NJ, Jason Aronson, 1979

Kagan J: Continuity and change in the opening years of life, in Continuities and Discontinuities in Development. Edited by Emde RN, Harmon RJ. New York, Plenum, 1984, pp 15–39

Kagan J, Moss A: Birth to Maturity. New York, John Wiley, 1962

Kernberg OF: Borderline Conditions and Pathological Narcissism. Northvale, NJ, Jason Aronson, 1976

Kernberg OF: The diagnosis of borderline conditions in adolescence, in Adolescent Psychiatry, Vol 6. Edited by Feinstein S, Giovacchini P. Chicago, IL, University of Chicago Press, 1978, pp 298–319

Kernberg PF: Psychoanalytic profile of the borderline adolescent, in Adolescent Psychiatry, Vol 7. Edited by Feinstein S, Giovacchini P. Chicago, IL, University of Chicago Press, 1979, pp 234–256

Kernberg PF: Hysterical personality in child and adolescent analysis, in Three Further Clinical Faces of Childhood. Edited by Anthony EJ. Jamaica, NY, Spectrum Publications, 1981, pp 27–58

Kernberg PF: Borderline conditions: child and adolescent aspects, in The Borderline Child: Approaches to Etiology, Diagnosis and Treatment. Edited by Robson KS. New York, McGraw-Hill, 1983a, pp 101–119

Kernberg PF: Issues in the psychotherapy of borderline conditions in children, in The Borderline Child: Approaches to Etiology, Diagnosis and Treatment. Edited by Robson KS. New York, McGraw-Hill, 1983b, pp 224–234

Kernberg PF: Children with borderline personality organization, in Handbook of Clinical Assessment of Children and Adolescents, Vol 2. Edited by Kestenbaum CJ, Williams DT. New York, New York University Press, 1988, pp 604–625

Kernberg PF: Narcissistic personality disorder in childhood. Psychiatr Clin North Am 12:671–694, 1989

Kestenbaum C: The concept of the borderline child as a child at risk for major psychiatric disorder in adult life, in The Borderline Child: Approaches to Etiology, Diagnosis and Treatment. Edited by Robson KS. New York, McGraw-Hill, 1983, pp 49–82

Korner A: Significance of primary ego and drive endowment for later development in the exceptional infant, in The Normal Infant, Vol 1. Edited by Helmuth J. New York, Brunner/Mazel, 1964, pp 192–207

Leichtman M, Nathan S: A clinical approach to the psychological testing of borderline children, in The Borderline Child: Approaches to Etiology, Diagnosis and Treatment. Edited by Robson KS. New York, McGraw-Hill, 1983, pp 121–170

Lewis M: Personality and personality disorder, in Psychiatry, Vol 2. Edited by Michels R, Cavenar JO Jr, Brodie HKH, et al. New York, Basic Books, 1986, p 108

Looney JG, Kramer J, Milich R: The hyperactive child grows up: prediction of symptoms, delinquency, and achievement at follow-up, in Psychosocial Aspects of Drug Treatment for Hyperactivity. Edited by Gadow K, Looney J. Boulder, CO, Westview Press, 1981, pp 212–241

Mahler M, Kaplan L: Developmental aspects in the assessment of narcissistic and so-called borderline personalities, in Borderline Personality Disorders: the Concept, the Syndrome, the Patient. Edited by Hartocollis P. New York, International Universities Press, 1977, pp 71–86

Martin WE: Singularity and stability of profiles of social behavior, in Readings in Child Behavior and Development. Edited by Stendler DB. New York, Harcourt, Brace, and World, 1964, pp 92–117

Masterson J: From Borderline Adolescent to Functioning Adult: The Test of Time. New York, Brunner/Mazel, 1980

McGlashan TH, Heinssen RK: Narcissistic, antisocial and non-comorbid subgroups of borderline disorder. Psychiatr Clin North Am 12:653–670, 1989

Metcalf A: Childhood process to structure, in Hysterical Personality. Edited by Horowitz MJ. Northvale, NJ, Jason Aronson, 1977, pp 223–282

Moss HA, Susman EJ: Longitudinal study of personality development, in Constancy and Change in Human Development. Edited by Brim OG Jr, Kagan J. Cambridge, MA, Harvard University Press, 1980, pp 530–595

Pedersen E, Faucher TA, Eaton WW: A new perspective on the effects of first grade teachers on children's subsequent adult status. Harvard Educational Review 48:1–31, 1978

Petti AT: Imipramine treatment of borderline children: case reports with a controlled study. Am J Psychiatry 138:515–518, 1981

Petti AT, Law W: Borderline psychotic behavior in hospitalized children: approaches to assessment and treatment. Journal of the American Academy of Child Psychiatry 21:197–202, 1982

Pfeffer CR: Clinical observations of suicidal behavior in a neurotic, a borderline and a psychotic child: common processes of symptom formation. Child Psychiatry Hum Dev 13:120–133, 1983

Pine F: On the borderline concept in children. Psychoanal Study Child 29:341–368, 1974

Pine F: A working nosology of borderline syndromes in children, in The Borderline Child: Approaches to Etiology, Diagnosis and Treatment. Edited by Robson KS. New York, McGraw-Hill, 1983, pp 83–100

Plakun EM: Narcissistic personality disorder: a validity study and comparison to borderline personality disorder. Psychiatr Clin North Am 12:3, 1989

Rapoport JL, Ismond DR: DSM-III-R Training Guide for Diagnosis of Childhood Disorders. New York, Brunner/Mazel, 1990

Richman N, Stevenson J, Graham P: Preschool to School: A Behavioral Study. London, Academic Press, 1982

Rinsley DB: Notes on the developmental pathogenesis of narcissistic personality disorder. Psychiatr Clin North Am 12:695–707, 1989

Rockland LH: Supportive Therapy: A Psychodynamic Approach. New York, Basic Books, 1989

Rosenfeld K, Sprince M: An attempt to formulate the meaning of the concept "borderline." Psychoanal Study Clin 18:603–635, 1963

Rutter M: Stress, coping and development: some issues and some questions. J Child Psychol Psychiatry 22:323–356, 1981

Rutter M: Continuities and discontinuities in socio-emotional development: empirical and conceptual perspectives, in Continuities and Discontinuities in Development. Edited by Emde RN, Harmon RJ. New York, Plenum, 1984 pp 41–68

Rutter M: Psychopathology and development: links between childhood and adult life, in Child and Adolescent Psychiatry: Modern Approaches. Edited by Rutter M, Hersov L. Oxford, UK, Blackwell Scientific, 1985, pp 720–739

Rutter M, Garmezy N: Developmental psychopathology, in Handbook of Child Psychology, Vol 4: Socialization, Personality and Social Development. Edited by Hetherington EM. New York, John Wiley, 1983, pp 775–991

Rutter M, Graham P: Psychiatric disorder in the young adolescent: a follow-up study. Proceedings of the Royal Society of Medicine (London) 66:1226–1229, 1973

Sandler V, Rosenblatt B: The concept of the representational world. Psychoanal Study Child 17:128–145, 1962

Scheidlinger S: Focus on Group Psychotherapy: Clinical Essays. New York, International Universities Press, 1982

Shapiro ER, Zinner J, Shapiro RL: The influence of family experience on borderline personality development. International Review of Psychoanalysis 2:399–412, 1975

Shields J: Some recent developments in psychiatric genetics. Arch Gen Psychiatry 22:347–360, 1975

Shulsinger F: Psychopathy: heredity and environment. Journal of Mental Health 1:190–206, 1972

Weil AM: Certain severe disturbances of ego development in childhood. Psychoanal Study Child 8:271–286, 1953

Weissman MM, Prusoff BA, Klerman GL: Personality and the prediction of long-term outcome of depression. Am J Psychiatry 135:797–800, 1978

Wiener JM: Diagnosis and Psychopharmacology of Childhood and Adolescent Disorders. New York, John Wiley, 1985

Yang RK, Moss HA: Longitudinal study of personality development, in Constancy and Change in Human Development. Edited by Brim OG Jr, Kagan J. Cambridge, MA, Harvard University Press, 1978, pp 530–595

Chapter 49

Forensic Psychiatry

John B. Sikorski, M.D.

The emergence of child and adolescent forensic psychiatry (Schetky and Benedek 1980, 1985) reflects not only the growth and maturation of child and adolescent psychiatry as a medical speciality with its own data base, knowledge, and clinical skills (Hirschberg 1966), but also the evolving social and cultural changes focusing on individual rights, changing family systems, and the role of governmental and other social institutions vis-à-vis children and families. Society's concern for children's rights (Harvard Educational Review 1974), family rights and responsibilities, and the interests of the state has a long tradition.

The first White House Conference on Children and Youth, called forth by President Theodore Roosevelt in 1909, focused concern on the plight of children and families in the changing American culture of the turn of the century and promoted, among other things, a more humane rehabilitative treatment of youth in a separately developing juvenile justice system.

The White House Conference on Children and Youth (U.S. Government Printing Office 1960) articulated the rights and needs of children:

1. To be wanted.
2. To be born healthy.
3. To live in a healthy environment.
4. To have their basic needs and rights met.
5. To have continuous loving care.
6. To acquire the intellectual and emotional skills necessary to achieve individual aspirations and to cope effectively in our society.

7. To receive care and treatment through facilities that are appropriate to their needs.
8. To keep children as close as possible within their normal social setting.

It is the intent of this chapter 1) to highlight the need for awareness and involvement in this arena of children's rights; 2) to introduce an overview of relevant forensic psychiatry concepts; 3) to highlight some major areas of particular concern and activity within the purview of child and adolescent psychiatry practice; and 4) to provide some direction and reference for further study.

The American Academy of Child Psychiatry (1983) called for increasing training to meet the needs for involvement in the juvenile justice and other forensic areas. Implementation of a "supervised essential experience" in the forensic area was made a special requirement for child psychiatry residency training programs in July 1988 (Accreditation Council for Graduate Medical Education 1988).

Demographic data compiled by governmental sources (University of California 1989; U.S. House of Representatives 1989) and reports from the National Council of Juvenile and Family Court Judges (1986, 1988) document the increasing numbers and percentages of children, youth, and families at risk for mental and emotional disorders and highlight the involvement of the legal and judicial processes in their care, treatment, and disposition (Congress of the United States 1986).

The child and adolescent psychiatrist must become knowledgeable and involved in forensic issues, at least as they impinge on particular aspects of patient care and clinical practices.

Definition

Forensic psychiatry generally refers to the interface between psychiatry and law, including not only the legal requirements on the practice of the clinical profession of psychiatry, but also the applicability of psychiatric knowledge, practice, and theory to the requirements of the legal process. The field has been defined by the American Board of Forensic Psychiatry and incorporated into its ethical guidelines by the American Academy of Psychiatry and Law as follows (Rosner 1989):

> Forensic psychiatry is a subspecialty of psychiatry in which scientific and clinical expertise is applied to legal issues in legal contexts, embracing civil, criminal, correctional or legislative matters; forensic psychiatry should be practiced in accordance with guidelines and ethical principles enunciated by the profession of psychiatry. (p. 323)

Although textbooks of psychiatry provide extensive discussion of the development of the field of forensic psychiatry (Diamond 1988; Gutheil 1989; Wettstein 1988), there has generally been minimal discussion of the more specific areas of interest and activity of the child and adolescent psychiatrist. Familiarity and knowledge of forensic psychiatry in general will facilitate the child psychiatrist's work in the juvenile and family court, as well as other areas at this interface.

Overview

In our society, law is not static, but rather is an ever-evolving organiclike system of rules and prohibitions reflecting the changing values, needs, and perceptions of our culture and society. Law in the formal sense is generated through legislative enactment and appellate court decision, as well as by government regulation or directive as authorized by the legislature, or by direct vote of the people as in election propositions. At any given time, the law may reflect the tension and conflict between legislated law, case or appellate court law, and a consensus of an ever-evolving social order.

In a somewhat oversimplified, pragmatic view, a law is anything that a court of competent jurisdiction will enforce, and what the courts enforce are claims on someone else's goods, services, or money or the deprivation or enhancement of someone's liberty or freedom of action. Court systems are empowered and defined by federal and state statutes for specific functions and operate under enabling statutes and the local rules of procedure.

In terms of the judicial process, it is the court that provides the mechanism for decision making. Courts in the person of the judge or jury are "triers of fact" and operate on evidence. Evidence is of two types: 1) fact, that is, what the court decides is a legal fact; and 2) expert opinion. (The court must qualify the expert as an expert in that particular technical field before such opinion can be considered as "expert evidence.")

The law also provides for different levels of confidence in the evidence presented, or "standards of proof" in the judicial decision-making process. The standard of proof in civil cases (e.g., injury, malpractice) is "preponderance of evidence." A higher standard of proof, as required by law, for example in involuntary civil commitment cases (*Addington v. Texas* 1979) and in cases of termination of parental rights (*Santosky v. Kramer* 1982), is "clear and convincing evidence."

The highest standard of proof, as required by law in criminal cases, including juvenile court delinquency proceedings (*In re Winship* 1970), is "beyond a reasonable doubt." The clinician should understand the legal reasoning and standards of proof in his or her particular case to evaluate the clinical data relative to that specific standard.

The Practitioner and the Process

A child psychiatrist may become involved in a legal matter arising subsequent to the evaluation or treatment of a child prior to some event such as an accident or trauma. The child psychiatrist then may be required to testify as to the child's prior condition, treatment, and prognosis, because the privilege of confidentiality has been waived or because the therapist has been legally required to report or testify, as for example, when a case falls under the requirements of child abuse reporting laws or when a patient's mental health has been placed at issue in a civil suit.

In another example, the child psychiatrist may become involved in a legal matter as a court-appointed expert to evaluate and make recommendations to the court concerning some specific legal purpose or issue, such as in child abuse, child custody, and visitation determinations; out-of-home placement or treatment alternatives; or termination of parental rights proceedings.

In developing the relevant evidence to be presented to a court, a physician's records may be subpoenaed. The subpoena is a valid court order requiring the production of records to a court or to an attorney or requiring participation in a deposition.

If a written report is required, the report should reflect five basic elements:

1. How one was referred or entered the case.
2. What was the purpose or issue to be addressed.
3. What did one do (e.g., interviews, record reviews, collateral information).
4. What were the observations and findings.
5. What is the conclusion, opinion, or recommendation, and what is the basis of that opinion relative to the law or legal guidelines, if any, appropriate to the legal matter under consideration.

Information or questions about the relevant laws or legal guidelines should be clarified with the court if one is court appointed, with the attorney involved in the case if that is appropriate, or with one's own attorney if further information or clarification is needed.

In writing a forensic report, the report should be comprehensive enough to document what was done, supporting the conclusions and reflecting the clinical judgment and reasoning, but not so long or jargonistic as to be unintelligible to the court.

If the child psychiatrist is selected and appointed by stipulation or court order, the order should specify: 1) the authority to proceed with the evaluation; 2) the scope and purposes of the evaluation, including the person or persons to be evaluated; 3) the method and person to whom the report is to be made; and 4) the method of payment of fees for the evaluator's professional services. Psychiatrists working in the forensic area are entitled to reasonable professional fees for their professional services, and such fee schedules and methods of payment should be arranged in advance of the work provided.

When one is appointed as an expert for evaluation of a person in a legal matter, it is essential that the person being examined clearly understand the nature and purpose of the interview and evaluation, the fact that it is not a confidential or otherwise private interview, and what the likely procedures to be followed in the reporting of the evaluation will be.

Ethical Issues

Child and adolescent psychiatrists are particularly challenged by ethical considerations because of their patients' age and vulnerability, as well as obligations to the parents or legal guardians who seek services on behalf of their children. The code of ethics of the American Academy of Child Psychiatry (1980) delineated these issues and stated in part: "The issues of consent, confidentiality, professional responsibility, authority and behavior must be viewed within the contexts of the overlapping and potentially conflicting rights of the child or adolescent, of the parents and of society" (p. 3).

The Practitioner and the Law

Clinical practice is a licensed privilege, governed by specific statutes in each state or jurisdiction that define and regulate the nature of the practice, as well as the duties and responsibilities of the practitioner (California Medical Association 1990). States also vary according to statute as well as appellate court rulings in regard to laws (Neinstein 1987) governing such issues as confidentiality and privileged communication, informed consent, age and conditions of consent to types of treatment, as well as refusal of treatment and special conditions for treatment, such as the use of medications for children in public custody (Barnum 1989).

Confidentiality as an ethical issue has a long tradition in the healing arts, going back to its codification in the Oath of Hippocrates. Confidentiality and privileged communication are considered to be the keystones of a trusting therapeutic relationship. The therapist is bound to hold in confidence the patient's privileged communication, and the legal right of the privilege is held by the patient. When the patient is a minor, it is clear that parental or legal guardian consent is required for evaluation, treatment, or release of information for the minor child, unless there are statutory or appellate court exceptions, which are numerous and varied in the different states.

In general, most states provide that the categories of "emancipated minors," those living away from parents and economically self-sufficient, and "mature minors," defined largely by case law, can consent to their own treatment, provided the minor has sufficient understanding of the treatment and will benefit from the treatment. The several states vary widely in their provisions to these minors for the authority to consent to various categories of their own care and treatment without parental consent. There is a wide variation in age of consent (e.g., age 12 in California for treatment of sexually transmitted diseases, age 14 in Washington State for similar treatment, age 16 in Idaho for the treatment of substance abuse), as well as specific type of condition or care that may be permissible.

Since generalizations as to permissibility may become misleading in this complex area, and states may quickly change statutes and appellate decisions under changing political conditions, it is prudent for the practitioner to consult with state or local medical or psychiatric organizations or his or her own counsel for the specific laws and guidelines in his or her jurisdiction.

The issue of informed consent by minors is almost always problematic because minors may not have sufficient maturity or worldly exposure to make an informed judgment about potential consequences. As a practical matter, most psychiatric evaluation and treatment with children and adolescents occur with the involvement and consent of the parents and the child. There should be an explanation of the nature and necessity for privileged communication between therapist and patient, and, where indicated, an articulation of the legal requirements wherein the privilege must be broken and information reported by the therapist to specific persons or agencies under specific conditions. The child psychiatrist, particularly dealing with adolescents, traverses the troubled waters between allying with the growth-enhancing aspects of the child and recognizing the stability, integrity, and legitimate caring of a functioning family.

In particular circumstances, the therapist may be in a position to enhance the best interests of the child, as well as the therapeutic alliance, by assisting and supporting a child in disclosing aspects of behavioral problems and real needs for family care and support to his or her parents.

Authorization for release of information about children from other sources should be discussed and obtained in writing from the parent(s) or legal guardian and should be specific as to the nature of the communication, the person with whom the communication is authorized, and the time frame of the authorization. In some specific cases, courts may, on proper legal justification, require the disclosure of certain information that is relevant to a specific legal issue before the court. States have varying laws reflecting the circumstances and conditions of such disclosure, and it must be kept in mind that the physician has no right to claim absolute privilege.

Concerning the use of medications, informed consent must be obtained from parents or legal guardians before administration of psychotropic medications to minors. This informed consent should include indications for use relative to the patient's condition, potential short- and long-term effects and side effects, and consent for administration of the medication.

The past two decades also have seen significant appellate court and legislative action, particularly in the area of prediction of dangerousness, duty to warn, and mandatory reporting of various diseases or conditions. These laws require licensed professionals to break their traditional obligation to confidentiality. The California Supreme Court, in the landmark "duty to warn" case (*Tarasoff v. Regents of the University of California* 1976), affirmed that psychotherapists have a legal duty to breach confidence and warn a third party if there is a serious danger of violence to that party by their patient. Subsequent appellate court and various state statutes have defined the nature and predictability of that dangerousness and the procedures for warning and reporting that dangerousness. The trend has been not to require a therapist to predict dangerousness in general, but rather to require a therapist to warn potential victims and local police authorities of specific threats of violence against specific identifiable individuals. These legislative and appellate court judgments represent continuing efforts to balance the rights of patients for confidentiality against the need for disclosure to protect the public. In reference to the behavior of minors in this regard, a California appellate court (*Thompson v. County of Alameda* 1980) indicated that a history of delinquent or violent behavior reflecting nonspecific threats against nonspecific victims does not constitute a duty to warn or a duty to report to the community.

Other chapters in this text focus on the areas of physical and sexual abuse (Chapters 44 and 45), AIDS (Chapter 46), and suicide (Chapter 47), but the clinician should be sufficiently familiar with these content areas to relate them to legal and ethical duties in regard to standards of care and community practice or seek further consultation in these areas in specific problem cases.

The past two decades have seen an alarming increase in reports and incidents of child neglect and abuse (National Council of Juvenile and Family Court Judges 1986) across all strata of American society. In response to federal initiatives as well as community and children's rights organizations, all states by the early 1980s passed more extensive and complex child abuse and neglect reporting statutes (Ten Bensel et al. 1985). These statutes tend to be very specific in regard to the definition of reportable behavior, including sexual abuse, sexual assault, sexual exploitation, neglect, willful cruelty or unjustifiable punishment of a child, unlawful corporal punishment or injury, abuse in out-of-home care, and child abuse. These statutes (e.g., California Penal Code number 11166) tend to be very specific as to the duty of observers to report what they observe or "know or reasonably suspect" to the local child protection agency immediately or as soon as practically possible, and further specify the mode of reporting of the suspected neglect or abuse and the procedures and duties of the various parties and agencies. There are usually provisions (e.g., California Penal Code number 11172) specifying the immunity to the professional regarding the mandatory reporting. Civil suits for failure in the duty to report also have occurred.

The particular and specialized child and adolescent psychiatric evaluation (American Academy of Child and Adolescent Psychiatry 1988), police and social service investigation procedures (Ten Bensel et al. 1985), and subsequent court proceedings (Edwards 1987) in these neglect and abuse cases can become exceedingly complex and require a knowledge and experience base, as well as a familiarity with statute and case law, that are beyond the scope of this chapter.

When a child is a victim of neglect or physical or sexual abuse or is a witness to a civil or criminal action, the child may be permitted or required to participate in the formal judicial proceedings, including testifying in court as a witness. There has been considerable debate in the past decade about this complex area, including the role and function of the child's evaluator (Terr 1986), the competency and credibility of the child as a witness (Benedek and Schetky 1986; Nurcombe 1986), and the effect of the process on the child witness, as well as attempts and recommendations to modify or reform the system and procedures for the best interests of the child, the constitutional rights of the accused, and the interests of justice (Arthur 1986; California Child Victim Witness Judicial Advisory Committee

1988). The landmark U.S. Supreme Court ruling in this area (*Wheeler v. United States* 1895) indicated that a 5-year-old boy "was not by reason of his youth, as a matter of law, absolutely disqualified as a witness" and that the question of competency "depends on the capacity and intelligence of the child, his appreciation of the difference between truth and falsehood, as well as his duty to tell the former." The clinician working in this area must be aware of the state and local jurisdiction rulings, as well as current standards of assessment relative to the child witness.

Practitioners should be aware that the confluence of children's rights, parental rights, and the interests of the state has generated some of the most tenacious and bitterly contested conflicts in several relevant areas during the past two decades. It follows that societal and professional consensus about these issues and their consequences has not yet firmly consolidated, and that modifications and changes can be expected in these areas in the foreseeable future.

A major area of ongoing concern and legal development involves the hospitalization of children and youth, which brings into conflict their rights to liberties and self-determination with the rights, responsibilities, and/or duties of parents, legal guardians, and state agencies. In the landmark case in this area (*Parham v. J.R.* 1979), the U.S. Supreme Court affirmed the parents' basic right to seek and secure hospital treatment for their minor children, provided independent medical review (not necessarily an adversarial due-process legal review) confirms the nature of the illness and likelihood of benefit from the proposed treatment. This independent medical review must have the power to deny admission if medical standards and legal requirements are not met, and the youth has the right to periodic reviews of treatment procedure and confinement. Civil commitment (Arthur 1987) and involuntary hospitalization require more rigorous due-process procedures, which may be specified and vary among the different states and various local jurisdictions.

Another area of significant societal conflict is reflected in the variety of state laws and appellate decisions regarding contraceptive information, sexually transmitted disease treatment, and ultimately consent for abortion for minors. The U.S. Supreme Court (*Bellotti v. Baird* 1979) defined the constitutionality of abortion rights for minors without parental consent and outlined a procedure of obtaining an expeditious independent judicial hearing concerning the minor's maturity and best interests. State laws may define the procedures whereby the minor provides her own consent or obtains the judicial hearing within the U.S. Supreme Court guidelines. The intensity and politicalization of the prolife-prochoice controversy will make this a problematic area for the foreseeable future.

The issue of a civil suit in the form of a malpractice claim may be raised against a psychiatrist (Schetky and Cavanaugh 1982) on the basis of breach of duty, negligence, abandonment, failure to follow established or community standards of care, or other alleged violations of law or practice procedures. Following precedents with the rest of medical practice and tort law, the issues involve the nature of the physician-patient relationship and the legal duties therein, evidence of breach of duty, the occurrence of injury or damage to the patient, and the demonstration that the breach of duty resulted in the specific damages. The demonstration of and the defense against such allegations require expert testimony on the standard of care relative to the particular allegations. Attentiveness to the physician's statutory duties, standards of care, and appropriate documentation in the clinical record are among the best methods of minimizing liability.

Dependency, Delinquency, and the Juvenile Court

The reform movements concerned with the condition and treatment of children in the changing American society of the beginning of the 20th century assisted in the creation of an innovative legal system for handling juvenile matters outside of the adult criminal court system. This specialized court system established through state-enabling legislation the local county courts with original jurisdiction over the care, treatment, rehabilitation, and disposition of minors who came to the attention of the courts by reason of 1) dependency, neglect, or abuse; 2) incorrigibility, now called "status offenses"; or 3) delinquency offenses (i.e., violation of criminal law). This system was based on the *parens patriae* concept of the civil authority exercising responsibility for children or those who are unable to care for themselves. The juvenile courts (Guyer 1985), as established in each state, had wide latitude and discretion to act in a rather informal, highly individualized fashion, creating and augmenting their procedures to intervene in the care, rehabil-

itation, and "reform" of the neglected, abandoned, incorrigible, or delinquent child.

Those youths deemed to be beyond the rehabilitation or reform capabilities of the juvenile court probation or "reform school" facilities were transferred or waived to the jurisdiction of the adult criminal court system. It was around this issue that the U.S. Supreme Court first intervened in a significant way concerning the rather informal functioning of the juvenile courts. In this decision (*Kent v. United States* 1966), the Supreme Court held that the decision of the juvenile court to transfer or waive jurisdiction to the adult criminal court is "critically important" and therefore requires a due-process-type hearing, including assistance of counsel with access to the social service records and a written record, including statement of reasons for the transfer so that it may be reviewed on appeal.

In the landmark decision that brought considerable reform in the operation of the juvenile court proceedings (*In re Gault* 1967), the U.S. Supreme Court held that "due process" and "procedural justice" apply to all stages of a trial for adjudication as delinquents. The U.S. Supreme Court articulated these elements to include:

1. Adequate notice of trial at all stages.
2. Right to counsel.
3. Right to confront witnesses in cross-examination.
4. Privilege against self-incrimination, both pretrial and during trial.
5. Proper appellate review, including the right to transcripts of the proceedings.

Subsequent U.S. Supreme Court decisions held that the standard of proof required for juvenile delinquency adjudication is the higher standard of "beyond a reasonable doubt" (*In re Winship* 1970), that there is no constitutional right to a jury trial in juvenile delinquency adjudication hearings (*McKeiver v. Pennsylvania* 1971), and that state statutes may provide for pretrial detention of a juvenile when there is "serious risk" that the juvenile "may before the return date, commit an act which, if committed by an adult, would constitute a crime" (*Schall v. Martin* 1984).

Child psychiatrists and other mental health professionals providing evaluation and treatment to individuals and families or consultative services to aspects of the juvenile justice system must acquaint themselves with the complexities and cross-currents of that system (Schwartz 1989), as well as aspects of the law (Thornton et al. 1987), processes (Mershon 1982), and dispositions that have developed in these areas and are relevant in their particular states and jurisdictions.

Child Custody Issues and Family Law

There is perhaps no issue at the interface of psychiatry and law that has burgeoned in volume, complexity, detail, and perhaps conflict in the past two decades more than the law in regard to domestic relations, divorce, and child custody (Hyde 1984). This rapid increase has followed changes in societal and family institutions; sharpened social consciousness about individual rights; and newly obtained social science research data on children, families, and the consequences of divorce during these past two decades (Hetherington 1979, 1989; Kelly 1988; Wallerstein 1980, 1985).

Concerning the legal standards for claims of custody of minor children, the long precedent of father's prima facie right and duty changed into a "maternal presumption" or "tender years doctrine" by the early 20th century. From a long process of legal and social science examination of claims and needs, not only of children involved in custody disputes (Derdeyn 1976; Watson 1969) but also of children in need of care and parenting (Goldstein et al. 1973), the concept of "best interests of the child" emerged. This has become the overriding legal concept codified in general terms in some states (e.g., California Civil Codes 4600-4608) or specifically defined in terms of the elements of that standard in other states (Group for the Advancement of Psychiatry 1980).

California Civil Code Number 4608 provides that the court's determination of what constitutes the child's best interests shall include but not be limited to considerations of the health, safety, and welfare of the child, including any history of abuse of the child, and the nature and amount of contact between the child and each parent. States that have provided minimal statutory definition have seen an abundance of litigation, expert testimony, and appellate court attempts at definition and resolution in generating public policy.

The Washington State legislature has taken an innovative approach in the Parenting Act of 1987 (1987 Wash. Laws, Ch. 460, RCW 26.09), mandating that each parent file a proposed permanent parenting plan along with all petitions and responses for dissolution. The Parenting Act defines the policy of best interests of the child; defines parenting functions; accounts for dispute resolution and allocation of decision-making authority; encourages parental agreements; and provides, among other things, for professional personnel to provide advice in writing to the court. It is too soon to assess the results of this statewide innovation, but it does represent a legislative attempt to minimize, rather than enhance, parental conflict over children.

The complexities of clinical evaluation and the variable legal considerations in different states and jurisdictions render a more definitive discussion of child custody evaluation (Ash and Guyer 1986) and consultation (American Psychiatric Association 1982), including assessment of parenting capacity (Steinhauer 1983), considerations of the type of custody arrangements, and other special considerations (Schetky and Benedek 1985), beyond the scope of this introductory chapter.

In conclusion, clinicians working at the interface of law and psychiatry are encouraged to proceed with caution, a current knowledge base, awareness of the relevant laws in the local jurisdiction, good clinical judgment, and perhaps, if in doubt, the consultation of experienced colleagues and/or the advice of one's own counsel if further information is needed.

References

Accreditation Council for Graduate Medical Education: Revision of Special Requirements to Directors, Residency Training in Child Psychiatry. Chicago, IL, Accreditation Council for Graduate Medical Education, 1988

Addington v Texas, 441 US 418, 99 S Ct 1804, 1979

American Academy of Child and Adolescent Psychiatry: Guidelines for the clinical evaluation of child and adolescent sexual abuse: position statements of the American Academy of Child and Adolescent Psychiatry. J Am Acad Child Adolesc Psychiatry 27:655–657, 1988

American Academy of Child Psychiatry: Code of Ethics. Washington, DC, American Academy of Child Psychiatry, 1980

American Academy of Child Psychiatry: Child Psychiatry: A Plan for the Coming Decades. Washington, DC, American Academy of Child Psychiatry, 1983

American Psychiatric Association: Child Custody Consultation: A Report of the Task Force on Clinical Assessment in Child Custody. Washington, DC, American Psychiatric Association, 1982

Arthur LG: Child sexual abuse: improving the system's response. Juvenile and Family Court Journal 37(2):1–75, 1986

Arthur LG: Civil commitment. Juvenile and Family Court Journal 38:1–58, 1987

Ash P, Guyer M: Child psychiatry and the law: the functions of psychiatric evaluation in contested child custody and visitation cases. Journal of the American Academy of Child Psychiatry 25:554–561, 1986

Barnum R: The regulation of psychopharmacological treatment for children in public custody in Massachusetts. Massachusetts Family Law Journal 7:22–31, 1989

Bellotti v Baird, 443 US 622, 99 S Ct 3035, 1979

Benedek EP, Schetky DH: The child as a witness. Hosp Community Psychiatry 37:1225–1229, 1986

California Child Victim Witness Judicial Advisory Committee: Final Report. Sacramento, CA, California Attorney General's Office, 1988

California Medical Association: California Physician's Legal Handbook. San Francisco, CA, California Medical Association, 1990

Congress of the United States: Children's mental health: problems and services. Congress of the United States, Office of Technology Assessment. Washington, DC, U.S. Government Printing Office, 1986

Derdeyn AP: Child custody contests in historical perspective. Am J Psychiatry 133:1369–1376, 1976

Diamond BL: Forensic psychiatry, in Review of General Psychiatry. Edited by Golman HH. Norwalk, CT, Appleton & Lange, 1988, pp 640–650

Edwards LP: The relationship of family and juvenile courts in child abuse cases. Santa Clara Law Review 27:201–278, 1987

Goldstein J, Freud A, Solnit AJ: Beyond the Best Interests of the Child. New York, Free Press, 1973

Group for the Advancement of Psychiatry, Committee on the Family: Divorce, Child Custody and the Family (Vol 10, No 106). San Francisco, CA, Jossey-Bass, 1980

Gutheil TG: Forensic psychiatry, in Comprehensive Textbook of Psychiatry V, Vol 2. Edited by Kaplan HI, Sadock BJ. Baltimore, MD, Williams & Wilkins, 1989, pp 2107–2124

Guyer MJ: Commentary: the juvenile justice system, in Emerging Issues in Child Psychiatry and the Law. Edited by Schetky DH, Benedek EP. New York, Brunner/Mazel, 1985, pp 159–179

Harvard Educational Review: The Rights of Children (Harvard Educational Review Reprint No 9). Cambridge, MA, Harvard Educational Review Publications, 1974

Hetherington EM: Divorce: a child's perspective. Am Psychol 34:851–858, 1979

Hetherington EM: Coping with family transitions: winners, losers and survivors. Child Dev 60:1–4, 1989

Hirschberg JC: The basic functions of a child psychiatrist in any setting. Journal of the American Academy of Child Psychiatry 5:360–366, 1966

Hyde LM: Child custody: divorce. Juvenile and Family Court Journal 35:1–72, 1984

In re Gault, 387 US 1, 87 S Ct 1428, 1967

In re Winship, 397 US 358, 90 S Ct 1068, 1970

Kelly JB: Longer term adjustment in children of divorce: converging findings and implications for practice. Journal of Family Psychology 2:119–140, 1988

Kent v United States, 383 US 541, 86 S Ct 1045, 1966

McKeiver v Pennsylvania, 403 US 528, 91 S Ct 1976, 1971

Mershon JL: Juvenile Justice: The Adjudicatory Process (Juvenile Justice Textbook Series). Reno, NV, National Council of Juvenile and Family Court Judges, 1982

National Council of Juvenile and Family Court Judges: Deprived children: a judicial response. Reno, NV, National Council of Juvenile and Family Court Judges, 1986

National Council of Juvenile and Family Court Judges: Drugs: the American family in crisis—a judicial response. Reno, NV, National Council of Juvenile and Family Court Judges, 1988

Neinstein LS: Consent and confidentiality laws for minors in the western United States. West J Med 147:218–224, 1987

Nurcombe B: The child as witness: competency and credibility. Journal of the American Academy of Child Psychiatry 25:473–480, 1986

Parham v J.R., 442 US 584, 99 S Ct 2463, 1979

Rosner R: Forensic psychiatry: a subspeciality. Bull Am Acad Psychiatry Law 17:323–333, 1989

Santosky v Kramer, 455 US 745, 102 S Ct 1388, 1982

Schall v Martin, 467 US 253, 104 S Ct 2402, 1984

Schetky DH, Benedek EP (eds): Child Psychiatry and the Law. New York, Brunner/Mazel, 1980

Schetky DH, Benedek EP (eds): Emerging Issues in Child Psychiatry and the Law. New York, Brunner/Mazel, 1985

Schetky DH, Cavanaugh JL: Child psychiatry perspective: psychiatric malpractice. Journal of the American Academy of Child Psychiatry 21:521–526, 1982

Schwartz IM: (In)Justice for Juveniles: Rethinking the Best Interests of the Child. Lexington, MA, Lexington Books, 1989

Steinhauer PD: Assessing for parental capacity. Am J Orthopsychiatry 53:468–481, 1983

Tarasoff v Regents of the University of California, 17 Cal 3rd 425, 1976

Ten Bensel RW, Arthur LG, Brown L, et al: Child Abuse and Neglect (Juvenile Justice Textbook Series). Reno, NV, National Council of Juvenile and Family Court Judges, 1985

Terr LC: The child psychiatrist and the child witness: traveling companions by necessity, if not by design. Journal of the American Academy of Child Psychiatry 25:462–472, 1986

Thompson v County of Alameda, 167 Cal Rptr 70, 1980

Thornton WE, Voight L, Doerner WG: Juvenile law and the juvenile court, in Deliquency and Justice, 2nd Edition. New York, Random House, 1987, pp 309–339

University of California: Conditions of children in California: policy analysis for California education. Berkeley, CA, School of Education, University of California, 1989

U.S. Government Printing Office: The Golden Anniversary White House Conference on Children and Youth. Washington, DC, U.S. Government Printing Office, 1960

U.S. House of Representatives: U.S. children and their families: current conditions and recent trends, 1989 (The Select Committee on Children, Youth and Families, U.S. House of Representatives). Washington, DC, U.S. Government Printing Office, 1989

Wallerstein JS, Kelly JB: Surviving the Breakup. New York, Basic Books, 1980

Wallerstein JS (ed): Children of divorce: recent research. Journal of the American Academy of Child Psychiatry 24:515–589, 1985

Watson AS: The children of Armageddon: problems of custody following divorce. Syracuse Law Review 21:55–86, 1969

Wettstein RM: Psychiatry and the law, in The American Psychiatric Press Textbook of Psychiatry. Edited by Talbott JA, Hales RE, Yudofsky SC. Washington, DC, American Psychiatric Press, 1988, pp 1059–1084

Wheeler v United States, 159 US 523 S Ct, 1895

Section XI

Treatment

Chapter 50

Psychopharmacology

Joseph Biederman, M.D.

The field of pediatric psychopharmacology has shown limited progress over the last 40 years beyond the use of stimulants. Relatively little of the information regarding the use of psychotropics in children and adolescents has been grounded on empirically based studies. Despite this limitation, psychotropics have been widely used in pediatric patients, often without clear indications or adequate monitoring (Biederman and Jellinek 1984). Pharmacotherapy should be part of a treatment plan in which consideration is given to all aspects of the child's or adolescent's life. It should not be used instead of other interventions or after other interventions have failed. Realistic expectations of pharmacotherapy based on knowledge of what it can and cannot do, as well as careful definition of target symptoms, are major ingredients for a successful intervention. The use of psychotropics should follow a careful evaluation of the child and the child's family, including psychiatric, social, cognitive, and educational evaluations. Diagnostic information should be gathered from the child, from the parents or caregivers, and whenever possible, from the teachers. This evaluation should arrive at a multiaxial diagnostic evaluation based on DSM-III-R (American Psychiatric Association 1987). Careful attention should be paid to differential diagnosis, including medical and neurologic as well as psychosocial factors contributing to the clinical presentation. Since psychiatric disorders of children and adolescents can be associated with additional cognitive deficits and learning difficulties, which may not respond to psychotropics, it is imperative that the child undergo a careful neuropsychological evaluation aimed at pinpointing deficits and defining remedial interventions. This evaluation may help in the design and implementation of an educational plan tailored to the needs of the child.

Early therapeutic intervention is important before complications, chronicity, and social incapacitation occur, which can make treatment and a restabilization of functional life habits more difficult. In addition to pharmacotherapy, treatment requires a variety of methods, including psychotherapy, family therapy, and behavioral therapy. In severe cases, hospitalization may be required. Before treatment with a psychotropic is initiated, the family and the child need to be made familiar with the risks and benefits of such intervention, the availability of alternative treatments, and the likely adverse effects, including short-term, long-term, and withdrawal adverse effects. Certain adverse effects can be anticipated based on known pharmacologic properties of the drug (e.g., the anticholinergic effects of tricyclic antidepressants); others, generally rare, are unexpected (idiosyncratic) and are difficult to anticipate based on the properties of the drug. Short-term adverse effects can be minimized by introducing the medication at low initial doses and titrating slowly. Long-term side effects require monitoring of anticipated adverse effects (e.g., growth when using stimulants; kidney and thyroid function when using lithium carbonate). Idiosyncratic adverse effects require drug discontinuation and selection of alternative treatment modalities.

Treatment should be started at the lowest possible dose, which usually is the lowest manufactured dose. Once pharmacotherapy is initiated, frequent (i.e., weekly) contact with the patient and family is necessary during the initial phase of treatment to monitor carefully response to the intervention and adverse effects. Evaluation of adverse effects should include both subjective reports from the patient and family (e.g., stomachaches, appetite changes) and appropriate evaluation of objective measurements (e.g., heart rate, blood pressure changes). Following a sufficient period of clinical stabilization (i.e., 6–12 months), it is prudent to reevaluate the need for continued psychopharmacologic intervention. Withdrawal symptoms should be distinguished from the exacerbation of the disorder for which the psychotropic was prescribed. To minimize withdrawal reactions, it is important to discontinue medications gradually. Since most psychiatric disorders are chronic or recurrent conditions, a mechanism for timely follow-up after drug discontinuation is necessary. In this chapter, the major clinical considerations will be reviewed first, followed by descriptions of the major drug classes.

Diagnostic Categories and Clinical Considerations

Developmental Disorders

This class of disorders is coded in DSM-III-R in Axis II and includes mental retardation, pervasive developmental disorders (autistic and autistic-like disorders), and the specific developmental disorders (learning disabilities) (Table 50-1). The syndrome of autism is discussed in detail by Tsai and Ghaziuddin in Chapter 17 (this volume). No specific treatment alters the natural history of this syndrome. The specific developmental disorders (learning disabilities) represent a mixed group of cognitive dysfunctions in the context of no overall intelligence deficit and adequate educational opportunities.

Children with mental retardation and pervasive developmental disorders often have psychiatric disorders and behavioral problems, including hyperactive, aggressive, distractible, and self-abusive behaviors. They also often manifest multiple neurologic abnormalities. Psychotropics are primarily used in this population for the treatment of agitation, aggression, and self-injurious behaviors. Antipsychotics have been traditionally used to con-

trol these symptoms. Few studies support the use of one type of antipsychotic drug over another. While a more sedating phenothiazine (e.g., chlorpromazine, thioridazine) may be beneficial for the more agitated patient, a more potent phenothiazine (e.g., perphenazine, trifluoperazine) or the butyrophenone haloperidol may be helpful in the withdrawn, inactive child. Beta-blockers (and clonidine) have been increasingly reported to be useful in developmentally disordered patients for the management of agitation, aggression, and self-abusive behaviors (Mattes 1986). Considering the relatively low toxicologic profile of these drugs compared with the antipsychotics, they are the preferred first treatment for the management of these complications.

Antidepressant drugs and lithium carbonate can be effective in controlling affective symptoms and disorders, and stimulants may improve the symptoms of attention-deficit hyperactivity disorder (ADHD) in children and adolescents with mental retardation. Antianxiety agents should be used with caution in the management of developmentally disordered children because they tend to produce disinhibition, which may result in increased restlessness and more disturbed behavior. The anorexigenic drug fenfluramine has been reported to have a beneficial effect in some children with autism; however, more recent studies reported equivocal results (Campbell et al. 1988a; Stubbs et al. 1986). An open report by Realmuto et al. (1989) found behavioral benefits in symptoms of aggression and hyperactivity associated with the nonbenzodiazepine antianxiety drug buspirone in four autistic children. In an open study, Campbell et al. (1988b) reported on the efficacy and safety of naltrexone, a potent and long-acting opioid antagonist in the treatment of autistic children, using daily doses of 1–2 mg/kg.

The treatment of specific developmental disorders (learning disabilities) is largely remedial and supportive. Although psychotropics have not been effective in altering the basic course of the disorder, Wilsher et al. (1987) reported on the apparent efficacy of piracetam in improving the reading ability and reading comprehension of reading-disabled children in a double-blind, placebo-controlled study. Piracetam is structurally similar to gamma-aminobutyric acid (GABA) and is purported to improve selectively the efficiency of higher cognitive functions. Children with learning disabilities and ADHD or major depressive disorder can benefit from the treatment approaches directed at treating the associated psychiatric disorder.

Table 50-1. **Developmental disorders**

Disorder	Main characteristics	Pharmacotherapy

Mental retardation	Coded as Axis II diagnoses
	Significant subaverage global intellectual functioning plus deficit in adaptive functioning
		No specific pharmacotherapy for the core disorder; pharmacotherapy of complications:
		For aggression and self-abuse:
		  Beta-blockers (e.g., propranolol)
		  Clonidine
		  High-potency benzodiazepines (e.g., clonazepam)
		  Lithium
		  Opiate antagonist
		  Antipsychotics
		Other Axis I disorders (e.g., ADHD, major depressive disorder, psychosis, anxiety): treat the underlying disorder as in individuals without mental retardation

Pervasive developmental disorders	Qualitative impairment in social interactions, acquisition of cognitive, language, and motor skills; it can be global, or in specific or multiple areas	Same as mental retardation
Specific developmental disorders (learning disabilities)	Inadequate development of specific academic, language, and motor skills not due to physical, neurologic disorder, pervasive developmental disorder, or deficient educational opportunities No specific treatment for core disorder	No specific pharmacotherapy for the core disorder; main treatment remains remedial help and special education Piracetam? Other Axis I disorders (e.g., ADHD, major depressive disorder, anxiety): treat the underlying disorder

Note. ADHD = attention-deficit hyperactivity disorder.

Disruptive Behavior Disorders

DSM-III-R includes in this class of disorders ADHD, conduct disorder, and oppositional disorders (Table 50-2) (see Chapters 23–27, this volume). ADHD is one of the major clinical and public health problems in the United States in terms of morbidity and disability in children and adolescents, and perhaps in adults. Its impact on society is enormous in terms of financial cost, the stress to families, the impact on schools, and the damaging effects on self-esteem. Data from cross-sectional, retrospective, and follow-up studies indicate that children with ADHD are at risk for developing other psychiatric disorders in childhood, adolescence, and adulthood, such as antisocial behaviors, psychosis, alcoholism, and substance abuse, as well as depressive symptoms and depressive disorders. A child with ADHD requires a comprehensive treatment plan addressing family, educational, and social factors. The pharmacologic component of treatment, although not curative, and limited in terms of helping educational achievement, can decrease some of the most disturbing symptoms of this disorder. Pharmacotherapy of ADHD children can help not only abnormal behaviors in school but, equally important, the child's social and familial life (Gittelman-Klein 1987).

Stimulants have been used widely in the treatment of ADHD, yet as many as 30% of children so treated do not improve (Barkley 1977). Since stimulants are short-acting drugs, their use is compli-

Table 50-2. Disruptive behavioral disorders

Disorder	Main characteristics	Pharmacotherapy
Attention-deficit hyperactivity disorder	Inattentiveness, impulsivity, hyperactivity 50% will continue to manifest the disorder into adulthood	Stimulants (70% response; for uncomplicated ADHD; contra-indicated in patients with tics) Tricyclic antidepressants (70% response, second line for uncomplicated cases; first line for patients with comorbid MDD or anxiety disorders, and for patients with ADHD + tics) Clonidine (second line for uncomplicated cases; for patients with ADHD + tics) Bupropion (third line for treatment-resistant cases) MAOIs (third line for treatment-resistant cases) Combined pharmacotherapy for treatment-resistant cases

Conduct disorder	Persistent and pervasive patterns of aggressive and antisocial behaviors
	Often associated with ADHD and MDD
		No specific pharmacotherapy available for core disorder
		Behavioral therapy
		Stimulants? Tricyclic antidepressants?
		For agitation, aggression, and self-abuse:
		  Beta-blockers (e.g., propranolol)
		  Clonidine
		  High-potency benzodiazepines (e.g., clonazepam)
		  Lithium
		  Opiate antagonist
		  Antipsychotics
		Other Axis I disorders (e.g., ADHD, MDD, psychosis, anxiety): treat the underlying disorder

Note. ADHD = attention-deficit hyperactivity disorder. MDD = major depressive disorder. MAOIs = monoamine oxidase inhibitors.

cated by the need to take medicine in school and the troublesome rebound of symptoms in the evening hours at home. In addition, insomnia, dysphoric mood, and, during development, some slowing of growth in weight and height may occur (Gittelman-Klein 1987). These problems encourage the search for pharmacologic alternatives in the treatment of ADHD. An important aspect of the search for alternatives to stimulant treatment is the need to define an effective and acceptable treatment for adolescents with ADHD. Although it is clear that the ADHD syndrome persists into ado-

lescence and adulthood in many patients who manifested ADHD as children (Gittelman and Mannuzza 1988; Gittelman et al. 1985; Weiss et al. 1985), there is very limited information regarding appropriate pharmacotherapy in the older age groups. Several open and controlled studies have reported beneficial effects of stimulants in adolescents with ADHD-like symptoms (Biederman 1988; Varley 1985). However, concerns about treating adolescents with stimulant medication include the hypothetical risk of abuse and dependence by the patient (or the patient's associates), concerns about growth suppression, and, in general, the common dislike by adolescents of the subjective effects of stimulant medication.

Tricyclic antidepressants (TCAs), mainly imipramine, have been proposed as an alternative treatment for ADHD. Possible advantages of TCAs over stimulants include a longer duration of action and the feasibility of once-daily dosing without symptom rebound or insomnia, greater flexibility in dosage, the option of monitoring plasma drug levels, and minimal risk of abuse or dependence. Controlled studies show that, in general, TCAs are superior to placebo, although not always superior to methylphenidate. Desipramine, a major active metabolite of imipramine, has relatively selective neuropharmacologic actions on noradrenergic neurotransmission and, like other TCAs, eventually enhances the functional availability and activity at alpha-adrenergic receptors. Because of its pharmacologic properties, desipramine is associated with a lesser risk of adverse effects, such as sedation, dry mouth, and impairment in cognition, commonly encountered with imipramine and other tertiary amine TCAs. Several open and controlled studies have reported beneficial effects of desipramine in children and adolescents with ADHD using daily doses ranging from 2 to 5 mg/kg (Biederman et al. 1989a, 1989b; Donnelly et al. 1986; Garfinkel et al. 1983; Gastfriend et al. 1985). In these reports, desipramine was well tolerated without clinically significant cardiovascular effects despite relatively high doses (Biederman et al. 1985).

In addition to TCAs, other compounds have been evaluated in the treatment of ADHD. In a 12-week double-blind, crossover trial using monoamine oxidase inhibitors (MAOIs) in 14 children, Zametkin et al. (1985) reported significant and rapid reduction in ADHD symptoms with minimal adverse effects. In an open trial with adults with ADHD, Wender et al. (1983) reported a 60% response to pargyline (Eutonyl). Using a crossover, double-blind study design, Hunt et al. (Hunt 1987; Hunt et al. 1985, 1986) reported the beneficial effects of the alpha-adrenergic stimulating agent clonidine in the treatment of children with ADHD with daily doses of up to 4–5 μg/kg. Clonidine was well tolerated, and the main adverse effect was sleepiness, which tended to subside after 3 weeks of continued treatment. More recently, the novel antidepressant bupropion was found to be superior to placebo and was well tolerated in the treatment of 30 ADHD children in a 6-week, parallel-group, placebo-controlled, double-blind study in daily doses of 3–6 mg/kg (Casat et al. 1989). Beta-blockers (propranolol) have been reported to be helpful in treatment of adults with ADHD and severe impulsive and dyscontrol symptoms (Mattes et al. 1984). Several other compounds found to be ineffective in the treatment of ADHD include dopamine agonists (amantadine and L-dopa) (Gittelman-Klein 1987) and amino acid precursors (DL-phenylalanine and L-tyrosine) (Reimherr et al. 1987). More recently, a controlled study failed to find therapeutic benefits in ADHD for the antiserotonergic, anorectic drug fenfluramine (Donnelly et al. 1989).

There is no specific pharmacotherapy for conduct disorder. In a large controlled investigation, Platt et al. (1984) found both haloperidol and lithium carbonate to be superior to placebo in reducing aggression in conduct-disordered children. Studies have shown a significant decrease in aggressive behaviors as a result of treatment using some form of behavioral management, whether focused on the child's coping skills or the parents' management skills (Quay 1986). When conduct disorder co-occurs with ADHD, mood disorders, or anxiety disorders, the treatment of the comorbid disorder can result in substantial clinical stabilization and facilitate the psychosocial treatment approach for the conduct-disordered child.

Tic Disorders

The best known of the tic disorders is Tourette's syndrome, a severe neuropsychiatric syndrome of childhood onset and lifelong duration that consists of multiform motor and phonic tics and other behavioral and psychological symptoms (Table 50–3). Affected patients commonly have spontaneous waxing, waning, and symptomatic fluctuation. Tourette's syndrome is commonly associated with ADHD (in about 50% of cases) and obsessive-compulsive disorder (in about 30% of cases) (Pauls et al. 1986a, 1986b). In many cases, the comorbid disorders are the major source of distress and disability rather than the tic disorder. The association with ADHD is particularly problematic since it appears earlier in life than the tics, and since the use of stimulants appears to be detrimental. The antipsychotic drugs, particularly haloperidol, continue to be considered the drugs of choice in Tourette's syndrome. However, antipsychotics have limited effects on the frequently associated comorbid disorders and carry a risk for the development of tar-

Table 50-3. Tic disorders

Disorder	Main characteristics	Pharmacotherapy
Tourette's syndrome	Multiple motor and one or more vocal tics Frequently associated with ADHD and obsessive-compulsive disorder	Clonidine Tricyclic antidepressants Clonazepam Beta-blockers Antipsychotics Combined pharmacotherapy for treatment-resistant cases

Note. ADHD = attention-deficit hyperactivity disorder.

dive dyskinesia when administered chronically (Golden 1985). Clonidine (Leckman et al. 1985) has proven to be effective in some children with this disorder. In addition, clonazepam, beta-blockers, and desipramine (Hoge and Biederman 1986; Riddle et al. 1988) have been reported to be helpful in some children with Tourette's syndrome. Clonidine and TCAs can be particularly helpful in patients with Tourette's syndrome and ADHD. Patients with comorbid obsessive-compulsive disorder may need additional pharmacotherapy with serotonergic blocking drugs, such as clomipramine or fluoxetine.

Childhood Anxiety Disorders

DSM-III-R includes a subclass of three disorders of childhood or adolescence in which anxiety that is not due to psychosocial stressors is the predominant feature (Table 50-4). These are separation anxiety disorder, avoidant disorder, and overanxious disorder. Childhood anxiety disorders are relatively common disorders that bear striking similarities to the adult anxiety disorders and in many cases persist into adult life. In addition to the juvenile anxiety disorders, adult anxiety syndromes commonly emerge and can be diagnosed in childhood and adolescence. These include panic disorder with and without agoraphobia, social phobia, generalized anxiety disorder, obsessive-compulsive disorder, and posttraumatic stress disorder, as well as the atypical anxiety disorders termed anxiety disorders not otherwise specified. Only fairly recently has the literature documented that the diagnosis of panic disorder can be made in juveniles (Biederman 1990; Leonard and Rapoport 1989).

Although TCAs, MAOIs, and benzodiazepines have been found to be effective in the treatment of adult anxiety disorders—mainly panic disorder with and without agoraphobia (Rickels and Schweizer 1987)—very little is known about the pharmacotherapy of juvenile anxiety disorders. This situation may be partly due to the existing diagnostic confusion, which limits the use of therapeutic strategies that have been proven successful for the adult anxiety disorders. Gittelman and Klein (1971) reported that a high dose of imipramine was superior to placebo in children with school phobia. Berney et al. (1981) did not find that a low dose of clomipramine was superior to placebo in a small number of children with school phobia. Flament et al. (1985) reported the results of clomipramine treatment of 19 children and adolescents with severe obsessive-compulsive disorder. They reported a significant improvement in the children receiving clomipramine when compared with placebo. However, anticholinergic symptoms, such as dry mouth, constipation, and blurred vision, were common; one child had a grand mal seizure. Clomipramine is thought to be effective in obsessive-compulsive disorder because of its effects in blocking the reuptake of serotonin in the brain. A deficit in serotonin neurotransmission has been suggested as a possible etiology of this disorder (Rapoport 1988). Leonard et al. (1989) compared clomipramine with desipramine in the treatment of juvenile obsessive-compulsive disorder, showing that clomipramine had specific antiobsessional effects. Swedo et al. (1989) reported on the beneficial effects of clomipramine in the treatment of trichotillomania (hair pulling). Although trichotillomania is classified in DSM-III-R as an impulse control disorder, it may have some association with obsessive-compulsive disorder. As in obsessive-compulsive disorder, the beneficial effects were specific to clomipramine and did not occur with desipramine.

Bernstein et al. (1987) reported preliminary results of an ongoing three-arm study comparing al-

Table 50-4.   Anxiety disorders

Disorder	Main characteristics	Pharmacotherapy
Childhood anxiety disorders		
Separation anxiety disorder	Excessive anxiety on separation from caregivers or familial surroundings Inability to separate from the parent or from major attachment figures Similar to agoraphobia	High-potency benzodiazepine (clonazepam) Tricyclic antidepressants MAOIs Buspirone? Combined pharmacotherapy for therapy-refractory patients or patients with comorbid diagnosis (e.g., MDD, ADHD)
Overanxious disorder	Excessive or unrealistic worry about future events (similar to generalized anxiety disorder)	Same as for separation anxiety disorder
Avoidant disorder	Persistent and severe shrinking from contact with strangers that interferes with psychosocial functioning (bears similarities to social phobia)	Same as for other anxiety disorders?
Adjustment disorder with anxious mood (severe)	Maladaptive short-term reaction to a severe stressor	Short-acting benzodiazepine (lorazepam)
Adult-like anxiety disorders		
Panic disorder (with and without agoraphobia)	Recurrent discrete periods of intense fear (panic attacks) Frequent comorbidity with MDD (50%) and ADHD (30%)	High-potency benzodiazepine (clonazepam) Tricyclic antidepressants MAOIs Buspirone? Combined pharmacotherapy for therapy-refractory patients or patients with comorbid diagnosis (e.g., MDD, ADHD)
Agoraphobia	Fear of being in places or situations with limited escape (e.g., school), and as a result of this fear, the adolescent restricts travel or needs a companion (e.g., parent) when away from home or caregiver (e.g., at school)	Same as panic disorder
Social phobia	Fear of social situations in which the person may be exposed to scrutiny by others or fears humiliation	Same?
Generalized anxiety disorder	Excessive or unrealistic worry about future events	Same
Obsessive-compulsive disorder	Recurrent, severe, and distressing obsessions and/or compulsions	Clomipramine Fluoxetine

Note.   MAOIs = monoamine oxidase inhibitors. MDD = major depressive disorder. ADHD = attention-deficit hyperactivity disorder.

prazolam, imipramine, and a placebo in 25 school-phobic children; both active medications were superior to the placebo ($P < .05$). Biederman (1987) reported on the use of clonazepam in the treatment of children with panic-like symptomatology in doses of 0.5–3.0 mg/kg. Clonazepam is a high-potency long-acting 1,4-benzodiazepine with antiepileptic properties that has been reported to be efficacious in the treatment of adults with panic disorder and agoraphobia (Pollack et al. 1986).

Despite the limited literature, adolescents with anxiety disorders can respond to the same pharmacologic approaches as the adult patients. Although TCAs and MAOIs can be effective in the treatment of most anxiety disorders, they are associated with substantial adverse effects, and the MAOIs require serious dietetic restrictions. When TCAs are used, careful monitoring with serum levels and electrocardiograms is necessary. The serotonergic antidepressant clomipramine has been found to be effective in the treatment of juvenile obsessive-compulsive disorder. Other newer antidepressants such as fluoxetine (Prozac) that have the property of enhancing serotonin effects in the central nervous system also appear to be effective in the treatment of obsessive-compulsive disorder. Because of their relatively benign adverse effects profile, high-potency benzodiazepines are the drug of choice for uncomplicated juvenile anxiety disorders (Biederman 1987, 1990). Clonazepam may be particularly useful in the treatment of adolescent patients because of its high potency and long duration of action. When the anxiety disorder presents with comorbid major depression or ADHD, treatment with an antidepressant may be preferable. In some cases, combined pharmacotherapy may be necessary.

Mood Disorders

Juvenile mood disorders are recognized by DSM-III-R as disorders with core symptoms similar to those found in adult mood disorders and with developmentally specific associated features, such as school difficulties, school refusal, negativism, aggression, and antisocial behavior (Table 50-5). The depressive disorders should be carefully differentiated from feeling states, such as unhappiness or disappointment, which commonly occur during childhood. The juvenile symptom complex of mania should be differentiated from ADHD, conduct disorder, and psychotic disorders. There has been a paucity of information regarding the psychopharmacology of juvenile mood disorders. To date, there are only a few studies, reporting equivocal results, that have addressed the effectiveness of TCAs in treatment of juvenile major depressive disorder, and no studies have evaluated

the efficacy of MAOIs or lithium carbonate. Although the initial pharmacologic literature tended to suggest that children with well-defined major depressive disorder can respond favorably to antidepressant therapy when adequate serum levels are attained (Preskorn et al. 1982), a more recent controlled investigation (Puig-Antich et al. 1987) failed to find a significant difference between imipramine and a placebo. Puig-Antich et al. found high levels of response in imipramine-treated and placebo-treated prepubertal children with major depressive disorder using high doses (5 mg/kg) and attaining good serum levels. Ryan et al. (1986) examined the relationship between maintenance plasma levels of imipramine plus desipramine and antidepressant effect at 6 weeks in a sample of 34 adolescents with major depressive disorder. On average daily doses of 4.5 mg/kg of imipramine and average total plasma concentrations of 284 ng/ml, only 44% of the subjects responded, and no relationship was detected between plasma levels and clinical response.

The suggested pharmacologic approaches for children and adolescents with mood disorders are based on available data from adults as well as on clinical experience and anecdotal information (Kashani and Sherman 1989; Youngerman and Canino 1978). In juveniles with nonbipolar major depressive disorder, treatment with conventional antidepressants (TCAs or MAOIs) is recommended. If there is no response to an adequate trial (in dose and time) of a conventional antidepressant, or if the patient cannot tolerate the drug, subsequent trials with novel antidepressants (fluoxetine, bupropion) are recommended. For bipolar disorders, manic-type treatment with lithium carbonate is recommended. If there is no response to an adequate trial (in dose and time) to lithium, or if the patient cannot tolerate the drug, subsequent trials with anticonvulsants are recommended (carbamazepine, valproic acid). In manic patients with psychotic symptoms, additional antipsychotic treatment is recommended. In bipolar disorder, depressed type, combined treatment with lithium carbonate and an antidepressant is indicated. Bipolar disorder, mixed type requires an aggressive treatment approach combining the therapeutic recommendation outlined earlier for the manic and depressive subtypes.

There is some evidence that juvenile mood disorders may be more refractory to pharmacologic intervention than the adult disorders (Ryan et al. 1986). In depressive adults, bipolarity, atypicality,

Table 50-5.   Mood disorders

Disorder	Main characteristics	Pharmacotherapy
Major depressive disorder	Similar to the adult disorders with age-specific associated features Sad or irritable mood and associated vegetative symptoms occurring together for a period of time	Tricyclic antidepressants New antidepressants MAOIs Antidepressants + antipsychotics when psychosis develops Adjunct strategies for therapy-refractory patients Antidepressants + low-dose Li + BZDs + T_3 + stimulants Electroconvulsive therapy
Bipolar disorder: depressed	Same as major depressive disorder	Li + strategies for major depressive disorder

Bipolar disorder: manic	Elevated or severely irritable/angry mood
	More frequent psychotic symptoms in juvenile mania
		Lithium
		Li + antipsychotics if psychosis develops
		Tegretol
		Valproic acid
		For therapy-refractory patients:
		    Li + carbamazepine;
		    Li + adjunct antipsychotics,
		    Li + high-potency BZDs,
		    Li + clonidine

Bipolar disorders: mixed	Mixed depressed and manic symptoms Most common presentation of bipolar disorder in juveniles Usually very severe clinical picture	Li + antipsychotics Li + antidepressants Li + high-potency BZDs Electroconvulsive therapy

Note.   MAOIs = monoamine oxidase inhibitors. Li = lithium. BZDs = benzodiazepines.

and psychotic symptoms are associated with poor response to TCAs (Biederman 1988). TCA nonresponders may benefit from treatment strategies that include 1) the use of higher doses of the TCA in patients without adverse effects and with a relatively low plasma concentration of the TCA; 2) adjunct treatment approaches such as a low dose of lithium carbonate, stimulants, thyroid hormone (T_3), or antianxiety medications; and 3) MAOIs for TCA nonresponders with atypical depression (Biederman 1988). It is reasonable to expect lithium carbonate to be effective in the treatment and prophylaxis of adolescents with bipolar disorder. However, rapid cycling and prepubertal onset are considered to be poor prognostic factors for lithium responsiveness. Adolescent bipolar patients receiving lithium therapy alone may benefit from the addition of antipsychotics when manic, and the addition of antidepressants when depressed. For lithium nonresponders, carbamazepine therapy could be considered.

Other Disorders

Psychotic disorders. The term *psychosis* is used in DSM-III-R to describe abnormal behaviors of individuals with grossly impaired reality testing (see Campbell et al., Chapter 20, this volume). The term *psychosis* is also used when the individual's behavior is grossly disorganized and when it can be inferred that reality testing is impaired. The diagnosis of psychosis requires the presence of either delusions or hallucinations (Table 50-6). Psychotic disorders in children, as in adults, can be "functional" or "organic." Functional psychotic syndromes include schizophrenia and related disorders and the psychotic forms of mood disorders. Organic psychosis can develop secondary to lesions to the central nervous system as a consequence of medical illnesses, trauma, or drug use, both licit and illicit.

The mainstay of treatment of psychoses is the antipsychotic medications. In cases in which the psychotic process occurs in the context of a mood

Table 50-6. Other disorders

Disorder	Main characteristics	Pharmacotherapy
Psychotic disorders	Delusions and hallucinations	Antipsychotics (risk for tardive dyskinesia) High-potency benzodiazepines for agitation *For treatment-resistant cases:* *Clozapine* Antipsychotics + lithium Antipsychotics + carbamazepine Antipsychotics + beta-blockers Antipsychotics + benzodiazepines
Enuresis	Bed wetting	Behavioral therapy Tricyclic antidepressants DDAVP

Note. DDAVP = desmopressin.

disorder, the concomitant use of specific treatments for mood disorders is crucial for clinical stabilization. In cases in which the clinical picture of psychosis is associated with severe agitation, the adjunct use of high-potency benzodiazepines, such as lorazepam and clonazepam, can facilitate the management of the patient and may lead to the use of lower doses of antipsychotics. The extent to which antiparkinsonian agents should be used prophylactically when antipsychotics are introduced is controversial. Whenever possible, antiparkinsonian agents should be reserved until extrapyramidal symptoms emerge. Extrapyramidal reactions can be prevented in many cases by avoiding rapid neuroleptization or the use of high-potency antipsychotics such as haloperidol. When a child or an adolescent on antipsychotics develops an acutely agitated clinical picture with associated inability to sit still and with aggressive outbursts, the possibility of akathisia should be rapidly considered in the differential diagnosis. If suspected, the dose of the antipsychotic may need to be lowered. Beta-blockers (e.g., propranolol) have been found helpful in relieving symptoms of antipsychotic-induced akathisia in adults and may help relieve similar symptoms in juveniles (Ananth and Lin 1986). In recent years, the syndrome of postpsychotic depression has received increasing attention. Initial trials with antidepressant drugs added to the antipsychotic treatment appear to be promising in relieving patients from associated depression, thus fostering rehabilitation efforts. Postpsychotic depression should be distinguished from akinesia,

which is an adverse extrapyramidal effect that can respond to antiparkinsonian agents.

Enuresis. Children with functional enuresis usually respond to nonpharmacologic therapies (e.g., behavior modification, psychotherapy), and these treatments should be considered first. When an immediate therapeutic effect is necessary, an antidepressant drug, commonly imipramine, may be used. In most cases, symptoms reappear after the drug is withdrawn. Antidepressant therapy should not be continued for a period of more than 6 months; enuresis may remit spontaneously. Recently, the Food and Drug Administration approved the synthetic antidiuretic hormone desmopressin (DDAVP) for the treatment of enuresis.

Major Drug Classes Used in Pediatric Psychiatry

Stimulants

Stimulant drugs were the first class of compounds to have been reported as effective in the treatment of the behavioral disturbances that are evident in children with ADHD (Gittelman-Klein 1987). Stimulants are sympathomimetic drugs structurally similar to endogenous catecholamines. The most commonly used compounds in this class include methylphenidate (Ritalin), *d*-amphetamine (Dexedrine), and magnesium pemoline (Cylert) (Table

50-7). These drugs are thought to act both in the central nervous system and peripherally by preventing reuptake of catecholamines into presynaptic nerve endings, and thus preventing their degradation by monoamine oxidase. Methylphenidate and *d*-amphetamine are both short-acting compounds with an onset of action within 30–60 minutes and a peak clinical effect usually seen between 1 and 3 hours after administration. Therefore, multiple daily administrations are required for a consistent daytime response. Slow-release preparations, with a peak clinical effect between 1 and 5 hours, are available for methylphenidate and *d*-amphetamine and can often allow for a single dose to be administered in the morning that will last during the school day. Typically these compounds have a rapid onset of action so that clinical response will be evident when a therapeutic dose has been obtained. Magnesium pemoline is a longer-acting compound with a duration of action that is greater than 24 hours, thus allowing for a single daily dose. The onset of action, however, can often be delayed for as long as 2–8 weeks, and it is considered to be a less reliably effective medication.

The primary indication for the use of stimulants is in the treatment of ADHD. Stimulants diminish motor overactivity and impulsive behaviors seen in ADHD and allow the patient to sustain attention. Stimulants can also be effective in children and adolescents with ADHD in whom hyperactivity is not a significant symptom (Safer and Krager 1988), as well as in the treatment of mentally retarded patients with ADHD. Finally, as in adults, stimulants can be helpful as an adjunct treatment for refractory mood disorders (depressive disorders).

Because of their short half-life, the short-acting stimulants should be given in divided doses throughout the day, typically 4 hours apart. The total daily dose ranges from 0.3 mg/kg to 2 mg/kg/day. Starting dose is generally 2.5–5 mg/day given in the morning, with the dose being increased if necessary every few days by 2.5–5 mg in a divided dose schedule. Because of the anorectic effects of the stimulants, it may be beneficial to administer the medicine after meals. Being longer acting, magnesium pemoline is typically given as a single daily dose in the morning, at a dose ranging from 1 to 3 mg/kg/day. The typical starting dose of pemoline is 18.75–37.5 mg, with increments in doses of 18.75 mg every few days thereafter until desired effects occur or side effects preclude further increments. The concern that optimal clinical efficacy is attained at the cost of impaired learning ability has not been confirmed (Gittelman-Klein 1987). The literature on the association between clinical benefits in ADHD and plasma levels of stimulants has been equivocal and complicated by large inter- and intraindividual variability in plasma levels at constant oral doses (Gittelman-Klein 1987).

Table 50-7.   Stimulants

Drug	Main indications	Daily dose (mg/kg)	Daily dosage schedule	Common adverse effects
Dextroamphetamine	ADHD Mental retardation + ADHD	0.3–1.5	Twice or three times	Insomnia, decreased appetite, weight loss Depression psychosis (rare, with very high doses)
Methylphenidate	Adjunct therapy in refractory depression	1.0–2.0		Increase in heart rate and blood pressure (mild) Possible reduction in growth velocity with long-term use Withdrawal effects and rebound phenomena
Magnesium pemoline		1.0–3.0	Once	Same as other stimulants Abnormal liver function tests

Note.   ADHD = attention-deficit hyperactivity disorder.

The most commonly reported side effects associated with the administration of stimulant medication are appetite suppression and sleep disturbances. The sleep disturbance that is commonly reported is delay of sleep onset and usually accompanies late afternoon or early evening administration of the stimulant medications. Although less commonly reported, mood disturbances ranging from increased tearfulness to a full-blown major depression-like syndrome can be associated with stimulant treatment (Klein et al. 1980). Other infrequent side effects include headaches, abdominal discomfort, increased lethargy, and fatigue. Although the adverse cardiovascular effects of stimulants beyond heart rate and blood pressure have not been examined, mild increases in pulse and blood pressure of unclear clinical significance have been observed (Brown et al. 1984). A stimulant-associated toxic psychosis has been observed, usually in the context of either a rapid rise in the dosage or very high doses. The reported psychosis in children in response to stimulant medications resembles a toxic phenomenon (e.g., visual hallucinosis) and is dissimilar from the exacerbation of the psychotic symptoms present in schizophrenia. The development of psychotic symptoms in a child exposed to stimulants requires careful evaluation to rule out the presence of a preexisting psychotic disorder. Administration of magnesium pemoline has been associated with hypersensitivity reactions involving the liver accompanied by elevations in liver function studies (serum glutamic-oxaloacetic transaminase [SGOT] and serum glutamic-pyruvic transaminase [SGPT]) after several months of treatment. Thus baseline liver function studies and repeat studies are recommended with the administration of this compound.

The precipitation or exacerbation of tic disorder following stimulant administration is a concern (Lowe et al. 1982). Evidence indicates that children with a personal or family history of tic disorders are at greater risk for developing a chronic tic disorder when exposed to stimulants; the tic disorder can persist after discontinuation of the stimulant. Although it is unknown whether the same child would have spontaneously developed a tic disorder, until more information is available, the administration of stimulants should be avoided in children at risk for tic disorders. Sallee et al. (1989) reported that acute treatment with pemoline was associated with choreoathetoid movements of the face, limbs, and trunk, which subsided after drug discontinuation in some ADHD children.

Concerns also have centered on the effect of long-term administration of stimulants on growth. The initial report by Safer et al. (1972), based on a small number of cases, suggested that there is a decrease in growth velocity in children who have been treated with stimulants. However, more recent studies do not support this contention (Gittelman and Mannuzza 1988; Mattes and Gittelman 1983). In general, the consensus is that stimulants can produce a small, negative (deficit) impact on growth velocity that can be offset by drug holidays (Mattes and Gittelman 1983). Careful monitoring of growth is indicated during stimulant therapy, and if a decrease in growth occurs, consideration should be given to a drug holiday or alternative treatment options. A transient behavioral deterioration can occur on the abrupt discontinuation of stimulant medications in some children. The prevalence of this phenomenon and the etiology are unclear. Rebound phenomena can also occur in some children between doses, creating an uneven, often disturbing clinical course. In those cases, consideration should be given to alternative treatments.

Antidepressant Drugs

There are two main families of antidepressant medications: the imipramine-like drugs, usually referred to as TCAs, and the MAOIs (Table 50-8). Although well established in the psychopharmacologic armamentarium of adult psychiatric disorders, their use in pediatric psychiatry has been rather limited and almost exclusively focused on the use of imipramine. There is no adequate information regarding the efficacy and toxicity of either the MAOIs (e.g., phenelzine, tranylcypromine) or the newer antidepressants (e.g., maprotiline, trazodone, and amoxapine) in the treatment of childhood psychiatric disorders. More recently, the novel antidepressant bupropion has been found to be superior to placebo in the treatment of ADHD in children (Casat et al. 1989).

TCAs are structurally similar to the phenothiazines but have a different spectrum of clinical and adverse effects. Several TCAs are currently available, including the tertiary amines amitriptyline, imipramine, doxepin, and trimipramine, and the secondary amines desipramine, nortriptyline, and protriptyline. Although the precise mechanism of therapeutic action for the TCAs remains unknown, it may be due to the blocking effects of these drugs on the reuptake of brain neurotransmitters, espe-

Table 50-8.   Antidepressants

Drug	Main indications	Daily dose (mg/kg)	Daily dosage schedule	Common adverse effects
Tricyclic antidepressants (e.g., imipramine, desipramine, amitriptyline, nortriptyline)	Major depressive disorder Enuresis ADHD Tic disorder + obsessive-compulsive disorder Anxiety disorders	2.0–5.0 (1.0–3.0 for nortriptyline) Dose adjusted according to serum levels (Therapeutic window for nortriptyline)	Once or twice	Anticholinergic (dry mouth, constipation, blurred vision) Weight loss Cardiovascular (mild increase) diastolic blood pressure and ECG conduction parameters with daily doses >3.5 mg/kg. Treatment requires serum levels and ECG monitoring
Clomipramine	Obsessive-compulsive disorder			No known long-term side effects Withdrawal effects can occur (severe gastrointestinal symptoms, malaise) Overdoses can be fatal
Monoamine oxidase inhibitors (e.g., phenelzine, tranylcypromine)	Major depressive disorder Atypical depression ADHD Anxiety disorders	0.5–1.0	Twice or three times	Severe dietary restrictions (high-tyramine foods) Hypertensive crisis with dietetic transgression or with certain drugs Weight gain Drowsiness Changes in blood pressure Insomnia Liver toxicity (remote)
New antidepressants Fluoxetine	Major depressive disorder Obsessive-compulsive disorder	0.5–1.0	Once (in the A.M.)	Irritability Insomnia Gastrointestinal symptoms Headaches
Bupropion	ADHD Major depressive disorder	3–6	Three times	Irritability Insomnia Drug-induced seizures (in doses >6 mg/kg) Contraindicated in bulimic patients

Note.   ADHD = attention-deficit hyperactivity disorder. ECG = electrocardiogram.

cially norepinephrine and serotonin (5-hydroxy-tryptamine [5-HT]). However, a causal relationship between any known effect of antidepressants and clinical improvement remains to be discovered. Although antidepressants have similar spectra of ac-tion, their inhibitory effects on transmitter reuptake and their anticholinergic effects vary (Hyman 1988).

Early reports in the 1970s raised concerns regarding possible pharmacokinetic differences for TCAs in children compared with adults (Rapoport and Potter 1979). These studies suggested that TCAs may be more toxic in children than in adults. This concept was based on two premises. First, children have a smaller adipose compartment than adults, which could affect the uptake, redistribution, and storage of these drugs in the body. Second, children have decreased binding of TCAs to plasma albumin, which may result in a greater amount of circulating free drug. Although these concerns may apply to very young children, available evidence derived from multiple reports as well as wide clinical experience in the use of TCAs over the last decade supports similarities rather than differences in efficacy and toxicity between the use of TCAs in the treatment of psychiatric disorders in children and adolescents (Biederman et al. 1989a, 1989b).

TCAs are long-acting drugs with half-lives in children that may range from 10 to 17 hours. Since the response to antidepressants is seen more rapidly in children with enuresis or ADHD than in children treated for mood disorders, a different mechanism of action has been postulated for these disorders. Because of the slow onset of antidepressant action, investigators have been concentrating on slow-onset neurobiological effects of antidepressants, such as their ability to decrease the sensitivity of beta$_1$- and alpha$_2$-adrenergic and perhaps 5-HT$_2$ receptors.

Established indications for TCAs in pediatric psychiatry include the treatment of enuresis (Klein et al. 1980), ADHD (Biederman et al. 1989a, 1989b), and major depression (Kashani and Sherman 1989). Other possible applications for TCAs include the treatment of Tourette's syndrome (Hoge and Biederman 1986; Riddle et al. 1988) and childhood anxiety disorders (Leonard and Rapoport 1989). Dosage should be individualized in an attempt to use the lowest effective dose. For imipramine, an upper dose limit of 5 mg/kg has been suggested for children. However, this absolute dosage limit has little meaning, since a substantial interindividual variability in the metabolism and elimination of TCAs has been demonstrated in children. Therefore, some children tolerate only low doses, and others may require doses above such a ceiling. High doses (up to 5 mg/kg) of imipramine and desipramine have been used to treat school phobia, major depressive disorder, and ADHD in children (Biederman et al. 1989a, 1989b). The use of such high doses of imipramine or desipramine in the treatment of childhood psychiatric disorders reflects the emerging impression that children are relatively efficient in metabolizing and eliminating TCAs.

Treatment with a TCA should be initiated with a 10-mg or 25-mg dose, depending on the size of the child (approximately 1 mg/kg), and increased slowly every 4–5 days by 20%–30%. When a daily dose of 3 mg/kg (or a lower effective dose) is reached, steady-state serum levels and an electrocardiogram should be obtained. Most TCAs are available in tablet or capsule form. Nortriptyline is also available in a liquid preparation. Widely varying drug concentrations may be obtained in different patients on the same dose, potentially leading to markedly different outcomes, ranging from no response to improvement, or to iatrogenic toxicity. TCA serum level monitoring is useful not only to predict clinical response, but also to determine the limits of serum TCA concentration associated with adverse cardiovascular effects. In contrast, subjective adverse effects such as dry mouth or dizziness are unrelated to drug serum levels. Since the clinical effectiveness and toxicity of TCAs appear to be dose related, and since there is a wide interindividual variability in serum levels attained at a given dose, monitoring serum levels of TCAs may be more pertinent to maximizing benefits and avoiding toxicity than the daily dose per se, even if based on body size.

Common short-term adverse effects of the TCAs include anticholinergic effects such as dry mouth, blurred vision, and constipation. However, there are no known deleterious effects associated with chronic administration of these drugs. Gastrointestinal symptoms and vomiting may occur when these drugs are discontinued abruptly. Since the anticholinergic effects of TCAs limit salivary flow, they may promote tooth decay in some children. Regular dental supervision may be advisable in children receiving long-term TCA treatment.

Concerns have been raised regarding the possible cardiac toxicity of TCAs in young children, especially at daily doses above 3.5 mg/kg. For example, it has been reported consistently that children tend to have small but statistically significant elevations in diastolic blood pressure induced by imipramine and desipramine. Sinus tachycardia (>100 bpm) was also reported in studies of TCAs in children. In young children, tachycardia is not in itself abnormal or of hemodynamic significance. In older children or adolescents, however, a persistent heart rate above 130 bpm is of greater concern and may require further noninvasive evaluation of cardiac function (Biederman et al. 1989b). TCA-induced electrocardiographic abnormalities (conduction defects) also have been consistently reported in children at TCA doses higher than 3.5 mg/kg (Biederman et al. 1989b). Although of unclear hemodynamic significance, the development of conduction defects in patients receiving TCA treatment deserves closer electrocardiographic and clinical monitoring, especially when relatively high doses of TCA are used. In the context of cardiac disease, however, conduction defects have potentially more serious implications. When in doubt about the cardiovascular state of the patient, a complete (noninvasive) cardiac evaluation is indicated before initiating treatment with a TCA to help determine the risk-benefit ratio of such an intervention (Biederman et al. 1989b).

Although overdoses of TCAs are serious and potentially lethal events, these drugs are relatively safe when used at therapeutic doses with adequate monitoring. Clinical signs of an overdose include dry axilla, redness of skin, tachycardia, widening of the QRS, arrhythmias, seizures, and coma. Management depends on rapid recognition and intervention, support of vital functions, and a clear understanding of the pharmacology of the drug. Emptying the gastrointestinal tract with ipecac or lavage with activated charcoal is extremely important. Cardiac arrythmias generally respond to sodium bicarbonate, and seizures to benzodiazepines (Braden et al. 1986).

The available information on clinical uses of MAOIs in pediatric psychiatry is extremely limited. This class of drugs include the hydrazine (phenelzine) and nonhydrazine (tranylcypromine) compounds. Major general limitations for the use of MAOIs in children and adolescents are the dietetic restrictions of tyramine-containing foods (e.g., most cheeses), pressor amines (e.g., sympathomimetic substances), or drug interactions (e.g., most cold medicines, amphetamines), which can induce a hypertensive crisis. Drug interactions are one of the most serious risks with MAOIs. There are no known established indications for the use of MAOIs in pediatric psychiatry. MAOIs can be helpful in the treatment of depressive disorders (atypical types with reverse endogenous features) and anxiety disorders (mainly panic disorder). One controlled study in a small group of patients suggested the usefulness of MAOIs in ADHD (Zametkin et al. 1985). Short-term adverse effects include the potential for hypertensive crisis (treatable with phentolamine) associated with dietetic transgressions or drug interactions, orthostatic hypotension, weight gain, drowsiness, and dizziness. There is no information on long-term adverse effects of MAOIs in children.

Extrapolating from the adult literature, those may include hypomania, hallucination, confusion, and hepatotoxicity (rare). Pediatric dose ranges have not been established. Daily doses should be carefully titrated based on response and adverse effects and range from 0.5 to 1.0 mg/kg.

Two recently marketed novel antidepressants, fluoxetine and bupropion, are chemically unrelated and pharmacologically distinct from TCAs and other available antidepressants. Fluoxetine is a straight chain phenylpropylamine with a selective inhibitory effect of serotonin reuptake in the central nervous system. In addition to its antidepressant properties, it has been found to be effective in the treatment of obsessive-compulsive disorder in adults and juveniles in open clinical trials. Fluoxetine and its active metabolite have a half-life of 7–9 days. Common adverse effects include irritability, insomnia, gastrointestinal symptoms, and headaches. It comes in capsules of 20 mg. Daily doses are approximately 0.5–1.0 mg/kg. Bupropion hydrochloride is a novel-structured antidepressant of the aminoketone class, pharmacologically distinct from known antidepressants (Casat et al. 1989). Although bupropion seems to have an indirect dopamine agonist effect, its specific site or mechanism of action remains unknown. Bupropion is rapidly absorbed, with peak plasma levels usually achieved after 2 hours, with an average elimination half-life of 14 hours (8–24 hours). Bupropion is indicated in the treatment of depressive disorder. Bupropion has also been reported to be effective in the treatment of ADHD (Casat et al. 1989). This finding has not yet been confirmed. Side effects include edema, rashes, nocturia, irritability, anorexia, and insomnia. It appears to have a somewhat higher (0.4%) rate of drug-induced seizures relative to other antidepressants, particularly in daily doses higher than 6 mg/kg. It should be avoided in patients with seizure disorders. Because of the limited knowledge of its use, treatment with bupropion should be limited to patients who failed to respond to or could not tolerate more conventional treatments.

Antipsychotics

The major classes of antipsychotic drugs used clinically are: 1) phenothiazines, which include the low-potency compounds (requiring high mg/day dosages) such as chlorpromazine and thioridazine, and the high-potency compounds such as trifluoperazine and perphenazine; 2) butyrophenones (haloperidol and pimozide); 3) the thioxanthenes (thiothixene); 4) indolone derivatives (molindone); and 5) the dibenzoxazepines and dibenzodiazepines (loxapine and clozapine). These chemically varied drugs, which are remarkably similar pharmacologically, generally yield comparable benefit when given in equivalent doses and induce a similar variety of adverse effects (Table 50-9). In addition, those with low potency (e.g., chlorpromazine and thioridazine) are particularly likely to induce unwanted autonomic side effects, such as hypotension and sedation.

Both their in vitro receptor-binding properties and their in vivo effects confirm that the antipsychotic drugs in current use block the binding of dopamine at its D_2 receptor. The best evidence that

the observed D_2 receptor antagonism is relevant to the therapeutic effects of the antipsychotic drugs (in psychotic disorders) is the finding that their rank order of clinical potency (e.g., haloperidol > perphenazine > chlorpromazine) reproduces their rank order of in vitro binding affinity for the D_2 receptor, but not for other receptors. Even if the D_2 receptor is the primary site of action of the antipsychotic drugs, much remains to be learned. In particular, the afferents and efferents of the mesolimbic dopamine projections and the role of dopaminergic transmission in normal as well as psychotic individuals must be better understood before we understand what D_2 receptor blockade actually accomplishes. Since most psychotic pa-

Table 50-9. Antipsychotics

Drug	Main indications	Daily dose (mg/kg)	Daily dosage schedule	Common adverse effects
Phenothiazines Low-potency (e.g., chlorpromazine, thioridazine)	Psychosis Mania	3–6	Once or twice	Anticholinergic (dry mouth, constipation, blurred vision, more common with low-potency agents)
High-potency (e.g., fluphenazine, perphenazine)	As last resource for hyperaggressive behavior, severe agitation, severe insomnia, severe self-abuse Tourette's syndrome	0.1–0.5		Weight gain (lower risk with molindone) Extrapyramidal reactions (dystonia, rigidity, tremor akathisia; higher risk with high potency) Drowsiness
Butyrophenones (e.g., haloperidol)				Risk for tardive dyskinesia with chronic administration
Thioxanthenes (e.g., thiothixene)		1–3		Withdrawal dyskinesia
Molindone (indolone derivative)				
Clozapine Dibenzodiazepine atypical antipsychotic with serotonergic, adrenergic, histaminergic activity	Treatment-refractory psychosis	3–5	Two or three times	Low incidence of extrapyramidal adverse effects; does not induce dystonia Low risk for tardive dyskinesia Granulocytopenia/ agranulocytosis (treatment requires constant monitoring of blood count) Higher risk of seizures (dose related)

tients often improve over a period of days to weeks, it is likely that blockade of the D_2 receptor initiates an as yet undiscovered slow-onset change in some other component of the synaptic machinery or in the postsynaptic neuron (Hyman 1988). Molindone, although structurally distinct, exhibits many similarities to other neuroleptics, including dopamine receptor blockade, antipsychotic effects, and anticholinergic adverse effects (Owen and Cole 1989). Clozapine, a new, recently available, atypical but apparently effective antipsychotic agent has relatively strong antagonistic interaction with central alpha$_1$-adrenergic receptors, lacks acute extrapyramidal adverse effects, and exerts only weak antagonism of dopaminergic transmission in the basal ganglia and the limbic forebrain. The highly specific dopamine-blocking antipsychotic drug pimozide has been used in the treatment of Tourette's syndrome with equivocal results (Shapiro et al. 1987). Prolongations of ECG QT interval corrected by rate (QTc) of unclear clinical significance have been reported with pimozide treatment. Pimozide in doses of up to 0.3 mg/kg is recommended for use in the treatment of patients with Tourette's syndrome who fail to respond to more conventional treatments.

Antipsychotics are indicated in the treatment of childhood psychotic disorders. However, they are prescribed for a variety of other disorders, such as severe agitation, aggression, self-abuse, and insomnia, when seen as complications of pervasive developmental disorders and mental retardation. This class of drugs is also used in the treatment of Tourette's syndrome and ADHD, as well as in the management of juveniles with aggressive forms of conduct disorder. The target symptoms that most commonly respond to antipsychotics include excessive motor activity (agitation), aggressiveness, tics, stereotypies, delusions, and hallucinations. Antipsychotic agents should not be used for the treatment of anxiety or for sedation, conditions for which antianxiety medication can be highly effective.

The usual oral dosage of antipsychotic drugs ranges between 3 and 6 mg/kg/day for the low-potency phenothiazines and between 0.1 and 0.5 (up to 1.0) mg/kg/day for the high-potency phenothiazines, butyrophenones, thioxanthenes, and indolone derivatives. Antipsychotic drugs have a relatively long half-life (2–38 hours in adults), and therefore they should be administered not more than twice daily. Most antipsychotic preparations are available in either tablet or capsule form. In addition, at least one compound from each class

of antipsychotics is available in a liquid concentrate form. Several compounds, including chlorpromazine, haloperidol, and fluphenazine (Prolixin), are available in an injectable form for intramuscular administration.

Common short-term adverse effects of antipsychotic drugs are drowsiness, increased appetite, and weight gain. Anticholinergic effects such as dry mouth, nasal congestion, and blurred vision are more commonly seen with the low-potency phenothiazines. Extrapyramidal effects such as acute dystonia, akathisia (motor restlessness), and parkinsonism (bradykinesia, tremor, facial inexpressiveness) are more commonly seen with use of the high-potency compounds (phenothiazines, butyrophenones, and thioxanthenes). Receptor-binding assays have been extremely successful in helping to understand some of the side effects. For example, it has been found that the rank order of binding affinities for cyclic antidepressants at the muscarinic cholinergic receptor parallels the potency of their clinical anticholinergic effects. Among the antipsychotics, thioridazine has the highest affinity for the muscarinic receptor (Hyman 1988). It has been suggested that molindone has less tendency to cause weight gain (Owen and Cole 1989).

As in adults, the long-term administration of antipsychotic drugs in children and adolescents may be associated with tardive dyskinesia (Gualtieri et al. 1982), although children appear to be generally less vulnerable than adults. The potentially irreversible tardive dyskinesia should be distinguished from the more common, generally benign withdrawal dyskinesia associated with the abrupt cessation of these drugs that tends to subside after several months of drug discontinuation. A behavioral syndrome of deteriorating behavior ("tardive dysbehavior," "supersensitivity psychosis") has also been reported to be part of the withdrawal phenomena associated with antipsychotic drug discontinuation (Gualtieri et al. 1982). This behavioral syndrome seems to be qualitatively different from the target symptoms for which the drug was initially prescribed and usually ceases spontaneously after a few weeks. In children with mental retardation and pervasive developmental disorders, tardive dyskinesia should be differentiated from the commonly occurring stereotypies (Meiselas et al. 1989). One approach to minimize withdrawal reactions is to taper antipsychotic drugs *very* slowly over several months. Little is known about the potentially lethal neuroleptic malignant syndrome in juveniles.

Prevention (appropriate use, clear indication, clear target symptoms, periodic drug discontinuation to assess need for drug use) and early detection (with regular monitoring) are the only available treatments for tardive dyskinesia. Reduction of dose or drug discontinuation (if clinically feasible) should be undertaken rapidly once tardive dyskinesia has been detected. Other, short-term, adverse effects of antipsychotics are more easily managed. Excessive sedation can be avoided by using less-sedating antipsychotics and managed by prescribing most of the daily dose at night. Drowsiness should not be confused with impaired cognition and can usually be corrected by adjusting the dose and timing of administration. In fact, there is no evidence that antipsychotics adversely affect cognition when used in low doses. Anticholinergic adverse effects can be minimized by choosing a medium- or high-potency compound. Extrapyramidal reactions can be avoided in most cases by slow titration of the antipsychotic dose. Antiparkinsonian agents (i.e., anticholinergic drugs, antihistamines, amantadine) should be avoided unless strictly necessary because of the added adverse effects that these drugs may produce. Akathisia may be particularly problematic in young patients because of common underrecognition. It should be considered in the differential diagnosis of agitation and anxiety in a patient receiving antipsychotic therapy. The centrally acting beta-adrenergic antagonist propranolol (Ananth and Lin 1986) and the high-potency benzodiazepine clonazepam (Kutcher et al. 1989) are helpful in treating this bothersome adverse effect.

Antimanic Agents

Lithium carbonate. Lithium is a simple solid element that bears chemical similarities to sodium, potassium, calcium, and magnesium. As with other psychotropic agents, the precise cellular mechanism of action by which lithium produces its beneficial effect is unknown. Lithium has diverse cellular actions that alter hormonal, metabolic, and neuronal systems. It is unknown if lithium-induced changes in these systems are the cause or the effect of the illness. Based on its putative biological and biochemical actions, proposed theories of lithium's mechanism of action include neurotransmission (i.e., interaction with catecholamine, indolamine, cholinergic, and endorphin systems; inhibition of beta-adrenoreceptors), endocrine system (i.e., blocking release of thyroid hormone and the synthesis of testosterone), circadian rhythm (i.e., normalization of altered sleep-wake cycles), and cellular processes (i.e., ionic substitution, inhibition of adenylate cyclase). However, until more is known about the pathophysiology of the psychiatric disorders for which lithium is used, it is not possible to determine which of lithium's effects is responsible for the therapeutic actions of this agent.

Despite its wide and clearly documented use in adult psychiatry, there is very limited empirical evidence documenting the uses of lithium in pediatric psychiatry (Biederman and Jellinek 1984; Campbell et al. 1984; Cohen et al. 1989; DeLong and Aldershof 1987). Based on the experience in adult psychiatry, the main use of lithium is in the acute and prophylactic treatment of juvenile bipolar disorder, manic type (Table 50-10). Lithium can also be effective in the treatment and prophylaxis of major depression (bipolar and nonbipolar) and schizoaffective disorders and as an adjunct treatment of schizophrenia and refractory depression (Ryan et al. 1988). Although lithium has been shown in clinical studies to have an antiaggressive effect in certain populations, its clinical usefulness in treating aggressive or explosive behavior has not been established. Nevertheless, lithium may be a viable treatment consideration for patients with episodic aggressive behavior, particularly those who have not been responsive to other treatments. It also has been suggested that lithium may be effective in the treatment of a wide range of behavioral disorders in children of lithium-responsive bipolar-disordered adults (Biederman 1988; Ryan and Puig-Antich 1987).

In adults, the elimination half-life of lithium is approximately 24 hours, and it takes 5–7 days to reach steady state. Thus there is no need to obtain serum lithium levels more often than once a week unless there is concern about toxicity. Since work done to determine therapeutic ranges of lithium has been based on a 12-hour sampling interval, blood samples for serum lithium determination should always be drawn 12 hours after the last dose. Micromethods for lithium serum level determinations are available and permit samples to be obtained using the fingerstick technique. Data suggest that lithium determination in the saliva correlates with serum lithium levels and may facilitate the monitoring of therapy in young children in which venipuncture may be problematic (Perry et al. 1984).

Because of the complex relationship between lithium and sodium excretion, dose versus serum level associations can be variable and require care-

Table 50-10.   Antimanic agents

Drug	Main indications	Daily dose (mg/kg)	Daily dosage schedule	Common adverse effects
Lithium carbonate	Bipolar disorder, manic Prophylaxis of bipolar disorder Major depressive disorder Hyperaggressive behavior Adjunct therapy in refractory major depressive disorder	10–30 Dose adjusted with serum levels	Once or twice	Polyuria, polydipsia Tremor, nausea, diarrhea Weight gain, drowsiness, skin abnormalities Possible effects on thyroid and renal functioning with chronic administration Therapy requires monitoring of lithium levels, thyroid and renal tests. Lithium toxicity (level >2 meq/l) can be life threatening.
Carbamazepine	Complex partial seizures Bipolar disorder Adjunct therapy in refractory major depressive disorder	10–20 Dose adjusted with serum levels	Twice	Bone marrow suppression (requires baseline and close monitoring of blood counts) dizziness, drowsiness, rashes, nausea Liver toxicity (uncommon)

ful monitoring. In general, the pharmacokinetics of lithium in children seem to have the same features as in adults, with a trend toward a shorter elimination half-life and shorter total clearance (Vitiello et al. 1988). The usual lithium starting dosage ranges from 10 to 30 mg/kg in divided doses once or twice a day. There is no known therapeutic serum lithium level in pediatric psychiatry. Based on the adult literature, suggested guidelines include serum levels of 0.8–1.5 meq/liter for acute episodes and levels of 0.6–0.8 meq/liter for maintenance therapy. Nevertheless, as with any other intervention, the lowest effective dose/serum level should always be used.

Lithium preparations include standard lithium carbonate, 300 mg (tablets or capsules). Scored tablets permit the introduction and titration of smaller doses (by permitting the breaking of the tablets into quarters or halves). Slow- or controlled-release lithium carbonate preparations (Lithobid [300 mg], Eskalith [450 mg]) are available. The slow-release preparations are more gradually absorbed, reaching peak serum levels about 3 hours later than the regular preparations. Although there does not appear to be a clear advantage to using the standard or the slow-release preparations, some individuals may tolerate one better than the other. Lithium is also available in a liquid preparation (lithium citrate), containing 8 meq of lithium per 5 cc (the same amount of lithium contained in 300 mg of lithium carbonate), which may facilitate its intake in young patients unable or unwilling to take pills.

Common short-term adverse effects include gastrointestinal symptoms such as nausea and vomiting; renal symptoms such as polyuria and polydipsia; and central nervous system symptoms such as tremor, sleepiness, and memory impairment. The chronic administration of lithium may be associated with metabolic (decreased calcium metabolism, weight gain), endocrine (decreased thyroid functioning), and possible renal damage. Data collected over the last 10 years, however, suggest that maintenance lithium therapy does not lead to serious nephrotoxicity, at least in adults (Gelenberg et al. 1987). It is imperative that children be screened for renal function (blood urea nitrogen, creatinine), thyroid function (triiodothyronine [T_3], thyroxine [T_4], and thyroid-stimulating hormone [TSH]), and calcium metabolism (Ca, P) before lithium treatment is started, and that these tests should be repeated at least every 6 months. Particular caution should be exercised when lithium is used in patients with neurologic, renal, and cardiovascular disorders.

Anticonvulsants: Carbamazepine. Carbamazepine is structurally related to the TCAs. It is the drug of choice in the treatment of temporal lobe epilepsy (complex partial seizures) (Table 50-10). There are no clear indications for the use of carbamazepine in the treatment of juvenile psychiatric disorders in the absence of clear seizure activity. Carbamazepine may be useful as a second-line treatment for juvenile bipolar disorder, manic type. In clinical practice, despite lack of adequate scientific evidence, anticonvulsants have been used in the treatment of nonspecific behavioral disturbances, particularly those associated with aggressive outbursts, impulsiveness, and restlessness in the absence of clinical or electroencephalographic evidence for seizure activity. The plasma half-life after chronic administration is between 13 and 17 hours. The therapeutic plasma concentration is variably reported at 4–12 μg/ml, and recommended daily doses in children range from 10 to 20 mg/kg administered twice a day. Since the relationship between dose and plasma level is variable and uncertain with marked interindividual variability, close plasma level monitoring is recommended. Common short-term side effects include dizziness, drowsiness, nausea, vomiting, and blurred vision. Idiosyncratic reactions, such as bone marrow suppression, liver toxicity, and skin disorder, have been reported but appear to be rare. However, given the seriousness of these reactions, careful monitoring of blood counts and liver and renal function is warranted during treatment.

Antianxiety Drugs

There is little information available regarding the efficacy and toxicology of antianxiety agents in pediatric psychiatry. The most important agents in this class are the benzodiazepines (Table 50-11). Other available compounds include barbiturates, several compounds structurally related to alcohol (e.g., chloral hydrate, paraldehyde, and meprobamate), and sedative antihistamines (e.g., diphenhydramine, hydroxyzine, and promethazine). Buspirone is a new, atypical nonbenzodiazepine antianxiety drug. Because of their pharmacologic (clinical effects) and toxicologic (comfortable mar-

gin of safety) properties and their minimal pharmacokinetic interactions with other drugs, benzodiazepines, along with other sedatives, hypnotics, and antihistamines, are perhaps the most widely used psychoactive drugs in children used mostly to treat poorly diagnosed symptoms of agitation and insomnia (Quinn 1986). Most benzodiazepines are lipophilic and are highly bound to plasma membranes; most have active metabolites that dominate their course of activity. Most benzodiazepines are absorbed at an intermediate rate, with peak plasma levels appearing 1–3 hours after ingestion. Benzodiazepines and related sedative drugs can produce tolerance (and cross-tolerance with other benzodiazepines) and dependence (physiologic [addiction] and psychological [habituation]).

The primary site of action of benzodiazepines in the central nervous system is at GABA$_A$ receptors. GABA$_A$ receptors are the primary site of action not only of benzodiazepines but also of barbiturates, and of some of the intoxicating effects of ethanol. Benzodiazepines and barbiturates act at separate binding sites on the receptor to potentiate the inhibitory action of GABA. Barbiturates and ethanol, but not benzodiazepines, can also independently open the Cl$^-$ channel within the receptor. The fact that benzodiazepines, barbiturates, and ethanol all have related actions on a common receptor type explains their pharmacologic synergy and cross-tolerance. Although benzodiazepines have their primary actions at GABA$_A$ receptors, it is not yet clear how they function as anxiolytics. Based on animal models, it is generally believed that the anxiolytic properties of benzodiazepines reflect their actions on the limbic system, including the hippocampus and the amygdala. Their anticonvulsant actions may be primarily cortical, and their sedative actions may be primarily mediated in the brain stem. Neurons inhibited by benzodiazepines to produce anxiolysis may include serotonin (5-HT) and noradrenergic neurons. For buspirone, the pharmacologic effects include inhibition of serotonin neurons and decrease of striatal levels of serotonin-binding sites.

There are no established indications for the use of antianxiety agents in pediatric psychiatry. Since the pharmacologic profile of antianxiety drugs includes behavioral disinhibition and since many childhood psychiatric disorders are characterized by behavioral disinhibition, the use of these agents in the absence of a specific indication carries the risk of worsening the clinical picture (Biederman

Table 50-11. Antianxiety drugs

Drug	Main indications	Daily dose (mg/kg)	Daily dosage schedule	Common adverse effects
High-potency benzodiazepines				
Clonazepam (long-acting)	Anxiety disorders Adjunct in therapy-refractory psychosis Adjunct in mania Severe agitation Tourette's syndrome Severe insomnia Major depressive disorder + anxiety	0.01–0.04	Once or twice	Drowsiness, disinhibition, agitation Confusion Depression Withdrawal reactions Potential risk for abuse and dependence Less risk for rebound and withdrawal reactions
Alprazolam (short-acting)	Same as clonazepam	0.02–0.06	Three times	Same as other benzodiazepines Higher risk for rebound and withdrawal reactions
Lorazepam (short-acting)	Same as other high-potency benzodiazepines Temporary use in severe adjustment disorder with anxious mood	0.04–0.09	Three times	Same as other benzodiazepines Higher risk for rebound and withdrawal reactions

1987). Possible indications for the use of antianxiety agents in pediatric psychiatry include the treatment of childhood anxiety symptoms and disorders (Leonard and Rapoport 1989). In recent years, the high-potency benzodiazepines alprazolam and clonazepam have received increasing attention as effective and safe treatment for adult panic disorder with and without agoraphobia (Biederman 1990; Herman et al. 1987). It has been suggested that children also can manifest adult-type anxiety disorders, such as panic disorder and agoraphobia, which may also respond to high-potency benzodiazepines (Biederman 1987). Possible additional uses of benzodiazepines include their use as an adjunct treatment in acute psychotic episodes, in treating refractory schizophrenia, and for the treatment of neuroleptic-induced akathisia (Kutcher et al. 1989). The chlorinated benzodiazepines clonazepam and clorazepate may be particularly helpful in the treatment of complex partial seizures. Lorazepam and oxazepam do not have active metabolites and do not tend to accumulate in tissue, making them preferable for short-term symptomatic use. When long-term use is anticipated, longer-acting benzodiazepines, such as clonazepam, are

preferable. It has been suggested that buspirone is beneficial in treating agitated states such as those encountered in developmentally disordered patients (Realmuto et al. 1989).

In general, the clinical toxicity of the benzodiazepines is low. The most commonly encountered short-term adverse effects are sedation, drowsiness, and decreased mental acuity. When given high doses, patients can become confused. In adults, benzodiazepines have been reportedly associated with depressogenic adverse effects. With the exception of the potential risk for tolerance and dependence (risk suspected but not well studied in adults, risk unknown in children), there are no known long-term adverse effects associated with benzodiazepines. Adverse withdrawal effects can occur, and benzodiazepines should always be tapered slowly.

Buspirone is a novel nonbenzodiazepine anxiolytic without anticonvulsant, sedative, or muscle relaxant properties. It is thought that the anxiolytic effects of buspirone may relate to reduction in serotonergic neurotransmission (Eison 1989). Clinical experience with this drug suggests limited antianxiety efficacy. Daily dose is estimated to range from 0.3 to 0.6 mg/kg. It has been suggested that buspirone may be effective in the treatment of aggressive behaviors in children with pervasive developmental disorders (Realmuto et al. 1989).

Other Drugs

Clonidine. Clonidine is an imidazoline derivative with alpha-adrenergic agonist properties that has been primarily used in the treatment of hypertension (Table 50-12). At low doses, it appears to stimulate inhibitory, presynaptic autoreceptors in the central nervous system. Established indications in psychiatry include the treatment of withdrawal syndromes, Tourette's syndrome, and, more recently, ADHD. Possible additional indications include the treatment of self-injurious and aggressive behaviors. Anecdotal reports suggest that clonidine may be efficacious in affective disorders, obsessive-compulsive disorder, anxiety disorders, tardive dyskinesia, and psychosis.

Clonidine is a relatively short-acting compound with a plasma half-life ranging from approximately 5.5 hours (in children) to 8.5 hours (in adults). Daily doses should be titrated and individualized. Usual daily dose ranges from 3 to 10 μg/kg given generally in divided doses, bid or tid. Therapy is usually initiated at the lowest manufactured dose of a full or half tablet of 0.1 mg, depending on the size of the child (approximately 1–2 μg/kg) and increased depending on clinical response and adverse effects. Initial dosage can more easily be given in the evening hours or before bedtime because of sedation.

The most common short-term adverse effect of clonidine is sedation. It can also produce, in some cases, hypotension, dry mouth, depression, and confusion. Clonidine is not known to be associated with long-term adverse effects. In hypertensive adults, abrupt withdrawal of clonidine has been associated with rebound hypertension. Thus it requires slow tapering when discontinued. Clonidine should not be administered concomitantly with beta-blockers since adverse interactions have been reported with this combination. In summary, clonidine is a new and welcome addition to the pharmacotherapy of juvenile psychiatric disorders for conditions and symptoms in which antipsychotics have been previously used. Since it has a relatively low side-effect profile compared with that of the antipsychotic compounds, it should be considered first for those indications in which both drug classes are recommended. Clonidine offers a clear treatment alternative for Tourette's syndrome and perhaps for ADHD, especially when the other agents are either ineffective or poorly tolerated.

Beta-adrenergic blocking agents: Propranolol. Propranolol is a nonselective (it affects both beta$_1$ and beta$_2$ receptors) beta-adrenergic antagonist. It has received considerable attention with regard to its potential use for psychiatric disorders, including drug-induced akathisia, anxiety disorders, schizophrenia, and aggressive and self-abusive behavioral disorders (Table 50-12) (Ananth and Lin 1986; Sorgi et al. 1986). Propranolol's effects are mediated through its ability to block beta-adrenergic receptors at multiple sites in the body. It also crosses the blood-brain barrier; this probably accounts for some of its efficacy in psychiatric disorders, but it also contributes to concerns regarding potential central nervous system toxicity. It is unclear whether the benefits obtained from propranolol are primarily due to peripheral or central effects of the drug. As much as a 20-fold variability in interindividual hepatic elimination can occur. The half-life after chronic administration is about 4 hours. There are no current established indications for the use of beta-blockade in the treatment of child and adolescent psychiatric disorders, but there are possible indications currently under investigation. At present, investigation centers around the use of propranolol in the management of severe aggressive and self-injurious behaviors. Propranolol represents an alternative in the pharmacologic management of aggressive behavioral disorders, offering the benefit of a relatively low side-effect profile, and it should be tried first for indications other than psychosis shared with antipsychotic drugs. The dose range used in pediatric disorders requiring propranolol is approximately 2–8 mg/kg/day.

Short-term adverse effects of propranolol are usually not serious and generally abate on cessation of drug administration. Nausea, vomiting, constipation, and mild diarrhea have been reported. Psychiatric side effects appear to be relatively infrequent but can occur and include vivid dreams, depression, and hallucinations. Allergic reactions manifested by rash, fever, and purpura are infrequent but have been reported and warrant discontinuation of the drug. Propranolol can cause bradycardia and hypotension as well as increased airway resistance and is contraindicated in asthmatic and in certain cardiac patients. There are no

Table 50-12.   Other drugs

Drug	Main indications	Daily dose	Daily dosage schedule	Common adverse effects

Clonidine	Tourette's syndrome
	ADHD
	Aggression/self-abuse
	Severe agitation
	Anxiety disorders?
	Adjunct in mania and
	    schizophrenia
	Withdrawal syndromes
		3–10 μg/kg	Two or three times	Sedation (very frequent)
				Hypotension (rare)
				Dry mouth
				Confusion (with high dose)
				Depression
				Rebound hypertension
				Localized irritation with
				    transdermal preparation

Propranolol	Tourette's syndrome
	ADHD
	Aggression/self-abuse
	Severe agitation
	Akathisia
		2–8 mg/kg	Twice	Similar to clonidine
				Higher risk for bradycardia
				    and hypotension (dose
				    dependent) and rebound
				    hypertension
				Bronchospasm
				    (contraindicated in
				    asthmatic patients)
				Rebound hypertension on
				    abrupt withdrawal

Fenfluramine	Pervasive
	    developmental
	    disorders?
		1–2 mg/kg	Two or three times	Anorexia, irritability,
				    drowsiness, weight loss,
				    insomnia (when
				    discontinued)

Naltrexone	Self-abuse	1–2 mg/kg	Once or twice	Long-acting opioid antagonist Minimal adverse effects Hepatotoxicity (rare)
Desmopressin	Enuresis	3–10 μg/kg (0.1–0.2 ml)	Intranasally once or twice	Headache Nausea

Note.   ADHD = attention-deficit hyperactivity disorder.

known long-term effects associated with chronic administration of propranolol. Since abrupt cessation of this drug may be associated with rebound hypertension, gradual tapering is recommended.

Fenfluramine.   Fenfluramine is a sympathomimetic amine related to the amphetamines utilized as an appetite suppressant. Fenfluramine has been shown to decrease blood and brain serotonin concentrations in animals. The finding that 30%–40% of patients with the syndrome of autism have elevated blood serotonin levels prompted investigation of this agent in the treatment of autism (Biederman 1985). Follow-up studies have been unable to document any efficacy for fenfluramine in autism (Aman and Kern 1989; Campbell et al. 1988a).

Opiate antagonists: Naltrexone.   Naltrexone is a potent, long-acting opioid antagonist with fast on-

set of action that has been used in the treatment of children with pervasive developmental disorders and of those with self-abuse in daily doses of 1–2 mg/kg (Table 50-12) (Lienemann and Walker 1989). Although it is relatively free of serious adverse effects, there have been some rare reports of hepatotoxicity.

Desmopressin (DDAVP).   DDAVP is a synthetic antidiuretic hormone peptide analogue, recently approved by the Food and Drug Administration for the treatment of enuresis (Table 50-12). Daily doses are 0.1–0.2 ml by intranasal spray given at bedtime. Although it effectively suppresses urine production for 7–10 hours, it lacks the pressor effects of antidiuretic hormone. Adverse effects are minimal. Its safety has been established in patients requiring long-term therapy (Rew and Rundle 1989).

Conclusions

Although the origins of pediatric psychopharmacology began more than 50 years ago, the long-term outlook for pediatric psychopharmacology is dependent on careful clinical applications and future research. As we have stated, it is essential to apply a careful differential diagnostic assessment that assesses psychiatric, social, cognitive, educational, and medical-neurologic factors that may contribute to the child's clinical presentation and, therefore, to consider the use of pharmacotherapy as part of a broader treatment plan that encompasses all aspects of a child's life.

Pharmacotherapy should be integrated into this treatment plan as an adjunct to psychoeducational-behavioral interventions and careful medical management, rather than as an alternative to these other interventions or only when these other interventions have failed. In defining the role of pharmacotherapy in the treatment plan, realistic expectations of pharmacotherapeutic interventions, careful definition of target symptoms, and careful assessment of the potential risks and benefits of this type of intervention for psychiatrically disturbed children are major ingredients for a successful pharmacologic intervention. The lack of Food and Drug Administration approval for many of the medications, although a restriction on general use, does permit the careful introduction of innovative therapy. Hopefully there will be an increasing number of referral centers that will explore the appropriate use of psychopharmacologic agents in pediatric psychiatry through high-quality research protocols.

References

Aman MG, Kern RA: Review of fenfluramine in the treatment of the developmental disabilities. J Am Acad Child Adolesc Psychiatry 28:549–565, 1989

American Psychiatric Association: Diagnostic and Statistical Manual of Mental Disorders, 3rd Edition, Revised. Washington, DC, American Psychiatric Association, 1987

Ananth H, Lin K: Propranolol in psychiatry. Neuropsychobiology 15:20–27, 1986

Barkley RA: A review of stimulant drug research with hyperactive children. J Child Psychol Psychiatry 18:137–165, 1977

Berney T, Kolvin I, Bhate SR: School phobia: a therapeutic trial with clomipramine and short-term outcome. Br J Psychiatry 138:110–118, 1981

Bernstein GA, Garfinkel B, Borchart C: Imipramine versus alprazolam for school phobia. Paper presented at the annual meeting of the American Academy of Child and Adolescent Psychiatry, Washington, DC, October 1987

Biederman J: Fenfluramine (Pondimin) in autism. Biological Therapies in Psychiatry 8:25–28, 1985

Biederman J: Clonazepam in the treatment of prepubertal children with panic-like symptoms. J Clin Psychiatry 48:38–41, 1987

Biederman J: Pharmacological treatment of adolescents with affective disorders and attention-deficit disorder. Psychopharmacol Bull 24:81–87, 1988

Biederman J: The diagnosis and treatment of adolescent anxiety disorders. J Clin Psychiatry 51 (5, suppl):20–26, 1990

Biederman J, Jellinek MS: Current concepts: psychopharmacology in children. N Engl J Med 310:968–972, 1984

Biederman J, Gastfriend D, Jellinek MS, et al: Cardiovascular effects of desipramine in children and adolescents with attention deficit disorder. J Pediatr 106:1017–1020, 1985

Biederman J, Baldessarini R, Wright V, et al: A double-blind placebo controlled study of desipramine in the treatment of attention-deficit disorder, I: efficacy. J Am Acad Child Adolesc Psychiatry 28:777–784, 1989a

Biederman J, Baldessarini R, Wright V, et al: A double-blind placebo controlled study of desipramine in the treatment of attention-deficit disorder, II: serum drug levels and cardiovascular findings. J Am Acad Child Adolesc Psychiatry 28:903–911, 1989b

Braden NJ, Jackson JE, Walson PD: Tricyclic antidepressant overdose. Pediatr Clin North Am 33:287–297, 1986

Brown RT, Wynne ME, Slimmer LW: Attention deficit disorder and the effect of methylphenidate on attention, behavioral, and cardiovascular functioning. J Clin Psychiatry 45:473–476, 1984

Campbell M, Perry R, Green WH: Use of lithium in children and adolescents. Psychosomatics 25:95–101, 1984

Campbell M, Adams P, Small AM, et al: Efficacy and safety of fenfluramine in autistic children. J Am Acad Child Adolesc Psychiatry 27:434–439, 1988a

Campbell M, Adams P, Small AM, et al: Naltrexone in infantile autism. Psychopharmacol Bull 24:135–139, 1988b

Casat CD, Pleasants DZ, Schroeder DH, et al: Bupropion in children with attention-deficit disorder. Psychopharmacol Bull 25:198–201, 1989

Cohen LS, Heller VL, Rosenbaum JF: Treatment guidelines for psychotropic drug use in pregnancy. Psychosomatics 30:25–33, 1989

DeLong GR, Aldershof AL: Long-term experience with lithium treatment in childhood: correlation with clinical diagnosis. J Am Acad Child Adolesc Psychiatry 26:389–394, 1987

Donnelly M, Zametkin AJ, Rapoport JL, et al: Treatment of childhood hyperactivity with desipramine: plasma drug concentration, cardiovascular effects, plasma and urinary catecholamine levels, and clinical response. Clin Pharmacol Ther 39:72–81, 1986

Donnelly M, Rapoport JL, Potter WZ, et al: Fenfluramine and dextroamphetamine treatment of childhood hyperactivity. Arch Gen Psychiatry 46:205–212, 1989

Eison MS: The new generation of serotonergic anxiolytics: possible clinical roles. Psychopathology 22:13–20, 1989

Flament MF, Rapoport JL, Berg CJ, et al: Clomipramine treatment of childhood obsessive-compulsive disorder: a double-blind controlled study. Arch Gen Psychiatry 42:977–983, 1985

Garfinkel BD, Wender PH, Sloman L, et al: Tricyclic antidepressant and methylphenidate treatment of attention-deficit disorder in children. Journal of the American Academy of Child Psychiatry 22:343–348, 1983

Gastfriend DR, Biederman J, Jellinek MS: Desipramine in the treatment of attention-deficit disorder in adolescents. Psychopharmacol Bull 21:144–145, 1985

Gelenberg AJ, Wojcick JD, Falk WE: Effects of lithium on the kidney. Acta Psychiatr Scand 75:29–34, 1987

Gittelman R, Klein DF: Controlled imipramine treatment of school phobia. Arch Gen Psychiatry 25:204–207, 1971

Gittelman R, Mannuzza S: Hyperactive boys almost grown up, III: methylphenidate effects on ultimate height. Arch Gen Psychiatry 45:1131–1134, 1988

Gittelman R, Mannuzza S, Shenker R: Hyperactive boys almost grown up. Arch Gen Psychiatry 42:937–947, 1985

Gittelman-Klein R: Pharmacotherapy of childhood hyperactivity: an update, in Psychopharmacology: The Third Generation of Progress. Edited by Meltzer HY. New York, Raven, 1987, pp 1215–1224

Golden GS: Tardive dyskinesia in Tourette syndrome. Pediatr Neurol 1:192, 1985

Gualtieri CT, Breuning SE, Schroeder SR, et al: Tardive dyskinesia in mentally retarded children, adolescents, and young adults: North Carolina and Michigan studies. Psychopharmacol Bull 18:62–65, 1982 [Retracted by Gualtieri CT: Psychopharmacol Bull 23:588, 1987]

Herman JB, Rosenbaum JF, Brotman AW: The alprazolam to clonazepam switch for the treatment of panic disorder. J Clin Psychopharmacol 7:175–178, 1987

Hoge SK, Biederman J: A case of Tourette's syndrome with symptoms of attention-deficit disorder treated with desipramine. J Clin Psychiatry 47:478–479, 1986

Hunt RD: Treatment effects of oral and transdermal clonidine in relation to methylphenidate: an open pilot study in ADD-H. Psychopharmacol Bull 23:111–114, 1987

Hunt RD, Minderaa RB, Cohen DJ: Clonidine benefits children with attention-deficit disorder and hyperactivity: report of a double-blind placebo-crossover therapeutic trial. Journal of the American Academy of Child Psychiatry 24:617–629, 1985

Hunt RD, Minderaa RB, Cohen DJ: The therapeutic effect of clonidine in attention-deficit disorder with hyperactivity: a comparison with placebo and methylphenidate. Psychopharmacol Bull 22:229–236, 1986

Hyman SE: Recent developments in neurobiology, Parts I–III. Psychosomatics 29:157–165, 254–263, 373–378, 1988

Kashani JH, Sherman DD: Mood disorders in children and adolescents, in Psychiatry Update: American Psychiatric Association Annual Review, Vol 8. Edited by Tasman A, Hales RE, Frances AJ. Washington, DC, American Psychiatric Press, 1989, pp 197–216

Klein DF, Gittelman R, Quitkin F, et al: Diagnosis and drug treatment of childhood disorders, in Diagnosis and Drug Treatment of Psychiatric Disorders: Adults and Children. Baltimore, MD, Williams & Wilkins, 1980, pp 590–775

Kutcher S, Williamson P, MacKenzie S, et al: Successful clonazepam treatment of neuroleptic-induced akathisia in older adolescents and young adults: a double-blind, placebo controlled study. J Clin Psychopharmacol 9:403–407, 1989

Leckman JF, Detlor J, Harcherik DF, et al: Short- and long-term treatment of Tourette's syndrome with clonidine: a clinical perspective. Neurology 35:343–351, 1985

Leonard HL, Rapoport JL: Anxiety disorders in childhood and adolescence, in Psychiatry Update: American Psychiatric Association Annual Review, Vol 8. Edited by Tasman A, Hales

RE, Frances AJ. Washington, DC, American Psychiatric Press, 1989, pp 162–179

Leonard HL, Swedo SE, Rapoport JL, et al: Treatment of obsessive-compulsive disorder with clomipramine and desipramine in children and adolescents: a double-blind crossover comparison. Arch Gen Psychiatry 46:1088–1092, 1989

Lienemann J, Walker F: Naltrexone in treatment of self-injury (letter). Am J Psychiatry 146:1639–1640, 1989

Lowe TL, Cohen DJ, Detlor J: Stimulant medications precipitate Tourette's syndrome. JAMA 247:1168–1169, 1982

Mattes JA: Propranolol for adults with temper outbursts and residual attention-deficit disorder. J Clin Psychopharmacol 6:299–302, 1986

Mattes JA, Gittelman R: Growth of hyperactive children on maintenance regimen of methylphenidate. Arch Gen Psychiatry 40:317–321, 1983

Mattes JA, Rosenberg MA, Mays D: Carbamazepine versus propranolol in patients with uncontrolled rage outbursts: a random assignment study. Psychopharmacol Bull 20:98–100, 1984

Meiselas KD, Spencer EK, Oberfield R, et al: Differentiation of stereotypies from neuroleptic-related dyskinesias in autistic children. J Clin Psychopharmacol 9:207–209, 1989

Owen RRJ, Cole JO: Molindone hydrochloride: a review of laboratory and clinical findings. J Clin Psychopharmacol 9:268–276, 1989

Pauls DL, Hurst CR, Kruger SD, et al: Gilles de la Tourette's syndrome and attention-deficit disorder with hyperactivity: evidence against a genetic relationship. Arch Gen Psychiatry 43:1177–1179, 1986a

Pauls DL, Towbin KE, Leckman JF, et al: Gilles de la Tourette's syndrome and obsessive-compulsive disorder: evidence supporting a genetic relationship. Arch Gen Psychiatry 43:1180–1182, 1986b

Perry R, Campbell M, Grega DM, et al: Saliva lithium levels in children: their use in monitoring serum lithium levels and lithium side effects. J Clin Psychopharmacol 4:199–202, 1984

Platt JE, Campbell M, Green WH, et al: Cognitive effects of lithium carbonate and haloperidol in treatment-resistant aggressive children. Arch Gen Psychiatry 41:657–662, 1984

Pollack MH, Tesar GE, Rosenbaum JF: Clonazepam in the treatment of panic disorder and agoraphobia: a one-year follow-up. J Clin Psychopharmacol 6:302–304, 1986

Preskorn SH, Weller EB, Weller RA: Depression in children: relationship between plasma imipramine levels and response. J Clin Psychiatry 43:450–453, 1982

Puig-Antich J, Perel JM, Lupatkin W: Imipramine in prepubertal major depressive disorders. Arch Gen Psychiatry 44:81–89, 1987

Quay HC: Conduct disorder, in Psychopathological Disorders of Childhood. Edited by Quay HC, Werry JS. New York, John Wiley, 1986, pp 35–73

Quinn DM: Prevalence of psychoactive medication in children and adolescents. Can J Psychiatry 31:575–580, 1986

Rapoport JL: The neurobiology of obsessive-compulsive disorder. JAMA 260:2888–2890, 1988

Rapoport JL, Potter WZ: Tricyclic antidepressants and children. Paper presented at the National Institute of Mental Health conference The Influence of Age on the Pharmacology of Psychoactive Drugs. Washington, DC, NIMH, 1979

Realmuto GM, August GJ, Garfinkel BD: Clinical effect of buspirone in autistic children. J Clin Psychopharmacol 9:122–125, 1989

Reimherr FW, Wender PH, Wood DR, et al: An open trial of L-tyrosine in the treatment of attention-deficit disorder, residual type. Am J Psychiatry 144:1071–1073, 1987

Rew DA, Rundle JS: Assessment of the safety of regular DDAVP therapy in primary nocturnal enuresis. Br J Urol 63:352–353, 1989

Rickels K, Schweizer EE: Current pharmacotherapy of anxiety and panic, in Psychopharmacology: The Third Generation of Progress. Edited by Meltzer HY. New York, Raven, 1987, pp 1193–1203

Riddle MA, Hardin MT, Cho SC, et al: Desipramine treatment of boys with attention-deficit hyperactivity disorder and tics: preliminary clinical experience. J Am Acad Child Adolesc Psychiatry 27:811–814, 1988

Ryan ND, Puig-Antich J: Pharmacological treatment of adolescent psychiatric disorders. J Adolesc Health Care 8:137–142, 1987

Ryan ND, Puig-Antich J, Cooper T, et al: Imipramine in adolescent major depression: plasma level and clinical response. Acta Psychiatr Scand 73:275–288, 1986

Ryan ND, Meyer V, Dachille S, et al: Lithium antidepressant augmentation in TCA-refractory depression in adolescents. J Am Acad Child Adolesc Psychiatry 27:371–376, 1988

Safer DJ, Krager JM: A survey of medication treatment for hyperactive/inattentive students. JAMA 260:2256–2258, 1988

Safer DJ, Allen RP, Barr E: Depression of growth in hyperactive children on stimulant drugs. N Engl J Med 287:217–220, 1972

Sallee FR, Stiller RL, Perel JM, et al: Pemoline-induced abnormal involuntary movements. J Clin Psychopharmacol 9:125–129, 1989

Shapiro AK, Shapiro E, Fulop G: Pimozide treatment of tic and Tourette disorders. Pediatrics 79:1032–1039, 1987

Sorgi PJ, Ratey JJ, Polakoff S: Beta-adrenergic blockers for the control of aggressive behavior in patients with schizophrenia. Am J Psychiatry 143:775–776, 1986

Stubbs EG, Budden SS, Jackson RH, et al: Effects of fenfluramine on eight outpatients with the syndrome of autism. Dev Med Child Neurol 28:229–235, 1986

Swedo SE, Leonard HL, Rapoport JL, et al: A double-blind comparison of clomipramine and desipramine in the treatment of trichotillomania (hair pulling). N Engl J Med 321:496–501, 1989

Varley CK: A review of studies of drug treatment efficacy for attention-deficit disorder with hyperactivity in adolescents. Psychopharmacol Bull 21:216–221, 1985

Vitiello B, Behar D, Malone R, et al: Pharmacokinetics of lithium carbonate in children. J Clin Psychopharmacol 8:355–359, 1988

Weiss G, Hechtman L, Milroy T, et al: Psychiatric status of hyperactives as adults: a controlled prospective 15-year follow-up of 63 hyperactive children. Journal of the American Academy of Child Psychiatry 24:211–220, 1985

Wender PH, Wood DR, Reimherr FW, et al: An open trial of pargyline in the treatment of attention-deficit disorder, residual type. Psychiatry Res 9:329–336, 1983

Wilsher CR, Bennett D, Chase CH, et al: Piracetam and dyslexia: effects on reading tests. J Clin Psychopharmacol 7:230–237, 1987

Youngerman J, Canino IA: Lithium carbonate use in children and adolescents: a survey of the literature. Arch Gen Psychiatry 35:216–224, 1978

Zametkin A, Rapoport JL, Murphy DL, et al: Treatment of hyperactive children with monoamine oxidase inhibitors, I: clinical efficacy. Arch Gen Psychiatry 42:962–966, 1985

Chapter 51

Psychoanalysis and Psychodynamic Therapy

Jules Bemporad, M.D.

The psychoanalytic treatment of children evolved as an application of this form of therapy with adults. Although modifications in technique have been recommended to fit in with the child's developmentally immature psychological state, the primary therapeutic agent, as with adults, is the analyst's interpretation of unconscious content so as to bring such material (and its behavioral and emotional derivatives) under greater control of the "ego."

Forays into child treatment were attempted early in the evolution of psychoanalysis: Sigmund Freud's (1909/1955) own treatment of little Hans via the child's father; Ferenczi's (1913/1950) single consultation with Arpad, a 5-year-old boy who was obsessed with and phobic of chickens; and the more systematic treatment of children by Hug-Helmuth (1920), utilizing drawings and games. However, it was not until the late 1920s that child analysis became established under the guidance of two pioneers: Melanie Klein and Anna Freud, whose respective influence continues to dominate the field after well over a half century. Klein and Freud each developed greatly disparate systems of treatment based on different theoretical modifications of psychoanalytic formulations derived from the treatment of adults, resulting in an unfortunate animosity between the two theorists and between their disciples. A detailed description of the metapsychological directions in which Klein took psychoanalytic theory, as opposed to the more traditional Freudian approach (and the latter's modification as an ego psychology), is beyond the scope of this chapter. Anna Freud's system is more prevalent in this country. However, Kleinian child analysis is cur-

rently a vital and popular form of treatment (particularly in Europe and South America), and a brief presentation of its principles is warranted.

Kleinian Child Psychoanalysis

Melanie Klein's technique is based on three fundamental principles: 1) play as the child's mode of free association, 2) the existence of transference in children, and 3) the restriction of the role of the analyst solely to interpreting unconscious sources of anxiety (Segal 1972). Klein maintained that play is the natural mode of expression for children and that through this medium the patients symbolize their inner wishes, fears, and internalized relationships. Play is therefore a suitable substitute for the free association of adults. Continuing this analogy, Klein maintained that inhibitions in the ability to play (and subsequently in the ability to learn) demonstrate a fear of letting one's imagination run freely lest it uncover disagreeable or terrifying fantasies. Comfort with free, unrestricted play is a sign of psychological health just as the ability of the adult to free-associate truly indicates a lack of repression or pathologic defenses (Klein 1932).

Klein also maintained that children are capable of transference neurosis despite their still largely dependent and interactive relationship with their actual parents. Transference is possible even in very young children, according to Klein, because they project onto the therapist aspects of their past internalized parents, with all their inherent distortions, rather than their actual current parents.

Finally, Klein insisted on strict neutrality on the

part of the analyst, who is to refrain from reassurance, guidance, or any deviation from supplying only interpretations. The analyst may participate in a game at the child's request, but he or she is to keep the participation to the barest minimum; the analyst may help a child perform tasks beyond the child's age capacity (e.g., sharpen a pencil) but may not help in the actual production of play or drawings. Support or reassurance, for Klein, was sufficiently derived by the child through the child's relief from anxiety as the therapy progresses. It is in this manner that the child realizes that the analyst is helpful, and not by the latter's nurturance or encouragement. In a brief retrospective account of her career, published in 1955, Klein described how she was, at first, timid about interpreting to the child what she perceived to be the basis for the child's anxiety. When she did so, the child experienced a momentary increase in anxiety as the child became aware of true, if repressed, motives, but then felt calmer and reassured as the child was able to integrate these wishes into his or her conscious life and no longer live in fear of them.

The purpose of Kleinian analysis is for children to differentiate what is internal and what is external to their psyche so that they no longer confuse significant others in their environment with projections of past internalized objects. By clarifying unconscious fantasies, which are symbolized in play, and bringing these to consciousness, children can realize their own feelings of envy, hatred, greed, lust, or jealousy and no longer need to project them onto others. Similarly, they can discover the sense of guilt over these feelings that causes them to fail or to be victimized in their everyday life. The actual technique of therapy is to explain that the child has come to sessions to play. Children are presented with an assortment of materials that are entirely their own and kept separately from those of other patients. Klein suggested dolls (child, adult, and animal), toy houses, cars, trains, fences and various containers, scissors, string, balls, paper, pencils, clay, and glue. These are to be as nondescript as possible so as to allow the freest use of the child's imagination. The therapy is conducted in a safe, plain room without breakable items so that children can freely vent their aggression. A chair and table (e.g., used for drawings) and a couch for occasional verbal free association are also included. A thorough history is obtained from the parents or others so that the analyst has some idea of problem areas and uses this information as the basis for interpretation. Starting with the child's initial visit, the analyst begins to interpret as indicated by the play or transference behavior of the child in order for the child to understand that the relationship to the analyst is different from the child's interchange with other adults. Sessions last about an hour and are scheduled five times per week.

Klein (1932) published detailed accounts of her analysis of children, providing the interested reader an almost verbatim narrative of the process. She first interpreted to the child that the play figures actually represent significant people in the child's psychic reality. Then, depending on what the child does with the figures in play, interpretations are directed at the latent meaning beneath the manifest behavior. For example, Peter, a boy 3 years and 9 months old, whose analysis Klein described, was referred for inability to play, poor frustration tolerance, and other difficulties. His behavior had deteriorated after a summer holiday, when he shared his parents' bedroom and, ostensibly, had witnessed his parents having intercourse. In the first session, Peter had two horse dolls bump into each other, after which Peter proclaimed that they were dead. Then he lined up toy cars and smashed them. Klein eventually interpreted the former play as the child's representation of parental coitus and the latter as his damaging his father's genitalia, an act that he feared would subsequently cause damage to himself. She related that these interpretations produced more play material, which in turn was interpreted, thus expanding his awareness of his repressed thoughts and wishes. In this process, according to Klein, the child came to understand those emotions and anxieties that he previously had to keep repressed but that restricted his psychic existence and distorted his appreciation of the external world.

Freudian Child Psychoanalysis

Anna Freud's system of treatment varies markedly from that of Klein, although Freud also considered interpretations of unconscious content as the major therapeutic agent. While basing her system on the traditional psychoanalysis of adults, Freud took great care in detailing how a child in analysis is quite different from an adult analysand (Freud 1965). Among these differences are that 1) children do not seek out therapy on their own and may have little motivation for cure; 2) children tend to deny problems and try to externalize their causes, rather than accept responsibility for them; 3) children will run away from discomfort and so will not easily relinquish fantasy for reality; and 4) children prefer the mode of acting to that of talking.

Perhaps more pertinent characteristics of child analysis, which reveal the disparity of Freud's system from that of Klein, are Freud's questioning if a child can really free-associate and her refusal to accept play as a substitute for free association. Therefore, Freud also differs from Klein in regarding a mastery of speech as a prerequisite for child analysis, and therefore she did not recommend this form of treatment for very young children (Freud 1945). Also, Freud doubted that a child can form a true transference neurosis, with a true reliving of a past relationship toward the analyst, although transference reactions are indeed manifest. In fact, Freud considered these transference reactions to be immediately evident in the overt behavior toward the analyst and contend that they should be interpreted as representing modes of relating to past significant others. These manifestations are of prime importance for Freud and may crowd out most other analytic material so that, in children, they replace dreams as the "royal road to the unconscious." (Freud 1965, p. 37). While expressing transferential repetitions of older relationships, the child also uses the analyst as a new "object" in a thirst for novelty and new experience. The analyst must know how to differentiate these healthier modes of relating from the aggressive and libidinal transferential behaviors, since cure results largely from encouraging the former and interpreting the latter as each occurs in the analytic session. The key to the Freudian system of child analysis is therefore to create a new relationship and to bring to consciousness the automatic repetition of prior relationships that impede the child's normal urge to complete development. This inherent maturational drive is seen as the most important ally of the analyst in the curative process and separates the analysis of children from that of adults.

Finally, Freud listed other modifications of analytic technique that are often necessary with children. These include the analyst's verbalization and clarification of preconscious material so as to prepare the child for an interpretation and to lessen the anxiety that may accompany the uncovering process, the use of suggestion and educational efforts, and the reassuring of the child as part of a trusting relationship with an adult. Also, given the role of the analyst as an important new figure in the child's life, the child patient will frequently misuse the therapy as a "corrective emotional experience" rather than benefit only from interpretations.

In summary, Anna Freud developed a system of child analysis that varies greatly in technique from that of adults but that is still based on the interpretation of transference and resistance, and the widening of consciousness at the expense of the unconscious, with the consequent increase in ego dominance (Freud 1965).

Psychodynamic Psychotherapy

This form of treatment is a derivative of child analysis, and it is often difficult to differentiate from analytic therapy, particularly when one considers those modifications in technique that Anna Freud suggested. Children in psychotherapy are not usually seen five times a week. There is often a greater involvement of the parents in treatment. In addition, indications are more general, encompassing a variety of conditions beyond neurosis.[1] Furthermore, children in psychotherapy are given more active support and practical guidance than children in analysis, where there is an almost exclusive reliance on the curative role of interpretations. Corrective emotional experiences are encouraged rather than viewed as obstacles to self-awareness. However, it would be a grave error to consider psychodynamic psychotherapy as a "watered down" or lesser form of treatment than child analysis, to be recommended only when constraints over time or money or the limited availability of a more highly trained therapist forces one to opt for a "second rate" form of treatment. Actually, most psychodynamic therapy has its own inherent logical consistency, techniques, and goals, although frequently and extensively utilizing psychoanalytic concepts. The similarities and distinctions between these forms of treatment may be made clearer by an examination of how psychodynamic psychotherapy conceptualizes play, the role of the therapist, and specific curative factors.

---

[1] This last criterion may not be completely valid, for although the ideal patient for Freudian child analysis would be one who possesses a strong ego that can easily integrate knowledge of unconscious forces, as Nagera (1980) commented, all too often this form of intensive treatment is sought as a last resort for very sick children who have not responded to other interventions. Also, Kleinians would consider most nonorganic childhood disorders as responsive, to some degree, to analysis.

In psychodynamic psychotherapy, the play of a young child, and the drawings of an older child, are viewed as the patient's manner of revealing his or her total life situation. Children do project their inner life into the play activity, but also reveal their reality situation. In essence, play is taken as the child's description of his or her perception of the universe, combining actual events and the particular distortions of developmental limitations or of a specific psychopathologic attitude. Play is not utilized predominantly as a substitute for free association, nor for its possible symbolism of unconscious drives or superego sanctions, but as a child's mode of communicating the totality of his or her current life. Play is selected as the medium for gathering information because it is the natural activity of the child, who often lacks the verbal ability to describe events via the spoken word. However, play affords an additional advantage, for it allows children to present their predicament "in displacement," as if it did not particularly pertain to themselves. Jacob Conn (cited in Kanner 1940) described a method of "play interview" in a series of papers in the 1930s in which he indicated how the child's feelings and wishes were projected (displaced) onto doll figures and thus could be expressed without fear or guilt. Conn wrote:

> It is not the child but the doll who is afraid of the dark. It is not he who is envious or hates but the doll character. Therefore, he can give an account of the motives and imaginations which explain the doll's behavior and consequently his own. (cited in Kanner 1940, p. 14)

The play activity can be used to gather information just by observing the situations and characters created by the child, or the therapist may join in the play by assuming the role of one or more of the child's characters to obtain more data. The therapist may also offer suggestions for solving problems or supply interpretations in the guise of a play character to the play figure that represents the child patient. This last technique represents the use of play as treatment, with the therapist confronting the child's usual manner of doing things or the therapist interpreting the child's motives or feelings without breaking down the defensive displacement. The play activity of the child is geared to the appropriate developmental level: younger children may prefer the use of dolls to represent their life situation; older children reveal their personal style of interacting through drawings or through games and other shared activities; and pre-

adolescents may dispense with any therapeutic props and insist on describing their circumstances verbally. The mode of communication varies with the age and the cognitive capacites of the child patient. However, there are no fixed rules regarding the medium of therapy; an older child may on occasion wish to draw or play a game to help in the revelation of his or her life, and, pari passu, a very young child may interrupt play for a significant verbal interchange. Overall, the activity of therapy should be geared to the capacities and limitations of the child's developmental state.

Another view of play is as a means of obtaining information, both in terms of the content of the play as well as from its form in the child's interactions with the therapist. Play is viewed as a familiar activity that fosters a relationship to the therapist; the way play is used in the relationship helps to define the task of therapy. This type of treatment, usually termed *relationship therapy*, was extensively described by Allen (1942) in the 1930s and 1940s and constitutes the framework for much of the child psychotherapy that is currently practiced. For Allen, the patient "must find new values in himself, not in isolation, but in the relation to another human being" (p. 57). Therapy becomes an active interchange in which at first the patients use the therapist according to their experiences with prior relationships, and gradually are allowed the freedom to relate in a more autonomous and creative fashion. If the therapist is sufficiently empathic and does not impose his or her values into the therapeutic situation, according to Allen, the patients will sense the potentially liberating atmosphere and will express themselves with increasing authenticity and a willingness to share themselves. In fact, Allen commented that the therapeutic value of talking lies less in the particular content expressed and more in the freedom to talk.

The curative factor in Allen's form of psychotherapy would appear to be a type of corrective emotional experience in which a new adult reacts to the child in a manner different from past significant others to supply the child with a new sense of self in the context of a trusting and liberating relationship. Although all psychotherapists would endorse Allen's emphasis on establishing a therapeutic relationship as the basis for therapy, most would consider it only a necessary but not entirely sufficient condition for the entire process. The creation of a close, trusting relationship has value in and of itself, but it also serves to facilitate the child's receptivity to interpretations regarding maladaptive behaviors and distortions of others as well as the child's acceptance of guidance in finding more productive ways to solve problems.

In summary, psychodynamic psychotherapy does not restrict itself to interpreting derivatives of the unconscious as these appear in play, transference repetitions, or other manifest activities. It tends to deal with the patient's total situation and uses a variety of means to create a therapeutic alliance. The therapist uses a position of influence to allow the child to experience himself or herself in a freer, more realistic fashion and to work actively with the child to solve reality-based problems, whether these stem from internalized conflicts or deviations of personality, environmental obstacles to psychological growth, or limiting organic or genetic deficits. The therapeutic experience is more similar to the child's activities outside the office as the therapist tries to create a real but influential relationship. As a result, techniques are more varied and less codified. Some therapists utilize play, others drawings, and others joint activities, from playing catch to building model airplanes. Gardner (1986), in particular, developed a series of games and techniques, which, while appealing to the child's natural attraction to play and fun, allow for the investigation and correction of psychological problems. As stated above, the selection of therapeutic activities parallels the child's developmental level, usually progressing from play to drawing and games to verbal interaction.

In further contrast to analysis, in which the child is largely left responsible for the unfolding of psychological material, the psychotherapist may bring up specific problems when it is believed that the child is ready to deal with them. These should be expressed in a manner that the child can comprehend according to the child's ontogenetic status. At times, the material can be presented in the play itself with a young child or as part of the style of mutual game playing in a latency-aged child. Finally, with a preadolescent, problem areas can be discussed verbally while taking into consideration the child's still immature appreciation of reality. Frequency of sessions is not specified and, aside from fiscal and time constraints, may depend on the child's ability to generalize from the therapy sessions to everyday life. Some children can apply what they gain from only one session per week to the rest of their waking hours, whereas others require more frequent meetings to reinforce a problem-solving attitude.

Parents, siblings, and other adults who affect the psychological life of the child (e.g., teachers, coaches) may be involved at various points during the therapeutic process. Termination usually occurs after the child is relatively free from presenting symptoms; has developed age-appropriate interests, behaviors, and modes of coping; and is progressing along normal developmental paths in a nonpathogenic environment.

Conclusions

In the preceding description of treatments, differences have been accentuated and similarities minimized for expository purposes. Actually, in practice, all of these systems have a great deal in common. Analysts realize the curative value of a close, trusting relationship, and psychotherapists, of whatever persuasion, appreciate the essential role of their patients' past and of motivating forces that are outside awareness in causing current problems. In each of these modes of therapy, the practitioner works to remove the blockages to normal psychological growth and to restore the child to his or her own optimal developmental path.

References

Allen FH: Psychotherapy With Children. New York, WW Norton, 1942

Ferenczi S: A little chanticleer (1913), in Sex and Psychoanalysis. New York, Robert Brunner, 1950, pp 240–252

Freud A: Indications for Child Analysis (1945), in The Writings of Anna Freud, Vol 4. New York, International Universities Press, 1968, pp 3–38

Freud A: Normality and Pathology in Childhood: Assessments of Development. New York, International Universities Press, 1965

Freud S: Analysis of a phobia in a five-year-old boy (1909), in The Standard Edition of the Complete Psychological Works of Sigmund Freud. Translated and edited by Strachey J. London, Hogarth Press, 1955, pp 1–149

Gardner RA: The Psychotherapeutic Techniques of Richard A Gardner. Cresskill, NJ, Creative Therapeutics, 1986

Hug-Helmuth H: On the technique of the analysis of children. Int J Psychoanal 1:361–362, 1920

Kanner L: Play investigation and play treatment of children's behavior disorders. J Pediatr 17:3–16, 1940

Klein M: Psychoanalysis of Children. London, Hogarth Press, 1932

Klein M: The psychoanalytic play technique. Am J Orthopsychiatry 25:223–237, 1955

Nagera H: Child psychoanalysis, in Emotional Disorders in Children and Adolescents. Edited by Sholevar GP, Benson RM, Blinder BJ. New York, Spectrum, 1980, pp 17–23

Segal H: Melanie Klein's technique of child analysis, in Handbook of Child Psychoanalysis. Edited by Wolman BB. New York, Van Nostrand Reinhold, 1972, pp 401–414

Chapter 52

Behavior Modification

Alan E. Kazdin, Ph.D.

Behavior modification or behavior therapy consists of an approach toward treatment that emphasizes the empirical evaluation of clinical problems.[1] When behavior modification first emerged as a formal movement in the 1950s, the focus of treatment on overt behavior, the absence of concern with presumed etiology, and the rejection of intrapsychic determinants were a few of the characteristics promoted (see Kazdin 1978). Many of these characteristics were proposed as a reaction to prevailing views of intrapsychic forces and provided the basis for devising behavior modification as an alternative approach toward treatment. Embedded in this broader movement were manifold theories, approaches, and treatment techniques. The diversity and sources of conflict among constituent theories and treatments were ignored in favor of promoting a larger movement. Even the initial characteristics proposed to define behavior modification at the inception of the movement could be challenged as untrue of major segments of behavioral treatments. In the last 40 years, behavior therapy has become even more diverse. Although it is meaningful to discuss behavior modification as an approach toward treatment, the characteristics and unique features are somewhat nonspecific. In this chapter, the approach and the scope of conceptual views, treatments, and applications are identified. Outcome evidence and treatment approaches are illustrated by description of quite different techniques. Finally, the critical issues and limitations of behavioral treatments are presented.

Characteristics of Behavior Modification

Primacy of Behavior

Within behavior modification, overt behavior plays a major part in the assessment and treatment of clinical dysfunction. Whenever possible, symptoms or groups of several symptoms that go together (syndromes or disorders) are operationalized in terms of overt behavioral referents. Although emphasis is placed on overt behavior, how people feel (affect) and think (cognition) also are important and are often central to the specific problems brought to treatment. For example, depressed persons often feel sad (affect), believe they cannot do anything right (cognition), and engage in few activities (behavior) in their everyday lives. Although affect, cognition, and behavior are important, behavioral treatments give primary attention to behavior as a means of altering the clinical problem. To continue the example, in the treatment process, a depressed patient may be encouraged to engage in specific activities involving interactions with others and in setting goals for accomplishing tasks. Increases in activity and completion of tasks are some of the

Completion of this chapter was facilitated by support of a Research Scientist Award (MH-00353) from the National Institute of Mental Health.

[1]The terms *behavior modification* and *behavior therapy* are used synonymously in the present chapter. Historically, these terms have been delineated on the basis of theoretical approaches, constituent treatment techniques, the manner in which the techniques are applied, and the countries in which the techniques have emerged (Franzini and Tilker 1972; Keehn and Webster 1969; Krasner 1971). The distinction, however, has not been applied in a consistent fashion.

behaviors found to alter depressive symptoms, including the many feelings and thoughts that comprise depression. Consequently, the approach often focuses on behavior both as an end in itself and as a means of changing affect and cognition.

Importance of Learning

An assumption of behavior modification is that behaviors of interest can be altered by providing new learning experiences. Behavioral treatments are designed to provide special learning experiences that alter deviant or clinically maladaptive behavior and increase adaptive behavior. Proponents of behavior modification do *not* adhere to the view that all behaviors are learned or that all behaviors can be changed through learning. Diverse biological, behavioral, social, cultural, and other factors converge to influence behavior. The key feature of the approach is recognition of the plasticity of behavior or the amenability of behavior to change when systematic learning experiences are provided. Whether providing new learning experiences will effectively alter behavior can be determined only empirically.

The psychology of learning within experimental psychology has provided a rich conceptual and empirical literature and has aided the explanation of the development of dysfunction. Learning paradigms, concepts, and methods of evaluation have been extended to develop and evaluate treatment techniques. For example, treatment of anxiety disorders in children and adults can be traced to animal laboratory work on conditioning, extensions of conditioning paradigms in demonstrations with humans, and the development of specific treatments (e.g., systematic desensitization, flooding) from these extensions (see Kazdin 1978). Thus laboratory research has served an important heuristic function.

Directive and Active Treatments

Behavioral techniques usually rely on directive and active treatments. This means that explicit training experiences are prescribed in treatment. Treatment sessions are frequently used as the context in which actions for change are planned. Often the actions or activities are assigned to persons as "homework" in which specific activities are carried out to help achieve the desired changes. For example, parents, teachers, and peers often assist the child

at home and at school in activities designed to promote therapeutic change. Treatment is conceptualized as *learning new behaviors* that are to be performed in everyday life. Activities by which learning takes place and the assistance of others in these settings serve as the basis for developing new behaviors.

Focus on Current Determinants of Behavior

Treatments focus on current rather than past influences on behavior. The significance of past influences (e.g., family processes, early experiences in psychologically sensitive periods of development) is widely recognized. Even if specific causes could be identified (e.g., sexual abuse of a child as the primary basis for depression as an adolescent), whether a historical focus (e.g., working through the past) is the most effective point of intervention is unclear. Historical influences and periods serve as the basis of initial discussion or history taking. Current influences and experiences serve as the basis for developing new patterns of behaving.

Importance of Assessment and Evaluation

A central characteristic of behavior modification is a commitment to assessment and evaluation of alternative treatments. In research, behavior modification places major emphasis on measuring outcome and evaluating treatment in controlled studies to decide if alternative treatments are effective and which variations of treatment are more effective than others. Proponents of behavior modification often view the emphasis on outcome research as the hallmark of the approach.

In clinical work with individual cases, evaluation also is very important to monitor the progress or its absence during the course of treatment. Evaluation of treatment in clinical work begins with assessment of the presenting symptoms or behaviors. The assessment may consist of direct observation of how the children perform at home and at school, evaluations by significant others (parents, peers), and evaluations by the children themselves (see Mash and Terdal 1988). The evaluation tends to focus on details of the symptoms or behaviors, the conditions associated with their performance (e.g., setting, antecedents, consequences), and resources in the child's repertoire and environment that might be mobilized in specific treatment strategies. Once treatment is implemented, assessment is likely to continue at several different points to determine if the desired outcomes are obtained. Specific measures and evaluation strategies are often used with the individual case to assess the effects of treatment and the extent to which clinically important changes have been achieved (Barlow et al. 1984; Kazdin 1982a). Evaluation of progress in treatment is also facilitated by having clearly specified goals and procedures.

Use of Persons in Everyday Life

Behavioral techniques often are carried out at home, at school, and in the community, rather than or in addition to a therapist's office. Persons who are responsible for the care, management, and education of children (e.g., parents, teachers, relatives, peers, and siblings) are often utilized to help with the behavior change program. Parents and teachers in particular often have access to critical influences that can be mobilized to alter child behavior under those conditions in which the problems emerge. For example, unmanageable child behavior at home is likely to be addressed by training parents to respond in ways to alter behavior.

General Comments

The previously stated characteristics are rather general. However, an effort to sharpen the characteristics immediately excludes major segments of behavior modification. For example, one might claim that behavioral approaches focus on consequences of behavior (e.g., rewards) to achieve therapeutic change. Although several interventions focus on consequences, very many techniques do not or do so only in an ancillary fashion. One might also pose that behavioral techniques view behaviors (e.g., presenting symptoms) as the appropriate treatment focus. That is often true. However, many techniques, particularly those based on cognitive-behavioral procedures, would not be represented by this view. The reason for characterizing behavior modification in somewhat general terms can be conveyed better by noting the range of conceptual views and applications.

Scope of Behavior Modification

Conceptual Views

Child behavior modification draws heavily on diverse theories to understand affect, cognition, and behavior and the factors that account for their emergence, maintenance, and alteration. Two general conceptual positions capture the diverse theoretical approaches and are referred to as *mediational* and *nonmediational* views. The mediational view emphasizes constructs such as affect and cognition that mediate or serve as underpinnings of behavior. A critical role is accorded such cognitive processes as plans, goals, beliefs, attributions, and self-statements. Cognitive-behavioral theories and treatments derived from them fall within a mediational view (e.g., Bandura 1977a; Beck et al. 1979).

The nonmediational view focuses on direct (i.e., nonmediated) connections between environmental or situational events and behavior. Operant conditioning, which views behaviors as a function of antecedents (e.g., prompts, cues) and consequences (e.g., reactions of others), represents a nonmediational view. Child problems are viewed as deficits or excesses in performance and altered directly by applying antecedent and consequent events (e.g., Cooper et al. 1987).

The dominant view within child behavior modification, referred to as social learning theory, reflects a broad orientation that attempts to integrate both cognitive and environmental influences (e.g., Bandura 1977b). Emphasis is accorded cognitive processes that underlie the acquisition and persistence of behavior. The primacy of cognitive mechanisms is by no means uniformly endorsed within the field.

Intervention Techniques

The vast range of intervention techniques within behavior modification is due to the diverse conceptual views and the quite varied clinical problems and child and adolescent populations to which they are applied. Indeed, 160 behavioral techniques and treatment variations have been identified (Bellack and Hersen 1985). Often a given technique is identified in ways that mask an extremely large number of variations. For example, contingency management is occasionally referred to as a specific intervention in which various rewarding and punishing consequences are utilized to alter behavior. The intervention refers generally to the alteration of antecedents (e.g., prompts, cues, instructions, and discriminative stimuli) and consequences (e.g., reinforcers, schedules of their delivery) in relation to child behavior. Treatments based on contingency management vary in the parameters and types of reinforcers (praise, tokens), the persons who administer treatment (parents, teachers, peers, siblings, the children themselves), and settings in which they are conducted (clinic, home, school, institutions). The variation has allowed application of this one class of treatment to children with a broad range of diagnoses (see Kazdin 1989).

Treatment Focus

Behavior modification has been applied to diverse child and adolescent areas of functioning. First and perhaps foremost, behavioral techniques have been applied to clinical dysfunctions, as reflected in the domains of disorders included in the DSM-III-R (American Psychiatric Association 1987). Thus behavior modification is applied to children with autism, mental retardation, anxiety disorders, disruptive behavior disorders, eating disorders, encopresis and enuresis, academic skills disorders, tics, stuttering, and others (see Bellack et al. 1990; Bornstein and Kazdin 1985; Mash and Barkley 1989). Within a given clinical dysfunction, the scope of applications is broad. For example, for children with pervasive developmental disorders, behavioral techniques have been quite useful in developing language, self-care, interpersonal, educational, and vocational skills (e.g., Schreibman et al. 1990).

Second, behavioral techniques have addressed several domains of child and adolescent functioning in everyday life in areas that would not necessarily be regarded as evidence of clinical dysfunction (Kazdin 1989). For example, behavioral techniques have focused on social interaction among withdrawn children, subclinical fears, academic performance, classroom deportment, toilet training, parent-child relations, home behaviors of latchkey children, and others. Some of these areas reflect mild versions of problems that are seen clinically. Thus parent-adolescent conflict might well fall within the clinical realm of dysfunction (e.g., oppositional defiant disorder or a V code) (Foster and Robin 1989). However, strained parent-adolescent relations may serve as the focus when the level would be disturbing but not within the realm of diagnosis. More broadly, many applications of behavior modification focus on performance, development, parenting, and teaching in the absence of clinical impairment.

Third, behavioral techniques are applied to domains in which children are victims, including physical and sexual abuse and neglect. These areas are obviously worthy of intervention on a variety of grounds, not the least of which are their likely long-term psychiatric sequelae. Intervention programs for children and parents who mistreat children have evaluated their impact on functioning of both parents and children (e.g., Azar and Wolfe 1989).

Fourth, behavior modification has been applied extensively to child and adolescent health-related domains. Behavior modification techniques are often used to increase adherence to medical (e.g., in the control of diabetes) or rehabilitation (e.g., to increase mobility and functioning of youth with physical disability, handicap, or chronic disease) regimens (Van Hasselt et al. 1990). Behavioral techniques also are used as adjuncts, as in the control of pain associated with disease, injury, or side effects of assessment or treatment (e.g., among children with severe burns, bone marrow aspirations, chemotherapy side effects) (e.g., Dolgan and Jay 1989). Often behavioral treatments have been provided as primary intervention for such problems as obesity, pediatric migraine, recurrent abdominal pain, and ruminative vomiting in infants, to mention a few. Health applications represent a major area of clinical activity and research.

The Effectiveness of Behavior Modification

The scope of treatment techniques, clinical problems, and populations to which these techniques have been applied precludes even a scant presentation of the outcome research.[2] Evaluation of the empirical evidence requires review of specific techniques separately by clinical dysfunction (see Bornstein and Kazdin 1985; Kratochwill and Morris 1991;

---

[2]Outcome research in behavior modification is dispersed through many journals in clinical psychology, psychiatry, education, and child services. In addition, several specialty journals within the field serve as an outlet for outcome research. Primary among these are *Behavior Therapy, Behavior Modification, Behavior Research and Therapy, Child and Family Behavior Therapy, Cognitive Therapy and Research*, the *Journal of Applied Behavior Analysis*, and the *Journal of Behavior Therapy and Experimental Psychiatry*.

Mash and Barkley 1989). The types of approaches, evidence, and limitations of contemporary research can be illustrated by focusing on one problem area as a "case study" of outcome research. For present purposes, behavioral treatments for conduct problems are described here to highlight the overall approach.

The term *conduct problems* has no uniform definition within behavior modification, but is often used to embrace the full range of disruptive behaviors, including antisocial, aggressive, and oppositional behaviors, tantrums, excessive whining, overactivity, teasing, and others. Aggressive and oppositional behaviors have served as a focus of different behavioral techniques. Five classes of treatment are highlighted: operant conditioning techniques, social skills training, problem-solving skills training, parent management training, and functional family therapy.

Operant Conditioning Techniques

The principles of operant conditioning have generated a large number of interventions (Cooper et al. 1987; Kazdin 1977). The techniques can be distinguished on the basis of whether they attempt to increase the frequency of appropriate (e.g., nonaggressive) behavior or to decrease the frequency of inappropriate behavior. A large number of demonstrations are available in which positive reinforcement is used to increase specific behaviors. Merely providing incentives for behavior is not likely to be very effective. Several parameters of administration (e.g., frequency, immediacy, contingent delivery, and schedule of delivery) are critically important and directly influence effectiveness.

Punishment procedures are also used in behavioral programs to suppress or eliminate conduct problem behaviors. The punishment procedures differ from the usual consequences applied to behavior in everyday life; they are also implemented somewhat differently. Punishment procedures in the context of treatment typically consist of the withdrawal of reinforcers. Procedures such as time-out from reinforcement (removal of positive reinforcers for a brief period of time), response cost (the loss of a positive reinforcer such as a token or privilege), and overcorrection (correcting the environmental effects of the inappropriate behavior and practicing appropriate performance) are three commonly used methods. There are many examples in which variations of reinforcement and pun-

ishment techniques are used to reduce conduct problems in children and adolescents at home and at school (see Kazdin 1989).

Illustrations. Large-scale programs combine several reinforcement and punishment contingencies to change behavior. Perhaps the most well known of these is the program at Achievement Place (in Kansas), which is conducted for youths (ages 10–16) who have been adjudicated for a variety of offenses, primarily felonies. Diverse diagnoses have been applied to the population, including personality disorder, adjustment reaction, and conduct disorder. The program is conducted in a home-style situation in which a small number of boys or girls (usually six to eight) live with a specially trained married couple. The children participate in a token economy in which a variety of self-care (e.g., room cleaning), social (e.g., communicating with peers, participating in group activity), and academic (e.g., reading, completing homework) behaviors are reinforced with points. The points can be exchanged for several rewards and privileges such as allowance; access to television, games, and tools; and permission to go downtown or to stay up late. Points can be lost for failure to meet particular responsibilities (e.g., to maintain passing grades in school) or violation of rules (e.g., being late in returning home, lying, stealing). In addition to reinforcement and punishment techniques, several other procedures are included, such as training children in specific skill areas (e.g., vocational training), self-government in which children decide many of the consequences of their behavior, a close interpersonal relationship with the teaching parents, and a structured family situation (e.g., Wolf et al. 1976, 1987). Several studies have demonstrated the effects of reinforcement and punishment contingencies on such behaviors as aggressive statements, completion of homework and chores, keeping up on current events, and communication skills (e.g., Phillips et al. 1973; Werner et al. 1975). In addition, while the youths were in the program, the gains were reflected in a reduction in criminal offenses in the community and significantly fewer criminal offenses than others in community-based or more traditional institutional programs (Kirigin et al. 1982). However, measures of offenses and reinstitutionalization from 1 to 3 years after participation in the program are no different for youths who complete the program from those of youths who participate in more traditional programs (Jones et al. 1981; Kirigin et al. 1979, 1982). Thus the evidence has been relatively consistent in showing gains during treatment but not thereafter.

Evaluation. Many other operant conditioning programs have been evaluated for a wide range of youths with conduct problems. The work has encompassed different settings, age groups, and levels of severity of conduct problems as reflected in programs in correctional institutions, (e.g., Hobbs and Holt 1976), elementary schools (e.g., Walker et al. 1981), summer camps (e.g., Hughes 1979), and the community (e.g., O'Donnell et al. 1979), to mention a few. These and other operant conditioning–based interventions can reduce aggressive behavior and increase prosocial behavior. There are limitations in what the studies have shown. First, the programs tend to focus on one or a few target behaviors, rather than on the larger constellation of behaviors in which that behavior may be embedded. Thus the often dramatic effects achieved with a particular behavior are tempered by the absence of information on related behaviors that may not have been addressed. Second, long-term follow-up is rarely assessed. Because of the recalcitrance of severe conduct problem behaviors to change, return and continuation of the behaviors are likely. Consequently, demonstrations of long-term impact are greatly needed.

Social Skills Training

Social skills training refers to a behavioral treatment approach that has been widely applied to children, adolescents, and adults (Kelly 1982; Michelson et al. 1983). Training focuses on the verbal and nonverbal behaviors that affect social interactions. Specific behaviors are developed to enhance the child's ability to influence his or her environment, to obtain appropriate outcomes, and to respond appropriately to demands of others. The underlying rationale for social skills training is drawn from the notion that conduct problems in children are basically interpersonal problems. Children are often identified as in need of treatment because their behaviors have a deleterious impact on others, as evident in aggressive acts, property destruction, noncompliant behavior, negativism, and tantrums. Several maladaptive patterns of social interaction among children have been implicated in clinical dysfunction. For example, asocial behavior, social isolation, and unpopularity in childhood are risk factors for childhood psychopathology, delinquency and conduct problems, dropping out of school, and antisocial behavior in adulthood (see Kazdin 1987a).

Social skills training develops a variety of interpersonal skills, usually in the context of individual treatment sessions. Typically, training consists of several procedures, including instructions, modeling by the therapist, practice by the child, corrective feedback, and social reinforcement (praise) for appropriate performance. The sequence of these procedures is enacted with several interpersonal situations, such as in interactions with parents, siblings, and peers. In each situation, the child and therapist role-play the appropriate behaviors. Instructions convey what the child is to do, the overall purpose, and salient features of the behavior. Modeling by the therapist shows exactly how the behavior should be performed. Feedback from the therapist conveys how the child's responses might be improved. The therapist may model what the child has done and may show the child how the action may be done differently. The child reenacts the desired behaviors. If they are appropriate, the therapist provides social reinforcement. The general sequence is continued until the child's responses are appropriate in particular situations and across a large number of different situations.

Illustration. As an example, Elder et al. (1979) used social skills training with four adolescents who had been hospitalized (from 2 months to 5 years). Each had a history of verbal and physical aggressiveness. Based on the behavior checklist ratings and interviews with the youth, the following behaviors were selected for treatment: interrupting others, responding to negative provocation, and making requests of others. Role-play situations were devised in which training was conducted. Training was carried out in a group in which each person had an opportunity to role-play and to observe others enact the situation. Treatment was evaluated in a multiple-baseline design in which the behaviors were trained in sequence using instructions, modeling, practice, and feedback, as highlighted earlier. Social skills training altered the specific skills that were trained; improvements also were associated with increases in social behaviors on the ward and with decreases in the frequency of seclusion for inappropriate behavior. Three of the four subjects were discharged and maintained their gains up to 9 months later.

Evaluation. Several studies have demonstrated that social skills can be developed in aggressive and conduct-problem children and adolescents (see Kazdin 1985). In such studies, the focus is usually on specific behaviors in simulated social situations. These behaviors include hostile tone of voice, eye contact, content of verbal statements, making appropriate requests of others, and responding appropriately to unreasonable requests. Evidence for effectiveness of training with conduct-problem children comes mainly from studies with small samples of only one or a few children. Also, the effects of social skills training on adjustment in the community and over the course of follow-up have been infrequently evaluated (e.g., Gross et al. 1980). Thus apart from changes in highly specific behaviors within the treatment setting, the therapeutic impact of this method is difficult to evaluate.

Problem-Solving Skills Training

Alternative interventions have focused on the child's cognitive processes (perceptions, self-statements, attributions, and problem-solving skills) that are presumed to underlie maladaptive behavior. Cognitive processes are frequently accorded a major role in aggressive behavior (Berkowitz 1977; Novaco 1978). Aggression is triggered not merely by environmental events, but rather through the way in which these events are perceived and processed. The processing refers to the child's appraisals of the situation, anticipated reactions of others, and self-statements in response to particular events. Clinic and nonreferred children identified as aggressive have shown a predisposition to attribute hostile intent to others, especially in social situations where the cues of actual intent are ambiguous (Dodge 1985). Understandably, when situations are initially perceived as hostile, children are more likely to react aggressively. The ability take the perspective of, or to empathize with, other persons is also related to aggressive behavior (Ellis 1982; Feshbach 1975).

The relation between cognitive processes and behavioral adjustment has been evaluated extensively by Spivack and Shure (Shure and Spivack 1978; Spivack and Shure 1982; Spivack et al. 1976). These investigators have identified different cognitive processes of interpersonal cognitive problem-solving skills that underlie social behavior (see Table 52-1). The ability to engage in these processes is related to behavioral adjustment, as measured, for example, in teacher ratings of disruptive behavior and social withdrawal. Disturbed children

Table 52-1.   Interpersonal cognitive problem-solving skills

1. Alternative solution thinking—the ability to generate different options (solutions) that can solve problems in interpersonal situations.
2. Means-end thinking—awareness of the intermediate steps required to achieve a particular goal.
3. Consequential thinking—the ability to identify what might happen as a direct result of acting in a particular way or choosing a particular solution.
4. Causal thinking—the ability to relate one event to another over time and to understand why one event led to a particular action of other persons.
5. Sensitivity to interpersonal problems—the ability to perceive a problem when it exists and to identify the interpersonal aspects of the confrontation that may emerge.

Note.   Adapted from Spivack et al. 1976.

tend to generate fewer alternative solutions to interpersonal problems, to focus on ends or goals rather than the intermediate steps to obtain them, to see fewer consequences associated with their behavior, to fail to recognize the causes of other people's behavior, and to be less sensitive to interpersonal conflict.

Problem-solving skills training consists of developing interpersonal problem-solving skills in which conduct-problem children are considered to be deficient. Many variations of problem-solving skills training have been applied to conduct-problem children (Camp and Bash 1985; Kendall and Braswell 1985; Spivack et al. 1976). The variations share many characteristics. First, the emphasis is on *how* children approach situations. Although it is obviously important that children ultimately select appropriate means of behaving in everyday life, the primary focus is on the thought processes rather than the outcome or specific behavioral acts that result. Second, children are taught to engage in a step-by-step approach to solve interpersonal problems. They make statements to themselves that direct attention to certain aspects of the problems or tasks that lead to effective solutions. Third, treatment utilizes structured tasks involving games, academic activities, and stories. Over the course of treatment, the cognitive problem-solving skills are increasingly applied to real-life situations. Fourth, the therapist usually plays an active role in treatment. The therapist models the cognitive processes by making verbal self-statements, applies the sequence of statements to particular problems, provides cues to prompt use of the skills, and delivers feedback and praise to develop correct use of the skills. Finally, treatment usually combines several different procedures, including modeling and practice, role-playing, and reinforcement and mild punishment (loss of points or tokens).

Case Study. The application of problem-solving skills training can be illustrated more concretely in a case application. Cory was a 10-year-old boy who was hospitalized on a short-term children's inpatient unit to begin a treatment regimen designed to control his aggressive, antisocial, oppositional, and disruptive behavior at home and at school. He had been caught on three occasions playing with matches and setting fires in his room. Before coming for treatment, he was suspended from school for assaulting a classmate and choking him to the point that the child almost passed out.

Problem-solving skills training was begun and completed while Cory was in the hospital because his parents said they could not return for treatment on an outpatient basis once hospitalization ended. Cory received 20 individual sessions of problem-solving training with two to three sessions each week. The sessions began by teaching Cory the problem-solving steps. These consist of specific self-statements, with each treatment representing a step for solving a problem. The steps or self-statements include 1) What I am supposed to do; 2) I have to look at all my possibilities; 3) I have to concentrate and focus in; 4) I need to make a choice and select a solution; and 5) I need to find out how I did.

In the first session, Cory was taught the steps so they could be recalled without special reminders or cues from the therapist. In the next several sessions, the steps were applied to simple problems involving various academic tasks (e.g., arithmetic problems) and board games (e.g., checkers). In each of these sessions, Cory's task was to identify the goal, the alternative choices or options and their consequences, the best choice in light of these consequences, and so on. In the sessions, Cory and the therapist took turns using the steps to work on the task. In these early sessions, the focus was on teaching the steps and training Cory to become facile in applying them to diverse but relatively simple situations. After session 8, the games were withdrawn, and the steps were applied to problems that were related to interactions with parents, teachers, siblings, peers, and others.

Cory was also given assignments outside of treatment. The assignments initially were to identify "real" problems (e.g., with another child on the inpatient service) for he could use the steps. When he brought one of these situations to the session, he described how the steps could have been used. He earned points for bringing in such a situation, and these points could be exchanged for small prizes. As the sessions progressed, he received points for using the steps in the actual situations. His use of the steps was checked by asking him exactly what he did, role-playing the situation within the session, and asking other staff on the ward if the events were portrayed accurately.

The majority of treatment consisted of applying the steps in the session to situations in which Cory's aggressive and antisocial behaviors had emerged. To illustrate this process, a portion of session 17 follows:

Therapist: Well, Cory today we are going to act out some more problem situations using the steps. You have been doing so well with this that I think we can use the steps today in a way that will make it even easier to use them in everyday life. When you use the steps today, I want you to think in your mind what the first steps are. When you get to step 4, say that one out loud before you do it. This will let us see what the solution is that you have chosen. Then, step 5, when you evaluate how you did, can also be thought in your mind. We are going to do the steps in our heads today like this so that it will be easier to use them in everyday life without drawing attention to what we are doing. The same rules apply as in our other sessions. We still want to go slowly in using the steps, and we want to select good solutions.

OK. Today I brought in a lot of difficult situations. I think it is going to be hard to use the steps. Let's see how each of us does. I have six stacks of cards here. You can see the stacks are numbered from 1 to 6. We will take turns rolling the die and take a card from the stack with the same number. As we did in the last session, we are going to solve the problem as we sit here, then we will get up and act it out as if it is really happening. OK, why don't you go first and role the die.

Cory (rolls the die): I got a 4.

Therapist: OK. Read the top card in that stack (therapist points to fourth stack).

Cory (reads the card): "The principal of your school is walking past you in the hall between classes when he notices some candy wrappers that someone has dropped on the floor. The principal turns to you and says in a pretty tough voice, 'Cory, we don't litter in the halls at this school! Now pick up the trash!'"

Therapist: This is a tough one—how are you going to handle this?

Cory: Well, here goes with the steps. (Cory holds his first finger up and appears to be saying step 1 to himself; he does this with steps 2 and 3 as well. When he gets to step 4 he says out loud) I would say to him that I did not throw the wrappers down and I would keep walking.

Therapist: Well, it was *great* that you did not get mad and talk back to him. He was sort of accusing you, and you hadn't really thrown the papers down. But, if you just say, "I didn't do it" and walk away, what might happen?

Cory: Nothing. Because I *didn't* do it.

Therapist: Yeah, but he may not believe you—maybe especially because you got into trouble before with him. Also, he asked you for a favor and you could help a lot by doing what he asked. Try going through the steps again and see if you can turn your pretty good solution into a great one.

Cory: (goes through steps 1, 2, and 3 again; at step 4 he says) I would say to him that I did not throw the wrappers down but that I would gladly pick 'em up and toss them in the trash.

Therapist (with great enthusiasm): That's great— that's a wonderful solution! OK. Go to step 5; how do you think you did.

Cory: I did good because I used the steps.

Therapist: That's right, but you did more than that. You nicely told the principal that you did not do it *and* you did the favor he asked. What do you think he will think of you in the future? Very nicely done. OK. Now let's both get up and act this out.

The treatment session continues as this situation is enacted through role-play and several other situations are presented. When the child does especially well, the situation may be made a little more difficult or provocative to help him or her apply the steps under more challenging circumstances.

Evaluation. A number of researchers have conducted programmatic series of studies showing the efficacy of problem-solving skills training (see Kendall and Braswell 1985; Spivack and Shure 1982). In several studies with impulsive or aggressive children and adolescents, cognitively based treatment has led to significant changes in behavior at home, at school, and in the community, with gains evident up to 1 year later (Arbuthnot and Gordon 1986; Kazdin et al. 1987, 1989; Kendall and Braswell 1982; Lochman et al. 1984). However, the magnitude of the changes needs to be greater than those currently achieved to return children to normative or adaptive levels of functioning at home and at school. Some evidence has suggested that the greater the level of child aggression, the less effective treatment is (Kendall and Braswell 1985). Duration of treatment has influenced outcome in one study with longer treatment (>18 sessions), leading to greater change than was evident in shorter treatment

(Lochman 1985). In general, the factors that contribute to treatment outcome have been infrequently studied in the treatment of aggressive children.

Parent Management Training

Parent management training refers to procedures in which a parent or parents are trained to interact differently with their children. Parents of conduct-problem youth, particularly those youth with aggressive behavior, engage in several practices that promote antisocial behavior and suppress prosocial behavior, including the inadvertent and direct reinforcement of aggressive behavior, frequent use of commands, nonreinforcement of prosocial behaviors, and others (Patterson 1982). Parent management training alters the interchanges between parent and child so that prosocial, rather than aggressive, behavior is directly fostered within the family.

Although many variations of parent management training exist, several common characteristics can be identified. First, treatment is conducted primarily with the parent or parents who directly implement several procedures in the home. There usually is no direct intervention of the therapist with the child. Second, parents are trained to identify, define, and observe problem behavior in new ways. The careful specification of the problem is essential for the delivery of reinforcing or punishing consequences and for evaluating if the program is achieving the desired goals. Third, the treatment sessions cover social learning principles and the procedures that follow from them, including positive reinforcement (e.g., the use of social praise and tokens or points for prosocial behavior), mild punishment (e.g., use of time-out from reinforcement, loss of privileges), negotiation, and contingency contracting. Fourth, the sessions provide opportunities for parents to see how the techniques are implemented, to practice using the techniques, and to review the behavior change programs in the home. The immediate goal of the program is to develop specific skills in the parents. As the parents become more proficient, the program can address the child's most severely problematic behaviors and encompass other problem areas (e.g., school behavior).

Case Illustration. The application of parent management training can be illustrated by a case of a 7-year-old boy named Shawn, referred for treatment because of his aggressive outbursts toward his two younger sisters at home and his peers at school. He argued and had severe tantrums at home, stayed out late at night, and occasionally stole from his mother's live-in boyfriend. At school, he fought with peers, argued with the teacher, and disrupted the class. Parent management training was provided to the mother. The boyfriend was unable to attend all of the meetings regularly because of his work as a trucker and his extended periods away from the home. The overall goal of treatment was to train the mother to behave differently in relation to Shawn and her other children. Specifically, she was to be trained to identify concrete problematic and prosocial behaviors, to observe these behaviors systematically, to implement positive reinforcement programs, to provide mild punishment as needed, and to negotiate such programs directly with the child.

The contents of the 16 sessions provided to the parent(s) are highlighted in Table 52-2. Each session lasted about 2 hours. In each session, the therapist reviewed the previous week's observations and implementation of the program. Queries were made to review precisely what the parents did (e.g., praise, administer points or tokens, send the child to time-out) in response to the child's behavior. The therapist and parent(s) role-played situations at home in which the parent might have responded more effectively. Parents practiced delivering the consequences and received feedback and reinforcement for this behavior from the therapist. Any problems in the programs, ambiguity of the observation procedures, or other facets were discussed. After the program was reviewed, new material was taught, as outlined in Table 52-2.

Shawn's mother and the therapist developed a program to increase Shawn's compliance with requests. Simple chores were requested (e.g., cleaning his room, setting the table) in the first few weeks of the program to help the parents apply what they had learned. Time-out from reinforcement was introduced to provide mild punishment for fighting. Over time, several behaviors were incorporated into a program in which Shawn earned points that could purchase special privileges (e.g., staying up 15 minutes beyond bedtime, having a friend sleep over, small prizes, time to play his video game). About halfway through treatment, a home-based reinforcement program was developed to alter behaviors at school. Two teachers at the school were contacted and asked to identify behaviors to be developed in class. The program was explained in which they were asked to initial cards that Shawn carried to indicate how well he behaved in class and whether he completed his homework. Based on daily teacher evaluations, Shawn earned additional points at home.

After approximately 5 months, Shawn improved greatly in his behavior at home. He argued very little with his mother and sisters. His parents felt they were much better able to manage him. At school, Shawn's teachers reported that he could remain in class like other children. Occasionally, he would not listen to the teacher or precipitated heated arguments with his peers. However, he was less physically aggressive than he had been prior to treatment.

Evaluation. The effectiveness of parent management training has been evaluated extensively with behavior-problem children varying in age and degree of severity of dysfunction (see Kazdin 1985). The work of Patterson and his colleagues (see Patterson 1986), spanning more than 25 years, exemplifies the ongoing development of a conceptual model and outcome research on parent training with antisocial youths. More than 200 families have been seen that include primarily aggressive children (ages 3–12 years) referred for outpatient treatment (see Patterson 1982). Several controlled studies have demonstrated improvements in child behavior at home and at school over the course of treatment. Moreover, these changes surpass those achieved with variations of family-based psychotherapy, attention-placebo (discussion), and no-treatment conditions. Parent management training has brought the problematic behaviors of treated children within the normative levels of their peers who are functioning adequately. Improvements often remain evident 1 year after treatment (e.g., Fleischman and Szykula 1981); the continued benefits of treatment have been evident with noncompliant children up to as many as 4.5 years (Baum and Forehand 1981) and 10 years later (Forehand and Long 1988).

Several characteristics of treatment administration contribute to outcome, including the duration of treatment, providing parents with in-depth knowledge of social learning principles, and utilizing time-out from reinforcement in the home (see Kazdin 1987b). Parent and family characteristics also relate to treatment outcome. As might be expected, families characterized by multiple risk factors associated with childhood dysfunction (e.g., marital

Table 52-2.   Parent management training sessions for the case of Shawn: session, topic, and brief description

1. Introduction and overview—This session provides the parents with an overview of the program and outlines the demands placed on them and the focus of the intervention.

2. Defining and observing—This session trains parents to pinpoint, define, and observe behavior. The parents and trainer define specific problems that can be observed and develop a specific plan to begin observations.

3. Positive reinforcement—This session focuses on learning the concept of positive reinforcement, factors that contribute to the effective application, and rehearsal of applications in relation to the target child. Specific programs are outlined in which praise and points are to be provided for the behaviors observed during the week.

4. Review of the program and data—Observations of the previous week as well as application of the reinforcement program are reviewed. Details about the administration of praise, points, and back-up reinforcers are discussed and as needed enacted so that the trainer can identify how to improve parent performance. Changes are made in the program as needed.

5. Time-out from reinforcement—Parents learn about time-out and the factors related to its effective application. The use of time-out is planned for the next week for specific behaviors.

6. Shaping—Parents are trained to develop behaviors by reinforcement of successive approximations and to use prompts and fading of prompts to develop terminal behaviors.

7. Review and problem solving—The concepts discussed in all prior sessions are thoroughly reviewed. The parent is asked to apply these concepts to hypothetical situations presented during the session. Areas of weakness in understanding the concepts or their execution in practice serve as the focus.

8. Attending and ignoring—Parents learn about attending and ignoring and choose undesirable behavior that they will ignore and a positive opposite behavior to which they will attend. These procedures are practiced during the session.

9. School intervention—Plans are made to implement a home-based reinforcement program to develop school-related behaviors. Prior to this session, discussions with the teachers and parents have identified specific behaviors to focus on in class (e.g., deportment) and at home (e.g., homework completion). These behaviors are incorporated into the reinforcement system.

10. Reprimands—Parents are trained in effective use of reprimands.

11. Family meeting—At this meeting, the child and parent(s) are brought into the session. The programs are discussed along with any problems. Revisions are made as needed to correct misunderstandings or to alter facets that are possibly not being implemented in a way that is likely to be effective.

12. Review of skills—Here the programs are reviewed along with all concepts about the principles. Parents are asked to develop programs for a variety of hypothetical everyday problems at home and at school. Feedback is provided regarding program options and applications.

13. Negotiating and contracting—The child and parent(s) meet together to negotiate new behavior programs and to place these in contractual form.

14. Low-rate behaviors—Parents are trained to deal with low-rate behaviors such as fire setting, stealing, or truancy. Specific punishment programs are planned and presented to the child as needed for behaviors characteristic of the case.

15, 16, & 17. Review, problem solving, and practice—Material from other sessions is reviewed in theory and practice. Special emphasis is given to role-playing application of individual principles as they are enacted with the trainer. Parents practice designing new programs, revising ailing programs, and responding to a complex array of situations in which principles and practices discussed in prior sessions are reviewed.

discord, parent psychopathology, social isolation, and socioeconomic disadvantage) tend to show fewer gains in treatment and are less likely to maintain therapeutic gains (e.g., Dumas and Wahler 1983; Strain et al. 1981). Thus variables beyond the specific parent-child interactions need to be considered in treatment.

Many issues regarding the effects of parent management training remain. The treatment cannot be applied to many cases of conduct-problem children in need of treatment. The requirement of active participation on the part of a parent makes the treatment inapplicable to some cases in which parent dysfunction and unwillingness cannot be surmounted. In cases in which treatment can be applied, further follow-up data are needed. With antisocial youths referred for aggressive behavior, follow-up typically has been completed up to 1 year. Given the recalcitrance of severe antisocial behavior, evidence is needed to assess the long-term impact. Notwithstanding the potential limitations, parent management training is one of the more well-developed and researched techniques for aggressive child behavior.

Functional Family Therapy

Functional family therapy reflects an integrative approach to treatment that has relied on a systems and behavioral view of dysfunction. Clinical problems are conceptualized from the standpoint of the functions they serve in the family as a system, as well as for individual family members. The assumption is made that problem behavior evident in the child is the only way some interpersonal functions (e.g., intimacy, distancing, support) can be met among family members. Maladaptive processes within the family are considered to preclude a more direct means of fulfilling these functions. The goal of treatment is to alter interaction and communication patterns in such a way as to foster more adaptive functioning. Treatment is also based on learning theory and focuses on specific stimuli and responses that can be used to produce change. Behavioral concepts and procedures identifying specific behaviors for change and reinforcing new adaptive ways of responding and empirically evaluating and monitoring change are included in this perspective. More recent formulations of functional family therapy have added cognitive processes to broaden the focus (Morris et al., in press). This perspective focuses on the attributions, attitudes, assumptions, expectations, and emotions of the family. Family members may begin treatment with attributions that focus on blaming others or themselves. New perspectives may be needed to help serve as the basis for developing new ways of behaving.

Functional family therapy requires that the family see the clinical problem from the relational functions it serves within the family. The therapist points out interdependencies and contingencies between family members in their day-to-day functioning and with specific reference to the problem that has served as the basis for seeking treatment. Once the family sees alternative ways of viewing the problem, the incentive for interacting more constructively is increased.

The main goals of treatment are to increase reciprocity and positive reinforcement among family members, to establish clear communication, to help specify behaviors that family members desire from each other, to negotiate constructively, and to help identify solutions to interpersonal problems. The family members read a manual that describes social learning principles to develop familiarity with the concepts used in treatment. In therapy, family members identify behaviors they would like others to perform. Responses are incorporated into a reinforcement system in the home to promote adaptive behavior in exchange for privileges. However, the primary focus is on the treatment sessions in which family communication patterns are altered directly. During the sessions, the therapist provides social reinforcement (verbal and nonverbal praise) for communications that suggest solutions to problems, clarify problems, or offer feedback to other family members.

Illustration. The technique requires understanding of several types of functions that behaviors can serve within the family.[3] These functions include behaviors that family members perform to sustain contact and closeness (merging), to decrease psychological intensity and dependence (separating), and to provide a mixture of merging and separating (midpointing). These processes are intricate because they usually involve the relations of all family members with each other. Also, the behaviors of a given family member may serve multiple and opposing functions in relation to different individuals within the family. Thus a behavior that may draw one family member close may distance another member. Finally, several different behaviors (e.g., the fighting of a child with a sibling, getting into trouble at school, running away from home overnight) may serve quite similar functions (e.g., bring the mother and father together). During the course of treatment, all family members meet. The focus of treatment is to identify consistent patterns of behavior and the range of functions they serve and messages they send. Specific techniques are enumerated and illustrated in Table 52-3.

Other strategies employed during the course of treatment include not blaming individuals; relabeling thoughts, feelings, and behaviors to take into account relational components; discussing the implications of symptom removal; changing the

---

[3]An illustration of the entire process of functional family therapy is difficult to convey because of the complex set of techniques, their relation to the nature of family functioning, and their dependence on individual features of the family. The techniques are well illustrated elsewhere, where guidelines are provided for therapists (Alexander and Parsons 1982). Selected features of the techniques can be described and illustrated to convey the manner in which the set of techniques operates.

Table 52-3.   Selected therapy techniques in functional family therapy: technique, goal, and illustration

Asking questions—To help focus on the relationships raised by the issue or problem. Example: After a description of an event involving the child (e.g., named Ginger) and the mother, the therapist may ask the father, "How do you fit into all of this?"

Making comments—To help identify and clarify relationships. Example: The therapist may say to the father, "So you are drawn into this argument when your wife gets upset?"

Offering interpretations—To go beyond the obvious observations by inferring possible motivational states, effects on others, and antecedents. Example: The therapist may say, "So when you have an argument, you believe that this is a message that you are needed. But at the same time, you feel pushed away."

Identifying sequences—To point to the relations among sequences or patterns of behavior to see more complex effects of interactions (i.e., several functional relations over time). Example: The therapist says, "It seems to me that the arguments between Ginger and you [to mother] make both you and your husband upset. This leads to everyone arguing for a while about who did what and what has to be done and no one agrees. But after the dust settles, you both [to mother and father] have something to talk about and to work on. This brings you both together at least for a little while. And this may help you a lot too Ginger, because you don't get to see your mother and father talking together like this very often."

Using the therapist as a direct tool—To have the therapist refer to his or her relation to the family within the session and what functions this could serve. Example: The therapist says, "I feel as if I am still being asked to choose sides here because it may serve a function similar to the one that Ginger serves: that is, to help bring you two together. That's not good or bad. But we need to see how we can get you two together when there is no argument or battle with a third party."

Stopping and starting interaction—To intervene to alter interactions between or among family members. The purpose may be to endue new lines of communication, to develop relations between members not initiating contact, or to point out functions evident at the moment. Example: The therapist says to Ginger and father (without asking the mother to comment here), "What do you two have to say about the effect that this has on each of you?"

context of the symptom to help alter the functions it may have served; and shifting the focus from one problem or person to another. Functional family therapy is designed not merely to identify functional relations but also to build new and more adaptive ways of functioning. Communication patterns are altered and efforts are made to provide families with concrete ways of behaving differently both in the sessions and at home (see Alexander and Parsons 1982).

Evaluation. The few available outcome studies of functional family therapy have produced relatively clear effects. The initial study included male and female delinquent adolescents referred to juvenile court for such behaviors as running away, truancy, theft, and unmanageability (Alexander and Parsons 1973). In comparison to other treatments (e.g., client-centered or psychodynamically oriented family treatment) and control conditions (e.g., attention-placebo, no treatment), functional family therapy has fared well. For example, functional family therapy, relative to other treatments, has shown greater improvement on family interaction measures and lower recidivism rates from juvenile court records up to 18 months after treatment (Alexander and Parsons 1973). Follow-up data ob-

tained 2½ years later indicated that the siblings of those who received functional family therapy showed significantly lower rates of referral to juvenile courts (Klein et al. 1977).

From the few available studies, several statements can be supported. First, the effectiveness of treatment is influenced by the relationship (e.g., warmth, integration of affect and behavior) and structuring (e.g., directiveness) skills of the therapist (Alexander et al. 1976). Second, process measures of family interactions at posttreatment are related to subsequent recidivism (Alexander and Parsons 1973). This finding lends credence to the model from which treatment was derived. Finally, in the outcome studies, client-centered and psychodynamically oriented forms of family-based therapies have not achieved the positive effects of functional family therapy. Thus treatment of the clinical problem at the level of the family per se does not appear to be sufficient to alter antisocial behavior.

General Comments

The discussion above highlighted selected treatments for conduct problems to illustrate behavioral interventions and their effects. The treatments illustrate the diversity noted earlier. The focus on specific, concrete behaviors (social skills training) or cognitive processes that underlie behavior (problem-solving skills training) illustrates treatment that is usually conducted in individual treatment sessions with the child. The approach with parents (parent management training) or families as a whole (functional family therapy) conveys a broader focus in which the child may or may not play a major part. Finally, other interventions (operant conditioning techniques) often make an effort to restructure contingencies in diverse settings in which the child may function, including home, school, the community, and institutional settings. Even with these different approaches, the full range of behavioral treatments has not been fairly represented (see Bellack and Hersen 1985).

Current Issues and Limitations

A number of issues are noteworthy in relation to the development of effective treatments. Already mentioned was the need for long-term follow-up evaluation of treatments that have been shown to produce change. Several other issues can be identified as critical to further developments of behavioral treatments.

Understanding Dysfunction

Behavioral treatments begin with the assumption that many dysfunctions and problematic behaviors can be altered by providing new learning experiences. The amenability to change of many clinical dysfunctions supports this assumption as a general point of departure. However, a long-term investment in developing effective treatments requires an understanding of the determinants of disorder and the points at which intervention is likely to be optimally effective. Theoretical views and alternative models of dysfunction need to be developed and tested. Broad views of disorder derived from a single conceptual model (e.g., psychodynamic, learning) focus attention on important levels of understanding. However, their breadth has often limited ability to generate testable hypotheses regarding the development of specific disorders.

Within contemporary research, there is an effort to develop models of dysfunction that address the relation of specific influences and how they may operate to produce clinical dysfunction. These efforts might be referred to as "minimodels" because they consider a circumscribed set of influences and their effects. Because they are restricted in scope, these minimodels are more likely to provide testable hypotheses to illuminate the emergence, course, and influences for specific types of disorders. The development of minimodels of dysfunction, and of development more generally, has profited from the use of alternative statistical techniques, such as path analysis and structural equation modeling. The analyses provide useful tools to test hypotheses about concurrent and longitudinal influences and the interrelations among diverse domains of influence that might be operating simultaneously (e.g., Newcomb and Bentler 1988).

For example, Patterson (1986) devised models to explain the development and maintenance of antisocial behavior of children. Separate models incorporate multiple influences, including parental discipline, modeling, maternal dysfunction, child verbal and physical aggression, and other factors. Each of these can be measured and evaluated to determine their temporal priority and likely direction of influence in relation to each other and child antisocial behavior. The direction of influence and the strength of the connections among alternative variables can generate hypotheses about points in the process at which interventions are feasible and likely to be effective. Further work on the evaluation and testing of alternative models is critically important to the development of treatments and represents the basic research underlying empirically based treatments.

Classification of Dysfunction

Behavior modification focuses primarily on presenting problems, often at the level of individual symptoms. A limitation resulting from this approach has been the absence of a consistent way of delineating and diagnosing child and adolescent dysfunction. This limitation has led to the accumulation of research in which the sample is not always clear. Ironically, the assessment of child dysfunction before, during, and after treatment is often exemplary in terms of the usual assessment desiderata (e.g., the use of multiple measures, from multiple domains, and assessment over time) (Mash and Terdal 1988). At the same time, no uniform methods of diagnostic assessment are systematically used to permit communication of characteristics in a consistent way.

Proponents of behavioral techniques have eschewed psychiatric diagnosis because in large part of the conceptual models on which early versions of contemporary diagnosis (e.g., the earlier DSMs) were based. Contemporary diagnosis (e.g., DSM-III [American Psychiatric Association 1980], DSM-III-R) emphasizes presenting symptoms rather than presumed etiologies and would make the use of diagnosis compatible with behavioral methods (Kazdin 1983). Nevertheless, there has been reluctance to draw on contemporary diagnosis as a way of describing samples included in treatment research or to develop an alternative diagnostic system that could serve as a way to compare samples across studies. Consequently, the accumulation of a knowledge base has been hampered by difficulties in discerning who the sample consists of and the scope, severity, and duration of their clinical dysfunction.

Diagnosis does not resolve many issues in the search for consistency in delineating dysfunction because the diagnostic criteria have undergone periodic revisions. An alternative is the use of standardized measures such as parent and teacher checklists. For example, the Child Behavior Checklist (Achenbach and Edelbrock 1983) assesses multiple symptom domains, broad scales (internalizing, externalizing), and prosocial behavior (participation in activities, social interaction, progress at school). The measure permits evaluation of these characteristics in relation to same-age peers who are functioning adequately in everyday life. The normative basis of this and similar measures also would be helpful for better specifying the treated population. At this point, a basic priority is the need to specify operationally and in greater detail the nature of the child's dysfunction. Better specification will help identify the children for whom treatments are effective.

Focusing on the Constellation of Behaviors

An important issue for many behavioral interventions is the focus of treatment. Often one or two salient behaviors serve as the target focus. A demonstration that behavior such as fighting in the classroom or obeying parents at home is altered dramatically is noteworthy. Yet additional assessment is needed to evaluate functioning in class (e.g., deportment or other measures, academic function-

ing), at home (e.g., compliance with parents, interactions with others), and in the community (e.g., staying out overnight, stealing with peers). Effectively altering one or a few behaviors may have no clear impact on the overall functioning of the child across other relevant behaviors and situations.

There is broad agreement that clinical problems (symptoms) come in packages. The co-occurrence of symptoms is part of a broader phenomenon in which behaviors, whether or not they are symptoms, tend to occur in clusters (see Kazdin 1982b; Voeltz and Evans 1982). How behaviors emerge as clusters, how these clusters change across situations and over time, and where to intervene to optimize behavior change remain to be evaluated. For example, Wahler (1975) carefully observed children over extended periods in the home and at school and found that groups of specific behaviors consistently go together. As an illustration, for one child, behaviors such as engaging in self-stimulation, socially interacting with adults, and complying with adult instructions tended to go together. Treatment that focused on one of the behaviors that was part of the cluster altered other behaviors as well. The spread of treatment effects to different behaviors could not be explained by the similarity of the behaviors.

The tendency of responses to change together or as a cluster has been referred to as response covariation. A number of studies have demonstrated that changing one of the behaviors in the cluster alters other behaviors as well (Kazdin 1982b). As yet, the applied implications of broad clusters have yet to be exploited in the development or application of treatment (see Wahler and Fox 1980). This may be particularly important in behavior modification, in which the specification of concrete and isolated behaviors can neglect broader domains of functioning.

Conclusions

Behavior modification represents a broad approach to treatment that encompasses diverse conceptual views, techniques, and applications. Behavioral treatments share a common commitment to operationalization, assessment, and evaluation. As noted previously, more than 160 different behavioral treatments and treatment variations have been identified. To illustrate the diversity of techniques, I have highlighted variations of operant conditioning, social skills training, problem-solving skills training, parent management training, and functional family therapy in this chapter. These techniques convey the diverse foci in the context of conduct problems.

Proponents of behavior modification have viewed the commitment to treatment research as the hallmark of the approach. It is clear that there is broad movement within child and adult psychotherapy to increase research and to operationalize critical facets of treatment (Goldfried et al. 1990; Kazdin 1990). The development of process measures and specification of treatments in manual form reflect attempts to improve treatment research well beyond the confines of behavior modification.

In the child and adolescent psychotherapy literature, outcome research is dominated by behavioral treatments. Traditional and widely practiced interventions (e.g., psychodynamic, individual, family-based therapy) with children and adolescents are less frequently subjected to empirical evaluation (Casey and Berman 1985; Kovacs and Paulauskas 1986; Tuma and Sobotka 1983; Weisz et al. 1987). Hopefully, the broader emphasis on outcome research and specification and assessment of processes will increase the empirical attention accorded all approaches to treatment.

References

Achenbach TM, Edelbrock CS: Manual for the Child Behavior Checklist and Revised Child Behavior Profile. Burlington, VT, University Associates in Psychiatry, 1983

Alexander JF, Parsons BV: Short-term behavioral intervention with delinquent families: impact on family process and recidivism. J Abnorm Psychol 81:219–225, 1973

Alexander JF, Parsons BV: Functional Family Therapy. Monterey, CA, Brooks/Cole, 1982

Alexander JF, Barton C, Schiavo RS, et al: Systems-behavioral intervention with families of delinquents: therapist characteristics, family behavior, and outcome. J Consult Clin Psychol 44:656–664, 1976

American Psychiatric Association: Diagnostic and Statistical Manual of Mental Disorders, 3rd Edition. Washington, DC, American Psychiatric Association, 1980

American Psychiatric Association: Diagnostic and Statistical Manual of Mental Disorders, 3rd Edition, Revised. Washington, DC, American Psychiatric Association, 1987

Arbuthnot J, Gordon DA: Behavioral and cognitive effects of a moral reasoning development intervention for high-risk behavior-disordered adolescents. J Consult Clin Psychol 54:208–216, 1986

Azar ST, Wolfe DA: Child abuse and neglect, in Treatment of Childhood Disorders. Edited by Mash, EJ, Barkley RA. New York, Guilford, 1989, pp 451–489

Bandura A: Self-efficacy: toward a unifying theory of behavioral change. Psychol Rev 84:191–215, 1977a

Bandura A: Social Learning Theory. Englewood Cliffs, NJ, Prentice-Hall, 1977b

Barlow DH, Hayes SC, Nelson RO: The Scientist-Practitioner: Research and Accountability and Research in Clinical and Educational Settings. Elmsford, NY, Pergamon, 1984

Baum CG, Forehand R: Long-term follow-up assessment of parent training by use of multiple outcome measures. Behavior Therapy 12:643–652, 1981

Beck AT, Rush AJ, Shaw BF, et al: Cognitive Therapy of Depression. New York, Guilford, 1979

Bellack AS, Hersen M: Dictionary of Behavior Therapy Techniques. Elmsford, NY, Pergamon, 1985

Bellack AS, Hersen M, Kazdin AE: International Handbook of Behavior Modification and Therapy, 2nd Edition. New York, Plenum, 1990

Berkowitz L: Situational and personal conditions governing reactions to aggressive cues, in Personality at the Crossroads: Current Issues in Interactional Psychology. Edited by Magnusson D, Endler NS. Hillsdale, NJ, Lawrence Erlbaum, 1977, pp 165–171

Bornstein PH, Kazdin AE (eds): Handbook of Clinical Behavior Therapy With Children. Homewood, IL, Dorsey, 1985

Camp BW, Bash MAS: Think Aloud: Increasing Social and Cognitive Skills: A Problem Solving Program for Children. Champaign, IL, Research Press, 1985

Casey RJ, Berman JS: The outcome of psychotherapy with children. Psychol Bull 98:388–400, 1985

Cooper JO, Heron TE, Heward WL: Applied Behavior Analysis. Columbus, OH, Merrill, 1987

Dodge KA: Attributional bias in aggressive children, in Advances in Cognitive-Behavioral Research and Therapy, Vol 4. Edited by Kendall PC. Orlando, FL, Academic, 1985, pp 73–110

Dolgan MJ, Jay SM: Pain management in children, in Treatment of Childhood Disorders. Edited by Mash EJ, Barkley RA. New York, Guilford, 1989, pp 383–404

Dumas JE, Wahler RG: Predictors of treatment outcome in parent training: mother insularity and socioeconomic disadvantage. Behavior Assessment 5:301–313, 1983

Elder JP, Edelstein BA, Narick MM: Adolescent psychiatric patients: modifying aggressive behavior with social skills training. Behav Modif 3:161–178, 1979

Ellis PL: Empathy: a factor in antisocial behavior. J Abnorm Child Psychol 10:123–134, 1982

Feshbach N: Empathy in children: some theoretical and empirical considerations. Counseling Psychology 5:25–30, 1975

Fleischman MJ, Szykula SA: A community setting replication of a social learning treatment for aggressive children. Behavior Therapy 12:115–122, 1981

Forehand R, Long N: Outpatient treatment of the acting out child: procedures, long-term follow-up data, and clinical problems. Advances in Behavior Research and Therapy 10:129–177, 1988

Foster SL, Robin AL: Parent-adolescent conflict, in Treatment of Childhood Disorders. Edited by Mash EJ, Barkley RA. New York, Guilford, 1989, pp 493–528

Franzini LR, Tilker HA: On the terminological confusion between behavior therapy and behavior modification. Behavior Therapy 3:279–282, 1972

Goldfried MR, Greenberg LS, Marmar C: Individual psychotherapy: process and outcome. Annu Rev Psychol 41:659–688, 1990

Gross AM, Brigham TA, Hopper C, et al: Self-management and

social skills training: a study with predelinquent and delinquent youths. Criminal Justice Behavior 7:161–184, 1980

Hobbs TR, Holt MM: The effects of token reinforcement on the behavior of delinquents in cottage settings. J Appl Behav Anal 9:189–198, 1976

Hughes HM: Behavior change in children at a therapeutic summer camp as a function of feedback and individual versus group contingencies. J Abnorm Child Psychol 7:211–219, 1979

Jones RR, Weinrott MR, Howard JR: The National Evaluation of the Teaching Family Model. Rockville, MD, National Institute of Mental Health, Center for Studies in Crime and Delinquency, 1981

Kazdin AE: The Token Economy. New York, Plenum, 1977

Kazdin AE: History of Behavior Modification: Experimental Foundations of Contemporary Research. Baltimore, MD, University Park Press, 1978

Kazdin AE: Single-Case Research Designs: Methods for Clinical and Applied Settings. New York, Oxford University Press, 1982a

Kazdin AE: Symptom substitution, generalization, and response covariation: implications for psychotherapy outcome. Psychol Bull 91:349–365, 1982b

Kazdin AE: Psychiatric diagnosis, dimensions of dysfunction, and child behavior therapy. Behavior Therapy 14:73–79, 1983

Kazdin AE: Treatment of Antisocial Behavior in Children and Adolescents. Homewood, IL, Dorsey Press, 1985

Kazdin AE: Conduct Disorder in Childhood and Adolescence. Newbury Park, CA, Sage, 1987a

Kazdin AE: Treatment of antisocial behavior in children: current status and future directions. Psychol Bull 102:187–203, 1987b

Kazdin AE: Behavior Modification in Applied Settings, 4th Edition. Pacific Grove, CA, Brooks/Cole, 1989

Kazdin AE: Psychotherapy for children and adolescents. Annu Rev Psychol 41:21–54, 1990

Kazdin AE, Esveldt-Dawson K, French NH, et al: Problem-solving skills training and relationship therapy in the treatment of antisocial child behavior. J Consult Clin Psychol 55:76–85, 1987

Kazdin AE, Bass D, Siegel T, et al: Cognitive-behavioral treatment and relationship therapy in the treatment of children referred for antisocial behavior. J Consult Clin Psychol 57:522–535, 1989

Keehn JD, Webster CD: Behavior therapy and behavior modification. Can J Psychol 10:68–73, 1969

Kelly JA: Social Skills Training: A Practical Guide for Interventions. New York, Springer, 1982

Kendall PC, Braswell L: Cognitive-behavioral self-control therapy for children: a components analysis. J Consult Clin Psychol 50:672–689, 1982

Kendall PC, Braswell L: Cognitive-Behavioral Therapy for Impulsive Children. New York, Guilford, 1985

Kirigin KA, Wolf MM, Braukmann CJ, et al: Achievement Place: a preliminary outcome evaluation, in Progress in Behavior Therapy With Delinquents. Edited by Stumphauzer JS. Springfield, IL, Charles C Thomas, 1979, pp 118–145

Kirigin KA, Braukmann CJ, Atwater JD, et al: An evaluation of teaching-family (Achievement Place) group homes for juvenile offenders. J Appl Behav Anal 15:1–16, 1982

Klein NC, Alexander JF, Parsons BV: Impact of family systems intervention on recidivism and sibling delinquency: a model of primary prevention and program evaluation. J Consult Clin Psychol 45:469–474, 1977

Kovacs M, Paulauskas S: The traditional psychotherapies, in Psychopathological Disorders of Childhood, 3rd Edition. Edited by Quay HC, Werry JS. New York, John Wiley, 1986, pp 496–522

Krasner L: Behavior therapy. Annu Rev Psychol, Vol 22, 1971

Kratochwill TR, Morris RJ (eds): The Practice of Child Therapy, 2nd Edition. Elmsford, NY, Pergamon, 1991

Lochman JE: Effects of different treatment lengths in cognitive behavioral interventions with aggressive boys. Child Psychiatry Hum Dev 16:45–56, 1985

Lochman JE, Burch PR, Curry JF, et al: Treatment and generalization effects of cognitive-behavioral and goal-setting interventions with aggressive boys. J Consult Clin Psychol 52:915–916, 1984

Mash EJ, Barkley RA (eds): Treatment of Childhood Disorders. New York, Guilford, 1989

Mash EJ, Terdal LG (eds): Behavioral Assessment of Childhood Disorders, 2nd Edition. New York, Guilford, 1988

Michelson L, Sugai DP, Wood RP, et al: Social Skills Assessment and Training With Children. New York, Plenum, 1983

Morris SB, Alexander JF, Waldron H: Functional family therapy: issues in clinical practice, in Handbook of Behavior Therapy. Edited by Falloon IRH. New York, Guilford (in press)

Newcomb MD, Bentler PM: Consequences of Adolescent Drug Use: Impact on the Lives of Young Adults. Newbury Park, CA, Sage, 1988

Novaco RW: Anger and coping with stress: cognitive behavioral intervention, in Cognitive Behavioral Therapy: Research and Application. Edited by Foreyt JP, Rathjen DP. New York, Plenum, 1978, pp 135–173

O'Donnell CR, Lydgate T, Fo WSO: The buddy system: review and follow-up. Child Behavior Therapy 1:161–169, 1979

Patterson GR: Coercive Family Process. Eugene, OR, Castalia, 1982

Patterson GR: Performance models for antisocial boys. Am Psychol 41:432–444, 1986

Phillips EL, Phillips EA, Wolf MM, et al: Achievement Place: development of the elected-manager system. J Appl Behav Anal 6:541–561, 1973

Schreibman L, Koegel RL, Charlop MH, et al: Infantile autism, in International Handbook of Behavior Modification and Therapy, 2nd Edition. Edited by Bellack AS, Hersen M, Kazdin AE. New York, Plenum, 1990, pp 763–789

Shure MB, Spivack G: Problem-Solving Techniques in Child-Rearing. San Francisco, CA, Jossey-Bass, 1978

Spivack G, Shure MB: The cognition of social adjustment: interpersonal cognitive problem solving thinking, in Advances in Clinical Child Psychology, Vol 5. Edited by Lahey BB, Kazdin AE. New York, Plenum, 1982, pp 323–372

Spivack G, Platt JJ, Shure MB: The Problem-Solving Approach to Adjustment. San Francisco, CA, Jossey-Bass, 1976

Strain PS, Young CC, Horowitz J: Generalized behavior change during oppositional child training: an examination of child and family demographic variables. Behav Modif 5:15–26, 1981

Tuma JM, Sobotka KR: Traditional therapies with children, in Handbook of Child Psychopathology. Edited by Ollendick TH, Hersen M. New York, Plenum, 1983, pp 391–426

Van Hasselt VG, Ammerman RT, Sisson LA: Physically disabled persons, in International Handbook of Behavior Modification and Therapy, 2nd Edition. Edited by Bellack AS, Hersen M, Kazdin AE. New York, Plenum, 1990, pp 831–855

Voeltz LM, Evans IM: The assessment of behavioral interrelationships in child behavior therapy. Behavioral Assessment 4:131–165, 1982

Wahler RG: Some structural aspects of deviant child behavior. J Appl Behav Anal 8:27–42, 1975

Wahler RG, Fox JJ: Solitary toy play and time out: a family treatment package for children with aggressive and oppositional behavior. J Appl Behav Anal 13:23–29, 1980

Walker HM, Hops H, Greenwood CR: RECESS: research and development of a behavior management package for remediating social aggression in the school setting, in The Utilization of Classroom Peers as Behavior Change Agents. Edited by Strain PS. New York, Plenum, 1981, pp 261–303

Weisz JR, Weiss B, Alicke MD, et al: Effectiveness of psychotherapy with children and adolescents: meta-analytic findings for clinicians. J Consult Clin Psychol 55:542–549, 1987

Werner JS, Minkin N, Minkin BL, et al: "Intervention package": an analysis to prepare juvenile delinquents for encounters with police officers. Criminal Justice Behavior 2:55–83, 1975

Wolf MM, Phillips EL, Fixsen DL, et al: Achievement Place: the teaching-family model. Child Care Quarterly 5:92–103, 1976

Wolf MM, Braukmann CJ, Ramp KA: Serious delinquent behavior as part of a significantly handicapping condition: cures and supportive environments. J Appl Behav Anal 20:347–359, 1987

Chapter 53

Focused Time-Limited Psychotherapy and Crisis Intervention

James C. Harris, M.D.

The place of long-term psychodynamic psychotherapy is changing in general psychiatric training (Mohl et al. 1990) and practice. It is now one of several treatment skills that psychiatrists are expected to possess. Focused time-limited psychotherapy, 2–20 sessions, is the more commonly practiced form of treatment with adults, and this can be expected to become the case in childhood, although longer-term approaches are often preferred by practitioners (Silver and Silver 1984). Approaches to psychotherapy may be described overall in regard to the type and acuteness of problems, treatment orientation, frequency of sessions, or as a focused approach to a specific disorder. The approach is best individualized to the specific case.

Although the terms *short-term* and *brief psychotherapy* have been proposed when the number of sessions is limited by intent, necessity, or special circumstance, it is conceptually clearer to speak of the categories of crisis intervention (Bolman and Bolian 1987; Caplan 1964, 1980; Hobbs 1984), focal psychotherapy, and time-limited psychotherapy (Budman and Stone 1983; Chess 1981; Davanloo 1980; Dulcan 1984; Lester 1968; Mackay 1967; MacKenzie 1988; MacLean et al. 1982; Malan 1979; Mann and Goldman 1987; Sifneos 1987). The time-limited treatment may be directed toward the child (Proskaer 1969, 1971) or the family (Bentovim and Kinston 1978), or, in crisis intervention, the family member most in need (MacLean et al. 1982). The focus may be on adaptation or readaptation, as in the treatment of adjustment disorders and crises,

on interpersonal issues, or on particular target symptoms in a clinical condition. The treatment is characterized as having specific and limited, but well-defined, aims (Lester 1968). The therapy is chosen to fit the patient's current needs and recognizes a commitment to provide an immediate intervention that takes into account the child's current life circumstances in the community.

A limitation on time and the designation of target symptoms requires active engagement, cooperation, and an intensity of purpose; therefore, clarity in patient selection is of considerable importance. The approach is present-centered and specifically focused, with the therapist assuming an active and empathic role in helping to define the parameters of treatment. These approaches are often seen as derivative of longer-term psychotherapy (Mohl et al. 1990; Sifneos 1989; Winnicott 1970), in that longer-term therapeutic experiences may be needed to develop the depth of psychodynamic understanding and to master the techniques necessary to facilitate change. However, this form of treatment also benefits from clinical experiences with crisis intervention in which a traumatic event provides an opportunity for an individual to mobilize energy for rapid change. In a crisis, the therapist may witness psychological decompensation and a subsequent restitution of function, which demonstrates what can be accomplished psychologically in a short time frame—a recovery process observed in microcosm. Both types of clinical treatment experiences inform focused time-limited approaches.

There is considerably more research experience

in this area with adults (Davanloo 1980; Malan 1979; Mann and Goldman 1987; Sifneos 1987); however, time-limited approaches are frequently utilized with children and adolescents individually, in groups, or as members of a family. In this chapter, I will review assessment, case selection, and methods of intervention. First I will address crisis intervention and then focal treatment and time-limited psychotherapeutic approaches.

Historical Background

Historically, the first experiences with focal and short-term psychotherapy were in the child guidance clinics. These clinics were the outgrowth of the "new psychology" espoused through the mental hygiene movement, which emphasized psychological causes and developmental issues in children's behavior (Witmer 1946). This new psychology emphasized the importance of the individual who was adapting to his or her environment or clinical disorder. To guide the family and the child, the psychiatrist relied on an individualized approach to correct maladaptation, which was initially stimulated by the psychobiology of Adolph Meyer, an early exponent of the prevention of disorders through intervention in childhood. Witmer noted that with respect to children, it was Meyer's viewpoint and his theories that underlay the practices of the first child guidance clinics. This approach addressed the child's development level, environmental circumstances, physical and mental capacities, feelings, and desires. Parents were given advice on child rearing, and interventions were often focused and time limited. This original approach to guidance was gradually modified with the introduction of psychodynamic approaches aimed at understanding the "movement of development" as a dynamic process and understanding the interventions needed to facilitate the unfolding and differentiation of the child's personality (Allen 1942). Family dynamics also began to receive greater emphasis. With increasing emphasis on psychodynamics, the duration of treatment began to increase, and there was greater selectivity in who was chosen for treatment. Increasingly longer-term treatments were introduced. Winnicott (1970) suggested that the motto be "How little need be done" in working with a child rather than "How much will one be allowed to do?" He emphasized the importance of applying psychodynamic understand-

ing in the most efficient period of time and in some instances offered therapy "on demand."

Approaches to guidance (parent training) and more efficient utilization of psychodynamic principles in working with the child and with the family system are current hallmarks of time-limited forms of psychotherapy (Dulcan 1984). An appreciation of ego psychology and learning theory further informs these treatment approaches. The time-limited approaches are particularly suited to dealing with crises and with addressing the mastery of developmental tasks.

Theoretical Focus

From its beginning in the early part of this century, practitioners of psychotherapy have debated the methods of psychotherapy in regard to treatment focus (past- or present-centered), length of therapy, how psychological regression should be handled, how active the therapist should be in structuring sessions, whether a "real relationship" should be encouraged, how transference or parataxic distortion should be handled and whether it should be encouraged, who should be seen, and finally which criteria (intelligence, openness, conscientiousness, motivation, past adaptation, type of symptom) are to be used to decide who is to be considered for which form of psychotherapy. Among these methods, time-limited therapy emphasizes present-centeredness, motivation for change, intensity of contact, capacity for relatedness, capacity to utilize interpretations of the meaning of interpersonal experience, ability to participate in problem solving, and ability to reflect on experience. A variety of theoretical perspectives are involved in its application. Classic psychoanalysis, ego psychology, analytical psychology, existential therapy, interpersonal approaches, learning theory, and family systems approaches all have useful perspectives to offer.

Ego Psychology

Ego psychology has been particularly important in the development of crisis intervention. Ego functions as they relate to such concepts as psychic determinism, the conflict-free sphere of the ego, epigenetic stages of development, and expression of coping strategies are applicable (Hartman 1958). The mastery of interpersonal developmental tasks was emphasized by Erikson (1965), who suggested that each phase of an epigenetically emerging, developmental life cycle presents a potential maturational crisis. These crises are presented as a series of polarities, which are often posed most clearly as questions asked by adolescents as they search for identity. The resolution of each of these crises leads to new perspectives or internal qualities.

Learning Theory

Learning theorists (Lazarus 1966) have investigated coping responses, including 1) the problem-solving basis of coping; 2) regression to prior behavioral patterns previously utilized to deal with stress; 3) behavior related to denial of the current danger; 4) the appearance of inertia-inactivity when the individual is unable to act; and 5) the expression of affect (Bancroft 1986). Affect may be appropriate, inappropriate, or exaggerated in regard to the situation. Bancroft noted that coping requires the mobilization of an affective response that is appropriate to the situation. The affective response may help resolve the situation, or it may hinder the coping process.

Existential Approach

The issue of time has been addressed specifically by existential therapists (May 1958) who emphasize the experiences "in time" of anxiety, depression, and joy. They suggest that the most crucial fact about existence is its emergence in time and highlight the processes of being and developing "in time." For example, existentialists point out that in depression there may be a lack of hope, a sense of discontinuity with the future, and a distorted attitude toward the future. Time binding—that is, bringing the past into the present and having the capacity to act in the light of a long-term future—is said to be the "essence of mind." It is suggested that the ability to project oneself through self-conscious imagination is an important feature in therapy that allows one to bring forth the past. They indicate that the capacity to see one's experience in time, in regard to the past and to the future, and to act and react to these suppositions is unique to human development and gradually develops in childhood.

May (1958) further suggested that recall of significant events depends on decisions about the future. For the existentialist, if material brought up from the past is tedious and flat, it is because there is a lack of commitment to the present and future. Commitment to the future is necessary in regard to overcoming anxiety or other symptoms and is necessary before uncovering the past will have importance. Finally, the existentialist emphasizes the "pregnant moment," the understanding of the meaning of an event from the past or a realization of hope for the future, as experienced in the present, in a moment of heightened awareness. In time-limited therapy, the emphasis on time and on the intensity of the encounter may be appreciated in an existential framework.

Analytical Psychology

The analytical psychologist (Jung 1913/1961) addresses symptoms specifically as they occur in the actual present and argues that the onset of psychological symptoms is not the result of fixation on infantile conflicts but the consequence of adaptive failure in the present. Symptoms emerge at a moment when a new psychological adaptation or adjustment is demanded. Preoccupation with the past may be an attempt to utilize past maladaptive approaches to solve current problems. Rather than fixation, personality traits or aspects of temperament make current adaptation difficult. An emphasis on enhancing transference is discouraged, since transference is seen as an unconscious process that interferes with interpersonal relationships in the here and now. This present-centered orientation provides another framework for time-limited approaches, since a present focus is maintained throughout the treatment, and it is expected that mastery of current tasks may lead to long-term improvement, since the cause of the disorder is an adaptive failure in the present, and symptoms are not necessarily caused by a reactivation of past unresolved conflicts.

Family Systems

Family systems approaches focus attention on observable interactions among family members and on their effects among family members and between them and the therapist (Weakland et al. 1974), instead of emphasizing past experience or inferred mental processes. Disturbed or difficult behavior is viewed as one aspect of a system and reflects dysfunction in that system. Treatment emphasizes changes in the system. Time-limited therapy and focal family therapy (Bentovim and Kinston 1978; Kinston and Bentovim 1978; Weakland et al. 1974) are present centered, provide active interventions, and have time-limited forms.

Crisis Support and Intervention

In medicine, the term *crisis* has traditionally been used to indicate a turning point where the individual would either mobilize his or her defenses and recover or succumb to the illness. In psychiatry, the term *crisis* is used in regard to the response to stress when critical situations, sometimes catastrophic events, occur. The crisis is not simply the experience of adversity but describes the response of an individual, family, or group to that experience. Some individuals are more vulnerable to stress than others, so the same event may be responded to differently as a result. As individual responses are better understood, crisis intervention, in addition to crisis support, has been developed as an approach in psychiatry. To understand approaches to crisis management, crisis theory, the natural history and characteristics of crisis events, crisis support, and crisis intervention will be reviewed. A crisis, although experienced as threatening to the individual, may provide an opportunity for change and lead to an increased resilience to future stressful events. In the Chinese language, the same ideograph used for the word *crisis* (or *danger*) is also used for the word *opportunity*. It is this therapeutic opportunity that must be kept in mind.

Origins of a Theory of Crisis

Crisis theory has its origins in ego psychology, social psychiatry, and learning theory. It also draws on existential theory and present-centered forms of psychotherapy. Thomas (1909) offered an early sociological definition of crisis as "a threat, a challenge, a call to new action, which may have the germ of a new organization." He suggested that it may act as a catalyst for personal development by disturbing old habits and evoking new responses. The classic approach to adult crisis theory and practice derives from Lindemann's (1944) study of grief following a fire at the Coconut Grove Night Club in Boston in 1942. He described grief as a normal response following a distressing situation, outlined

its manifestations, and identified pathologic outcomes when grief was not resolved. Lindemann recognized the importance of early intervention to facilitate acknowledgment of the death of the loved person, the need to mourn, and the need to identify and master psychological and everyday practical tasks following loss. Bereavement represents the archetypal situation of crisis. Bereavement counseling has lead to classic models of crisis intervention.

There is an initial direct effect or impact in a stressful situation, with the appearance of fear, agitation, grief, or inactivity, followed by recoil (Hobbs 1984). When the acute stressful event subsides, responses may be regressive and often are idiosyncratic. There is a subsequent posttraumatic awareness when the individual appreciates what has happened and may begin to take appropriate action. Delay in the phase of recoil may be associated with a mental disorder.

Caplan's (1964) contribution to crisis theory has been of particular importance in child psychiatry. He emphasized "emotional homeostasis" and adaptation. The acute state of heightened susceptibility may provide an opportunity for realignment of internal boundaries. His work on the importance of early intervention resulted in an emphasis on preventive intervention in crisis management programs. Caplan (1964) described four phases of crisis: 1) phase 1, increasing arousal and an increase in attempts at problem-solving behavior; 2) phase 2, with increased arousal, "tension," impairment of function occurs with distress and disorganization; 3) phase 3, both internal and external emergency resources are tried, and novel approaches to cope are instituted; and 4) phase 4, ongoing failure to resolve the problem results in a further deterioration in function, with exhaustion and decompensation. The degree of arousal may hinder rather than promote adaptation.

More recently, Caplan (1980) suggested that all children and families do not respond in the same way to a crisis or to critical events. For each person there are risk factors and vulnerabilities that need to be considered. The resonance or dissonance between genetic, temperamental, and personality traits; brain dysfunction; and harmful psychosocial events produces an individual impact on the person that may lead to a mental disorder. Since all children do not respond in the same way, intervening or mediating processes must be considered. These processes are on a scale of competencies or vulnerabilities.

Crisis Situations

Critical situations that lead to crisis may be accidental, situational and unexpected, or developmental and normative in nature (critical events in development). The developmental stage is not in itself a crisis, but at those times a child may be more vulnerable to change. Accidental events include natural disasters, loss (e.g., death of a parent), or physical events (e.g., injury or illness). Developmental crises include identity issues described by Erikson (1965), transitions (e.g., school entry, divorce), and interpersonal events (e.g., the birth of a sibling). Crises are often a mixture of events and frequently involve unexpected stresses at times of developmental vulnerability. Of particular importance in childhood is the loss of self-esteem, the loss of social role mastery, or the loss of nurturance. Vulnerability factors include developmental losses, as the child sacrifices an earlier, more dependent level of adaptation when new developmental tasks present themselves; coexistent physical and social stresses; absence of family and social supports; cultural isolation or alienation from meaningful and customary supportive social rituals; and intrapsychic factors, particularly maladaptive residua of previous psychic trauma. There are also protective factors. These include emotional support from family members and previous experience with the mastery of similar crises.

The following are characteristics of crisis situations (Hobbs 1984). One, crises are self-limited in time. Some resolution occurs in 4–6 weeks, but the time frame is complicated by the experience of multiple stressors. Two, the expression of new dependency needs must be recognized. In children, a disruption in social support may be followed by disruptive behavior. Three, an individual may develop symptoms from a crisis within the family or social group when collective coping fails. One person may manifest symptoms for the whole group; the person presenting in crisis is the one family member who is most vulnerable psychologically or the member chosen symbolically to carry the burden, a scapegoat. For intervention, the family and indeed the social network are targets. Four, the crisis may provide an opportunity for psychological growth as new methods of coping are mastered. Five, a crisis may provide an opportunity for the mastery of old conflicts that are the residua of previous crises. Conflicts out of awareness may be activated along with their associated feelings. This "action replay" of an old crisis in the context of current concerns may lead to further complications. For example, if a suicide attempt led to rescue in the past, there is the risk of its recurrence. These reenactments may further complicate crisis recovery.

The following areas are important to consider in crisis management.

The experience of loss. The most common crises result from loss. The most striking form is that of bereavement, which is characteristically expressed as a grief response following the death of a loved one. Symptoms are both physical and psychological. Loss is also experienced with a separation, the loss of self-esteem, the loss of bodily function (e.g., gymnastic accidents, physical trauma), or the loss of financial security. Phases of loss are well documented. Special crises for the family include a terminal illness in a child and the birth of a handicapped child. There is an initial phase of disorganization that is associated with shock, denial of reality, and feelings of grief.

Life change events. Rather than loss, a new condition presents as a change in role (e.g., school entry or the specific maturation issues described by Erikson [1965]). Here there is usually a potentially threatening challenge to be met. Becoming ill also is considered a change event as it relates to the so-called sick role, which also includes an element of loss.

Interpersonal and family crises. Interpersonal problems among family members can create major stresses. Living in a home without interpersonal warmth or one that is physically hostile can increase susceptibility to other stressful life events. Major crisis events in childhood include physical abuse, sexual abuse, kidnapping (Terr 1987), and the experience of war or terrorism.

Major family crises may develop with the birth of a handicapped child or when a child has a severe illness. Critical times for handicapped and chronically ill children include 1) the establishment of a diagnosis and the discussion of its implications; 2) living with the child at home and participating in the specific management program; 3) time of school entry; 4) entry into adolescence; 5) dealing with loss of function and deterioration; and 6) future family planning.

Richmond (1972) outlined several psychological processes in parents in adapting to the handicapped child. He suggested phases of denial, projection, guilt, and dependency that must be worked through. Futterman (1975) expanded this model when dealing with the anticipated loss of a terminally ill child. He focused on the phases of parental anticipatory mourning and identified five processes: 1) acknowledgment, 2) grieving, 3) reconciliation, 4) memorialization, and 5) detachment. These were particularly associated with adaptational processes that focused on the maintenance of confidence. Adaptational processes included search for factual information about the illness and participation in the physical care of the child. Futterman noted the importance of balancing several contrasting perspectives (e.g., acknowledgment and hope, maintenance of everyday activities and grief, confidence and doubt). Interventions are aimed at understanding these processes and helping the individual to be able to experience, express, and work through his or her loss.

Assessment for Crisis Intervention

To facilitate early intervention, crisis services operate on a self-referral basis rather than through established waiting lists for treatment. The child and family are included in the assessment process. The first stage is to determine the degree of decompensation using the approach outlined above from Caplan (1964). Second, the nature of the stressor or stressors is established. The full emotional significance of the trauma must be understood and this understanding communicated to the child and family. Finally, the intensity of the crisis, the individual's adaptive behavioral reserves, and previous ability to cope are noted. Assessment is followed by a formulation that may utilize several of the theoretical frameworks described. A psychiatric diagnosis, psychodynamic formulation, and a formulation of the current crisis, which establish the previous psychological equilibrium, the critical events precipitating the crisis, and how the crisis is manifested in the individual, are developed. For children at risk, the emphasis is on developing competence.

Clarification and cognitive appraisal of the situation including the crisis, encouraging appropriate emotional expression, recognizing willingness to be helped, and mobilizing coping resources are considered. The steps are to review the threat, redefine the problem to achieve cognitive understanding of its origins, and identify the tasks to be mastered in the present.

There are many questions to consider in assessment. What is the crisis? Whom does it affect? Why is it disorganizing? What were the prior resources for coping before the crisis? How can issues related to the crisis be opened? What are the unspoken issues? What strengths can be mobilized? How can the individuals be mobilized in their own behalf? What tasks need to be carried out for resolution of the crisis? What specific help is needed? How can gains be consolidated? Does the person have a preexisting psychiatric disorder and is it being treated? It is often the case that crisis occurs in the most poorly organized families and those with preexisting disorders.

Crisis Intervention and Support

Crisis intervention is an approach taken for the prevention and treatment of acute psychological decompensation. The intervention attempts to maximize the individual's potential for psychological growth and maturation as the crisis is mastered. In this way, mastery of the situation has a potentially protective effect for coping with future crises, a strengthening or steeling effect. On the other hand, failure in coping, particularly in regard to catastrophic events, may have a sensitizing effect. Crisis intervention provides a conceptual framework to approach these situations.

The principles of crisis intervention follow from the concepts of crisis theory, although there is disagreement in regard to specific methods. However, there is agreement that it is a short-term approach. Crisis support and crisis intervention can be differentiated along a continuum of services from emergency treatment, to crisis support, to crisis intervention, to short-term therapy (Davanloo 1980). Because those in crisis are in a state of flux, psychodynamic principles can be applied effectively to treatment. Psychiatric emergency services are used for those whose adaptive capacities have already broken down; crisis support for those with limited coping capacities in danger of decompensating and with a history of poor adaptation; and crisis intervention for those in danger of decompensating, but who have sufficient coping ability and a past history of good adaptive functioning.

Selection Criteria

The type of intervention depends on previous life adaptation. Those who are most vulnerable with both temperamental and psychosocial risk factors present require crisis support with anxiety reduction or suppression procedures. For others with better premorbid adjustment, the choice is crisis intervention.

Efforts are made to overcome the crisis as rapidly as possible and to return the individual to preexisting levels of emotional functioning. Anxiety is high, and efforts are made to reduce it. Efforts are made to remove the sources of crisis while supporting the individual. Crisis support eliminates stressors, supports the child and family, provides practical guidance, and considers medication, if it is indicated.

Outcome of Crisis Support

One seeks evidence of crisis resolution and an ability to discuss symptoms meaningfully. The ability to plan for the future, to turn back to routine activities with friends and family, and to complete schoolwork successfully are measures of successful outcome.

Crisis Intervention

For crisis intervention, the criteria for selection are based on a history of a specific stressor of recent origin that has resulted in anxiety. The event is clearly defined, and the patient is highly motivated to overcome the crisis. The person has the ability to recognize psychological reasons for the current crisis.

Techniques

Therapist and patient agree on the issues that led to the crisis; the patient is actively involved rather than only a recipient of support. The length is from one or two sessions to several interviews over 1–2 months. The sequence of events that led to the crisis is reviewed, and the maladaptive reactions are identified, but the focus remains only on the crisis. Interventions should not arouse resistance or exacerbate conflicts that will lead to further decompensation. The healthiest part of the ego is enlisted in the goal to reach achievable ends. Positive

feelings toward the therapist are utilized for new learning aimed at avoiding situations that may lead to future crises. Intervention is terminated when the crisis is resolved and the patient understands the steps that led to the crisis and its resolution.

Crisis intervention includes both anticipatory guidance and preventive intervention. Anticipatory guidance is the approach taken when a crisis can be predicted. Preventive intervention is a method of guidance for parents and children during the crisis itself. This approach recognizes the patient's increasing dependency and provides continuing support during the crisis. Help is provided by facilitating communication among family members and by discussion of their concerns and their plans for coping. During these discussions, the physicians should point out that negative feelings are normal, sympathize with the family's frustration, and encourage the sharing of tasks among family members in recognition of the fatigue that may develop. Interview sessions should focus on present problems and not emphasize discussion of past failures. Identification of psychological needs and the development of confiding relationships among family members are both essential in preventive intervention.

With the handicapped or chronically ill child, the way families cope depends on the support that family members can offer one another and the ability of each to adapt to loss, both potential and actual. It is the physician's first responsibility to convene a support group at the time of diagnosis. In the circumstances, the first step is to counsel both parents together, rather than either parent alone, and then to assist the family in finding local resources through extended family, recognized parent support groups for the given condition, community agencies, and religious organizations. If family support systems are inadequate, additional help in the form of support groups and organizations is essential. Individuals in crisis show signs of stress that elicit care from others, be they relatives, friends, neighbors, or professionals. If this does not occur spontaneously, it is appropriate for the professionals involved to arrange active support. Bringing together parents who face similar crises can be particularly helpful.

Time-Limited Interventions

The time-limited treatments may also be primarily supportive or provide potentially anxiety-eliciting interventions. This form of psychotherapy most clearly places the focus on the experience and meaning of time. In some instances, a set number of sessions is recommended; in others, a set termination date without a set number of sessions is established; or it is agreed that there will be a time limit but the specific number of sessions is not established in advance and a specific date is not set. With a time limitation, a struggle between wishes for nurturance versus awareness of finite time suggests a limitation on the degree to which one's wishes can be gratified.

The same principles apply to working with children and adolescents as are applied in working with adults. However, some modifications are necessary in working with the child (Petti 1989). Three issues complicate the approach: 1) children do not request treatment directly; 2) the parents must be engaged in the therapeutic process; and 3) the therapist must be more actively engaged in the treatment with the child. However, engagement into short-term therapy may be less difficult than into long-term therapy. In stressful situations, it may be more apparent to the child that help is needed. Children may not have a fully developed sense of time, so aids may be necessary to help them appreciate the time-limited nature of treatment. Both child and parent may be more amenable to a time-limited approach.

Assessment for Time-Limited Intervention

Approaches to brief therapy begin with an initial assessment of the entire family, the formulation of dynamic focal hypotheses, selection of the specific goals for treatment (MacLean et al. 1982), and identification of who will participate in the treatment. Goals are chosen based on current specific target symptoms, behaviors, and attitudes that are addressed as "here-and-now" problems. How these foci are approached will depend on the model utilized, be it a brief supportive or dynamic intervention (Sifneos 1989), focused time-limited therapy (Proskaer 1969, 1971), short-term group therapy (Fine et al. 1989; Parmenter et al. 1987), or focal individual or family treatment (Bentovim and Kinston 1978; Lesse and Dare 1975; Rosenthal 1982; Selinger and Barcai 1981). The choice of who should be treated is of particular importance; one asks who is it crucial to treat. Aspects of the family system that are most in need of change and that are most amenable to treatment must be addressed. Who is engaged in treatment will vary from family to family. Regardless of who is involved, the focus is as a child advocate with a primary concern for the child, although it may be the individual parent or both parents together who are seen rather than the child.

Selection Criteria

Motivation for change is more important than severity of symptomatology. The factor that is reported to correlate best with improvement is motivation for change or for insight. This motivation may override chronicity and pervasiveness of symptoms. Recent onset is not necessarily correlated with good outcome (Malan 1979). The need for a capacity for rapid effective therapeutic involvement and the capacity for disengagement at termination are important considerations.

For adults, at least one meaningful relationship with another person in the past, a capacity for basic trust, an emotional crisis, ability to interact with the evaluating psychiatrist (to think in psychological terms) and to express feeling, and motivation to work hard on a specific chief complaint are important for a good outcome (Sifneos 1989). Additional selection criteria for children include evidence of an intact and supportive family and evidence of motivation to change within the family system (Schulman et al. 1977). Psychotherapy is presented as a joint venture between therapist and patient. There must be an aim that both the patient and therapist agree is the same for them both.

Some indications for focused therapy in childhood include school refusal, adjustment disorder, mild dysthymic disorder, anxiety states, unresolved grief (complicated bereavement), less severe antisocial disorder (antisocial tendency), parent-child conflicts (often associated with oppositional behavior), marital discord or pending divorce, and management of learning problems with associated inadequacy and low self-esteem (Leaverton et al. 1977; Wilson and Herzog 1985).

Technique

A central focus is chosen, and issues in regard to termination as an experience of eventual separation and loss are considered from the onset. The use of drawings and stories may be helpful in establishing a focus (Proskaer 1969). Asking the child about three wishes for things they would like to change in their lives (e.g., at school, at home, and in themselves) can also be utilized to elicit areas the child wishes changed, which may serve as a focus for short-term intervention. To maintain this focus, there is the need for a strong therapeutic alliance, with basic trust and some capacity for intimacy. As termination nears, the child may elaborate on imagined self-defeating interpersonal consequences following the end of treatment. The meaning of termination may be distorted in terms of the child's negative self-esteem. A therapist must concurrently deal with the child's discomfort about the meaning of the approaching termination (Lester 1975, 1986; Madger 1980; McDermott and Char 1984).

Establishing Contact

The rapid establishment of rapport is necessary to establish a therapeutic alliance in short-term therapy. In children, the use of special techniques to establish contact and choose a treatment focus often is necessary (Kestenbaum 1985). This entails the use of drawings, stories, and other imaginal techniques. Winnicott (1970) introduced the "squiggle game" as a means of establishing contact with the child, exploring psychodynamic issues, and helping to define a focus. Fantasies about the therapist as a helpful or nonhelpful person are elicited in early sessions. As Frank (1974) noted, expectancy and belief in the therapist play an important role in any therapeutic endeavor. How the child experiences the session and makes use of it outside the session is the important thing. Often children surprise themselves as they proceed to complete drawings and see their situation in a new way. Winnicott (1970) looked for the use the child made of any new understandings. Whether the parents are able to provide a normally expectable supportive environment that could facilitate therapy and lead to internalization of positive supportive inner figures is an important goal. The ability to establish therapeutic contact can be assessed, using imaginal techniques. A determination is then made to establish if the child could proceed with a time-limited approach or requires longer-term intervention (management or therapy). The parents' ability to make the necessary nurturant environmental provision can also be assessed by observing their responses to the child's drawings. Parental confidence in the physician is necessary. Contraindications include adverse environmental factors and inability of the parent to "meet" the child psychologically and support the necessary changes in the child that are expected in treatment.

In the squiggle game, the therapist makes a spontaneous line. The child makes a drawing; patient and therapist alternate pictures as the therapist observes the child and identifies themes for treatment.

Another means of making contact with the child, gathering information on psychotherapeutic issues and finding themes for short-term treatment, is by therapeutic communication through use of the mutual storytelling technique (Gardner 1971).

Time-limited therapy, then, initially establishes a positive therapeutic alliance. There may be limited interpretation of transference; however, identification with the therapist is more often an aspect of treatment. Emphasis is placed on clarification of internal feeling states and interpersonal difficulties. Limit setting, encouragement, reassurance, and direction may be offered.

Outcome

MacLean et al. (1982) noted that favorable outcome in their treatment program depended on 1) warmth between family members; 2) a positive feeling of hope on the part of the therapist toward the family; 3) the ability of the family to engage themselves as active agents and their recognition of the time-limited nature of the treatment; 4) the ability to define a clear treatment focus, which might be denial of feelings related to the death of a parent, stealing to gain attention, displacement of anger between parents onto a child; 5) the ability to choose a functional unit for treatment, the person most strategic to treat; 6) assignment of one therapist to the case rather than splitting the case between two; and 7) acknowledgment that the time frame will be recognized and adhered to. A family might return later with a different presentation or with different goals.

There has been considerable interest in outcome research regarding short-term psychotherapy (Koss and Butcher 1986; Koss et al. 1986; Leventhal and Weinberger 1975; Shaffer 1984). Focal time-limited therapy has been found to be an efficient and effective approach. In an extensive review, Koss and Butcher concluded that studies comparing brief with unlimited therapy show essentially no difference in results. Both these authors and Shaffer commented on the need for more sophisticated research designs with clearer specification of patients. Shaffer noted that such studies should include specific therapy with the child and not the parent alone. Future research requires that rather than ask whether short-term therapy works, investigators must answer the question for whom and for what kind of problems is time-limited therapy effective (Shaffer 1984).

References

Allen FH: Psychotherapy With Children. New York, WW Norton, 1942

Bancroft J: Crisis intervention, in An Introduction to the Psychotherapies, 2nd Edition. Edited by Bloch S. Oxford, UK, Oxford University Press, 1986, pp 113–132

Bentovim A, Kinston W: Brief focal family therapy when the child is the referred patient, I: clinical. J Child Psychol Psychiatry 19:119–143, 1978

Bolman WM, Bolian GC: Crisis intervention as primary or secondary prevention, in Basic Handbook of Child Psychiatry, Vol 4. Edited by Berlin IN, Stone LA (Noshpitz JD, Editor-in-Chief). New York, Basic Books, 1987, pp 225–254

Budman SH, Stone J: Advances in brief psychotherapy: a review of recent literature. Hosp Community Psychiatry 34:939–946, 1983

Caplan G: Principles of Preventative Psychiatry. New York, Basic Books, 1964

Caplan G: An approach to preventative intervention in child psychiatry. Can J Psychiatry 25:671–682, 1980

Chess S: Selectivity of treatment modalities. Can J Psychiatry 26:309–315, 1981

Davanloo H: Short-Term Dynamic Psychotherapy. Northvale, NJ, Jason Aronson, 1980

Dulcan MK: Brief psychotherapy with children and their families: the state of the art. Journal of the American Academy of Child Psychiatry 23:544–551, 1984

Erikson E: Childhood and Society. London, Penguin, 1965

Fine S, Gilbert M, Schmidt L, et al: Short term group therapy with depressed adolescent outpatients. Can J Psychiatry 34:971–1002, 1989

Frank JD: Psychotherapy: the restoration of morale. Am J Psychiatry 131:271–274, 1974

Futterman EH: Studies of family adaptational responses to a specific threat, in Explorations in Child Psychiatry. Edited by Anthony EJ. New York, Plenum, 1975, pp 287–301

Gardner RA: Therapeutic Communication With Children: The Mutual Story Telling Technique. New York, Science House, 1971

Hartman H: Ego Psychology and the Problem of Adaptation. London, Imago, 1958

Hobbs M: Crisis intervention in theory and practice: a selective review. Br J Med Psychol 57:23–34, 1984

Jung CG: Psychoanalysis and neurosis (1913), in Collected Works of CG Jung, Vol 4: Freud and Psychoanalysis. Translated by Hull RF. New York, Pantheon, 1961, pp 243–251

Kestenbaum CJ: The creative process in child psychotherapy. Am J Psychother 39:479–489, 1985

Kinston W, Bentovim A: Brief focal family therapy when the child is the referred patient, II: methodology and results. J Child Psychol Psychiatry 19:119–143, 1978

Koss M, Butcher JN: Research on brief psychotherapy, in Handbook of Psychotherapy and Behavior Change, 3rd Edition. New York, John Wiley, 1986

Koss M, Butcher JN, Strupp H: Brief psychotherapy methods in clinical research. J Consult Clin Psychol 54:60–67, 1986

Lazarus R: Psychological Stress and the Coping Process. New York, McGraw-Hill, 1966

Leaverton DR, Rupp JW, Poff MG: Brief therapy for monocular hysterical blindness in childhood. Child Psychiatry Hum Dev 74:254–263, 1977

Lesse S, Dare C: A classification of interventions in child and conjoint family therapy. Psychother Psychosom 25:116–125, 1975

Lester EP: Brief psychotherapies in child psychiatry. Canadian Psychiatric Association Journal 13:301–309, 1968

Lester EP: Language behaviour and child psychotherapy. Canadian Psychiatric Association Journal 20:175–181, 1975

Lester EP: On transference: developmental and clinical considerations. Can J Psychiatry 31:146–153, 1986

Leventhal T, Weinberger G: Evaluation of a large-scale brief therapy program for children. Am J Orthopsychiatry 45:119–132, 1975

Lindemann E: Symptomatology and management of acute grief. Am J Psychiatry 10:141–148, 1944

Mackay J: The use of brief psychotherapy with children. Canadian Psychiatric Association Journal 12:269–279, 1967

MacKenzie KR: Recent developments in brief psychotherapy. Hosp Community Psychiatry 39:742–752, 1988

MacLean G, MacIntosh BA, Taylor E: A clinical approach to brief dynamic psychotherapies in child psychiatry. Can J Psychiatry 27:11–38, 1982

Madger D: The Wizard of Oz: a parable of brief psychotherapy. Can J Psychiatry 25:564–568, 1980

Malan DH: Individual Psychotherapy and the Science of Psychodynamics, 2nd Edition. London, Butterworth, 1979

Mann J, Goldman R: A Casebook in Time-Limited Psychotherapy. Washington, DC, American Psychiatric Press, 1987

May R: Existence. New York, Basic Books, 1958

McDermott JF, Char WF: Stage related models of psychotherapy with children. Journal of the American Academy of Child Psychiatry 23:537–543, 1984

Mohl PC, Lomax J, Tasman A, et al: Psychotherapy training for the psychiatrist of the future. Am J Psychiatry 147:7–13, 1990

Parmenter G, Smith JC, Cecic NA: Parallel and conjoint short-term group therapy for school age children and their parents: a model. Int J Group Psychother 37:239–254, 1987

Petti TA: Child psychiatry: psychiatric treatment, in Comprehensive Textbook of Psychiatry V, Vol 2. Edited by Kaplan HI, Sadock BJ. Baltimore, MD, Williams & Wilkins, 1989, pp 1910–1926

Proskaer S: Some technical issues in time-limited psychotherapy with children. Journal of the American Academy of Child Psychiatry 8:154–159, 1969

Proskaer S: Focused time-limited therapy with children. Journal of the American Academy of Child Psychiatry 10:619–639, 1971

Richmond JB: The family and the handicapped child. Clinical Proceedings of the Children's Hospital National Medical Center 8:156–164, 1972

Rosenthal PA: Short-term family therapy and pathological grief resolution with children and adolescents. Fam Process 19:15–19, 1982

Schulman JL, DeLafuente ME, Suran BG: An indicator for brief psychotherapy: the fork in the road phenomenon. Bull Menninger Clin 41:553–562, 1977

Selinger D, Barcai A: Brief family therapy may lead to deep personality change. Am J Psychother 31:302–309, 1981

Shaffer D: Notes on psychotherapy research among children and adolescents. Journal of the American Academy of Child Psychiatry 23:552–561, 1984

Sifneos PE: Short-Term Dynamic Psychotherapy, 2nd Edition. New York, Plenum, 1987

Sifneos PE: Brief dynamic and crisis therapy, in Comprehensive Textbook of Psychiatry V, Vol 2. Edited by Kaplan HI, Sadock BJ. Baltimore, MD, Williams & Wilkins, 1989, pp 1562–1567

Silver LB, Silver BJ: Clinical practice of child psychiatry: a survey. J Am Acad Child Adolesc Psychiatry 22:573–579, 1984

Terr LC: Treatment of psychic trauma in children, in Basic Handbook of Child Psychiatry, Vol 5. Edited by Call JD, Cohen RL, Harrison SI, et al. (Noshpitz JD, Editor-in-Chief). New York, Basic Books, 1987, pp 414–421

Thomas W: A Source Book of Social Origins. Boston, MA, R Gadger, 1909

Weakland JH, Fisch R, Watzlawick P, et al: Brief therapy: focused problem resolution. Fam Process 13:141–168, 1974

Wilson P, Herzov L: Individual and group psychotherapy, in Child and Adolescent Psychiatry: Modern Approaches, 2nd Edition. Edited by Rutter M, Herzov L. London, Blackwell Scientific, 1985, pp 826–838

Winnicott DW: Therapeutic Consultations in Child Psychiatry. New York, Basic Books, 1970

Witmer HL: The nature of child guidance, in Psychiatric Interviews With Children. Edited by Witmer HL. New York, The Commonwealth Fund, 1946, pp 3–15

Chapter 54

Family Therapy

Charles A. Malone, M.D.

For more than 30 years, family therapy as a modality and the family systems conceptual model have had a far-reaching impact on clinical practice. As a therapeutic modality, family therapy has added to the range, depth, and effectiveness of our capacity to diagnose and treat childhood psychopathology and to manage a variety of clinical tasks. Research based on a family systems conceptual model enriches and modifies our understanding of intergenerational developmental issues and the meaning of symptoms and disorders in children and adolescents (Malone 1983). Family studies and the clinical observations on which they are based provide us with a new conception of mental illness, one that focuses on the role of symptoms and disorder in maintaining family integrity and stability, however troubled (Reiss 1983). These studies reframe such fundamental conceptual issues as who is the patient, what is the target of intervention, and what are the pathways of therapeutic change and repair.

Despite the far-reaching nature of the impact of family therapy, however, the full integration of the family systems model into child and adolescent psychiatric practice has, unfortunately, not occurred. In the years since McDermott and Char (1974) "declared" the undeclared war between child psychiatry and family therapy, there has been limited progress in bringing the two fields together (Malone 1979). Although only a small minority of child psychiatrists reported that they never use family interviews in diagnosis and treatment (Malone 1979), a survey of practicing child psychiatrists (Silver and Silver 1983) revealed that only a small part of their clinical time is spent in family sessions.

Similarly, Grunebaum and Belfer (1986) reported that child psychiatrists view children and families very differently than do family therapists.

Certainly there are understandable historical and current conceptual family therapy issues, such as the indications-contraindications controversy (Malone 1983; McDermott 1981) and the conflict between the family systems circular causality model and the linear causality model of medical diagnosis, that may account for the delay in the integration of family therapy and the family systems model into child and adolescent psychiatry. Nevertheless, it remains a regrettable irony that at the same time the family systems model has demonstrated and continues to demonstrate its usefulness in understanding and treating children's mental disorders, the full integration of family therapy into child and adolescent psychiatric practice continues to lag.

Lest this line of thinking appear to be too pessimistic, let me quickly add that there are a number of encouraging developments and reasons for optimism that significant convergence between child psychiatry and family therapy has occurred and is continuing to occur. Increasingly, for example, child psychiatrists accept the proposition that a child or an adolescent cannot be assessed accurately or treated successfully apart from or in isolation from their family life and social context. Therefore, intrapsychic dynamics and interpersonal transactions and the interventions related to them are seen as interrelated and interdependent. Clinical experience has convinced many child psychiatrists and other child mental health professionals that transactions within the family play a critical role in determining what in a child's early experience endures and what opportunities to change prevail. Consequently, there is a growing emphasis on family therapy training in child and adolescent psychiatric education.

Family therapists concerned about the argumentation and fragmentation that is occurring within the field of family therapy around issues such as gender (Goldner 1988; Hare-Mustin 1988),[1] violence (Dell 1989), and purity of technique (Keeney 1983) are urging their colleagues to take a more holistic integrated approach (Kantor and Neal 1985). Theory-anchored schema of classification of family therapy (e.g., Levant 1984) also propose a more integrated view that emphasizes the similarities and overlap between schools and models of therapy. More importantly, Reiss's (1989) conceptualization of family continuity in terms of the *represented* family perspective and the *practicing* family perspective not only identifies the major roots of family therapy in psychoanalytic and general systems and cybernetics theory, but also provides a framework for examining, interrelating, and, possibly, integrating models of family therapy based on these theories. The central concept in the represented family perspective is that relationships are not only represented by inner working models (Bowlby 1969), but also coherence and stability of the relationships themselves are located in and conserved over time by such internal structures (i.e., the family) (Reiss 1989). In the practicing family perspective, the coherence and stability of family relationship processes do not reside within individuals but rather in the coordinated practices of the family as a whole (Reiss 1989).

This latter development is particularly encouraging because most of the difficulties that child psychiatrists have had in taking a family systems perspective in clinical practice stem from their sense that systemic family therapy approaches are overly focused on family process and structure, as observed in transactional patterns, and overlook or ignore the child's intrapsychic life and individual development. Reiss's (1989) conceptualization of family stability and coherence across time coupled with research methodological developments now provides empirical means for studying the relationship between a child's (or adult's) inner world of working models and the outer world of family

transactional patterns and coordinated practices (Malone 1988). These encouraging developments now make it possible to study aspects of developmental psychopathology (Sroufe and Rutter 1984), and to explore the relationship between the influence of childhood experience on a patient's inner working model of parent-child relationship and how that model is expressed in actual parent-child interaction (Zeanah and Zeanah 1989), which become part of and, consequently, are supported by the enduring coordinated practices of ongoing family life (Malone 1988). These developments offer a promising means for interrelating and eventually integrating a psychoanalytic object-relations attachment theory perspective and a family systems perspective in assessing, treating, and studying childhood mental and behavioral disorders. While a number of family therapists (e.g., Kantor 1983; Malone 1979, 1983; Scharff and Scharff 1987; Slipp 1984) have been attempting this type of conceptual integration in clinical practice for a number of years, through the pioneering efforts of a group of family researchers (Gottman 1979; Main and Goldwyn 1984; Patterson 1982, 1988; Reiss 1981, 1989; Steinglass et al. 1987) we now have the research methodology that will provide a sound basis for the empirical studies that will support such an integration (Wamboldt and Reiss 1989) and become a powerful impetus for convergence between child and adolescent psychiatry and family therapy.

This introduces the central theme of this chapter: the current state of affairs in family therapy, with particular emphasis on the promising directions that have emerged from family research that have significant implications for the practice of child and adolescent psychiatry in the 1990s. Let us begin with the status of assessment and diagnosis and the models of family therapy, and then consider the issue of efficacy before moving on to the promising new directions that are being opened up by family research.

Family Assessment and Therapy Models

The process of family therapy begins with an assessment that focuses on evaluating family functioning (Minuchin 1974) and process (Stanton 1981). The focus of diagnosis and treatment is the family system, including the identified child patient, who is regarded as the most manifest part of a pathologic process involving the entire family. Symptoms and dysfunction are seen as being fully

---

[1] The research of Wamboldt and Reiss on early marital relationship (1989) confirms the view that the field and practice of family therapy has ignored important gender differences and their implications in family life and family interventions.

integrated into enduring, complex patterns of family interaction. The clinician is particularly interested in wholeness, organization, and patterning (Papp 1983) and in determining the connection between the presenting problems and the family system. In this assessment process, it is essential to appreciate the role of ethnocultural values in the clinical presentation (McGoldrick et al. 1982) and to identify the family's convictions about itself and its relationship to social reality (Kantor and Lehr 1975; Reiss 1981) in formulating the diagnosis and deciding on treatment strategies and methods. Diagnosis and treatment of the family that do not take into account ethnocultural issues and the family's beliefs about itself and its convictions about social reality will not be accurate or effective. For example, therapists proposing an egalitarian negotiation model (Malone 1983) for family decision making around the oppositional, at times, defiant independence-seeking behavior of an adolescent daughter to a traditional closed system (Kantor and Lehr 1975) or New England "Yankee" family (McGoldrick et al. 1982) will run into powerful resistance and probably will be ineffective. Such an approach may also run the risk of labeling as "pathology" traits or characteristics of family life that reflect ethnocultural influence.

In the family assessment process, child mental health professionals have found evaluation of the family's developmental stage and appreciation of the importance of preparatory transition between stages (Carter and McGoldrick 1980) particularly informative. The integration of individual and family developmental perspectives is particularly valuable in the process of understanding and treating the presenting problems of children and adolescents. Many family therapists believe that the appearance of symptoms in children frequently reflects the fact that the family is stuck and unable to move successfully through a developmental stage transition. For example, a family presented at my office when one of two adolescent daughters began running away, abusing alcohol, and placing herself in danger following the mother's remarriage. During evaluation, it became apparent that this new family had never successfully reconstituted and that each parent "secretly" believed the family would be better off without the unruly, defiant daughter. Once we identified the source of the "adolescent's problem," intervention was considerably easier. The family developmental models that are most informative in the family diagnostic process are those of Carter and McGoldrick (1988), Combrinck-

Graham (1985), Wynne (1988), and Zilbach (1989). These models are particularly useful in viewing individual and family development as reciprocal interactive processes.

Evaluation of families is essentially a matter of systematic clinical interviewing. However, structured interviews, clinical rating scales, and family self-report methods (Beavers and Voeller 1983; Epstein et al. 1978, 1982) can be used for clinical and research diagnostic purposes. Combining the data from structured as well as unstructured clinical interviews with family self-report and observer clinical rating scales improves the accuracy and thoroughness of assessment and identifies specific focal goals and objectives for intervention. Nevertheless, these adjunctive methods of evaluation are rarely used in clinical practice outside of research protocols.

Historically, the adiagnostic or even antidiagnostic stance of many family therapists has been troublesome for child psychiatrists and other child mental health professionals. Child-oriented clinicians have not always understood the theoretical and practical reasons for the family therapist's resistance to diagnosis and insistence on appreciating the family homeostatic function of a child's symptoms, and hence the need to understand the *connection between* the presenting symptoms and the family system. Consequently, they have not always appreciated why family therapists express to a family their concern about what would happen to the family system if the child's symptoms were removed (Papp 1983). Individual children, including their symptoms, are important in family therapy; however, understanding the linkage between the child's dysfunction and the family system provides a critically important perspective on the meaning of symptoms in the context of the family.

The difficulty that practicing child mental health professionals have had in appreciating the family therapist's orientation to diagnosis has been compounded by the lack of a unified theory of family therapy and an agreed-on family diagnostic schema that have made it difficult to achieve order in relation to the multiple, diverse, and, at times, contradictory approaches used in family therapy. As a result, in the past, various efforts to classify family therapy models (Beels and Farber 1969; Haley 1962) have struggled with the experimentation in therapeutic techniques that has characterized the field, the powerful identificatory influence of charismatic family therapy leaders who have evoked loyalty from their followers, and a tendency to polarize rather than integrate different perspectives. More recently, however, classificatory efforts appropriately have placed emphasis on the similarities between and interrelatedness of family therapy models (Levant 1984; Nichols 1984). Following Ackerman's lead (1972), these classificatory schemas (Grunebaum and Chasin 1980; Levant 1984) recognize that the multiple treatment approaches that characterize the family therapy field do not always represent pure or distinct forms of treatment. Consequently, the significant overlap between family therapy approaches (and the concepts utilized to explain these particular approaches) is emphasized.

It is particularly useful to organize models of family therapy according to the principal theory that informs the therapeutic method (Levant 1984; Nichols 1984). The theory that organizes and drives the therapy model determines such important treatment issues as the focus and presumed mechanisms of therapeutic change, the role of the therapist, and the model's orientation to history and time. Therefore, therapists vary as to whether they emphasize the present or the past and as to whether they focus on underlying structure or transactional patterns. The theory that informs the treatment even determines how the therapist defines a family system. In clinical practice, most family therapists evaluate a family system in terms of what they believe is causing the problem and how they plan to intervene. As a result, therapists using the Bowen *multigenerational model* assess a family system in terms of an intergenerational separation-individuation process and the continuation in nuclear families of unresolved family-of-origin issues through emotional cutoff, triangulation, and the family projection process. Therapists using a *structural model* evaluate a family in terms of its adaptive or maladaptive structure, particularly in relation to hierarchical power-authority organization, boundaries, and preferred transactional patterns that reflect structural imbalance. *Strategic model* therapists assess families in terms of process and maladaptive problem-solving efforts and the balance between the forces for and against change in the family, especially during periods of family developmental transition.

Using the theoretical perspective, which informs the therapeutic approach as the key to classification and differentiation (Levant 1984), the many models of family therapy can be grouped into three clusters: First, the *historical-dynamic therapeutic model*, informed by psychoanalytic theory, emphasizes history, intergenerational transmission, and the process of becoming more adaptive through understanding the dominant influence of introjected objects (internal working models) and unresolved issues from the past. Second, the *process-structural therapeutic model*, influenced by general systems and learning theories, which focuses on the family as a social organization, is concerned only with the history of the presenting problem and problem-solving efforts, and attempts therapeutically to alter patterns and structure through transformational directive or paradoxical methods. Third, the *experiential therapeutic model*, influenced by phenomenalism and existentialism, emphasizes identification and affective experience in the present, utilizes active encountering methods, and attempts to enhance the current quality of life for the family and its members.

Most child psychiatrists find the historical-dynamic model appealing because it emphasizes intergenerational transmission and fits well with their medical history–anchored orientation. Some gravitate to and are able to master the techniques of the experiential model of family treatment (Satir 1972; Whitaker 1976). A significant group are attracted to the process-structural model because it offers effective access to the diagnostic and therapeutic power of a systems approach, even though it involves the challenge of integrating it with their traditional concern about the development, psychology, and needs of individual child and adolescent patients (Malone 1983; Pinsof 1983).

Whatever family therapy model within one of these larger theoretical orientations a child psychiatrist or mental health professional chooses and masters, he or she will be far better equipped to address the complexity of most child-family mental health problems, which require a flexible combination of individual, subsystem, and family perspectives and interventions. In evaluating and treating complex child-family presenting problems, the child mental health professional must diagnose the relationship between individual child symptoms and dysfunctional patterns and structural imbalance within the family. This presents the challenge of how to combine family, subsystem, and individual interviewing to explore effectively the interplay between levels within the family system and to determine whether family, subsystem, and individual treatment is indicated separately or in combination, at one time or in stages over time (Malone 1983). Child psychiatrists equipped with a family systems assessment and treatment model can meet this challenge and can also more effectively deal with the dialectic between change (transformation) and stability (homeostasis) that characterizes family response to therapeutic efforts (Papp 1983). Having the capacity to diagnose and treat the relationship between a child's symptoms and the family system enables the practicing clinician to counteract the family forces that contribute to and maintain the child's presenting problems and to involve effectively the entire family in the therapeutic effort.

Review of Outcome Research

Family therapy outcome research reveals, rather convincingly, that family and marital therapies lead to positive outcomes. In their exhaustive view of the literature, Gurman et al. (1986) concluded that family therapy no longer needs to justify itself on empirical grounds. Family and marital therapies are clearly superior to no treatment and lead to beneficial outcomes in two-thirds of cases, usually in treatment of short duration. Not unexpectedly, increased communication skills (Berman 1983; Gottman 1979; Wamboldt and Reiss 1989) are consistently empirically related to success in marital therapy (Birchler and Spinks 1980; Jacobson 1978), and conjoint behaviorally oriented treatment is considered the therapy of choice for sexual dysfunction (Gurman and Kniskern 1981). In a rather guarded statement, however, Gurman et al. (1986) concluded that family therapy is probably as effective as, and possibly more effective than, many commonly offered treatments for problems attributed to family conflicts.

Interestingly, family variables such as quality of family interaction, family constellation, and identified patient diagnosis and developmental level have not been found to affect treatment outcomes significantly. This counterintuitive conclusion perhaps reflects limitations in research methodology rather than the true state of affairs. Not surprisingly, sophisticated and refined therapist relationship skills appear necessary to achieve positive clinical outcomes. Importantly, research on family therapy outcomes appropriately suggests caution in that inexperienced or unskilled therapists who provide little structuring and also confront highly charged emotional issues within the family, particularly early in treatment, may be more harmful than helpful to families (Gurman et al. 1986).

Although efficacy research on particular family treatment methods is less well developed, it is nevertheless clear that no school or model of family therapy has established evidence of overall, let alone superior, effectiveness. However, six models (structural, strategic, behavioral, problem-centered, psychodynamic, and multigenerational) have shown at least moderate efficacy with at least one clinical disorder (Gurman et al. 1986). There are four disorders (i.e., schizophrenia, substance abuse, conduct disorder and juvenile delinquency, marital discord) for which we now have at least moderately positive evidence of the efficacy of more than one method of family treatment (Gurman et al. 1986). The research methodological limitations of outcome research with specific diagnostic entities, other than schizophrenia, conduct disorder and juvenile delinquency, and substance use disorder, however, preclude any further conclusions or generalizations at this time. These methodological limitations include unclear inclusion criteria, the representative character of subjects, the definition and measurement of change, the "purity" of technique, the role of nonspecific therapeutic factors, and the relative contribution of therapeutic method and the personal qualities of the therapist.

New Directions for Clinical Practice

In recent years, family research has opened up exciting new prospects for clinical work and provided an impetus for convergence between family therapy and child and adolescent psychiatry. Among a number of exciting areas of research that have important implications for child and adolescent psychiatry, there are four lines of programmatic research that suggest exciting new directions for clinical practice: the studies of Main (Main et al. 1985), Reiss (1989), Patterson (1982, 1989), and Goldstein (1987) and their colleagues. Importantly, the major themes of these four lines of programmatic research not only suggest new directions and areas for exploration in clinical practice, but also provide an empirical and theoretical framework for examining, interrelating, and, eventually, integrating models of family therapy derived from the two root theories (psychoanalytic and general systems) of family therapy and the two corresponding perspectives (represented and practicing) on family continuity (Reiss 1989). The research of the Reiss, Patterson, and Goldstein groups, for example, fits well with the practicing family perspective and with the family assessment and treatment models related to this perspective (structural, strategic, systemic, problem-centered, and behavioral). On the other hand, the studies of the Main group are congruent with the represented family perspective and the family assessment and treatment models related to this perspective (psychodynamic, intergenerational, and contextual).

Although each group is pursuing quite different research agendas, there are important points of convergence and significant conceptual and theoretical interrelationships among the four lines of investigation. The most important point of convergence for the child mental health clinician is the fact that all four lines of research are concerned with family factors in intergenerational transmission and in the exacerbation and maintenance of psychopathology. For example, the studies of Main and her associates demonstrate that transmission of patterns of relating across generations, including abuse and maltreatment, is mediated by an individual's internal working models (Zeanah and Zeanah 1989). The Reiss group's investigations of alcoholism (Steinglass et al. 1987) indicate that transmission across generations is influenced by the degree to which an alcoholic individual's drinking behavior is included in critical family rituals, which are important expressions of family identity (Wolin et al. 1980). Patterson (1982, 1988) and his colleagues have identified and traced the mechanisms by which a coercive family process initiates and maintains conduct disorder in boys. Finally, the Goldstein group has studied the strong association between the presence of high expressed emotion and marked communication deviance and the development of schizophrenia and schizophrenia spectrum disorders in a group of adolescents first identified in a psychiatric outpatient setting (Doane et al. 1981; Goldstein 1987).

To illustrate the new directions and areas for exploration in clinical practice suggested by family research, I will now summarize components of the work of two of the groups, Main's and Reiss's, in greater detail.

The Main Group

Although not focusing on clinical issues per se, the line of research conducted by Main sheds considerable light on the psychological issues involved in the question of intergenerational transmission of abuse and other forms of aggression and violence (Malone 1988). As one of the leading proponents of attachment theory research, Main and her colleagues have investigated the social interactions of young abused (George and Main 1979) and rejected nonabused children and attempted to relate these behaviors to mother-child relationship patterns, which in turn are associated with the mother's own relationship history, as evaluated by a structured interview (Main and Goldwyn 1984).

George and Main (1979) conducted the first controlled study of the social interactive behavior of abused young children. They found that abused 1–3-year-old children frequently physically assaulted their peers. They "harassed" their caregivers and were the only children who assaulted or threatened to assault their caregivers. Thus even at a young age, abused children are physically aggressive with peers and caregivers and behave in ways that invite punitive responses from others and that tend to repeat or recreate experiences that are congruent with their maltreatment relationship history. Main (1983) found similar behavior patterns in nonabused toddlers who had been rejected by their mothers.

To relate parent-child relationship patterns systematically to the parent's relationship history, George et al. (unpublished) developed the Berkeley Adult Attachment Interview. This interview was designed to measure individual differences in relationship history at the level of internal representation by systematically inquiring about early relationships, separations, losses, or other traumatic experiences; specific supportive or contradictory memories; and assessments of relationships in childhood and current relationships (Main and Goldwyn 1984).

Using the Adult Attachment Interview, a number of investigators have found strong associations between "parent-child" relationship patterns and the parent's own relationship history, and a high degree of congruence (75%–82%) between a parent's working model of attachment and his or her child's attachment classification measured independently 1–5 years earlier (Eichberg 1986; Main et al. 1985). As Zeanah and Zeanah (1989) pointed out, the striking similarities in how parents organize and *represent* their relationship history and how their own children respond to and interact with them provide valuable insights into the process by which organizing relationship patterns (inner working models) are carried forward across generations.

The attachment studies of Main and Goldwyn (1984) make it clear that abusive parents are not all alike in their caregiving behaviors. Some are rejecting, distant, unavailable, and punitive; some combine an underlying rejection with an apparent closeness and role reversal with the child; some are simply unpredictable and are alternately accepting and rejecting; and some are very depressed and extremely anxious and behave in frightening or frightened ways with their children. The retrospective reports of parents who were abused in childhood point to three major patterns of parent-child relationship associated with a parental abuse history (Zeanah and Zeanah 1989). Each pattern is characterized by a different organizing theme of the dyadic relationship and is associated with a different pattern of parental behavior toward the child. To date, this line of research has disclosed patterns of rejection, role reversal and ambivalence, and fear as organizing themes of abusive relationships across generations. The research of Main and her associates thus reframes the issue of intergenerational transmission of abuse. What appears to be repeated across generations in the abused-abusing cycle is not so much a specific type of abuse, but rather an organizing theme of parent-child relationship and a way of living and experiencing that theme: the inner working model (Zeanah and Zeanah 1989).

Clearly this line of research provides strong suggestive evidence for the importance of inner working models and the *represented family* perspective in the intergenerational transmission of organizing relationship themes that are associated with abuse. However, this line of research does not consider how the organizing relationship themes contained in a parent's inner working model become expressed and elaborated in the parent's actual ongoing relationship with his or her own child. To understand this aspect of intergenerational transmission, we must turn from the represented family perspective to the *practicing family* perspective (Malone 1988).

The parent-child relationship that may give rise to abuse is embedded in other relationship systems (Belsky 1980). As can repeatedly be seen in clinical practice, child abuse by a mother or a father, however it might begin, cannot continue without the support (collusive or not) of the spouse or parenting partner and the family. While a number of factors—such as isolation and lack of social support; distressing and burdening infant or child characteristics; chronic intrafamilial conflict, particularly marital discord; and stressful life events, especially relationship loss—may singly or in combination

precipitate the expression of actual abuse, sustained expression in repeated and persistent child abuse cannot take place without the support of the social context in which the abuse takes place. Importantly, the transactional patterns within the family that support the intergenerational expression of abuse are aspects of the abusing parent's practicing family. Therefore, efforts to diagnose and treat intergenerational transmission of abuse or other forms of aggression and violence must take into account the interrelationship between the abusing parent's represented family of inner working models shaped by childhood abuse and rejection experiences and the coordinated practices and transactional patterns of his or her practicing family (Malone 1988).

This line of research suggests to child mental health clinicians that early diagnosis and treatment of child abuse requires a combination of individual, couple, and family system interventions. These interventions should identify and therapeutically address the parent's vulnerability to abuse and his or her tendency distortedly to attribute aggressive, violent, victimizing intent to the behaviors of a spouse or child (projective identification) and the spouse's or child's complementary tendency to become involved in abusive acts. Also to be addressed is how these acts are subsequently supported by transactional patterns and coordinated practices (e.g., storytelling) in ongoing family life. Such a combination of interventions would, of necessity, involve utilization of methods based on psychodynamic intergenerational diagnostic and therapeutic models and approaches based on family systems assessment and treatment models. Such a combination of interventions would also involve a systematic integration of evaluation and treatment methods based on these two orientations.

Interestingly, in studying parents who had been maltreated in childhood, Main and Goldwyn (1984) also found that when mothers who were rejected, deprived, or abused in childhood could express anger about these experiences and had a clear perspective about and could discuss their childhood relationships in a coherent nonidealizing fashion, they were not abusive but rather were able to provide reliable nurturant care for their children. This confirms the clinical studies of Fraiberg (1975) and suggests that parents (fathers as well as mothers) can, through the positive effects of later corrective relationships or through treatment, contain the negative effects of an abusive, depriving, or rejecting childhood. Consequently, preventive intervention efforts aimed at interrupting the maltreated-maltreating cycle should be focused on assisting parents who were maltreated in childhood to gain access to the feelings that are associated with the maltreatment and to be able to put their family of origin relationship experiences into a coherent perspective.

The research of the Main group, which operationalizes Bowlby's (1969, 1973, 1980) object-relations and attachment theory construct of internal working models in children and adults, makes it possible to study aspects of intergenerational transmission and opens up exciting possibilities for understanding more clearly and specifically the role of early childhood experience in the pathogenesis of mental disorders. Stimulated by this line of research, other investigators have begun to study intergenerational transmission issues in relation to failure to thrive (Benoit et al. 1989), childhood psychopathology in general (Crowell and Feldman 1988), and child abuse (Zeanah and Zeanah 1989). Other researchers are studying the relationship between attachment patterns and anorexia and bulimia (Hirshberg and Zeanah, unpublished). Still other investigators are attempting to evaluate treatment outcome by studying the effects of treatment on patterns of attachment in children and adults (Lieberman and Birch 1985).

The Reiss Group

Just as the attachment theory research of Main and her associates operationalizes important psychoanalytic theoretical constructs and makes it possible to study the represented family and intergenerational transmission, the investigations of Reiss (1989) have identified a range of coordinated family practices through which family integrity and stability are maintained across time, and have developed methods that now make study of the practicing family and of the relationship between coordinated family practices and clinical outcomes possible. From the various aspects of family research conducted by this group, I have chosen to focus on their studies of family convictions or paradigms, chronic illness, and alcoholism to illustrate the new directions for clinical practice suggested by this line of programmatic research.

Family paradigms. The Reiss group has shown that a family's response to a card-sorting task reveals its beliefs about the laboratory setting and reflects the family's enduring convictions about ambiguous social settings (Reiss 1981). The problem-solving laboratory procedure has been used to predict a family's conceptions and convictions about treatment modalities. For example, the procedure was used to predict family response to a family-oriented inpatient program for adolescents. In this study (Costell et al. 1981), it was found that two dimensions of family performance—coordination and configuration—successfully predicted family engagement in the treatment program. Coordination is measured by the amount of coordination and agreement the family shows as it works on the card-sorting task. Configuration is measured by the amount of information and detail on the cards the family uses in its solution. Families high in coordination participated more actively in therapeutic activities, attended therapy more regularly, and were better liked by other families. Within the group of high-coordination families, however, an important difference appeared along the configuration dimension. Families high in configuration were open to a variety of relationships and seemed available and accessible to change through their interactions with staff and other families. By contrast, low-configuration families had rigid boundaries, withdrew from relationships, and were less open to change.

The implications of this type of research for therapists and treatment agencies are considerable. Clearly, clinicians and therapeutic modalities must understand and be sensitive and adaptive to the family's underlying belief about itself and its constructions of its social reality: its paradigm. Otherwise, a treatment program may be designed or conducted in such a way that its likelihood of success has been jeopardized by its failure to take the family's paradigm into account (Constantine 1986; Kantor and Neal 1985; Reiss 1983).

Family role in chronic illness. Reiss et al. (1986) have used the same laboratory problem-solving situation in studies of the family's role in the course of chronic illness. For example, in studying a group of 23 families, each containing a patient with end-stage renal disease who was being treated by hemodialysis, they encountered unexpected and surprising results. In sharp contrast to predictions based on previous research, high scores on the problem-solving variable coordination, as well as on the measures of family accomplishments and intactness, predicted early death rather than survival. Furthermore, they also found that a testing-the-limits type of noncompliance accounted for most of the association between family variables and 3-year survival.

In attempting to account for the results, Reiss et al. (1986) put forward an interesting three-step explanation: 1) the paradoxical vulnerability of "strong" families; 2) exclusion of the ill member as a last-stage family coping effort; and 3) medical compliance as acceptance, by the patient, of exclusion. In this view, high coordination, while adaptive in the acute phase of illness, may make the family vulnerable in the long run in *chronic* severe illness. In high-coordination families, members remain highly engaged with each other and overly focused on the needs of the chronically ill member, to the detriment of family coherence and the developmental needs of other members and the family as a unit. Families enduring long-term distress react with an extreme coping mechanism, the reorganization of the family, which takes the form of excluding a member (Boss 1980). In the end stages of the illness, the excluded member is the patient, an exclusion in which the patient participates. This is considered to lead to medical compliance, which reflects the patient's attitude of resignation to the dire implications of his or her illness and an acceptance of family exclusion.

Based on this study and on 8 years of research and observation of families with a member who has a chronic disabling medical illness, the Reiss group (Gonzalez et al. 1989) developed a family-focused intervention, the multiple-family discussion group (MFDG). This short-term (eight-session) psychoeducationally oriented intervention brings four to six families (including the medically ill child or adult) together to discuss illness-related family issues in a structured format. The MFDG intervention is an adaptation to a chronic medical illness population of the recently developed psychoeducational family interventions that have been used so successfully in the treatment of chronic psychiatric illness (McFarlane et al. 1983).

Through discussing their issues in a supportive nonblaming atmosphere, in the presence of other families facing similar challenges, families learn that the stresses and painful feelings they experience are normative for families with a severely chronically ill member. Families are encouraged to reexamine their typical coping styles, with the goal of avoiding an illness-centered family organization, and to balance illness management demands with the needs of well family members and family growth and development. Thus they avoid the dilemma of

the high-coordination families noted above in the end-stage renal disease study. Preliminary results suggest that the MFDG is an effective means of assisting families with a severely chronically ill member to adjust adaptively to the protean demands that confront them over time. It seems highly likely that studies of family paradigms in other chronic medical or psychiatric illness among youth will provide an understanding of factors that predict successful or unsuccessful outcome, which in turn will provide valuable guidelines for psychosocial interventions. Using a supportive, nonjudgmental, psychoeducational, multifamily group format such as the MFDG may be a particularly effective type of intervention. Similar positive results with this kind of intervention have been reported with other chronic, relatively intractable conditions, such as encopresis (Stark et al. 1990).

Family patterns of alcoholism across generations. The studies on the intergenerational transmission of alcoholism are particularly informative. The "transmission study" focuses attention on the role of family identity, as most clearly expressed in family rituals, in the transmission of alcoholism across generations (Wolin et al. 1980). The investigators noted that families that contain one or more alcoholic members differ strikingly according to whether or not the alcoholic individual's drinking behavior is included in or excluded from family rituals (Wolin and Bennett 1984). Families that allow the alcoholic's drinking to intrude on, disrupt, and become a part of family ritual life are predicted to be at greatest risk of transmitting alcoholism to subsequent generations. In these families, the alcoholism has become a central part of the family's identity (Reiss 1983). Offspring from such families who wish to maintain continuity with their origin family are likely to include alcoholic behavior in the rituals and identity of their nuclear families, either by becoming alcoholics or by marrying alcoholics. To test out this hypothesis, Wolin et al. (1980) conducted a retrospective study of 25 families and found that families that included the drinking behavior of an alcoholic parent in key family rituals were far more likely to transmit alcoholism to the next generation. The single trait that most dramatically set nontransmitter families apart from transmitter families was their uniform overt rejection of the alcoholic parent's drinking or intoxicated behavior during family rituals.

In a prospective study, Steinglass et al. (1987) attempted to determine the factors that predict which offspring in an alcoholic family will later become alcoholics themselves or marry an alcoholic. In this study, a factor termed *deliberateness* proved to be a very powerful predictor of alcoholism transmission. Deliberateness refers to the conscious decision made by a late adolescent or young adult child of an alcoholic family to shape and organize rituals in his or her developing nuclear family along specific lines that are different from his or her family of origin and do not include excessive use of alcohol. Thus the key issue in this prospective study of the transmission of alcoholism is whether or not the vulnerable youth can make a deliberate decision to disengage selectively from the family rituals and identity of the family of origin (heritage) containing an alcoholic parent.

What is particularly interesting about both of these studies are the implications they have for clinical practice. These studies suggest that in the treatment of alcoholic families, the critical issue is the need to develop clear, overt opposition of family members to the inclusion of the alcoholic parent in family rituals when he or she is drinking or intoxicated. In addition, in the prevention of transmission to the next generation, another key issue appears to be the capacity of the late adolescent and young child of an alcoholic family to make a deliberate, conscious decision to disengage selectively from the identity and rituals of the family of origin in the process of forming his or her new family.

The capacity for deliberateness in making this critical decision would appear to require that the vulnerable young person have a clear and cohesive perspective on the impact of the parent's alcoholism on him or her during childhood. Such a cohesive perspective undoubtedly requires access to feelings about the alcoholic parent and having witnessed episodes of heavy drinking and intoxication and the impact of alcoholism on family life. This type of cohesive perspective may be similar to the kind of perspective Main and Goldwyn (1984) found was necessary for parents who had been abused or rejected in childhood to *contain* the negative effects of that maltreatment experience and not to repeat it in their subsequent relationships with their own children.

This line of research and conceptualization suggests that practicing child and adolescent psychiatrists should develop ways of incorporating family, couple, and individual intervention aimed at promoting access to feelings about a parent's alcoholism and a clear cohesive perspective on the impact

of alcoholism on relationships and on family life, especially family rituals, in their clinical work with alcoholic families and with the children of alcoholic families.

Conclusions

Despite the regrettable historical lag in the *full* integration of the family systems model into child and adolescent psychiatric practice, there have been a number of encouraging developments, particularly in family research, that indicate that a significant convergence of family therapy and child and adolescent psychiatry has begun and is likely to become an increasingly strong trend in the future. The challenges of complex child-family pathology coupled with the insights that are emerging from clinical and research efforts organized by a family systems perspective are paving the way for increasing integration of family therapy assessment and treatment models into clinical practice.

The encouraging developments noted in this chapter include 1) the proposal by Reiss (1989) of two empirically driven concepts of family stability and coherence across time (the represented and the practicing family perspectives), which reflect the influence of the two root theories (psychoanalytic and general systems) of family therapy; 2) the appearance of theory-based classification schemas of family therapy models, which emphasize the similarities and overlap between treatment methods and the concepts that underlie them; and 3) the promising directions that have emerged from research, which have significant implications for the practice of child and adolescent psychiatry in the 1990s.

The areas of family research that suggest new directions for clinical practice are concerned with family factors in intergenerational transmission and in the exacerbation and maintenance of psychopathology. These lines of research and the methodology to which they have led also offer the exciting prospect of allowing us to examine, to interrelate, and eventually to integrate models of family therapy. Thus recent family research not only suggests novel directions for clinical practice, but also provides a significant impetus for the convergence of the fields of family therapy and child and adolescent psychiatry.

Reiss's conceptualization of family stability and coherence across time, coupled with recent methodological developments derived from family research, now provides empirical means for studying developmental psychopathology, specifically in terms of the relationship between a child's (or adult's) inner world of working models and the outer world of family transactional patterns and coordinated practices. These developments offer a promising means for interrelating a psychoanalytic object-relations attachment theory perspective and a family systems perspective in evaluating, treating, and studying childhood mental disorders.

References

Ackerman NW: The growing edge of family therapy, in Progress in Group and Family Therapy. Edited by Sager CJ, Kaplan HS. New York, Brunner/Mazel, 1972, pp 440–456

Beavers WR, Voeller MN: Family models: comparing and contrasting the Olson circomplex model with the Beavers systems model. Fam Process 22:85–98, 1983

Beels CC, Farber A: Family therapy: a view. Fam Process 8:280–332, 1969

Belsky J: Child maltreatment: an ecological integration. Am Psychol 35:320–335, 1980

Benoit D, Zeanah CH, Barton ML: Maternal attachment disturbances in mothers of failure-to-thrive infants. Infant Mental Health Journal 10:185–202, 1989

Berman E: The treatment of troubled couples, in Psychiatry Update: The American Psychiatric Association Annual Review, Vol 2. Edited by Grinspoon L. Washington, DC, American Psychiatric Press, 1983, pp 215–228

Birchler GR, Spinks SH: Behavioral-systems marital and family therapy: integration and clinical applications. American Journal of Family Therapy 8:6–28, 1980

Boss PG: The relationship of psychological father presence, wife's personal qualities and wife/family dysfunction in families of missing fathers. Journal of Marriage and the Family 42:541–549, 1980

Bowlby J: Attachment and Loss, Vol 1: Attachment. New York, Basic Books, 1969

Bowlby J: Attachment and Loss, Vol 2: Separation. New York, Basic Books, 1973

Bowlby J: Attachment and Loss, Vol 3: Loss. New York, Basic Books, 1980

Carter EA, McGoldrick M: The family life cycle and family therapy, in The Family Life Cycle. Edited by Carter EA, McGoldrick M. New York, Gardner Press, 1980, pp 3–20

Carter EA, McGoldrick M (eds): The Changing Family Life Cycle. New York, Gardner Press, 1988

Combrinck-Graham L: A model of family development. Fam Process 24:139–150, 1985

Constantine LL: Family Paradigms. New York, Guilford, 1986

Costell R, Reiss D, Berkman H, et al: The family meets the hospital: predicting the family's perception of the treatment program from its problem-solving style. Arch Gen Psychiatry 38:569–577, 1981

Crowell J, Feldman S: The effects of mother's internal models of relationships and children's behavioral and developmental status on mother-child interaction. Child Dev 59:1273–1285, 1988

Dell PF: Violence and the systemic view: the problem of power. Fam Process 28:1–13, 1989

Doane JA, West KL, Goldstein MJ, et al: Parental communication deviance and affective style. Arch Gen Psychiatry 38:679–685, 1981

Eichberg C: Security of attachment in infancy: contribution of mother's representation of her own experience and childhood attitudes. Unpublished doctoral dissertation, University of Virginia, Charlottesville, VA, 1986

Epstein NB, Bishop DS, Levin S: The McMaster model of family functioning. Journal of Marriage and Family Counseling 4:29–31, 1978

Epstein NB, Bishop DS, Baldwin LM: McMaster model of family functioning: a view of the normal family, in Normal Family Processes. Edited by Walsh F. New York, Guilford, 1982, pp 115–141

Fraiberg S, Adleson E, Shapiro V: Ghosts in the nursery: a psychoanalytical approach to problems of impaired infant-mother relationships. Journal of the American Academy of Child Psychiatry 14:387–421, 1975

George C, Main M: Social interactions of young abused children: approach, avoidance and aggression. Child Dev 50:306–318, 1979

Goldner V: Generation and gender: normative and covert hierarchies. Fam Process 27:17–31, 1988

Goldstein MJ: Family interaction patterns that antedate the onset of schizophrenia and related disorders: a further analysis of data from a longitudinal prospective study, in Understanding Major Mental Disorder: The Contribution of Family Interaction Research. Edited by Hahlweg K, Goldstein MJ. New York, Family Process Press, 1987, pp 11–32

Gonzalez S, Steinglass P, Reiss D: Putting the illness in its place: discussion groups for families with chronic medical illnesses. Fam Process 28:69–87, 1989

Gottman JM: Marital Interaction: Experimental Investigations. New York, Academic, 1979

Grunebaum H, Belfer ML: What family therapists might learn from child psychiatry. Journal of Marriage and Family Therapy 12:415–423, 1986

Grunebaum H, Chasin R: Thinking like a family therapist, in The Challenge of Family Therapy. Edited by Flomenhaft K, Christ AE. New York, Plenum, 1980, pp 54–74

Gurman AS, Kniskern DP (eds): Handbook of Family Therapy. New York, Brunner/Mazel, 1981

Gurman AS, Kniskern DP, Pinsof WM: Research on the process and outcome of marital and family therapy, in Handbook of Psychotherapy and Behavior Change, 3rd Edition. Edited by Garfield SL, Bergin AE. New York, John Wiley, 1986, pp 565–624

Haley J: Wither family therapy? Fam Process 1:69–100, 1962

Hare-Mustin RT: Family change and gender differences: implications for theory and practice. Family Relations 27:36–41, 1988

Jacobson NS: A review of the research of the effectiveness of marital therapy, in Marriage and Marital Therapy. Edited by Paolino TJ, McCrady BS. New York, Brunner/Mazel, 1978, pp 395–444

Kantor D: The structural-analytic approach to the treatment of family developmental crisis, in Family Life Cycle: Implications for Clinicians. Edited by Hausen JC, Liddle HA. Rockville, MD, Aspen, 1983, pp 12–30

Kantor D, Lehr W: Inside the Family. San Francisco, CA, Jossey-Bass, 1975, pp 13–30

Kantor D, Neal J: Integrative shifts for the theory and practice of family systems therapy. Fam Process 24:13–30, 1985

Keeney DP: Aesthetics of Change. New York, Guilford, 1983

Levant RF: Family Therapy: A Comprehensive Overview. Englewood Cliffs, NJ, Prentice-Hall, 1984

Lieberman AF, Birch M: The etiology of failure to thrive: an interactive developmental approach, in New Directions in Failure to Thrive: Implications for Research and Practice. Edited by Drotar D. New York, Plenum, 1985, pp 259–279

Main M: Exploration, play and cognitive functioning related to infant-mother attachment. Infant Behavior and Development 6:167–174, 1983

Main M, Goldwyn R: Predicting rejection of her infant from mother's representation of her own experience: implications for the abused-abusing intergenerational cycle. Child Abuse Negl 8:203–217, 1984

Main M, Kaplan N, Cassidy J: Security in infancy, childhood and adulthood: a move to a level of representation, in Growing Points in Attachment Theory and Research. (Society for Research in Child Development Monograph 50, Nos 1–2, No 209.) Edited by Bretherton I, Walters E. Chicago, IL, University of Chicago Press, 1985, pp 66–104

Malone CA: Child psychiatry and family therapy: an overview. Journal of the American Academy of Child Psychiatry 18:1–21, 1979.

Malone CA: Family therapy and childhood disorder, in Psychiatry Update: The American Psychiatric Association Annual Review, Vol 2. Edited by Grinspoon L. Washington, DC, American Psychiatric Press, 1983, pp 228–241

Malone CA: Child abuse and conduct disorder: family perspectives on intergenerational transmission of aggression and violence, in Conduct Disorders and Their Family Contexts. Edited by Sholevar PG. Washington, DC, American Academy of Child and Adolescent Psychiatry, 1988

McDermott J Jr: Indications for family therapy. Journal of the American Academy of Child Psychiatry 20:409–419, 1981

McDermott JF, Char WF: The undeclared war between child and family therapy. Journal of the American Academy of Child Psychiatry 13:422–436, 1974

McFarlane WR, Beels CC, Rosenheck S: New developments in the family treatment of the psychotic disorders, in Psychiatry Update: The American Psychiatric Association Annual Review, Vol 2. Edited by Grinspoon L. Washington, DC, American Psychiatric Press, 1983, pp 242–256

McGoldrick M, Pearce JK, Giordano J: Ethnicity and Family Therapy. New York, Guilford, 1982

Minuchin S: Families and Family Therapy. Cambridge, MA, Harvard University Press, 1974

Nichols MP: Family Therapy: Concepts and Methods. New York, Gardner Press, 1984

Papp P: The Process of Change. New York, Guilford, 1983

Patterson GR: Coercive Family Process. Eugene, OR, Castalia, 1982

Patterson GR: Coercive family processes and evolution of aggression in children: theoretical consideration, in Conduct Disorders and Their Family Context. Edited by Sholevar PG.

Washington, DC, American Academy of Child and Adolescent Psychiatry, 1988, pp 1–48

Pinsof WM: Integrative problem-centered family therapy: toward the synthesis of family and individual psychotherapies. Journal of Marriage and Family Therapy 9:19–35, 1983

Reiss D: The Family's Construction of Reality. Cambridge, MA, Harvard University Press, 1981

Reiss D: Family studies: reframing the illness, the patient and the doctor, in Psychiatry Update: The American Psychiatric Association Annual Review, Vol 2. Edited by Grinspoon L. Washington, DC, American Psychiatric Press, 1983, pp 172–185

Reiss D: The represented and practicing family: contrasting visions of family continuity, in Early Relationship Disorders. Edited by Sameroff AJ, Emde RM. New York, Basic Books, 1989, pp 191–220

Reiss D, Gonzalez S, Kramer N: Family process, chronic illness, and death. Arch Gen Psychiatry 43:795–804, 1986

Satir V: Peoplemaking. Palo Alto, CA, Science and Behavior Books, 1972

Scharff DE, Scharff JS: Object Relations Family Therapy. Northvale, NJ, Jason Aronson, 1987

Silver LB, Silver BJ: Clinical practice of child psychiatry: a survey. Journal of the American Academy of Child Psychiatry 22:573–579, 1983

Slipp S: Object Relations: A Dynamic Bridge Between Individual and Family Treatment. Northvale, NJ, Jason Aronson, 1984

Sroufe LA, Rutter M: The domain of developmental psychopathology. Child Dev 55:17–29, 1984

Stanton MD: Strategic approaches to family therapy, in Handbook of Family Therapy. Edited by Gurman AS, Kniskern DP. New York, Brunner/Mazel, 1981, pp 361–402

Stark LJ, Owens-Stively J, Spirito A: Group behavioral treatment of retentive encopresis. J Pediatr Psychol 15:659–671, 1990

Steinglass P, Bennett LA, Wolin SJ, et al: The Alcoholic Family. New York, Basic Books, 1987

Wamboldt FS, Reiss D: Defining a family heritage and a new relationship identity: two central tasks in the making of a marriage. Fam Process 28:317–334, 1989

Whitaker CA: The hindrance of therapy in clinical work, in Family Therapy: Theory and Practice. Edited by Guerin PJ. New York, Gardner Press, 1976, pp 154–164

Wolin SJ, Bennett LA: Family rituals. Fam Process 23:401–420, 1984

Wolin SJ, Bennett LA, Noonan DL, et al: Disruptive family rituals: a factor in the intergenerational transmission of alcoholism. J Stud Alcohol 41:199–214, 1980

Wynne LC: An epigenetic model of family processes, in Family Transitions. Edited by Falicov CJ. New York, Guilford, 1988, pp 81–106

Zeanah CH, Zeanah PD: Intergenerational transmission of maltreatment: insights from attachment theory and research. Psychiatry 52:177–196, 1989

Zilbach JJ: The family life cycle: a framework for understanding children in family therapy, in Children in Family Contexts. Edited by Combrinck-Graham L. New York, Guilford, 1989, pp 46–66

Chapter 55

Group Therapy

Steven L. Jaffe, M.D.
Bernard Kahan, M.D.

Children and adolescents live, play, study, and work with peers in numerous group settings. Group treatment offers unique opportunities and challenges to use these normal processes for therapeutic advantage. In this chapter, the usual developmental division separating children and adolescents is used.

Child Group Therapy

A large variety of group treatment approaches are currently available for work with children. Groups simulate aspects of the family and school environment and closely approximate a child's daily experiences and challenges. Bender and Woltman (1936) described the use of puppet shows as a therapeutic method for psychiatrically hospitalized children. They noted that "the value of group discussion lies partly in the fact that the children will actually discuss more freely in groups than they will alone" (p. 353). In 1934, Slavson pioneered the notion of treating small numbers of carefully selected latency-aged children in groups over a long-term period. Although activity group therapy in its pure form is uncommonly practiced at this time, Slavson's contributions form the cornerstone of most current group therapy approaches.

Classification of Child Therapy Groups

Groups for children may be classified along various dimensions, such as theoretical framework and technique, group composition, goals, physical set-ting, or treatment duration. The recent proliferation of group approaches is in part a response to an increasing focus on treatment planning, namely, the match between a patient's needs and the specific type of therapy selected.

Activity therapy groups. Activity group therapy, which was first developed by Slavson in 1945, is a psychoanalytically oriented, nondirective, noninterpretive small group treatment in which four to eight latency-aged (8–12 years old) children are seen for 2 years or more (Slavson and Schiffer 1975). To be eligible for this type of group therapy, children must have the potential capacity to relate to others and also have the ability to change attitudes and conduct through corrective experiences. The types of problems appropriate for treatment with activity group therapy include withdrawal, constriction, anxiety, infantilization, social fears, overprotection, and mildly disordered behaviors. Contraindications would include psychosis, conduct disorder, mental retardation, and excessive aggression. Patients and therapists are usually of the same sex, and patients are within a 1- to 2-year age range of each other.

The therapist, through a position of neutrality and permissiveness, creates an atmosphere in which controlled regression and subsequent working through can occur. Patients are selected to achieve a dynamic balance such that the group cycles between periods of overactivity and disequilibrium (nodal behavior) and quiescence (antinodal behavior). Children with a generally positive, mobilizing effect on the group are referred to as "positive instigators"; those promoting disharmony and hostility are called "negative instigators."

This nondirective nature of activity group therapy allows for virtually unrestricted freedom of choice and action, which is initially unexpected, unfamiliar, and anxiety provoking. As the children begin to overcome their isolation, individual relationships develop into an awareness of the group as a whole. Distinct from analytically oriented groups, where each individual in turn becomes the center of group attention, the dynamic interactions of the group in activity group therapy serve as the central therapeutic force, or in Slavson's terms, lead to "therapy through the group" rather than therapy of the individual in the group. With continued exposure to corrective reexperiences in activity group therapy, maladaptive behavior patterns are left behind and new patterns are permanently integrated.

Modifications to activity group therapy. Activity-interview group psychotherapy was developed as an extension of activity group therapy for children who require active limit setting and guidance but who are not so disturbed as to lack the capacity for relatedness (Slavson and Schiffer 1975). Activity-interview group psychotherapy involves groups of four to six children, who may be mixed with respect to sex. Activity materials are selected to promote acting out of internal conflicts. The therapist focuses attention during the group by individual interviews with specific children. Additionally, a group interview is conducted following the activity portion of the session. Issues discussed include why each child attends the group and what events occurred earlier in the group session.

Kinetic psychotherapy (Schacter 1974) is a form of activity-interview group psychotherapy specifically developed for children who have difficulty with the verbal expression of emotion. Playground-type interactive games are used to catalyze emotional responses, at which time the therapist freezes the action and facilitates identification and verbalization of feelings.

A modified form of activity group therapy suitable for severely impaired or deprived children involves guidance, limit setting, and reality testing by the therapist (Scheidlinger 1960, 1965). Activity therapy for younger children (ages 4–6 years) necessitates significantly more therapist involvement than for older groups. This method, called *play group therapy*, requires modifications in the setting and procedural methods of the therapist. Play group

therapy groups consist of four to five children of similar age, with group balance and mixing of boys and girls. Materials are chosen to facilitate symbolic play and projection of fantasy, and include dolls, puppets, and toy figures. Therapists involve themselves in dyadic interaction, verbal or physical limit setting, and the provision of explanations and educational information.

Although activity therapy groups are usually conducted by a single therapist, cotherapy allows mutual support, which buffers countertransference reactions (Semonsky and Zicht 1974).

Interpretive groups. Interpretive group psychotherapy involves the facilitation of conflicts, defenses, and fantasies via play and verbalization. An interpretive model is appropriate for latency-aged children with psychosomatic symptoms, anxiety, intense sibling rivalry, or behavioral disturbances. The therapist's role is to be friendly and informal, initially attempting to facilitate group interactions around play. As defensive or transference material arises, interpretive methods are used when appropriate. The group setting, unlike the large, well-stocked activity group room, may consist of a typical office playroom (Charach 1983; Sugar 1974).

Short-term group therapy. Short-term treatments emphasize patient strengths and avoid excessive dependence. Short-term group approaches focus on current behavior, adaptation, coping, and growth to promote change (Scheidlinger 1984).

Diagnostic groups were an early form of short-term therapy conceived by Redl (1944). A series of group diagnostic contacts may be useful to observe in-group behavior, provide intrinsic therapeutic value, and avoid the artificiality of the dyadic interview. Sands and Golub (1974) developed a 10-session "talking club," which utilized the group process itself, including such issues as quarrels over seating or mutual determining of group rules, as the essential material of therapy. The process whereby each child finds a place in the group constitutes the intervention.

Specific techniques to mobilize involvement with the group process are often needed in short-term groups. Genograms may be helpful with children from fragmented and disorganized families (Davis et al. 1988), and video playback of the group interactions facilitates engagement (Mallery and Navas 1982). Smith et al. (1985) developed a short-term "clown club" in which structured fantasy and drama facilitated expression and resolution of internal conflict.

Cognitive-behavioral groups. Development of good peer relationships during childhood is often seen as a predictor of subsequent adjustment during adolescence and adulthood. Behavioral groups utilize the principles of learning theory to facilitate and reinforce the development of appropriate social behavior. Clement et al. (1970) conducted a 20-session group consisting of socially withdrawn second- and third-grade boys in which tokens were used to reinforce verbalizations or social interactions. There were comparison groups: one group used verbal reinforcers in place of tokens, another group met without a therapist, and a third had the boys engaging in solitary play. Although improvements were modest, the token group proved superior to the verbal group or the control groups. A "star-chart" system using positive reinforcement of specific assigned therapeutic tasks combined activity and verbal therapy (Dannefer et al. 1975). Rose and Edleson (1987) described a structured multimethod approach to group therapy. Systematic assessment and goal setting identify the targets for intervention. Interpersonal skills, cognitive coping abilities (eliminating self-defeating cognitions), active coping skills (including the ability to use relaxation or avoidance during stress), and self-management are used within the group meetings. Treatment modalities in the small group setting include modeling, operant conditioning and stimulus control, cognitive restructuring, problem-solving methods, sociorecreational procedures, relaxation training, and environmental modification. These strategies have the ultimate goal of behavioral change in situations external to the group context.

Specialized groups. While heterogenous groups may be preferred for long-term intensive therapy, homogenous groups are advantageous when the goal is specifically short-term support or symptomatic relief. Homogenous groups attain cohesion more rapidly, have less conflict, and offer more immediate support.

Chronic illness groups. In 1951, Dubo proposed groups for children with heart disease, diabetes, or various allergic conditions in an effort to reduce anxiety and potentially to ameliorate disease symptomatology. Child, parent, and sibling group approaches have been devised for various medical conditions, including diabetes (Tattersall et al. 1985), cystic fibrosis (Farkas and Schwachman 1973), and cancer (Adams and Deveau 1988). Group approaches range from play groups for preschoolers to verbal or behavioral groups. Peer identification facilitates acceptance of chronic illness and the required medical management. Williams and Baeker (1983) described a school-based, short-term, structured group for children with a variety of chronic illnesses. Group sharing of factual information about the diseases and the requirements of treatment, feelings about their condition, and perceived family reactions, together with other expressive activities, contributed to emotional gains in all group members. Although homogenous groups have generally been recommended, Kennedy (1989) described grouping physically healthy but emotionally disturbed children together with chronically ill patients. Benefits of this approach were the acceptance of the chronically ill children by their healthy peers, an understanding of the universal nature of emotions like anger and disappointment, and mutual correction of distorted stereotypes about illness or health.

Obesity groups. Brownell et al. (1983) described a structured group approach to obesity involving both didactic material and discussions regarding family issues, feelings about being overweight, and weight control strategies. Three experimental group designs were conducted; separate, concurrent groups for parents and children; groups for parents and children together; and children-only groups. Outcome was most favorable for the separate parent and child groups, which allowed for freer expression of emotional issues.

Divorce groups. Group interventions for children of divorce have become increasingly popular, particularly in school settings, as part of preventive intervention. Kalter et al. (1984) identified appropriate goals for these interventions: to normalize the condition of being a child of divorce, to provide a forum for experiencing and reworking feelings, to develop coping strategies, and to provide feedback to parents.

Groups for children of alcoholics. Latency-aged children are at particular risk as a result of family denial of the reality of addiction; impermeable family boundaries to contain the secret; inappropriate guilt and self-blame; and family chaos, including neglect, abuse, divorce, and impoverishment. Group

approaches provide opportunities for healthy social interactions with peers and adults, facilitate
identification and expression of feelings, establish
a sense of predictability and order, and convey appropriate education about addiction (Bingham and
Bargar 1985).

Groups for abused children. Group treatment
approaches for the sequelae of physical and sexual
abuse have included short-term experiences with
expressive and educational activities structured
around a weekly theme (Kitchur and Bell 1989);
open-ended groups with a recurrent, structured
cycle of themes (Gilbert 1988); developmental play
therapy groups (Mitchum 1987); and long-term play
group therapy (Steward et al. 1986). Although data
regarding efficacy of treatment approaches in this
population are incomplete, group therapy is increasingly being viewed as the primary treatment
modality because of its power in alleviating the
common themes of isolation and guilt.

Postdisaster groups. Group counseling is increasingly being utilized with children as a prevention intervention following catastrophic events,
such as plane crashes, kidnappings, floods, or
earthquakes. Eth et al. (1985) illustrated a group
crisis consultation to a preschool following the
murder of a mother and child. Although children
typically rely on their families or school environment to provide outlets for expression and working
through of stress, this process may be compromised when individuals or groups in these settings
are reacting to the collective trauma.

Inpatient psychiatric groups. Lev (1983) described modified activity group therapy in a hospital setting in which lengths of stay averaged several
months. Such methods are considered appropriate
for long-term treatments of selected children and
would seem difficult to apply to short-term settings
with highly variable populations. As inpatient programs are faced with decreasing lengths of stay and
higher-acuity populations, experimentation with
alternate models is essential. Short-term, structured modalities such as psychodrama or role-playing groups are proving useful in some inpatient
settings.

Parental Involvement in Groups

Numerous models exist for conjoint work with the
parents of children being seen in groups. Oberfield

and Ciliotta (1983) described a model for treating
school-age boys with behavioral disorders together
with their single mothers. The boys met together
biweekly, alternating with conjoint mother-son
groups. Issues of mutual support and modeling of
parenting skills were profitably raised, as were feelings of isolation and conflicted emotions regarding
males. Training of parents to deal with behavioral
disorders in their children is increasingly being done
in group formats. For example, Pevsner (1982)
demonstrated superior outcome and greater efficiency of parent training plus group behavior therapy over individual family behavior therapy.

Outcome of Child Group Therapy

Abramowitz (1976) conducted a comprehensive review of outcome data and noted numerous limitations in research across the various types of groups.
Existing evidence regarding efficacy appeared inconclusive, with equal numbers of studies yielding
positive, mixed, and null findings. A trend favored
behavioral as opposed to other approaches. This
may be a reflection of better study design and more
reliable outcome measures rather than actual methodological superiority.

Adolescent Group Therapy

Adolescence begins with the physical changes of
puberty. Peer relationships take on an intense, almost desperate quality, as the irrational emotional
swings of early adolescence are moderated by the
safety net of a same-sex peer group. Thus the adolescent seeks and is nurtured by the developmentally normal groups of the teenage years. Group
relationships foster social skills and self-esteem,
mediate the emotional separation-individuation
process from parental units, and enhance the development of a sense of identity. Since group influences and affiliations are so important in
adolescent development, adolescent groups are a
"natural" for therapy. Some investigators (Scheidlinger 1985) feel that group therapy is the treatment
of choice for most disturbed adolescents.

Betty Gabriel in 1939 appears to have been the
first clinician to use interview group therapy after
an adolescent girls group preferred to ask questions
and talk rather than do activities (Rachman and
Ravbolt 1984). Slavson, considered the father of
adolescent group therapy, extended his develop-

ment of activity groups for children into verbal groups for adolescents (Slavson and Schiffer 1975). Through the years, modifications of psychoanalytic technique have been the standard for all who work with adolescents. This has been called the *para-analytical approach*. Brandes (1973) attributed this term to Slavson and described this method as a process to "allow the psychotherapist the freedom to interpret the present dynamics of the members of the group in terms of the past, and also, in the group session, . . . [to allow the therapist] to teach, direct, support, reassure, coax, argue and be a real person" (p. 73).

Classification of Adolescent Therapy Groups

There is an almost endless variety of "helping" groups for adolescents. To clarify this confusing field, Scheidlinger (1985) proposed the following classification: 1) group psychotherapy, 2) therapeutic groups, 3) human development and training groups, and 4) self-help and mutual help groups. Using this basic classification system, each category will be further defined and characterized, with differences between categories highlighted (see Table 55-1).

Para-analytic group psychotherapy for adolescents. This category is primarily composed of the long-term outpatient psychodynamically oriented (with modified parameters for adolescents) groups led by a trained mental health professional. Each patient has had a diagnostic evaluation, and suitability of this patient for this specific group is carefully considered. There is a clear therapeutic contract individually defined, with specific goals of relief of distress and improved psychosocial functioning. Groups usually consist of 8–12 patients who meet weekly for approximately 1½ hours. Early adolescents tend to function better in same-sex groups; middle and late adolescents are usually seen in mixed-sex groups (Ackerman 1955; Sugar 1975). Pubertal and early adolescent groups need activities in addition to the sitting and talking; middle-late adolescent groups can function verbally. Some snacks and drinks are often used in both. Patients may be seen concurrently in individual or family therapy. These groups tend to be long term, with participation lasting 6 months to 2 years.

Indications for para-analytic group psychotherapy are many; it is "generally the treatment of choice for adolescents" (Scheidlinger 1985, p. 109). Contraindications are few and include overt psychosis

and severe "narcissism" (Berkowitz and Sugar 1975). Schiedlinger (1985, p. 109) excluded adolescents in "crisis, sociopathic, overt sexual perverts, acute psychotics and all paranoids." Of most difficulty is the clinical decision of the suitability of a specific patient to a specific group so that a workable balance is achieved. Group cohesion while maintaining individual working alliances must be developed. Kraft (1989) referenced Holmes in describing the dropout rate from these groups to be 20%–40%. One must also be aware of the possible negative peer influences from the groups when mixing sexually active and/or drug-using adolescents with nonacting-out adolescents. Firm rules of no extra-group relationships with members of the group help decrease this danger. These groups are often most helpful for those teenagers with specific problems in social skills and self-esteem areas.

Para-analytic outpatient adolescent therapy groups tend to move through specific stages having common characteristics to the early, middle, and end phases. This was described more than 20 years ago (MacLennan and Felsenfeld 1968, p. 14): "In therapy groups, adolescents have been described as going through phases of initial politeness and good behavior; griping, testing, and acting out; dependency and demandingness; and ultimately mature problem-solving and separation to lead a more independent and self-reliant life." Scheidlinger (1985) similarly described an early phase characterized by anger at authority figures and testing the leader and other group members in establishing trust and a working alliance. The middle phase is where the real therapeutic work is done, as deeper feelings are shared and appropriate confrontations, clarifications, and interpretations are made by the leader and especially by the other group members. The termination phase involves looking at what one did and did not gain from the group, as well as saying good-bye, and raises the painful issues of mourning and loss.

In defending against the group's purpose to share feelings and work on problems, adolescents in group therapy use a litany of individual and group resistances. The individual resistances include silence, inconsequential chattering, obsessing, complaining, fighting, not coming, monopolizing, vacillating, listing irrelevant events, demanding, boasting, withholding, and helping others in order to avoid focusing on one's own problems (MacLennan and Felsenfeld 1968). The group resistances include mutual admiration, fighting, physical or verbal diversionary tactics, competing, scapegoating, set-

Table 55-1. Comparison of categories of adolescent groups

Type of group:	Para-analytic group psychotherapy	Therapeutic group	Educational and sensitivity groups	Self-help groups
Leader	Trained mental health professional	Trained mental health professional or counselor	Variable	"Recovering" group member
Participants	Have had diagnostic evaluation and match patient to group	Diagnostic evaluation or screening but less specificity of patient to group	No evaluation	Only criterion: desire to stop addictive behavior
Therapeutic contract	Yes	Yes	No	Yes
Goals	Define specific individual goals	Goals more defined by nature of group	"Personal growth" or developmental problem focus	All have same goal: to achieve abstinence
Group frequency	Weekly	Variable	One or a few times	Every day
Duration (hours)	1½	1–2	Varies	1–2
Course	Long term (6 mo– >2 yrs)	Short term (i.e., inpatient) (weeks to a few months) or longer term, supportive	One time to few weeks	For life
Process	Individual dynamics interface with group dynamics	Varies with group purpose but more ego supportive or skill focused	Directive leadership style	"Working" of the 12 steps

ting up cliques, playing secrets, and uniting against the leader. These resistances may account for why many mental health professionals avoid or choose other therapeutic modalities for adolescents. The group therapist must be skilled at limit setting as well as empathic caring. As Phelan (1974, p. 244) described: "The therapist working with adolescent groups needs occasionally to fill some of the functions of a parent, often to be literally a teacher, and always to provide the analytic atmosphere which leads to insight and understanding."

Long-term groups in residential settings and the long-term outpatient groups defined by diagnosis (e.g., eating disorder) or negative experience (e.g., sexual abuse) would also be placed into this category, provided the leader is a trained professional, a diagnostic evaluation is conducted, and a therapeutic contract is enacted. The group process

should involve individual psychodynamics interacting with the group process, including parent and sibling transference interpretations, catharsis, and corrective cognitive/emotional experiences.

Therapeutic groups for adolescents. Groups included in this category are those that are conducted by a mental health professional for patients who have had a diagnostic evaluation, but the group course is usually short term (i.e., inpatient) or long-term supportive. The individual's goals for the group are more determined by the overall group purpose. Also, there is less emphasis on the group process and transference development and more emphasis on the here-and-now. Within this category are numerous types of inpatient and outpatient therapy groups.

Inpatient therapy groups. There are many types of adolescent inpatient groups, which are dependent on and interface with the program milieu. The control of aggressive and destructive behavior is crucial for survival of an adolescent hospital program (Beskind 1962). Others have described that establishing a firm structure and setting of limits by staff was related to the controls needed by patients and preceded the development of a positive therapeutic milieu in which positive relationships between staff and patients were formed (Jaffe and Manis 1974).

Adolescents in a hospital inpatient program live in the various therapy groups of the program. These groups include community meetings, school groups, recreation, art, music, and dance groups as well as more focused groups. "Boys' groups" tend to focus on sexual issues and aggressive-authority issues; "girls' groups" frequently examine their experiences with rape and incest. Assertive training groups focus on role playing of assertive, rather than aggressive, expressions of angry feelings. There may also be social skills training groups; nutrition groups for patients with eating disorders; and chemical dependency groups, which utilize more confrontative approaches because of the lying and denial of drug-abusing adolescents. Community meetings often combine administrative and limit settings, as well as therapeutic functions, of the milieu.

Two other types of groups include a positive group, developed by Rogeness and Stewart, in which only positive comments can be made, and an early A.M. group therapy, developed by Rosenstock, Gale, and Levy, held every 3–4 weeks to deal with high group resistance (Stein and Kymissis 1989). A fishbowl format (Flvet et al. 1980), where group members take turns observing the group and then join the discussion, enhances constructive feedback. Stein and Kymissis (1989) defined the present challenge of inpatient group therapy to be to enhance meaningful commitment to the group process during briefer periods of hospitalization.

Outpatient therapy groups. This subcategory includes the short-term groups at mental health clinics (e.g., diagnostic groups, crisis-oriented groups) as well as the support groups for teenagers with medical illnesses (Walker 1985). Longer-term support groups for adolescents with severe mental disorders (e.g., mental retardation, schizophrenia), as well as adolescents with eating disorders and victims of abuse, would be categorized here if the emphasis is more ego supportive and not on in-

trapsychic or group dynamics. The group counseling of junior and senior high schools, which must be adapted to the school administrative organization, would also be placed here. The goals of these groups include improvement in behavior, school performance, and mild emotional problems (Berkowitz 1989).

Group therapy is seen as especially helpful with treatment of minority teenagers (Constantino et al. 1988) and Southeast Asian refugee adolescents (Lee 1988). With adolescents who have been sexually abused, group therapy is often considered an essential part of a treatment program (Knittle and Tuana 1980).

Educational and sensitivity groups. This category includes all those school- and church-sponsored nontherapeutic educational groups. Often these groups focus on a specific area (e.g., sex education, drug prevention, suicide prevention) or a normal developmental transition (e.g., entering senior high school). These groups involve cognitive learning but also try to explore affective issues related to the specific developmental problem. The sensitivity groups (personal growth groups), so popular in the 1960s and early 1970s, have largely disappeared, but some of their techniques involving exploration, confrontation, emotional expressions, and self-disclosure related to a here-and-now focus are used in present-day communication workshops (Yalom 1985). One- or two-day group seminar workshops to help adolescents deal with common family problems (e.g., divorce and reconstituted families) are readily available in many communities.

Self-help groups. The growth of self-help groups has been the strongest group movement of the 1980s. Alcoholics Anonymous has almost two million members in 63,000 groups (Robertson 1988), and its membership is doubling every 10 years. The only criteria for membership is the desire to stop using alcohol and/or drugs. Since addicts presumably cannot moderate their use of alcohol or drugs, the goal of participation is abstinence. The core of the program is the "working" of the 12 Steps. These involve a complex psychosocial-spiritual treatment path leading to a life without alcohol or drugs. Since the recovering addict is considered always susceptible to relapse, the 12 Steps are expected to be a life-long process.

Because of the importance of these steps to addiction treatment, they will be described in some detail. The first step involves examining one's life and realizing that one could not control or moderate alcohol or drug use. Facing that one's life was unmanageable and that life-threatening self-destructive behavior occurred indicates the need for abstinence. Although this is especially difficult for adolescents, admitting powerlessness over alcohol and drugs gives them the power to begin having a real life (Jaffe 1990a, 1990b). The second and third steps involve developing a positive spiritual belief system. The fourth step involves taking an honest detailed moral inventory, and the fifth step consists of the cathartic experience of verbalizing this inventory to another person. Steps 6 through 12 involve changing behavior, making amends, continuing the personal inventory, and enhancing spirituality. These 12 steps are discussed and "worked" at daily meetings and also through the guidance and support of other recovering members who take on special role-modeling functions as contacts and sponsors. For adolescents recovering from alcoholism or drug addiction, the group cohesion, support, and relationships give them a peer group of nonusing adolescents that is essential for their sobriety.

The 12 Steps are used for Narcotics Anonymous and Cocaine Anonymous as well as in the self-help groups for other addictions (e.g., Gamblers Anonymous). Codependency groups for the relatives of addicts (e.g., Alanon, Alateen, Adolescent Children of Alcoholics) (Bogdaniak and Piercy 1987) frequently use a modified version of the 12 Steps. Overeater's Anonymous similarly uses the 12-step structure, adapting it based on the addiction being the abuse of food. This model views anorexia nervosa and bulimia as addictive diseases, and many treatment programs will integrate the Overeaters Anonymous groups into the recovery program of adolescents with severe chronic eating disorders.

Research and Outcome Studies of Adolescent Group Therapy

Tramontana (1980) reviewed 33 independent studies on adolescent individual, group, and family therapy. Of the 15 controlled experimental studies, the study of Redfering on group therapy and the study by Persons (1966), which combined individual and group methods, were sufficiently well designed and rigorously executed to demonstrate convincing evidence of the superiority of psychotherapy over no therapy conditions. Verleur et al.

(1986) did a controlled study using rating scales, behavioral observations, and a daily log with adolescent female incest victims. The intervention of group therapy and sexual education resulted in a significant increase in positive self-esteem and knowledge of human sexuality. Corder et al. (1981), using Yalom's categories of curative factors (which Yalom changed to therapeutic factors in 1985) and a Q-sort method, found that adolescents identified catharsis, interpersonal learning, and existential factors categories as most helpful in group psychotherapy. Unlike adults, adolescents rated the insight category as least helpful. Azima and Dies (1989) stressed that, in addition to using appropriate control groups, reliable valid objective measures of clinical functioning, and detailed diagnostic evaluations, group therapy research needs to study the difficult issue of how and what group processes and dynamics induce therapeutic change.

References

Abramowitz CV: The effectiveness of group psychotherapy with children. Arch Gen Psychiatry 33:320–326, 1976

Ackerman NW: Group psychotherapy with a mixed group of adolescents. Int J Group Psychother 5:249–260, 1955

Adams DW, Deveau EJ: Coping With Childhood Cancer: Where Do We Go From Here? Hamilton, Ontario, Kinbridge Publications, 1988

Azima FJC, Dies KR: Clinical research in adolescent group psychotherapy: status, guidelines and directions, in Adolescent Group Psychotherapy. Edited by Azima FJC, Richmond LH. Madison, CT, International Universities Press, 1989, pp 193–223

Bender L, Woltmann AG: The use of puppet shows as a psychotherapeutic method for behavior problems in children. Am J Orthopsychiatry 6:341–354, 1936

Berkowitz IH: Secondary schools: application of group therapy in secondary schools. in Adolescent Group Psychotherapy. Edited by Azima FJC, Richmond LH. Madison, CT, International Universities Press, 1989, pp 99–123

Berkowitz IH, Sugar M: Indications and contraindications for adolescent group psychotherapy, in The Adolescent in Group and Family Therapy. Edited by Sugar M. New York, Brunner/Mazel, 1975, pp 3–36

Beskind H: Psychiatric inpatient treatment of adolescents. Compr Psychiatry 3:354–369, 1962

Bingham A, Bargar J: Children of alcoholic families. Journal of Psychosocial Nursing 23:13–15, 1985

Bogdaniak RC, Piercy FP: Therapeutic issues of adolescent children of alcoholics (AdCA) groups. Int J Group Psychother 37:569–588, 1987

Brandes NS: Outpatients, in Group Therapy for the Adolescent. Edited by Brandes NS, Gardner ML. New York, Jason Aronson, 1973, pp 63–81

Brownell KD, Kelman JH, Stunkard AJ: Treatment of obese children with and without their mothers: changes in weight and blood pressure. Pediatrics 71:515–523, 1983

Charach R: Brief interpretive group psychotherapy with early latency-age children. Int J Group Psychother 33:349–364, 1983

Clement PW, Fazzone RA, Goldstein B: Tangible reinforcers and child group therapy. Journal of the American Academy of Child Psychiatry 9:409–427, 1970

Constantino G, Malgady RG, Rogler LH: Folk hero modeling therapy for Puerto Rican adolescents. J Adolesc 11:155–165, 1988

Corder BF, Whiteside L, Haizlip TM: A study of curative factors in group psychotherapy with adolescents. Int J Group Psychother 31:345–354, 1981

Dannefer E, Brown R, Epstein N: Experience in developing a combined activity and verbal group therapy program with latency-age boys. Int J Group Psychother 25:331–337, 1975

Davis L, Geike G, Schamess G: The use of genograms in a group for latency age children. Int J Group Psychother 38:189–209, 1988

Dubo S: Opportunities for group therapy in a pediatric service. Int J Group Psychother 1:235–242, 1951

Eth S, Silverstein S, Pynoos RS: Mental health consultation to a preschool following the murder of a mother and child. Hosp Community Psychiatry 36:73–76, 1985

Farkas F, Schwachman H: Psychological adaptation to chronic illness: a group discussion with cystic fibrosis patients. Am J Orthopsychiatry 43:259–260, 1973

Flvet NR, Holmes GR, Gordon LC: Adolescent group psychotherapy: a modified fishbowl format. Adolescence 15:75–82, 1980

Gilbert CM: Sexual abuse and group therapy. J Psychosoc Nurs Ment Health Serv 26(5):19–23, 1988

Jaffe SL: The Step Workbook for Adolescent Chemical Dependency Recovery: A Guide to the First Five Steps. American Academy of Child and Adolescent Psychiatry. Washington, DC, American Psychiatric Press, 1990a

Jaffe SL: Staff Guidelines for Using the Step Workbook for Adolescent Chemical Dependency Recovery. American Academy of Child and Adolescent Psychiatry. Washington, DC, American Psychiatric Press, 1990b

Jaffe SL, Manis R: The formation of a milieu on an adolescent inpatient ward. Journal of the American Academy of Child Psychiatry 13:699–706, 1974

Kalter N, Pickar J, Lesowitz M: School-based developmental facilitation groups for children of divorce: a preventive intervention. Am J Orthopsychiatry 54:613–623, 1984

Kennedy JF: The heterogeneous group for chronically ill and physically healthy but emotionally disturbed children and adolescents. Int J Group Psychother 39:105–125, 1989

Kitchur M, Bell R: Group psychotherapy with preadolescent sexual abuse victims: literature review and description of an inner-city group. Int J Group Psychother 39:285–310, 1989

Knittle BJ, Tuana SJ: Group therapy or primary treatment for adolescent victims of intrafamilial sexual abuse. Clinical Social Work Journal 8:236–242, 1980

Kraft I: A selective overview, in Adolescent Group Psychotherapy. Edited by Azima FJC, Richmond LH. Madison, CT, International Universities Press, 1989, pp 55–68

Lee E: Cultural factors in working with Southeast Asian refugee adolescents. J Adolesc 11:167–179, 1988

Lev EL: An activity therapy group with children in an inpatient psychiatric setting. Psychiatr Q 55:55–64, 1983

MacLennan BW, Felsenfeld N: Group Counseling and Psychotherapy With Adolescents. New York, Columbia University Press, 1968

Mallery B, Navas M: Engagement of preadolescent boys in group therapy: videotape as a tool. Int J Group Psychother 32:453–467, 1982

Mitchum NT: Developmental play therapy: a treatment approach for child victims of sexual molestation. Journal of Counseling and Development 65:320–321, 1987

Oberfield R, Ciliotta C: A school-age boys/single mothers group. Journal of the American Academy of Child Psychiatry 22:375–381, 1983

Persons R: Psychological and behavioral change in delinquents following psychotherapy. J Clin Psychol 22:337–340, 1966

Pevsner R: Group parent training versus individual family therapy: an outcome study. J Behav Ther Exp Psychiatry 13:119–122, 1982

Phelan J: Parent, teacher or analyst: the adolescent group therapist's trilemma. Int J Group Psychother 24:238–244, 1974

Rachman A, Raubolt R: The pioneers of adolescent group psychotherapy. Int J Group Psychother 34:387–413, 1984

Redl F: Diagnostic group work. Am J Orthopsychiatry 14:53–67, 1944

Robertson N: Getting Better: Inside Alcoholics Anonymous. New York, William Morrow, 1988

Rose SD, Edleson JS: Working With Children and Adolescents in Groups: A Multimethod Approach. San Francisco, CA, Jossey-Bass, 1987

Sands RM, Golub S: Breaking the bonds of tradition: a reassessment of group treatment of latency-age children. Am J Psychiatry 131:662–665, 1974

Schacter RS: Kinetic psychotherapy in the treatment of children. Am J Psychother 28:430–437, 1974

Scheidlinger S: Experiential group treatment of severely deprived latency-age children. Am J Orthopsychiatry 30:356–368, 1960

Scheidlinger S: Three group approaches with socially deprived latency-age children. Int J Group Psychother 15:434–445, 1965

Scheidlinger S: Short-term group psychotherapy for children: an overview. Int J Group Psychother 34:573–585, 1984

Scheidlinger S: Group treatment of adolescents: an overview. Am J Orthopsychiatry 55:102–111, 1985

Semonsky C, Zicht G: Activity group parameters. Journal of the American Academy of Child Psychiatry 13:166–179, 1974

Slavson SR, Schiffer M: Group Psychotherapies for Children: A Textbook. New York, International Universities Press, 1975

Smith JD, Walsh RT, Richardson MA: The clown club: a structured fantasy approach to group therapy with the latency-age child. Int J Group Psychother 35:49–64, 1985

Stein MD, Kymissis P: Adolescent inpatient group psychotherapy, in Adolescent Group Psychotherapy. Edited by Azima FJC, Richmond LH. Madison, CT, International Universities Press, 1989, pp 69–84

Steward MS, Farquhar LC, Dicharry DC, et al: Group therapy: a treatment of choice for young victims of child abuse. Int J Group Psychother 36:261–277, 1986

Sugar M: Interpretive group psychotherapy with latency children. Journal of the American Academy of Child Psychiatry 13:648–666, 1974

Sugar M: The structure and setting of adolescent therapy groups, in The Adolescent in Group and Family Therapy. Edited by Sugar M. New York, Brunner/Mazel, 1975, pp 42–48

Tattersall RB, McCulloch DK, Aveline M: Group therapy in the treatment of diabetes. Diabetes Care 8:180–188, 1985

Tramontana MG: Critical review of research on psychotherapy

outcome with adolescents: 1967–1977. Psychol Bull 88:429–450, 1980

Verleur D, Hughes RE, deRios MD: Enhancement of self-esteem among female adolescent incest victims: a controlled comparison. Adolescence 21:843–854, 1986

Walker L: Adolescent analysands in group therapy. Social Casework 66:21–29, 1985

Williams K, Baeker M: Use of small group with chronically ill children. School Health 3:205–207, 1983

Yalom ID: The Theory and Practice of Group Psychotherapy, 3rd Edition. New York, Basic Books, 1985

Chapter 56

Hypnosis

Daniel T. Williams, M.D.

The history of psychotherapy preceding the advent of hypnosis abounds with dramatic reports of healing involving altered states of consciousness. These trance states were believed over many centuries to result from invoking of divine or other spiritual intervention by spiritual healers. Efforts to conceptualize these phenomena in more secular, scientific terms led to a variety of formulations during the 18th and 19th centuries and to the emergence of the term *hypnosis* to describe them (Ellenberger 1970). An interesting developmental pattern has subsequently emerged; namely, episodic fascination by certain clinicians and segments of the population with the sometimes dramatic effects observed with hypnosis, followed by disillusionment when its ineffectiveness or apparent untoward effects are encountered.

As the clinical use of hypnosis in psychotherapy has matured, a sophisticated understanding of its benefits has moved beyond the long-standing tradition of glowing, uncontrolled clinical case reports. More recent efforts to conceptualize the therapeutic use of trance experience in contemporary psychological terms have come to focus on the intrinsic human trance capacity, which can be seen retrospectively as having been tapped in different ways in different cultures and in different eras. Hypnosis in this context has come to be understood as a potentially powerful means of actively facilitating therapeutic change that draws on the patient's trance capacity. This is done in a manner now understood to be distinctly different from the nonspecific effects of placebo and suggestion, although hypnosis also draws on those important nonspecific influences, as do all psychotherapeutic modalities.

Furthermore, hypnosis as a specific means of augmenting psychotherapeutic intervention is a resource that the vast majority of children and adolescents are capable of utilizing. Once one understands its rationale, the range of its clinical usefulness, its techniques of application, and its limitations, hypnosis can be a valuable addition to the child/adolescent psychiatrist's armamentarium.

Definition

Even sophisticated contemporary researchers who agree that hypnosis is an important therapeutic modality may differ in those features of hypnosis that they choose to emphasize in its definition. Thus Spiegel (1988) emphasized the features of absorption, dissociation, and suggestibility. Absorption connotes the characteristic state of attentive, receptive, focal concentration that is essential to hypnosis. Dissociation connotes the relative suspension of peripheral awareness that is a by-product of absorption. Inherent in this feature of dissociation is that less cathected perceptions, which would ordinarily be part of consciousness, become split off from consciousness during the trance experience. Suggestibility connotes the tendency to accept instructions uncritically in trance, a reflection of the receptive, trusting rapport, which is another key feature of hypnosis. In slight contrast, Orne and Dinges (1989) defined hypnosis as a state in which the individual is able to respond to appropriate suggestions by experiencing changes of perception, memory, or mood.

Implicit in both of the above definitions, overt

behavior (as in a hypnotic induction procedure) may be one useful indicator of the trance state, but requires associated inquiry into the subjective experience of the patient to document that a trance state exists. Also implicit in both of the above formulations, when hypnosis is applied in a clinical setting, is the relevance of positive transference. This refers to the tendency of the patient to develop subjective elaborations of the therapy transaction based both on prior life experiences and on hopes and expectations regarding the therapy relationship. In contrast to the psychoanalytic approach, in which the transference is gradually fostered nondirectively and then analyzed gradually, hypnosis actively and directively exploits the therapeutic leverage inherent in the transference, with a view to expediting therapeutic change (Williams 1988).

The areas of consensus regarding the contemporary definition of hypnosis dispel the common misconception of hypnosis as a form of sleep. In sleep, contraction of peripheral awareness is part of a general withdrawal of attention from the environment. In hypnosis, peripheral awareness contracts insofar as this enhances heightened focal concentration (Spiegel and Spiegel 1978).

Historically, it is noteworthy that Freud's early experiences with hypnosis played an important role in the conceptualization of repression and associated unconscious processes (Freud 1925[1924]/1955). Interestingly, Freud explained his early abandonment of hypnosis as being in part due to the emergence of rather intense (erotic) transference reactions. This was puzzling and disconcerting to him at a juncture preceding his fuller formulation of psychodynamic theory and an operational method of handling such transference reactions. In subsequent years, however, he came to see that public health needs would reactivate a role for hypnosis to allow more widespread and expeditious therapeutic applications of psychoanalytic insights than the protracted and expensive method of psychoanalysis could permit (Freud 1919[1918]/1955).

Assessing Hypnotizability

Another reason cited by Freud and other psychotherapists for abandoning hypnosis after initial enthusiasm about its use was their discovery that not all patients can be hypnotized. When viewed in the mesmeric tradition, hypnotizing the subject constituted a tribute to the therapist's charismatic personality and/or skillful therapeutic prowess;

failure to do so would signify a failure by the therapist, with ensuing narcissistic injury.

A major contribution to our understanding of hypnosis in more recent years has been the emergence of objective, reproducible measures of hypnotizability (Frankel 1987). It is clear that hypnotizability reflects a psychological capacity of an individual subject, similar to intellectual capacity; it is not a "spell," "projected" onto the subject by the mesmeric hypnotist. The common finding of large sample studies using different standard measures of hypnotizability is that there is a broad range of hypnotizability within the population, with a normal distribution approximating a typical bell-shaped curve. Thus a minority of subjects will be not at all hypnotizable, another minority at the other end of the distribution scale will be very highly hypnotizable, and the rest of the population will be normally distributed in the midrange in between. This replicated finding has had important implications. From a research standpoint, it has spawned productive studies elucidating specific effects of hypnosis by allowing comparison of highly hypnotizable and nonhypnotizable subjects. From a clinical standpoint, the degree of hypnotizability allows for appropriate selection of patients for the therapeutic application of hypnosis.

Space limitations preclude a detailed discussion of hypnotic induction procedures here, but two scales applicable for children and adolescents will be noted. The particular induction technique employed is relatively unimportant clinically, as long as it is aesthetically and emotionally acceptable to the patient. Of primary importance, by contrast, is the tacit expectation by both the patient and therapist that the ceremonious transaction between them will lead to a change in the patient's subjective experience. The prerequisite for establishing this shared expectation is the creation of a trusting rapport during the course of initial diagnostic assessment. If this has been achieved, the induction procedure constitutes a formal signaling to the patient to shift into a state of heightened concentration and receptivity to the therapist's further comments and suggestions.

Morgan and Hilgard (1979) developed the Stanford Hypnotic Clinical Scale for Children, which can be administered in 20 minutes. The form for older children (6–16 years old) is based on an eye closure-relaxation induction followed by seven test items. The form for younger children (4–8 years old) contains six test items and is based on an active imagination induction, since younger children often are resistant to suggestions for eye closure.

The Hypnotic Induction Profile (Spiegel and Spiegel 1978) can be administered in 5–10 minutes, making it particularly convenient in clinical settings. It measures and correlates the subject's pattern of response to instructions for eye roll, dissociation, posthypnotic arm levitation, and posthypnotic subjective experiences. The wording of its instructions can readily be modified according to the age and cognitive level of a given child or adolescent (Williams 1988).

Aside from ascertaining the patient's hypnotizability, formal measurement has the additional advantage of providing the patient with a "practice exposure" to hypnosis without associated concern about its concomitant therapeutic application. Once hypnotizability has been established, there is a demonstrated new resource with which to tackle the presenting problem. This approach is supported by findings that hypnotizability is correlated with relative psychological intactness. Spiegel et al. (1982) found that, in contrast to the normal distribution referred to in sampling nonclinical populations, severely impaired patient groups, including those with anxiety disorders, affective disorders, and particularly schizophrenic disorders, have a significant skewing of scores in the direction of nonhypnotizability.

Special Considerations With Children and Adolescents

Surveys of hypnotizability with children and adolescents, using adaptations of adult scales, indicate that children and adolescents are generally more hypnotizable than adults. Morgan and Hilgard (1973), assessing 1,232 subjects at various ages, found increases in hypnotic responsivity between the ages of 5 and 10, a peak in the preadolescent years (11–12), and a gradual decline during adolescence, becoming relatively stable through early adulthood, then tailing off again in the older population. One of the reasons for the presumed lesser hypnotic responsivity of younger children (below 6) may be the inappropriateness of existing scales to assess this capacity at these younger ages (Olness and Gardner 1988). The consensus of many studies is that there are no overall differences between the sexes in hypnotizability at any age. Furthermore, there is no correlation between hypnotizability and either socioeconomic background or intelligence, as long as the subject has sufficient intellectual capacity to understand the given instructions for trance induction.

Developmental aspects of hypnotizability were explored by Morgan (1973), who looked at genetic and environmental influences by studying 140 twin pairs, 5–22 years old. In a controlled study, involving independent testing of each twin, she found significant positive correlations of hypnotizability for monozygotic twins but not for dizygotic twins, suggesting a genetic contribution to hypnotizability. Morgan further found, however, that personality resemblance as rated by parents on a standardized questionnaire was positively related to hypnotizability score similarity for either-sexed child and the like-sexed parent. No such correlation was found with the opposite-sexed parent. Morgan interpreted these findings as suggesting an environmental contribution to hypnotizability, based on the child's identification with the like-sexed parent and emulation of the latter's emotional-cognitive affinity for trance experience. There is thus evidence that hypnotizability, as an indicator of trance capacity, derives from both genetic and environmental influences.

Reasoning from clinical experience and theoretical considerations, Gardner (1974) postulated that the greater hypnotizability of children compared with adults was due in part to children's propensity for a narrower cognitive focus. She noted Piaget's observations of the child's tendency toward concrete, literal thinking as helping to explain the child's greater ease in affiliating with the ceremony of hypnosis. Indeed, as is evident cross-culturally in the practice of transmitting religious traditions and concepts through ceremony, children give less consideration than adults to theoretical questions and logical complexities if the experience of the authoritatively sanctioned ceremony is emotionally palatable. As adolescents develop more sophisticated cognitive perspectives, some demonstrate more critical and skeptical styles that may be a source of resistance to hypnosis. However, a therapist's preparedness to respond effectively to questions raised in search of clarification may well defuse such resistance.

Emotional factors postulated by Gardner (1974) as contributing to the greater hypnotizability of children include their general openness to new experience, their emotional malleability, their intrinsic orientation to learning new skills, and the greater ease with which they can accept regressive phenomena. Indeed, psychoanalytic reformulations of hypnosis have viewed it as a circumscribed, guided "regression in the service of the ego" in the psychotherapy setting (Gill and Brenman 1959). In this spirit, the child's greater propensity for trusting responsiveness to suggestions from a respected adult authority is part of a natural developmental progression toward achieving mastery and autonomy.

Enlisting parental understanding and support is essential for the success of any child-centered treatment technique, and this certainly applies to the use of hypnosis. This frequently requires dispelling misconceptions about hypnosis and explaining how it can play a safe and useful part in the overall treatment strategy. The same principle applies in the hospital setting, including the involvement of other physicians and nurses.

Indications and Applications

As documented comprehensively by Olness and Gardner (1988), hypnosis has been used in a wide array of psychiatric and medical disorders in children and adolescents. The contemporary standard of demonstrated efficacy for pharmacologic agents requires double-blind, controlled studies to rule out the influence of placebo and suggestion. Such controlled studies have been much more difficult to mount regarding psychotherapeutic interventions for a variety of methodological reasons (Karasu et al. 1984). Suffice it to say that the measurability of trance capacity with standardized scales has afforded us a unique model for being able to assess the specificity of psychotherapeutic intervention in a variety of psychiatric and medical disorders. What follows constitutes a brief outline of some of the indications for hypnosis with children and adolescents about which there is some consensus among contemporary workers in the field.

Pain

This is one of the best established and most systematically studied indications for hypnosis. It is clear that an individual's perception of pain represents both the cortical registration of pain deriving from tissue injury and the ensuing psychological reaction to it. Furthermore, the individual's psychological reaction will be influenced by many variables, including preexisting and ongoing affective state, personality, cognitive level, and the changing patterns of social reinforcement, which are contingent on pain-related behavior. Taking all of these into consideration, hypnosis can facilitate alteration of the subjective experience of pain.

Using the paradigm of comparing highly hypnotizable and essentially nonhypnotizable patients, McGlashan et al. (1969) demonstrated that hypnotic analgesia is clearly different from placebo in highly hypnotizable subjects and is significantly more effective for them. By contrast, in nonhypnotizable subjects, the ceremony of hypnosis functions as the equivalent of placebo. Further amplification of the distinction between hypnotic analgesia and the placebo effect has been made possible by the finding that placebo-induced analgesia is mediated by endogenous opioids and can be blocked by naloxone. Studies with both adult volunteers (Goldstein and Hilgard 1975) and adult patients in chronic pain (Spiegel and Albert 1983) have shown that hypnotic analgesia is not blocked or reversed by a substantial dose of naloxone given in double-blind, crossover fashion. In this context, both Zelter and Le Baron (1982), as well as Kuttner et al. (1988), demonstrated that hypnosis is superior to an attentional control condition for children with cancer undergoing painful procedures.

The techniques most often employed for children undergoing painful procedures involve focusing the patient's attention on engrossing imagery that provides a distraction from, and hence a diminution of, the painful sensation. Selection of appropriate imagery is geared to the favorite activities, television programs, or current cultural heroes of the child. For example, the child may be guided in trance to the image of huddling with his favorite football team in a championship game and receiving encouragement from the quarterback to disregard temporary pain as the child focuses on helping the team to score the game-winning touchdown. A variety of other strategies and examples are cited by Olness and Gardner (1988).

Operationally, the rationale for hypnosis is initially presented to both the parents and the patient. In lay terminology, hypnosis may be usefully explained as a "relaxation exercise" that can "harness the power of imagination" to help the patient develop a new strategy to diminish and overcome pain as well as the associated anxiety that can worsen pain. The initial assessment of hypnotizability and development of an individualized hypnosis exercise is then generally best done with the patient alone, free from the distracting presence of the parents. Inherent in this format is the implication that the patient is being taught a new technique (i.e., self-hypnosis). The therapist has been the teacher, but the newly developed skill resides within the patient, implicitly imparting a newfound sense of mastery with which to confront the challenge of pain. Providing the patient with either an audiotape or written instructions for the self-hypnosis exercise is often helpful in encouraging the patient's sense of autonomy regarding its use. Once this format has been imparted, however, particularly with younger children, it is often helpful to review the exercise conjointly with the parents so that they can supportively further review and reinforce it in the absence of the therapist.

In clinical situations involving chronic pain, it becomes extremely important to take account of the contingencies of social reinforcement that interact with pain-related behavior and deal with these in one's overall treatment strategy. If a state of invalidism (somatization) that provides a refuge from other life problems has been inadvertently fostered, one must address the constellation of pathogenic life influences contributing to this state before launching into a treatment strategy centered on the pain (Williams and Hirsch 1988).

Psychological Factors Affecting Physical Conditions

Current understanding has clarified the capacity of psychological state potentially to influence the course and certainly to influence the subjective experience of virtually any medical disorder. It is not surprising that hypnosis has been reported anecdotally to be beneficial in a large array of medical disorders in both adults and children. In many respects, principles of application are similar to those outlined above regarding pain. Aside from the mechanisms demonstrated to be operative with diminished pain perception, however, the presumed mechanism of action of hypnosis in this group of disorders involves the element of relaxation. This is postulated to attenuate or reverse the emotionally based hyperaroused state in response to stress that is thought to mediate a wide variety of psychophysiologic disorders. Only a few representative examples are cited here. An important precaution, as with pain, is to avoid having one's enthusiasm about addressing presumed psychogenic contributants obscure the need to identify and treat possible underlying organic contributants to the patient's condition.

Seizure disorders. The clinical literature on epilepsy contains many references to the role of psychogenic stress as an excitant of paroxysmal electroencephalographic activity and as a precipi-

tant of seizures (Williams 1982). This also has been demonstrated under controlled conditions in experimental animals (Lockard et al. 1972). There have been a number of reports pointing to the value of hypnosis as a psychotherapeutic adjunct in improving the control of psychogenically precipitated neurogenic seizures (Williams et al. 1978, 1979, 1987). It is important to distinguish the above seizure type from both "pure" neurogenic seizures and from purely psychogenic seizures (pseudoseizures), which may coexist (Williams and Mostofsky 1982). The above distinction is particularly important, because uncontrolled seizures tend to elicit aggressive pharmacologic anticonvulsant treatment with substantial potential side effects, and failing such intervention, surgery in selected cases (Williams et al. 1991).

Gastrointestinal disorders. These often present similar complexities in diagnosis and treatment at the medical-psychiatric interface. Clinical reports abound of the useful application of hypnosis with children and adolescents having a variety of gastrointestinal problems (Olness and Gardner 1988; Williams and Singh 1976); two recent controlled studies with adults deserve mention. Colgan et al. (1988) reported a controlled trial of hypnotherapy in relapse prevention of duodenal ulceration. After 30 patients had rapidly relapsing ulcers healed with medication, they were divided into two randomly selected groups who either did or did not receive hypnotherapy. After 1 year, only 8 (53%) of the hypnotherapy patients relapsed, versus 15 (100%) of the control subjects. Further evidence pointing to the capacity of hypnosis to modulate gastric secretion was presented by Klein and Spiegel (1989). In highly hypnotizable healthy volunteers, they demonstrated the ability of specific hypnotic suggestion either to increase acid secretion (by 89%) or to reduce it (by 39%) compared with basal acid secretion. Clearly, the capacity of hypnosis to modulate pain perception would also be clinically pertinent in this area.

Headache. Much clinical literature supports the potential efficacy of hypnosis in treating a variety of types of headache in both children and adolescents (Olness and Gardner 1988) as well as in adults (Brown and Fromm 1987; Davidson 1987). A study by Olness et al. (1987) compared self-hypnosis, placebo, and propranolol in the treatment of juvenile classic migraine. Among 28 children completing the study, there was a significantly greater reduction in headache frequency with self-hypnosis training than with either propranolol or placebo. Insofar as the pathophysiology of migraine remains obscure, the mechanism of impact of hypnosis in this as in other types of headache remains speculative as well.

Asthma. The pathophysiology of asthma is also complex and multidetermined, including genetic vulnerability, allergic sensitivity, infections, and emotional stress (Avery 1989). Here again, the clinical literature suggests the efficacy of hypnosis in controlling apparent psychogenic contributants (Brown and Fromm 1987; Olness and Gardner 1988). Kohen (1986) reported a prospective study of 28 children with asthma who were randomized into groups who either learned self-hypnosis techniques or served as controls. Although there were no differences between experimental and control groups with regard to pulmonary function tests from the initial to the postintervention period, there were dramatic improvements after 1 and 2 years of follow-up. Further support for this observation of benefit is offered by a systematic, although uncontrolled, study by Morrison (1988). After 1 year of hypnotherapy, 16 chronic asthmatic patients whose condition had previously been inadequately controlled by medications experienced a dramatic and significant drop in frequency and duration of hospital admissions, as well as a significant reduction in use of prednisolone.

Somatoform Disorders

Somatoform disorders are characterized by physical symptoms suggesting physical disorder for which there are no demonstrable organic findings or known physiologic mechanisms, and for which there is positive evidence, or a strong presumption, that symptoms are linked to psychological factors or conflicts (American Psychiatric Association 1987). The symptom production in somatoform disorders is not under voluntary control, implying the involvement of an unconscious mechanism dissociation in symptom formation.

Effective clinical treatment of somatoform disorders in children and adolescents is often multimodal, corresponding to the multifactorial etiologies that have been discerned as pertinent to this group of disorders (Williams and Hirsch 1988). Freud saw the limitations of hypnosis when applied by his contemporaries to these disorders, which were then subsumed under hysteria. Hypnosis was then limited to a narrow focus of authoritative suggestion of symptom removal, without the dynamic understanding of symptom formation that Freud was subsequently to develop (Freud 1919[1918]/1955). When used in the more enlightened manner that Freud and others later came to advocate, hypnosis can be the vehicle for actively imparting to the patient a summary formulation of the psychodynamics of symptom formation. This then becomes the basis of an emotional-cognitive reorientation, in which the therapist supportively suggests to the patient guidelines for a more adaptive mode of coping with ongoing life stresses.

Implicitly, pathologic dissociation is a key phenomenological feature of somatoform disorders. It can be quite helpful to a patient and the family to understand through the use of hypnosis that dissociation is a psychological attribute that can be channeled, under therapeutic auspices, in the service of symptom alleviation. What had been a mechanism of maladaptive self-victimization thus becomes transformed into a vehicle for self-reparation and mastery. Further considerations and illustrations of this have been outlined elsewhere (Williams 1988).

Dissociative Disorders

It would be expected from the above that hypnosis should also have application with youngsters having dissociative disorders. The most common currently described form of dissociative disorder is multiple personality disorder, which is now recognized often to have documentable antecedents in childhood physical and sexual abuse (Braun and Sachs 1985; Kluft 1985). One way of understanding a central feature of this disorder is that children come to use this pathologic dissociation as a defense, distancing themselves from the terrifying experience of abuse, but paying a heavy psychological price for this escape (Spiegel 1986). Multiple personality disorder is thus conceptualized as a posttraumatic stress disorder that arises in response to repeated trauma imposed by sadistic and double-binding parenting figures.

It follows that a host of psychotherapeutic considerations pertain in treating children and adolescents with these disorders (Kluft 1986; Putnam 1989). For many patients with multiple personality disorder, memories of repressed traumas may be accessible initially only in the context of certain dissociated states. Hypnosis can be a useful facilitator in this regard, in helping patients recognize the phenomenon of dissociation in a more balanced, supportive frame of reference. Hypnosis may then become a vehicle to help penetrate amnestic barriers, an aid in abreaction, and a resource in the psychotherapeutic endeavor of reintegration.

Anxiety Disorders

In a controlled study, Spiegel et al. (1982) demonstrated that adult patients with generalized anxiety disorder are markedly less hypnotizable than normal control subjects. When such patients are treated with benzodiazepines, they test as more hypnotizable than those who are untreated (Spiegel 1980). No comparable studies have been done as of this writing with children or adolescents. Clinical experience suggests, however, that hypnosis may be a useful adjunct to both behavioral and psychodynamic therapy, including serving as a facilitator of systematic desensitization and as a facilitator of restructuring the cognitive and emotional response to feared stimuli or situations. When antianxiety medication is needed and is effective, the ceremony of hypnosis can concretize for the child and family those behavioral and psychological strategies of reorientation geared to eventually obviating the need for medication.

Habit Disorders

Childhood habit disorders is a generic term including enuresis, encopresis, thumb sucking, nail biting, and a host of other disorders. Clearly, enuresis (Shaffer 1988) and encopresis (Pawl 1988) have possible organic etiologies, and these must be evaluated before embarking on any psychotherapeutic or behavioral intervention. Although Olness and Gardner (1988) have reviewed many clinical reports suggesting the potential value of hypnosis for many forms of habit disorder in children and adolescents, well-controlled studies are sorely lacking in this area. Olness and Gardner outlined a number of guidelines for integrating hypnosis with traditionally advocated behavioral measures for this group of disorders.

Neurophysiologic Considerations

The role of the reticular formation in the central nervous system appears to be that of a selective information modulator that filters out stimuli of less interest to the organism, thus accentuating attention to those stimuli that are of more significance (Kelly 1985). This capacity provides a plausible conceptual model for understanding the neurophysiologic basis of focal attention (absorption) and dissociation, two key phenomenological features of hypnosis.

Empirical support for the above formulation is evident in two elegant studies evaluating the capacity of hypnosis to modify cortical evoked responses in highly hypnotizable individuals, using low hypnotizable subjects as controls (Spiegel et al. 1985, 1989). These findings provide evidence that hypnotically induced subjective changes such as anesthesia or visual hallucinations involve alterations in neurophysiologic processing. They also provide a model for conceptualizing the mechanism of intervention of hypnosis in the varied conditions outlined above.

Precautions and Limitations

Already noted is the need for differential diagnostic caution in one's approach to pain, psychological factors affecting a physical condition, and presumptive somatoform disorders. It is crucial to consider here the possible presence of undiagnosed organic pathology before zealously embarking on psychotherapeutic endeavor, with or without hypnosis. This is especially true when evident psychopathology and plausible psychodynamic formulations tempt one to premature diagnostic closure (Williams 1988; Williams and Hirsch 1988).

Conversely, the presence of documented organic disorder in no way precludes the coexistence of secondarily superimposed somatoform disorder, factitious disorder, malingering, or psychological factors affecting a primary organic disorder. In those cases in which the diagnosis is initially unclear, it is often useful to pursue a clinical trial of psychotherapeutic intervention, including hypnosis, in close liaison with those physicians responsible for evaluation and treatment of the apparent organic disorder. Such a combined assessment, if thorough on both organic and psychological fronts, will generally clarify whether the presenting problem is primarily organic, primarily psychogenic, or a substantial combination of the two (Fahn and Williams 1988; Williams and Mostofsky 1982).

Hypnosis is generally not appropriate for treatment of patients with psychotic disorders. As previously noted, patients with schizophreniform disorders are predominantly nonhypnotizable (Spiegel et al. 1982). Because hypnosis implicitly involves a relatively intense, trusting rapport with an implicit temporary transfer of executive control of the patient's subjective experience to the therapist, such an experience may be quite threatening to a paranoid patient and is best avoided. Severely depressed or manic patients are also predominantly nonhypnotizable. A seeming exception in this domain is that of "hysterical psychosis" (Spiegel and Fink 1979), which on closer inspection turns out phenomenologically to be a dissociative disorder and not a true psychosis.

One must note the contraindication to using hypnosis coercively rather than collaboratively with the patient. Overzealous attempts at rushing removal of a psychodynamically based symptom that has served a defensive function, for example, without helping the patient and family restructure their perspectives for more adaptive coping strategies, will fail. Such misguided, heavy-handed interventions, even if transiently effective, undermine the patient's confidence in the therapist and lead to symptom recurrence or symptom substitution. These quagmires can be avoided by a thorough diagnostic assessment that allows fashioning of a treatment plan sensitive to individual and family dynamics and to the pace at which the patient and family can achieve designated goals. Symptoms may recur even after relinquished via appropriate application of hypnosis if excessive adverse life stresses recur or if psychotherapeutic support needed to consolidate gains is terminated prematurely. These observations apply, however, to any psychotherapeutic intervention, whether or not hypnosis is used.

Treatment strategies geared to effective and sustained relief of symptoms must deal with secondary gain features of the symptoms (Feldman 1988). This may be accomplished by parental counseling, environmental restructuring, or a behavior modification program. Integration of this consideration is crucial to the success of any intervention using hypnosis. If one sees no symptomatic improvement in a hypnotizable patient after two to three sessions of treatment with hypnosis, there has probably been some error or omission in either diagnostic assessment or treatment formulation, often including appreciation of the role of secondary gain factors. A reassessment and reformulation in these areas is then in order. On the other hand, if one sees partial, gradual indications of improvement, which is often the case, this points to the

patient's communicating both a positive response to treatment and a call for continued support to help "work through" the therapeutic reorientation. In this context, self-hypnosis serves as both a "cognitive restructuring homework exercise" between sessions and an opportunity to incorporate emotionally the healthier and "more mature" mode of adaptation suggested by the therapist. Clearly, the therapist should judge the need for frequency and duration of further treatment based on the needs of the individual patient and family.

Conclusions

Studies have established that the vast majority of children and adolescents are hypnotizable. Hypnosis constitutes a specific and potentially powerful facilitator of therapeutic change, provided that a thorough diagnostic assessment and comprehensive treatment formulation have delineated the appropriate role that hypnosis is to play. The effectiveness of hypnosis then depends on the capacities of the patient and family to respond to therapeutic suggestions, on the severity of pathogenic environmental stressors, and on the skill of the therapist in integrating hypnosis with other elements of a well-formulated treatment plan to foster a more healthy mode of adaptation.

References

American Psychiatric Association: Diagnostic and Statistical Manual of Mental Disorders, 3rd Edition, Revised. Washington, DC, American Psychiatric Press, 1987

Avery ME: Pulmonology, in Pediatric Medicine. Edited by Avery ME, First LR. Baltimore, MD, Williams & Wilkins, 1989, pp 217–300

Braun BG, Sachs RG: The development of multiple personality disorder: predisposing, precipitating, and perpetuating factors, in Childhood Antecedents of Multiple Personality. Edited by Kluft RP. Washington, DC, American Psychiatric Press, 1985, pp 37–64

Brown DP, Fromm E: Hypnosis and Behavioral Medicine. Hillsdale, NJ, Lawrence Erlbaum, 1987

Colgan SM, Faragher EB, Whorwell PJ: Controlled trial of hypnotherapy in relapse prevention of duodenal ulceration. Lancet 1:299–300, 1988

Davidson P: Hypnosis and migraine headache: reporting a clinical series. Australian Journal of Clinical and Experimental Hypnosis 15:111–118, 1987

Ellenberger HI: The Discovery of the Unconscious. New York, Basic Books, 1970

Fahn S, Williams DT: Psychogenic dystonia. Adv Neurol 50:431–455, 1988

Feldman RS: Behavior therapy, in Handbook of Clinical Assessment of Children and Adolescents, Vol 2. Edited by Kestenbaum CJ, Williams DT. New York, New York University Press, 1988, pp 1111–1128

Frankel FH: Significant developments in medical hypnosis during the past 25 years. Int J Clin Exp Hypn 35:231–247, 1987

Freud S: Lines of advance in psycho-analytic therapy (1919 [1918]), in The Standard Edition of the Complete Psychological Works of Sigmund Freud, Vol 17. Translated and edited by Strachey J. London, Hogarth Press, 1955, pp 157–168

Freud S: An autobiographical study (1925 [1924]), in The Standard Edition of the Complete Psychological Works of Sigmund Freud, Vol 20. Translated and edited by Strachey J. London, Hogarth Press, 1955, pp 1–74

Gardner G: Hypnosis with children. Int J Clin Exp Hypn 22:20–38, 1974

Gill M, Brenman M: Hypnosis and Related States. New York, International Universities Press, 1959

Goldstein E, Hilgard E: Failure of opiate antagonist naloxone to modify hypnotic analgesia. Proc Natl Acad Sci USA 72:2041–2043, 1975

Karasu TB, Conte HR, Plutchik R: Psychotherapy outcome research, in The Psychosocial Therapies. Edited by Karasu TB. Washington DC, American Psychiatric Association, 1984, pp 831–872

Kelly J: Cranial nerve nuclei, the reticular formation and biogenic amine containing neurons, in Principles of Neural Science, 2nd Edition. Edited by Kandel ER, Schwartz JH. New York, Elsevier, 1985, pp 539–561

Klein KB, Spiegel D: Modulation of gastric acid scretion by hypnosis. Gastroenterology 96:1383–1387, 1989

Kluft RP: Childhood multiple personality disorder: predictors, clinical findings, and treatment results, in Childhood Antecedents of Multiple Personality. Edited by Kluft RP. Washington, DC, American Psychiatric Press, 1985, pp 167–196

Kluft RP: Treating children who have multiple personality disorder, in Treatment of Multiple Personality Disorder. Edited by Braun BG. Washington, DC, American Psychiatric Press, 1986

Kohen DP: Applications of relaxation/mental imagery to the management of asthma: report of behavioral outcomes of a two-year, prospective controlled study (abstract). Am J Clin Hypn 28:196, 1986

Kuttner L, Bowman M, Teasdale M: Psychological treatment of distress, pain, and anxiety for young children with cancer. J Dev Behav Pediatr 9:374–381, 1988

Lockard JS, Wilson WL, Uhlir V: Spontaneous seizure frequency and avoidance conditioning in monkeys. Epilepsia 13:437–444, 1972

McGlashan T, Evans F, Orne M: The nature of hypnotic analgesia and placebo responses to experimental pain. Psychosom Med 31:227–246, 1969

Morgan A: The heritability of hypnotic susceptibility in twins. J Abnorm Psychol 82:55–61, 1973

Morgan A, Hilgard E: Age differences in susceptibility to hypnosis. Int Clin Exp Hypn 21:78–85, 1973

Morgan A, Hilgard JR: The Stanford Hypnotic Clinical Scale for Children. Am J Clin Hypn 21:148–155, 1979

Morrison JB: Chronic asthma and improvement with relaxation induced by hypnotherapy. J R Soc Med 81:701–704, 1988

Olness K, Gardner G: Hypnosis and Hypnotherapy With Children, 2nd Edition. Philadelphia, PA, Grune & Stratton, 1988

Olness K, MacDonald JT, Uden DL: Comparison of self-hypnosis and propranolol in the treatment of juvenile classic migraine. Pediatrics 79:593–597, 1987

Orne MT, Dinges DF: Hypnosis, in Comprehensive Textbook of Psychiatry V, Vol 2. Edited by Kaplan HI, Sadock BJ. Baltimore, MD, Williams & Wilkins, 1989, pp 1501–1516

Pawl GA: Encopresis, in Handbook of Clinical Assessment of Children and Adolescents, Vol 2. Edited by Kestenbaum CJ, Williams DT. New York, New York University Press, 1988, pp 711–721

Putnam FW: Diagnosis and Treatment of Multiple Personality Disorder. New York, Guilford, 1989

Shaffer D: The clinical management of bedwetting in children, in Handbook of Clinical Assessment of Children and Adolescents, Vol 2. Edited by Kestenbaum CJ, Williams DT. New York, New York University Press, 1988, pp 689–710

Spiegel D: Hypnotizability and psychoactive medication. Am J Clin Hypn 22:217–222, 1980

Spiegel D: Dissociation, double binds, and posttraumatic stress in multiple personality disorder, in Treatment of Multiple Personality Disorder. Edited by Braun BG. Washington, DC, American Psychiatric Press, 1986, pp 61–77

Spiegel D: Hypnosis, in The American Psychiatric Press Textbook of Psychiatry. Edited by Talbott JA, Hales RE, Yudofsky SC. Washington, DC, American Psychiatric Press, 1988, pp 907–928

Spiegel D, Albert L: Naloxone fails to reverse hypnotic alleviation of chronic pain. Psychopharmacology (Berlin) 81:140–143, 1983

Spiegel D, Fink R: Hysterical psychosis and hypnotizability. Am J Psychiatry 136:777–781, 1979

Spiegel D, Detrick D, Frischholz E: Hypnotizability and psychopathology. Am J Psychiatry 139:431–437, 1982

Spiegel D, Cutcomb S, Ren C, et al: Hypnotic hallucination alters evoked potentials. J Abnorm Psychol 94:249–255, 1985

Spiegel D, Bierre P, Rootenberg J: Hypnotic alteration of somatosensory perception. Am J Psychiatry 146:749–754, 1989

Spiegel H, Spiegel D: Trance and Treatment: Clincial Uses of Hypnosis. New York, Basic Books, 1978

Williams DT: The treatment of seizures: special psychotherapeutic and psychobiological techniques, in Epilepsy: A Handbook for the Mental Health Professional. Edited by Sands H. New York, Brunner/Mazel, 1982, pp 58–74

Williams DT: Hypnosis, in Handbook of Clinical Assessment of Children and Adolescents, Vol 2. Edited by Kestenbaum CJ, Williams DT. New York, New York University Press, 1988, pp 1129–1146

Williams DT, Hirsch G: The somatizing disorders: somatoform disorders, factitious disorders, and malingering, in Handbook of Clinical Assessment of Children and Adolescents, Vol 2. Edited by Kestenbaum CJ, Williams DT. New York, New York, University Press, 1988, pp 743–768

Williams DT, Mostofsky DI: Psychogenic seizures in childhood and adolescence, in Pseudoseizures. Edited by Riley T, Roy A. Baltimore, MD, Williams & Wilkins, 1982, pp 169–184

Williams DT, Singh M: Hypnosis as a facilitating therapeutic adjunct in child psychiatry. Journal of the American Academy of Child Psychiatry 15:326–342, 1976

Williams DT, Spiegel H, Mostofsky DI: Neurogenic and hysterical seizures in children and adolescents. Am J Psychiatry 135:82–86, 1978

Williams DT, Gold AP, Shrout P, et al: The impact of psychiatric intervention on patients with uncontrolled seizures. J Nerv Ment Dis 167:626–631, 1979

Williams DT, Pleak R, Hanesian H: Neuropsychiatric disorders of childhood and adolescence, in The American Psychiatric Press Textbook of Neuropsychiatry. Edited by Hales RE, Yudofsky SC. Washington, DC, American Psychiatric Press, 1987, pp 365–383

Williams DT, Pleak RR, Hanesian H: Neurological disorders, in Child and Adolescent Psychiatry: A Comprehensive Textbook. Edited by Lewis M. Baltimore, MD, Williams & Wilkins, 1991, pp 629–646

Zelter L, Le Baron S: Hypnosis and nonhypnotic techniques for reduction of pain and anxiety during painful procedures in children and adolescents with cancer. J Pediatr 101:1032–1035, 1982

Index

*Page numbers that appear in italics refer to tables
that are separated from the discussion of the subject in text*